SELECTED MEDICAL DIAGNOSES

Adjustment disorders, 670
Agoraphobia without panic attacks, 332
Anorexia nervosa, 396, 462, 474, 965
Attention deficit-hyperactivity disorder, 862
Autism, 862
Bipolar disorder, 438, 475
Borderline personality disorder, 396, 515, 862
Bulimia nervosa, 396, 463, 474
Conduct disorder, 554, 889
Conversion disorder, 362
Cyclothymia, 438
Delirium, 581
Delusional disorders, 554
Delusional (paranoid) disorder, 554
Dementia, 579, 581
Dependent personality disorder, 515
Depersonalization disorder, 396
Developmental disorder, 862
Disruptive behavior disorder, 554, 862
Dissociative disorder, 396
Dysthymia, 438
Elimination disorders, 862
Gender identity disorder, 646
Generalized anxiety disorder, 334
Hypochondriasis, 362, 893, 964
Idiopathic pain disorder, 362
Major depression, 438, 475
Mental retardation, 861
Multiple personality disorder, 396

Narcissistic personality disorder, 396
Noncompliance with medical treatment, 475
Obsessive-compulsive disorder, 333
Oppositional defiant disorder, 554
Organic mental disorders, 581
Organic personality syndrome (explosive type), 554
Panic disorder, 332
Paranoid personality disorder, 515, 554
Personality disorder, 513-515
Pervasive developmental disorder, 862
Pica, 862
Post-traumatic stress disorder, 334
Psychoactive substance dependence, 616
Psychoactive substance-induced organic mental disorders, 614
Psychogenic amnesia, 396
Psychogenic fugue, 396
Schizoid personality disorder, 513
Schizophrenia, 513, 862
Separation anxiety disorder, 862
Sexual disorders, 646
Sexual dysfunctions, 647
Simple phobia, 333
Social phobia, 333
Somatization disorder, 362
Somatoform disorders, 362
Tic disorders, 862
Tourette's disorder, 862

PRINCIPLES
AND
PRACTICE
OF
PSYCHIATRIC NURSING

FOURTH EDITION

PRINCIPLES

AND

PRACTICE

OF

PSYCHIATRIC NURSING

GAIL WISCARZ STUART, Ph.D., R.N., C.S.

Professor, College of Nursing, Associate Professor, College of Medicine;
Chief of the Division of Psychiatric Nursing,
Department of Psychiatry and Behavioral Sciences,
Medical University of South Carolina,
Charleston, South Carolina

SANDRA J. SUNDEEN, R.N., M.S., C.N.A.A.

Chief Psychiatric Nurse, Mental Hygiene Administration, Maryland Department of
Health and Mental Hygiene, Baltimore, Maryland; Adjunct Assistant Professor,
University of Maryland School of Nursing, Baltimore, Maryland;
Adjunct Assistant Professor, Salisbury State University,
Salisbury, Maryland

with illustrations

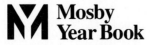
Mosby
Year Book

St. Louis   Baltimore   Boston   Chicago   London   Philadelphia   Sydney   Toronto

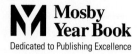
Mosby
Year Book
Dedicated to Publishing Excellence

Editor: Linda Duncan
Developmental Editors: Linda Stagg, Teri Merchant
Project Manager: Patricia Gayle May
Book and Cover Design: Gail Morey Hudson

Artwork for the part and chapter openers is by M.C. Escher.
Reprinted with permission of John W. Vermeulen on behalf of the Escher heirs.
Photographs courtesy National Gallery of Art, Washington, D.C.

FOURTH EDITION

Mosby–Year Book, Inc.
11830 Westline Industrial Drive, St. Louis, Missouri 63146

Library of Congress Cataloging in Publication Data

Principles and practice of psychiatric nursing/ [edited by] Gail
  Wiscarz Stuart, Sandra J. Sundeen—4th ed.
      p. cm.
    Includes bibliographical references and index.
    ISBN 0-8016-5885-3
    1. Psychiatric nursing. I. Stuart, Gail Wiscarz
  II. Sundeen, Sandra J.
    [DNLM: 1. Psychiatric Nursing. WY 160 P957]
  RC440.P69 1990
  610.73'68—dc20
  DNLM/DLC   90-13567
  for Library of Congress   CIP

CL/VH 9 8 7 6 5 4 3 2

CONTRIBUTORS

BEVERLY A. BALDWIN, R.N., Ph.D.

Associate Professor and Coordinator, Graduate Major in Gerontological/Geriatric Nursing, University of Maryland School of Nursing, Baltimore, Maryland

E. SUSAN BATZER, M.S., R.N., C.S.

Psychotherapist and Consultant, Fallston, Maryland; Program Coordinator, Psychiatric Emergency Service, Baltimore County, Maryland

RUTH WILDER BELL, R.N., D.N.Sc.

Assistant Professor, University of Maryland School of Nursing, Baltimore, Maryland

SANDRA E. BENTER, D.N.Sc., R.N., C.S.

Director of Clinical Programs, Division of Psychiatric Nursing, University of Maryland Medical System, Baltimore, Maryland; Psychotherapist and Consultant, Owings Mills, Maryland

DIANE E. BOYER, R.N., M.S.

Program Director, Residential Rehabilitation, Region 10 Community Services Board, Charlottesville, Virginia

JACQUELINE C. CAMPBELL, R.N., Ph.D., F.A.A.N.

Associate Professor, Wayne State University College of Nursing, Detroit, Michigan

PATRICIA E. HELM, M.S.N., R.N., C.S.

West Haven Veterans Administration Medical Center, West Haven, Connecticut

JEANETTE LANCASTER, R.N., Ph.D., F.A.A.N.

Dean and Professor, University of Virginia School of Nursing, Charlottesville, Virginia

ARTHUR J. LaSALLE, Ed.D., C.C.M.H.C.

Consultant, Training and Counseling, LaSalle Associates, Ellicott City, Maryland

PAULA CHELES LaSALLE, M.S., R.N., C.S., C.C.M.H.C.

Psychiatric Nurse Consultant, Department of Infectious Disease, The Johns Hopkins University, Baltimore, Maryland; Psychotherapist, Consultant, and Trainer, LaSalle Associates, Ellicott City, Maryland

MICHELE T. LARAIA, R.N., M.S.N.

Assistant Professor and Nursing Director of Research, Department of Psychiatry and Behavioral Sciences, Medical Unviersity of South Carolina, Charleston, South Carolina

RITA J. LAUTZ, Ph.D., R.N., C.S.

Psychotherapist, Bel Air, Maryland; Consultant, Psychiatric Emergency Service, Baltimore County, Maryland

FRANCES G. LEHMANN, M.S.N., R.N., C.S.

Frances G. Lehmann Health Consultants, Indianapolis, Indiana

BARBARA PARKER, R.N., Ph.D.

Associate Professor, University of Maryland School of Nursing, Baltimore County Campus, Catonsville, Maryland

HELEN R. PEDDICORD, M.S., R.N., C.S.

Director of Residential Services, Regional Institute for Children and Adolescents, Rockville, Maryland

SUSAN G. POORMAN, Ph.D., R.N., C.S., C.S.E.

Assistant Professor, School of Nursing, University of Pittsburgh; Psychotherapist and Consultant, Pittsburgh, Pennsylvania

AUDREY REDSTON-ISELIN, M.A., R.N., C.S.

Clinical Specialist, Children's Service, Soundview Throgs Neck Community Mental Health Center, Albert Einstein College of Medicine, Yeshiva University, Bronx, New York; Psychotherapist and Consultant, White Plains and New York, New York

RITA L. RUBIN, M.S., R.N., C.S.

Human Development Center of Pasco New Port, Richey, Florida

KAY SIENKILEWSKI, M.S., R.N., C.N.A.A.

Director of Nursing, Sheppard and Enoch Pratt Hospital, Towson, Maryland

PREFACE

In many ways the fourth edition of this text reflects the process of separation-individuation being experienced by the discipline of psychiatric nursing. More than a decade has passed since the first edition of our book was published. At that time we felt much like pathfinders traveling unexplored frontiers, since the idea for this text was both a departure and an evolution. It was a departure in that other texts in the field were being organized around the medical model and its classifications of psychiatric illnesses. At the same time, it was an evolution in that our first edition attempted to identify and refine, for psychiatric nurses, the distinct body of knowledge that is nursing. The second and third editions continued to travel on unexplored territory. They attempted to consolidate and synthesize the expanding knowledge in the field, while continuing to use a nursing model as the basis for defining and describing the practice of psychiatric nursing.

Now, our fourth edition emerges in the decade of the 1990s. In this decade, psychiatric nursing will begin to mature and become better differentiated from our related disciplines in health care. In this decade also, psychiatric nurses will better articulate the essence of what we do as "caring," "holism," and "science." Thus these three threads are woven throughout the fourth edition of this text. The "caring" art of the nursing process continues to be the organizing framework for the text. The "holism" of nursing practice is further developed in the nursing conceptual model, as it describes the integration of biological, psychological, and sociocultural aspects contributing to the continuum of health-illness behavior. And the "science" of nursing knowledge is consolidated and synthesized in the nursing interventions described in each chapter. The task has been formidable, but the product is greater self-definition for psychiatric nursing.

Most of the strengths of the previous editions of this text have been retained and further developed. New developments in the biological and behavioral aspects of psychiatry and psychiatric nursing have been included in each chapter. The text also continues to interrelate the NANDA nursing diagnoses with the DSM-III-R diagnoses in an attempt to clarify the way in which they work together to complement patient care. Prevention, rehabilitation, and health education also continue to be emphasized, and a new chapter has

been added on psychological responses to physical illness. Perhaps the hardest task for us, however, was to simplify the language of the text whenever possible to make the content clearer, more easily understood, and thus more readily applied by the reader.

Part One, Principles of Psychiatric Nursing, has a sharpened focus on the professional dimensions of psychiatric nursing practice. It presents a refined analysis of our conceptual model of health-illness phenomena that provides a framework for the nursing therapeutic process. Unit I defines concepts and theories of care. Chapter 1 critically analyzes the roles and functions of psychiatric nurses from the many perspectives of historical evolution, contemporary practice, levels of performance, and issues of professional autonomy. Chapter 2 continues to explore models of psychiatric care, while introducing the medical model and a brief perspective of the nursing model used in this text. Chapter 3 describes a nursing model of health illness phenomena that is inclusive and holistic, yet discrete and relevant to nursing practice. This model views health and illness as a continuum of adaptation and provides an organizing framework for the application of the nursing process. Chapter 4 presents a comprehensive analysis of the elements of the nurse-patient relationship, including the effective use of self, the therapeutic communication process, the phases of the nurse patient relationship, responsive and action dimensions, therapeutic impasses, and supervision. Chapter 5 describes the phases and needed documentation of the nursing process with application demonstrated in a clinical case analysis. The Standards of Psychiatric and Mental Health Nursing Practice are integrated throughout this discussion. Chapter 6 describes elements of the comprehensive psychiatric evaluation including the mental status examination, psychiatric examination, and new technological approaches to biological evaluation, while Chapter 7 presents legal and ethical aspects of psychiatric nursing care.

The first three chapters of Unit II describe primary, secondary, and tertiary prevention levels of nursing intervention. Chapters 11 through 21 have all been updated, and strengthened from a nursing perspective. Each explores a category of maladaptive coping responses, including the nursing problems of anxiety, psychophysiological illness, alterations in self-concept, disturbances of mood, self-destructive behavior, disruptions in relatedness, problems with the expression of anger, impaired cognition, substance abuse, variations in sexual response, and a new chapter on psychological responses to physical illness. At the beginning of each of these chapters, a continuum of adaptive and maladaptive coping responses is presented relative to the chapter's nursing problem. Each phase of the nursing process is then applied and synthesized with the conceptual model. A consistent approach is used in formulating nursing diagnoses and comparing them with relevant medical diagnoses. Nursing research is used to provide a rationale for nursing interventions. Principles and nursing actions for the interventions are clearly discussed and concisely summarized in each of these chapters. Evaluation is addressed in light of effectiveness, efficiency, and areas in need of further study. The strength of this integrated approach is that it can be applied in any nursing care setting to patients who are responding to any type of stressor, whether physical, psychological, or sociocultural. Thus it is as useful to nurses working on medical units of general hospitals, long-term care facilities, and community health agencies as it is to nurses working in psychiatric facilities. The last two chapters in Part One, Chapters 22 and 23, address updated analyses of somatic therapies and psychopharmacology.

Part Two, Practice of Psychiatric Nursing, has similarly been divided into two units. The first unit describes psychiatric nursing practice in specific settings including inpatient, community mental health, and the general hospital. Unit II addresses specialized treatment approaches including behavior modification, group and family approaches, child and adolescent psychiatric nursing, intervening with victims of abuse and violence, care of the chronic mentally ill, and gerontological psychiatric nursing. All of Part Two reflects the most current thinking on the treatment settings, modalities, and roles of psychiatric nursing.

We have also tried to clarify content and reinforce learning throughout the text. To this end, each chapter contains behaviorally stated learning objectives, expanded illustrations and tables, sample nursing care plans, health teaching formats, summaries of important points, directions for future nursing research, and suggested cross-references, updated references, and annotated suggested readings. This edition of our book is also accompanied by an instructor's manual, which is complete with learning objectives, lecture outlines, chapter glossaries, thought-provoking discussion questions, and multiple-choice test questions that include both theoretical aspects and clinical applications of the text's content.

Visually, this fourth edition continues to incorporate the artwork of M.C. Escher, which has become closely associated with our text. Over the past years his drawings have continued to stimulate and intrigue us, as we believe that they truly reflect the complexity of human behavior and one's own perceptual responses. We have come to identify with the precision, balance, and creative perspective of his work and hope to realize these same qualities in this latest edition of our text.

Gail Wiscarz Stuart
Sandra J. Sundeen

CONTENTS

ix

PRINCIPLES
OF PSYCHIATRIC NURSING

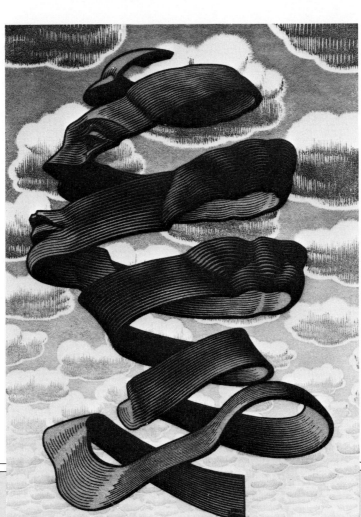

UNIT I
CONCEPTS AND THEORIES

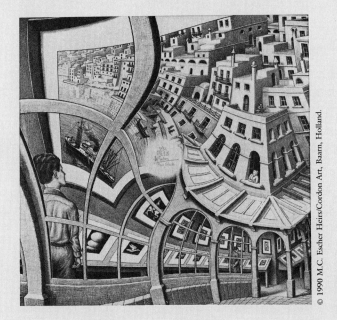

© 1990 M.C. Escher Heirs/Cordon Art, Baarn, Holland.

The philosophies of one age have become the absurdities of the next, and the foolishness of yesterday has become the wisdom of tomorrow.

Sir William Osler

CHAPTER 1

ROLES AND FUNCTIONS OF PSYCHIATRIC NURSES

After studying this chapter, the student should be able to:

- describe the early history of psychiatric nursing.
- discuss the evolution of a psychiatric nursing role, including the specific contributions of Peplau.
- explain the influence of the social environment on psychiatric nursing.
- describe the nature, scope, and setting of psychiatric nursing practice.
- identify direct and indirect psychiatric nursing care functions using the concepts of primary, secondary, and tertiary prevention.
- analyze factors that contribute to effective interdisciplinary team functioning.
- discuss the leadership skills needed by psychiatric nurses.

- analyze the way in which the psychiatric nurse's level of performance is affected by each of the following factors: laws, qualifications, practice setting, and personal competence and initiative.
- assess the purpose and importance of the American Nurses' Association Standards of Psychiatric—Mental Health Nursing Practice.
- evaluate the position of psychiatric nursing on the six characteristics of the scale of professionalization.
- critique problematic areas for psychiatric nursing and formulate recommendations for future growth.
- identify directions for future nursing research.
- select appropriate readings for further study.

Evolutionary perspectives

The function of nursing or caring for the sick has existed since the beginning of civilization. Family members, servants, friends, neighbors, and religious groups all have cared for the ill or infirm throughout the course of history. Before 1860 the emphasis in psychiatric institutions was on custodial care, and attendants were prepared to maintain control of the patients. Frequently these attendants were little more than jailers or cellkeepers with very little training, and psychiatric care was poor. Nursing, as a profession, began to emerge in the late nineteenth century.

Early history

In 1873 Linda Richards graduated from the New England Hospital for Women and Children in Boston. She developed better nursing care in psychiatric hospitals and organized nursing services and educational programs in state mental hospitals in Illinois. For these activities she is called the first American psychiatric nurse. Basic to Richards' theory of care was her

premise: "It stands to reason that the mentally sick should be at least as well cared for as the physically sick."[10]

The first school to prepare nurses to care for the mentally ill opened at McLean Hospital in Waverly, Massachusetts in 1882. It was a 2-year program, but few psychological skills were addressed; the care was mainly custodial. Nurses took care of the patients' physical needs, such as medications, nutrition, hygiene, and ward activities. Until the end of the nineteenth century little changed in the role of psychiatric nurses. They had limited special training in psychiatry, and they primarily adapted the principles of medical-surgical nursing to the psychiatric setting. At that time psychological care consisted of kindness and tolerance toward the patients.

One of Linda Richards' more important contributions was her emphasis on assessing both the physical and emotional needs of the patients. In this early period of nursing history, nursing education separated these two needs; nurses were taught either in the general hospital or in the psychiatric hospital. In 1913, Johns Hopkins became the first school of nursing to include a fully developed course for psychiatric nursing in the curriculum. Other schools soon began to do likewise. It was not until the late 1930s that nursing education recognized the importance of psychiatric knowledge in general nursing care for all illnesses.

An important factor in the development of psychiatric nursing was the emergence of various somatic therapies, including insulin shock therapy (1935), psychosurgery (1936), and electroconvulsive therapy (1937). These techniques all required the medical-surgical skills of nurses. Although these therapies did not foster the patient's insight, they did control behavior and make him more amenable to psychotherapy. Somatic therapies also increased the demand for improved psychological treatment for patients who did not respond.

As nurses became more involved with somatic therapies, they began the struggle to define their role as psychiatric nurses. An editorial in the *American Journal of Nursing*[12] in 1940 described the conflict between nurses and physicians as nurses tried to implement what they saw as appropriate care for psychiatric patients. This conflict continues to demand attention in current nursing practice. Another article published in 1933[34] noted that psychiatrists were looking for experienced psychiatric nurses. A superintendent of nursing from a state hospital identified the three most pressing needs at that time as (1) more nurses, (2) better prepared nurses, and (3) cooperation and understanding of the nursing organizations.

The period after World War II was one of major growth and change in psychiatric nursing. Because of the large number of service-related psychiatric problems and the increase in treatment programs offered by the Veterans Administration, psychiatric nurses with advanced preparation were in demand. The content of psychiatric nursing had now become an integral part of the generic nursing curriculum; its principles were applied to other areas of nursing practice, including general medical, pediatric, and public health nursing. Graduate nursing programs, however, were few in number.

In 1946 Congress passed the National Mental Health Act. The act authorized the creation of the National Institute of Mental Health (NIMH), located in Bethesda, Maryland, and a program for (1) training professional psychiatric personnel, (2) conducting psychiatric research, and (3) aiding the development of mental health programs at the state level. The purpose of NIMH is to research the origins of mental illness and possible methods of treatment. The agency also is the administrative body that distributes training funds and research grants. Psychiatric nursing was one of the professions specified in the act, which paved the way for federal funding of nursing education. Collegiate programs developed at both the undergraduate and graduate levels. At about the same time the nursing profession endorsed the idea of graduate programs that focused on clinical practice in nursing. By 1947 eight graduate programs in psychiatric nursing had been started.

Basic nursing programs, meanwhile, continued to grow and change. Many nursing leaders questioned the practice of having specialized hospitals offer training programs for a particular type of patient, such as psychiatric hospitals training psychiatric nurses. The trend was to combine the basic knowledge and various skills needed by nurses into one general education program.

In 1948 Brown's report on "Nursing for the Future" recommended eliminating basic schools of nursing in mental hospitals. The report suggested that such hospitals consider closing their schools and instead "make their clinical facilities more widely available for affiliating students (from general training schools)."[6:136] The report also recommended using the psychiatric hospitals in advanced courses for graduate nurse specialists. This report was given additional support in 1950 when the National League for Nursing (NLN) instituted the requirement that, to be accredited, a school had to provide experience in psychiatric nursing.

■ Role emergence

The role of psychiatric nursing began to emerge during this developmental period in the early 1950s. In 1947 Weiss[51] published an article in the *American Journal of Nursing* that reemphasized the shortage of psychiatric nurses and outlined the differences between psychiatric and general duty nurses. She described "attitude therapy" as the nurse's directed use of attitudes that contribute to the patient's recovery. In implementing this therapy the nurse observes the patient for small and fleeting changes, demonstrates acceptance, respect, and understanding of the patient, and promotes the patient's interest and participation in reality. Weiss stressed the need to treat each patient as an individual with unique problems. It was also her belief that only physicians should attempt to interpret the patient's behavior; the physician would then prescribe the appropriate attitude needed by the nurse, based on the patient's problem. More independent functions were described by Santos and Stainbrook[44] in 1949. They believed that nurses should perform "psychotherapeutic tasks" and should understand concepts related to therapy, such as transference. They were vague, however, about the exact nature of the nurse's functions.

An article by Bennett and Eaton[5] in the *American Journal of Psychiatry* in 1951 identified three problems affecting psychiatric nurses: (1) the scarcity of qualified psychiatric nurses, (2) the underutilization of their abilities, and (3) the fact that "very little real psychiatric nursing is carried out in otherwise good psychiatric hospitals and units." The authors listed the functions and responsibilities of the chief psychiatric nurse as:

1. To have policy-making authority independent of the psychiatric staff members, hospital administrators, and general nursing staff
2. To decide psychiatric nursing policies
3. To develop all rules and regulations of the department
4. To train an auxiliary staff of assistants to conform to his or her standards

Bennett and Eaton considered the role of the nurse in insulin treatment, electroconvulsive therapy, and lobotomy, as well as two additional areas—community activities and psychotherapy. These psychiatrists believed that the psychiatric nurse should join mental health societies, consult with welfare agencies, work in outpatient clinics, practice preventive psychiatry, engage in research, and help educate the public. They supported the nurse's participation in individual and group psychotherapy and stated, "Despite the fact that most psychiatrists seem to ignore the role of the psychiatric nurse in psychotherapy, all nurses in psychiatric wards do psychotherapy of one kind or another by their contacts with patients."[5:170] They urged that nurses, like psychologists and social workers, be used in "team psychotherapy." Many of the issues raised in the article would be debated years later.

■ **NURSING THERAPY.** The most controversial issue was that of nurses conducting psychotherapy. Mellow[30] wrote in the *American Journal of Nursing* of the work she did with schizophrenic patients at Boston State Hospital in 1951. She called these activities "nursing therapy" and delineated three phases in the treatment process. The task in phase 1 is to establish contact with the patient and enter his life as a partner in the establishment of a therapeutic symbiotic relationship. In phase 2 the nurse allows the patient to relive his symbiotic attachment to a maternal figure and helps him resolve it. The task of phase 3 is to help the patient manage his separation anxieties as he assumes more responsibility for his own life. In 1952 Tudor[50] published a study, "Sociopsychiatric Nursing Approach to Intervention in a Problem of Mutual Withdrawal on a Mental Hospital Ward," in which she described the nurse-patient relationships she established, which were characterized by unconditional care, few demands, and the anticipation of her patients' needs. These articles by Mellow and Tudor were some of the earliest descriptions by psychiatric nurses of the nurse-patient relationship and the nature of its therapeutic process.

As nurses engaged in these kinds of activities, many questions arose. Are these activities therapeutic or are they therapy? What is a therapeutic relationship or a one-to-one nurse-patient relationship? How does it differ from psychotherapy? These questions were addressed by Dr. Hildegard Peplau, a dynamic nursing leader whose ideas and beliefs shaped psychiatric nursing.

In 1952 Peplau[35] published a book, *Interpersonal Relations in Nursing,* in which she described the skills, activities, and role of psychiatric nurses. It was the first systematic, theoretical framework developed for psychiatric nursing. Peplau defined nursing as a "significant, therapeutic process." She believed that the nurse-patient relationship was characterized by four overlapping and interlocking phases—orientation, identification, exploitation, and resolution. As she studied the nursing process in nurse-patient situations, she saw nurses emerge in various roles, as a resource person, teacher, leader in local, national, and international situations, surrogate parent, and counselor. She wrote, "Counseling in nursing has to do with helping the patient remember and to understand fully what is happening to him in the present situation, so that the experience can be integrated with rather than dissociated from other experiences in life."[35:64]

The use of the nursing process in defining a role for psychiatric nurses was further explored in 1953 when the National League for Nursing published, "A Study of Desirable Functions and Qualifications for Psychiatric Nurses."[36] This report identified the following desirable functions:

1. Collecting significant data that help identify problems (e.g., observing behavior, recording observations).
2. Making inferences and/or judgments based on these data and leading to action (e.g., interpreting the behavior of the patient, seeking to understand patients' needs)
3. Acting or intervening on the basis of inferences (e.g., clarifying with a patient the meaning of a procedure, discussing and acting to solve problems in a work situation)

Evolutionary Timeline in Psychiatric Nursing

Social environment		Psychiatric nursing
	1873	Linda Richards graduated from the New England Hospital for Women and Children
	1882	First school to prepare nurses to care for the mentally ill opened at McLean Hospital in Massachusetts
American Journal of Nursing first published	1900	
Clifford Beer's book, *A Mind That Found Itself,* published	1908	
Florence Nightingale died	1910	
	1913	Johns Hopkins was first school of nursing to include a course on psychiatric nursing in its curriculum
	1920	First psychiatric nursing textbook, *Nursing Mental Disease* by Harriet Bailey, published
Electroconvulsive therapy developed	1937	
National Mental Health Act passed by Congress, creating National Institute of Mental Health (NIMH) and providing training funds for psychiatric nursing education	1946	
	1950	National League for Nursing (NLN) required that to be accredited schools of nursing must provide an experience in psychiatric nursing
	1952	Hildegard Peplau published *Interpersonal Relations in Nursing*
Maxwell Jones published *The Therapeutic Community*	1953	
Development of major tranquilizers	1954	
	1962	Hildegard Peplau published "Interpersonal Techniques: The Crux of Psychiatric Nursing"
Community Mental Health Centers Act passed	1963	*Perspectives in Psychiatric Care* published; *Journal of Psychiatric Nursing and Mental Health Services* published
	1973	*Standards of Psychiatric-Mental Health Nursing Practice* published; Certification of psychiatric mental health nurse generalists established by the American Nurses' Association
Report of the President's Commission on Mental Health	1978	
	1979	*Issues in Mental Health Nursing* published; Certification of psychiatric mental health nurse specialists established by the American Nurses' Association
Mental Health Systems Act passed	1980	*Nursing: A Social Policy Statement* published by the American Nurses' Association
Mental Health Systems Act repealed	1981	
	1982	*Revised Standards of Psychiatric and Mental Health Nursing Practice* published
National Center for Nursing Research created in National Institute of Health (NIH)	1985	*Standards of Child and Adolescent Psychiatric and Mental Health Nursing Practice* published
National Institute of Mental Health (NIMH) Task Force on Nursing created	1987	*Archives of Psychiatric Nursing* published; *Journal of Child and Adolescent Psychiatric and Mental Health Nursing* published
	1988	Coalition of Psychiatric Nursing Organizations (COPNO) established
National Mental Health Leadership Forum formed	1989	

4. Evaluating the process based on whether identified problems have been solved (e.g., mutually evaluating experiences and learning)

As nurses continued to describe their qualifications, skills, activities, and responsibilities, the role of the psychiatric nurse began to gain substance.

Two significant developments in psychiatry in the 1950s affected nursing's role for years to come. The first was Jones' publication of *The Therapeutic Community: A New Treatment Method in Psychiatry*[21] in 1953. It encouraged using the patient's social environment to provide a therapeutic experience. The patient was to be an active participant in his own care and become involved in the daily problems of the community. All patients were to help solve problems, plan activities, and develop the necessary rules and regulations. Their independence was increased as they gained control over many of their personal activities. The environment fostered trust, self-direction, and individual dignity, and patients became aware of how their behavior affected others. Therapeutic communities became the preferred environment for psychiatric patients.

Gregg explored the implications of this development in an 1954 article.[17] She wrote that the role of the psychiatric nurse was to help create an environment in which the patient could develop new behavior patterns that would allow a more mature adjustment to life. Achieving this goal involved "nurse-patient relationships that promote emotional growth and are consistent with the therapeutic plan of the doctor-patient relationship." Gregg contrasted such an environment to those that are custodial or protective and those that emphasize conformity and acceptable routines. To establish a therapeutic environment, she wrote the patient had to be allowed to express conflict, the staff had to try to understand him, and there had to be an opportunity for learning and growth through the development of interpersonal relationships.

The idea of the therapeutic community received support in the second significant development in psychiatry in the early 1950s—the use of psychotropic drugs. With these drugs more patients became treatable, and fewer environmental constraints such as locked doors and straightjackets were required. Also more personnel were needed to provide therapy, and the roles of various psychiatric practitioners were expanded, including the nurse's role.

■ **EMERGING FUNCTIONS.** An article by Maloney[25] published in 1962 questioned whether the psychiatric nurse should have independent functions. Maloney reviewed the spectrum of nursing philosophies and the descriptions of roles and functions. One clear area of independent functioning was identified in the management and supervision of the patient's environment. However, this function could be either therapeutic or mechanical and clerical, depending on the nurse's goals in implementation.

Hays[18] reviewed the literature in 1958 and reported the following functions of psychiatric nurses: dealing with patients' problems of attitude, mood, and interpretation of reality; exploring disturbing and conflicting thoughts and feelings; using the patient's positive feelings toward the therapist to bring about psychophysiological homeostasis; counseling patients in emergencies, including panic and fear; and strengthening the well part of patients. Hayes reported that the nurse-patient relationship was referred to by a variety of terms, including "therapeutic nurse-patient relationship," "psychiatric nursing therapy," "supportive psychotherapy," "rehabilitation therapies," and "nondirective counseling." The distinction between these terms and the exact nature of the nurse's role remained hazy.

Once again Peplau[37] clarified psychiatric nursing's position and directed its future growth. In "Interpersonal Techniques: The Crux of Psychiatric Nursing," published in 1962, she identified the heart of psychiatric nursing as the role of counselor or psychotherapist. Other functions such as mother surrogate, technician, manager, socializing agent, and health teacher were seen as subroles. In her article Peplau differentiated between (1) general practitioners who were staff nurses working on psychiatric units, and (2) psychiatric nurses who were specialists and expert clinical practitioners with graduate degrees in psychiatric nursing.

Thus, from an undefined role involving primarily physical care, psychiatric nursing was evolving into a role of clinical competence based on interpersonal techniques and use of the nursing process. The expanding ideas and clinical experiences of psychiatric nurses received an even larger forum with publication of two new nursing journals in 1963—*Perspectives in Psychiatric Care* and the *Journal of Psychiatric Nursing and Mental Health Services*. These journals continue to explore elements of psychiatric nursing practice. (The name of the latter journal was changed in 1981 to the *Journal of Psychosocial Nursing and Mental Health Services*.) In 1979, a third journal, *Issues in Mental Health Nursing*, and in 1987 two additional journals, *Archives of Psychiatric Nursing*, and *Journal of Child and Adolescent Psychiatric and Mental Health Nursing* were published, providing nurses with additional means for exploring the emerging role of psychiatric nursing.

■ **Social-environmental influences**

An evolutionary perspective on psychiatric nursing would be incomplete without a discussion of its relationship to the larger social environment. A major factor in this relationship is the 35 years of federal support for psychiatric nursing education; this support advanced the practice of psychiatric–mental health nursing in the United States. Programs started with federal funds increased the number of new master's degree psychiatric nursing programs, thus providing greater numbers in practice; baccalaureate nursing programs placed greater emphasis on the integration of mental health concepts into their curricula; and many continuing education programs that focus on psychiatric–mental health content have been developed.

In the 1960s the focus of psychiatric nursing was on primary prevention and implementing care and consultation in the community. This focus was stimulated by the Community Mental Health Centers Act of 1963, which made federal money available to states to plan, construct, and staff community mental health centers. This legislation was prompted by growing awareness of the value of treating people in the community and of preventing hospitalization whenever possible. It also encouraged the formation of multidisciplinary treatment teams by joining the skills and expertise of many professions to alleviate illness and promote mental health. This team approach continues to be negotiated. The issues of territoriality, professionalism, authority structure, consumer rights, functioning, labeling, and the use of paraprofessionals are still being debated throughout the country.

The 1978 report of the President's Commission on Mental Health[43] tried to address some of the complex problems and inadequacies of the existing mental health services system. The report emphasized the continued need for community-based services that would provide the following:

1. A range of diagnostic, treatment, rehabilitative, and supportive services that would include long-term and short-term care
2. Easy access and continuity of care
3. Coordination with the network of other human services, such as education, health, income, and social services to provide comprehensive care
4. Adaptation to meet changing circumstances and the needs of special population groups
5. Adequate financing with public and private funds

The report focused on the need to broaden the base of knowledge about the nature and treatment of mental disabilities. It also called attention to several problems among mental health professionals that ultimately work to the disadvantage of the patient: (1) uneven geographic distribution, (2) similarities in function, and (3) interprofessional tension. Increased mental

health funding was proposed in an effort to solve some of these problems.

The Mental Health Systems Act of 1980 reaffirmed the goal of providing comprehensive mental health services for the United States. It focused on services for children, youths, the elderly, minorities, and the chronic mentally ill. The act was signed by President Jimmy Carter, who regarded it as landmark legislation, because it established a federal role in mental health in the 1980s.

■ **PRESENT CONSTRAINTS.** The federal role in mental health services seemed to become less certain, however, with the change to the Reagan administration in 1981. The Mental Health Systems Act was repealed almost immediately after President Reagan took office. In October of 1981, the new federal fiscal budget for 1982 went into effect, in which funds for psychological and social health services, as well as for the education of health care professionals, were severely cut. The remaining money was to be dispensed primarily through block grants to the states. Instead of the previous 25 categorical grants for health and human services, four block grants were awarded to each state:

1. Alcoholism, drug abuse, and mental health
2. Maternal and child care
3. Primary care
4. Prevention and health services

Nursing professionals have several major concerns about block grants:

1. Sufficient funds may not be available for the needed services, and states may not make up the deficits to support these essential programs.
2. Some health concerns are best handled through a national approach.
3. Lack of guidelines and responsibility may lead to inefficient use of funds, inadequate programs, and neglect of groups most in need.

These constraints have continued under the administration of President George Bush, and many people believe that mental health care is facing a crisis in the United States. Some of the most recent changes include further shifts in the level of government responsibility for the allocation of resources from the federal to the state level and from the state to the county level; shifts from institutional to community-based care but without the needed funds; increased influence by judges and legislators; development of a large mental health delivery sector made up of insurance companies, health maintenance organizations (HMOs), and third party payers; and the multiple needs of new target populations in this country, including the homeless mentally ill.

Thus the promise of "fewer services, economic constraints, and less federal regulation" has replaced that of "comprehensive care, right to health, and government subsidy." Consequently, the concern is that the most needy, who are least likely to receive equitable health care from state to state, will not have the advocacy that the federal government has historically provided as a basic right.

Partly as a response to these concerns, the National Mental Health Leadership Forum was formed in 1989 with funding from the National Institute of Mental Health. Over 20 organizations have joined the forum, representing consumers, mental health care delivery systems, and providers. A number of psychiatric nursing organizations are members of this forum. The goals of this group are to:

1. Establish mental illnesses as one of the nation's central and most pressing health care responsibilities.
2. Raise the national health care priority of mental illnesses to a level commensurate with their wide prevalence and the suffering and disability they cause.
3. Raise public awareness about mental illness and inform the public and policymakers about current knowledge and advances in research and treatment.
4. Galvanize a major national research and service effort to largely conquer mental illnesses by the year 2000.

It is fair to say that these are very ambitious goals.

■ Agenda for the 1990s

Since 1946 the social environment has changed greatly. Three current trends in the mental health field will have a great impact on the future of psychiatric nursing in the 1990s. The first trend is the increasing numbers of people who are experiencing mental illness, particularly the chronically mentally ill. Vulnerable groups include substance-exposed infants, children and adolescents with behavioral disorders, HIV-infected patients and their families, individuals with substance abuse problems, and elderly patients with psychiatric disorders.

A second major trend is the shift in the field of psychiatry to a more biological and neurochemical model of understanding and treating mental illness. This shift is reflected in all aspects of the field of psychiatry—from NIMH research priorities to medical

treatment protocols. For nurses this requires a more sophisticated understanding of biological and neurochemical processes, greater mastery of rapidly emerging technology, and expanded knowledge and diligence in administering and monitoring potent psychiatric drugs.

The third impact on psychiatric nursing is the change in the organization and delivery of mental health care. Patients who are hospitalized for psychiatric treatment are more acutely ill, present the nursing staff with complex management problems, and require greater amounts of nursing care. At the same time, early discharge, reimbursement issues, and public initiatives are moving less acute mental health care into the community at a rapid pace. Thus there are increasing demands for the services of psychiatric nurses in community mental health centers, home health agencies, and with the homeless mentally ill. These needs extend well beyond the present, limited supply of psychiatric nurses and the projections of nurses who will be entering the field in the near future.

■ **RECRUITMENT INTO THE FIELD.** Twenty years ago, psychiatric nursing educators were in the vanguard of nursing education. Graduate education for psychiatric nursing practice was well established. Federal funding of nursing programs and student traineeships was readily available. As a result of this progressive educational system, nurses were actively involved in the changes in the mental health care system that occurred in the 1960s and 1970s. However, since 1980, drastic changes have taken place. Funding for nursing education programs of all types has been drastically reduced. For psychiatric nursing, it is now necessary to compete for limited funds with other disciplines. Unfortunately, psychiatric nurses have never been able to compete effectively with the other mental health care disciplines. As a result, the graduate psychiatric nursing education system is in a precarious position.

Another trend with serious implications for psychiatric nursing in the future is the declining enrollment of students in schools of nursing. As more job opportunities are becoming open to women, fewer are choosing the traditionally female occupations, such as nursing. The image of the nurse as subservient to the physician, overworked, and underpaid does little to encourage young women to enter the field. At the same time, the identification of nursing as a "woman's profession" discourages men from entering schools of nursing in large numbers. Recently, the American Nurses' Association has recognized this problem and has launched a nationwide campaign to update the image of nursing. However, individual nurses must become more active in promoting a positive image to the public.

Although recruitment to nursing in general has declined, the percentage of nursing graduates who select psychiatric nursing as their area of practice has declined even more rapidly. Only about 5% of senior nursing students select psychiatry as their clinical setting, and only 7% of all nurses choose psychiatric nursing as a specialty area for their graduate degree. This is in contrast to the 40% of masters students who selected psychiatry in 1968. This specialty used to attract nurses who looked forward to independent practice and greater autonomy, but other nursing specialties, such as nurse midwifery and nurse practitioners of various types, now offer those same benefits and have done a better job of marketing their opportunities.

Nurse educators and administrators have proposed explanations for the waning interest in psychiatric nursing. One theory is that the integrated nursing curriculum separated psychiatric nursing out as a unique area of practice. Some students completed their nursing education program with no experience in an inpatient psychiatric setting and were therefore not attracted to that as a place of employment. Stereotypical images of mental hospitals remained unchallenged by personal experience. In addition, graduating students were routinely advised by faculty to "get basic medical-surgical nursing experience before you go into a specialty area like psych." This message is reinforced by nurse administrators who require medical-surgical nursing experience before employment in psychiatric settings. Although probably well meant, this advice is discouraging to new graduates who would otherwise consider exploring mental health nursing as a career option. It is time for psychiatric nursing leaders to reevaluate the integrated curriculum and approaches to career counseling so that sufficient numbers of nurses may be attracted to psychiatric nursing careers and to graduate education for advanced practice. Options such as concentrated clinical study in psychiatric settings and internships for new graduates should be expanded.

■ **PSYCHIATRIC NURSING PRACTICE.** Challenges also exist in the scope and characteristics of psychiatric nursing practice. While psychiatric nurses are prepared for the new decade with standards, credentials, advanced powers of observation, and communication skills, McBride suggests that two major readjustments need to be made.[27] First psychiatric nurses must begin to revalue biological knowledge in their clinical practice. This need is influenced by the complexity of the problem experienced by the mentally ill, and in the movement of consumer advocacy groups

who fully support the notion that mental illness is a disease of the brain. While this is a needed dimension of psychiatric nursing practice, it does not negate the need for psychosocial knowledge and intervention. It merely supports the idea that human behavior is a function of both nature (biology) and nurture (environment).

Second, psychiatric nurses must become reassociated with care and caring. This focus seems essential given the limited number of psychiatric cures and the large amount of continuing mental health problems experienced by most people. Caring behaviors can be directed toward an individual, a family system, or the larger health care delivery system. In many ways, care and caring represent the roots of psychiatric nursing and an appropriate balance to the high technology of current health care practices.

Another area for continued work is in describing the phenomena of concern to psychiatric nurses. The use of a standardized diagnostic system and nursing protocols will enhance reimbursement for psychiatric nursing care. In order to be paid for providing a service, one must be able to clearly describe the nature of it. Until now, nurses have been limited to trying to describe nursing services in medical terms. This has curtailed nursing's ability to receive reimbursement for the delivery of nursing services. This has also limited the ability to demonstrate the cost-effectiveness of psychiatric nursing intervention, thus handicapping nurse executives in their efforts to justify the employment of clinical nurse specialists. The present focus on cost containment in all health care settings mandates the documentation of cost-benefit data relative to psychiatric nursing practice.

Issues related to competition in the mental health care marketplace must also be addressed by mental health nurses. Free competition requires that equal reimbursement for services be available to all providers. At this time, this is not the case in most states. Psychiatric nurses, through their professional oragnization, must continue to lobby federal and state legislators to extend full reimbursement to psychiatric nurse specialists. In addition, vigilance is required to be sure that the Federal Trade Commission retains its jurisdiction over professional practice in order to prevent attempts to restrain or limit practice of some disciplines. In recent sessions of Congress, the American Medical Association has promoted legislation to revoke this FTC power. A coalition of the other health care disciplines has been successful thus far in blocking this effort.

Consumers must also be assured that the providers of psychiatric nursing care are well qualified. The profession has a responsibility to set and maintain standards of practice. Certification for specialty practice and peer review for quality assurance are responsibilities of all nurse specialists. There has been a steady increase in the number of mental health nurses who are certified at the specialist and generalist levels. This trend must continue in order to elicit public confidence in nurses as mental health care providers.

■ **POLITICAL ACTION.** In order for nurses to accomplish the level of influence that they need relative to these issues and trends, they must become a recognized force in the political system. The numbers are there. The question is, is the will there also? Political action and accountability are the only routes to acquiring professional autonomy and leadership in mental health care. Nurses must become educated in the legislative and regulatory process. They must be involved in political campaigns, and they must testify in legislative hearings. In coalition with other mental health care providers and consumers, they must lobby for government budgets that provide adequate funding for mental health service delivery, professional education, and research. Psychiatric nurses must then assert their right to an equitable share of the resources, given the value of the services they provide. Passive acceptance of decisions made by legislators, bureaucrats, and other health care providers will lead to the decline of psychiatric nursing as an important influence on the future of the mental health care system. Senator Daniel Inouye of Hawaii has said, "You nurses, you can have whatever you want, you can control the health care system, you have more power than any other group, including all the oil lobbyists, but you will go to your graves with 'docile' written on your tombstones."[23] This challenge by one of our staunchest supporters must be met. For psychiatric nurses, this means that the days of reaction are past. Proaction is the key to meeting the challenges of psychiatric nursing in the 1990s.

Contemporary practice

Psychiatric nursing is an interpersonal process that promotes and maintains behavior that contributes to integrated functioning. The patient may be an individual, family, group, organization, or community. The American Nurses' Association Division on Psychiatric and Mental Health Nursing defined psychiatric and mental health nursing as*:

---

*Quotations in this chapter are from the American Nurses' Association, Division on Psychiatric and Mental Health Nursing Practice: Statement on psychiatric and mental health nursing pratice, Kansas City, Mo., 1976. Reprinted by permission.

... a specialized area of nursing practice employing theories of human behavior as its science and purposeful use of self as its art. It is directed toward both preventive and corrective impacts upon mental disorders and their sequelae and is concerned with the promotion of optimal mental health for society, the community, and those individuals who live within it.[2:5]

The National Institute of Mental Health officially recognizes psychiatric and mental health nursing as one of the four core mental health disciplines. (The other three are psychiatry, psychology, and social work.) The current practice of psychiatric nursing is based on a number of underlying premises or beliefs. Some of the major philosophical beliefs of psychiatric nursing practice are described in the accompanying box.

■ Roles and activities

The psychiatric nurse uses knowledge from the psychosocial and biophysical sciences and theories of personality and human behavior. From these sources the nurse derives a theoretical framework on which to base his or her practice. The choice of a conceptual model and theoretical framework is an individual one. Various theories of psychiatric care are briefly described in Chapter 2, and a nursing model of health-illness phenomena is presented in Chapter 3.

Some nurses might base their practice on a psychoanalytical framework; others might adopt a family systems orientation; still others may use a behavioral theoretical model. The nurse's choice of a model depends on personal philosophy, educational background, setting, and experience in working with patients. Powers[42] believes that the selected theoretical framework should encompass the following commonalities of nursing models:

1. A holistic view of people, with usually three major interdependent components (i.e., biopsychosocial)
2. People as systems in dynamic interaction with the environment
3. People developing over time
4. People adapting continuously to both internal and external forces or variables

The theoretical model selected by the nurse can then be used as a framework for nursing practice.

■ **PRACTICE SETTINGS.** Psychiatric nurses may practice in settings that vary widely in purpose, type, location, and administration. They may be employed by an agency or self-employed in a private practice. Nurses employed by an agency are paid for their services on a salaried or fee-for-service basis. Most nurses

Philosophical Beliefs of Psychiatric Nursing Practice

- The individual has intrinsic worth and dignity. Each person is worthy of respect by his nature and presence alone.
- The goal of the individual is one of growth, health, autonomy, and self-actualization.
- Every individual has the potential to change and the desire to pursue personal goals.
- The person functions as a holistic being who acts on, interacts with, and reacts to the environment as a whole person. Each part affects the total response, which is greater than the sum of each separate component.
- All people have common, basic, and necessary human needs. Maslow[29] defined these needs as physical, safety, love and belonging, esteem, and self-actualization. Physical needs include physiological requirements such as food, water, and air. Safety needs pertain to the necessity of a secure physical environment that is free from threat. Love and belonging needs include the desire for intimacy and relatedness. Esteem needs refer to the desire for self-respect and recognition from others that one is a worthwhile and valuable person. Self-actualization needs include the desire for self-fulfillment as one concentrates on realizing one's own potential.
- All behavior of the individual is meaningful. It arises from personal needs and goals and can be understood only from the person's internal frame of reference and within the context in which it occurs.
- Behavior consists of perceptions, thoughts, feelings, and actions. These occur in a sequential manner; from one's perceptions thoughts arise, emotions are felt, and actions are conceived. Disrup-

tions may occur in any of these areas and be evident in distorted perceptions, impaired thought processes, alterations in the expression of emotions, and maladaptive or inappropriate actions.
- Individuals vary in their coping capacities, which depend on genetic endowment, environmental influences, nature and degree of stress, and available resources. All individuals have the potential for both health and illness.
- Illness can be a growth-producing experience for the individual. The goal of nursing care is to maximize the person's positive interactions with his environment, promote his level of wellness, and enhance his degree of self-actualization.
- All people have a right to an equal opportunity for adequate health care regardless of sex, race, religion, ethics, or cultural background. Nursing care is based on the needs of individuals, families, and communities and mutually defined goals and expectations.
- Mental health is a critical and necessary component of comprehensive health care services.
- The individual has the right to participate in decision making regarding his physical and mental health. The person has the right to self-determination. This right allows the individual the choice of changing present behavior or continuing it without modification. It is the decision of the individual to pursue health or illness.
- An interpersonal relationship has the potential for producing change and growth within the individual. It is the vehicle for the application of the nursing process and the attainment of the goal of nursing care.

work in such organized settings. The administrative policies of these organizations can either foster or limit full use of the nurse's potential. Nurses who are self-employed are paid for their services through third-party payment and direct patient fees. Some self-employed specialists maintain staff privileges with institutional facilities.

The settings in which nurses work can focus on either acute or long-term care. Settings include psychiatric hospitals, community mental health centers, general hospitals, community health agencies, outpatient clinics, homes, schools, prisons, health maintenance orga-

nizations, private organizations, crisis care units, day and night care centers, offices, camps, and industrial centers.

FUNCTIONS. Within these care settings, psychiatric nurses may assume various roles. They may be staff nurses, administrators, consultants, in-service educators, clinical practitioners, researchers, or program evaluators. Thus the settings of practice range from institutional to community-based to independent practice. The corresponding roles can include both direct and indirect nursing functions. The American Nurses' Association has identified nine major activities in-

---

Psychiatric Nursing Activities Identified by the American Nurses' Association*

1. Providing a therapeutic milieu
2. Working with the here-and-now problems of clients
3. Using the surrogate parent role
4. Caring for the somatic aspects of the client's health problems
5. Teaching factors related to emotional health
6. Acting as a social agent
7. Providing leadership to other personnel
8. Conducting psychotherapy
9. Engaging in social and community action related to mental health

*American Nurses' Association, Division on Psychiatric and Mental Health Nursing Practice: Statement on psychiatric and mental health nursing practice, Kansas City, Mo, 1976, The Association.

---

volved in the practice of psychiatric nursing.[2] (See the box above.)

The various functions or activities engaged in by psychiatric nurses can be classified as direct or indirect. "**Direct nursing care functions** presume that the nurse's actions and reflections are focused on a particular client or family and that the nurse has personal responsibility and is accountable to the client or family for the outcome of such actions."[2:15] **Indirect nursing care functions** are those in which some other person actually carries out the patient's care. All of the direct and indirect nursing functions are actions for which the nurse is directly responsible. They are done whether or not the patient is under medical care and in any setting agreed on by the nurse and the patient.

In projecting future roles of psychiatric nurses, Slavinsky envisions the creation of a new primary care role for psychiatric nurses developed in liaison with community health nurses, using a system of mutual referral and consultation.[45] This primary care role would involve three functions: assessment, direct patient care, and case management. Such a role would combine both the direct and indirect care functions previously described.

■ **PRIMARY PREVENTION.** The concepts of primary, secondary, and tertiary prevention provide a framework for discussing psychiatric nursing activities. Primary prevention is a community concept. It involves lowering the incidence of illness in a community by changing causative factors before they can do harm. It is a concept that precedes disease and is applied to a generally healthy population. It includes health promotion, illness prevention, and protection against disease. Within this area lie many of nursing's independent functions, which have as their goal to decrease the vulnerability of individuals to illness and to strengthen their capacity to withstand stressors. Direct nursing care functions in this area include:

1. Health teaching regarding principles of mental health
2. Affecting changes in improved living conditions, freedom from poverty, and better education
3. Consumer education in such areas as normal growth and development and sex education
4. Making appropriate referrals before mental disorder occurs, based on assessment of potential stressors and life changes
5. Assisting patients in a general hospital setting to avoid future psychiatric problems
6. Working with families to support family members and group functioning
7. Becoming active in community and political activities related to mental health

■ **SECONDARY PREVENTION.** Secondary prevention involves reducing actual illness by early detection and treatment of the problem. Direct nursing care functions in this area include:

1. Intake screening and evaluation services
2. Home visits for preadmission or treatment services
3. Emergency treatment and psychiatric services in the general hospital
4. Providing a therapeutic milieu
5. Supervising patients receiving medication
6. Suicide prevention services
7. Counseling on a time-limited basis
8. Crisis intervention
9. Psychotherapy with individuals, families, and groups of various ages ranging from children to older adults
10. Intervening with communities and organizations based on an identified problem

■ **TERTIARY PREVENTION.** Tertiary prevention involves reducing the residual impairment or disability resulting from an illness. Direct nursing care functions in this area include the following:

1. Promoting vocational training and rehabilitation
2. Organizing aftercare programs for patients discharged from psychiatric facilities to ease their transition from the hospital to the community
3. Providing partial hospitalization options for patients

In addition to direct nursing care functions, psychiatric nurses engage in indirect activities that affect all three levels of prevention. These activities include training nursing personnel in various educational programs; administrating in mental health settings to help provide optimal nursing care; supervising nursing personnel to improve the quality of nursing services; consulting with colleagues, other professionals, consumer groups, community care givers, and local and national agencies; and researching clinical nursing problems.

■ Interdisciplinary mental health teams

An essential part of contemporary practice is to work with other health care providers. Nurses may be members of three different types of teams: *unidisciplinary,* having all team members of the same discipline; *multidisciplinary,* having members of different disciplines who each provide specific services to the patient; and *interdisciplinary,* having members of different disciplines involved in a formal arrangement to provide patient services while maximizing educational interchange. Most organized mental health settings employ an interdisciplinary team approach, which requires highly coordinated and frequently interdependent planning based on the separate and distinct roles of each team member (Fig. 1-1).

- Physicians carry the medical responsibility for diagnosis, medical orders, medication, admission, and discharge, and the accountability for medical treatment. They may or may not be the team leaders.

- Activity therapists are accountable and responsible for activity programming, sometimes sharing aspects of it with nurses.
- Social workers are accountable and responsible for family casework and social placement.
- Psychologists are accountable and responsible for psychological assessment and testing.
- Nurses are accountable and responsible for the patient's milieu and for implementing the nursing process. This includes assessment and diagnosis, planning care, implementing nursing interventionsproviding a safe environment, dealing with the daily activity of patients, and evaluating the outcome of nursing care.

■ **BARRIERS TO TEAM FUNCTIONING.** Interdisciplinary collaboration does not always proceed smoothly. Given and Simmons describe seven barriers to interdisciplinary team formation: (1) educational preparation, (2) role ambiguity and incongruent expectations, (3) authority, (4) power, (5) status, (6) autonomy, and (7) personal characteristics of members.[16] Benfer has identified three specific problems related to team functioning: (1) problems identifying roles and functions; (2) difficulties in resolving overlapping roles; and (3) communication problems within the team.[4]

If the roles and functions of the various team members are not clarified and agreed on, confusion, crossing of boundaries, resentment, and underutilization of health professionals are likely to occur. Some overlapping of roles and functions among psychiatric professionals is to be expected, since all mental health disciplines have access to the same body of knowledge on which professional education is based. Thus all members of the mental health team may be competent in providing psychotherapy, although some may prefer group therapy, others individual therapy, and still oth-

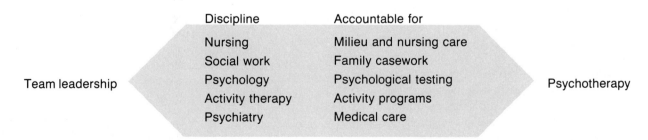

Fig. 1-1. Roles assumed by mental health team members. (Modified from Benfer B: Perspect Psychiatr Care 18(4):167, 1980.)

```
┌──────────────────────────────────────────────────────────────────────────┐
│                              TABLE 1-1                                      │
│                  ANALYSIS OF INTERDISCIPLINARY TEAMS                        │
└──────────────────────────────────────────────────────────────────────────┘
```

Personal qualities vital to interdisciplinary team function	Activities necessary for interdisciplinary team function
Accept differences/perspectives of others	Establish new professional interaction patterns
Function interdependently	Accept changes in authority and status
Negotiate role with other team members	Develop modes of conflict resolution and decision making
Form new values, attitudes, and perceptions	Accept shared authority and responsibility
Tolerate constant review and challenge of ideas	Tolerate risk-taking behavior
Possess personal identity and integrity	
Accept team philosophy of care	

From Given B and Simmons S: Nurs Forum 16(2):165, 1977.

ers family therapy. Only team members with the necessary education, experience, and credentials can be considered qualified to handle ethically responsible psychotherapy. For nurses, psychotherapy should be undertaken only by a psychiatric clinical nurse specialist educated at the master's level.

The issue of various team members moving toward an individual psychotherapy approach has many implications. It can lead to unhealthy competition among team members to establish equally significant relationships with the patient. It might also lead to a disruption of the psychotherapeutic process. At the least, it can be very confusing to a patient. Finally, Ruch suggests, when a patient has several close relationships with team members, the patient is less likely to develop an effective therapeutic alliance. Ruch concludes that formal psychotherapy is best left to one member of the team who can coordinate other interpersonal interventions.

In addition to a discrete role description, certain personal characteristics are essential to teamwork. Professional members who can tolerate frustration and are flexible in their adjustment to new situations function better in team situations. Appropriate members and adequate time are also important to the interdisciplinary team functioning. Table 1-1 summarizes these elements.

■ **JOINT COMMISSION ON INTERPROFESSIONAL AFFAIRS.** Partly in response to vested interests among mental health professionals and lack of cooperation, the Joint Commission on Interprofessional Affairs (JCIA) was founded in 1974. The members are representatives of the American Nurses' Association, the American Psychiatric Association, the American Psychological Association, and the National Association of Social Workers. With three representatives from each organization, the commission meets three times a year. It discusses legislation, reimbursement, education, and patient care issues related to mental health. The commission's goal is to promote interprofessional trust, communication, and cooperation among mental health practitioners.

The commission recommends that a variety of methods be pursued to facilitate communication and resolution of problems at national, state, and local levels. These methods include joint meetings, regular exchange of information, exchange of formal liaison representatives, and organization of local and statewide interprofessional groups.

One of the commission's major efforts has been development of the following guidelines for interprofessional ethics:

1. Seek to achieve interprofessional unity and cooperation.
2. Recognize and respect the autonomy and specialized competency of each profession.
3. Know the facts before speaking or issuing public statements about interprofessional issues, and use the facts in a responsible and appropriate fashion.
4. Attempt to resolve issues through direct discussion, debate, and negotiation.
5. Pursue joint actions toward mutually acceptable goals.

Observing these guidelines should make each profession more effective in providing mental health services. The Joint Commission currently is working on a consumer document to help the public select appropriate insurance coverage for mental health services and a statement about the content and distinct characteristics of each of the four core mental health professions.

■ **Leadership skills**

Psychiatric nurses, individually and collectively, need knowledge and strategies that enable them to exercise leadership and management in their work. Such leadership has an effect on the care patients receive; it also strengthens and expands the contribution of psychiatric nursing to the larger health care system.

One might approach this area from two different perspectives: (1) examine the individual who holds a position of leadership or (2) explore leadership as a transactional process. The former approach would include the styles and functions of leadership. The latter would include the conditions and processes of leadership as a social role or transaction (Table 1-2).

Dumas has noted the following:

Those processes occurring in the groups in which or with which nurses work are of special significance. Pressures to conform to the image of the kind, nurturing, self-sacrificing

angel of mercy (the analogue of the good mother) pose a perplexing dilemma for nurse leaders. Those who conform often find themselves deluged by bids from subordinates and colleagues in other disciplines for special attention or assistance to help them deal with the stresses of organizational life. These demands often exceed the responsibilities of their formal positions and drain time and energy that should be used for work tasks. Those who resist run the risk of the opposite stereotype—the cold, rigid, inconsiderate authoritarian leader (the rejecting, depriving, bad mother). There are big prices to pay in either instance.[11:712-713]

■ **CHANGE AGENTS.** There is no question that psychiatric nurses must use their leadership skills and work as change agents to a greater degree than they are doing at present. Mental health consumers need adequate, humane, and socially acceptable care. To this end nurses can initiate change; assist in change by supporting, participating, or implementing it; engage in joint ventures for planned change; and evaluate completed change. To do so, the psychiatric nurse needs the following key characteristics[26]:

1. The ability to take risks. The nurse must develop the ability to calculate potential risks sur-

TABLE 1-2

THE NATURE OF EFFECTIVE LEADERSHIP

Conditions of effective leadership	Social processes underlying effective leadership	Styles of leadership	Functions of effective leadership
Recipient of communication must be able to understand it	Respect expressed *by* leader breeds respect *for* leader	Authoritarian style characterized by firmness, self-assurance, and domination of others	Leaders are alert to unanticipated consequences of previous collective action
Person must have resources and ability to comply with directive	Leader must demonstrate competence in performing own roles	Democratic style characterized by responsiveness, participation, and mutual interaction	Leaders represent group to its environment
Person must believe action is consistent with personal beliefs and values	Leader should be in continuing touch with what is going on in work group	Bureaucratic style characterized by strict adherence to rules	Leaders evaluate resources and cope with problems of their allocation
Person must perceive directive as consistent with purposes and values of organization	Although leader has access to power that coerces, he or she seldom makes use of it	Laissez-faire style characterized by lack of direction and control	Leaders express group values and ideals and give people pride in their group identity
		Paternalistic style characterized by benevolent control	Leaders mediate inevitable conflicts that emerge in social interaction, so that most members of group believe justice has been done most of time

Modified from Merton R: Am J Nurs 69:2614, 1969.

rounding the implementation of the change and then decide whether these risks are indeed worth taking.

2. A commitment to the efficacy of the change. The change agent must develop a commitment to investigating the worth, value, effectiveness, and necessity of the change before initiating it.

3. Three areas of competence: (1) a knowledge of nursing that combines research findings and basic scientific information, (2) clinical competence, and (3) skill in interpersonal relationships and communication.

Communication at times requires confrontation, yet this is a skill that nurses have tended to avoid using. Confrontation can be justified only as a precursor to negotiations, which are a foundation for change. The process has two phases; the first phase requires an assault on the system to be changed; the second phase requires reconciliation to mend strained relationships or to create new ones. Smoyak believes:

Confrontations are in order when the goals are resolving an issue, improving health care systems, defining changing work roles, revamping licensing and practicing acts, gaining and keeping suitable salary schedules, attaining and maintaining control over professional practice, or any other professional issue, locally defined and carried out, on which there is consensus among nurses who are affected by the issue. They are in order when the group has gathered facts, may have tried other means, and has decided on collective action.[47:1635]

One result of the use of confrontation is that statutes governing licensing of nursing have undergone considerable change and scrutiny in the past decade. Although not all states have revised their nurse practice acts, those that have show nurses assuming responsibility for more complex patient care involving major independent decision making. Another positive sign was the publication in 1980 of the American Nurses' Association's *Nursing: A Social Policy Statement.*[3] This statement defines and establishes the scope of nursing practice and nursing's social responsibility.

Yet such statements and definitions are only words. They cannot actually determine the scope of practice, the relationships between nurses and other health professionals, the needs of the consumer, or the interaction between nursing and the government in formulating and implementing health-related policy. Only nurses working together through political processes can make these determinations. Although the impact nurses can have on the quality and quantity of health care may be phenomenal, it is largely untapped. Nurses have the potential to be significant forces in the process of shaping the health care future of our society. To do so, they must learn to use their power and resources in the political arena—truly one of the most important targets for nursing action.

Level of performance

The description of various nursing activities and functions indicates a wide variation in levels of performance. Not all psychiatric nurses can perform each of these functions. Individual nurses have primary responsibility and accountability for their own practice; one aspect of accountability is that nurses define and adhere to the legitimate scope of their practice. Four major factors—laws, qualifications, setting, and personal initiative—play a role in determining the level at which the nurse functions and the types of activities he or she engages in.

■ Laws

Laws are the primary factor affecting the level of nursing practice. Each state has its own nurse practice act, which regulates entry into the profession and defines the legal limits of nursing practice that must be adhered to by all nurses. Currently there are three general patterns of nurse practice acts: regulatory acts, expanded definition acts, and delegatory acts. Some acts recognize advanced practice of nurses; others do not. Nurses must be familiar with the nurse practice act of their state and define and limit their practice accordingly.

■ Qualifications

A nurse's qualifications include his or her education, work experiences, and certification status. The American Nurses' Association has identified two types of psychiatric nurse practitioners: (1) nurses who are generalists, called *psychiatric and mental health nurses,* and (2) nurses who are specialists, called *psychiatric and mental health nurse specialists.*[2]

■ **EDUCATION AND EXPERIENCE.** The recommended educational preparation for the generalist role is a baccalaureate degree in nursing. The nurse also must demonstrate the profession's standards of knowledge, experience, and quality of care through formal review processes. Most nurses working in psychiatry are generalists. They provide most of the care for most of the people served by nursing.

In contrast, specialization involves adding to the generic base of nursing practice a systematized body of knowledge and competencies within a discrete area of nursing. The specialist in psychiatric and mental health nursing has a graduate education, supervised clinical experience, and depth of knowledge, competence, and

TABLE 1-3

DOCTORAL PROGRAMS IN NURSING, 1988-1989

	Institution	Degree		Institution	Degree
AL	U. of Alabama in Birmingham Birmingham, AL 35294	D.N.S.	NY	State University of New York at Buffalo Buffalo, NY 14212	D.N.S.
AZ	U. of Arizona Tucson, AZ 85721	Ph.D.	NY	Adelphi University Garden City, NY 11530	Ph.D.
CA	U. of California, Los Angeles Los Angeles, CA 90024	D.N.S.	NY	New York University New York, NY 10003	Ph.D.
CA	U. of California, San Francisco San Francisco, CA 94143	Ph.D.	NY	Teachers College, Columbia University	Ed.D.
CA	U. of San Diego San Diego, CA 92110	D.N.S.		New York, NY 10027	
CO	U. of Colorado Denver, CO 80262	Ph.D.	NY	U. of Rochester Rochester, NY 14642	Ph.D.
DC	Catholic University of America Washington, DC 20064	D.N.S.	OH	Case Western Reserve University Cleveland, OH 44106	Ph.D.
FL	U. of Florida Gainesville, FL 32610	Ph.D.	OH	Ohio State University Columbus, OH 43210	D.N.S.
FL	U. of Miami Coral Gables, FL 33124	Ph.D.	OR	Oregon Health Sciences University Portland, OR 97201	Ph.D.
GA	Georgia State University Atlanta, Georgia 30303	Ph.D	PA	U. of Pennsylvania Philadelphia, PA 19104	Ph.D.
GA	Medical College of Georgia Augusta, GA 30912	Ph.D.	PA	U. of Pittsburgh Pittsburgh, PA 15261	Ph.D.
IL	Rush University Chicago, IL 60612	D.N.S.	PA	Widener University Chester, PA 19013	Ph.D.
IL	U. of Illinois Chicago, IL 60612	Ph.D.	RI	U. of Rhode Island Kingston, RI 02881	Ph.D.
IN	Indiana University Indianapolis, IN 46223	D.N.S.	SC	U. of S. Carolina Columbia, SC 29008	Ph.D.
KS	U. of Kansas Kansas City, KS 66103	Ph.D.	TX	Texas Woman's University Denton, TX 76204	Ph.D.
KY	U. of Kentucky Lexington, KY 40506	Ph.D.	TX	U. of Texas at Austin Austin, TX 78701	Ph.D.
LA	Louisiana State University New Orleans, LA 70112	D.N.S.	UT	U. of Utah Salt Lake City, UT 84112	Ph.D.
MA	Boston College Chestnut Hill, MA 02167	Ph.D.	VA	George Mason U. Fairfax, VA 22030	D.N.S.
MA	Boston University Boston, MA 02215	D.N.S.	VA	U. of Virginia Charlottesville, VA 22903	Ph.D.
MD	U. of Maryland Baltimore, MD 21201	Ph.D.	VA	Virginia Commonwealth University Richmond, VA 23298	D.N.S.
MI	U. of Michigan Ann Arbor, MI 48109	Ph.D.	WA	U. of Washington Seattle, WA 98195	Ph.D.
MI	Wayne State University Detroit, MI 48202	Ph.D.	WI	U. of Wisconsin-Madison Madison, WI 53792	Ph.D.
MN	U. of Minnesota Minneapolis, MN 55455	Ph.D.	WI	U. of Wisconsin-Milwaukee Milwaukee, WI 53201	Ph.D.

skill in practice. The nurse specialist can apply this added knowledge to the solution of mental health problems. The minimum level of preparation for the specialist is a master's degree in psychiatric nursing, which requires academically supervised clinical practice and study in the theoretical bases for therapeutic intervention.

Currently there are more than 60 master's degree programs in psychiatric nursing; more than 8000 psychiatric and mental health nurses have master's degrees. In addition, there are 45 doctoral programs in nursing (Table 1-3). They focus on either research and theory development in nursing or advanced development of the nurse-therapist role and specific clinical problems. The first type of program usually leads to a doctor of philosophy (Ph.D.) degree, whereas the second results in a doctor of nursing science (D.N.S.) degree. Doctorally prepared nurses contribute to the advancement of knowledge in the field of psychiatric and mental health nursing through research and scholarship.

Another qualification is the nurse's relevant work experience. Although work experience does not replace education, it does provide an added and necessary dimension to the nurse's level of competence and ability to function therapeutically. Gardner[15] believes that the nurse's role should be determined by his or her education, level of experience, and personal assets. She suggests defining the role of the psychiatric nurse in an ambulatory setting based on three levels of practice. Table 1-4 summarizes the requirements and responsibilities of each level of practice. The nurses identified in level 3 of this table are clinical nurse specialists, with master's degrees in psychiatric nursing. They have advanced knowledge and expertise in psychiatric care and principles of supervision and consultation.

■ **CERTIFICATION.** The certification process is a formal review of the clinical practice of nurses that has

TABLE 1-4

LEVELS OF PRACTICE FOR PSYCHIATRIC NURSES IN AMBULATORY SETTINGS

	Level 1	Level 2	Level 3
Educational requirements	No formal education is necessary other than current state licensure	Baccalaureate degree in nursing	Master's degree in psychiatric nursing
Experience requirements	Minimum of 1 year experience in acute psychiatric nursing care	Minimum of 2 years of experience in acute psychiatric care settings	Advanced knowledge and expertise in psychiatric care and principles of supervision and consultation
Nature of practice	Supportive treatment	Supportive treatment	Insight treatment
Therapeutic functions	Communicating with other professionals and agencies relative to patient care	Primary responsibility for supportive therapy	Primary responsibility for insight-oriented psychotherapy
	Assisting in assessment and data collection	Assessment of patient functioning	Responsibility for patients cared for by nurses in levels 1 and 2 of practice
	Assisting patient to use environmental resources	Initiation and attendance at all conferences regarding patients	Assessment of patient pathology
			Supervision of other health team members
	Assisting in community primary prevention programs	Assignment to interdisciplinary teams responsible for delivery of primary mental health care in ambulatory units	Participation in primary community prevention programs
			Responsibility for obtaining supervision consultation
			Responsible for assumption of nursing leadership

Modified from Gardner K: J Psychiatr Nurs 15:26, 1977.

evolved within the American Nurses' Association.

The objectives of this process, as described by Tousley, are to:

1. Assure the public of quality care
2. Provide credentials to expedite employment and third-party reimbursement for services rendered
3. Expand opportunities for vertical and horizontal mobility and career advancement
4. Attain greater prestige and peer recognition for achieving clinical expertise
5. Improve clinical practice[49]

As was mentioned previously, psychiatric nursing has two levels of certification: the **generalist** who may be a staff nurse, and the **specialist** who specializes in either adult or child and adolescent psychiatric nursing. As of October 1989, there were 12,140 certified nurse generalists, 3,362 certified nurse specialists in adult psychiatric mental health nursing, and 385 certified nurse specialists in child and adolescent psychiatric mental health nursing.

To become a *certified generalist* the psychiatric nurse must demonstrate expertise in practice, knowledge of theories concerning personality development and behavior patterns in treating mental illness, and the relationship of such treatments to nursing care. Special requirements include:

1. Practice as a psychiatric and mental health nurse a minimum of 1600 hours within 2 of the last 4 years.
2. Current work in psychiatric and mental health nursing for a minimum of 8 hours per week.

Certification as a *specialist* requires that the nurse show a "high degree of proficiency in interpersonal skills, in the use of the nursing process, and in psychiatric, psychological, and milieu therapies."[2:11-12] Following are six requirements for certification as a specialist in psychiatric and mental health nursing:

1. Current involvement in psychiatric and mental health nursing practice at least 4 hours per week
2. A master's or higher degree in nursing, with a specialization in psychiatric and mental health nursing *OR* a nurse may apply for individual consideration if he or she has a master's or higher degree in nursing or a mental health field with a minimum of 24 graduate academic credits in psychiatric and mental health theory and supervised training in two psychotherapeutic treatment modalities.

3. Practice in psychiatric and mental health nursing after receiving a master's degree with direct patient/client contact for either 8 hours a week for 2 years *OR* 4 hours a week for 4 years
4. Access to clinical supervision or consultation
5. Experience in at least two different treatment settings
6. At least 100 hours of supervision by or consultation with a certified member of the core mental health disciplines (clinical specialist in psychiatric and mental health nursing, psychiatrist, psychologist, or psychiatric social worker) after receiving a master's degree

On successful completion of the certification examination and written documentation, the nurse is identified as certified (C.) if a generalist or as a certified specialist (C.S.) in psychiatric mental health nursing. Although any specialist nurse may be certified, it is expected that the nurse who is self-employed in the practice of psychotherapy will obtain certification to assure the public of his or her ability to perform as a competent nurse psychotherapist.

■ **Practice Setting**

The setting in which he or she practices also influences the psychiatric nurse's level of performance. According to Peplau, the role the nurse assumes in any psychiatric mental health setting depends on the following:

1. The competence brought to work as a consequence of basic or post-basic nursing education
2. The definition of mental illness that prevails in a given setting
3. The extent of consensus about whether each profession should have discrete and unique roles or whether there can be overlap
4. The cost of certain kinds of care, the difference in status and salary levels, and the number of persons needed and available to provide certain kinds of care.[38]

A basic consideration is the philosophy of the particular health care system—the way in which the setting defines mental illness. From this definition emerges the work of the patient and the role of the nurse as illustrated in Table 1-5. If the setting is that of an organization, additional constraints may be imposed on the nurse as a result of administrative policies, staff norms, or nursing service expectations.

A study done by Sloboda[46] determined that inpatient nurses ranked their functions as primarily those of a "nurse clinician," followed by "change agent," and

---

TABLE 1-5

DIFFERENT DEFINITIONS OF MENTAL ILLNESS AND THEREFORE OF THE WORK OF THE PATIENT AND THE ROLE OF THE NURSE

Definition	Work of the patient	Role of the nurse
Socially unacceptable behavior of the patient has previously been "rewarded"; he has unfortunately been "conditioned" to behave in these ways	Submit to treatment using behavior modification (reconditioning) techniques	Surveillance of patient following treatment plan; pass out rewards; general nursing routine care
Unacceptable behavior is the result of genetic inheritance	Submit to whatever ameliorative treatment of symptoms is ordered	Surveillance and custody; reporting; general nursing routine care
Unacceptable behavior is caused by a biochemical imbalance	Submit to tests and prescribed treatment drugs to rectify the imbalance	Surveillance; reporting; pass medications such as tranquilizers, stimulants, lithium, hormones, etc.; observe effects; general nursing routine care
Unacceptable behavior is caused by some unknown but adverse brain activity	Submit to prescribed treatment (electrostimulation, electroshock, lobotomy, etc.)	Surveillance; reporting; pretreatment and posttreatment "preparation"; general nursing (and surgical nursing) care
Unacceptable behavior reflects problems in living with people and lack in intellectual and interpersonal competencies to understand and solve those problems	Participate in psychotherapy sessions and in ad hoc talking sessions with the available professionals, to investigate, understand, and resolve those problems and in the process gain new intellectual and interpersonal competencies on an experiential/educative basis	Use all "activities of daily living" as a basis for observation, discussion, and intervention in ways that enhance the patient's intellectual and interpersonal competencies to change his own behavior; also general nursing care Using "situational counseling" to aid patients involved in disputes, violence, and other grossly unacceptable behavior to investigate the problem inherent in the acting-out situation Referral for other professional services such as clergy and coordination and follow-up on discharge
The unacceptable behavior is caused by "lack of insight" into intrapsychic causes	Seek psychoanalysis for those who can afford it	

From Peplau H: Int Nurs Rev 25(2):45, 1978.

---

finally "therapist." Nurses in outpatient settings ranked all three functions fairly equally. Lieb, Underwood, and Glick[24] suggest that inpatient staff nurses are limited in providing primary therapy because of the ready supply of other professionals and a concern for appropriate preparation. The nurse's relationship with other health professionals thus emerges as an important influence on level of functioning.

Traditional settings for psychiatric nurses include psychiatric facilities, community mental health centers, the general hospital, and private practice. With the movement toward early discharge and increased community care, however, alternative treatment settings are emerging. Such settings include home health care agencies, business and industry, and health maintenance organizations.

Wojdowski and Hartnett describe a formal acute psychiatric service within a large health maintenance organization (HMO), in which psychiatric nurse clinicians were valued for their special expertise.[52] The nurses noted that the new service reduced the overload on the more traditional outpatient facility and increased patient satisfaction. In addition, the HMO had a low psychiatric hospitalization rate once the service was in operation; this low rate contributed to the overall cost effectiveness of the organization.

The current economic environment of the health care system in the United States suggests that new opportunities will emerge for psychiatric nurses in nontraditional settings. Nurses should assess mental health needs and practically and creatively identify settings and strategies that will be most effective in promoting health and preventing illness.

■ Personal initiative

The personal competence and initiative of the individual nurse determine how he or she interprets the nursing role and the success of its implementation. The importance of this final factor should not be ignored; without a realization of clinical competence and the assumption of professional initiative, the nurse is significantly limited in performance.

■ **BURNOUT AND SUPPORT.** In recent years the nursing literature has described a phenomenon known as job burnout. It is defined as a "syndrome of physical and emotional exhaustion, involving the development of negative self-concept, negative job attitudes, and loss of concern and feeling for clients."[40] Burnout may lead to physical illness, irritability, cynicism, fatigue, and withdrawal from work. At the extreme it may produce harmful patient contact through physical or verbal abuse or nontherapeutic communication.

Burnout results from prolonged stress that causes depletion of a nurse's personal resources. Some common sources of stress for psychiatric nurses are:

- conflict with supervisors or co-workers
- job dissatisfaction
- heavy patient load
- high patient acuity
- authority not equal to responsibility
- lack of participation in decisions affecting work
- inadequate staff support
- lack of promotion potential
- low salary
- lack of autonomy
- numerous organizational constraints

One study of stress among nurses in four specialty areas reported that psychiatric nurses experienced intense interpersonal involvement and frequent conflicts with patients, families, physicians, and colleagues.[8] They also experienced less social affirmation and recognition than intensive care nurses and less assistance than operating room nurses. These findings are noteworthy, especially in view of the fact that psychiatric nurses are expected to provide psychosocial assistance and support to their patients and, to some degree, to their peers.

Another recent study measured specific aspects of occupational stress as perceived by psychiatric nurses.[9] The study found that stressors inherent in the nursing role produced low levels of stress, but that stressors inherent in the organizational system produced high levels of stress. In fact, 50% of the high stresses and all the top 10 identified stresses were organizational in nature. The single most stressful experience involved not being notified of changes before they occurred.

Given the seriousness of the problem, it is important to plan and implement stress management strategies for psychiatric nurses. Evans and Lewis claim that the best cure for burnout is prevention.[13] They suggest that measures be instituted to provide a supportive environment for psychiatric nurses. Attention should be paid to

- the number and mix of staff
- delegation of nonessential paperwork
- open communication
- recognition of nurses' contributions
- opportunity to influence the work context
- involvement in unit decision making
- encouragement of professional activities
- provision of new work roles or responsibilities.

Evans and Lewis believe that "support, understanding, receptivity, and flexibility are all keys to providing an environment in which professional practice and personal growth can flourish."[16:173]

A final strategy for enhancing the personal growth and competence of the psychiatric nurse is the use of support groups both to prevent and to alleviate staff burnout. Such groups have been described in the nursing literature for both staff nurses and clinical nurse specialists. One model of a professional support group developed by Johnson and co-workers has as its major purposes to provide practical help to one another, stimulate ideas, share professional experiences, and share relevant information.[20] Possible group activities are described in Table 1-6.

As just discussed, the four major factors affecting nursing performance together account for variations in levels of nursing practice. Specifically, these variations are evident in regard to the following:

- Assessment and data collection
- Analysis of data
- Application of theory
- Breadth and depth of knowledge base, especially clinical, psychosocial, and pathophysio-

```
┌─────────────────────────────────────┐
│            TABLE 1-6                 │
│                                      │
│   PROFESSIONAL SUPPORT GROUP         │
│           ACTIVITIES                 │
```

Purposes	Related activities
Practical help	Case presentations
	Evaluating record-keeping methods
	Interventions for staff performance problems
	Standardized nursing care plan development
	Position title changes
Stimulation of ideas	Educational meeting reports
	Individual role components discussion
Sharing of experiences	Discussion of difficult work experiences
	Description of successful interventions
Sharing information	Exchange of continuing education brochures
	Distribution of articles
	Update on new laws
	Sharing of institutional policies
	Suggestions of resources for additional information for problem solving

From Johnson R et al: J Psychosoc Nurs Ment Health Serv 20(2):9, 1982.

logical theories relating to nursing diagnosis and treatment
- Range of nursing techniques
- Need for, kind, and extent of supervision by other nurses in practice
- Evaluation of effects of practice
- Identification of relationships among phenomena, nursing actions, effects (outcomes for the patients)[3:19-20]

All nurses practicing with patients are expected to address the phenomena that form the core of nursing practice. These are identified and described in the *Standards of Psychiatric and Mental Health Nursing Practice,* on the following pages.

The question of professional autonomy

Psychiatric nurses as a group displayed certain personal qualities in a study reported by Mlott.[31] He found that they had adequate defenses, a good self-concept, adequate but flexible impulse control, the ability to trust others, and tolerance. They viewed events as products of their own actions and sought information relevant to problems they encountered. He also reported that they were better adjusted and more active, striving, independent, effective, self-confident, persevering, and determined than other subspecialty nurses. His study paints a rather rosy picture of psychiatric nurses as competent, effective, and confident mental health professionals. However, are they truly professionalized?

The professional status of nursing has been a long-debated issue, both within nursing and among observers and scholars outside of nursing. Nursing literature often carries defensive assertions or soothing assurances that yes, indeed, nursing really is a profession. However, outside the field nursing is described as a semiprofession, subprofession, or marginal profession. There is no consensus, and the question is far from resolved. It is helpful, however, to analyze psychiatric nursing's present position on the professionalization continuum. In so doing, conflicts and roadblocks to future growth can be identified.

Viewed as a continuum, professionalization is the evidence of a continuous attempt of a group to gain more and more control over certain resources related to an occupational area. The attainment of professional status very often involves a struggle. Society alone has the power to grant it, and consensus for it must exist in the body politic. Moore[32] identified six characteristics of the scale of professionalization. Comprehensive in scope and developmental in nature, they suggest the following process of professionalization:

1. **Occupation.** The requirement that the work be a full-time undertaking by a group of individuals.
2. **Calling.** A personal commitment or intention to pursue a stable career in the occupation. It incorporates socialization into the culture of the profession with its values, norms, and symbols.
3. **Organization.** The formation of an association by members because of common occupational interests. The organization concerns itself with the occupation's status as a profession, the tasks of its members, the ways to raise the quality of applicants, and political action.
4. **Education.** Preparation by intense study of a systematic "body of theory." This body of theory is a system of abstract propositions that describe in general terms the phenomena that make up the profession's focus of interest. The-

STANDARDS OF PSYCHIATRIC AND MENTAL HEALTH NURSING PRACTICE

INTRODUCTION

The purpose of *Standards of Psychiatric and Mental Health Nursing Practice* is to fulfill the profession's obligation to provide a means of improving the quality of care. The standards reflect the current state of knowledge in the field and are therefore provisional, dynamic, and subject to testing and subsequent change. Since standards represent agreed-upon levels of practice, they have been developed to characterize, to measure, and to provide guidance in achieving excellence in care.*

The standards presented here are a revision of the standards enunciated by the Division on Psychiatric and Mental Health Nursing Practice in 1973. They apply to any setting in which psychiatric and mental health nursing is practiced, and to both generalists and specialists in psychiatric and mental health nursing. Standards V-F (psychotherapy) and X (community health systems) apply specifically to the specialist. The standards are written within the framework of the nursing process, which includes data collection, diagnosis, planning, treatment, and evaluation.*

The treatment or intervention phase of the nursing process is elaborated upon in order to highlight the specific interventions or nursing care activities commonly carried out by psychiatric and mental health nurses: therapeutic interventions, health teaching, activities of daily living, somatic therapies, therapeutic environment, and psychotherapy. In addition to the standards concerned with the nursing process are standards that address professional performance, such as use of theory, peer review, continuing education, interdisciplinary team collaboration, community health systems, and research. Accountability of the provider to the client, client rights, and client advocacy are implicit throughout the standards.

A rationale is provided for each standard, and criteria are developed to measure each standard. The criteria are divided into *structure, process,* and *outcome.* They are intended to provide a means by which attainment of the standard may be specifically measured. The criteria for each standard are not exhaustive.

Standards of Psychiatric and Mental Health Nursing Practice should be used in conjunction with the following ANA publications: (1) *Standards of Nursing Practice,* (2) *Statement on Psychiatric and Mental Health Nursing Practice,* (3) *Nursing: A Social Policy Statement,* and (4) *Code for Nurses with Interpretive Statements.*

PROFESSIONAL PRACTICE STANDARDS

STANDARD I. THEORY
The nurse applies appropriate theory that is scientifically sound as a basis for decisions regarding nursing practice.
Rationale

Psychiatric and mental health nursing is characterized by the application of relevant theories to explain phenomena of concern to nurses, and to provide a basis for intervention and subsequent evaluation of that intervention. A primary source of knowledge for practice rests on the scholarly conceptualizations of psychiatric and mental health nursing practice and on research findings generated from intradisciplinary and cross-disciplinary studies of human behavior. The nurse's use of selected theories provides comprehensive, balanced perceptions of clients' characteristics, diagnoses, or presenting conditions.

From American Nurses' Association, Division on Psychiatric and Mental Health Nursing Practice: Standards of psychiatric and mental health nursing practice, Kansas City, Mo., 1982, The Association. Reprinted by permission.
*From American Nurses' Association: A plan for implementation of the standards of nursing practice, Kansas City, Mo., 1974, The Association, p. 4.

Continued.

STANDARDS OF PSYCHIATRIC AND MENTAL HEALTH NURSING PRACTICE—cont'd

STANDARD II. DATA COLLECTION
The nurse continuously collects data that are comprehensive, accurate, and systematic.
Rationale

Effective interviewing, behavioral observation, and physical and mental health assessment enable the nurse to reach sound conclusions and plan appropriate interventions with the client.

STANDARD III. DIAGNOSIS
The nurse utilizes nursing diagnoses and/or standard classification of mental disorders to express conclusions supported by recorded assessment data and current scientific premises.
Rationale

Nursing's logical basis for providing care rests on the recognition and identification of those actual or potential health problems that are within the scope of nursing practice.

STANDARD IV. PLANNING
The nurse develops a nursing care plan with specific goals and interventions delineating nursing actions unique to each client's needs.
Rationale

The nursing care plan is used to guide therapeutic intervention and effectively achieve the desired outcomes.

STANDARD V. INTERVENTION
The nurse intervenes as guided by the nursing care plan to implement nursing actions that promote, maintain, or restore physical and mental health, prevent illness, and effect rehabilitation.
Rationale

Mental health is one aspect of general health and well-being. Nursing actions reflect an appreciation for the hierarchy of human needs and include interventions for all aspects of physical and mental health and illness.

STANDARD V-A. INTERVENTION: PSYCHOTHERAPEUTIC INTERVENTIONS
The nurse uses psychotherapeutic interventions to assist clients in regaining or improving their previous coping abilities and to prevent further disability.
Rationale

Individuals with and without mental health problems often respond to health problems in a dysfunctional manner. During counseling, interviewing, crisis or emergency intervention, or daily interaction, nurses diagnose dysfunctional behaviors, engage clients in noting such behaviors, and assist the client in modifying or eliminating those behaviors.

STANDARD V-B. INTERVENTION: HEALTH TEACHING
The nurse assists clients, families, and groups to achieve satisfying and productive patterns of living through health teaching.
Rationale

Health teaching is an essential part of the nurse's role with those who have mental health problems. Every interaction can be utilized as a teaching-learning situation. Formal and informal teaching methods can be used in working with individuals, families, groups, and the community. Emphasis is on understanding principles of mental health as well as on developing ways of coping with mental health problems. Client adherence to treatment regimens increases when health teaching is an integral part of the client's care.

STANDARD V-C. INTERVENTION: ACTIVITIES OF DAILY LIVING
The nurse uses the activities of daily living in a goal-directed way to foster adequate self-care and physical and mental well-being of clients.
Rationale

A major portion of one's daily life is spent in some form of activity related to health and well-be-

STANDARDS OF PSYCHIATRIC AND MENTAL HEALTH NURSING PRACTICE—cont'd

ing. An individual's developmental and intellectual levels, emotional state, and physical limitations may be reflected in these activities. Nurses are the primary professional health care providers who interact with clients on a day-to-day basis around the tasks of daily living. Therefore, the nurse has a unique opportunity to assess and intervene in these processes in order to encourage constructive changes in the client's behavior so that each child, adolescent, and adult can realize his potential for growth and health or maintain that level previously achieved.

STANDARD V-D. INTERVENTION: SOMATIC THERAPIES
The nurse uses knowledge of somatic therapies and applies related clinical skills in working with clients.
Rationale

Various treatment modalities may be needed by clients during the course of illness. Pertinent clinical observations and judgments are made concerning the effect of drugs and other somatic treatments used in the therapeutic program.

STANDARD V-E. INTERVENTION: THERAPEUTIC ENVIRONMENT
The nurse provides, structures, and maintains a therapeutic environment in collaboration with the client and other health care providers.
Rationale

The nurse works with clients in a variety of environmental settings such as inpatient, residential, day care, and home. The environment contributes in positive and negative ways to the state of health or illness of the client. When it serves the interest of the client as an inherent part of the overall nursing care plan, the setting is structured and/or altered.

STANDARD V-F. INTERVENTION: PSYCHOTHERAPY
The nurse utilizes advanced clinical expertise in individual, group, and family psychotherapy, child psychotherapy, and other treatment modalities to function as a psychotherapist, and recognizes professional accountability for nursing practice.
Rationale

Acceptance for the role of psychotherapist entails primary responsibility for the treatment of clients and entrance into a contractual agreement. This contract includes a commitment to see a client through the problem presented or to assist the client in finding other appropriate assistance. It also includes an explicit definition of the relationship, the respective role of each person in the relationship, and what can be realistically expected of each person.

STANDARD VI. EVALUATION
The nurse evaluates client responses to nursing actions in order to revise the data base, nursing diagnoses, and nursing care plan.
Rationale

Nursing care is a dynamic process that implies alterations in data, diagnoses, or plans previously made.

PROFESSIONAL PERFORMANCE STANDARDS

STANDARD VII. PEER REVIEW
The nurse participates in peer review and other means of evaluation to assure quality of nursing care provided for clients.
Rationale

Evaluation of the quality of nursing care through examination of the clinical practice of nurses is one way to fulfill the profession's obligation to ensure that consumers are provided excellence in care. Peer review and other quality assurance procedures are utilized in this endeavor.

Continued.

STANDARDS OF PSYCHIATRIC AND MENTAL HEALTH NURSING PRACTICE—cont'd

STANDARD VIII. CONTINUING EDUCATION

The nurse assumes responsibility for continuing education and professional development and contributes to the professional growth of others.

Rationale

The scientific, cultural, social, and political changes characterizing our contemporary society require the nurse to be committed to the ongoing pursuit of knowledge that will enhance professional growth.

STANDARD IX. INTERDISCIPLINARY COLLABORATION

The nurse collaborates with other health care providers in assessing, planning, implementing, and evaluating programs and other mental health activities.

Rationale

Psychiatric nursing practice requires planning and sharing with others to deliver maximum mental health services to the client and the community. Through the collaborative process, different abilities of health care providers are utilized to communicate, plan, solve problems, and evaluate services delivered.

STANDARD X. UTILIZATION OF COMMUNITY HEALTH SYSTEMS

The nurse participates with other members of the community in assessing, planning, implementing, and evaluating mental health services and community systems that include the promotion of the broad continuum of primary, secondary, and tertiary prevention of mental illness.

Rationale

The high incidence of mental illness in our contemporary society requires increased effort to devise more effective treatment and prevention programs. Nurses must participate in programs that strengthen the existing health potential of all members of society. Such concepts as primary prevention and continuity of care are essential in planning to meet the mental health needs of the community. The nurse uses organizational, advisory, advocacy, and consultative skills to facilitate the development and implementation of mental health services.

STANDARD XI. RESEARCH

The nurse contributes to nursing and the mental health field through innovations in theory and practice and participation in research.

Rationale

Each professional has responsibility for the continuing development and refinement of knowledge in the mental health field through research and experimentation with new and creative approaches to practice.

ory construction through systematic research is a distinctive professional activity, as characterized in the role of researcher-theoretician. In this way the profession creates, organizes, and transmits its knowledge. The minimum educational requirement is the baccalaureate degree, although many professions have considerably longer educational requirements. A spirit of rationality prevails among the members, as shown in the ongoing commitment to learning and the assumption of a critical attitude toward theory and knowledge base.

5. **Service orientation.** Characterized by rules of competence, conscientious performance, and loyalty or service. Rules of competence require the accreditation of educational programs, establishment of a licensing system, and maintenance and improvement of standards through continuing education. Rules of conscientious performance refer to self-discipline and self-regulation. Rules of service require that professionals serve the client's interest first, placing it over personal gain or commercial profit.

6. **Autonomy.** Legitimate control over one's own work. Autonomy is the ultimate value for professionals, characterized by professional authority. The outcome of autonomy and authority is power, prestige, and status accorded by society, which in turn expects exemplary behavior from the profession.

Psychiatric nursing has amply met the first two characteristics. The remaining four, however, appear to be problematic.[48]

■ Organization

The American Nurses' Association was founded in 1896. It is the major professional organization, but only about 25% of all licensed nurses belong to it. Members of the association represent various educational backgrounds and, consequently, various interpretations of the tasks and roles of nursing. They disagree on the uniqueness of their contribution as members of the health care team, their educational programs, and their legal rights and responsibilities.[1] The American Nurses' Association has a specialty subgroup, the Council on Psychiatric and Mental Health Nursing. In 1973 the council published the *Standards of Psychiatric and Mental Health Nursing Practice* and revised them in 1982. The *Statement on Psychiatric and Mental Health Nursing Practice*[2] was published in 1976. It defines psychiatric nursing, identifies types of practitioners, and describes the scope of practice.

These publications have served to clarify and refine the roles, tasks, and functioning of psychiatric nurses.

Since 1948, the American Nurses' Association has had an economic security program. One of its goals is to upgrade the economic position of registered nurses. To do this, the association engages in collective bargaining activities. Most nurses appear to accept the validity and necessity of collective action to attain economic goals. What remains in conflict are the mechanism and scope of issues appropriately covered by collective bargaining agreements. Specific items of conflict are the inclusion of patient care issues in negotiations and the leadership dilemma of a professional organization functioning as a collective bargaining agent.

Underlying the position of the American Nurses' Association toward collective bargaining is the conviction that nurses must speak for nursing. This issue is more fundamental than the single aspect of salary or scheduling. It is the basis for the difference between a professional organization and a union, and it has particular significance for nursing because of nursing's long history of domination by other groups. No one group represents a majority of nurses; neither is the economic security program the primary purpose of the American Nurses' Association. However, unless nursing accepts its responsibility to control its own practice and to have nurses speak for nursing, the economic security issue may end up being the end, not just the means.

Cleland[7] has described a professional collective bargaining model. She believes that the labor contract can become the legal instrument through which the profession can implement standards of care. To do so, the labor contract should include negotiated clauses relating to wages, hours, and conditions of work. To gain control of nursing practice, Cleland believes, the contract should contain provisions on shared governance, individual accountability, and collective professional responsibility. Clearly, the model she advocates is a professional one that would require the active participation and support of nurses. Before it can be widely undertaken, however, nurses as a group must decide if they wish to be professionals.

■ **NETWORKING AND NURSING.** Nursing would also benefit from another strategy—networking. Networks are groups of individuals drawn together by common concerns to support and help one another. Networks range from informal friendships to small groups providing contacts and advancement to large, open groups providing emotional support.

Nursing's prevailing inbreeding, infighting, and impotence have been noted in the literature. The history of nursing documents the profession's preoccupation with internal disagreements, inconsistencies, and deficiencies. Furthermore, nurses often feel alienated from nursing peers in other positions. This feeling frequently results in conflict among nurse administrators, educators, practitioners, and researchers. To counter this phenomenon, nurses need to identify with their peers, feel trusted by their colleagues, and pledge loyalty to other members of their own profession.

Forming networks can help nurses to unite and to value their profession. Meisenhelder believes that nursing networking is needed on three levels.[29] Networking at the grass roots or staff nurse level is crucial to the unity and survival of the profession. It would help nurses work toward caring for one another and having an influence on their work environment. She believes that a supportive staff network can extend beyond affirmation of the members and become an influential force in managing daily nursing care.

The next level of networking is at the leadership level, where nursing leaders can unite for a common goal of increased power in the health care system. Nurses at this level are in a position to make a significant contribution to the self-esteem of their fellow nurses through support and affirmation of their abilities and potential. The final level includes informational networks that are a requisite for effective political action. Herein lies a dormant element of nursing power that often is described but seldom activated.

■ Education

A major challenge to psychiatric nursing in the area of education is the need for a well-defined body of nursing knowledge. The question "Is psychiatric nursing unique?" has preoccupied the profession for some time now.

McMurrey explores the subject of unique nursing knowledge by posing three questions: (1) What is unique knowledge? (2) Does nursing have a unique knowledge base? and (3) Is a unique knowledge base essential to nursing?[28] She argues that knowledge becomes unique because of the unique perspective of the discipline in which that knowledge is incorporated. She further cautions that if nursing does not define its focus, it cannot become an autonomous profession, and one of two things will occur. Either the functions that have been associated with nursing will be taken over by others or, in their search for definition, nurses will assume roles within other disciplines such as psychology or medicine. There is some evidence that both of these trends are already taking place in the field of psychiatric nursing.

Nursing's contribution is an outcome of a unique manner of problem conceptualization, the use of theoretical models to explain behavior, and a process approach to individuals, families, and communities. The existence of this psychiatric nursing textbook is evidence of the distinct body of knowledge that is nursing. This book incorporates existing nursing research, is organized around a nursing model of health-illness phenomena, and views the nursing process as the basis for practice. It is the combination of this knowledge base, clinical skills, holistic viewpoint, and behavioral focus that makes the psychiatric nurse's contribution a valuable and unique one.

■ **NURSING RESEARCH.** The development of conceptual models further attests to the validity of viewing nursing as a unique profession. These theoretical models contribute to the knowledge base of nursing education, the framework for nursing practice, and the direction for nursing research. More than half of the federally supported nursing research projects deal with investigations into nursing practice. The development of doctoral programs in nursing also suggests that the science of nursing is coming of age. The momentum in nursing research is steadily increasing. Evidence of that momentum includes:

- the establishment of a National Center for Nursing Research in the National Institutes of Health
- the development of programs for the preparation of nurse scientists (see Table 1-3)
- the increasing support of federal and interstate agencies
- increased acceptance of long-term, research-oriented goals toward enlarging nursing's body of knowledge
- the development of centers for nursing research
- a rise in the number of consortia and collaborative efforts
- a change in the nature and number of avenues for reporting research changes in the direction of research from a limited number of studies on curricula, administration, and personal attributes of nurses to more extensive clinical studies that apply the new nursing science to practice.

The most recent statement regarding the overall need for psychiatric nurse researchers was provided by the NIMH Task Force on Nursing Report in 1988.[33] It developed a working definition of psychiatric nursing research that focused on three areas:

1. Improving the understanding, treatment, and rehabilitation of the mentally ill; preventing mental illness; and fostering mental health.
2. Improving the continuous care of persons who are acutely or chronically mentally ill or who are at risk for mental illness, as well as the supportive care of their families.
3. Designing, implementing, and evaluating new and existing models of service delivery, especially those related to nursing care.

Along with these advances, however, have emerged a number of problems identified by Feldman[14]:

1. The need for financial support often outweighs available money.
2. As the number of doctoral programs has increased, the quality may have suffered.
3. There are still too few research journals, and too few research papers accepted.
4. A rush to produce research has led to inferior quality in some cases.
5. Many nurses do not appreciate research, are unable to interpret research findings, and do not use those findings in practice.
6. Some nurses do not participate in research because they view it as costly, time consuming, and demanding in preparation, or because they have poor self-images and are reluctant to ask for help and expose themselves to possible criticism.

Rather than simply identifying problems, Feldman[14] offers possible solutions to enhance nursing's growth in this area. All of the following are applicable to psychiatric nursing:

1. **Funding.** If the nursing profession truly supports nursing science, it must contribute to nursing's evolution. Hospital nursing services, professional nursing organizations, and educational facilities should encourage research by contributing a percentage of their income to this endeavor. Also, positions should exist for nurse researchers in clinical and educational settings.
2. **Collaboration.** Collaboration takes many forms and may occur in developing research questions, designing and implementing studies, providing forums for developing theory and reporting investigative work, and establishing networks for sharing all kinds of information. Symposia must continue to increase, involving nurses at all levels and in all types of practice. A nationwide research network could be established using computers; the technology is available to set up an international network by satellite.
3. **Education.** The process of educating nurses to perform research must be stepped up to meet the demands of a developing science. This involves additional recruitment but not at the expense of quality.

Preparation for participation in research occurs to various degrees within different educational programs. Table 1-7 summarizes the expecta-

TABLE 1-7

NURSING RESEARCH PARTICIPATION BASED ON EDUCATION

Educational preparation	Research involvement
Associate Degree in Nursing	Help identify clinical problems in nursing practice; assist in data collection within a structured format; use research findings in practice with supervision
Baccalaureate Degree in Nursing	Identify clinical problems in need of research; help experienced investigators gain access to clinical sites; influence the selection of appropriate methods of data collection; participate in data collection and implementation of research findings
Master's Degree in Nursing	Collaborate in proposal development, data collection, data analysis, and interpretation; appraise the clinical relevance of research findings; provide leadership for integrating findings into practice
Doctoral education	Develop nursing knowledge through research and theory development; conduct funded independent research projects; develop and coordinate funded research projects; disseminate research findings to the scientific community

tion for nurse participation in research based on the various educational levels. Still, all nurses need to take an active role in generating scientific knowledge through research while they also incorporate that knowledge into practice.

Doctoral programs in nursing must have a core of productive nurse scientists who can serve as role models and mentors in the study of specific problems. Encouraging greater concentration on concerns of highest priority would enhance theory development. It would also involve students in the research process in such a way that their enthusiasm and creativity would be nurtured. However, doctoral preparation for research is just the beginning. Postdoctoral work would enable the scientist to pursue particular areas of need and interest and to more fully develop the researcher role.

4. **Marketing.** Enhancing the usefulness of nursing research requires changing the present climate. Increased receptivity to and involvement in the process and outcomes of research studies will be required. To accomplish this, Feldman proposes an intensive effort in "marketing" nursing research. She describes the strategies useful in marketing products as segmenting the market, identifying common characteristics within each of the target segments, identifying the needs of those markets, and developing a marketing plan to appeal to the target markets. She then describes how this approach can be adapted to the problem of increasing receptivity to research among nursing professionals.

5. **Reporting.** There needs to be increased reporting of research in journals designed for that purpose. However, new ideas are needed about ways to communicate findings in a fashion acceptable to clinical practitioners. Additionally, prestige must be given to the replication of selected studies, and replication studies must be reported as readily as originals.

The importance of this final suggestion, reporting, should not be minimized. To attain full professional status, the body of nursing knowledge must be accepted as legitimate by other professionals, as well as by society. Many people outside nursing and some within nursing still have no concept of this body of knowledge nor of the unique expertise of nursing. To overcome this, psychiatric nurses need to write and publish more and in a greater variety of journals and texts, including multidisciplinary

journals and consumer publications. A study by Kalisch and Kalisch examined the quality of news about psychiatric nurses in the nation's newspapers.[22] The study found inadequate dissemination of psychiatric nursing information to the public via the news media and deficiencies in the quality of reported information.

Nurses should also increase their visibility by attending and presenting papers at the meetings of their colleagues, including psychiatrists, psychologists, and social workers. A more assertive and self-confident public stance is both necessary and appropriate for the psychiatric nurse. Knowledge of the role of psychiatric nurses has been found to be correlated with an accepting attitude and greater utilization among other mental health professionals. The gradual implementation of each of these proposed solutions by psychiatric nurses will promote the creation, organization, and transmission of the distinct body of science that is nursing.

■ Service orientation

Nursing is characterized by clear rules of competence and strong rules of loyalty or service. The rules of performance, however, apply to self-regulation and accountability for practice that must be shown individually and collectively. Accountability means to be answerable to someone for something. It focuses responsibility on the individual nurse for his or her actions, or perhaps, lack of actions:

Organized nursing services and the professional association carry the leadership responsibility for development, implementation, and evaluation of nursing care systems, which assure relevant, high quality nursing to consumers. Individual nurses have primary responsibility and accountability for their own practice, and thus activities to monitor and improve the quality of nursing care form an intrinsic part of the individual's practice.

In the field of psychiatric and mental health nursing, nurses have a particular obligation to define, supervise, and evaluate nursing care. Nursing standards provide authoritative measures for determining the quality of nursing care a client receives, whether services are provided solely by a professional nurse or by a professional nurse and nursing assistants.[2:2]

The preconditions of accountability, therefore, include ability, responsibility, and authority. Finally, accountability includes formal review processes and requirements, but also an attitude of integrity and vigilance—"a quality of the heart and mind of those professionals who are competent and determined that every psychiatric patient will have the best problem-resolving assistance possible."[39]

The mechanisms of regulation and accountability within psychiatric nursing include state licensing, certification, primary nursing as a mode of staffing, nursing audit, implementation of standards of practice, and peer review. Sometimes these mechanisms appear more structural than functional. The division between nursing theory and nursing practice is somewhat addressed in the literature; it is implied in the sometimes adversarial roles of nursing educators and administrators. Often what is learned in theory is not put into practice. For example, direct and indirect psychiatric nursing care functions, although impressive, are often carried out sporadically and inconsistently.

One study examined what functions psychiatric nurses working in an inpatient setting considered to be important and how well nurses were able to perform them.[41] The results indicated the following five functions as the most important of the 46 listed:

1. To assess patients' emotional needs
2. To respond to patients' crises
3. To intervene to reduce panic of disturbed patients
4. To make sure patients' rights are safeguarded
5. To assess the effect of somatic therapies on patients

Although these functions implied the use of the nursing process, the items to "develop a nursing care plan" and "implement a nursing care plan" were ranked as numbers 18 and 15, respectively. Items related to leadership functions ranked low—providing leadership was ranked number 9, initiating improvements was 11, participating in policy making was 24, and political involvement was 29. Psychotherapy activities were numbered 34, 36, and 38, and research activities were 32, 41, and 46. The ability ratings corresponded closely with the importance ratings. The same questionnaire was given to a group of psychiatrists and psychologists. Significantly, they gave a lower ranking than did the nurses to nurses' ability to assess emotional needs and to develop and implement a nursing care plan. This study raises many questions about the role of the nurse and the contrast between theory and practice.

Traditionally, one response to this perceived dichotomy was to place blame. Complaints about "ivory-tower" educators, the "nonsupportive" nurse administrators, or the "impersonal" hospital organization were heard. However, this type of response is characterized by passivity and a noticeable lack of accountability. What is currently needed is for psychiatric nurses to assume an active posture of accountability—to oneself, one's patients, one's colleagues, one's profession, the public, and nurse administrators.

■ Autonomy

Autonomy implies self-determination, independence, shared power, and authority. Professionals are not likely to achieve autonomy without having met the previous characteristics of professionalization. It is the condition that allows for definition of and control over a work domain. For psychiatric nursing, attaining autonomy means being able to define the domain of nursing and being able to exercise control over psychiatric nursing practice.[56] This idea of shaping destiny, rather than letting outside forces be in control, is power viewed as a positive force and the capacity to attain goals. Power can be viewed as both a means to an end and a product—the instrument used to attain full professional status and the outcome of achieving professionalization. It involves a conscious decision to identify goals, plan strategy, assume responsibility, exercise authority, and be held accountable.

Autonomy, at an individual level, has two major and interrelated components. The first is **control over nursing tasks,** which means:

1. Having the opportunity for independent thought and action
2. Having use of one's time, skills, and ability by being able to eliminate, refuse, and delegate nonnursing tasks
3. Having the authority and responsibility for implementing goals related to quality nursing care
4. Being able to initiate changes and innovations in one's practice

The second component of autonomy is **participation in decision making.** It requires the nurse's participation in the following:

1. Determining and implementing standards of quality nursing care
2. Making decisions affecting one's nursing job context, including salary, staffing, and professional growth
3. Setting institutional policies, procedures, and goals

This second component of participation of autonomy in decision-making is particularly problematic for nursing. Most nurses are employed in hospitals in which authority rests primarily with administrators, physicians, and trustees. Furthermore, nurses often are expected to do tasks they are overqualified for, such as housekeeping and dietary and clerical duties. This results in underutilization of their many important skills. Nurses are thus caught in the crosswind. They staff the units around the clock, make important clinical decisions, and shoulder major responsibility for coordinating and managing the patient care units; but they lack legitimate decision-making authority as to the allocation of hospital resources. Because nurses are not compensated on a fee-for-service basis, they are not viewed as a source of revenue by hospital administrators and therefore lack a most critical base for power. It is not surprising that if nurses do not have a role in hospital decision making, they will have only a limited ability to exercise control of their practice.

Recommendations from two national studies of nursing, the Special Committee on Nursing sponsored by the American Hospital Association and the Commission on Nursing sponsored by the U.S. Department of Health and Human Services, reflect this problem. Both studies were completed in 1988. They call for increased decision-making authority for nurses and collaborative relationships with physicians in providing care. In addition, the Joint Commission on Accreditation of Hospitals (JCAH) Nursing Service Standards extend the current provision for nursing staff communication with a hospital's governing body to include communication "with those levels of management involved in policy decisions affecting patient care services in the hospital."[19]

However, nurses should not expect that autonomy and power will be given to them. It is obtained in a negotiated process with other health professionals, consumers, and society at large. It requires increased access to resources, demonstration of expertise, and acknowledgement by other professionals, as shown in interdependent collaboration. Nurses are not yet fully accepted as professionals by other disciplines and often do not function at their full potential. Yet psychiatric nursing is practiced largely in collaboration, coordination, and cooperation with a variety of other professionals working with and on behalf of the patient. Nurses will progress in this area as they are able to communicate with other professionals and as their clinical skills demand recognition and respect. As nurses view themselves in a positive way, they will increase their ability to assert themselves and function effectively.

Benfer[4] has some specific suggestions in this regard. She believes that psychiatric nurses must first assess patients based on their own reading of the patient's emotional difficulties, rather than first checking with the psychiatrist or other team members for their evaluation. When the nurse has completed her assessment, she must then be able to articulate that information both orally and in writing. This requires an asser-

tiveness in putting forth ideas, observations, and beliefs about treatment. Benfer does not believe nurses have done very well in explaining their framework for practice and communicating to other mental health team members what the nursing process is and how it is utilized. Unless psychiatric nurses define their own role, others will define it for them.

Nurses also have a team teaching function. They can share their knowledge, experience, and perceptions with other team members so that the result is more skilled practitioners. Although nurses often have taught interns and residents, this teaching seldom has been given adequate recognition and importance. Furthermore, some nurses may feel threatened at the thought of teaching other professionals. However, teaching and learning are continuous experiences in life, and nurses have a contribution to make in this area.

DIRECTIONS FOR FUTURE RESEARCH

The following are some of the nursing research problems raised in Chapter 1 that merit further study by psychiatric nurses:

1. Factors associated with the recruitment of nursing students into the field of psychiatric nursing
2. The amount of nursing care in the areas of primary, secondary, and tertiary prevention performed by psychiatric nurses relative to their qualifications, roles, and settings
3. Structural and process characteristics of effective mental health teams
4. The perceptions by other mental health professionals and the public of the doctoral degree in nursing
5. The level of public understanding of certification, the types of psychiatric nurse practitioners, and their functions
6. The nontraditional settings and the parameters of practice of psychiatric nurses
7. The extent of and factors contributing to psychiatric nursing "burnout" and ways to effectively deal with this phenomenon
8. The manner in which the *Standards of Psychiatric and Mental Health Nursing Practice* are implemented in various psychiatric settings
9. The effectiveness of mechanisms to assure accountability in psychiatric nursing practice
10. The degree to which psychiatric nurses exercise control over their nursing tasks and participate in the decision-making structure of the organizations in which they work

Finally, for interdisciplinary teams to function well, the members must view themselves as equals. Benfer believes that this is one of the most elusive and difficult issues affecting nurses. They must be helped to strengthen their self-concept by identifying their expertise and the ways in which they can contribute to the common purpose of the team.

Thus the movement toward professionalization contains complex issues for all psychiatric nurses. Many of these issues are interwoven, and all of them are familiar, since they have been repeatedly addressed by nurses over many decades. The prize is professional autonomy, but its attainment remains in question.

■ SUGGESTED CROSS-REFERENCES ■

This chapter serves as a foundation for formulating principles of psychiatric nursing and implementing psychiatric nursing practice. As such, it is related to all other chapters of this text.

■ SUMMARY ■

1. Nursing began to emerge as a profession in the nineteenth century. Linda Richards was the first American psychiatric nurse, and the first school for psychiatric nurses opened in 1882. A critical development within the profession occurred with the publication of Peplau's book in 1952 in which she presented a theoretical framework for psychiatric nursing. By 1962 psychiatric nursing had evolved a role of clinical competence based on interpersonal techniques and use of the nursing process. Counseling was a primary nursing function.

2. Psychiatric nursing is an interpersonal process that strives to promote and maintain behavior that contributes to integrated functioning. The patient or client may be an individual, family, group, organization, or community.

3. Essential parts of contemporary practice are cooperation and collaboration with other health care providers. The role functions of various team members and barriers to effective team functioning were discussed.

4. The development of knowledge and strategies enabling nurses to exercise leadership and management in the settings in which they work is essential. Characteristics of psychiatric nurses as change agents and the nature of effective leadership were described.

5. Four major factors that help to determine the levels of function and types of activities a nurse engages in are (a) the law; (b) qualifications, including education, work experience, and certification status; (c) practice setting; and (d) personal competence and initiative.

6. The *Standards of Psychiatric and Mental Health Nursing Practice* as identified by the American Nurses' Association were presented.

7. The question of whether psychiatric nurses are truly professionalized was addressed. The following problematic areas were explored:

   a. Organization, including lack of support for the American Nurses' Association, disagreement over tasks and roles, questions related to collective bargaining issues, and the need for the formation of networks that can help nurses to unite and to value their profession
   b. Education, specifically the need for a well-defined body of nursing knowledge, problems and advances in nursing research, and the need for greater visibility of psychiatric nurses through publishing and presentations
   c. Service orientation, focusing on the issues of self-regulation, accountability, and the theory-practice dichotomy
   d. Autonomy, with its elements of self-determination, power, authority, and status as evidenced in control over nursing tasks and participation in decision making in nursing care, job context, and institutional policies and goals

■ REFERENCES ■

1. American Nurses' Association: Educational preparation for nurse practitioners and assistants to nurses: a position paper, New York, 1965, The Association.
2. American Nurses' Association, Division on Psychiatric and Mental Health Nursing Practice: Statement on psychiatric and mental health nursing practice, Kansas City, Mo, 1976, The Association.
3. American Nurses' Association: Nursing: a social policy statement, Kansas City, Mo, 1980, The Association.
4. Benfer B: Defining the role and function of the psychiatric nurse as a member of the team, Perspect Psychiatr Care 18(4):166, 1980.
5. Bennett A and Eaton J: The role of the psychiatric nurse in the newer therapies, Am J Psychiatry 108:167, 1951.
6. Brown E: Nursing for the future, New York, 1948, Russell Sage Foundation.
7. Cleland V: The supervisor in collective bargaining, J Nurs Adm 4(4):33, 1974.
8. Cronin-Stubbs D and Brophy E: Burnout: can social support save the nurse? J Psychosoc Nurs Ment Health Serv 23(7):9, 1985.
9. Dawkins J, Depp F, and Selzer N: Stress and the psychiatric nurse, J Psychosoc Nurs Ment Health Serv 23(11):9, 1985.
10. Doona M: At least as well cared for . . . Linda Richards and the mentally ill, Image 16(2):51, 1984.
11. Dumas R: Expanding the theoretical framework for effective nursing, Nurs Clin North Am 13(4):707, 1978.
12. Editorial, Am J Nurs 40:23, 1940.
13. Evans C and Lewis S: Nursing administration of psychiatric-mental health care, Rockville, Md, 1985, Aspen Systems Corp.
14. Feldman H: Nursing research in the 1980's: issues and implications, Adv Nurs Sci 3(1):85, 1980.
15. Gardner K: Levels of psychiatric nursing practice in an ambulatory setting, J Psychiatr Nurs 15:26, Sept 1977.
16. Given B and Simmons S: The interdisciplinary health-

care team: fact or fiction? Nurs Forum 16(2):165, 1977.

17. Gregg D: The psychiatric nurse's role, Am J Nurs 54:848, 1954.

18. Hays D: Suggested clinical practice of psychiatric nurses recorded in the literature between 1946 and 1958. In Psychiatric nursing 1946 to 1974: a report on the state of the art, New York, 1975, American Journal of Nursing Co.

19. JCAH Perspectives, 1985. 5,4,4.

20. Johnson R et al: The professional support group: a model for psychiatric clinical nurse specialists, J Psychosoc Nurs Ment Health Serv 20(2):9, 1982.

21. Jones M: The therapeutic community: a new treatment method in psychiatry, New York, 1953, Basic Books, Inc.

22. Kalisch P and Kalisch B: Psychiatric nurses and the press: a troubled relationship, Perspect Psychiatr Care 22(1):5, 1984.

23. Lang N: Nurse-managed centers, will they survive? Am J Nurs, 83:1290, 1983.

24. Leib A, Underwood P, and Glick I: The staff nurse as primary therapist: a pilot study, J Psychiatr Nurs 14:11, 1976.

25. Maloney E: Does the psychiatric nurse have independent functions? Am J Nurs 62:61, 1962.

26. Mauksch IG and Miller MH: Implementing change in nursing, St Louis, 1981, The CV Mosby Co.

27. McBride A: Psychiatric nursing in the 1990s, Archiv Psych Nurs, 4:21, 1990.

28. McMurrey P: Toward a unique knowledge base in nursing, Image 14(1):12, 1982.

29. Meisenhelder J: Networking and nursing, Image 14(3):77, 1982.

30. Mellow J: Nursing therapy, Am J Nurs 68:2365, 1968.

31. Mlott S: Personality correlates of a psychiatric nurse, J Psychiatr Nurs 14(2):19, 1976.

32. Moore W: The professions: roles and rules, New York, 1974, Russell Sage Foundation.

33. National Institute of Mental Health: NIMH task force on nursing report, Bethesda, Maryland, 1987.

34. Noyes A: Nursing needs in the state mental hospitals, Am J Nurs 33:787, 1933.

35. Peplau H: Interpersonal relations in nursing, New York, 1952, GP Putnam's Sons.

36. Peplau H: Historical development of psychiatric nursing. A preliminary statement on some facts and trends, 1956. (Mimeographed.)

37. Peplau H: Interpersonal techniques: the crux of psychiatric nursing, Am J Nurs 62:53, June 1962.

38. Peplau H: Psychiatric nursing: role of nurses and psychiatric nurses, Int Nurs Rev 25(2):41, 1978.

39. Peplau H: The psychiatric nurse—accountable? To whom? For what? Perspect Psychiatr Care 18(3):128, 1980.

40. Pines A and Maslach C: Characteristics of staff burnout in mental health settings, Hosp Community Psychiatry 29:233, 1978.

41. Plutchik R, Conte H, Wells W, and Karasu T: Role of the psychiatric nurse, J Psychiatr Nurs 14(9):38, 1976.

42. Powers M: Universal utility of psychoanalytic theory for nursing practice models, J Psychiatr Nurs 18(4):28, 1980.

43. Report to the president from the President's Commission on Mental Health, vol 1, Washington, DC, 1978, US Government Printing Office.

44. Santos E and Stainbrook E: Nursing and modern psychiatry, Am J Nurs 49:107, 1949.

45. Slavinsky A: Psychiatric nursing in the year 2000: from a nonsystem of care to a caring system, Image 16(1):17, 1984.

46. Sloboda S: What are mental health nurses doing? J Psychiatr Nurs 14:24, 1976.

47. Smoyak S: The confrontation process, Am J Nurs 74(9):1632, 1974.

48. Stuart G: How professionalized is nursing? Image 13(1):18, 1981.

49. Tousley M: Certification as a credential: what are the issues? Perspect Psychiatr Care 20(1):23, 1982.

50. Tudor G: Sociopsychiatric nursing approach to intervention in a problem of mutual withdrawal on a mental hospital ward, Psychiatry 15(2):193, 1952.

51. Weiss MO: The skills of psychiatric nursing, Am J Nurs 47:174, 1947.

52. Wojdowski P and Hartnett K: The HMO question: can a large health maintenance organization deliver acute psychiatric nursing services? J Psychosoc Nurs Ment Health Serv 23(9):23, 1985.

■ ANNOTATED SUGGESTED READINGS ■

*American Nurses' Association, Division on Psychiatric and Mental Health Nursing Practice: Statement on psychiatric and mental health nursing practice, Kansas City, Mo, 1976, The Association.

Official statement of the American Nurses' Association, which includes a definition and description of setting, types of practitioners, and list of functions. A resource pamphlet for all psychiatric nurses.

*American Nurses' Association, Division on Psychiatric and Mental Health Nursing Practice: Standards of psychiatric and mental health nursing practice, Kansas City, Mo, 1982, The Association.

Presents the standards of psychiatric nursing, each of which is accompanied by a rationale and structure, process, and outcome criteria. Lists the means by which attainment of the standards may be specifically measured.

*Bushy A and Smith T: Lobbying: the hows and wherefores, Nursing Management 21(4):39, 1990.

Details the steps involved in lobbying activities in order to help nurses become politically active. Practical, thorough, and needed information for all nurses.

*Church O: From custody to community in psychiatric nursing, Nurs Res 36(1):48, 1987.

*Asterisk indicates nursing reference.

Excellent review of the history of psychiatric nursing. Provides perspective and insight into current practice issues.

*Critchley D and Maurin J: The clinical specialist in psychiatric mental health nursing: theory, research and practice, New York, 1985, John Wiley & Sons, Inc.

Intended for clinical nurse specialists, this book presents more advanced discussions of theory and practice in the field.

*England D: Collaboration in nursing, Rockville, Md, 1986, Aspen Systems Corp.

Overview of the process and structure of collaborative nursing practice. Nurses, consumers, and health professionals are all considered as potential collaborators.

*Evans C and Lewis S: Nursing administration of psychiatric-mental health care, Rockville, Md, 1985, Aspen Systems Corp.

Provides guidelines and assistance to nurses responsible for the administration of psychiatric-mental health nursing care. The only book to do so in psychiatric nursing, with much to offer all employed nurses, not just those in administration.

*Jones J: Stress in psychiatric nursing. In Payne R and Firth-Cozens J, editors: Stress in health professionals, New York, 1987, John Wiley and Sons.

Literature is reviewed and summarized that addresses sources of stress for the psychiatric nurse. Presents current, inclusive, and good analysis of existing research in this area.

*Lancaster J. and Lancaster W: Concepts for advanced nursing practice: the nurse as change agent, St Louis, 1982, The CV Mosby Co.

Identifies and describes practical ways for dealing with key issues currently facing nursing. Collected articles divided into three major sections, all of which serve to conceptualize the role of the nurse as an agent of change.

*Lynaugh J and Fagin C: Nursing comes of age, Image: J Nurs Scholar, 20(4):184, Winter 1988.

Five enduring dilemmas affecting nursing are explored, with a focus on the evolution of nursing to its present state. An excellent overview of the progression of the profession.

*McBride A: Psychiatric nursing in the 1990s, Arch Psych Nurs 4(1):21, 1990.

Reviews accomplishments and notes some limitations of psychiatric nursing. Includes recommendations for future growth of the specialty.

Mechanic D: Evolution of mental health services and areas for change. In Improving mental health services: what the social sciences can tell us, San Francisco, 1987, Jossey-Bass.

Good review of current mental health services. Suggests that appropriate care for the most seriously mentally disabled will require an improved framework for public-sector services, Medicaid reforms, systems of managed care, and effective advocacy.

*Mechanic D: Nursing and mental health care: expanding future possibilities for nursing services. In Aiken L, editor: Nursing in the 80s: crises, opportunities, challenges, Philadelphia, 1982, JB Lippincott Co.

Written by a sociologist who has studied nursing. Suggests many areas where nursing may potentially contribute a great deal to the development of a progressive mental health care delivery system.

*Milio N: Promoting health through public policy, Philadelphia, 1981, FA Davis Co.

Describes how public policy evolves and its consequences for the health of Americans. Excellent documentation throughout. Its depth and substance make this a valuable book for all nurses to read.

*Peplau H: Future directions in psychiatric nursing from the perspective of history, J Psychosoc Nurs, 27(2):18, 1989.

Review of historical factors that are integrated into present perspectives of psychiatric nursing from one of its early leaders.

*Peplau H: Interpersonal relations in nursing, New York, 1952, GP Putnam's Sons.

Presents the first theoretical framework for the practice of psychiatric nursing. Describes phases and roles in psychiatric nursing, psychological tasks, influences in nursing situations, and methods for studying nursing as an interpersonal process. A "classic" in nursing literature.

*Puetz B: Networking for nurses, Rockville, Md, 1983, Aspen Systems Corp.

Describes strategies for networking, personal growth, and mentoring. Any nurse interested in career advancement or in encouraging others toward that goal will find this book helpful.

*Smoyak S and Rouslin S, editors: A collection of classics in psychiatric nursing literature, Thorofare, NJ, 1982, Slack, Inc.

A truly classic collection of 37 articles written by luminaries in psychiatric nursing. Provides a clear sense of the field's early history.

Stein L, Watts D, and Howell T: The doctor-nurse game revisited, N Engl J Med 322(8):546, 1990.

Addresses major changes in the doctor-nurse relationship over the past two decades. Reviews past behavior and superbly summarizes present interactions. Highly recommended.

*Stuart G: An organizational strategy for empowering nursing, Nurs Econ 4(2):35, 1986.

A new approach for empowerment advocates nurses acting as a unified group and the impact they can have on the organizations in which they work. Challenging and timely perspective.

*Tilbury M: Marketing and nursing: a contemporary view, Owings Mills, Md, 1989, National Health Publishers.

Addresses the need for nurses to market their skills and contributions to health care. Proactive and suggested reading for all nurses.

*Tornquist E and Funk S: How to write a research grant proposal, Image: J Nurs Scholar 22(1):45, 1990.

Provides clear and complete guidelines for writing all of the standard parts of a research proposal.

*Wieczoiek R: Power, politics and policy in nursing, New York, 1985, Springer Publishing Co, Inc.

Numerous perspectives on nursing and power. An important contribution to our professional literature with implications for all nurses.

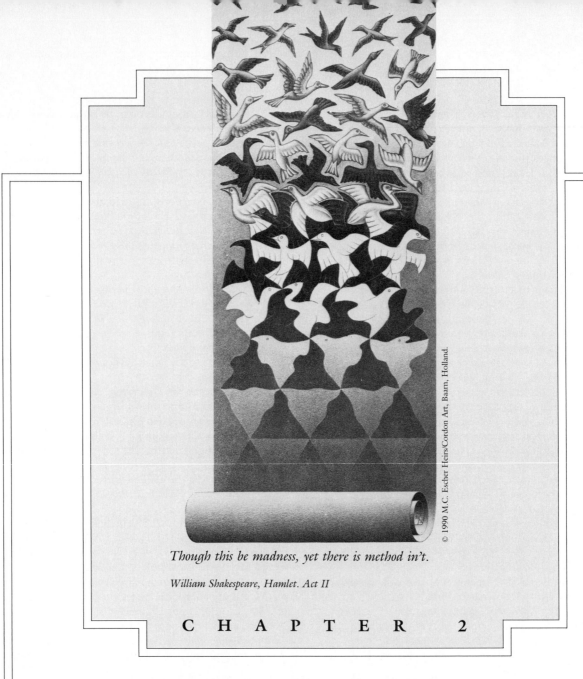

Though this be madness, yet there is method in't.

William Shakespeare, Hamlet. Act II

C H A P T E R 2

CONCEPTUAL MODELS OF PSYCHIATRIC CARE

LEARNING OBJECTIVES

After studying this chapter, the student should be able to:

- discuss the concepts of mental health and mental illness.

- describe the purpose of using a conceptual model as a framework for professional practice.

- compare and contrast eight models of mental health care: psychoanalytical, interpersonal, social, existential, communication, behavioral, medical, and nursing.

- identify major theorists associated with each model.

- describe the roles of the therapist and the patient in the context of each model.

- analyze the therapeutic process as it is experienced in each of the models.

- critique the advantages and disadvantages of the various models.

- compare and contrast the nursing diagnosis and the medical diagnosis.

- identify directions for future nursing research.

- select appropriate readings for further study.

Most people believe that they can recognize normal and abnormal behavior in themselves and others. This is true to an extent. Although people may be unwilling or unable to admit to a serious disturbance of feelings or behavior, most are aware of feeling "nervous" or "irritable" or "depressed" from time to time. This awareness comes from comparing current behavior to an internalized norm or behavioral self-expectation. Mild or transient disruptions in behavior or feelings usually are experienced as anxiety. These disruptions are resolved by using coping mechanisms. Each person learns these adaptive mechanisms during the developmental process. Some mechanisms are consciously recognized and selected, as when an angry person goes for a walk to "cool down" before confronting another person. Other mechanisms are unconscious and come into play without the person's being aware of it. An example of this is displacement of anger to a spouse, when the person really is angry at a supervisor at work. A more complete discussion of conscious and unconscious means of coping with anxiety is found in Chapter 11.

Personal coping mechanisms are not always adequate to control anxiety. When a person is unable to cope alone, he faces the difficult decision of whether to seek help from another person. The helping person may be a friend or relative, a nonprofessional counselor, or a mental health professional. The choice may depend on the severity of the problem. A young girl wondering how to act on her first date may discuss her concerns with her mother, her older sister, her best friend, or her favorite teacher. On the other hand, a woman who is so frightened of crowds that she refuses to leave her house needs to seek professional help. Frequently, significant others help the troubled person identify what type of help to consider. Seriously disturbed people may not recognize their need for help. Others may be frightened of the need to see a psychiatrist or other health professional, thinking that they will be labeled as "crazy." These people need encouragement and support to reach out for help.

Normalcy may be defined on the basis of the person's own feelings of anxiety or discomfort. It may also be defined on the basis of the cultural mores, norms, and value system in the person's society. Observable behavior that differs from the norm may be labeled deviant or sick. Social pressure may convince the person to seek help. In this case "help" means modifying behavior to comply with social norms. Clinical example 2-1 gives a brief description of normal behavior that at first appeared deviant.

Behavior may also be defined as normal or deviant for political reasons. Thomas Szasz[25] is a theorist who believes that certain types of behavior are labeled "crazy" for the convenience of society and the political system, even though the behavior may be acceptable to

---

CLINICAL EXAMPLE 2-1

Early in the fall semester a black male exchange student from Africa was brought to the psychiatric emergency room. He had been walking around the campus carrying a spear and had been apprehended by the university security patrol. His speech was heavily accented and they could not understand his explanation of his behavior. Later evaluation revealed that in his culture one never went walking at night without a spear to defend against attack by wild beasts or hostile neighboring tribes. He was sent back to his dormitory after being convinced that his spear was not appropriate to the culture of the American college campus.

---

the person involved. For example, the hospitalization of a woman who walked nude through her neighborhood could be seen as the political system's response to the neighbors' discomfort. In the Soviet political system, citizens who criticized the government were labeled mentally ill and hospitalized; their behavior was considered deviant.

These examples show that defining normal behavior is not simple or obvious. Does normality mean conformity? Does it mean controlling anxiety? Does it mean acceptability to significant others? Depending on a person's background, it could mean any, all, or none of these. Currently, perhaps the most generally accepted definition of normal behavior is behavior that enables a person to function adequately in activities of daily living and to feel reasonably satisfied with his lifestyle. This is far from precise, but human behavior varies greatly, and an exact description of normal behavior is impossible. Behavior must be viewed on a continuum, with a wide variation of what is accepted as normal. Otherwise individual behavior could be unreasonably restricted, limiting creativity and personal growth. Mental health nurses must try to understand the patient's view of his behavior and help him change unsatisfactory behavior.

Most mental health professionals practice within the framework of a conceptual model. A model is a means of organizing a complex body of knowledge, such as concepts related to human behavior. Models help the practitioner function rationally and allow for evaluation of his or her effectiveness as a therapist. Organization of data also facilitates much-needed research into human behavior.

Currently, scientific knowledge about behavior is limited. Therefore it is difficult to view any particular conceptual model as right or wrong. Unfortunately, adherents of one model or another sometimes become embroiled in conflicts about which framework is most accurate. However, the only measure of the value of any approach to mental health care is the satisfaction of the person who receives the care. It has not been proved whether the patient's response to care results from the theoretical model used or from the relationship with the therapist.

The remainder of this chapter presents an overview of several conceptual models commonly used by contemporary mental health professionals. These models include psychoanalytical, interpersonal, social, existential, communication, behavioral, medical, and nursing models. The chapter discusses information relative to each model, including the definition of behavioral deviations, the therapy process, the role of the patient, and the role of the therapist, and identifies representative theorists. Because it is impossible to explore these complex theories thoroughly in a single chapter, the reader is referred to the list of annotated suggested readings at the end of the chapter. This list includes several basic references for each theoretical framework.

Psychoanalytical model

The psychoanalytical theory was first conceptualized by Sigmund Freud in the late nineteenth and early twentieth centuries. It encompassed the nature of deviant behavior and proposed an entirely new perspective on human development. Many of Freud's ideas were controversial, particularly in the Victorian society into which they were introduced. Sexuality was a central concept in his developmental theory. For some time the emotional response to the assertion that children are sexual beings overshadowed the broader implications of Freudian theory. Objective observation of human behavior was a great contribution of the early psychoanalysts, as was the identification of a mental structure. Such concepts as id, ego, superego, and ego defense mechanisms are still widely accepted and used by many therapists. Most people readily accept the existence of an unconscious level of mental functioning. Because of space limitations the psychoanalytical theory of psychosexual development is not presented here. Rather, the focus is on the analytical method of intervening in deviant behavior, based on an understanding of the norm. Readers interested in exploring psychoanalytical theories of psychosocial development are referred to the works of Freud and Erik Erikson, a contemporary psychoanalytical theorist, and to the discussion in Chapter 30.

■ Psychoanalytical view of behavioral deviations

Psychoanalysts trace disrupted behavior in the adult to earlier developmental stages. Each stage of development has a task that must be accomplished. For instance, the child at the anal stage must learn to accept limits on his behavior and become more independent. If undue emphasis is placed on any stage or if unusual difficulty arises in dealing with the associated conflicts, psychological energy (libido) becomes fixated in an attempt to deal with anxiety. Since energy maintains repression of early conflicts, this leaves less libido available to the ego for other tasks. When the anxiety level rises, the person may regress behaviorally to the level of the fixation, using the defenses that were effective at that time. Unfortunately, these are childhood defenses that are not appropriate to the adult situation. Since the childhood conflict was not resolved, the adult is not free to use mature problem-solving techniques.

For example, a young woman was unable to resolve her competitive feelings toward her mother for her father's attention. She repressed this conflict from the phallic stage of development. She was angry and jealous of her mother and could not relate to her openly. As an adult, she was unable to develop close relationships with other women, because she suspected that they were always competing with her for the attention of men. At the same time, her relationships with men were dependent and childlike. She constantly demanded that they prove their devotion to her. She was lonely and unhappy.

Psychoanalysts say that neurotic symptoms arise when so much energy must be invested to control anxiety that there is serious interference with functional ability. Everyone is neurotic to some extent, according to this conceptual model. Everyone carries the burden of childhood conflicts and is influenced in adulthood by childhood experiences. Psychoanalysts in training must undergo a personal analysis so that their neurotic behavior does not hinder their objectivity as therapists.

According to psychoanalytic theory, symptoms are symbols of the original conflict. For instance, compulsive hand washing may represent the person's attempt to cleanse himself of impulses that his mother labeled unclean during the anal stage of development. Neurotic symptoms arise when the ego uses mechanisms of condensation and displacement. Thus the meaning of the behavior is hidden from the conscious awareness of the person, who usually is upset about these uncontrollable thoughts, actions, and feelings.

Freud developed most of his theories around neurotic symptoms. His theory is less well formulated in the area of psychosis, and it was found that people with psychotic behavior were not responsive to classical psychoanalytical therapy. This position has been modified by psychoanalytical theorists such as Harold Searles and Frieda Fromm-Reichmann, who have successfully worked with psychotic patients. The psychotic symptom occurs when the ego must invest most or all of the libido to defend against primitive id impulses. This leaves little, if any, energy to deal with external reality and leads to symbolization and the lack of reality testing ability seen in psychosis.

■ Psychoanalytical process

Psychoanalysis, as developed by Freud, uses free association and dream analysis to reconstruct the personality. Free association is the verbalization of thoughts as they occur without any conscious screening or censorship. Of course, there is always unconscious censorship of thoughts and impulses that threaten the ego. The psychoanalyst searches for patterns in verbalizations and in the areas that are unconsciously avoided. The latter areas are identified by comparison to the therapist's knowledge of basic themes of human conflict. Conflictual areas that the patient does not discuss or recognize are identified as resistances. Analysis of the patient's dreams can provide additional insight into the nature of the resistances, since dreams symbolically communicate areas of intrapsychic conflict.

The therapist helps the patient recognize intrapsychic conflicts by using interpretation. Interpretation involves explaining to the patient the meaning of dream symbolism and the significance of the issues that are discussed or avoided. However, the process is complicated by transference, which occurs when the patient develops strong positive or negative feelings toward the analyst. These feelings are unrelated to the analyst's current behavior or characteristics; they represent the patient's past response to a significant other, usually a parent. The therapist's response to the patient is called countertransference. Transference provides the motivation for a patient to work in therapy. Strong positive transference causes the patient to want to please the therapist and to accept interpretations of his behavior. Strong negative transference may impede the progress of therapy as the patient actively resists the therapist's interventions. Countertransference can also interfere with therapy if the analyst is unaware of it or unable to deal with it.

Since the therapist can temporarily replace the significant other of the patient's early life experience, previously unresolved conflicts can be brought into the therapeutic situation. These conflicts can be worked through to a healthier resolution. This releases previously invested libido for mature adult functioning. The person can conduct his life according to an accurate assessment of external reality, uninhibited by neurotic conflicts in relating to others. Psychoanalytical therapy is a long-term proposition. The patient usually is seen five times a week for several years. This approach is therefore time consuming and expensive.

■ Roles of the patient and the psychoanalyst

The roles of the patient and the psychoanalyst were explicitly defined by Freud. The patient was to be an active participant, freely revealing all thoughts exactly as they occurred and describing all dreams. The patient often lies down during therapy to induce relaxation, which facilitates free association. This also places the patient in a vulnerable position vis-a-vis the therapist, helping to recreate the childhood situation.

The psychoanalyst is a shadow person. Whereas the patient is expected to reveal all his thoughts and feelings, the analyst reveals nothing personal. This allows the transference to develop uncontaminated by the reality of the therapist as a person. The analyst usually is out of the patient's sight to ensure that nonverbal responses do not influence the patient's verbalizations. Verbal responses are brief and noncommittal for the most part to prevent interference with the associative flow. For instance, the analyst might respond with "Uh huh," "Go on," or "Tell me more." The therapist departs from this communication style when interpreting behavior. Interpretations are presented for the patient to accept or reject, but rejections imply an area of resistance. Likewise, frustration that the patient expresses toward the analyst is interpreted as transference. All the patient's behavior can be defined within the context of the psychoanalytical therapy model. By the end of therapy, the patient should be able to view the analyst realistically as another adult, having worked through his conflicts and dependency needs.

■ Other psychoanalytical theorists

Much of Freud's basic theory is still used by psychotherapists. The theorists who followed him have modified and built on the original psychoanalytical theories. Even some of Freud's contemporaries who later severed relationships with him reveal the basic influence of psychoanalytical theory in their own work. Most prominent among those who left Freud to form their own schools are C.G. Jung, who developed the idea of the "collective unconscious," and Alfred Adler, who evolved the concept of the "inferiority complex."

The following is a list of several contemporary psychoanalytical theorists and a brief statement identifying the major contributions of each:

- Erik Erikson—expanded Freud's theory of psychosocial development to encompass the entire life cycle; identified an epigenetic progression of developmental tasks; described behavioral disturbances resulting from failure to accomplish developmental tasks
- Anna Freud—expanded psychoanalytical theory in the area of child psychology; further developed the concept of the mechanisms of defense
- Melanie Klein—extended the use of psychoanalytical techniques to work with young children through development of play therapy
- Karen Horney—focused on psychoanalytical theory relative to neurotic behavior; related behavior to cultural and interpersonal factors; rejected Freud's view of feminine sexuality
- Frieda Fromm-Reichmann—used psychoanalytical techniques with psychotic individuals; expanded the psychoanalytical theory of psychotic behavior
- Karl Menninger—applied the concept of dynamic equilibrium to mental functioning; expanded the concept of coping; developed levels of dysfunction

The unique contributions of these theorists can best be understood by reading their works. This will also foster an appreciation for the continuing relevance of many aspects of psychoanalytical theory.

Interpersonal model

The origin of the interpersonal model of psychotherapy can be traced to psychoanalytical thought. Karen Horney, Erich Fromm, and Wilhelm Reich are the first theorists who tried to incorporate sociocultural influences on human behavior into the psychoanalytical model.[8] However, the theorist presented here as most representative of the interpersonal model is Harry Stack Sullivan, a twentieth-century American therapist. In addition, attention is given to the interpersonal nursing theory of Hildegard Peplau. Her work represents a milestone in the conceptualization of the psychotherapeutic role of the nurse in the context of the interpersonal relationship.

■ Interpersonal view of behavioral deviations

Interpersonal theorists believe that behavior evolves around interpersonal relationships. Whereas Freudian theory emphasizes a person's intrapsychic experience, interpersonal theory emphasizes social or interpersonal experience. Sullivan, like Freud, traced a progression of psychological development. In fact, the psychoanalytical influence can be seen in some of Sullivan's terminology. For instance, the "self-system" resembles the "ego."

Sullivan also emphasizes early life experiences as extremely influential in the person's later mental health. He believes that anxiety is first experienced empathically when the infant perceives the anxiety of the mothering person. Later, anxiety is associated with disapproval from significant others. The self-system develops in the context of approval and disapproval. Disapproval causes anxiety, because it includes a threat of rejection by the significant other. Security operations are developed to deal with anxiety-provoking areas of disapproval. The most anxiety-laden experiences are dissociated, meaning that they are excluded from the awareness of the self. Note the similarity to the psychoanalytical concept of repression.

If a child is given only disapproving messages about the self, a negative self-system develops. Interestingly, Sullivan states that ". . . one can find in others only that which is in the self."[12:310] Therefore a person who sees himself as untrustworthy views others with suspicion. The person is burdened with a lack of self-approval and is handicapped in establishing supportive relationships with others that could help modify his self-concept.

Sullivan's theory states that the person bases his behavior on two complex drives: the drive for satisfaction and the drive for security. Satisfaction refers to the basic human drives, including hunger, sleep, lust, and loneliness.[12] Security relates to culturally defined needs such as conformity to the social and value system of one's ethnic group. Sullivan states that when the nature of a person's self-system interferes with his ability to attend to his needs for either satisfaction or security, he is mentally ill.[12]

When Peplau defined nursing as an interpersonal process, she also discussed the importance of basic human needs. Needs must be met if a healthy state is to be achieved and maintained. Health is defined as "forward movement of personality and other ongoing human processes in the direction of creative, constructive, productive, personal and community living."[20:2] Lack of growth, for whatever reason, implies impaired health. The two interacting components of health are physiological demands and interpersonal conditions.[16] These may be viewed as parallel to the drives of satisfaction and security identified by Sullivan. Clinical example 2-2 clarifies this perspective on behavioral deviation.

CLINICAL EXAMPLE 2-2

Ms. Y, an attractive 26-year-old woman, appeared at a psychiatric outpatient clinic requesting therapy. She described her problem as "I can't get close to people." She said that her childhood was happy; that she had loving parents and liked her sister. Her family were devout members of a fundamentalist Protestant church, so most of her activities were church related. She had many friends during childhood and then one close girl friend in early adolescence. She thought that her fear of closeness began when she slept over at her friend's house. During the night her friend began to fondle her in a way that she interpreted as sexual. She became very frightened and felt guilty about this. She did not tell her parents because of her guilt and, in fact, had told no one before entering therapy. Although she attended college, she never dated and would participate only in superficial social contacts. She realized that this was not healthy young adult behavior and, as the behavior continued into her twenties, Ms. Y decided that she needed to seek help.

From an interpersonal perspective, Ms. Y was unable to fulfill her needs for friendship and sexual love. Proponents of Sullivan's theory would perceive the unfulfilled lust dynamism as a lack of satisfaction and her fear that she had deviated from the norm as a lack of security. Her anxiety stemmed from her conviction that her parents would disown her if they heard what had happened. This belief was based on their earlier responses to childhood sexual play. The therapist decided that Ms. Y first needed to experience intimacy at a nonsexual level. This was approached in therapy. When she began to feel comfortable sharing closeness with the therapist, she gradually explored friendships and later began dating.

■ Interpersonal therapeutic process

The interpersonal therapist, like the psychoanalyst, explores the patient's life history. This exploration focuses on the person's progress through the developmental stages of learning to relate productively to others. Components of the self-system are identified, including the security operations used to defend the self. The therapist also notes areas the patient avoids or claims to have forgotten, since this material may have been dissociated.

The crux of the therapeutic process is the corrective interpersonal experience. The premise is that by experiencing a healthy relationship with the therapist, the patient can learn to have more satisfying interpersonal relationships. The therapist actively encourages the development of trust by relating authentically to the patient. The therapist must share feelings and reactions with the patient. The process of therapy is a process of reeducation. The therapist helps the patient identify interpersonal problems and then encourages him to try more successful styles of relating. For example, patients often have a fear of intimacy. The therapist allows the patient to become close while clearly showing that there is no threat of sexual involvement. It is believed that closeness within the therapeutic relationship builds trust, facilitates empathy, enhances self-esteem, and fosters growth toward healthy behavior. Peplau[20] describes this process as "psychological mothering," which includes the following steps:

1. The patient is accepted unconditionally as a participant in a relationship that fully satisfies his needs.
2. There is recognition of and response to the patient's readiness for growth, as initiated by the patient.
3. Power in the relationship shifts to the patient as he is able to delay gratification and to invest energy in goal achievement.

Therapy is ended when the patient can establish satisfying human relationships, thereby meeting his basic needs. Termination is a significant part of the relationship that must be experienced and shared by both the therapist and the patient. The patient learns that leaving a significant other involves pain but can also be an opportunity for growth.

■ Roles of the patient and the interpersonal therapist

The patient-therapist dyad is viewed as a partnership by practitioners of interpersonal therapy. Sullivan describes the therapist as a "participant observer," who should not remain detached from the therapeutic situation.[24] The therapist's role is to engage the patient, establish trust, and empathize. There is an active effort to provide the patient with consensual validation, which helps him realize that his perceptions and concerns are similar to those of others. An atmosphere of uncritical acceptance encourages the patient to speak openly. The therapist interacts as a real person who also has beliefs, values, thoughts, and feelings. The patient's role is to share his concerns with the therapist and to participate in the relationship to the best of his ability. The relationship itself is meant to serve as a model of interpersonal relationships. As the patient

matures in his ability to relate, he can enhance his other life experiences with people outside the therapeutic situation.

Interpersonal nursing roles have been identified by Peplau.[20] They include the following:

1. Stranger—the role assumed by both nurse and patient when they first meet
2. Resource person—provider of health information to a patient who has assumed the consumer role
3. Teacher—assisting the patient as learner to grow and learn from his experience with the health care system
4. Leader—assisting the patient as follower to participate in a democratically implemented nursing process
5. Surrogate—assuming roles that have been assigned by the patient, based on his significant past relationships, similar to the psychoanalytical concept of transference
6. Counselor—helping the patient integrate the facts and feelings associated with an episode of illness into his total life experience

These roles may be assumed by the nurse or assigned to others. The practitioner helps the patient meet the goals of therapy: need satisfaction and personal growth. In addition, the therapist experiences growth as she learns about herself through her role performance. Self-awareness is essential to success as an interpersonal therapist.

Social model

The two preceding models focused on the individual and his intrapsychic processes and interpersonal experiences as the most significant factors to be considered in psychiatric care. The social model moves beyond the individual to consider the social environment as it affects the person and his life experience. Psychoanalytical theory has been criticized as being heavily influenced by Freud's Victorian, Viennese, upper middle-class, Jewish background. Concepts such as the Oedipus complex, castration anxiety, and penis envy might not extend to other cultures and times. Likewise, Freud's view of women reflects his culture and times. This view has been repeatedly challenged, particularly by feminists.

Some recent theorists believe that the culture itself is useful in defining mental illness, prescribing the nature of therapy, and determining the patient's future. The following sections discuss the theories of Thomas Szasz and Gerald Caplan. In addition, the community mental health plan of the 1960s is presented as an example of a governmental effort to respond to the philosophy of the social theorists.

■ Social view of behavioral deviations

According to the social theorists, social conditions are largely responsible for deviant behavior. Deviancy is culturally defined. Behavior considered normal in one cultural setting may be eccentric in another and psychotic in a third. An example is the African exchange student mentioned in Clinical example 2-1. With this point of view, Szasz[25] writes of the "myth of mental illness." He believes that society must find a way of managing "undesirables," so it labels them as mentally ill. People who are so labeled usually are unable or refuse to conform to social norms, and this behavior usually leads to institutionalization. If the person then conforms to social expectations, he is considered to be recovered and is allowed to return to the community. Institutionalization, then, performs the dual function of removing deviant members from the community and exerting social control over their behavior. Szasz states, "Mental illness is coercion concealed as loss of self-control; institutional psychiatry is countercoercion concealed as therapy."[26:100]

The first part of Szasz' statement recognizes that the person is responsible for his behavior. The person has control over whether to conform to social expectations. The person labeled mentally ill may be a scapegoat, but he participates in the scapegoating process by inviting it or by allowing it to occur. Szasz objects strongly to describing deviant behavior as "illness." He believes that illness can occur in the body and that diseases of the body can influence behavior (e.g., brain tumors), but that no physiological disruption can be demonstrated to cause most deviancy.[25] He distinguishes between the biological condition that is central to illness and the social role that is the focus of deviancy.

Caplan also has studied deviant behavior from a social perspective. He has extended the public health model of primary, secondary, and tertiary prevention to the mental health field. Primary prevention is the avoidance of the occurrence of disease, secondary prevention is the reduction of the duration of the illness episode, and tertiary prevention is the limitation of impairment resulting from a disease process.[9] Caplan has focused particularly on primary prevention, since much attention has been given in the past to the secondary and tertiary levels. Lack of understanding of the cause of deviant behavior has hindered the development of primary prevention techniques.

Caplan believes that social situations can predispose a person to mental illness. Such situations include poverty, family instability, and inadequate education. Deprivation throughout the life cycle results in limited ability to cope with stress. The person has few available environmental supports. The result is a predisposition to use pathological means of coping.

Crises are possible precipitating causes of deviant behavior. A person is vulnerable during a crisis. If internal coping mechanisms or external supports are inadequate, the person may exhibit pathological behavior. If adequate resources are available to help the person learn from the experience and improve coping mechanisms, a crisis may be an opportunity for growth. The supports must be available through the social system.

■ Social therapeutic process

Theorists who see behavioral deviation as intertwined with the social environment believe that therapy is also influenced by this dimension. Szasz advocates freedom of choice for psychiatric patients. The person should be allowed to select his own therapeutic modality and therapist without coercion. This also implies a well-informed consumer who can base this decision on knowledge of available modes of therapy.[12] Szasz does not believe in involuntary hospitalization of the mentally ill. He said, "Involuntary mental hospitalization is like slavery. Refining the standards for commitment is like prettifying the slave plantations. The problem is not how to improve commitment, but how to abolish it."[26:89] He questions whether any psychiatric hospitalization is truly voluntary. Szasz disapproves of the community mental health trend that purports to place mental health care within the reach of every American. He questions government involvement in what he views as a private concern.

Caplan, on the other hand, supports community psychiatry. In 1963 President John F. Kennedy announced the government's intention to become involved in the improvement of mental health care. Caplan saw this as a challenge to psychiatry. He predicted a new focus on a reduction of the frequency of mental health problems, which prompted his elaboration of primary prevention theories.[9] Caplan sees the mental health professional as using consultation to combat societal problems. Possible future psychiatric patients would benefit indirectly from positive social change.

The mental health consultant indirectly helps socially deprived people at risk for developing a mental illness. Such people include the poor or minorities. People in crisis are also at risk. They include mothers of premature babies, or husbands or wives who have recently lost a spouse. The consultant may intervene on many levels. Consultee-centered case consultation focuses on an individual client and that person's problems. This approach has relatively narrow impact. Consultee-centered administrative consultation provides advice on program development or on the interpersonal relationships of agency workers. Consultation must focus on the work situation rather than on the workers' personal problems. Program-centered administrative consultation focuses on a broader perspective of the program of an agency or a group of related agencies.[7]

■ Roles of the patient and the social therapist

Szasz believes that a therapist can help the patient only if the patient requests help. The patient, then, initiates therapy and defines the problem to be solved. The patient also has the right to approve or reject the recommended therapeutic intervention. Therapy is successfully completed when the patient is satisfied with the changes that he has chosen to make in his lifestyle. The therapist collaborates with the patient to promote change. This includes making recommendations to the patient about possible means of effecting behavioral change, but it does not include any element of coercion, particularly the threat of hospitalization if the patient does not conform to the therapist's recommendations. The therapist's role also may involve protecting the patient from social demands that he be treated against his will. Szasz feels strongly that the therapist has moral and ethical obligations toward the patient.

Caplan, too, takes a moral approach to therapy. However, he believes that society itself has a moral obligation to provide a wide range of therapeutic services covering all three levels of prevention. The patient has a consumer role and selects the appropriate level of help from a wide array of available services. Ideally, effective primary preventive services forestall the need for secondary or tertiary care. The client never becomes a patient. For example, a recently widowed woman is seen by her clergyman, who has received consultative training in counseling techniques. Concerned about the course of her grief process, he may refer her to a crisis intervention clinic. There she receives brief psychotherapy from a mental health professional. Crisis intervention services provide short-term support while coping mechanisms and environmental supports are strengthened. The widow may then be referred to a community group of widows who help each other adjust to the shock of widowhood.

Therapists may be professionals or nonprofessionals with professional consultation. People such as clergy, police, bartenders, and beauticians can be trained to listen and to refer people who need professional help to appropriate resources. The therapist in the social context is not tied to the office but is involved in the community. Activities may include home visits, lectures to community groups, or consultation with other agencies. The rationale for this approach is that the more involved therapists are in the community, the greater the impact on the community's mental health. Community involvement also enhances the therapist's understanding of patients who live in that environment.

■ Community mental health

Community mental health became a significant movement of the 1960s. It marked the vigorous entry of the federal government into mental health care, a development that proved to be a mixed blessing. The inadequacies of mental health care for most people were brought to public attention. Public funding created new facilities and trained additional mental health professionals. Care systems were examined and modified. For instance, a broader range of services was to be established, increasing their availability to the community. Emphasis was placed on making services available to groups previously neglected, including the mentally retarded, children, the poor, alcoholics, and drug abusers.

Critics of community mental health point to the enormous amount of money that was spent with no apparent significant impact on the incidence of mental illness. These critics view the community approach as a bandwagon used by some agencies to acquire new physical facilities with little or no commitment to community mental health. There was pressure to deinstitutionalize chronically hospitalized patients without adequate social skills. These patients then entered communities lacking adequate resources to help them adjust. In some cases the use of nonprofessional mental health workers led to the fear of yet another type of second-rate care.

Community mental health has had an impact on the provision of psychiatric care. It is still too soon to evaluate the total effect objectively. However, the very scrutiny of psychiatric services is a healthy development, despite some unmet expectations.

Existential model

The existential model of psychiatric care and its theorists are heavily influenced by the work of such philosophers as Sartre, Heidegger, and Kierkegaard. They are also in agreement with the theory of the I-thou relationship as described by the religious philosopher Martin Buber. This theory focuses on the person's experience in the here and now, with much less attention to the person's past than in other theoretical models. Among the earliest existentialistic psychiatric thinkers were Karl Jaspers and Ludwig Binswanger. Many contemporary theorists also advocate this model, including Frederick S. Perls, founder of gestalt therapy; William Glasser, founder of reality therapy; Albert Ellis, proponent of rational-emotive therapy; Carl Rogers, particularly in his later work with encounter groups; and R.D. Laing, who combines existentialist philosophy with an iconoclastic view similar to that of Szasz.

■ Existentialist view of behavioral deviations

Existentialist theorists believe that behavioral deviations result when the individual is out of touch with himself or his environment. This alienation is caused by inhibitions or restrictions that the person has placed on himself. He is not free to choose from among all alternative behaviors. Deviant behavior frequently is a way of avoiding more socially acceptable, more responsible behavior.

The person who is alienated from himself feels helpless, sad, and lonely. Lack of self-awareness and self-approbation prevents participation in authentic, rewarding relationships with others. Theoretically, the person has innumerable choices in terms of behavior. However, Heidegger[10] noted that people tend to avoid being real and instead yield to tradition and the demands of others. This belief has been accepted by the existentialist practitioners of mental health care.

Black[6] has described the psychiatric patient as a person who has lost or who never found the values that can give meaning to his existence. Hence the world seems absurd to him, and its demands seem invalid. Rather than accept the painful realities of life, he gives up. His lack of commitment may lead to a hazy identity and a sense of unreality that extends to his perception of other people.

■ Existential therapeutic process

There are several existential therapies, including logotherapy and gestalt, rational-emotive, reality, and encounter group therapy. All of these assume that the patient must be able to choose freely from what life has to offer. Although the approaches are somewhat different, the goal is to return the patient to an authentic awareness of his being. Laing[19] describes the process of going mad and then returning to sanity. Going mad is compared to death, movement backward, an altered sense of time, self-absorption, and a return to the womb. Recovery is compared to return to life, forward movement, restoration of temporal meaning, the growth of a new ego, and "an existential rebirth." It is the work of therapy for the patient, with the help of the therapist, to find his way from the alienation of madness to the relatedness of a full life.

The existential therapeutic process focuses on the encounter. The encounter is not merely the meeting of two or more people; it also involves their appreciation of the total existence of each other. As Binswanger has stated, "encounter is a being-with-others in *genuine presence*, that is to say, in the present which is altogether continuous with the *past* and bears within it the possibilities of a *future*."[12:377] This temporal orientation, which notes the patient's life as a process of becoming, is basic to most existential theories. Through the encounter the patient is helped to accept and understand his past, to live fully in the present, and to look forward to the future.

The actual process of therapy differs somewhat, depending on the specific theory being practiced. Following are several of the better-known existentially based theories, with a brief statement about the therapeutic process of each. For further information, the reader is encouraged to explore the writings of these theorists.

- Rational-emotive therapy (Albert Ellis)—an active-directive, cognitively oriented therapy. Confrontation is used to force the patient to assume responsibility for his behavior. The patient is encouraged to accept himself as he is, not because of what he does. He is taught to take risks and to try out new behavior. Action is emphasized for both the patient and the therapist.[13]
- Logotherapy (Viktor E. Frankl)—a future-oriented therapy; "the patient is actually confronted with and oriented toward the meaning of his life."[14:153] This search for meaning *(logos)* is viewed as a primary life force. This includes meaning in the spiritual sense. Without a sense of meaning, life becomes an "existential vacuum." The aim of therapy is to help the patient become aware of his responsibleness. In essence, the patient is guided to take control of his own life and to determine its meaning for himself.
- Reality therapy (William Glasser)—central themes are the need for identity reached by loving, feeling worthwhile, and behaving responsibly. The patient is helped to recognize his life goals and the way he keeps himself

from accomplishing his goals. He is made aware of the alternatives available to him. Another focus of therapy is development of the capacity for caring, through the warm acceptance of the therapist. Temporal orientation is to the present. The patient is directed to talk about any topic but to focus on behavior rather than feelings.[16]

- Gestalt therapy (Frederick S. Perls)—emphasizes the here and now. The patient is encouraged to identify feelings by enhancing self-awareness. There is focus on body sensations as they reflect feelings. The increased awareness makes the patient more sensitive to other aspects of his existence. Self-awareness is expected to lead to self-acceptance. The patient is assisted in dealing with unfinished business by becoming aware of the totality of his responses. More attention is focused on the "how" and "what" of behavior rather than the "why."[16]

- Psychosynthesis (Roberto Assagioli)—focuses on the self as "an inner center of awareness and peace."[4] Three developmental stages are described: The prepersonal in which the individual asks, "Do I exist?"; the personal, "I exist, who am I?"; and the transpersonal, "I know who I am. What is the meaning of my life?" The therapist helps the person use techniques such as guided imagery and meditation to achieve self-awareness and control over the course of his life.[27]

- Encounter group therapy (William C. Schutz, Carl Rogers)—focuses on the establishment of intimate interactions in a group setting. Therapy is oriented to the here and now. The patient is expected to assume responsibility for his own behavior. Feeling is stressed; intellectualization discouraged. Group exercises in relating are frequently used. Group members are encouraged to honestly and openly share their thoughts and feelings, thus becoming more self-aware.[16]

■ Roles of the patient and the existential therapist

The existential theorists emphasize that the therapist and the patient are equal in their common humanity. The therapist acts as a guide to the patient, who has gone astray in his search for authenticity. The therapist is direct in pointing out areas where the patient should consider changing. However, caring and warmth are also emphasized. The therapist and the patient are to be open and honest. The therapeutic experience is a model for the patient; he can test new behaviors before risking them in his daily life.

The patient is expected to assume and accept responsibility for his behavior. Dependence on the therapist generally is not encouraged. The patient is treated as an adult. Frequently illness is deemphasized. The patient is viewed as a person alienated from himself and others, but for whom there is hope if he can trust and follow the directions of the therapist. The patient is always active in therapy, working to meet the challenge presented by the therapist.

Communication model

A sophisticated system of communication is one of the characteristics that distinguish human beings from lower orders of animal life. According to communication theorists, all behavior communicates something. Understanding the meaning of behavior is based on the clarity of communication between the actor (sender) and observer (receiver). Disruptions in behavior may be viewed as disturbances in the communication process. This point of view is appealing in an information-oriented culture such as the United States. Frequent use of the media to spread information demonstrates the increasing use of communication techniques. Breakdown in successful transmission of information causes anxiety and frustration.

Theorists who have emphasized the importance of communication are Eric Berne, the founder of transactional analysis, Richard Bandler and John Grinder, who developed neurolinguistic programming, and Paul Watzlawick and his associates, who have studied the pragmatics of human communication.

■ Communications view of behavioral deviations

All behavior is communication, whether verbal or nonverbal. Therefore deviant behavior may be viewed as an attempt to communicate. The message may be masked or distorted; the route may be indirect, but the end result of behavior is still the transmission of a message to others who are able to perceive it.

According to Berne,[5] people communicate from the perspective of one of three ego states: parent, adult, or child. These terms do not refer to actual status in life but to the concept that the person acts like a parent, for instance. A communication unit is referred to as a transaction. *Complementary transactions* occur when the message that is sent from one ego state to another is responded to as expected. The ego state that is addressed actually responds: For instance, the sender's parent addresses the receiver's child and then the

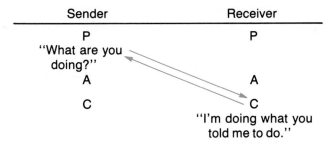

receiver's child responds to the sender's parent. Problems occur when transactions are crossed. As an example, the sender's adult may address the receiver's adult but receive a response from the receiver's parent to the sender's child. An example would be, "Bring me a glass of milk, please" followed by "Get it yourself, I'm busy." This type of transaction results in a communication block. The four most common crossed communications are the following:

1. Adult to adult—child to parent (the transference reaction)

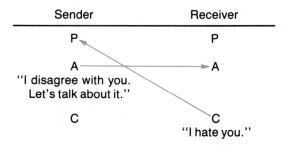

2. Adult to adult—parent to child (countertransference)

3. Child to parent—adult to adult (exasperating)

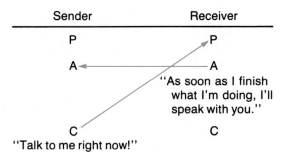

4. Parent to child—adult to adult (impudent)

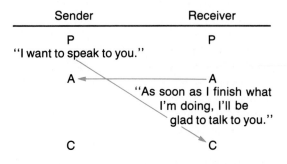

In some transactions an ulterior motive is operating. For example, the adult may appear to be addressing the other's adult but may expect a response from the parent or child. In other transactions superficial social and deeper psychological levels of meaning may be operating at the same time. According to Berne, the basis of transactional analysis is "rigorous analysis of single transactions into their component specific ego states."[5:20]

Berne further believes that people respond to three drives or hungers: (1) stimulus hunger—the need for sensation, (2) recognition hunger—the need for special interpersonally experienced sensations, and (3) structure hunger—the need to organize. The last drive leads the person to structure his time. He describes six basic types of social behavior that help provide the needed structure: (1) withdrawal; (2) rituals, which are responses to custom and characterized by strokes or units of recognition; (3) activities or work; (4) pastimes; (5) games; and (6) intimacy.[5] Two of these in particular, games and intimacy, require further elaboration. Berne describes games as "sets of ulterior transactions, repetitive in nature, with a well-defined psychological payoff." "Payoff" refers to the feelings aroused by the game. Each participant receives a payoff, although the feelings may differ. The other elements of the game are the "con," or bait, which involves the other player; the "switch," in which the initiator changes the rules or the character of the game; and the "cross-up," in which the other player feels confused and becomes aware of the switch. All of these factors are necessary for a game to be played. Intimacy refers to an open relationship in which game playing is avoided. Structure is also accomplished by way of a script, which Berne identifies as a " 'life plan' which derives from childhood ideas." Deviant behavior, then, indicates that the person is relating through game playing rather than intimacy and may be living out a script that is irrelevant to his adult life.

Bandler and Grinder based their formulation of neurolinguistic programming on an awareness of the importance of attending to choice of words and non-verbal communication.[18] Much of their theory builds on the work of Milton Erickson, a noted hypnotherapist. Erickson believed that people usually have the resources they need to manage their lives but for various reasons do not have access to their internal resources. He used hypnosis to help people identify and make use of their strengths. In addition, he gave his patients assignments of activities to carry out that would help them learn new behavior patterns.

Neurolinguistic programming focuses on the sensory channels through which people receive information. These include the visual, auditory, and kinesthetic channels. Each person develops a preference for one channel over the others. They habitually use the preferred channel for their own communication, and they feel most in tune with other people who use the same channel. The following are examples of the use of the three channels by nurses who see a patient crying:

Nurse A: "I *see* that you are upset." (visual)
Nurse B: "If you can *talk* about what is upsetting you, I would like to *listen*." (auditory)
Nurse C: "You *feel* upset right now." (kinesthetic)

By paying attention to the predicates that the person generally uses in conversation, the preferred channel can be identified. A list of representative predicates is presented in Table 2-1. Communication that uses the preferred channel is more congruent with the person's thoughts and feelings and is therefore more acceptable.

Another concept related to neurolinguistic programming is mirroring. This involves attending to the nonverbal aspects of communication such as body position, respiratory rate, and speed and volume of speech. These characteristics are then imitated in an unobtrusive way. The result of mirroring is also to increase the other person's comfort level.

Watzlawick[28] and other communications pragmatists believe that deviant behavior is based on disrupted communication patterns. They have identified several such patterns. The first is an effort not to communicate, which is self-defeating because it is impossible. A second disrupted communication pattern is a lack of congruity in levels of communication. In this case the focus is on the content of the message, but the real issue involves the relationship between the communicators. When a person makes a statement about himself, the other may confirm, reject, or disconfirm it. Disconfirmation denies the reality of the speaker.

Imperviousness is a situation in which each person assumes he understands and is understood, when this is not actually the case. Discrepancies in punctuation occur when one party has less information than the

TABLE 2-1

PREFERRED PREDICATES

Auditory	Kinesthetic	Visual
listen	feel	see
hear	knock out	behold
gripe	turn	observe
hassle	thin-skinned	view
attend	tender	witness
give ear to	stir	perceive
get	excite	discern
listen in	arouse	spy
eavesdrop	whet	sight
hang upon every word	sharpen	discover
tip	sore spot	notice
take in	itch	distinguish
overhear	creeps	recognize
register	sting	imagine
reach	thrill	catch sight of
listening	tingle	take in
hearsay	shudder	look

From Knowles RD: Building rapport through neurolinguistic programming, AJN 83:1010, 1983.
According to the NLP communication model, most people's speech reflects a preference for one of three sensory categories. The lists above suggest typical word choices in each group.

other but does not know it, leading to different perceptions of reality. The person who exhibits the self-fulfilling prophecy generally behaves as he expects others to respond to him, thus reinforcing his (usually negative) self-concept.

Human relationships are either symmetrical or complementary. Symmetry implies equality; complementarity implies difference. One disruption in this area is called symmetrical escalation, which occurs when the participants strive to be "more equal." A disruption of complementarity is folie à deux, in which each partner confirms the pathological condition of the other. For instance, a rigid, controlling mother and a passive, compliant child may depend on each other for role confirmation.[28]

■ Communications therapeutic process

Because communications theorists locate the disruption in behavior within the communication process, interventions are made in patterns of communication. This may take place with individuals, groups, or families. The communication pattern is first assessed and the disruption diagnosed. The patient is then helped to recognize his own disrupted communication. In this sense there is a definite education component to communication therapy.

Transactional analysts help patients to recognize ego states in themselves and others and to identify crossed transactions. Analysis of games is an important part of therapy. The patient sees what games he plays repeatedly. He is then assisted to find the elements of these games (i.e., What is the payoff for him? For the other person?). Games that arise during therapy are pointed out, and alternative behavior is presented. As with the existential therapies, the emphasis is on authenticity and responsibility for the self. In addition to the focus on games, the patient works to discover his script. Once identified, the script can be modified to meet the person's adult needs and to facilitate healthy relationships.

Neurolinguistic programming requires the therapist to be very observant of the patient and then to use various aspects of the patient's behavior to establish rapport. This increases the acceptability of the suggestions that are made by the therapist. Specific techniques are used to gain the patient's trust and involvement in the therapeutic process and to create change.

Conscious use of congruent predicates and mirroring of communication styles provide access to the patient. Behavior change may then be accomplished by the use of pacing. The therapist gradually modifies the mirrored characteristic that is to be changed. For instance, if an angry patient is speaking loudly and rapidly, the therapist initially would mirror that behavior by speaking in the same way. However, the therapist would then bit by bit speak more slowly and softly, leading the patient into more controlled behavior. Neurolinguistic programmers believe that this provides an opportunity to demonstrate to the patient that he can express his feelings in a more socially acceptable way, thus teaching him a new behavior pattern. Similarly, if the patient is depressed and reflecting this by sitting in a slumped, dejected position, the therapist can influence the person's feelings by first mirroring the body position and then, once communication is established, gradually sitting up straighter and establishing eye contact.

Neurolinguistic programming techniques must be used with respect and sensitivity. This approach may be viewed as manipulative, but if used properly it may also provide the therapist with a powerful tool for accessing the patient's strengths and helping him to use them productively. Advanced practitioners of this model use additional techniques, including the use of metaphor, story telling, and hypnosis. These require specialized training.

Watzlawick and his colleagues developed the technique of the therapeutic double bind. They contend that there are two ways to induce change in therapy.

One is to tell the person to change, which he probably would have done if he were able to do so. The other is to tell him not to change. This enhances his awareness of his behavior, increases tension, and may stimulate him to change. Telling the person to change by not changing creates a paradox. Any behavior is expected to result in a change. This is a difficult technique to master and should be attempted only by skilled therapists who can deal with the high level of anxiety that might result.

■ Roles of the patient and the communications therapist

The communications therapist induces change in the patient by intervening in the communication process. Feedback is given about the person's success at communicating. Effective communication is reinforced, and alternatives for ineffective communication are discussed. In group or family settings, patterns are analyzed on a more complex level. The therapist also demonstrates how to relate to others clearly, without playing games or using paradoxes. Nonverbal communication is also emphasized, particularly in terms of congruence with verbal behavior.

The patient must be willing to become involved in an analysis of his style of communicating. If in transactional analysis, he frequently will have to study the communication theory. He is then asked to participate in identifying ego states, games, and scripts. The responsibility for changing rests with the patient. Significant others often are included in communication therapy to deal with their response to change in the patient. Change in one participant in a communication system stimulates responses in the other members, and these responses generally are directed toward maintaining the status quo. Thus change is more lasting if it takes place at the system level.

Behavioral model

Behavior modification therapy is derived from learning theories. The focus is on the patient's actions, not on thoughts and feelings. Supporters of this theory believe that a change in behavior leads to a change in the cognitive and affective spheres. Behavior therapists emphasize the quantitative aspect of observable behavior. They believe that one of the strengths of this approach is the possibility of conducting research on the effectiveness of therapy. They contend that most other psychotherapies are not compatible with a scientific research process because of the high degree of subjectivity involved in defining the problem and identifying improvement. In addition, the therapeutic behavior of psychotherapists who use other models varies. Personality style individualizes therapy even among therapists who share the same theoretical framework. Behavior modification therapy, on the other hand, is structured and therefore more reproducible from therapist to therapist.

Prominent theorists of behavioral therapy include H.J. Eysenck, Joseph Wolpe, and B.F. Skinner.

■ Behavior theorists' view of behavioral deviations

Since the behavioral theorists believe that all behavior is learned, deviations from the norm are habitual responses that can be modified through application of learning theory. Learning occurs when a stimulus is presented, a response occurs, and the response is reinforced. The response is strengthened by repetition of the learning sequence. The desirability of the reinforcer to the learner is also important, although even painful (aversive) reinforcers enhance a behavior more than does no response at all.

From the behavioral point of view, deviations from behavioral norms occur when undesirable behavior has been reinforced. Clinical example 2-3 illustrates this theory.

■ Behavioral therapeutic process

Behavioral therapy, as described by Wolpe,[10] includes the technique of reciprocal inhibition. This is based on the premise that the observable behavior, or symptom, is a learned response to anxiety. The symptom is reinforced because it leads to a reduction of anxiety, even though it is not otherwise a productive behavior. Reciprocal inhibition substitutes a more adaptive behavior for the symptom through learning an alternative means of reducing the anxiety. One such approach is desensitization or the relaxation technique.

CLINICAL EXAMPLE 2-3

Ms. J was a 45-year-old woman who was brought to the mental health center at the insistence of her family. She was actively resisting her 20-year-old son's plan to move to his own apartment by threatening to kill herself. Each time she threatened, he agreed not to move for a few more weeks, thus reinforcing her behavior. The therapeutic plan was that the son would set a date to move and do so. At the same time, Mr. J would give his wife extra attention during the difficult time of their son's leaving.

The patient establishes a hierarchy of anxiety-provoking experiences from low to high levels of anxiety. He then either actually experiences or fantasizes each experience from lowest to highest. During the fantasy he may practice relaxation exercises with the help of the therapist. Sometimes the patient is hypnotized. The whole process takes several therapy sessions. The patient does not move on to the next level of the hierarchy until the anxiety associated with the lower level has been reduced. For further discussion of this technique and an example of a hierarchy, see Chapter 11.

Wolpe also advocates assertiveness training to alleviate anxiety. This is useful when the patient's anxiety arises from interpersonal relationships. Assertiveness implies the ability to stand up for one's own rights while not infringing on the rights of others. It is differentiated from passive behavior, which ignores the person's own rights. It is also differentiated from aggressive behavior, which violates the other's rights. In assertiveness training the patient identifies his usual mode of behavior. Through role play and practice he modifies his behavior toward increased assertiveness. This increases self-esteem and the sense of self-control. Interpersonally based anxiety is reduced.

Other behavior modification approaches include aversion therapy and the token economy system. Aversion therapy refers to the use of a painful stimulus, usually an electrical shock, to create an aversion to a stimulus. This approach has been tried as an attempt to change homosexual behavior.[10] There has been controversy over the moral-ethical aspects of using a method of therapy that deliberately induces pain to change behavior. However, therapists who use this approach believe the end justifies the means. Patients who accept aversion therapy generally do so of their own volition. This indicates that their emotional pain is so intense that physical pain is accepted to alleviate it.

Token economy systems are positive reinforcement programs. One use of this system is to encourage socially acceptable behavior in chronically hospitalized patients. The person is rewarded with a token, generally a poker chip, when the desirable behavior occurs. He is penalized by removal of tokens when undesirable behavior takes place. When enough tokens are accumulated, they may be spent for snacks, grounds passes, or whatever is meaningful to the patient. This pleasurable experience reinforces the future repetition of the desired behavior. For patients with good ability for abstract thinking, points may be substituted for tokens. The reward must be highly desirable to the patient. Sometimes a token economy system is helpful with children and acting-out adolescents.

■ Roles of the patient and the behavioral therapist

When a behavioral approach to treatment is used, the roles of patient and therapist are those of learner and teacher, respectively. The therapist is an expert in behavior who helps the patient unlearn his symptoms and replace them with more satisfying behavior. The therapist uses the patient's anxiety as a motivational force toward learning. Behavioral objectives are devised, and careful evaluation takes place.

As a learner, the patient is an active participant in the therapy process. He must produce fantasies or practice uncomfortable behavior. Although it is not necessary that the patient know the rationale for a therapy, the knowledgeable patient is a more cooperative patient. Homework assignments often are given to reinforce the teaching done in the therapeutic session. Significant others also may be trained to continue the therapy program at home. Therapy is complete when the symptoms are gone. No attempt is made to unearth an underlying conflict, and the patient is not encouraged to explore his past.

Medical model

The medical model refers to psychiatric care that is based on the traditional physician-patient relationship. It focuses on the diagnosis of a mental illness, and subsequent treatment is based on this diagnosis. Somatic treatments, including pharmacotherapy, electroconvulsive therapy, and occasionally psychosurgery, are important components of the treatment process. The interpersonal aspect of the medical model varies widely, from intensive insight-oriented intervention to brief, superficial medication-supervision sessions.

Much of modern psychiatric care is dominated by the medical model. Other health professionals may be involved in interagency referrals, family assessment, and health teaching, but physicians are viewed as the leaders of the team when this model is in effect. Elements of other models of care may be used in conjunction with the medical model. For instance, a patient may be diagnosed as schizophrenic and treated with phenothiazine medication. This patient may also be on a token economy program to encourage socially acceptable behavior.

Siegler and Osmond[23] believe that the medical model performs two functions. The first is treating the ill. The second is avoiding placing blame for deviant behavior. This second function is very important and may account for the wide acceptance of the medical model. When illness is attributed to disease and a cause is postulated that is external to the patient and his immediate social system, the focus can be put on healing rather than blaming. Viewing mental illness in this way removes some of the social stigma that it otherwise incurs.

Chamberlin, however, disputes the contention that the medical model reduces stigmatism. She believes that labeling behavior by giving a diagnosis is destructive to the patient, and that behavior takes place in the context of the social system and should be interpreted within that context. She asserts that a diagnosis of mental illness, particularly schizophrenia, creates fear and withdrawal of others from the patient.[11]

A positive contribution of the medical model has been the continuous exploration for causes of mental illness using the scientific process. Recently great strides have been taken in learning about the functioning of the brain and nervous system. This progress has led to a beginning of understanding of the probable physiological components of many behavioral disruptions and will lead to increasingly specific and sophisticated approaches to psychiatric care.

■ Medical view of behavioral deviations

Most adherents of the medical model believe that deviant behavior is a manifestation of a disorder of the central nervous system. As Andreasen writes, "Mental illness is truly a nervous breakdown—a breakdown that occurs when the nerves of the brain have an injury so severe that their own internal healing capacities cannot repair it."[3:219] She lists several types of brain disorders that could lead to mental illness: loss of nerve cells, excesses or deficits in chemical transmission, abnormal patterns of brain circuitry, problems in the command centers, and disruptions in the movement of messages along nerves.[3]

Currently the exact nature of the physiological disruption is not well understood. It is suspected that the psychotic disorders such as bipolar disorder, major depression, and schizophrenia involve an abnormality in the transmission of neural impulses. It is also believed that this difficulty occurs at the synaptic level and involves neurochemicals such as dopamine, serotonin, and norepinephrine.

Recently a new group of neurochemicals, called endorphins and enkephalins, has attracted a great deal of interest. These neurochemicals have been called natural opiates, because they bind to opiate receptors in the brain. Their role in determining behavior is being explored.

Much research currently is taking place so that the brain's involvement in emotional response can be better understood. Another branch of research focuses on stressors and the human response to stress. Researchers are asking, "Why do some people seem to tolerate great stress and continue to function well, and others fall apart when a small problem arises?" These researchers suspect that humans may have a physiological stress threshold that may be genetically determined. These areas of research are intriguing but currently not well enough explored to provide definitive guidelines for therapy.

Environmental and social factors are also considered in the medical model. They may be either predisposing or precipitating factors in an episode of illness. For example, the person who is unemployed, lonely, and lives near a bar may be predisposed by these factors to develop a drinking problem. In combination with other possible genetic and physiological predispositions, this constellation of circumstances could result in alcoholism. In another instance an episode of illness in an alcoholic patient could be precipitated by the social event of separation from his wife.

■ **Medical therapeutic process**

The medical process of therapy is well defined and familiar to most patients. The physician's examination of the patient includes the history of the present illness, past history, social history, medical history, review of systems, physical examination, and mental status examination. Additional data may be collected from significant others, and past medical records are reviewed if available. A preliminary diagnosis is then formulated, pending further diagnostic studies and observation of the patient's behavior. This process may take place on an ambulatory or an inpatient basis, depending on the patient's condition.

The diagnosis is stated and classified according to the Diagnostic and Statistical Manual of Mental Disorders, Third Edition, Revised (DSM-III-R)[2] of the American Psychiatric Association. The names of the various illnesses are accompanied by a description of diagnostic criteria that have been tested for reliability on a group of psychiatric practitioners. Changes in the manual reflect changes in the medical model of psychiatric care; DSM-III-R is the most up-to-date edition.[2]

According to Andreasen, one DSM-III innovation was detailed discussion of each disorder, followed by a definition that included a specific set of diagnostic criteria. This edition also reorganized the classification system, adding many more classifications than were present in DSM-II. The changes included:

1. The use of more objective and descriptive terminology
2. Increased focus in the diagnostic interview
3. A clearer and more objective diagnostic process

Andreasen also describes limitations in DSM-III. She said that it failed to completely reflect a medical model by focusing on disorders, not diseases; that causation was not discussed; and that although the manual could help in the formulating of a more reliable diagnosis, it did not help the clinician in predicting treatment, course, or outcome.[3] DSM-III-R[2] attempts to resolve these problems by including more specific diagnostic criteria and descriptions of the course of the illness.

One way DSM-III-R[2] differs from earlier diagnostic manuals is in its use of the concept of multiaxial diagnosis. Five axes are presented for consideration in formulating a psychiatric diagnosis. (These five axes are presented in their entirety in Chapter 3.) Axes I and II include the mental disorders. The diagnostic categories of Personality Disorders and Specific Developmental Disorders are assigned to axis II; all other diagnoses are included in axis I. In this way the axis II diagnoses would not be overlooked if they occurred in conjunction with the frequently more dramatic axis I conditions.[2] Axis III is used for documentation of coexisting physical conditions. These three axes make up the diagnosis that is documented for all patients who receive psychiatric care. Specialized clinical settings or individuals who conduct psychiatric research may include axes IV and V as well. Axis IV documents the severity of psychosocial stressors on a scale of one to seven.[2] Axis V rates the patient's highest level of adaptive functioning in the last year.[2] Information from axes IV and V is not routinely included in the medical diagnosis, and this illustrates an important difference between psychiatry and psychiatric nursing: such information is important when formulating a nursing diagnosis.

After the diagnosis is formulated, treatment is instituted. The physician-patient relationship is developed to foster trust in the physician and compliance with the treatment plan. If indicated, the therapist helps the patient face the stressful situation in his life and his style of coping. Other health team members may contribute their expertise. Response to treatment is evaluated on the basis of the patient's subjective assessment of how he feels, and the therapist's objective observations of symptomatic behavior. In some cases therapy is terminated when the patient returns to a satisfactory functional level. For instance, the person who has experienced an adjustment disorder with depressed mood may be able to return to his usual life-style after a short course of medication and supportive therapy. Other patients require long-term follow-up therapy, often including pharmacotherapy. For example, the patient with bipolar disorder may need to take lithium carbonate indefinitely. He also may need to see a therapist for observation of behavior and periodic laboratory studies. Other patients may receive long-term insight-oriented therapy to learn improved methods of coping with stressors.

■ Roles of the patient and the medical therapist

The roles of physician and patient have been well defined by tradition and apply in the psychiatric setting. The physician, as the healer, identifies the patient's illness and institutes a treatment plan. The patient may have some say about the plan, but the physician prescribes the therapy. Patients are not encouraged to question the physician's decision.

The role of the patient involves admitting that he is ill, which can be a problem in psychiatry. Patients sometimes are not aware of their disturbed behavior and may actively resist treatment. This is not congruent with the medical model. The patient is expected to comply with the treatment program and to try to get well. If observable improvement does not occur, caregivers and significant others often suspect that the patient is not trying hard enough. This can be frustrating to a patient who is trying to get well and is disappointed at his own lack of progress. The patient also may have difficulty letting people take care of him while he tries to help himself. It may be difficult to meet both expectations. The patient who cannot respond to the therapy offered may be transferred to another physician, another mental health professional, or to a long-term custodial institution, where his deviant behavior will be tolerated.

Nursing model

Since nursing is still coming of age as a profession, no universally accepted theoretical model for nursing care has emerged. However, nursing theorists have proposed several models that currently are being explored and refined. These include models based on general systems theory, developmental theories, and interaction theory.[21] These nursing models have some general similarities. They all incorporate a holistic approach to the individual, addressing biological, psychological, and sociocultural needs. Providing nursing care is a collaborative effort, with both the nurse and the patient contributing ideas and energy to the therapeutic process. The focus is on the caring functions of nurses, which are distinct from but complementary to the curing functions of physicians.

Shaver points out that the medical model does not

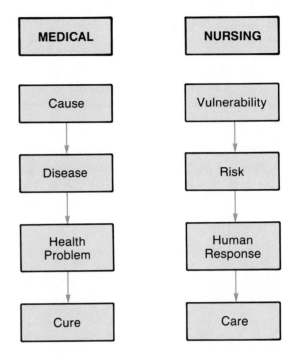

Fig. 2-1. Shaver's comparison of the biomedical and nursing models of care.

fit well with nursing. A human ecological model works much better; in this model the focus is on personal behavior, the environment, and host factors.[22] Fig. 2-1 illustrates the difference between the nursing and medical models as described by Shaver.

Hall also discusses the contrast between the medical and nursing models.[15] She describes the medical model as having a monocausal orientation. The medical diagnosis treats abstract conditions as if they are real and is unreliable and overdetermined. The medical model also fails to give adequate attention to external influences on the person. Nursing models are criticized as not being holistic enough. Hall believes that a nursing model should be a holistic or "field" one, which recognizes that the person exists within a context that determines health status.

Nurses are experts at observing and interpreting a patient's behavior. They also help the patient assess his behavior, identify unfulfilling behavior, and undertake behavioral change. Nurses are concerned with the patient's emotional response to a problem and use comfort measures to ease his pain, emotional as well as physical. To understand the patient as a whole person, the nurse must spend time talking with him and establishing a therapeutic nurse-patient relationship. The nurse is a patient advocate, interpreting his needs to significant others and to health team members.

TABLE 2-2

NURSING MODELS THAT RELATE CLOSELY TO SELECTED MAJOR PSYCHOSOCIAL MODELS

Psychosocial model	Nursing model
Psychoanalytical/interpersonal (Freud, Sullivan, Erikson)	Interpersonal (Peplau) Self-care (Orem)
Behavioral (Watson, Skinner)	Adaptation (Roy)
Communication (Bateson, Weakland, Watzlawick)	Systems (King)
Humanistic (Maslow)	Unitary man (Rogers)

Modified from Johnston RL: Individual psychotherapy: relationship of theoretical approaches to nursing conceptual models. In Fitzpatrick JJ, Whall AL, Johnston RL, and Floyd JA: Nursing models and their psychiatric mental health applications, Bowie, Md, 1982, Robert J Brady Co.

Nursing theorists who have been developing models for providing nursing care include Ida Jean Orlando, Hildegard Peplau, Imogene King, Dorothea Orem, Joan Riehl, Sister Callista Roy, and Martha Rogers. The works of these leaders are recommended for those who want to gain a broad appreciation of the current issues in nursing. Johnston compares the congruency of nursing with other psychosocial models to clarify similarities and differences, hoping that research related to theory-based practice will result. Johnston compares the person, the environment, and health.[17] Table 2-2 shows which nursing models are most closely related to selected major psychosocial models. The remainder of this chapter reflects our philosophy of nursing; this nursing model is discussed in detail in Chapter 3.

■ Nursing view of behavioral deviations

Nursing focuses on the individual's response to potential or actual health problems.[1] The defining characteristics of nursing, as related to this focus, include: (1) the *health-illness phenomena* that are encountered, (2) the *theory base* for nursing care, (3) the *nursing actions* that are carried out, and (4) the *effects* that are identified as resulting from nursing intervention.[1]

Behavior is viewed on a continuum from healthy, adaptive responses to maladaptive responses that indicate illness. The behavior observed is the result of many factors. Each individual is predisposed to respond to life events in unique ways. These predisposi-

tions are biological, psychological, and sociocultural, the sum of the person's heritage and past experiences. Behavior is the result of combining the predisposing factors with precipitating stressors. Stressors are life events that the individual perceives as challenging, threatening, or demanding. The nature of the behavioral response depends on the person's primary appraisal of the stressor and his secondary appraisal of the coping resources available to him. The continuum of coping responses may include actual health problems that lead to a medical diagnosis or potential health problems. Nursing intervention may take place at any point on the continuum. Nursing diagnoses may focus on behavior associated with a medical diagnosis or other health behavior that the patient wishes to change. A nurse may practice primary prevention by intervening in a potential health problem, secondary prevention by intervening in an actual acute health problem, or tertiary prevention by intervening to limit the disability caused by actual chronic health problems.

Under the nursing model, human behavior is viewed from a holistic perspective. A stressor that has primary impact on physiological functioning also affects the person's psychological and sociocultural behavior. For instance, a man who has had a myocardial infarction may also become severely depressed, because he fears he will lose his ability to work and to satisfy his wife sexually. On the other hand, the patient who enters the psychiatric inpatient unit with a major depression may be suffering from malnutrition and dehydration because of a refusal to eat or drink. The holistic nature of nursing encompasses all of these facets of behavior and incorporates them into patient care planning.

■ Nursing therapeutic process

Psychiatric nurses base their care of patients on the nursing process. This involves collecting data, formulating the nursing diagnosis, and planning, implementing, and evaluating nursing care. Data collection includes eliciting a complete health history. The nurse learns the patient's perception of his problems and their causes and assesses the strengths and weaknesses of the patient system and the social system. The nurse attempts to identify the predisposing factors and the precipitating stressors in the immediate problem. The nurse also assesses the patient's biopsychosocial behavior in terms of norms for a person of the patient's age, sex, and sociocultural background and consults professional literature. Inferences are validated with the patient to limit bias. Other resources for data collection include the patient's health records, significant others, and other health professionals who have cared for the patient. Data are collected more systematically when the nurse uses a data collection tool that incorporates information about the individual's total health status.

The nursing diagnosis is formulated from the collected data. It is a statement of the patient's nursing problem that incorporates the behavioral disruption and the stressor or stressors contributing to the actual or potential disruption. The nursing diagnosis provides the focus for nursing care and requires the patient's input and concurrence when possible. Noting the patient's medical diagnosis and using that as a basis for nursing care is not sufficient. Each patient is unique and although some needs may be common to the medical and nursing diagnoses, there also will be individual needs related to that person's own life experience.

Nursing care goals are formulated from the nursing diagnosis. Generally both long-term and short-term goals are developed. Long-term goals describe the health behavior to be accomplished when the identified problem is considered resolved; short-term goals contribute to achievement of the long-term goal.

Nursing actions are planned and implemented on the basis of nursing care goals combined with knowledge and review of nursing theory. Nursing care goals must incorporate the patient's own goals for his health care. Goals should be stated in behavioral terms. Priorities for the nursing care goals must be agreed on by the nurse and the patient to avoid fragmentation in providing nursing care.

Nursing actions may be dependent, based on the physician's order. For example, administering medication is a dependent nursing function. Other nursing actions are independent, such as deciding to approach a patient who appears upset and allowing him to express his feelings. There are also interdependent nursing functions, such as asking the social worker to obtain information for the patient about his medical insurance and reinforcing the social worker's explanation. All of these levels of nursing should be incorporated into the written nursing care plan. All are important to the patient's total well-being. Nursing actions should also take advantage of the patient's strengths to build on the healthy aspects of his behavior. All patients have strengths; it is a nursing challenge to discover and capitalize on them. Well-planned nursing intervention helps the patient to develop insight and to carry out a plan of positive action.

Nursing actions may include psychotherapeutic modalities of care, depending on the nurse's level of professional experience and education. Nurses with advanced psychiatric preparation may be qualified to conduct individual, group, or family psychotherapy,

psychodrama, assertiveness training, behavior modification, or other specialized therapies. Many of these therapeutic modalities were mentioned earlier in this chapter. The nursing model does not preclude any care modality as long as the nurse is skilled in its application and is adequately supervised. Nursing care respects the rights and dignity of the patient, a troubled person who deserves concern and caring. To ensure the highest quality patient care, the nursing care plan takes into account the potential contributions of the entire health care team. The patient's preferences, wants, and needs are particularly important.

Nursing care is continuously evaluated and modified by the patient and the nurse as the nursing process is used. The nursing care plan is modified on the basis of the evaluation. The most important factor in the evaluation process is the patient's reaction to the nursing care; therefore the patient must be an active participant. Validation with the patient ensures that the nurse's inferences are correct. Ongoing evaluation can add flexibility to nursing care. It allows the nurse and the patient to explore alternatives and to choose the most helpful interventions.

Nursing care is terminated mutually by the patient and the nurse. Termination usually is based on successful accomplishment of the identified goals. At other times it results because the patient or the nurse must leave the care system or because the patient chooses not to comply with the identified plan. Whatever the reason for termination, a final evaluation of the nursing care episode is necessary, since this serves as a learning and growth experience for the patient and the nurse.

■ **Roles of the patient and the nurse**

The nurse-patient relationship is based on mutuality. The needs of the patient are the focus of the relationship, and the emphasis is on the patient's strengths as a person and his growth potential. The patient actively participates in the nursing care and is asked for feedback about the effectiveness of that care. The nurse and patient then collaborate to modify the care plan. The patient is the learner. The nurse strives to make him aware of his health needs and to help him understand the nature of his health problems.

The nurse coordinates the patient's health care experience and elicits his needs. When necessary the nurse interprets these needs to other members of the mental health team. The nurse applies his or her knowledge of nursing theory and the biological and social sciences to the patient's health problem, using this knowledge to devise a sophisticated plan of care. The nurse also is responsible for making sure that the patient understands this plan. If the patient seems puzzled or is not complying with the care plan, the nurse explores his understanding of it and explains it as needed. Most important, the nurse cares for the patient, in the fullest sense of caring. He or she listens to the patient's problems nonjudgmentally, empathizes, and helps the patient identify and articulate feelings. The nurse is accessible at the time a need arises and conveys a sense of availability to the patient. He or she engenders trust by being consistent and reliable and by maintaining confidentiality. The nurse encourages the patient to be as independent as possible but also allows dependency when this is necessary. By applying psychomotor and interpersonal skills, the nurse helps the patient to grow and to reach maximum functional capabilities.

■   **SUGGESTED CROSS-REFERENCES**   ■

The nursing model of health-illness phenomena, which describes nursing and medical diagnoses, is discussed in Chapter 3. The elements of the nursing process are discussed in Chapter 5 and integrated into the other chapters of the book. Medical diagnostic categories are integrated into Chapters 8 through 22. Primary intervention strategies based on the medical and behavioral models are discussed in Chapter 8. Community mental health is discussed in Chapter 25. For further discussion of crisis intervention and the consultation process, see Chapters 9 and 26. Behavior modification is discussed in Chapter 27.

DIRECTIONS FOR FUTURE RESEARCH

The following are some of the nursing research problems raised in Chapter 2 that merit further study by psychiatric nurses:

1. The relationship between various stressors, anxiety levels, and behavioral deviations
2. Measurement of patient behavioral outcomes related to the application by nurses of psychotherapeutic techniques based on various conceptual models
3. Exploration of the ability of nurses to identify and describe the conceptual model or models that constitute the theoretical base for their practice
4. The relationship between preference for a particular conceptual model and other characteristics, such as sociocultural background, personality characteristics, and educational level
5. Conceptual models that are incorporated into curricula of graduate programs in psychiatric nursing
6. Characteristics of team relationships when members of interdisciplinary teams are homogeneous or heterogeneous in terms of preferred conceptual models of psychiatric care
7. Consumer awareness of the characteristics of various therapeutic approaches and the extent to which choice of therapist is based on understanding of the therapist's frame of reference
8. Portrayal of various therapeutic approaches in the media and how this portrayal influences the public's perception of psychiatric care

SUMMARY

Model (major theorists)	View of behavioral deviation	Therapeutic process	Role of patient and therapist
Psychoanalytical (S Freud, Erikson, Adler, Jung, Searles, A Freud, Klein, Horney, Fromm, W Reich, Fromm-Reichmann, Menninger)	Based on early development and inadequate resolution of developmental conflicts. Ego defenses inadequate to control anxiety. Symptoms result as effort to deal with anxiety and are related to unresolved conflicts.	Psychoanalysis uses techniques of free association and dream analysis. Interprets behavior. Uses transference to revise earlier traumatic experiences. Identifies problem areas through interpretation of patient's resistances.	Patient verbalizes all thoughts and dreams; considers therapist's interpretations. Long-term commitment to frequent therapy sessions. Therapist remains remote to encourage development of transference. Interprets patient's thoughts and dreams in terms of conflicts, transference, and resistance.

SUMMARY

Model (major theorists)	View of behavioral deviation	Therapeutic process	Role of patient and therapist
Interpersonal (Sullivan, Peplau)	Anxiety arises and is experienced interpersonally. Symptoms occur when security operations are unable to protect the self from anxiety. Basic fear is fear of rejection. Person needs security and satisfaction that result from positive interpersonal relationships.	Relationship between therapist and patient builds feeling of security. Therapist helps patient experience trusting relationship and gain interpersonal satisfaction. Patient then assisted to develop close relationships outside therapy situation.	Patient shares anxieties and feelings with therapist as he is able. Therapist develops close relationship with patient. Uses empathy to perceive patient's feelings. Uses relationship as a corrective interpersonal experience.
Social (Szasz, Caplan)	Social and environmental factors create stress, which causes anxiety, resulting in symptom formation. Unacceptable (deviant) behavior is socially defined and meets needs of social and political system.	Patient helped to deal with social system. May use crisis intervention. Environmental manipulation and enlistment of social supports also employed. Peer support encouraged.	Patient actively presents problem to therapist and works with therapist toward resolution. Utilizes community resources. Therapist explores patient's social system and helps patient use resources available. Works to create new resources when needed.
Existential (Jaspers, Binswanger, Perls, Glasser, Ellis, Assagioli, Rogers, Laing, Frankl)	Life is meaningful when the person can fully experience and accept the self. Behavioral deviation is expression of the individual as he is thwarted in his effort to find and accept self. The self can be experienced through authentic relationships with other people.	Person aided to experience authenticity in relationships. Therapy frequently conducted in groups. Patient encouraged to explore and accept self. Patient helped to assume control of his behavior.	Patient assumes responsibility for behavior. Participates in meaningful experiences to learn about real self. Therapist helps patient recognize value of self. Clarifies realities of situation. Introduces patient to genuine feelings and expanded awareness.
Communication (Berne, Bandler, Grinder, Watzlawick)	Behavioral disruptions occur when messages are not clearly communicated. Language can be used to distort meaning. Messages may be transmitted simultaneously at several levels. Verbal and nonverbal messages may lack congruence. These conditions result in behavioral deviations.	Communication patterns analyzed. Feedback given to clarify problem areas. Family therapy frequently used to help modify lack of congruence or complementarity in communication. Transactional analysis focuses on games and learning to communicate directly without game playing.	Patient looks at communication patterns, including games. Works to clarify own communication and validate messages from others. Therapist interprets communication pattern to patient. Helps him improve communication with significant others. Teaches principles of good communication.
Behavioral (Eysenck, Wolpe, Skinner)	Behavior is learned. Deviations occur because person has formed undesirable behavioral habits. Since behavior is learned, it can also be unlearned. Deviant behavior may be perpetuated because it reduces anxiety. If so, another anxiety-reducing behavior may be substituted.	Therapy is educational process. Behavioral deviations not rewarded. More productive behaviors reinforced. Reciprocal inhibition involves substituting an acceptable behavior that reduces anxiety for deviance. Relaxation therapy and assertiveness training are behavioral approaches.	Patient practices behavioral technique used. Does homework and reinforcement exercises. Helps develop behavioral hierarchies. Therapist determines behavioral technique. Teaches patient about behavioral approach. Helps develop behavioral hierarchy. Reinforces desired behavior.

Continued.

SUMMARY

Model (major theorists)	View of behavioral deviation	Therapeutic process	Role of patient and therapist
Medical (Freud, Meyer, Kraeplin, Spitzer)	Behavioral disruptions result from disease process, probably originating in central nervous system. Symptoms result from a combination of physiological, genetic, environmental, and social factors. Deviant behavior relates to patient's tolerance for stress.	Diagnosis of illness is based on current condition and historical information plus diagnostic studies, and treatment is related to diagnosis. Frequently includes somatic therapies in addition to various interpersonal techniques. Treatment approach adjusted depending on symptomatic response. Other mental health professionals involved when their expertise is required.	Patient practices prescribed therapy regimen. Reports effects of therapy to physician. Complies with long-term therapy if necessary. Therapist uses combination of somatic and interpersonal therapies. Diagnoses illness and prescribes therapeutic approach. May teach patient about illness.
Nursing (Orlando, Peplau, King, Orem, Rogers, Riehl, Roy)	Person is biopsychosocial entity who responds to stress in an individualized way. Behavioral disruptions affect whole person. Observable behavior must be related to predisposing factors and precipitating stressors involved. Every person demonstrates strengths as well as weaknesses. Adaptive responses to stress (health) and maladaptive responses (illness) are on a continuum of potential behavior.	Nursing process includes collecting data, formulating a nursing diagnosis, and planning, implementation, and ongoing concurrent evaluation of care plan, resulting in modification of the plan. Plan is mutually formulated with patient. Nurse collaborates with other caregivers. Long-term and short-term goals specified.	Patient collaborates in development of nursing care plan. Participates in evaluation and modification of treatment. Therapist collaborates with patient and other health team members in developing plan of care. Modifies plan on the basis of patient feedback and own observations. May use many therapeutic modalities within nursing process framework, depending on education, experience, and available supervision.

■ REFERENCES ■

1. American Nurses' Association: Nursing: a social policy statement, Kansas City, Mo, 1980, The Association.
2. American Psychiatric Association: Diagnostic and statistical manual of mental disorders, ed 3, Revised (DSM-III-R), Washington, DC, 1987, The Association.
3. Andreasen NC: The broken brain, New York, 1984, Harper & Row, Publishers, Inc.
4. Assagioli R: Psychosynthesis, New York, 1976, Penguin Books, Inc.
5. Berne E: What do you say after you say hello? New York, 1972, Grove Press, Inc.
6. Black KM Sr: An existential model for psychiatric nursing, Perspect Psychiatr Care 6:185, 1968.
7. Brockopp DY: What is NLP? Am J Nurs 83:1012, 1983.
8. Brown JAC: Freud and the post-Freudians, Baltimore, 1961, Penguin Books, Inc.
9. Caplan G: Principles of preventive psychiatry, New York, 1964, Basic Books, Inc.
10. Cautela J: Behavior therapy. In Hersher L, editor: Four psychotherapies, New York, 1970, Appleton-Century-Crofts.
11. Chamberlin J: On our own, New York, 1978, McGraw-Hill Book Co.
12. Ehrenwald J: The history of psychotherapy, New York, 1976, Jason Aronson, Inc.
13. Ellis A: Rational-emotive therapy. In Hersher L, editor: Four psychotherapies, New York, 1970, Appleton-Century-Crofts.
14. Frankl V: Man's search for meaning, New York, 1959, The Beacon Press.
15. Hall BA: Specialty knowledge in psychiatric nursing: where are we now? Arch Psych Nurs 2:191, 1988.
16. Harper RA: The new psychotherapies, Englewood Cliffs, NJ, 1975, Prentice-Hall, Inc.
17. Johnston RL: Individual psychotherapy: relationship of theoretical approaches to nursing conceptual models. In Fitzpatrick JJ, Whall AL, Johnston RL, and Floyd JA: Nursing models and their psychiatric mental health applications, Bowie, Md, 1982, Robert J Brady Co.
18. Knowles RD: Building rapport through neuro-linguistic programming, Am J Nurs 83:1010, 1983.
19. Laing RD: The politics of experience, New York, 1967, Ballantine Books.

20. Peplau HE: Interpersonal relations in nursing, New York, 1952, GP Putnam's Sons.
21. Riehl JP and Roy C: Conceptual models for nursing practice, New York, 1974, Appleton-Century-Crofts.
22. Shaver JF: A biopsychosocial view of human health, Nurs Outlook 33:186, 1985.
23. Siegler M and Osmond H: Models of madness, models of medicine, New York, 1976, Harper Colophon Books.
24. Sullivan HS: The psychiatric interview, New York, 1954, WW Norton & Co, Inc.
25. Szasz TS: Ideology and insanity, Garden City, NY, 1970, Anchor Books, Doubleday Publishing Co.
26. Szasz TS: The second sin, Garden City, NY, 1974, Anchor Books, Doubleday Publishing Co.
27. Tuyn LK: Psychosynthesis: evolutionary framework for psychotherapy, Arch Psych Nurs 2:260, 1988.
28. Watzlawick P, Beavin JH, and Jackson DD: Pragmatics of human communication, New York, 1967, WW Norton & Co, Inc.

■ ANNOTATED SUGGESTED READINGS ■

The following selections are representative works of respected psychiatric theorists. All of these readings are recommended as resources of classical approaches to psychiatry.

Adler A: The practice and theory of individual psychology, New York, 1929, Harcourt, Brace & Co.

Bandler R and Grinder J: Frogs and princes: neuro-linguistic programming, Moab, Utah, 1979, Real People Press.

Bandler R and Grinder J: Reframing: neuro-linguistic programming and the transformation of meaning, Moab, Utah, 1982, Real People Press.

Berne E: Transactional analysis in psychotherapy, New York, 1961, Grove Press, Inc.

Berne E: Games people play, New York, 1964, Grove Press, Inc.

Caplan G: Principles of preventive psychiatry, New York, 1964, Basic Books, Inc.

Ellis A and Harper RA: A guide to rational living, Englewood Cliffs, NJ, 1961, Prentice-Hall, Inc.

Erikson E: Childhood and society, ed 2, New York, 1963, WW Norton & Co, Inc.

Frankl V: Man's search for meaning, New York, 1959, The Beacon Press.

Freud A: The ego and the mechanisms of defense, New York, 1966, International Universities Press.

Freud S: In Strachey J, editor: The standard edition of the complete psychological works of Sigmund Freud, London, 1953-1974, Hogarth Press.

Fromm-Reichmann F: Principles of intensive psychotherapy, Chicago, 1950, The University of Chicago Press.

Fromm-Reichmann F: In Bullard DM, editor: Psychoanalysis and psychotherapy, selected papers, Chicago, 1959, The University of Chicago Press.

Glasser W: Reality therapy: a new approach to psychiatry, New York, 1965, Harper & Row, Publishers.

Horney K: The collected works of Karen Horney, vols 1 and 2, New York, 1937-1950, WW Norton & Co, Inc.

Jung CG, Mayman M, and Pruyser P: The psychogenesis of mental disease, New York, 1960, Pantheon Books.

King M, Novik L, and Citrenbaum C: Irresistible communication: creative skills for the health professional, Philadelphia, 1983, WB Saunders Co.

Klein M: The psychoanalysis of children, London, 1949, Hogarth Press.

Laing RD: The politics of experience, New York, 1967, Ballantine Books.

Lankton SR: Elements and dimensions of an Ericksonian approach, New York, 1985, Brunner/Mazel Publishers.

Menninger KA: The vital balance, New York, 1963, Viking Press.

*Peplau HE: Interpersonal relations in nursing, New York, 1952, GP Putnam's Sons.

Perls FS: In and out of the garbage pail, Lafayette, Calif, 1969, Real People Press.

Rogers CR: Client-centered therapy, Boston, 1951, Houghton Mifflin Co.

Rogers CR: Carl Rogers on encounter groups, New York, 1970, Harper & Row, Publishers, Inc.

Schutz WC: Joy, New York, 1967, Grove Press, Inc.

Sullivan HS: In Perry HS and Gawel ML, editors: The interpersonal theory of psychiatry, New York, 1953, WW Norton & Co, Inc.

Sullivan HS: In Perry HS and Gawel ML, editors: The psychiatric interview, New York, 1954, WW Norton & Co, Inc.

Szasz T: The myth of mental illness, New York, 1961, Hoeber-Harper.

Watzlawick P, Beavin JH, and Jackson DD: Pragmatics of human communication, New York, 1967, WW Norton & Co, Inc.

Wolpe J: The practice of behavior therapy, ed 2, New York, 1973, Pergamon Press.

The following selections include anthologies of theoretical approaches to psychiatry. Also included are several selections of interest to the nurse who is developing a conceptual approach to psychiatry.

Andreasen NC: The broken brain, New York, 1984, Harper & Row, Publishers, Inc.

A readable book that provides valuable information about the anatomy and physiology of the brain, and then applies that information in discussions of the biological theories of psychiatric disorders. Recommended to students and to practicing nurses as a way of updating knowledge in this rapidly expanding area.

*Black K Sr: An existential model for psychiatric nursing, Perspect Psychiatr Care 6:178, 1968.

Discusses the concept of the existential encounter as it applies to the therapeutic nurse-patient relationship. Conveys a basic respect for the patient's dignity, illustrated with a clinical example.

Brown JAC: Freud and the post-Freudians, Baltimore, 1961, Penguin Books, Inc.

---

*Asterisk indicates nursing reference.

Presents a review of the works of the major post-Freudian theorists, allowing the reader to compare these theorists with Freud and each other.

*Burnard P: Existentialism as a theoretical basis for counselling in psychiatric nursing, Arch Psych Nurs 3:142, 1989.

Proposes an existential approach to counseling by nurses and contrasts it with Rogers' nondirective approach. The clearly presented contrast between the two models should stimulate thought and discussion.

*Clark CC: Combining therapeutic approaches, J Psychiatr Nurs 15:18, 1977.

Compares and contrasts two apparently incompatible approaches to psychotherapy: psychoanalysis and behavioral therapy. The author demonstrates that a combination of these approaches may be used very effectively with some patients. She also identifies several commonalities between these models.

*Clark MD: Carl Rogers revisited, Can J Psychiatr Nurs 22:14, 1981.

A concise review of the principles of Rogers' approach to counseling. A good example of the application of a theoretical frame of reference to the therapy process.

*Critchley DL: The adverse influence of psychiatric diagnostic labels on observation of child behavior, Am J Orthopsychiatry 49:157, 1979.

The author found that informing a student nurse of a psychiatric diagnosis for a child influenced the nurse's perception of the child's behavior. Children diagnosed as not normal were not perceived to behave normally, even if the child was not, in reality, mentally ill. This demonstrates the value of nursing research in model development and also points out the dangers inherent in labeling behavior. Critchley also points out the problems in focusing on pathological conditions rather than health, thereby reinforcing sick behavior.

Ehrenwald J: The history of psychotherapy, New York, 1976, Jason Aronson, Inc.

A fascinating description of the historical development of models of psychotherapy, including both mystical/religious and scientific approaches. Theories are illustrated with lengthy and informative quotes from the original theorist.

*Fitzpatrick JJ, Whall AL, Johnston RL, and Floyd JA: Nursing models and their psychiatric mental health applications, Bowie, Md, 1982, Robert J Brady Co.

Takes the important step of attempting to compare and correlate nursing models with mental health care models; provides much food for thought and should stimulate lively debate. Not a book for beginning students, as a thorough knowledge of the theories is needed to comprehend the condensed presentations in this text.

Frank JD: Persuasion and healing, Baltimore, 1973, The Johns Hopkins University Press.

Thought-provoking comparison of psychotherapy to other forms of persuasion such as religious revivalism and thought reform; considers several models of psychiatric care in terms of this frame of reference. Particularly useful for those engaged in psychotherapy.

Haley J: The art of psychoanalysis. In Haley J: The power tactics of Jesus Christ, New York, 1969, Avon Books.

Takes a provocative look at psychoanalysis as a power relationship that is set up to enhance the superior position of the therapist. Amusing reading, but very thought-provoking.

*Hall BA: Specialty knowledge in psychiatric nursing: where are we now? Arch Psych Nurs 2:191, 1988.

A provocative article that challenges psychiatric nurses to break away from limiting theoretical models, exemplified by the medical model. The author proposes a focus on holistic models that incorporate all the elements that influence the individual's health status and urges agreement on a nursing model for mental health nursing care.

*Mansfield E: A conceptual framework for psychiatric-mental health nursing, J Psychiatr Nurs 18:34, 1980.

Describes a conceptual model for a graduate program in psychiatric nursing. It incorporates theoretical concepts of general systems, human development, communication, and self-esteem into a nursing process model. Of particular interest are the author's suggestions about the utility of the model for generating nursing research.

Marriner-Tomey A: Nursing theorists and their work, ed 2, St Louis, 1989, The CV Mosby Co.

A readable book that presents the basic concepts of 28 nursing theorists, offering the reader an excellent opportunity to compare and contrast their approaches to nursing practice.

*Powers ME: Universal utility of psychoanalytic theory for nursing practice models, J Psychiatr Nurs 18:28, 1980.

Demonstrates that a nursing practice model can accommodate the adaptation of a particular theoretical concept. The author applies classical psychoanalytical theory to nursing in a way that challenges the reader to agree or disagree with her assertion.

Powers ME: Understanding psychological man: a state-of-the-science report, Psychol Today 16:5:40, 1982.

Several leading psychologists who represent most of the major schools of thought provide their views on the current state of psychology. Most of the models described in this chapter are represented, with applications to trends such as psychobiology and technological advances.

*Riehl JP and Roy C: Conceptual models for nursing practice, New York, 1974, Appleton-Century-Crofts.

An excellent discussion of the status of the development of models for nursing practice; presents several nursing models in a format that allows the reader to make comparisons. Highly recommended for nurses at all levels of experience and education.

Rosenhan DL: On being sane in insane places, Science 179:250, 1973.

A report of admission of several pseudopatients to psychiatric hospitals; raises interesting questions about the implications of labeling people as mentally ill. The experience of being a psychiatric patient is also recounted. Worthwhile reading for any nurse.

Scheff TJ: Being mentally ill: a sociological theory, Chicago, 1966, Aldine Publishing Co.

Discusses the definition of insanity from a sociological framework; presents interesting material on the experience of being a psychiatric patient and on society's role in defining the conditions of insanity.

*Shaver JF: A biopsychosocial view of human health, Nurs Outlook 33:186, 1985.

Compares the medical and nursing models of health care. The author describes a biopsychosocial nursing model and provides several examples of health care interventions based on this model. Scholarly and thought-provoking.

Siegler M and Osmond H: Models of madness, models of medicine, New York, 1976, Harper Colophon Books.

A comparison of the medical model to other models of psychiatric care; presents the case for continued use of the medical model as the most helpful framework for psychiatry.

*Slavinsky AT: Psychiatric nursing in the year 2000: from nonsystem of care to a caring system, Image 16:1:17, 1984.

From the perspective of the year 2000, the author analyzes the deficiencies of the current mental health system and proposes nursing roles to improve mental health care. She makes a convincing case for the pivotal role of mental health nurses in a caring system.

*Sundeen SJ et al: Nurse-client interaction, ed 4, St Louis, 1989, Mosby–Year Book, Inc.

Provides discussion of the nursing process and includes a clinical example of how this process can be used to organize nursing care planning.

Wolberg LR: The techniques of psychotherapy, parts I and II, ed 4, New York, 1988, Grune & Stratton, Inc.

A thorough presentation of basic theories of psychotherapy, followed by a discussion of the practice of psychotherapy. An excellent resource for the experienced practitioner of psychiatric nursing. Contains a discussion of psychosocial development, including the theories of Freud, Erikson, and Sullivan.

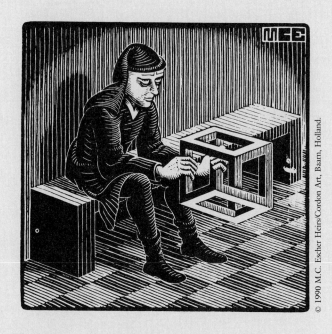

The highest wisdom has but one science, the science of the whole.

Leo Tolstoy, War and Peace

C H A P T E R   3

A NURSING MODEL OF HEALTH-ILLNESS PHENOMENA

- discuss why it is difficult to define mental health and the conditions and criteria associated with it.

- relate the dimensions and prevalence of mental and addictive disorders in the United States.

- identify developmental stages and tasks of individual and family life cycles.

- describe cultural relativism and ethnocentrism and the implications of each for psychiatric nursing care.

- analyze a nursing model of health-illness phenomena and the components of it that result in adaptive or maladaptive coping.

- critique the significance of stressful life events in precipitating illness.

- discuss primary appraisal of a stressor as it occurs on the cognitive, affective, physiological, behavioral, and social levels.

- describe various types of coping.

- discuss secondary appraisal of coping resources that involve cognitive, affective, physiological, behavioral, and social responses.

- distinguish between constructive and destructive coping mechanisms and between neurotic and psychotic disorders.

- compare and contrast coping responses, health problems, nursing diagnoses, and medical diagnoses.

- analyze the interrelationship between DSM-III-R medical diagnoses and NANDA nursing diagnoses.

- identify directions for future nursing research.

- select appropriate readings for further study.

Defining mental health and illness

Since the early 1940s, *mental health* and *mental hygiene* have appeared in the health care literature and in public policy statements. These terms are now common in everyday speech and thought. However, relatively few attempts have been made to define "mental health," and little consensus exists.

One of the few studies to examine mental health in Americans reported that men and women use the same six dimensions in evaluating their mental health: unhappiness, lack of gratification, strain, feelings of vulnerability, lack of self-confidence, and uncertainty.[5] Yet problems still exist for researchers and clinicians.

Mental health often is spoken of as a state of well-being such as happiness, contentment, satisfaction, or achievement. These are difficult terms to apply, and their meanings fluctuate according to different conditions. Happiness is a desirable consequence of mental health, but it poses problems if used as a criterion. Similar problems arise with viewing mental health sta-

tistically as the central tendency or mean of a group. What is derived in this way is "average," which may not necessarily mean "healthy."

In seeking the signs of mental health, Jahoda[22] suggested the following conditions:

1. The idea of any single criterion of mental health should be abandoned. Mental health cannot be refined to a simple concept, and a single item of behavior is not adequate.
2. The terms we use to define mental health should be reduced to definite operational procedures. We need scales and measures for each criterion.
3. Each of the criteria should be thought of as a continuum, since there are unhealthy trends in an otherwise healthy person.
4. These criteria of mental health indicate trends in the individual toward health or disease. Implicit in the criteria is the concept of gradients of mental health.

5. The criteria are regarded as relatively enduring attributes of the person. They are not merely functions of a particular situation the individual may find himself in.

6. These criteria are set up as the optimum of mental health. They are not absolute. The minimum standard for any individual has yet to be determined and may change with age. Each individual has limits, and no one reaches the ideal in all the criteria. However, most people can approach the optimum. Below a yet-to-be-determined minimum, most if not all people break down.

■ **Criteria of mental health**

The following six criteria were offered by Jahoda[22] as a recipe for mental health:

1. Positive attitudes toward self
2. Growth, development, and self-actualization
3. Integration
4. Autonomy
5. Reality perception
6. Environmental mastery

Positive attitudes toward self include an acceptance of self and self-awareness. A person must have some objectivity about the self and realistic aspirations that necessarily change with age. A healthy person must also have a sense of identity, a wholeness, belongingness, security, and meaningfulness.

Growth, development, and self-actualization have been the objects of considerable research. Maslow[32] and Rogers[40], for example, developed extensive theories on the development and realization of the human potential. Maslow describes the concept of "self-actualization," and Rogers emphasizes the "fully functioning person." Both theories focus on the entire range of human adjustment. They describe a self engaged in a constant quest, always seeking new growth, development, and challenges. These theories focus on the total person and whether he (1) is adequately in touch with his own self to free the resources that are there; (2) has free access to his feelings and can integrate them with his intellectual and cognitive functioning; (3) is immobilized by inner conflicts and stresses or can interact freely and openly with his environment; and (4) can share himself with other people and grow from such experiences. Maslow[32] identified 15 personality characteristics that distinguish "self-actualized" individuals—people moving in the direction of achieving their highest potential. Rogers[40] described seven essential personality traits of the "fully functioning per-

TABLE 3-1

THEORIES ON DEVELOPMENT AND REALIZATION OF HUMAN POTENTIAL

Maslow's "self-actualized" individual	Rogers' "fully functioning" person
Has accurate perception of reality	Moves away from facades that are not true to self
Has a high degree of acceptance of self, others, and human nature	Moves away from others' expectations of what he "ought to be"
Exhibits spontaneity	Moves away from pleasing others who impose artificial goals on him
Is problem-centered as opposed to self-centered	Moves toward becoming autonomous, self-directing, and self-responsible
Has need for privacy	Is open to change and exploring his potential
Demonstrates high degree of autonomy and independence	Is open to his own self and the lives of others
Has freshness of appreciation	Trusts and values himself and dares to express himself in new ways
Has frequent "mystic or peak" experiences	
Shows identification with mankind	
Shares intimate relationships with a few significant others	
Has democratic character structures	
Possesses strong ethical sense	
Demonstrates unhostile sense of humor	
Possesses creativeness	
Exhibits resistance to conformity	

son," who similarly is moving toward self-growth and fulfillment. See Table 3-1.

Integration is a balance between what is expressed and what is repressed, between outer and inner conflicts and drives, and a regulation of one's moods and emotions. It includes emotional responsiveness and control and a unified philosophy of life. This consistent set of values provides a framework for continuity in all responses. This criterion can be measured at least in part by the person's ability to withstand stress and cope with anxiety. A strong but not rigid ego enables the person to handle change and grow from it.

Autonomy involves self-determination, a balance between dependence and independence, and acceptance of the consequences of one's actions. It implies that the person is responsible for himself, including his decisions, actions, thoughts, and feelings. Consequently, the person can respect autonomy and freedom in others.

Reality perception is the individual's ability to test his assumptions about the world by empirical thought. The mentally healthy person can change his perceptions in the light of new information. This criterion includes empathy or social sensitivity, a respect for the feelings and attitudes of others.

Environmental mastery enables a mentally healthy person to feel success in an approved role in his society or group. He can deal effectively with the world, work out his problems of living, and obtain satisfaction from life. This criterion incorporates the idea of social competence as well. The person should be able to cope with loneliness, aggression, and frustration without being overwhelmed. The mentally healthy person can respond to others, love and be loved, and cope with reciprocal relationships. He can build new friendships and have satisfactory social group involvement.

Finally, a person should not be assessed against some vague or ideal notion of health. Rather, he should be seen in a group context, an age context, and an individual context. The issue is not how well someone fits an arbitrary age standard, but rather what is reasonable for a particular person. Is there continuity or discontinuity with the past? Does the person adapt to changing needs throughout his life cycle? Such a view incorporates the concept of **psychobiological resilience,** which proposes that humans must weather periods of stress and change throughout life. Successfully weathering each period of disruption and reintegration leaves the person better able to deal with the next change. This dimension equates mental health with adaptation and mental illness with maladaptation.

■ **Dimensions of mental illness**

The health-illness continuum is asymmetrical. The two poles of health and illness are not equally clear. Rather, the standards of mental health are less clear and less agreed on than those of mental illness. Whereas conceptions of mental health can be extended indefinitely, conceptions of mental illness are bounded by greater consensus of symptoms that can be specified and studied.

Mental disorders are a major contributor to the burden of illness in the United States. They attract less public attention than some other disorders for a number of reasons, including their relatively low mortality rate, the low social status of many of the mentally ill,

and the stigma that many people attach to mental disorders. Still, both the chronicity of some disorders and the problems that can arise from them cause great strain on affected individuals and on the larger health care system.

The prevalence of mental and addictive disorders for all age groups in the United States is approximately 15% to 22.5%. Thus mental disorders, alcoholism, and drug addiction profoundly disrupt the lives of 30 million to 45 million people in the United States each year. Furthermore, mental disorders and addictive states rank third for personal health care expenditures. Conservative estimates of annual expenditures for direct health care are placed at $20 billion and of total economic costs to society at $185 billion.[1]

Research has greatly improved drug and psychosocial therapies for some mental illnesses and addictions, but much work remains to be done on prevention, diagnosis, and treatment of these disabling conditions. Yet, since 1966 the real level of federal support for research in the area of mental illness and addictive disorders has dropped markedly, even as research opportunities and the number of available researchers have increased. For example, more than $300 is spent on research for every cancer patient, whereas the comparable figure for schizophrenia is $7. The Report of the Board on Mental Health and Behavioral Medicine, Institute of Medicine, has called for a marked expansion of research support for mental illness and addictive disorders. Emerging information about brain function and behavioral responses to stress gives hope that sustained research and clinical support will benefit the millions whose lives are touched by severe mental disorders, alcoholism, and drug addiction.

Developmental norms and stages

A knowledge of normal growth and development is essential for assessing a person's functioning, as well as for intervening with a nursing model for health-illness phenomena. Other sources[43] describe these stages in detail, and the nurse should be familiar with normative stages, tasks, and parameters to know what issues the person has faced in the past and what challenges lie ahead. Besides understanding the individual's development, the nurse must know about the family cycle. Many nursing interventions are directed at the family, from mobilizing their support of a patient to modifying dysfunctional family patterns.

Table 3-2 summarizes the developmental stages of the individual, using Erikson's theory[14] of psychosocial development and Duvall's stages[13] of the family life cycle. Streff[42] integrated Erikson's theory with Duvall's to define developmental tasks of the family paral-

TABLE 3-2

DEVELOPMENTAL STAGES AND TASKS OF THE INDIVIDUAL AND FAMILY UNIT

Erikson's stage of individual psychosocial development[14]	Developmental task of the individual[43]	Duvall's stage of the family life cycle[13]	Developmental task of the family identified by Streff[42]
Trust vs. mistrust (0-2 years)	Oral needs are of primary importance Adequate mothering is necessary to meet infant's needs Acquisition of hope	Premarital-married couple	Establishing relationship Defining mutual goals Developing intimacy Developing appropriate dependence, independence, interdependence pattern Establishing mutually satisfying relationship Negotiating boundaries of couple relationship and with individuals' families of origin Discussing issue of childbearing Making decision to conceive
Autonomy vs. shame (1½-3 years)	Anal needs are of primary importance Father emerges as important figure Acquisition of will	Childbearing	Working out authority and responsibility issues Working out caretaker roles Having children Forming new unit Facilitating child's establishment of trust Acknowledging need for personal time and space while sharing with each other and child
Initiative vs. guilt (3-6 years)	Genital needs are of primary importance Family relationships contribute to early sense of responsibility and conscience Acquisition of purpose	Preschool	Continuing individual development as couple, parent, and family Experiencing changes in energy and time for individual and couple needs Promoting continued growth in each other and the relationship while encouraging child to develop autonomy and retain self-esteem Establishing own family tradition with each other and children without guilt related to breaks with traditions of families of origin
Industry vs. inferiority (6-12 years)	Active period of socialization for child as he moves from family and into society Acquisition of competence	School age	One or both spouses establishing new roles in work settings or community or changes in child-rearing practices and gaining recognition for selves and children Children in school and after-school activities, relating with peers, self-esteem being enhanced or inhibited, and interfacing with activities in family
Identity vs. identity diffusion (13+ years)	Search for self, in which peers play important role Psychosocial moratorium is provided by society to aid adolescent Acquisition of fidelity	Teenage	Parents continue to develop roles in community and interests other than with children Children examine ways to experience freedom while expressing responsibility for actions

TABLE 3-2

DEVELOPMENTAL STAGES AND TASKS OF THE INDIVIDUAL AND FAMILY UNIT—cont'd

Erikson's stage of individual psychosocial development[14]	Developmental task of the individual[43]	Duvall's stage of the family life cycle[13]	Developmental task of the family identified by Streff[42]
			Struggles evolve with parents as emancipation process proceeds
			Family's value system may be challenged
			Couple's relationship may be strong or weak, depending on how members respond to each other's needs
Intimacy vs. isolation (adulthood)	Characterized by increasing importance of human closeness and sexual fulfillment Acquisition of love	Launching career	Parents launching young adults with rituals marking rites of passage
			Change in relationship with children who are becoming adults and/or in new living situations; change in couple's relationship because of children's absence and increased time with one another
Generativity vs. self-absorption (middle-age)	Characterized by productivity, creativity, parental responsibility, and concern for new generation Acquisition of care	Middle-age parents	Energy channeled into guiding next generation via family or community activities, or couple may now be dealing with issues of aging of their own parents
			Children of middle-age parents may be adolescent
Integrity vs. despair (old age)	Characterized by unifying philosophy of life and more profound love for mankind Acquisition of wisdom	Aging family members	Persons have achieved satisfying relationships and feel sense of accomplishment and desire to continue to live fully until death instead of existing in state of despair
			Aging members are coping with bereavement and may now be living alone

leling those of the individual. This integrated approach allows life to be viewed as stages marked by critical developmental tasks. This helps the nurse identify potential future stressors for an individual or family. By understanding and anticipating these stressors, the nurse can implement effective nursing care.

Cultural relativism

Mental health and illness emerge within a social context in which cultural relativism is particularly important. Cultural relativism refers to the differences in beliefs, feelings, behaviors, traditions, social practices, and technology that are found among the various peoples of the world. These differences are related because they arise from differences in culture.[15] Thus culture influences the most basic characteristics of people, in-

cluding their beliefs, emotions, sense of self, and even the illnesses to which they may be susceptible. Similarly, the content and form of mental health and mental illness vary greatly, since different cultures place varied stressors on people. They also vary in symbolic interpretation, acceptance of expression or repression, cohesion of social groups, and tolerance of deviation.

The problem of cultural relativism is particularly relevant to psychiatry because it is a field that emphasizes the whole person, including biological, psychological, and social components. So too, even if all psychiatric illnesses were found to be caused by biological imbalances, the social and emotional consequences of the illnesses would still exist and need to be addressed. In addition, over the centuries, psychiatry has been involved with problems that overlap with social issues and questions of conformity and deviance.

The search for a link between cultural factors and mental illness has significant roots. As early as 1897, Durkheim wondered about a connection between suicide and social conditions.[12] In the 1930s, Faris and Dunham suggested a causal relationship between schizophrenia and the living conditions in Chicago slums.[16] In 1959 Leighton and coworkers documented both an overall correlation between mental illness and social disarray and correlations between specific sociocultural settings and particular psychiatric disorders.[29] In the 1970's Dohrenwend and Dohrenwend found that although schizophrenia seemed to be present in all cultures, there was considerable discrepancy in the types of schizophrenia that dominated in different cultures.[11] More recently, Comas-Diaz and Griffith have summarized the expanding research and theoretical literature on this subject.[10]

The danger in ignoring cultural diversity and group norms is that deviance may be equated with illness. When social alternatives are equated with illness, an unusual life-style is regarded as sick, and aberrant behavior is taken as a sign of personal abnormality. For example, in one study that controlled for psychiatric condition and social class, it was found that nonwhite males were involuntarily hospitalized more often than white males, because the police brought the nonwhite males into treatment more often. The authors concluded that the more coercive conditions under which nonwhites enter treatment determine the health care system's more severe responses to nonwhites' deviance.[41]

This inaccuracy can be avoided if it is recognized that health-illness and conformity-deviance are independent variables. Combining them generates four patterns: the healthy conformist, the healthy deviant, the unhealthy conformist, and the unhealthy deviant (Fig. 3-1). A mental health professional must consider carefully the meaning of deviant behavior and its social context, since it may reflect an adaptation to realistic forces in a person's life or conformity to group norms.

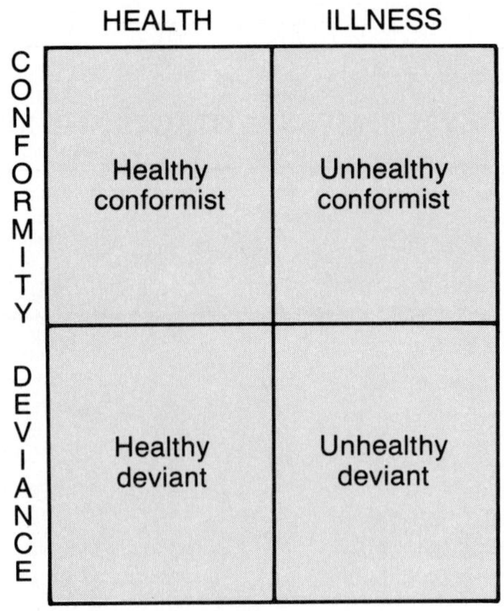

■ Ethnocentrism

Another challenge in assessing mental health and illness arises from ethnocentrism, which is marked by two assumptions:

1. "Others" should live by our own peculiar ethnic or national logic and mores.
2. One can influence "others" to change their way of life or philosophy.

If the nurse's own views and standards are imposed on others, misdiagnosis or a therapeutic impasse might re-

Fig. 3-1. Patterns of behavior.

sult. For example, it has been shown that the diagnoses of psychiatrists are influenced by such characteristics as the sex and race of the patient.[31] These biases can change society's perceptions of mental health, since white males represent the majority of psychiatrists in the United States, and their judgments play a dominant role in the definition of mental health and illness by other mental health professionals, the scientific community, and the lay public. When this principle operates among groups of people in a society, it becomes the foundation for nationalism or racism and can result in political friction between nations.

A related problem occurs when clinicians regard their theories or techniques as universally applicable in the absence of relevant research among other cultural groups. What is needed in this pluralistic world is an understanding of different peoples and of the social, cultural, and political forces that shape behavior.

These include, but are not limited to, one's race, ethnicity, nationality, gender, socioeconomic status, previous experience with the health care system, and social role.

Too often, nurses and physicians assume that patients' perceptions and goals are similar to their own, when the literature suggests that significant discrepancies persist in the perceptions of patients and health care providers.[35] These differences in perceptions often result in poor communication, poor compliance, inadequate or unnecessary treatment, and legal and ethical problems. Through the reflective process of analyzing his or her reactions to culturally diverse patients, the nurse will better meet the needs of all patients. Most important, the nurse must be able to view culturally diverse patients as individuals and seek a common ground of communication and understanding. In this way the nurse can share the fundamental human bond through which the nurse-patient relationship is established and maintained.

A final reason to consider racial and ethnic factors in psychiatric care has been identified through recent psychiatric research. Current findings suggest that cultural differences exist in the symptom presentations of psychiatric disorders. Racial differences have also been noted among proposed biological markers for various psychiatric disorders such as serum creatinine phosphokinase, platelet serotonin, and HLA-A2. Failure to control for race therefore would alter the interpretation of studies evaluating these markers. Finally, racial and ethnic differences in response to psychotropic medications, such as higher blood levels found among Asians, affect dosage requirements and potential side effects.[25] Sociocultural needs therefore should be incorporated when planning psychiatric care.

Nursing model of health-illness phenomena

Models serve many purposes. They help clarify relationships, generate hypotheses, and give perspective to an abstract idea or concept. Psychiatric nurses can practice more effectively if their actions are based on a model of health-illness phenomena that is inclusive and holistic, yet discrete and relevant. Such a model must recognize that health or illness is an outcome when several of a person's biological and personality characteristics interact with factors in the larger social environment.

This model of health and illness assumes that nature is ordered as a social hierarchy or continuum from the simplest unit to the most complex (Fig. 3-2). Each level within this hierarchy represents an organized whole with distinctive properties and a complex, integrated organization. The study of each level therefore requires unique criteria for explaining structure and function. Additionally, each level is a component of each higher level, so that nothing exists in isolation. Thus the individual is a component of family and community. Material and information flow across levels, and each level is influenced by all the others. For this reason one level of organization, such as the individual, cannot be characterized as a dynamic system without incorporating the other levels of the social hierarchy. The most basic level of nursing intervention is the individual level. An exploration of this level must focus on its unique aspects without forgetting its relation-

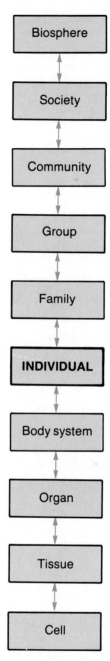

Fig. 3-2. Levels of organization that make up the social hierarchy.

ship to the whole, because "wholeness" is part of the essence of nursing.

The model that serves as the unifying perspective for this text is presented at the level of the individual in Fig. 3-3. It portrays a flow of events that result in adaptive or maladaptive coping responses, the basis for the health-illness continuum. This model also serves as the focus for the nursing process. Each element is im-

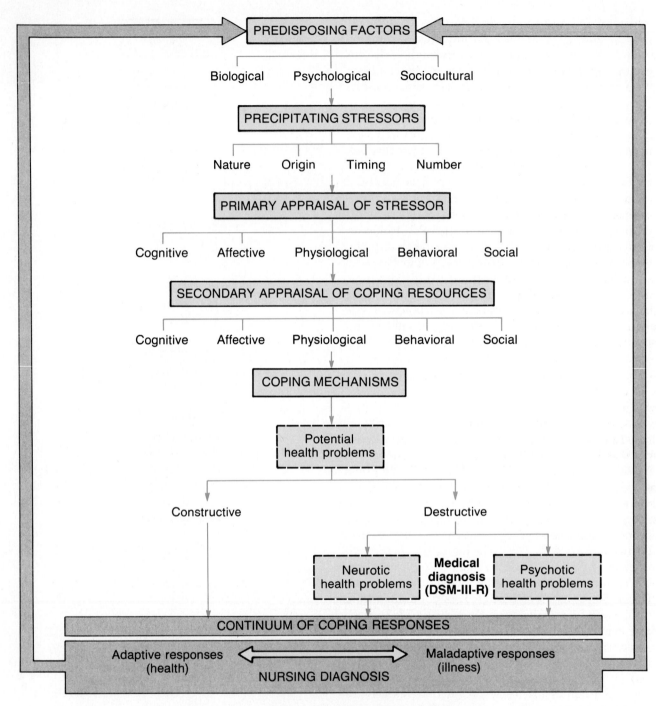

Fig. 3-3. Nursing model of health-illness phenomena.

portant, both in itself and in its relation to the larger hierarchy, and will now be discussed.

■ **Predisposing factors**

Predisposing factors are biological, psychological, and sociocultural in nature. They may be viewed as conditioning factors that influence both the type and

amount of resources the person can elicit to handle stress. Genetic background, nutritional status, biological sensitivities, general health, and exposure to toxins are examples of *biological* predispositions. *Psychological* factors include but are not limited to intelligence, verbal skills, morale, personality, past experiences, self-concept, motivation, psychological defenses, and locus of control, or a sense of mastery over one's own fate.

Sociocultural characteristics include age, education, income, occupation, social position, cultural background, religious upbringing and beliefs, political affiliation, socialization experiences, and level of social integration or relatedness. Together these factors provide a link with higher and lower levels of the hierarchy and a backdrop against which all current experiences are given meaning and value.

■ Precipitating stressors

Stressors are stimuli that the individual perceives as challenging, threatening, or demanding. They require excess energy and produce a state of tension and stress within the individual. They may be biological, psychological, or sociocultural in nature, and they may arise from the person's internal or external environment. Besides describing the *nature* and *origin* of a stressor, it is important to assess the timing of the stressor. This **timing** has many dimensions, such as when the stressor occurred, the duration of exposure to the stressor, and the frequency with which it occurs. A final factor to be considered is the **number** of stressors an individual experiences within a certain period of time, because events may be more difficult to deal with when they occur close together.

■ **STRESSFUL LIFE EVENTS.** One group of stressors that have received much attention in the health care literature are stressful life events. The relationship of stressful life events to the cause, onset, course, and outcomes of various psychiatric illnesses, such as schizophrenia, depression, and anxiety, has been the focus of much research.[34]

Holmes and Rahe[19] provided a systematic scale by measuring the correlation of major life events and physical and psychiatric illness. They developed the "Social Readjustment Rating Scale" (Table 3-3), which assigns a value to each life event on the basis of the coping behavior the event requires of the individual. As the score of the mean value increases, the likelihood of an illness is similarly hypothesized to increase.

Rahe[39] has also developed a questionnaire called the *"Schedule of Recent Experience,"* which assesses life events for the individual during specific periods. The schedule determines the degree of change in a given period by totaling the mean values of reported life events. Rahe suggests that the schedule is useful in identifying the degree and type of life change experienced.

More recent issues related to life events as stressors focus on the nature of the event and the magnitude of change it represents. There appear to be three ways of

TABLE 3-3

SOCIAL READJUSTMENT RATING SCALE

Rank	Life event	Mean value
1	Death of spouse	100
2	Divorce	73
3	Marital separation	65
4	Jail term	63
5	Death of close family member	63
6	Personal injury or illness	53
7	Marriage	50
8	Fired at work	47
9	Marital reconciliation	45
10	Retirement	45
11	Change in health of family member	44
12	Pregnancy	40
13	Sex difficulties	39
14	Gain of new family member	39
15	Business readjustment	39
16	Change in financial state	38
17	Death of close friend	37
18	Change to different line of work	36
19	Change in number of arguments with spouse	35
20	Mortgage over $10,000	31
21	Foreclosure of mortgage or loan	30
22	Change in responsibilities at work	29
23	Son or daughter leaving home	29
24	Trouble with in-laws	29
25	Outstanding personal achievement	28
26	Wife begin or stop work	26
27	Begin or end school	26
28	Change in living conditions	25
29	Revision of personal habits	24
30	Trouble with boss	23
31	Change in work hours/conditions	20
32	Change in residence	20
33	Change in schools	20
34	Change in recreation	19
35	Change in church activities	19
36	Change in social activities	18
37	Mortgage or loan less than $10,000	17
38	Change in sleeping habits	16
39	Change in number of family get-togethers	15
40	Change in eating habits	15
41	Vacation	13
42	Christmas	12
43	Minor violations of the law	11

Reprinted with permission from Holmes T and Rahe RJ: Psychosom Res 11:213, 1967, Pergamon Press, Ltd.

categorizing events reported in the literature. The first method is by social activity, which involves family, work, educational, interpersonal, health, financial, legal, or community crises. The second category includes the individual's social field. These events are defined as entrances and exits. An entrance is the introduction of a new person into the individual's social field; an exit is the departure of a significant other from the person's social field. A third way of classifying events is by relating them to social desirability. In terms of the currently shared values of American society, one group of events can be considered generally desirable, such as promotion, engagement, and marriage. In contrast, another and proportionately larger group of events can be viewed unfavorably, such as death, financial problems, being fired, and separation.

Unfortunately, conclusions about life events are far from definitive. Although they have been correlated with the onset of anxiety and disease symptoms, the methodological and theoretical aspects of research in this area have been the subject of much criticism. Intervening or mediating variables often are not taken into account in the design and execution of empirical studies. The use of unidimensional scales with questionable content validity, internal consistency, and test-retest reliability continues to be a problem. Also, the particular events in the scales may not be the most relevant to certain groups, such as students, working mothers, the elderly, or the poor.

It may be more helpful, therefore, to suggest that stressful life events act along a continuum to influence the development of psychiatric illness. On one end of the continuum, they may act as "triggers" to precipitate an illness in predisposed individuals who would have developed the illness eventually for one reason or another. At the other end of the continuum, stressful life events may have a "formative effect" in depleting one's resistance and coping resources and thus greatly advancing or bringing about psychiatric illness. Research has shown that social class and ethnic group affect the magnitude of the stress associated with various life events.[4] Also, the life-events approach provides no clues to the specific processes by which the events affect health. In retrospective studies, sources of error in measuring life events include selective memory, denial of certain events, and overreporting to justify a current illness. In prospective studies, subjective evaluation of the significance of the life event to the individual often has been neglected.

■ **LIFE STRAINS AND HASSLES.** Finally, life-events theory is built on the idea of change. However, much stress arises from chronic conditions such as boredom, continuing family tension, job dissatisfac-

tion, and loneliness. This aspect is reflected in the work of Pearlin and Schooler,[38] who wished to explore what people considered potential life strains. In their sample of 2,300 people, 18 to 65 years of age, the following four areas were delineated:

1. Marital strains
2. Parental strains associated with teenage and young adult children
3. Strains associated with household economics
4. Overloads and dissatisfactions associated with the work role

These findings suggest more long-term life dissatisfactions than major episodic events.

Research by Kanner and by Lazarus[27] indicates that small daily hassles or stresses may be more closely linked to and have a greater effect on a person's moods and health than do major misfortunes. These researchers define hassles as irritating, frustrating, or distressing incidents that occur in everyday life. Such incidents may include disagreements, disappointments, and unpleasant surprises such as losing a wallet, getting stuck in a traffic jam, or arguing with a teenage son or daughter. In Kanner and Lazarus' research, hassles turned out to be better predictors of psychological and physical health than were life events. The more frequent and intense the hassles people reported, the poorer their overall mental and physical health. Major events did have some long-term effects, and the authors suggest that these effects may be accounted for by the daily hassles they precipitate.

A certain amount of stress is necessary for survival, and degrees of it can challenge the individual to grow in new ways. However, too much stress at inappropriate times can place excessive demands on the individual and interfere with his integrated functioning. Stress does not reside within the particular life event itself or within the individual. Rather, it is in the interaction between the individual and situation. The questions that emerge therefore are "How much stress is too much?" and "What is a stressful life event?" These questions lead the person to explore the significance of the event for the individual's need-value system. The importance of the person's subjective appraisal in determining stress values has been documented and is crucially important to implementating therapy.

■ **Primary appraisal of a stressor**

Primary appraisal of a stressor refers to the processing and comprehension of the stressful situation that takes place on many levels for the individual. Specifically, it involves cognitive, affective, physiological, behavioral, and social responses. Primary appraisal is an evaluation of the significance of an event for one's well-being. The stressor assumes its meaning, intensity, and importance by the unique interpretation and affective significance assigned to it by the person at risk.

Cognitive appraisal is a critical part of this health-illness model. Lazarus[26] believes that cognitive factors play a central role in adaptation, that they affect the impact of stressful events, the choice of coping patterns used, and the emotional, physiological, and behavioral reactions. Cognitive appraisal mediates psychologically between the person and the environment in any stressful encounter. That is, the person evaluates damage or potential damage according to his understanding of the situation's power to produce harm and the resources he has available to neutralize or tolerate the harm.

Lazarus[26] describes three types of primary cognitive appraisals to stress:

1. *Harm/loss,* referring to damage that has already occurred
2. *Threat,* referring to anticipated or future harm
3. *Challenge,* in which the focus is placed positively on potential gain, growth, or mastery rather than on the possible risks

This last perception, of challenge, may play a crucial role in psychological hardiness or resistance to stress. This theory proposes that psychologically hardy individuals are less likely than nonhardy people to fall ill as a result of stressful life events. Three parts of a hardy personality have been described and researched.[21,24] First, hardy individuals are high in commitment—the ability to involve oneself in whatever one is doing. Second, hardy individuals are high in challenge—the belief that change rather than stability is to be expected in life, so that events are seen as stimulating rather than threatening. Finally, hardy individuals are high in control—the tendency to feel and believe that they influence events, rather than feeling helpless in the face of life's problems.

From this one can conclude that stress-resistant people have a specific set of attitudes toward life, an openness to change, a feeling of involvement in whatever they are doing, and a sense of control over events. Such differences in cognitive appraisal affect the person's response to events. Those who view stress as a challenge are more likely to transform events to their advantage and thus reduce their level of stress. This is in contrast to more passive, avoidance, and self-defeating tactics, in which the source of stress does not go away.

Among the most important factors affecting a person's cognitive appraisal are commitments and beliefs.[28] Commitments express what is important to the individual, and they underlie the choices a person makes. Commitments can thus guide people into or away from situations that threaten, harm, or potentially benefit. Beliefs also determine how a person evaluates events. Personal control and existential beliefs are particularly relevant to stress reduction, since they influence the person's emotional response and potential coping ability.

An **affective** response is the arousal of a feeling state. In the primary appraisal of a stressor, the predominant affective response is a nonspecific or generalized anxiety reaction. Consistent with this is the **physiological** response associated with the "fight-or-flight" response. This response stimulates the sympathetic division of the autonomic nervous system and increases activity of the pituitary-adrenal axis. The **behavioral** response is focused on the impact of the stressor. A range of behaviors may be evident, depending on the level of anxiety and physiological changes. These behaviors usually are reactive, rather than goal-directed at this time. Chapters 11 and 12 explore these responses in greater depth.

Finally, Mechanic[33] describes three aspects of a person's **social** response to stress and illness. The first aspect is the search for meaning, in which individuals seek information about their problem. This is a prerequisite for devising a coping strategy, because only through some formulation of what is occurring can a reasonable response be devised.

The second aspect of social response is social attribution, in which the person tries to identify the unique factors that contributed to the situation. Patients who view their problem as resulting from their own negligence may be blocked from an active coping response. They may view their problems as a sign of their personal failure and engage in self-blame and passive, withdrawn behavior. Thus the way cause is viewed by both patients and health professionals can greatly affect successful coping.

The third aspect of social response is social comparison, in which the individual compares his own skills and capacities with those of others with similar problems. How a person assesses himself depends very much on those around him with whom comparisons are made. In many situations feelings and self-esteem may depend as much on this comparison process as on objective coping capacities. The outcome is an evaluation of the need for support from the person's social network or social support system. Both the person's predisposing factors such as age, developmental level, and cultural background, and the characteristics of the precipitating stressor determine his perceived need for social support.

In summary, the way a person appraises an event is the psychological key to understanding his coping efforts and the nature and intensity of his stress response. Unfortunately, many nurses and other health professionals ignore this fact when they presume to know how certain stressors will affect an individual and thus render "routine" care. Not only does this depersonalize the individual, it also undermines the basis of nursing care. The patient's appraisal of life stressors with its cognitive, affective, physiological, behavioral, and social components must be an essential part of the nurse's assessment.

■ Secondary appraisal of coping resources

Secondary appraisal is the person's evaluation of his own coping resources, options, or strategies. It is a crucial feature of every stressful encounter, because the outcome depends on what, if anything, can be done, as well as what is at stake. Primary and secondary appraisals probably are not separate processes but often are integrated into the same overall evaluation.

■ **TYPES OF COPING RESOURCES.** Mechanic[33] identifies five coping resources that help individuals adapt to the stress of illness. These coping resources are economic assets, individual abilities and skills, defensive techniques, social supports, and motivational impetus. They incorporate all levels of the social hierarchy represented in Fig. 3-2. Interrelationships between the individual, family group, and society assume critical importance at this point of the model.

Lazarus and Folkman add to these the resources of health and energy, positive beliefs, problem-solving and social skills, and social and material resources.[28] The role played by physical well-being is well documented in the literature. Similarly, viewing oneself positively can serve as a basis of hope and can sustain a person's coping efforts under the most adverse of circumstances. Problem-solving skills include the ability to search for information, identify the problem, weigh alternatives, and implement a plan of action. Social skills facilitate the solving of problems involving other people, increase the likelihood of enlisting cooperation and support from others, and in general give the individual greater social control. Finally, material resources refer to money and the goods and services that money can buy. Obviously, monetary resources greatly increase a person's coping options in almost any stressful situation.

Much research is being done on these coping resources. Antonovsky is examining what he calls "generalized resistance resources"—characteristics of the person, group, or environment that can encourage more adaptive responses.[3] He believes that knowledge and intelligence offer such a resource, since they allow people to see different ways of dealing with their stress. Other resources he identifies are a strong ego identity, commitment to a social network, cultural stability, a stable system of values and beliefs derived from one's philosophy or religion, a preventive health orientation and genetic or constitutional strengths. Thus empirical research lends support to the relationship between predisposing factors and coping resources within a strong social community.

Like primary appraisal, secondary appraisal of coping resources involves cognitive, affective, physiological, behavioral, and social responses. A person's **cognitive** appraisal at this time concentrates on the availability and effectiveness of coping strategies. But secondary appraisal is more than a mere intellectual exercise in analyzing all the things that might be done. Rather, it is a complex process that takes into account which coping options are available, the likelihood that a given option will accomplish what it is supposed to, and the likelihood that the person can apply a particular strategy effectively.

Affectively, the general anxiety response becomes expressed as emotions. These may include joy, sadness, fear, anger, acceptance, distrust, anticipation, or surprise. Emotions may be further classified according to type, duration, and intensity—characteristics that change over time and events. For example, when an emotion is prolonged over time, it can be classified as a mood; when prolonged over a longer time, it can be considered an attitude.

Physiological responses reflect the interaction of several neuroendocrine axes involving growth hormone, prolactin, adrenocorticotropic hormone (ACTH), luteinizing and follicle-stimulating hormones, thyroid-stimulating hormone, vasopressin, oxytocin, epinephrine, norepinephrine, and insulin.

Behavioral responses reflect emotions and physiological changes as well as cognitive analysis of the stressful situation. Caplan[7] described four interdigitating phases or facets of an individual's responses to a stressful event.

■ Phase 1 is behavior that changes the stressful environment or enables the individual to escape from it.

■ Phase 2 is behavior to acquire new capabilities for action to change the external circumstances and their aftermath.

■ Phase 3 is intrapsychic behavior to defend against unpleasant emotional arousal.

■ Phase 4 is intrapsychic behavior to come to terms with the event and its sequelae by internal readjustment.

Conceptualizing the individual's response in terms of these phases may be helpful to the nurse.

A person's **social** response is that of evaluating the social support available. Numerous studies have documented increased rates of psychiatric disorder and of general medical morbidity and mortality among people who are socially isolated. So, too, research in the fields of medical sociology, epidemiology, organizational and social psychology, and experimental stress reveals that members of the social environment whom a stressed individual perceives as "significant others" help to protect or restore good health.

■ **SOCIAL SUPPORT SYSTEMS.** Social support for the individual begins in utero and is communicated in a variety of ways to the newborn baby, including in the way he is held, fed, and comforted. As life progresses, support is increasingly derived from other members of the family, then from peers at school, work, and in the community. At times of great need, support may be provided by nurses or other health professionals. Although social support systems or social networks are commonly understood terms, they reflect complex dimensions. It is not surprising, therefore, that social support is defined differently by various researchers and practitioners. These definitions indicate that different types of support may be provided by social support systems. Some of the functions of social networks that have been identified are shown in Table 3-4. Although phrased differently by each theorist, five common functions of social networks may be described as:

1. Emotional support
2. Task-oriented help
3. Feedback and evaluation

4. Social relatedness and integration
5. Access to new information

The value of social networks in providing emotional support has long been recognized. Some believe it is the primary function and equate support with love, affection, and nurturance. Although not minimizing this contribution of social support, Caplan[6] believes that the most important contribution is in the cognitive and educational areas and in helping the person with concrete tasks. Caplan states that a supportive group of family, friends, or community members helps the individual deal with his environment:

This group or network adds to his information; helps him improve his own data collection; aids him in evaluating the situation and working out a sensible plan; and assists him in implementing his plan, assessing its consequences, and replanning in line with the feedback information. It reminds him of his continuing identity and bolsters his positive feelings about himself; assures him that his discomforts are expectable and, although burdensome, can usually be tolerated; and maintains his hope in some form of successful outcome of his efforts, which is a prerequisite to his continuing them.

In effect, a supportive social network complements and supplements those specific aspects of the individual's functioning that are weakened by the effect of the stressful experience.[6:415]

Although the relative importance of social support may be subject to some variation, there is strong agreement with Caplan on its effect. It is particularly relevant in two areas: help seeking and psychological adaptation. Gourash[17] outlined the four ways that social networks influence help seeking:

1. Buffering the experience of stress that creates the need for help
2. Precluding the necessity for professional assistance through instrumental and emotional support

TABLE 3-4

FUNCTIONS OF SOCIAL SUPPORT SYSTEMS

Caplan[6]	House[20]	Walker et al[44]	Weiss[45]
Task-oriented assistance Communication of evaluation and expectation Sense of belonging	Emotional support Instrumental support Appraisal support Informational support	Emotional support Material aid and services Maintenance of social identity Access to new social contacts Diverse information	Attachment Exchange of services Guidance; social integration Sense of alliance; reassurance of worth Opportunity to provide nurturance

3. Acting as screening and referral agents to professional services
4. Transmitting attitudes, values, and norms about help seeking

These findings have implications for primary, secondary, and tertiary prevention.

The large number of studies that address psychological adaptation prevents discussion of each one here. However, five important review articles outline the historical context and scope of research in this area. In 1974, Cassel[8] explored the topic from an epidemiological perspective and concluded that social support was an important environmental factor affecting human resistance to disease. In 1976, Cobb[9] reviewed social support around the crises of the life cycle, including pregnancy and childhood, hospitalization, recovery from illness, extensive life changes, employment termination, bereavement, aging and retirement, and the threat of death. He suggests that social support functions as a moderating variable that facilitates coping with crises. Kaplan, Cassel, and Gore's[23] review in 1977 emphasized the importance of social support as protective of health but only in conjunction with certain circumstances that they believe need to be better conceptualized and researched. In 1980, Mueller[36] presented a comprehensive review of the literature on social support and psychiatric disorders. Finally, in 1982, Greenblatt and coworkers[18] reviewed the patterns of social networks that maintain health, explored the relationship between social networks and the outcome of treatment for mental illness, and described clinical network interventions that have facilitated patient care and maximized performance of former patients in the community.

What one can conclude from all these studies is that links do exist between social support and adaptive coping responses. However, a precise definition of social support, its determinants or conditions, its measurement, the nature of the support process, and the existence of a causal relationship between lack of social support and maladaptation have yet to be established in theoretical or empirical work.

■ **Coping mechanisms**

It is at this point in the nursing model of the health-illness phenomena that coping mechanisms and potential health problems emerge. Thus this is an important juncture for nursing activities directed toward primary prevention. Coping mechanisms can be defined as any efforts directed at stress management. There are three main types of coping mechanisms. The first type is a **problem-focused** coping mechanism; it

involves tasks and direct efforts to cope with the threat itself. Examples of this type include negotiation, confrontation, and seeking advice. In the second type, **cognitively-focused** coping mechanisms, the person attempts to control the meaning of the problem and thus neutralize it. Examples here include positive comparisons, selective ignorance, substitution of rewards, and the devaluation of desired objects. The third type of coping mechanism is **emotion-focused**; with this type the patient can be intrapsychic or oriented to moderating his emotional distress. Examples of this include the use of ego defense mechanisms such as denial, suppression, or projection. A more detailed discussion of coping and defense mechanisms appears in Chapter 11.

Coping mechanisms may also be constructive or destructive. They can be considered **constructive** when anxiety is treated as a warning signal and the individual accepts it as a challenge to resolve the problem. In this respect anxiety can be compared to a fever—both serve as warnings that the system is under attack. Once employed successfully, constructive coping mechanisms modify the way past experiences are used to meet future threats. **Destructive** coping mechanisms ward off anxiety without resolving the conflict, using evasion instead of resolution.

■ **MEDICAL DIAGNOSES.** Destructive coping mechanisms often are subject to medical evaluation and diagnosis. The medical diagnosis of a psychiatric health problem can be broadly differentiated as neurotic or psychotic. In the DSM-III-R, **neurotic disorders** are distinguished by the following characteristics[2]:

1. A symptom or group of symptoms is distressing and is recognized as unacceptable and alien to the individual.
2. Reality testing is grossly intact.
3. Behavior does not actively violate gross social norms (although functioning may be significantly impaired).
4. The disturbance is relatively enduring or recurrent without treatment and is not limited to a transitory reaction to stressors.
5. No demonstrable organic cause or factor is present.

In situations of severest conflict, however, the person may be powerless to cope with the threat by such patterns and may distort reality, as in **psychosis.** Psychosis consists of the following characteristics[2]:

1. A severe mood disorder
2. Regressive behavior

3. Personality disintegration
4. A significant reduction in level of awareness
5. Great difficulty in functioning adequately
6. Gross impairment in reality testing

This last characteristic is critical. When there is gross impairment in reality testing, the individual incorrectly evaluates the accuracy of his perceptions and draws incorrect inferences about external reality, even in the face of contrary evidence. According to the DSM-III-R, direct evidence of psychosis is the presence of either delusions or hallucinations without insight into their pathological nature. Psychotic health problems reflect the most severe level of illness and maladaptive coping responses.

Medical diagnoses are classified according to the *Diagnostic and Statistical Manual of Mental Disorders,* *3rd edition, Revised* of the American Psychiatric Association. The various illnesses are accompanied by a description of diagnostic criteria, tested for reliability by psychiatric practitioners. DSM-III-R uses a multiaxial system that gives attention to certain disorders, aspects of the environment, and areas of functioning that might be overlooked if the focus is exclusively on the presenting problem. The individual thus is evaluated on the following axes:

Axis I	Clinical syndromes and V Codes
Axis II	Developmental disorders and personality disorders
Axis III	Physical disorders and conditions
Axis IV	Severity of psychosocial stressors
Axis V	Global assessment of functioning

DSM-III-R Classification: Axes I and II Categories and Codes

All official DSM-III-R codes are included in ICD-9-CM. Codes followed by a * are used for more than one DSM-III-R diagnosis or subtype in order to maintain compatibility with ICD-9-CM. A long dash following a diagnostic term indicates the need for a fifth digit subtype or other qualifying term. The term *specify* following the name of some diagnostic categories indicates qualifying terms that clinicians may wish to add in parentheses after the name of the disorder. NOS means Not Otherwise Specified.

The current severity of a disorder may be specified after the diagnosis as:

Mild
Moderate — Currently meets diagnostic criteria
Severe

In partial remission (or residual state)
In complete remission

Disorders Usually First Evident in Infancy, Childhood, or Adolescence

Developmental Disorders

Note: These are coded on Axis II.

Mental Retardation

317.00	Mild mental retardation
318.00	Moderate mental retardation
318.10	Severe mental retardation
318.20	Profound mental retardation
319.00	Unspecified mental retardation

Pervasive Developmental Disorders

299.00	Autistic disorder
	Specify if childhood onset
299.80	Pervasive developmental disorder NOS

Specific Developmental Disorders

	Academic skills disorders
315.10	Developmental arithmetic disorder
315.80	Developmental expressive writing disorder
315.00	Developmental reading disorder

Language and speech disorders

315.39	Developmental articulation disorder
315.31*	Developmental expressive language disorder
315.31*	Devleopmental receptive language disorder
	Motor skills disorder
315.40	Developmental coordination disorder
315.90*	Specific developmental disorder NOS

Other Developmental Disorders

315.90*	Developmental disorder NOS

Continued.

DSM-III-R Classification: Axes I and II Categories and Codes—cont'd

Disruptive Behavior Disorders

314.01	Attention-deficit hyperactivity disorder
	Conduct disorder,
312.20	group type
312.00	solitary aggressive type
312.90	undifferentiated type
313.81	Oppositional defiant disorder

Anxiety Disorders of Childhood or Adolescence

309.21	Separation anxiety disorder
313.21	Avoidant disorder of childhood or adolescence
313.00	Overanxious disorder

Eating Disorders

307.10	Anorexia nervosa
307.51	Bulimia nervosa
307.52	Pica
307.53	Rumination disorder of infancy
307.50	Eating disorder NOS

Gender Identity Disorders

302.60	Gender identity disorder of childhood
302.50	Transsexualism
	Specify sexual history: asexual, homosexual, heterosexual, unspecified
302.85*	Gender identity disorder of adolescence or adulthood, nontranssexual type
	Specify sexual history: asexual, homosexual, heterosexual, unspecified
302.85*	Gender identity disorder NOS

Tic Disorders

307.23	Tourett's disorder
307.22	Chronic motor or vocal tic disorder
307.21	Transient tic disorder
	Specify: single episode or recurrent
307.20	Tic disorder NOS

Elimination Disorders

307.70	Functional encopresis
	Specify: primary or secondary type
307.60	Functional enuresis
	Specify: primary or secondary type
	Specify: nocturnal only, diurnal only, nocturnal and diurnal

Speech Disorders Not Elsewhere Classified

307.00*	Cluttering
307.00*	Stuttering

Other Disorders of Infancy, Childhood, or Adolesence

313.23	Elective mutism
313.82	Identity disorder
313.89	Reactive attachment disorder of infancy or early childhood
307.30	Stereotypy/habit disorder
314.00	Undifferentiated attention-deficit disorder

Organic Mental Disorders

Dementias Arising in the Senium and Presenium

	Primary degenerative dementia of the Alzheimer type, senile onset,
290.30	with delirium
290.20	with delusions
290.21	with depression
290.00*	uncomplicated
	(Note: code 331.00 Alzheimer's disease on Axis III)

Code in fifth digit:

	1 = with delirium, 2 = with delusions, 3 = with depression, 0* = uncomplicated
290.1x	Primary degenerative dementia of the Alzheimer type, presenile onset, _____
	(Note: code 331.00 Alzheimer's disease on Axis III)
290/4x	Multi-infarct dementia, _____
290.00*	Senile dementia NOS
	Specify etiology on Axis III if known
290.10*	Presenile dementia NOS
	Specify etiology on Axis III if known (e.g., Pick's disease, Jakob-Creutzfeldt disease)

Psychoactive Substance-Induced Organic Mental disorders

	Alcohol
303.00	intoxication
291.40	idiosyncratic intoxication
291.80	Uncomplicated alcohol withdrawal
291.00	withdrawal delirium
291.30	hallucinosis
291.10	amnestic disorder
291.20	Dementia associated with alcoholism
	Amphetamine or similarly acting sympathomimetic
305.70*	intoxication
292.00*	withdrawal

DSM-III-R Classification: Axes I and II Categories and Codes—cont'd

292.81*	delirium
292.11*	delusional disorder
	Caffeine
305.90	intoxication
	Cannabis
305.20*	intoxication
292.11*	delusional disorder
	Cocaine
305.60*	intoxication
292.00*	withdrawal
292.81*	delirium
292.11*	delusional disorder
	Hallucinogen
305.30*	hallucinosis
292.11*	delusional disorder
292.84*	mood disorder
292.89*	Posthallucinogen perception disorder
	Inhalant
305.90*	intoxication
	Nicotine
292.00*	withdrawal
	Opioid
305.50*	intoxication
292.00*	withdrawal
	Phencyclidine (PCP) or similarly acting arylcyclohexylamine
305.90*	intoxication
292.81*	delirium
292.11*	mood disorder
292.84*	organic mental disorder NOS
	Sedative, hypnotic, or aniolytic
305.40*	intoxication
292.00*	Uncomplicated sedative, hypnotic, or anxiolytic withdrawal withdrawal delirium
292.83*	amnestic disorder
	Other or unspecified psychoactive substance
305.90*	intoxication
292.00*	withdrawal
292.81*	delirium
292.82*	dementia
292.83*	amnestic disorder
292.11*	delusional disorder
292.12	hallucinosis
292.84*	mood disorder
292.89*	anxiety disorder
292.89*	personality disorder
292.90	organic mental disorder NOS

Organic Mental Disorders associated with Axis III physical disorders or condition, or whose etiology is unknown.

293.00	Delirium
294.10	Dementia
294.00	Amnestic disorder
293.81	Organic delusional disorder
293.82	Organic hallucinosis
293.83	Organic mood disorder
	Specify: manic, depressed, mixed
294.80*	Organic anxiety disorder
310.10	Organic personality disorder
	Specify if explosive type
294.80*	Organic mental disorder NOS

Psychoactive Substance Use disorders

	Alcohol
303.90	dependence
305.00	abuse
	Amphetamine or similarly acting sympathomimetic
304.40	dependence
305.70*	abuse
	Cannabis
304.30	dependence
305.20*	abuse
	Cocaine
304.20	dependence
305.60*	abuse
	Hallucinogen
304.50*	dependence
305.30*	abuse
	Inhalant
304.60	dependence
305.90*	abuse
	Nicotine
305.10	dependence
	Opioid
304.00	dependence
305.50*	abuse
	Phencyclidine (PCP) or similarly acting arylcyclohexylamine
304.50*	dependence
305.90*	abuse
	Sedative, hypnotic, or anxiolytic
304.10	dependence
305.40*	abuse
304.90*	Polysubstance dependence
304.90*	Psychoactive substance dependence NOS
305.90*	Psychoactive substance abuse NOS

Continued.

DSM-III-R Classification: Axes I and II Categories and Codes—cont'd

Schizophrenia

Code in fifth digit: 1 = subchronic, 2 = chronic, 3 = subchronic with acute exacerbation, 4 = chronic with acute exacerbation, 5 = in remission, 0 = unspecified.

	Schizophrinia,
295.2x	catatonic, _____
295.1x	disorganized, _____
295.3x	paranoid, _____
	Specify if stable type
295.9x	undifferentiated, _____
295.6x	residual, _____
	Specify if late onset

Delusional (Paranoid) Disorder

297.10	Delusional (Paranoid) disorder
	Specify type: erotomanic
	grandiose
	jealous
	persecutory
	somatic
	unspecified

Psychotic Disorders Not Elsewhere Classified

298.80	Brief reactive psychosis
295.40	Schizophreniform disorder
	Specify: without good prognostic features or with good prognostic features
295.70	Schizoaffective disorder
	Specify: bipolar type or depressive type
297.30	Induced psychotic disorder
298.90	Psychotic disorder NOS (Atypical psychosis

Mood Disorders

Code current state of Major Depression and Bipolar Disorder in fifth digit:

1 = mild
2 = moderate
3 = severe, without psychotic features
4 = with psychotic features (*specify* mood-congruent or mood-incongruent)
5 = in partial remission
6 = in full remission
0 = unspecified

For major depressive episodes, *specify* if chronic and *specify* if melancholic type.

For Bipolar Disorder, Bipolar Disorder NOS, Recurrent Major Depression, and Depressive Disorder NOS, *specify* if seasonal pattern.

Bipolar Disorders

	Bipolar disorder
296.6x	mixed, _____
296.4x	manic, _____
296.5x	depressed, _____
301.13	Cyclothymia
296.70	Bipolar disorder NOS

Depressive Disorders

	Major Depression,
296.2x	single episode, _____
296.3x	recurrent, _____
300.40	Dysthymia (or Depressive neurosis)
	Specify: primary or secondary type
	Specify: early or late onset
311.00	Depressive disorder NOS

Anxiety Disorders (or Anxiety and Phobic Neuroses

Panic disorder

300.21	with agoraphobia
	Specify current severity of agoraphobic avoidance
	Specify current severity of panic attacks
300.01	without agoraphobia
	Specify current severity of panic attacks
300.22	Agoraphobia without history of panic disorder
	Specify with or without limited symptom attacks
300.23	Social phobia
	Specify if generalized type
300.29	Simple phobia
300.30	Obsessive compulsive disorder (or Obsessive compulsive neurosis)
309.89	Post-traumatic stress disorder
	Specify if delayed onset
300.02	Generalized anxiety disorder
300.00	Anxiety disorder NOS

DSM-III-R Classification: Axes I and II Categories and Codes—cont'd

Somatoform Disorders

300.70*   Body dysmorphic disorder
300.11   Conversion disorder (or Hysterical neurosis, conversion type)
          Specify: single episode or recurrent
300.70*   Hypochondriasis (or Hypochondriacal neurosis)
300.81   Somatization disorder

Dissociative Dosorders

292.00*
307.80   Somatoform pain disorder
300.70*   Undifferentiated somatoform disorder
300.70*   Somatoform disorder NOS

(or Hysterical Neuroses, Dissociative Type)

300.14   Multiple personality disorder
300.13   Psychogenic fugue
300.12   Psychogenic amnesia
300.60   Depersonalization disorder (or Depersonalization neurosis)
300.15   Dissociative disorder NOS

Sexual Disorders

Paraphilias

302.40   Exhibitionism
302.81   Fetishism
302.89   Frotteurism
302.20   Pedophilia
          Specify: same sex, opposite sex, same and opposite sex
          Specify if limited to incest
          Specify: exclusive type or nonexclusive type
302.83   Sexual masochism
302.84   Sexual sadism
302.30   Transvestic fetishism
302.82   Voyeurism
302.90*   Paraphilia NOS

Sexual Dysfunctions

Specify: psychogenic only, or psychogenic and biogenic (Note: If biogenic only, code on Axis III)
Specify: lifelong or acquired
Specify: generalized or situational
          Sexual desire disorders
302.71   Hypoacive sexual desire disorder
302.79   Sexual aversion disorder

          Sexual arousal disorders
302.72*   Female sexual arousal disorder
302.72*   Male erectile disorder
          Orgasm disorders
302.73   Inhibited female orgasm
302.74   Inhibited male orgasm
302.75   Premature ejaculation
          Sexual pain disorders
302.76   Dyspareunia
306.51   Vaginismus
302.70   Sexual dysfunction NOS

Other Sexual Disorders

302.90*   Sexual disorder NOS

Sleep Disorders

Dyssomnias

          Insomnia disorder
307.42*   related to another mental disorder (nonorganic)
780.50*   related to known organic factor
307.42*   Primary insomnia
          Hypersomnia disorder
307.44   related to another mental disorder (nonorganic)
780.50*   related to a known organic factor
780.54   Primary hypersomnia
307.45   Sleep-wake schedule disorder
          Specify: advanced or delayed phase type, disorganized type, frequently changing type
          Other dyssomnias
307.40*   Dyssomnia NOS

Parasomnias

307.47   Dream anxiety disorder (Nightmare disorder)
307.46*   Sleep terror disorder
307.46*   Sleepwalking disorder
307.40*   Parasomnia NOS

Factitious Disorders

          Factitious disorder
301.51   with physical symptoms
300.16   with psychological symptoms
300.19   Factitious disorder NOS

Continued.

DSM-III-R Classification: Axes I and II Categories and Codes—cont'd

Impulse Control Disorders Not Elsewhere Classified

312.34	Intermittent explosive disorder
312.32	Kleptomania
312.31	Pathological gambling
312.33	Pyromania
312.39*	Trichotillomania
312.39*	Impulse control disorder NOS

Adjustment Disorder

	Adjustment disorder
309.24	with anxious mood
309.00	with depressed mood
309.30	with disturbance of conduct
309.40	with mixed disturbance of emotions and conduct
309.28	with mixed emotional features
309.82	with physical complaints
309.83	with withdrawal
309.23	with work (or academic) inhibition
309.90	Ajustment disorder NOS

Psychological Factors Affecting Physical Condition

316.00	Psychological factors affecting physical condition
	Specify physical condition on Axis III

Personality disorders

Note: These are coded on Axis II.

Cluster A

301.00	Paranoid
301.20	Schizoid
301.22	Schizotypal

Cluster B

301.70	Antisocial
301.83	Borderline

301.50	Histrionic
301.81	Narcissistic

Cluster C

301.82	Avoidant
301.60	Dependent
301.40	Obsessive compulsive
301.84	Passive aggressive
301.90	Personality disorder NOS

V Codes for Conditions Not Attributable to a Mental Disorder that are a Focus of Attention or Treatment

V62.30	Academic problem
V71.01	Adult antisocial behavior
V40.00	Borderline intellectual functioning (Note: this is coded on Axis II.)
V71.02	Childhood or adolescent antisocial behavior
V65.20	Malingering
V61.10	Marital problem
V15.81	Noncompliance with medical treatment
V62.20	Occupational problem
V61.20	Parent-child problem
V62.81	Other interpersonal problem
V61.80	Other specified family circumstances
V62.89	Phase of life problem or other life circumstance problem
V62.82	Uncomplicated bereavement

Additional Codes

300.90	Unspecified mental disorder (nonpsychotic)
V71.09*	No diagnosis or condition on Axis I
799.90*	Diagnosis or condition deferred on Axis I
V71.09*	No diagnosis or condition on Axis II
799.90*	Diagnosis or condition deferred on Axis II

Axes I and II constitute the entire classification of mental disorders plus V codes (conditions not attributable to a mental disorder that are a focus of attention or treatment). These are listed on pp. 79-84. The disorders listed on axis II, developmental disorders and personality disorders, generally have an onset in childhood or adolescence and usually persist in a stable form into adulthood. Axis III allows the clinician to identify any physical disorder potentially relevant to the understanding or treatment of the individual. These three axes make up the diagnosis to be documented for any patient receiving psychiatric care.

Specialized clinical settings or individuals conducting psychiatric research may choose to include axes IV and V as well. Axis IV documents the severity of psychosocial stressors on a scale of 1 to 7 (Table 3-5).

TABLE 3-5

SEVERITY OF PSYCHOSOCIAL STRESSORS SCALES (Axis IV)

Code	Term	Examples of stressors Acute events	Enduring circumstances
Adults			
1	**None**	No acute events that may be relevant ot the disorder	No enduring circumstances that may be relevant to the disorder
2	**Mild**	Broke up with boyfriend or girlfriend; started or graduated from school; child left home	Family arguments; job dissatisfaction; residence in high-crime neighborhood
3	**Moderate**	Marriage; marital separation; loss of job; retirement; miscarriage	Marital discord; serious financial problems; trouble with boss; being a single parent
4	**Severe**	Divorce; birth of first child	Unemployment; poverty
5	**Extreme**	Death of spouse; serious physical illness diagnosed; victim of rape	Serious chronic illness in self or child; ongoing physical or sexual abuse
6	**Catastrophic**	Death of child; suicide of spouse; devasting natural disaster	Captivity as hostage; concentration camp experience
0	**Inadequate information, or no change in condition.**		
Children and Adolescents			
1	**None**	No acute events that may be relevant to the disorder	No enduring circumstances that may be relevant to the disorder
2	**Mild**	Broke up with boyfriend or girlfriend; change of school	Overcrowded living quarters; family arguments
3	**Moderate**	Expelled from school; birth of sibling	Chronic disabling illness in parent; chronic parental discord
4	**Severe**	Divorce of parents; unwanted pregnancy; arrest	Harsh or rejecting parents; chronic life-threatening illness in parent; multiple foster home placements
5	**Extreme**	Sexual or physical abuse; death of a parent	Recurrent sexual or physical abuse
6	**Catastrophic**	Death of both parents	Chronic life-threatening illness
0	**Inadequate information, or no change in condition**		

Axis V allows the clinician to rate an individual's psychological, social, and occupational functioning on a continuum of mental health-illness. Ratings are made on a 9-point global assessment of functioning scale (see box on p. 86) for both current functioning and the highest level of functioning during the past year. Psychiatric nurses use all five axes of the DSM-III-R and integrate the axes with related nursing diagnoses.

■ Continuum of health-illness coping responses

An individual's response to stressors is based on specific conditioning factors, the quality of the stressor, his perception of the situation, and his analysis of resources and needs. His responses can be placed on a coping continuum of health and illness.

A nurse can evaluate health by measuring an indi-

Global Assessment of Functioning Scale (Axis V)

Consider psychological, social, and occupational functioning on a hypothetical continuum of mental health-illness. Do not include impairment in functioning due to physical (or environmental) limitations.

Code

90-81   Absent or minimal symptoms (e.g., mild anxiety before an exam), good functioning in all areas, interested and involved in a wide range of activities, socially effective, generally satisfied with life, no more than everyday problems or concerns (e.g., an occasional argument with family members).

80-71   If symptoms are present, they are transient and expectable reactions to psychosocial stressors (e.g., difficulty concentrating after family argument); no more than slight impairment in social, occupational, or school functioning (e.g., temporarily falling behind in school work).

70-61   Some mild symptoms (e.g., depressed mood and mild insomnia) or some difficulty in social, occupational, or school functioning (e.g., occasional truancy, or theft within the household), but generally functioning pretty well, has some meaningful interpersonal relationships.

60-51   Moderate symptoms (e.g., flat affect and circumstantial speech, occasional panic attacks) or moderate difficulty in social, occupational, or school functioning (e.g., few friends, conflicts with co-workers).

50-41   Serious symptoms (e.g., suicidal ideation, severe obsessional rituals, frequent shoplifting) or any serious impairment in social, occupational, or school functioning (e.g., few friends, unable to keep a job).

40-31   Some impairment in reality testing or communication (e.g., speech is at times illogical, obscure, or irrelevant) or major impairment in several areas, such as work or school, family relations, judgment, thinking, or mood (e.g., depressed man avoids friends, neglects family, and is unable to work; child frequently beats up younger children, is defiant at home, and is failing at school).

30-21   Behavior is considerably influenced by delusions or hallucinations or serious impairment in communication or judgment (e.g., sometimes incoherent, acts grossly inappropriately, suicidal preoccupation) or inability to function in almost all areas (e.g., stays in bed all day; no job, home, or friends).

20-11   Some danger of hurting self or others (e.g., suicide attempts without clear expectation of death, frequently violent, manic excitement) or occasionally fails to maintain minimal personal hygiene (e.g., smears feces) or gross impairment in communication (e.g., largely incoherent or mute).

10-1   Persistent danger of severely hurting self or others (e.g., recurrent violence) or persistent inability to maintain minimal personal hygiene or serious suicidal act with clear expectation of death.

vidual's potential and liability in three areas: (1) functional status (tasks and responsibilities of daily living), (2) psychological status (intellectual and emotional realms), and (3) clinical status (physical components). Functional status is the ability to carry out daily tasks and to fulfill the challenges of social roles. Psychological status includes the person's sense of well-being, mental and emotional state, perception of the quality of life, and integration of strengths and resources toward maximizing personal potential. Clinical status incorporates the physical dimensions of health, including risk factors such as cigarette smoking and pathological or disease processes. By assessing the patient's status in all three areas, the nurse can provide a holistic approach to the patient and better evaluate his coping responses. Responses that support integrated functioning are viewed as adaptive or healthy; they lead to growth, learning, and goal achievement. Responses that block integrated functioning are viewed as maladaptive or unhealthy; they take the form of impaired thought processes, alterations in the expression of emotions, physiological illness, inappropriate behavior, or problems in socialization.

■ **NURSING DIAGNOSES.** Responses to stress, whether actual or potential, are the subject of nursing diagnoses. A nursing diagnosis is a clinical judgment about individual, family, or community responses to stress. These problems may be overt, covert, existing, or potential, and the assessment should include both the behavioral disruption or threatened disruption and the contributing stressors. Like the diagnosis, treatment of these disruptions is a nursing function for which the nurse is accountable.

The accompanying box lists the nursing diagnoses

Alphabetical List of NANDA-Accepted Diagnoses

Activity intolerance
Activity intolerance, potential
Adjustment, impaired
Airway clearance, ineffective
Anxiety
Aspiration, potential for
Body image disturbance
Body temperature, altered, potential
Breastfeeding, effective
Breastfeeding, ineffective
Breathing pattern, ineffective
Cardiac output, decreased
Communication, impaired verbal
Constipation
Constipation, colonic
Constipation, perceived
Coping, defensive
Coping, family: potential for growth
Coping, ineffective family: compromised
Coping, ineffective family: disabling
Coping, ineffective individual
Decisional conflict (specify)
Denial, ineffective
Diarrhea
Disuse syndrome, potential for
Diversional acitivity deficit
Dysreflexia
Family processes, altered
Fatique
Fear
Fluid volume deficit (1)
Fluid volume deficit (2)
Fluid volume deficit, potential
Fluid volume excess
Gas exchange, impaired
Grieving, anticipatory
Grieving, dysfunctional
Growth and development, altered
Health maintenance, altered
Health seeking behaviors (specify)
Home maintenance management, impaired
Hopelessness
Hyperthermia
Hypothermia
Incontinence, bowel
Incontinence, functional
Incontinence, relfex
Incontinence, stress
Incontinence, total
Incontinence, urge
Infection, potential for
Injury, potential for

Knowledge deficit (specify)
Mobility, impaired physical
Noncompliance (specify)
Nutrition, altered: less than body requirements
Nutriton, altered: more than body requirements
Nutrition, altered: potential for more than body requirements
Oral mucous membrane, altered
Pain
Pain, chronic
Parental role conflict
Parenting, altered
Parenting, altered, potential
Personal identity disturbance
Poisoning, potential for
Post-trauma response
Powerlessness
Protection, altered
Rape-trauma syndrome
Rape-trauma syndrome: compound reaction
Rape-trauma syndrome: silent reaction
Role performance, altered
Self care deficit, bathing/hygiene
Self care deficit, dressing/grooming
Self care deficit, feeding
Self care deficit, toileting
Self-esteem disturbance
Self-esteem, chronic low
Self-esteem, situational low
Sensory/perceptual alterations (specify) (visual, auditory, kinesthetic, gustatory, tactile, olfactory)
Sexual dysfunction
Sexuality patterns, altered
Skin integrity, impaired
Skin integrity, impaired, potential
Sleep pattern disturbance
Social interaction, impaired
Social isolation
Spiritual distress (distress of the human spirit)
Suffocation, potential for
Swallowing, impaired
Thermoregulation, ineffective
Thought processes, altered
Tissue integrity, impaired
Tissue perfusion, altered (specify type) (renal, cerebral, cardiopulmonary, gastrointestinal, peripheral)
Trauma, potential for
Unilateral neglect
Urinary elimination, altered patterns
Urinary retention
Violence, potential for: self-directed or directed at others

From the Proceedings of the Ninth National Conference of the North American Nursing Diagnosis Association, March 1990 identified through the Ninth National Conference of the North American Nursing Diagnosis Association (NANDA). In addition, a task force of the Council on Psychiatric and Mental Health Nursing of the American Nurses' Association developed a classification system for human responses for psychiatric–mental health nursing practice. They are now working with NANDA to create one classification system that all nurses can use.

Coping responses to stress emerge whether or not a medical diagnosis has been made. If the individual has been diagnosed, the treatment will be primarily a medical function. It is here that the practice of medicine and nursing interrelate and become complementary, although each retains its distinct focus. A nurse may implement the nursing process for maladaptive responses *whether or not* a physician has diagnosed a psychiatric illness. However, all health professionals have an obligation to refer a patient to another practitioner when it is in the patient's best interests.

An additional aspect of nursing care is presented by Loomis and Wood[30] in their model of clinical nursing. The authors propose that the potential outcome of nursing is not limited to "care" alone but may include the possible "cure" of actual or potential health problems. The model presents four prototypes of health care situations to demonstrate this point.[31] The first prototype is typical of the medical model, in which a patient's health problem precedes his human responses. In this case nurses collaborate with physicians in treating the physiological response and with the patient in treating the emotional, cognitive, behavioral, and social responses. In the second prototype, human responses precede health problems; in this case nurses act to prevent health problems by education, environmental change, and supporting social systems. In the third prototype, health problems are defined as human responses; thus the nursing diagnosis is the same as the medical diagnosis, and nurses assume curative functions. In the fourth prototype, a patient's health problems are interactive with his human responses; in this case caring and curing may be synonymous as nurses mediate among medical treatments, health deviations, and life-style disruptions. Thus the overlap in health problems and human responses suggests the interdependence of nursing and medicine and the need for collaboration.

The final outcome of the model is the emergence of health and illness behaviors, which are seen as a continuum rather than as discrete entities. Volumes

TABLE 3-6

SUMMARY OF THE NURSING MODEL OF HEALTH-ILLNESS PHENOMENA

Component	Definition	Examples
Predisposing factors	Conditioning factors that influence both the type and amount of resources the individual can elicit to cope with stress	Age, education, marital status, social class
Precipitating stressors	Stimuli that the individual perceives as challenging, threatening, or demanding and that require excess energy for coping	Life events, injury, hassles, strains
Primary appraisal of a stressor	An evaluation of the significance of a stressor for a person's well-being, considering the stressor's meaning, intensity, and importance	Hardiness, perceived seriousness, anxiety, attribution
Secondary appraisal of coping resources	An evaluation of a person's coping resources, options, and strategies	Finances, social support, ego integrity, intelligence
Coping mechanisms	Any effort directed at stress management	Problem-solving, compliance, defense mechanisms, health goals
Continuum of health-illness responses	A range of human responses that reflect a person's health status	Social changes, physical and emotional health/illness

DIRECTIONS FOR FUTURE RESEARCH

The following are some of the nursing research problems raised in Chapter 3 that merit further study by psychiatric nurses:

1. Attitudes of psychiatric nurses regarding the health-illness and conformity-deviance conceptions of mental illness
2. The role of psychiatric nurses in the delivery of mental health care to cultural, sexual, and ethnic minorities
3. The prevalence of ethnocentrism among psychiatric nurses, and patient care outcomes associated with it
4. The validity and reliability of tools used to collect data about coping strategies used by healthy and ill individuals
5. Methods to evaluate the effectiveness of coping strategies
6. The direct and interactive effects related to the nature, origin, timing, and number of stressors
7. Variables that intervene between stressful life events and maladaptive coping responses
8. Stressful life events, chronic strains, and daily hassles relevant to various high-risk groups
9. The role of social attribution in an individual's response to threat
10. The types of coping resources associated with adaptive responses and their mechanism of action

have been written about each component of this model, but this brief description was presented to reveal the framework for this text (Table 3-6). Chapters 11 through 21 explore various maladaptive responses. Each chapter begins with a continuum of coping or health-illness, followed by a discussion of predisposing or conditioning factors, precipitating stressors, behaviors, and coping mechanisms. Each phase of nursing is applied to the maladaptive response. Medical diagnoses of health problems are presented when appropriate and when they are related to the nursing diagnoses. Through consistent use of this framework, the art and science of psychiatric nursing emerges.

■ SUGGESTED CROSS-REFERENCES ■

This chapter serves as a foundation for formulating and implementing psychiatric nursing. As such it is related to all other chapters in this text.

■ SUMMARY ■

1. Conditions and criteria of mental health were described, and the dimensions and prevalence of mental illnesses were discussed.
2. Developmental stages and tasks of individual and family life cycles were identified.
3. Cultural relativism was explored, because the content and form of mental illness vary greatly from one culture to another.
4. A nursing model of health-illness phenomena was presented at the individual level of the social hierarchy. This model serves as a focus for the nursing process. It portrays six components that result in adaptive or maladaptive coping; these are :
   a. Predisposing factors, which are biological, psychological, and sociocultural in nature.
   b. Precipitating stressors, which vary in nature, origin, timing, and number. (Research related to stressful life events was critiqued.)
   c. Primary appraisal of a stressor, which is evaluation of the significance of an event that takes place on the cognitive, affective, physiological, behavioral, and social levels.
   d. Secondary appraisal of coping resources, which is evaluation coping resources or strategies that involve cognitive, affective, physiological, behavioral, and social responses.
   e. Coping mechanisms, which are any efforts directed at stress management; they may be constructive or destructive. Destructive coping often is classified according to axes I through V of the *DSM-III-R*.
   f. The continuum of health-illness responses, which reflects health status. These responses to stress, whether actual or potential, are the subject of nursing diagnoses. The relationships among coping responses, health problems, medical diagnoses, and nursing diagnoses were explored.

■ REFERENCES ■

1. American Journal of Psychiatry: Research on mental illness and addictive disorders: progress and prospects 142(7), 1985.
2. American Psychiatric Association: Diagnostic and statistical manual of mental disorders, ed 3, revised, Washington, DC, 1987, The Association.
3. Antonovsky A: Health, stress and coping, San Francisco, 1979, Jossey-Bass.
4. Askenasy AR, Dohrenwend BP, and Dohrenwend BS: Some effects of social class and ethnic group membership on judgments of the magnitude of stressful life events: a research note, J Health Soc Behav 18(4):432, 1977.
5. Bryant F: Dimensions of subjective mental health in American men and women, J Health Soc Behav 25(2):116, 1984.

6. Caplan G: Support systems and community mental health, New York, 1974, Behavioral Publications.

7. Caplan G: Mastery of stress: psychosocial aspects, Am J Psychiatry 138(4):41, 1981.

8. Cassel J: Psychosocial processes and "stress": theoretical formulation, Int J Health Serv 4:471, 1974.

9. Cobb S: Social support as a moderator of life stress, Psychosom Med 38:300, 1976.

10. Comas-Diaz L and Griffith E: Clinical guidelines in cross-cultural mental health, New York, 1988, John Wiley & Sons, Inc.

11. Dohrenwend BP and Dohrenwend BS: Social and cultural influences on psychopathology, Annu Rev Psychol 7(25):417, 1974.

12. Durkheim E: Suicide: a study in sociology, Glencoe, Ill, 1951, Free Press. (Translated by J Spaulding and C Simpson.)

13. Duvall E: Marriage and family development, ed 5, Philadelphia, 1977, JB Lippincott Co.

14. Erikson E: Childhood and society, ed 2, New York, 1963, WW Norton & Co, Inc.

15. Fabrega H: Cultural relativism and psychiatric illness, J Nerv Ment Dis 177(7):415, 1989.

16. Faris R and Dunham H: Mental health in urban areas: an ecological study of schizophrenia and other psychoses, Chicago, 1939, University of Chicago Press.

17. Gourash N: Help-seeking: a review of the literature, Am J Community Psychol 6:499, 1978.

18. Greenblatt M, Becerra R, and Serafetinides E: Social networks and mental health: an overview, Am J Psychiatry 139(8):977, 1982.

19. Holmes T and Rahe R: The social readjustment rating scale, J Psychosom Res 11:213, 1967.

20. House J: Work stress and social support, Reading, Mass, 1981, Addison-Wesley Publishing Co, Inc.

21. Hull J, Van Treuren R, and Virnelli S: Hardiness and health: a critique and alternative approach, J Personality Social Psych 53(3):518, 1987.

22. Jahoda M: Current concepts of positive mental health, New York, 1958, Basic Books Publishers.

23. Kaplan B, Cassel J, and Gore S: Social support and health, Med Care 15(5)(suppl):47, 1977.

24. Kobasa S, Maddi S, and Kahn S: Hardiness and health: a prospective study, J Personality Social Psych 42(1):168, 1982.

25. Lawson W: Racial and ethnic factors in psychiatric research, Hosp Community Psychiatry 37(1):50, 1986.

26. Lazarus R: Psychological stress and the coping process, New York, 1966, McGraw-Hill, Inc.

27. Lazarus R: Little hazards can be hazardous to health, Psychology Today 15:58, 1981.

28. Lazarus R and Folkman S: Stress, appraisal and coping, New York, 1984, Springer Publishing Co.

29. Leighton A et al: Stirling County study of psychiatric disorder and sociocultural environment: my name is legion, vol 1, New York, 1959, Basic Books Publishers.

30. Loomis M and Wood D: Cure: the potential outcome of nursing care, Image 15(1):4, 1983.

31. Loring M and Powell B: Gender, race and DSM-III: a study of the objectivity of psychiatric diagnostic behavior, J Health Social Behav 29:(1), 1988.

32. Maslow A: Motivation and personality, New York, 1958, Harper & Row Publishers.

33. Mechanic D: Illness behavior, social adaptation, and the management of illness, J Nerv Ment Dis 165(2):79, 1977.

34. Miller T: Advances in understanding the impact of stressful life events on health, Hosp Community Psychiatry 39(6):615, 1988.

35. Molzahn A and Northcott H: The social bases of discrepancies in health/illness perceptions, J Adv Nurs 14:132, 1989.

36. Mueller D: Social networks: a promising direction for research on the relationship of the social environment to psychiatric disorder, Soc Sci Med 14A:147, 1980.

37. O'Toole A and Loomis M: Revision of the phenomena of concern for psychiatric mental health nursing, Arch Psych Nurs 3(5):288, 1989.

38. Pearlin LI and Schooler C: The structure of coping, J Health Soc Behav 19(3):2, 1978.

39. Rahe R: Life-change measurement as a predictor of illness, Proc R Soc Med 61:1124, 1968.

40. Rogers C: On becoming a person, Boston, 1961, Houghton Mifflin Co.

41. Rosenfield S: Race differences in involuntary hospitalization: psychiatric versus labeling perspectives, J Health Soc Behav 25(1):14, 1984.

42. Streff M: Examining family growth and development: a theoretical model, Adv Nurs Sci 3(4):61, 1981.

43. Sundeen S et al: Nurse-client interaction: implementing the nursing process, ed 4, St Louis, 1989, Mosby–Year Book, Inc.

44. Walker K, MacBride A, and Vachon M: Social support networks and the crisis of bereavement, Soc Sci Med 11:35, 1977.

45. Weiss R: The provisions of social relationships. In Rubin A, editor: Doing unto others, Englewood Cliffs, NJ, 1974, Prentice-Hall, Inc.

■ ANNOTATED SUGGESTED READINGS ■

American Journal of Psychiatry: Research on mental illness and addictive disorders: progress and prospects, 142(7), 1985.

Summary of the the latest findings, statistics, and progress in mental and addictive disorders. Makes an eloquent case for the need for more research funding in psychiatric care.

*Dean P: Expanding our sights to include social networks, Nurs Health Care 7:545, 1986.

Describes the importance of social networks and how nurses should assess them with implications for nursing practice.

*Derdiarian A: A valid profession needs valid diagnoses, Nurs Health Care 8:137, 1987.

Discusses the diagnostic process in nursing and why validation is important to practice, research, and education.

Elizur J and Minuchin S: Institutionalizing madness: families, therapy and society, New York, 1989, Basic Books.

Using case studies, this book explores patients, families, and insitiutions and the culture-bound way the mental health field responds to people labeled patients.

*Flaskerud J: Community mental health nursing: its unique role in the delivery of services to ethnic minorities, Perspect Psychiatr Care 20(1):37, 1982.

Reviews shared characteristics and values of various cultural groups and describes culture-related interventions that are most appropriate to the role of community mental health nurses.

Horwitz A: Help-seeking processes and mental health services. In Mechanic D, editor: New directions for mental health services, San Francisco, 1987, Jossey-Bass.

Excellent review of the cultural, social, and organizational factors that promote or inhibit contact with mental health professionals.

Jordan-Marsh M et al: Life-style intervention: a conceptual framework, Patient Educ Counsel 6(1):29, 1985.

An excellent paper presenting a conceptual framework that individuals can use to assess their life-styles and to plan for health-behavior changes. Can also be used by nurses who are developing programs to teach healthy life-style choices.

*Kane C: Family social support: toward a conceptual model, Adv Nurs Sci 10(2):18, 1988.

Presents a conceptual model of family social support, including family characteristics, interactional factors, antecedents, and consequences.

Klerman G et al: A debate on *DSM-III*, Am J Psychiatry 141(4):539, 1984.

Series of four brief articles debates the advantages and disadvantages of the DSM-III. Recommended reading for all psychiatric nurses who use the DSM-III in their practice.

Lazarus R and Folkman S: Stress, appraisal and coping, New York, 1984, Springer Publishing Co.

Compiles all of Lazarus' work on stress and coping into one understandable volume. Definitive reading for any nurse interested in mastering the area of stress and coping in practice or research.

Miller T: Advances in understanding the impact of stressful life events on health, Hosp Community Psychiatry 39(6):615, 1988.

Reviews research exploring the relationship between life stresses and illness. Describes efforts to develop objective tools to assess the degree of stress associated with specific life events.

*Minrath M: Breaking the race barrier, J Psychosoc Nurs Ment Health Serv 23(8):19, 1985.

Addresses specific issues in breaking the race barrier between white therapists and ethnic minority patients. One of the few psychiatric nursing articles to address this issue directly.

*Molzahn A and Northcott H: The social bases of discrepancies in health/illness perceptions, J Advanced Nurs 14:132, 1989.

Thought-provoking article that summarizes the literature pertaining to discrepancies in health/illness perceptions between patients and health care providers and social factors that may effect these perceptions, including culture, gender, socioeconomic status, experience, and role. Highly recommended reading for all nurses.

Ness R and Wintrob R: Folk healing: a description and synthesis, Am J Psychiatry 138(11):1477, 1981.

An excellent review of four systems of folk healing that have evolved in different cultural groups in the United States: faith healing, rootwork, curanderism, and espiritismo.

*Nymathi A: Comprehensive health seeking and coping paradigm, J Adv Nurs 14:281, 1989.

Presents a 12-dimension coping paradigm based on Lazarus' work and applies it to nursing. Reading for the advanced student.

*O'Toole A and Loomis M: Revision of the phenomena of concern for psychiatric mental health nursing, Arch Psych Nurs 3(5):288, 1989.

Provides information on the ANA's task force work on developing the phenomena of concern to psychiatric mental health nursing practice, and how it is being merged with the work of NANDA.

Sue D: Counseling the culturally different: theory and practice, New York, 1981, John Wiley & Sons, Inc.

Necessary reading for all psychiatric nurses working with patients from different cultures. One of the few texts devoted to this topic that approaches it from an integrated, conceptual framework. Specific chapters concern Asian-Americans, blacks, Hispanics, and American Indians.

*Sullivan G: Evaluating Antonovski's salutogenic model for its adaptability to nursing, J Adv Nurs 14:336, 1989.

Antonovsky's coping theory stressing the importance of generalized resistance resources and a sense of coherence are adapted to nursing in this article for the advanced student.

*Talley S: Basic health care needs of the mentally ill: issues for psychiatric nurses, Issues Mental Health Nurs 9:409, 1988.

Reviews the literature on the medical health care needs of psychiatric patients, with implications for psychiatric nurses. Essential reading.

Williams J, Karls J, and Wandrei K: The person-in-environment (PIE) system for describing problems of social functioning, Hosp Community Psychiatry, 40(11):1125, 1989.

Describes the new system for classifying problems of social functioning experienced by clients treated by social workers, including social role and environment problems.

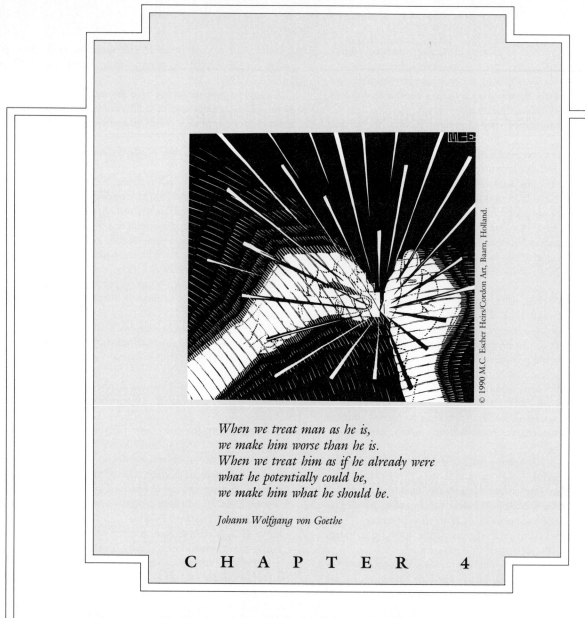

When we treat man as he is,
we make him worse than he is.
When we treat him as if he already were
what he potentially could be,
we make him what he should be.

Johann Wolfgang von Goethe

C H A P T E R   4

THE THERAPEUTIC NURSE-PATIENT RELATIONSHIP

After studying this chapter, the student should be able to:

- state the nature and goals of the therapeutic nurse-patient relationship.

- discuss six personal qualities a nurse needs to be an effective helper.

- describe the nurse's tasks and the problems that may arise in each of the four phases of the relationship process.

- explain the relevance of communication theory to nursing.

- compare and contrast the verbal and nonverbal levels of communication in types of behavior, effectiveness, factors limiting correct interpretation, and implications for nursing care.

- identify the three elements of the communication process.

- analyze the structural and transactional analysis models of the communication process with respect to the components of each and the communication problems they reveal.

- define and give examples of 12 therapeutic communication techniques.

- describe how each of the responsive dimensions of genuineness, respect, empathic understanding, and concreteness can be shown by the nurse in a therapeutic relationship.

- describe how confrontation, immediacy, nurse self-disclosure, catharsis, and role playing can be demonstrated by the nurse in a therapeutic relationship.

- define the following therapeutic impasses and identify nursing interventions that can deal with them: resistance, transference, and countertransference.

- discuss the goals of supervision and the ways in which therapy and supervision are parallel processes.

- demonstrate increasing effectiveness in using therapeutic relationship skills with psychiatric patients.

- identify directions for future nursing research.

- select appropriate readings for further study.

Nature of the relationship

The therapeutic nurse-patient relationship is a mutual learning experience and a corrective emotional experience for the patient. The observation, "We are all more human than otherwise," nicely describes the relationship. In this relationship the nurse uses personal attributes and clinical techniques in working with the patient to bring about insight and behavioral change. In general, the goals of a therapeutic relationship are directed toward the growth of the patient. These goals include the following:

1. Self-realization, self-acceptance, and an increased genuine self-respect
2. A clear sense of personal identity and an improved level of personal integration

3. An ability to form intimate, interdependent, interpersonal relationships with a capacity to give and receive love
4. Improved functioning and increased ability to satisfy needs and achieve realistic personal goals

To achieve these goals, various aspects of the patient's life experiences are explored during the nurse-patient relationship. The nurse allows the patient to express his thoughts and feelings and relates these to observed and reported actions. Areas of conflict and anxiety are clarified. The nurse identifies and maximizes the patient's ego strengths and encourages socialization and family relatedness. Communication problems are corrected, and maladaptive behavior patterns are modified as the patient tests new patterns of behavior and new coping mechanisms.

■ Characteristics

The nurse-patient relationship is characterized by mutual growth of two individuals who "dare" to discover love, growth, and freedom together. The uniqueness of each of the two is valued, and differing values are respected. The nurse and the patient find mutual satisfaction, and the world of each is enlarged and enriched by the other.

The two communicate through a dialogue or discussion, not a monologue. The patient's reality and worth are affirmed, allowing him to grasp and more fully define his ego identity. To achieve this the nurse must be open to experiences and willing to disclose aspects of his or her own being to the patient. In the following questions Rogers summarizes the characteristics of helping relationships that facilitate growth:

1. Can I *be* in some way that will be perceived by the other person as trustworthy, as dependable or consistent in some deep sense?
2. Can I be expressive enough as a person that what I am will be communicated unambiguously?
3. Can I let myself experience positive attitudes toward this other person—attitudes of warmth, caring, liking, interest, and respect?
4. Can I be strong enough as a person to be separate from the other?
5. Am I secure enough within myself to permit him his separateness?
6. Can I let myself enter fully into the world of his feelings and personal meaning and see these as he does?
7. Can I be acceptant of each facet of the other person that he presents to me? Can I receive him as he is? Can I communicate this attitude? Or can I only receive him conditionally, acceptant of some aspects of his feelings and silently or openly disapproving of others?
8. Can I act with sufficient sensitivity in the relationship that my behavior will not be perceived as a threat?
9. Can I free him from the threat of external evaluation?
10. Can I meet this other individual as a person who is in the process of *becoming,* or will I be bound by his past and my past?[51:50-51]

All nurses working with patients may ask themselves these questions; their answers largely determine the progress of the relationship. The therapeutic nurse-patient relationship is a complex one that can be analyzed in many different ways. Various elements and therapeutic dynamics of it merit further exploration, including the nurse as helper, the phases of the relationship, facilitative communication, responsive and action dimensions, therapeutic impasses, and the nurse's effectiveness. The interplay among the elements that produce a therapeutic outcome is shown in Fig. 4-1. The rest of this chapter analyzes these elements.

The nurse as helper

Helping others is a function of all concerned people; it is not limited to health professionals. Nor is there a cluster of traits that describes a helping person who is universally effective. Nurses, however, as helpers must be therapeutic in their care, since the goal of nursing is to enable the patient to adapt as a unique individual to the stress he is experiencing.

The key helping tool the nurse can use in practice is himself or herself. Thus self-analysis is the first building block in providing quality nursing care. Some feel that nurses as professionals have become impersonal and detached. Is it possible that nurses are alienated from their true selves and thus do not allow patients the freedom to express all aspects of themselves?

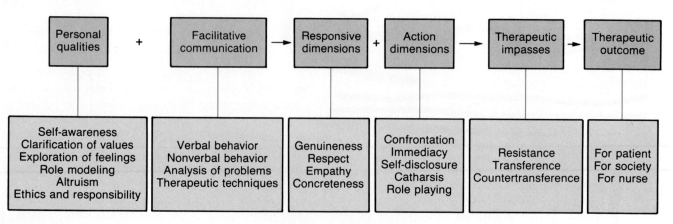

Fig. 4-1. Elements affecting the nurse's ability to be therapeutic.

Jourard believes that the socialization process into nursing destroys the nurse's spontaneity, and he or she becomes detached from the real self:

> Now, if a nurse is afraid or even ignorant of her own self, she is highly likely to be threatened by a patient's real-self expressions. . . . A nurse who is more aware of the breadth and depth of her own real self is in a much better position to empathize with her patients and to encourage (or at least not block) their self-disclosures.[32:184]

Research on counselor and teacher effectiveness suggests some essential qualities associated with being able to help others. These qualities can be viewed as necessary characteristics for all nurses who wish to be therapeutic. This section describes these qualities in some detail to help the nurse set goals for future growth.

■ **Awareness of self**

Theorists and practitioners universally agree that helpers must be able to answer the question "Who am I?" The nurse who cares for the biological, psychological, and sociocultural needs of patients sees a broad range of human experiences; he or she must learn to deal with anxiety, anger, sadness, and joy in helping patients at all intervals of the health-illness continuum.

Self-awareness is a key component of the psychiatric nursing experience. The nurse's goal is to achieve authentic, open, and personal communication. The nurse must be able to examine personal feelings and reactions as well as his or her actions as a provider of care. A firm understanding and acceptance of self allows the nurse to acknowledge a patient's differences and uniqueness.

Campbell has identified a holistic nursing model of self-awareness.[10] This model consists of four interconnected parts—the psychological, physical, environmental, and philosophical components.

1. The *psychological* component of self-awareness includes knowledge of one's emotions, motivations, self-concept, and personality. Being psychologically self-aware means being sensitive to one's feelings and to external elements that affect those feelings.
2. The *physical* component of the self is the knowledge of personal and general physiology, one's bodily sensations, one's body image, and one's physical potential.
3. The *environmental* aspect of the self consists of one's social environment, relationships with others, and knowledge of the relationship between humans and nature.
4. The *philosophical* component refers to the sense

that one's life has meaning. One's personal philosophy of life and death may or may not include a formulation of a superior being, but it does take into account the world in which one lives and the ethics of one's behavior.

Together these components provide a model that can be used to promote the self-awareness and self-growth of both nurses and the patients for whom they care.

■ **INCREASING SELF-AWARENESS.** No one ever completely knows his inner self. The Johari Window shown in Fig. 4-2 illustrates this idea.[41] Quadrant 1 is the open quadrant; it includes the behaviors, feelings, and thoughts known to the individual and those around him. Quadrant 2 is called the blind quadrant because it includes all those things that others know but that the individual does not know. Quadrant 3 is the hidden quadrant; it includes those things that only the individual knows about himself. Quadrant 4 is the unknown quadrant, containing aspects of the self unknown to the individual and to others. Taken together, these quadrants represent the total self. The following three principles may help clarify how the self functions in this representation:

1. A change in any one quadrant affects all other quadrants.
2. The smaller the first quadrant, the poorer the communication.
3. Interpersonal learning means that a change has taken place, so that quadrant 1 is larger and one or more of the other quadrants are smaller.[45:14]

The goal of increasing self-awareness is to enlarge the area of quadrant 1 while reducing the size of the other three quadrants. To increase knowledge of self, one begins by **listening to oneself.** This means allow-

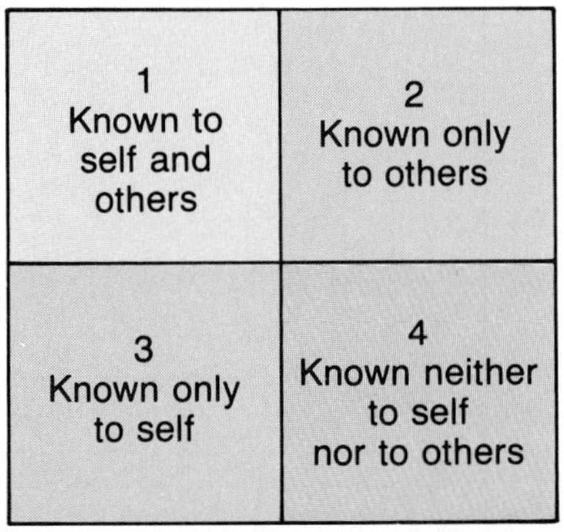

1 Known to self and others	2 Known only to others
3 Known only to self	4 Known neither to self nor to others

Fig. 4-2. Johari Window. Each quadrant, or windowpane, describes one aspect of the self. (From Sundeen SJ et al: Nurse-client interaction: implementing the nursing process, ed 4, St Louis, 1989, Mosby–Year Book, Inc.)

ing oneself to experience genuine emotions, identify and accept personal needs, and move one's body in free, joyful, and spontaneous ways. It includes exploring one's own thoughts, feelings, memories, and impulses:

I am most alive when I am open to all the many facets of my inner living—desires, emotions, the flow of ideas, body sensations, relationships, reasoning, forethought, concern for others, my sense of values and all else within me. I am most alive when I can let myself experience and genuinely realize all of these facets even as I am truly feeling and expressing my wholeness.[7:276]

The next step in the process is to reduce the size of quadrant 2 by **listening to and learning from others.** Knowledge of self is not possible alone. As we relate to others, we broaden our perceptions of self. But such learning requires active listening and openness to the feedback others provide. The final step involves reducing the size of quadrant 3 by **self-disclosing,** or revealing to others important aspects of oneself. Jourard states that no one "can come to know himself except as

an outcome of disclosing himself to another person. Self-disclosure is a symptom of personality health and a means of achieving healthy personality."[32:6]

Compare *A* and *B* of Fig. 4-3. *A* represents a person with little self-awareness. His behaviors and feelings are limited in variety and scope. *B,* however, shows an individual with great openness to the world. Much of his potential is being developed and realized. He has an increased capacity for experiences of all kinds—joy, hate, work, and love. He has few defenses and can interact more spontaneously and honestly with others. This configuration represents a worthy goal for the nurse to attain. The results of being attuned to the inward sense of self are greater integration of the many aspects of one's being, more vitality, readiness for action, more committed choices, and more authenticity in relationships.

■ **THE NURSE AND SELF-GROWTH.** People often assume that because a nursing education includes some courses in the behavioral sciences, a nursing student is able to use himself or herself in a therapeutic manner in the clinical setting. However, although most nursing textbooks include a paragraph or two stressing the importance of self-awareness in quality nursing care, the process and components of self-growth for the nurse are never described. A student who looked for this information would discover that the nursing literature has only a few references that develop in depth the concept of self-awareness and its application to the nurse. The self-concept of the patient is treated in a similarly cursory way. These omissions give an implicit message to the nursing student: Self-analysis is commendable, but a token assessment will suffice. This message is reinforced by the student's curriculum, which is burdened with tasks and reports that allow little time for quiet contemplation leading to self-growth.

Nurses need the time to explore and define the many facets of their personalities. If nursing does involve perceiving, feeling, and thinking, nursing students should have the time and opportunity to study their own experiences. Authenticity in relationships must be learned. For the nurse to do this, he or she must first experience openness and authenticity in relationships with instructors and supervisors. Rogers has stated that one might enhance another's personal growth by accepting the other as an individual and by viewing the world as it appears through his eyes.[51] The student and instructor can participate in a relationship that accepts and respects their individual differences. Acting as role models, instructors can help students by (1) facilitating students' self-awareness, (2) increasing their level of functioning, (3) stimulating

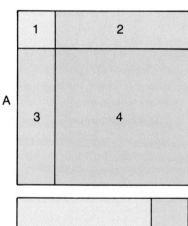
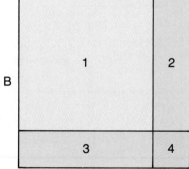

Fig. 4-3. Johari Windows showing varying degrees of self-awareness. **A,** Person with little self-understanding. **B,** Individual with great self-awareness. (From Sundeen SJ et al: Nurse-client interaction: implementing the nursing process, ed 4, St Louis, 1989, Mosby–Year Book, Inc.)

more self-direction, and (4) enabling students to cope more effectively with the stressors of life.

Authenticity also involves being open to exploring one's self: one's thoughts, needs, emotions, values, defenses, actions, communications, problems, and goals. In becoming a nurse, the student has many new experiences that provide opportunities for self-learning. Feelings about these expressions should be focused on and discussed. The student might enter clinical settings with high ideals and unrealistic images. Perhaps he or she views nurses as "miracle workers," who are all-knowing and all-caring. During initial encounters the student may feel fearful, anxious, and inadequate and may wonder how a nurse ever acquires the necessary knowledge. The student might devalue his or her ability and feel like an imposition on the patient. Both the nurse's expectations and abilities should be analyzed to raise self-esteem and reinforce capabilities. At another time the nurse may identify closely with the patient and feel anger at the impersonal system and unresponsive personnel. This anger should be identified, verbalized, and accepted. Only then can the nurse analyze how he or she expresses anger and how these feelings can be resolved in a constructive manner.

It is not easy to embark on a career in nursing while still in adolescence. As a nurse the student will be faced with many adult responsibilities, such as disease, bizarre behavior, complex problems, and even death, when most of one's friends are focusing on youth, enjoyment, and the future. This might alienate the nurse from some friends and trigger feelings of despair and self-doubt. These feelings of loneliness and sadness should be shared, so that the nurse can experience the benefit of an interpersonal relationship in working through his or her own needs.

The nurse must initiate the process of developing self-awareness. The nurse is an active participant in analyzing thoughts, communications, and relationships with others. Because it is difficult to be participant and observer at the same time, other ways of collecting data should be used. Tape recordings provide an opportunity for the student to review communications and study them more closely. Videotapes give feedback regarding nonverbal messages as well as tone and inflection. Maintaining a diary allows for the expression of feelings, the description of the student's self-concept, and comments on the student's level of self-esteem.

Introspection should also be accompanied by self-disclosure. Sharing perceptions with others allows the nurse to gain new information and evolve new insights. The analysis may be written in the form of a process recording.[61] The nurse looks beyond the obvious and takes the time to explore feelings. The instructor can review the recording with the student and identify areas that may have been overlooked or blocked.

Throughout the growing process the student needs the support and guidance of an instructor. Together they can analyze the student's behavior, and the student can then assess personal strengths and limitations. It is often helpful to share these experiences with a peer group. Because students are all in a similar situation, they can empathize, criticize, and support each other as together they learn more about themselves.

Finally, the process of self-awareness is a painful one. It is not easy or pleasant to examine one's self objectively, particularly when what one finds conflicts with one's self-ideal. However, like many painful experiences, discovering self-awareness presents a challenge: to accept these limitations of the self or to change the behaviors that support them. Choices such as this are the catalysts for growth and stimulate new responses to the question "Who am I?"

■ **Clarification of values**

Besides knowing who they are, nurses should be able to answer the question, "What is important to me?" Awareness helps the nurse to be honest with himself or herself and to avoid the unwarranted and unethical use of patients to meet personal needs. Although the nurse-patient relationship involves mutual growth and satisfaction, the patient's needs always come first. Nurses should have enough sources of satisfaction and security in their nonprofessional life to avoid the temptation to use patients for the pursuit of personal satisfaction or security. If nurses do not have sufficient personal fulfillment, they should realize it; their sources of dissatisfaction should then be clarified so that they do not interfere with the success of the nurse-patient relationship.

■ **VALUE SYSTEMS.** Values are the concepts that a person holds worthy. They are formed as a result of one's life experiences with family, friends, culture, education, work, and relaxation. The word "value" has positive connotations, since it denotes worth or significance. Yet values also imply negatives. If we value one thing, such as honesty, then it follows that we do not value its opposite, such as dishonesty. Areas in which people are likely to hold strong values include religious beliefs, family ties, sexual preferences, other ethnic groups, and sex role beliefs.

However, value systems are more than statements of what a person regards highly. They provide the framework, either consciously or unconsciously, for many of one's daily decisions and actions. By being aware of his or her value system, the nurse can more readily identify situations in which a value system conflict has arisen. Clarification of values also provides some insurance against the tendency to project one's values onto another. Many therapeutic relationships test the nurse's values. A patient may describe a sexual behavior that the nurse finds unacceptable. The patient may talk about divorce, whereas the nurse may strongly believe that marriage contracts should not be broken. Or the patient may be a "born-again" Christian, but the nurse may have no belief in God or religion. How does the nurse respond? Can he or she maintain personal values and still accept those of the patient? Can the nurse empathize with and help the patient solve a problem while being aware of personal values and natural tendencies to project those values?

■ **VALUE CLARIFICATION PROCESS.** Understanding one's values may be promoted by *value clarification*. It is a method developed by Raths, Harmin, and Simon[50] and adapted to nursing by Uustal.[63] Using this method, a person can discover one's own values by assessing, exploring, and determining what those values are and what priority they hold in one's decision making. It is a growth-producing process that promotes self-understanding and permits one to behave in ways appropriate to one's value priorities. Value clarification does not tell an individual what his values should be or what values he should live by. To avoid the imposition of values, value clarification focuses exclusively on the *process* of valuing, or on how people come to have the values they have.

Seven criteria are used to determine whether a person is actually holding a value. These criteria should be considered in relation to a person's strongest value and tested against one's own definition of a value. The criteria are broadly grouped into the following three steps:

Choosing	1. Freely
	2. From alternatives
	3. After thoughtful consideration of the consequences of each alternative
Prizing	4. Cherishing, being happy with the choice
	5. Willing to affirm the choice publicly
Acting	6. Doing something with the choice
	7. Repeatedly, in some pattern of life[55]

The first three criteria, those of **choosing,** rely on the person's cognitive abilities; the next two criteria, **priz-**ing, emphasize the emotional or affective level; the last two criteria, **acting,** have a behavioral focus.

Simple exposure to the value clarification process causes change in people. This change takes place when the person becomes disturbed emotionally as a result of realizing the existence of certain contradictions in his value system. To eliminate the inevitable self-dissatisfaction that follows such a realization, the person realigns his values to coincide with the new self-concept.

■ **THE MATURE VALUING PROCESS.** Rogers has described the valuing process in the mature person.[51] He does not view it as an easy or simple thing. Rather, the process is complex and the choices often perplexing and difficult. There is no guarantee that the choice made will prove to be self-actualizing. The valuing process in the mature person has the following characteristics[34]:

1. It is fluid and flexible, based on the particular moment and the degree to which the moment is experienced as enhancing, enriching, and actualizing. Values are not held rigidly but are continually changing.
2. The valuing experience is highly differentiated, that is, tied to a particular time and experience.
3. The locus of evaluation in the valuing process is firmly established within the person. It is one's own experience that provides the value information. Although the person is open to all the evidence that can be obtained from other sources, he views it as outside evidence that is not as significant as his own responses. The psychologically mature adult trusts and uses his own wisdom.
4. In the valuing process, the person is open to the immediacy of experiences, trying to sense and clarify all its complex meanings. However, the immediate impact of the moment is colored by experiences from the past and conjecture about the future. Thus past and future combine in the present and enter into the valuing process.

■ **Exploration of feelings**

It is often assumed that helping others requires complete objectivity and detachment from one's feelings. This is definitely not true. Complete objectivity and detachment from one's feelings describe someone who is unresponsive, false, unapproachable, impersonal, and alienated from oneself—qualities that impede or prohibit the establishment of a therapeutic relationship. What is desired is that the nurse be open to his or her feelings, aware of them, and in control of them so that they can be used to help patients.

Nurses, as people, are feeling all the time; these feelings serve an important purpose. They are barometers for feedback about themselves and their relationships with others. They are useful, serve adaptive purposes, and are part of a person's learning experience. Gaylin believes:

> Feelings are the instruments of rationality. . . . They are fine tunings directing the ways in which we will meet and manipulate our environment. . . . Mental illness is usually a mere disarray of the ingredients of survival. All that is necessary is rearrangement. Feelings are internal directives essential for human life.[21:3-7]

In helping others, nurses experience many feelings—elation at seeing a patient improve, disappointment when a patient regresses, distress when a patient refuses help, and anger when a patient is demanding or manipulative. Feelings of power can arise when patients express strong dependence on the nurse or indicate that the nurse has influence over them. When patients express profuse gratitude to the nurse, he or she must wonder if the patients believe they helped themselves or whether the nurse did it for them.

The nurse who is open to his or her own feelings has access to two important pieces of information: how he or she is responding to the patient, and how he or she appears to the patient. While talking to a patient, the nurse should be aware of his or her response. Despite the patient's words, the nurse might perceive a strong sense of despair or anger. The nurse's feelings are valuable clues to the patient's problems and should be incorporated into the nurse's care for the patient. So too, the nurse should be aware of the feeling he or she is conveying to the patient. Is the nurse's mood one of hopelessness or contempt? If the nurse views feelings as barometers and feedback instruments, his or her effectiveness as a helper will improve.

■ Ability to serve as model

Formal helping is a strong influence process, and nurses do function as models to their patients, whether they want to or not. Much research has shown the power of models for acquiring socially adaptive, as well as maladaptive, behavior. Thus a nurse has an obligation to model adaptive and growth-producing behavior. If a nurse has a chaotic personal life, such as one characterized by stormy intimate relationships, drug abuse, or conflictual parental ties, it will show in the nurse's work with patients. Not only will it decrease the effectiveness of care, it also will call into question the nurse's credibility as a helper and the validity of care. The nurse may object that he or she can separate the personal life from the professional life, but

in psychiatry this is not possible, because psychiatric nursing *is* the therapeutic use of self.

This is not to imply, however, that the nurse must conform totally to local community norms or must live an idyllic, placid life. What is suggested is that the effective nurse has a fulfilling and satisfying personal life that is not dominated by conflict, distress, or denial, and that his or her approach to life conveys a sense of growing and adapting.

■ Altruism

It is vital for nurses to have an answer to the question "Why do I want to help others?" The nurse need not extensively analyze his or her motives, but should be aware of acting for oneself as well as for the patient's good. Obviously, an effective helper is interested in people and tends to help out of a deep love for humanity, that is focused on a particular person or group of people. It is also true that everyone seeks a certain amount of personal satisfaction and fulfillment from his or her work. The goal is to maintain a balance between these two needs. Helping motives have the potential to become destructive tools in the hands of naive or zealous users.

Another danger lies in subscribing to an extreme view of altruism. Altruism is concern for the welfare of others. It does not mean that because one works with a sense of altruism, one should not expect adequate compensation and recognition. It does not mean that one must practice extreme denial or self-sacrifice. The desire to help humanity does not conflict with the desire for a satisfying life. In fact, only if the nurse's personal needs have been appropriately met can he or she expect to be maximally therapeutic.

Finally, a sense of altruism can also apply to more general social support and change motives. Altruism is necessary for society to survive. Activist helpers are needed who are primarily concerned with changing social conditions to meet human welfare needs. One goal of all helping professionals should be to create a people-serving and growth-facilitating society. As such, a legitimate and necessary role for the nurse is to work to change the larger structure and process of society in ways that will promote the individual's health and welfare.

■ Sense of ethics and responsibility

Personal beliefs about people and society can serve as conscious guidelines for action. When ethical principles are shared among helpers, they are written down and codified. The Code for Nurses (see Chapter 7) reflects common values regarding nurse-patient relationships and responsibilities and serves as a frame of reference for all nurses in their judgments about patient welfare and social responsibility.

For professional psychiatric nurses, decisions are a part of daily functioning. Responsible ethical choice involves accountability, risk, commitment, and justice. Sigman identifies the following elements of responsible ethical behavior for the nurse[59]:

1. A moral principle exists that involves a moral obligation or duty to do or to refrain from doing something that is within the power of the person to do or is such that the person can do otherwise.
2. Some source of responsibility is involved, as well as a source of reward, praise, or punishment for responsible actions.
3. The cause of the behavior is internal to the individual, and he or she is not compelled to act by others.
4. The behavior itself is not done through ignorance, is respectful of the laws, maintains one's integrity and freedom of choice, and attempts to do justice.

The concept of responsible ethical choice, therefore, involves a dynamic decision-making process for the nurse. It incorporates one's values, judgments, and actual choice.

Related to the nurse's sense of ethics is the need to assume responsibility for his or her own behavior. This involves knowing one's limitations and strengths and being accountable for them. As a member of a health care team, the nurse has the knowledge and expertise of other people readily available; these people should be used appropriately. Responsibility implies maturity and is an essential quality of an effective nurse.

Phases of the relationship

A vital characteristic of the nurse-patient relationship is the sharing of behaviors, thoughts, and feelings to establish a context of therapeutic intimacy. Coad-Denton[14] describes this intimacy as the use of the nursing process to support the patient as he explores areas of needs, solves problems, and acquires new coping skills. It is distinct from social superficiality and imposes specific expectations on the nurse. Table 4-1 identifies seven components of relationships in general and contrasts social superficiality and therapeutic intimacy with these components. This is not to assume, however, that these elements emerge simultaneously. Rather, they evolve as the nurse moves through the various phases of the therapeutic relationship with the patient.

Four sequential phases of the relationship process have been identified: preinteraction phase; introductory, or orientation, phase; working phase; and termination phase. Each phase builds on the preceding one and is characterized by specific tasks. While these phases are a well-accepted part of psychiatric nursing theory, there has been little research on them. In one of the few studies in this area, Forchuk and Brown[18]

TABLE 4-1

CONTRAST BETWEEN SOCIAL SUPERFICIALITY AND THERAPEUTIC INTIMACY

Components of relationship	Social superficiality	Therapeutic intimacy
Mutual self-disclosure	Variable	Patient: self-disclosure; nurse: self-disclosure in terms of response to patient only
Focus of conversation	Unknown to participants	Known to nurse and patient
Pertinence of topic	Social, business, generalized, impersonal	Personal and relevant to nurse and patient
Relationship of experiences to topic	Sense of uninvolvement and use of indirect knowledge	Sense of involvement and use of direct knowledge
Time orientation	Past and future	Present
Use of feelings	Sharing of feelings discouraged	Sharing of feelings encouraged by nurse
Recognition of individual worth	Not acknowledged	Fully acknowledged

From Coad-Denton A: Therapeutic superficiality and intimacy. In Longo D and Williams R, editors: Psychosocial nursing: assessment and intervention, New York, 1978, Appleton-Century-Crofts.

developed an instrument with initial validity and reliability to measure the phases of the nurse-patient relationship based on observed behaviors. They believe that if nurses can accurately assess the phase of the relationship, appropriate interventions are more likely to be selected.

The phases of the nurse-patient relationship are described as they apply to nurses working with psychiatric patients. Other sources present detailed information on basic elements of the relationship process.[69,70]

■ **Preinteraction phase**

■ **CONCERNS OF NEW NURSES.** The preinteraction phase begins before the nurse's first contact with the patient. The nurse's initial task is one of self-exploration, analyzing his or her own feelings, fantasies, and fears. In his or her first experience working with psychiatric patients, the nurse brings the misconceptions and prejudices of the general public. (See accompanying box for some common concerns of psychiatric nursing students.) Some of these feelings and fears are common to all novices. An overriding one usually is anxiety or nervousness, which is provoked by new experiences of any kind. A related feeling is ambivalence

---

Common Concerns of Psychiatric Nursing Students

- Acutely self-conscious
- Afraid of being rejected by the patients
- Anxious because of the newness of the experience
- Concerned about personally overidentifying with psychiatric patients
- Doubtful of the effectiveness of one's skills or coping ability
- Fearful of physical danger or violence
- Inadequacy in one's therapeutic use of self
- Suspicious of psychiatric patients stereotyped as "different"
- Threatened in one's nursing role identity
- Uncertain about one's ability to make a unique contribution
- Uncomfortable about the lack of physical tasks and treatments
- Vulnerable to emotionally painful experiences
- Worried about hurting the patient psychologically

---

or uncertainty; the nurse may see the need for working with these patients but feel unclear about his or her own ability or motivations.

There may also be a threat to the nurse's role identification, precipitated by the informal nature of psychiatric settings. Usually psychiatric patients do not wear hospital gowns or clothing, staff members do not wear uniforms, and the staff and patients mingle in a casual, relaxed, and apparently unstructured way. A common first reaction among students is a feeling of panic when they realize that they "can't tell the patients from the staff." The student's discomfort may be aggravated if one of the patients mistakes him or her for a newly admitted patient. Finally, it is unsettling for many students to give up their uniforms, stethoscopes, and scissors. Doing so dramatically emphasizes that, in this nursing setting, the most important tools are one's ability to communicate, empathize, and solve problems. Without a tangible physical illness to care for, new students are likely to feel acutely self-conscious and hesitant about introducing themselves to a patient and initiating a conversation.

Many nurses express feelings of inadequacy and fears of hurting or exploiting the patient. They worry about saying the wrong thing, which might drive the patient "over the brink." They wonder if, with their limited knowledge and experience, they will be of any value. They wonder how they can help or if they can really make a difference. Some nurses perceive the plight of psychiatric patients as hopeful; others perceive it as hopeless.

A common fear of nurses is related to the stereotype of psychiatric patients as abusive and violent. Because this is the picture portrayed by the media, many nurses are afraid of being physically hurt by a patient's outburst of aggressive behavior. Other nurses fear being psychologically hurt by a patient through rejection or silence. A final fear is related to the nurse's questioning of his or her own mental health. Nurses may fear mental illness and worry that exposure to psychiatric patients might cause them to lose their own grasp on reality. Nurses who are working on their own crises of identity and intimacy may fear overidentifying with patients and using patients to meet their own needs.

Clinical example 4-1 contains many of the feelings and fears expressed by one nursing student in the preinteraction phase of self-analysis, as reported in the notes from her diary of her psychiatric rotation.

Schoffstall has described a method that can be used in the classroom to assess and reduce the anxiety of students who are about to begin their clinical experience in psychiatric nursing.[56] The exercise has four purposes:

CLINICAL EXAMPLE 4-1

When first told that I would have a clinical psychiatric nursing experience, I received this information with a blank mind. Mental overload, denial, repression, or whatever it was made me hear the words but put off dealing with it. Then, when given a chance to sort through my thoughts and feelings, I thought more about what this experience would entail. Having never been personally involved with any people who were psychiatrically ill before, I was unable to rely on past personal experiences. I did, however, have quite a "pseudo-knowledge base" from my novels, television, and movie encounters. Do places like the hospital in "One Flew Over the Cuckoo's Nest" really exist? Was the portrayal of "Sybil" accurate? How could I possibly help someone who has so many problems, like the boy in "Ordinary People"? I'm afraid these thoughts have raised more questions in me than they have answered.

Three things scare me the most about this experience. First, I feel that the behavior of a psychiatric patient is quite unpredictable. Would they get violent or aggressive without any warning? Would this aggression be directed toward me? If so, would I be hurt? Did I provoke them and was I wrong in my actions that caused this sudden shift? The second, related to the first, is my feeling of inadequacy. I've been exposed to physically ill people and have learned how to respond to them. But, the psychologically ill are almost totally alien to me. How can I help? What if I do, or say, or infer something they could take offense to? Will I have the patience to persevere? I just don't know, and my not knowing makes me even more nervous. My third fear is how seeing and being in contact with the psychiatrically ill will affect me. Although I know it's not contagious, the more exposure and knowledge I acquire in this area, the more I may begin to doubt my own stability and sanity. I mean, adolescence hasn't been easy for me, and I feel like I'm just now beginning to see things more clearly and feel better about myself. Will this experience stir up any past fears and doubts and, if so, how will I handle it? I am beginning to realize that there is a fine line between sanity and insanity and that the psychiatric patients we'll meet have been unable to gather enough resources from within to cope with their problems. Help, reassurance, and understanding are their needs. I'm hoping I can help them . . . but I'm just not sure.

1. to identify student concerns and anxieties
2. to identify factors that influence the nurse-patient relationship
3. to provide information about the experience
4. to discuss the patient's subjective experiences related to hospitalization and the psychiatric diagnosis

In a group setting students were asked to anonymously write down a specific fantasy that they had about beginning their experience in psychiatric nursing. The fantasies were read aloud, and the group discussed the content and feelings in the responses. In a similar group discussion the students were then asked how they thought patients felt about being hospitalized. The exercise was found to be an effective way to handle the student's reluctance in expressing their concerns and to increase their empathy toward psychiatric patients.

■ **SELF-ASSESSMENT.** Experienced nurses benefit by analyzing additional aspects of their practice. They may ask themselves the following questions:

- Do I label patients with the stereotype of a group?
- Is my need to be liked so great that I become angry or hurt when a patient is rude, hostile, or uncooperative?
- Am I afraid of the responsibility I must assume for the relationship, and do I therefore limit my independent functions?
- Do I cover feelings of inferiority with a front of superiority?
- Do I require sympathy, warmth, and protection so much that I err by being too sympathetic or too protective toward patients?
- Do I fear closeness so much that I am indifferent, rejecting, or cold?
- Do I need to feel important and keep patients dependent on me?

The self-analysis that characterizes the preinteraction phase is a necessary task. To be effective, nurses should have a reasonably stable self-concept and an adequate amount of self-esteem. They should engage in constructive relationships with others and face reality to help patients do likewise. If they are aware of and in control of what they convey to their patients verbally and nonverbally, nurses can function as role models. To do this, however, some nurses abandon their own personal strengths and assume a facade of "professionalism." This facade is an alienation of their authentic self. Instead of increasing their effectiveness, it immobilizes them and acts as a barrier to establishing mutuality with patients.

All nurses have professional assets and limitations. Therapeutic use of self means using and maximizing one's assets or strengths and minimizing one's limitations. Promoting a patient's self-realization and self-acceptance is made possible when the nurse accepts himself or herself and behaves in ways congruent with his or her own personality. Nurses receive feedback from patients that can help them identify their strengths and assets. Self-analysis, peer review, and supervision also provide opportunities to explore feelings and fears and to develop useful insights into one's professional role. The effective nurse uses this information and relates to patients in a natural and relaxed manner.

Additional tasks of this phase include gathering data about the patient if information is available and planning for the first interaction with the patient. The nursing assessment is begun, but most of the work related to it is accomplished with the patient in the second phase of the relationship. The nurse reviews general goals of a therapeutic relationship and considers what he or she has to offer the patient.

■ Introductory, or orientation, phase

It is during the introductory phase that the nurse and patient first meet. One of the nurse's primary concerns is to find out why the patient sought help and if he did so voluntarily. Burgess and Burns[8] described six categories of reasons why people seek psychiatric help and identified an appropriate nursing approach for each (see Table 4-2). Determining the patient's reason directly influences the establishment of mutuality between the nurse and the patient. The reason for seeking help forms the basis of the nursing assessment and helps the nurse to focus on the patient's problem and to determine his motivation.

TABLE 4-2

ANALYSIS OF WHY PATIENTS SEEK PSYCHIATRIC HELP

Reasons for patients' seeking psychiatric care	Appropriate nursing approach	Sample response
Environmental change from home to hospital: They desire protection, comfort, rest, and freedom from demands of their usual home and work environments.	Emphasis should be placed on ability of environment to provide protection and comfort while healing process of mind occurs.	"Tell me what it was at home/on the job that made you feel so overwhelmed."
Nurturance: They wish for someone to care for them, cure their illnesses, and make them feel better.	Respond by acknowledging their nurturance needs and assuring them that help and caring are available to them.	"We're here to help you feel better."
Control: They are aware of their destructive impulses to themselves or others but lack internal control.	Offer person sources of internal control such as medication, if prescribed, and reinforce external controls available through services of staff.	"We're not going to let you hurt yourself. Tell us when these thoughts come to mind and someone will stay with you."
Psychiatric symptoms: They describe symptoms of depression, nervousness, or crying spells. They know they need psychiatric help and actively want to help themselves.	Ask for clarification of symptom and strive to understand life experiences of patient.	"I can see that you're nervous and upset. Can you tell me about how things are at home/on the job so I can better understand?"
Problem solving: They identify a specific problem or area of conflict and express desire to reason it out and change.	Help patient look at problem objectively, and utilize problem-solving process with him.	"How has drinking affected your life?"
Advised to come to hospital: Family member, friend, or health professional has convinced them to come to hospital. They may feel angry, ambivalent, or indifferent about being there.	Confirm facts surrounding his seeking of help and set limits appropriate to agency, ward, etc.	"I see that you're angry about being here. Perhaps as you become part of the ward community, you'll feel differently."

Modified from Burgess A and Burns J: Am J Nurs 73:314, 1973.

> ### Elements of a
> ### Nurse-Patient Contract
>
> - Names of individuals
> - Roles of nurse and patient
> - Responsibilities of nurse and patient
> - Expectations of nurse and patient
> - Purpose of the relationship
> - Meeting location
> - Time of meetings
> - Conditions for termination
> - Confidentiality

■ **FORMULATING A CONTRACT.** As the nurse relates to the patient in this phase of the relationship, the tasks are to (1) establish a climate of trust, understanding, acceptance, and open communication and (2) formulate a contract with the patient. The accompanying box lists the elements of a nurse-patient contract. The contract begins with the introduction of the nurse and patient, exchange of names, and explanation of roles. Too often this is omitted when the nurse has determined the patient's name from another source such as a chart, family member, or other clinician; the nurse then fails to introduce himself or herself because of anxiety, discomfort, or lack of recognition of the patient as an individual worthy of respect. An explanation of roles includes the responsibilities and expectations of the patient and nurse, with a description of what the nurse can and cannot do. This is followed by a discussion of the purpose of the relationship, in which the nurse emphasizes that the focus of it will be the patient, his life experiences, and areas of conflict. Because establishing the contract is a mutual process, it is a good opportunity to clarify misperceptions held by either the nurse or patient.

With the "who" and the "why" determined, the "where, when, and how long" are discussed. Where will the meetings be held? When and how often will they occur? How long will each be and how long will the series of meetings be? The conditions for termination should be reviewed and may include a specified length of time, attainment of mutual goals, or the discharge of the patient if he is hospitalized. The issue of confidentiality is an important one to discuss with the patient at this time. Confidentiality does not imply secrecy or the exclusive possession of information.

Rather, it involves the disclosure of certain information to another specifically authorized person. This means that information about the patient will be shared with people who are directly involved in his care in the form of verbal reports and written notes. This is important in providing for the continuity and comprehensiveness of patient care and should be clearly explained to the patient.

Establishing a contract is a mutual process in which the patient participates as fully as possible. In some cases, such as with the psychotic or severely withdrawn patient, the patient may be unable to fully participate, and the nurse must take the initiative in establishing the contract. As the patient's contact with reality increases, the nurse should review the elements of the contract when appropriate and strive to attain mutuality.

It is also possible to use a written contracting model to work therapeutically with patients and groups. Loomis describes a formal treatment contract as an openly negotiated, clearly stated set of mutual expectations that indicate what the nurse and patient expect of each other regarding the patient's health care.[40] Such a contract establishes a set of shared objectives as well as an understanding of the structure and process of arriving at mutually determined outcomes. This model identifies four levels of change contracts (see Table 4-3). Each higher level implies the inclusion of all lower level contracts.

Level I, or care contracts, involves provision of physical and emotional safety. Level II, or social contracts, deals primarily with behaviors and situations that can be brought under the patient's conscious control. Level III, or relationship contracts, focuses on the repetitive or cyclical nature of patient problems as shown in their day-to-day relationships. Level IV contracts involve structural change and require intensive psychotherapy. The emphasis here is on reworking the entire pathological structure, as well as the here-and-now relationship process. Nurse therapists entering into level IV contracts require master's degree preparation and perhaps even specialized training in the theory and application of structural change treatment approaches. Since the level of contract can change over time, this contracting model allows the nurse and patient to evaluate their progress over time, renegotiate their work together, and determine the termination of a treatment relationship.

■ **EXPLORING FEELINGS.** Both the nurse and patient may experience some degree of discomfort and nervousness in the introduction phase of the relationship because of its newness and the expectations each person brings to it. The nurse may be well aware of

TABLE 4-3

LEVELS OF CHANGE CONTRACTS

Level and type of contract	Focus of care	Nursing action
I Care contracts	Physical safety	Provide physical care
	Emotional safety	Protect from loss of functional abilities
	Avoid predictable negative outcomes	
II Social control contracts	Self-care activities	Crisis intervention
	Problem-solving ability	Brief therapy
	Alteration in time structuring	
	Alteration in reinforcement patterns	
III Relationship contracts	Relationship patterns	Insight work
	Life-script decisions	Cognitive restructuring
	Traumatic early scenes	Marital, family, or relationship counseling
IV Structural change contracts	Parental modeling	Script analysis
	Persistent early injunctions	Reparenting work
		Psychotherapy

From Loomis M: J Psychosoc Nurs Ment Health Serv 23(3):10, 1985.

personal anxieties and fears, but the difficulty inherent in the patient's role often is often overlooked. Receiving help can be difficult from the patient's point of view for the following reasons:

1. It may be hard to admit one's difficulties, first to oneself and then to another, and to see them clearly.
2. It is not easy to trust strangers and be open with them.
3. Sometimes problems seem too large, too overwhelming, or too unique to share them easily.
4. Sharing one's problems with another person can pose a threat to one's sense of independence, autonomy, and self-esteem. Some may view this sharing as a sign of weakness or failure.
5. It is very difficult to commit oneself to change. Solving a problem involves thinking about some things that may be unpleasant, viewing life realistically, deciding on a plan of action, and then, most important, carrying out whatever it takes to bring about a change. These activities place great demands on the patient's energy and commitment.

If this is the nursing student's first psychiatric experience, he or she may feel particularly stressed. Stacklum[60] identified a process that all new students go through in the beginning of their relationships. In the first stage, they experience a moderate to severe level of anxiety characterized by selective inattention to instructions, obsession with detail, dissociation of theory from practice, and avoidance behavior.

Stage two is characterized by the student's use of the defense mechanisms of denial of the patient's problems and strong identification with the patient. Social conversation with the patient predominates, and nursing actions tend to be concrete and simple. In stage three, the student questions his or her own ability and experiences feelings of anger and omnipotence. Hostility often is projected onto the staff.

From these early reactions students hopefully progress to a beginning adjustment stage, which marks the transition into the working phase of the relationship. Students now are truly able to hear what the patient is saying; their anxiety is decreased; their interactions show more depth and insight; and their nursing actions become more realistic. A therapeutic process has begun.

The tasks of the nurse in the orientation phase of the relationship are:

1. to explore the patient's perceptions, thoughts, feelings, and actions
2. to identify pertinent patient problems
3. to define with the patient, mutual, specific goals

It is not uncommon for patients to display manipulative or testing behavior during this phase as they explore the nurse's consistency and intent. Patients may also show temporary regressions during the sessions as reactions to a large amount of self-disclosure in a previous meeting or to the anxiety created by a particular topic.

■ Working phase

Most of the therapeutic work is carried out during the working phase. The nurse and the patient explore relevant stressors and promote the development of insight in the patient by linking his perceptions, thoughts, feelings, and actions. These insights should be translated into action and integrated into the individual's life experiences. The nurse helps the patient to master anxieties, increase independence and self-responsibility, and develop constructive coping mechanisms. Actual behavioral change is the focus of this phase of the relationship.

Patients usually display resistance behaviors during this phase of the relationship, because this phase encompasses the greater part of the problem-solving process. As the relationship develops, the patient panics when he recognizes his beginning feelings of closeness to the nurse, and he fears impending disintegration. He responds by clinging to his defensive structures, and he resists the nurse's attempts to move forward. An impasse or plateau in the relationship results. Since overcoming resistance behaviors is crucial to the progress of the therapeutic relationship, these behaviors are discussed in greater detail later in this chapter.

■ Termination phase

Termination is one of the most difficult but most critically important phases of the therapeutic nurse-patient relationship. However, little has been researched or written about the process and outcome of termination. Schiff has said:

Of all the phases of the psychotherapeutic process, the one which can produce the greatest amount of difficulty and create substantial problems for patient and therapist alike is the phase of termination. It is at this time when the impact of the meaning, in affective terms, of the course of therapy and the nature of the therapist-patient relationship is experienced most keenly, not only by the patient but also by the therapist.[55:77]

During the termination phase learning is maximized for both the patient and the nurse. It is a time to exchange feelings and memories and to evaluate mutually the patient's progress and goal attainment. Levels of trust and intimacy are heightened, reflecting the quality of the relationship and the sense of loss experienced by both nurse and patient. The accompanying box lists criteria identified by Campaniello that can

---

Criteria for Determining Patient Readiness for Termination[9]

1. The patient experiences relief from the presenting problem.
2. The patient's social function has improved, and his isolation has decreased.
3. The patient has strengthened his own ego functions and attained a sense of identity.
4. The patient employs more effective and productive defense mechanisms.
5. The patient has achieved the planned treatment goals.
6. An impasse has been reached in the therapist-patient relationship because of resistance or countertransference that cannot be worked through.

---

be used to determine whether the patient is ready to terminate.

Although agreement between the patient and the therapist is desirable in deciding when to terminate, this is not always possible. Sometimes the reason is beyond the control of either person, such as when it is the result of an institutional rule, the end of a clinical rotation, or the eventual move of the therapist.

Regardless of the reason, the nurse's tasks during this phase revolve around establishing the reality of the separation. Together the nurse and the patient review the progress made in therapy and the attainment of specified goals. Feelings of rejection, loss, sadness, and anger are expressed and explored. The patient's dependence on the nurse should decrease, and his interdependence with his environment and significant others should increase. It may be helpful to prepare the patient for termination by decreasing the number of visits, incorporating others into the meetings, or changing the location of the meetings. If a change is made, the reasons behind it should be clarified with the patient, so he does not interpret it as rejection by the nurse. It may also be appropriate to make referrals at this time for continued care or treatment.

One's understanding of the feelings that accompany termination can be enhanced by examining Fox, Nelson, and Bolman's comparison[20] of the phases in the termination process to the phases of grief work:

The first phase is a period of denial in which the person attempts to ward off either recognition of the loss or important feelings associated with it. The second, a phase that begins when the denial breaks down, is one of considerable emotional expression, usually of grief and sadness but often including anger and expressions of narcissistic hurt. The third phase is a prolonged period in which the reality of loss and the associated feelings of grief and anger are bit by bit worked through in the multitude of current life experiences that bring up memories of the lost person. To the extent that the mourner is able to perform this grief work successfully, he is gradually able to detach or free the emotional ties that are essential for finding new people or interests.*

In light of this comparison, it is evident that successful termination requires that the patient work through those feelings related to separation from emotionally significant people. The nurse can help the patient accomplish this by allowing him to experience and feel the effects of the anticipated loss, to express those feelings generated by the impending separation, and to relate his feelings to former symbolic or real losses.

■ **REACTIONS TO TERMINATION.** Patients may react to termination in a variety of ways. They may deny the separation or deny the significance of the relationship and impending separation. The inexperienced nurse, not seeing the reasons behind this denial, might feel rejected by the patient or believe that he or she has failed him. Patients may express anger and hostility, either overtly and verbally or covertly through lateness, missed meetings, or superficial talk. These patients may view the termination as personal rejection, which reinforces their negative self-concept. Patients who feel rejected by the nurse may terminate prematurely. By thus ending the relationship, they experience a sense of power and control and assert themselves by rejecting the nurse before she rejects them. It is also common to see the onset of symptoms and maladaptive behavior when termination approaches. In this way the patient regresses to his earlier behavior pattern and hopes to convince the nurse not to terminate because he still needs help.

The nurse who is aware of these possible reactions can anticipate them and discuss them with the patient if they occur. For some patients termination is a critical therapeutic experience, because many of their past relationships were terminated in a negative way that left them with unresolved feelings of abandonment, rejection, hurt, and anger. All these patient reactions have a similar goal—to cope with the anxiety about the separation and to delay the termination process.

Levinson[39] has identified five factors that can in-

fluence the patient's reaction of the patient to termination:

1. The greater the degree of involvement the patient has had in the treatment and with the therapist, the more intense will be the nature of the reaction to termination.
2. Reaction to termination will vary with the degree of success and satisfaction the patient feels with the treatment.
3. The greater the degree of transference involvement and wished-for gratification or fulfillment of childlike wishes, the more intense will be the nature of the patient's reaction to termination.
4. Patients who have sustained earlier losses of significant persons in their lives will reexperience, as termination approaches, the arousal of affects and conflicts from those earlier periods.
5. Whether the patient has experienced key losses or not, his reaction to termination will be influenced by the level at which he has mastered the early separation—individuation crisis.

The patient's response also will be significantly affected by the nurse's ability to remain open, sensitive, empathic, and responsive to the patient's changing needs. Helping the patient to work and grow through the termination process is an essential goal of each relationship. It is important therefore that the nurse does not deny the reality of it or allow himself or herself to be manipulated by the patient into repeated delays. Particularly in this phase of the relationship, as in the orientation phase, the patient will be testing the nurse's judgment, and the issues of trust and acceptance will again predominate.

During the course of the relationship and with the attainment of nursing goals, the nurse and the patient come to realize a growing sense of equality. The impending termination therefore can be as difficult for the nurse as for the patient. The nurse must deal with his or her reaction to the various aspects of termination to make this a positive learning experience for the nurse and patient. The nurse who can begin reviewing his or her thoughts, feelings, and experiences, will be more aware of personal motivation and more responsive to the patient's needs. Schultz states:

When the student shares her own feelings and explains how she, too, feels the pain and separation, the patient can learn it is not he alone who needs to be dependent on others and to cling to successful relationships, but that life is a series of making and breaking relationships. The student and the patient learn that to be involved with other human beings is part of living, often a very satisfying part, but there is a time to love and a time to leave. . . . That allowing another to

---

TABLE 4-4

NURSE'S TASKS IN EACH PHASE OF THE RELATIONSHIP PROCESS

Phase	Task
Preinteraction	Explore own feelings, fantasies, and fears
	Analyze own professional strengths and limitations
	Gather data about patient when possible
	Plan for first meeting with patient
Introductory or orientation	Determine why patient sought help
	Establish trust, acceptance, and open communication
	Mutually formulate a contract
	Explore patient's thoughts, feelings, and actions
	Identify patient's problems
	Define goals with patient
Working	Explore relevant stressors
	Promote patient's development of insight and use of constructive coping mechanisms
	Overcome resistance behaviors
Termination	Establish reality of separation
	Review progress of therapy and attainment of goals
	Mutually explore feelings of rejection, loss, sadness, and anger and related behaviors

---

mourn with you, to share the agony of separation unashamedly, could be an answer to bridging some of the gulf between human beings in need of one another.[57:41-42]

Learning to bear the sorrow of the loss while working positive aspects of the relationship into one's life is the goal of termination for both the nurse and the patient.

The major tasks of the nurse during each phase of the nurse-patient relationship are summarized in Table 4-4.

Facilitative communication

Communication can either facilitate the development of a therapeutic relationship or serve as a barrier to its development. Nurses should understand the elements of the communication process and use specific techniques that help the patient work through the problem-solving process. According to Carkhoff and Truax, "The central ingredient of the psychotherapeutic process appears to be the therapist's ability to *perceive and communicate,* accurately and with sensitivity, the feelings of the patient and the meaning of those feelings."[13:28]

Every individual communicates constantly from birth until death. As Watzlawick, Beavin, and Jackson[64] have stated, all behavior is communication and all communication affects behavior. This reciprocity is central to the communication process. One of the most widely respected communication theorists is Jur-

gen Ruesch. He has defined communication as "all those processes by which people influence one another."[53] These definitions focus on both behavioral change and interpersonal influence as factors in communication.

The relevance of communication theory to nursing practice is apparent. First, communication is the vehicle for establishing a therapeutic relationship, since it involves conveying information and exchanging thoughts and feelings. Second, communication is the means by which people influence the behavior of another. Thus it is critical to the successful outcome of nursing intervention. Finally, communication is the relationship itself, since without it, a therapeutic nurse-patient relationship is impossible.

■ Verbal communication

Communication takes place on two levels, verbal and nonverbal. Verbal communication occurs through the medium of words, spoken or written. Taken alone, verbal communication can convey factual information accurately and efficiently. It is a less effective means of communicating feelings or nuances of meaning, and it represents only a small segment of total human communication.

Another limitation of verbal communication is that words can change meanings with different cultural groups or subgroups. The reason is that words have both denotative and connotative meanings. The denotative meaning of a word is the concrete representation of it. For example, the denotative meaning of the word "bread" is "a food made of a flour or grain dough that is kneaded, shaped, allowed to rise, and baked." The connotative meaning of a word, in contrast, is its implied or suggested meaning. Thus the word "bread" can conjure up many different connotative or personalized meanings. Depending on a person's experiences, preferences, and present frame of reference, he may think of French bread, rye bread, a sesame seed roll, or perhaps pita bread. The phrase "Give me some bread" can even have another meaning. When used as slang, it may be commonly understood to mean "give me some money." Once again the characteristics of the speaker and the context in which the phrase is used influence the specific meaning of verbal language.

When communicating verbally, many people assume that they are "on the same wavelength" as the listener. But since words are only symbols, they seldom mean precisely the same thing to two people. And if the word represents an abstract idea such as "depressed" or "hurt," the chance of misunderstanding or misinterpretation may be great. In addition, many feeling states or personal thoughts cannot be put into words easily. A nurse who wishes to communicate effectively must be aware of the limitations and possible problems inherent with verbal language. The nurse should strive to overcome these obstacles by checking his or her interpretation and incorporating information from the nonverbal level as well.

■ **Nonverbal communication**

Nonverbal communication includes everything that does not involve the spoken or written word, including all of the five senses. It has been estimated that about 7% of meaning is transmitted by words; 38% is transmitted by paralinguistic cues, such as voice; and 55% is transmitted by body cues.[43] Nonverbal communication serves many functions in relating to others: supplementing, substituting, reinforcing, contradicting, and emphasizing verbal language; displaying emotion; and regulating the flow of information. This level of communication often is unconsciously motivated and may more accurately indicate a person's meaning than the words he is saying. People tend to verbalize what they think the receiver wants to hear, whereas less acceptable or more honest messages may be communicated simultaneously by the nonverbal route.

■ **TYPES OF NONVERBAL BEHAVIORS.** Various types of nonverbal behaviors have been identified. Following are brief descriptions of five categories of non-

verbal communication. **Vocal cues,** or paralinguistic cues, include all the noises and sounds that are extraspeech sounds. Some examples include pitch, tone of voice, quality of voice, loudness or intensity, rate and rhythm of talking, and unrelated nonverbal sounds such as laughing, groaning, and nervous coughing and sounds of hesitation ("um," "uh"). These are particularly vital cues of emotion and can be powerful conveyors of information.

Action cues are body movements, sometimes referred to as kinetics. They include automatic reflexes, posture, facial expression, gestures, mannerisms, and actions of any kind. Facial movements and posture can be particularly significant in interpreting the speaker's mood.

Object cues are the speaker's intentional and nonintentional use of all objects. Dress, furnishings, and possessions all communicate something to the observer about the speaker's sense of self. These cues often are consciously selected by the individual, however, and therefore may be chosen to convey a certain "look" or message. Thus they can be less accurate than other types of nonverbal communication.

Space provides another clue to the nature of the relationship between two people. Hall[24] extensively researched proxemics, the use of space between communicators, and identified the following four zones of space that are demonstrated interpersonally in North America:

1. Intimate space—up to 45.5 cm (18 inches). This allows for maximum interpersonal sensory stimulation.
2. Personal space—45.5 to 120 cm (18 inches to 4 feet). This is used for close relationships and touching distance. Visual sensation is improved over the intimate range.
3. Social-consultative space—270 to 360 cm (9 to 12 feet). This is less personal and less dependent. Speech must be louder.
4. Public space—360 cm (12 feet) and over. This is used in speech giving and other public occasions.

Observation of seating arrangements and use of space by patients can yield valuable information to the nurse, with implications for both the nurse's assessment of the patient and the way the nursing intervention should be implemented.

Touch involves both personal space and action. It is possibly the most personal of the nonverbal messages. A person's response to it is influenced by setting, cultural background, type of relationship, sex of communicators, ages, and expectations. Touch can have many meanings. It can express a striving to connect with another person as a way of meeting them or relating to them. It can be a way of expressing or conveying something to another, such as concern, empathy, or caring. Touch can also be used receptively as a way of sensing, perceiving, or allowing someone else to leave their imprint on another. Finally, Krieger[35] has developed the concept of "therapeutic touch," or the nurse's laying hands on or close to the body of an ill person for the purpose of helping or healing. Krieger believes touch to be the imprimatur of nursing and contends that the therapeutic, comforting effects of touch often have been overlooked in nursing.

Touch is a universal and basic aspect of all nurse-patient relationships. It is often described as the first and most fundamental means of communication. Nevertheless, relatively little is really known about touch as it relates to health.[66] This is clearly one area in which many questions exist and many aspects remain unexplored. For example, one recent study comparing nurse and patient perceptions of touch found that male patients interpreted touch from a female nurse more positively than did female patients; however, female nurses interpreted female patients' behavior as being more receptive to touch and therefore appeared to be more comfortable touching female rather than male patients.[37] These variables and the therapeutic value of touch merit further examination through nursing research.

■ **INTERPRETING NONVERBAL BEHAVIOR.**
All types of nonverbal messages are important, but interpreting them correctly can present numerous problems for the nurse. Body messages are rapid, often imprecise, and extremely complex. It is impossible to examine nonverbal messages out of context, and sometimes one's body reveals a number of different and perhaps conflicting feelings at the same time. Cultural background is also a major influence on the meaning of nonverbal behavior. In the United States, with its diverse ethnic communities, messages between people of different upbringing can easily be misinterpreted. Some people may have been taught to suppress hand and facial expressions; others may not show emotional response. For instance, Arabs tend to stand closer together when speaking, and Orientals tend to touch more; touching in the United States is often minimized because of perceived sexual overtones or one's Puritan heritage. Because the meaning attached to nonverbal behavior is so subjective, it is essential that the nurse check its meaning.

Nurses should respond to the variety of nonverbal behaviors displayed by the patient, particularly voice inflections, body movements, gestures, facial expres-

sion, posture, and physical energy levels. Incongruent behavior or contradictory messages are especially significant. The nurse should refer to the specific behavior observed and attempt to confirm its meaning and significance with the patient. If the nurse's words and tone of voice indicate that he or she is truly clarifying, suggesting, or validating, a defensive reaction usually is not evoked. The nurse may use three kinds of responses to the patient:

1. Questions or statements intended to increase the patient's awareness
2. Content reflections
3. Statements reflecting the nurse's responsiveness

These possible responses are illustrated in the following interaction.

PATIENT: **(Shifting nervously in his chair, eyes scanning the room and avoiding the nurse) What . . . what do you want to talk about today?**
NURSE: **I sense that you are uncomfortable talking to me. Could you describe to me how you are feeling?**
NURSE: **You're not sure what we should be talking about, and you want me to start us off?**
NURSE: **You look very nervous, and I can feel those same feelings in me as I sit here with you.**

The nurse's first possible response is a reflection and attempt to validate the patient's feelings. The purpose is to communicate to the patient the nurse's awareness of his feelings, to show acceptance of those feelings, and to request that he focus on them and elaborate on them. The nurse's second possible response deals with the content of the patient's message. The nurse here is clarifying what the patient is trying to say. The third possible response shares both the nurse's perception of her patient's feelings and the personal disclosure that she has some of those same feelings. This type of response may help the patient feel that the nurse accepts and understands him.

■ **IMPLICATIONS FOR NURSING CARE.** Besides responding to the patient's nonverbal behavior, the nurse should incorporate aspects of it into the patient's care. This may be most evident in the use of space in the nurse-patient relationship. A patient who resists closeness will recoil from entry into his intimate space. The close distance area of personal space may also be intolerable to a patient who fears closeness. The nurse can assess the patient's level of spatial tolerance by observing the distance the patient maintains with other people. The nurse can also be alert to the patient's response when he or she interacts with him. If the nurse sits next to him on the sofa, does he get up and move to a chair? If the nurse pulls her chair closer to him, does he move his chair away to reestablish the original space? Sometimes increasing the space between the nurse and an anxious patient can alleviate the anxiety enough to allow the interaction to continue. A decrease in the distance the patient chooses to maintain from others may indicate a decrease in interpersonal anxiety.

Territoriality is a concept related to those of personal distance and personal space. Territoriality is the drive to acquire and defend territory in order to assure species' survival. In analyzing territorial behavior among the chronically institutionalized mentally ill, Cooper found that territoriality can be measured by determining the prevalence and degree of the following behaviors:

- Attempting to consistently sit in the same area or chair
- Arranging concrete boundaries around one's body
- Rearranging body position to face away from others
- Avoiding eye contact
- Sitting side-by-side rather than face-to-face
- Increased sleeping or retreat into drugs, fantasies, etc.
- Various adornments of the body[15]

Cooper believes that whenever possible, the hospitalized patient should be allowed to control and enjoy personal possessions and private living space, no matter how small or seemingly insignificant. Specifically, residents should be allowed free access to their personal living quarters and, as soon as possible, free access out of doors or at least off the ward itself. Residents can also be encouraged to wear personal clothing and keep personal items. In summary, hospitalized patients' territorial behavior should be recognized and its free expression allowed, while at the same time attempting to decrease the crowding and high density that threatens it.

Argyle[3] enumerates other spatial parameters that are interpersonally significant. Height may communicate dominance and submission. Communication is made easier when both participants are at similar levels. Orientation of the participants' body positions is also significant. Face-to-face confrontation is more threatening than oblique (sideways) body positions. The physical setting also has spatial meaning. Ownership of a space affects the communication context. A patient may be more comfortable in his own room than in the therapist's office, unless the patient's room is also defined as bedroom. Control issues are minimized when communication takes place in a neutral area that belongs to neither participant. However,

people quickly identify their own turf, even in unfamiliar settings, and then begin to exert ownership rights over this area. A common example of this can be observed in most college classes. At the beginning of the semester, people seat themselves somewhat randomly, but the arrangement usually solidifies after a couple of classes. Students then feel vaguely annoyed if they arrive in class to find another person in "their seat." They are experiencing an invasion of personal space. Awareness of a patient's use of space can add a further dimension to the nurse's ability to understand the patient.

Touch also should be used judiciously. It is a powerful communicative tool. Patients who are sensitive to issues of closeness may experience a casual touch as an invasion or an invitation to intimacy, which may be even more frightening. Physical contact with a person of the same sex may be experienced by the patient as a homosexual advance and may precipitate a panic reaction. If procedures requiring physical contact must be carried out, careful explanations should be given both before and during the procedure. An efficient, impersonal, but caring approach to physical nursing care may be least threatening to a patient experiencing interpersonal anxiety.

The last point to be made here regarding nonverbal communication is that the nurse must not only be aware of the patient's nonverbal cues but must also be aware of his or her own. The nurse's nonverbal cues can communicate interest, respect, and genuineness or disinterest, lack of respect, and an impersonal facade. La Crosse[36] did a study of nonverbal behaviors to determine which promoted relating to someone else and which prohibited it. He concluded that affiliative nonverbal behavior included smiles, positive head nods, gestures, 80% eye contact, and a 20% forward body lean. Unaffiliative nonverbal behavior included 40% eye contact, a 20% reclining body lean, and none of the other categories. Furthermore, affiliative counselors were perceived to be more attractive and persuasive than unaffiliative ones. The implication of this type of research is that nurses, as therapeutic helpers, need to be aware of a spectrum of nonverbal behaviors in their patients and themselves and then incorporate them judiciously into their care.

The communication process

Human communication is a dynamic process influenced by the psychological and physiological conditions of the participants. Ruesch[54] has identified three elements of the process: perception, evaluation, and transmission. Perception occurs by activation of the sensory end organs of the receiver. The impulse is then transmitted to the brain. Human beings are most reliant on visual and auditory stimuli for communications. Vision is the primary means of perceiving nonverbal communication, and hearing primarily responds to verbal stimuli. However, if one of the primary senses is dysfunctional, the other functional senses accommodate to improve the person's perception. For instance, the deaf person can learn sign language and lip-reading, which rely on vision, to compensate for not being able to hear the verbal component of communication.

When the sensory impulse reaches the brain, evaluation takes place. The person analyzes and categorizes the message in terms of its meaning. Personal experience is the matrix within which new experience is evaluated. If the person encounters a new experience for which there is no frame of reference, confusion results. Evaluation results in two responses: a cognitive response and an affective response. The cognitive response relates to the informational aspect of the message, and the affective response relates to the relationship aspect of the message. Most messages stimulate both types of responses.

When the evaluation of the message is complete, transmission takes place. This is perceived by the sender as feedback, thereby influencing the continued course of the communication cycle. Transmission must take place once communication has been initiated. It is impossible not to transmit some kind of feedback. Even lack of any visible response is feedback to the sender that the message did not get through, was considered unimportant, was an undesirable interruption, or any of a number of other possible interpretations. Feedback stimulates perception, evaluation, and transmission by the original sender. The cycle continues un-

til the participants agree to end it or one participant physically leaves the setting.

Theoretical models of the communication process help one to visualize its dynamic nature. They show visual relationships more clearly and can aid in finding and correcting communication breakdowns or problems. Two models, the structural and transactional analysis models, are presented, since each gives a valuable but different perspective on the communication process.

■ **STRUCTURAL MODEL.** The structural model has five functional components in communication: the sender, the message, the receiver, the feedback, and the context[69] (Fig. 4-4). The **sender** is the originator of the message, which is then transmitted to the receiver. The **message** is the information that is transmitted from the sender to the receiver. The **receiver** is the perceiver of the message, which influences his behavior in some way. The verbal or behavioral response of the receiver is **feedback** to the sender. Feedback, as defined here, functions as described in general systems theory. Positive feedback promotes change within the system, and negative feedback promotes stability. An example of positive feedback might be the receiver unexpectedly telling the sender that the message made him angry, whereas negative feedback might be to respond exactly as the sender anticipated. When viewed structurally, communication is a circular process. The designation of sender and message and receiver and feedback is somewhat arbitrary once the cycle has begun, since feedback is also a new message initiated by the receiver, who then becomes the sender.

The fifth structural element of communication is the **context.** This is the setting in which the communi-

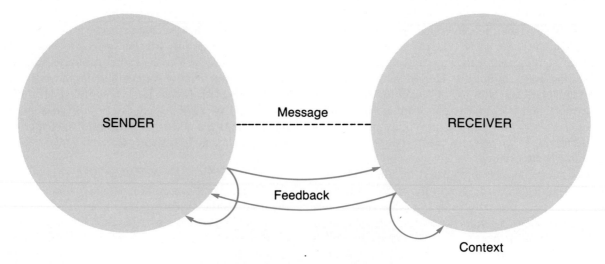

Fig. 4-4. Components of communication.

cation takes place. Knowledge of context is necessary to understand the meaning of the communication. For example, the phrase "I don't understand what you mean" may have different meanings in the context of a classroom or a courtroom. Context involves more than the physical setting for communication, however. It also includes the psychosocial setting, which includes the relationship between the sender and the receiver, their past experiences with each other, and past experiences with similar situations, and cultural values and norms. Consider again the meaning of "I don't understand what you mean" in the following contexts: two college students discussing a philosophy assignment, a wife responding to her husband's accusation of infidelity, and a Japanese tourist asking directions in San Francisco. Although the content of the message is the same, its meaning is different, depending on the context in which the communication takes place.

Related problems. If one evaluates the communication process with regard to the five structural elements, specific problems or potential errors become evident. These problems are summarized in Table 4-5. First, the sender must be communicating the same message on both the verbal and nonverbal levels. If he does this, the sender's communication is termed **congruent.** If, however, the levels are not in agreement, the communication is termed **incongruent,** which can be problematic.

CONGRUENT COMMUNICATION

VERBAL LEVEL: **I'm pleased to see you.**
NONVERBAL LEVEL: **Voice sounds warm; continuous eye contact maintained; smile.**

INCONGRUENT COMMUNICATION

VERBAL LEVEL: **I'm pleased to see you.**
NONVERBAL LEVEL: **Voice sounds cold and distant; eye contact avoided; neutral facial expression.**

Incongruent, or double-level, messages produce a dilemma for the listener; he does not know to which level he should respond, the verbal or nonverbal. Since he cannot respond to both, he is likely to feel frustrated, angry, or confused. This is a double-bind situation in which one is "damned if you do, and damned if you don't." Obviously, both patients and nurses can display incongruent communication if they are not aware of their internal feeling states and the nature of their communication.

Another problem initiated by the sender is that of inflexible communication. This is communication that is either too rigid or too permissive. A rigid approach is one of exaggerated control by the nurse; it may be evident in the overuse of a standardized history or assessment form. It does not allow the patient to spontaneously express himself, nor does it allow him to contribute to the flow or direction of the interaction. Exaggerated permissiveness, on the other hand, refers to a nurse who does not share personal thoughts or impressions with the patient; thus the interaction lacks direction and mutuality. The patient may interpret the nurse's behavior as lack of interest or incompetence.

The next element of the communication process, the message, can also pose problems. Basically, problem messages are ineffective, inappropriate, inadequate, or inefficient. Ineffective messages are not goal-directed or purposeful. They serve at least to distract

---

TABLE 4-5

SPECIFIC PROBLEMS ASSOCIATED WITH THE STRUCTURAL ELEMENTS OF THE COMMUNICATION PROCESS

Structural element	Communication problem	Definition
Sender	Incongruent communication	Lack of agreement between the verbal and nonverbal levels of communication
	Inflexible communication	Exaggerated control or permissiveness by the sender
Message	Ineffective messages	Messages that are not goal-directed or purposeful
	Inappropriate messages	Messages not relevant to the progress of the relationship
	Inadequate messages	Messages that lack a sufficient amount of information
	Inefficient messages	Messages that lack clarity, simplicity, and directness
Receiver	Errors of perception	Various forms of listening problems
	Errors of evaluation	Misinterpretation due to personal beliefs and values
Feedback	Misinformation	Communication of incorrect information
	Lack of validation	Failure to clarify and ratify understanding of the message
Context	Constraints of physical setting	Noise, temperature, or various distractions
	Constraints of psychosocial setting	Impaired previous relationship between the communicators

and at most to prevent the objectives of the nurse-patient relationship from being met. Inappropriate messages are not relevant to the progress of the relationship. They may include failures in timing, stereotyping the receiver, or overlooking important information. Inadequate messages lack a sufficient amount of information. The sender assumes that the receiver knows more than he actually does. Inefficient messages lack clarity, simplicity, and directness. Using more energy than is necessary, these messages confuse or complicate the information. The sender can do this consciously or unconsciously, possibly because of disease in the organ of communication (e.g., stuttering) or because of a lack of knowledge or poor use of language.

The third element, the receiver, is subject to the same problems as the sender plus some additional ones. The receiver may experience errors of perception in which he misses nonverbal cues, responds only to content and ignores messages of affect, is selectively inattentive to the speaker's message because of his own physical or psychological discomfort, is preoccupied with other thoughts, or has a physiological hearing impairment. All of these errors are fundamentally problems of listening. The receiver may also experience problems in evaluating the message. He may misinterpret the meaning of the message, because he views it in terms of his own value system rather than that of the speaker. In this case he is not being open to the speaker but is judging him on the basis of his own personal experiences and beliefs. He might also interpret a symbolic message literally or a literal one symbolically.

Errors in the feedback element include all of those that apply to the message. Feedback can also convey to the sender incorrect information about the message. Another serious error exists when the receiver fails to use feedback to validate his understanding of the message. Although feedback is the last step in the cyclical communication process, it has the potential for correcting previous errors and clarifying the nature of the communication.

The fifth element of context can also contribute to communication problems. The setting may be physically noisy, cold, or distracting to one or both parties. So, too, the psychosocial context, or past relationship between the communicators, may be one of mistrust or harbored resentment. This analysis shows the complexity of the communication process. It may even seem surprising that successful communication can occur, given all of these vulnerable areas. However, it can and does occur among those people who understand the process, have analyzed the elements of it, and use appropriate techniques.

■ **TRANSACTIONAL ANALYSIS MODEL.** Transactional analysis (TA) is the study of the communica-tion or transactions that take place between people; it uncovers the sometimes unconscious and destructive ways ("games") in which people relate to each other. This approach to personality was developed by Berne, a psychiatrist who made transactional analysis a popular theory through his book, *Games People Play: The Psychology of Human Relationships.*[4] It is a method of therapy, as well as a model of communication.

The cornerstone of Berne's theory is that each person's personality is made up of three distinct components called **ego states.** An ego state is a consistent pattern of feeling, experiencing, and behaving. The three ego states that make up one's personality are the parent ego state (parent); adult ego state (adult), and child ego state (child) (Fig. 4-5). It is as though each person actually has three "people" inside him: the "parent" incorporates all the attitudes and behavior the individual was taught (directly or indirectly) by his parents; the "child" contains all the feelings the individual had as a child; and the "adult" deals with reality in a logical, rational, computer-like manner. These three ego states are distinct, each having a consistent pattern of feeling, experiencing, and behaving.

The parent and child ego states are made up of the feelings, attitudes, and behaviors that are remnants of the past but can be reexperienced under certain conditions. The parent ego state consists of all the nurturing, critical, and prejudicial attitudes, behaviors, and experiences learned from other people, especially parents and teachers. The adult ego state is the reality-oriented part of the personality. It gathers and processes information about the world and is objective, emotionless, and intelligent in its approach to problem solving. The child ego state is the feeling part of the

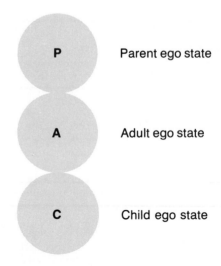

Fig. 4-5. Three ego states as described by Berne's theory of transactional analysis.

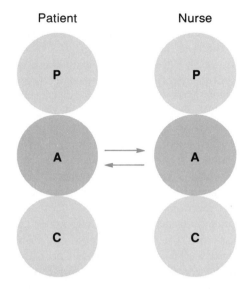

Fig. 4-6. Diagram of complementary transaction.

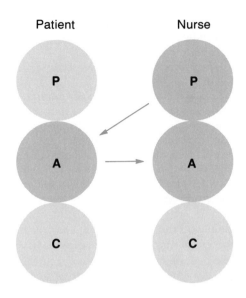

Fig. 4-7. Diagram of a crossed transaction.

personality. In it resides feelings of happiness, joy, sadness, depression, and anxiety.

Berne's model of communication allows one to diagram transactions using these ego states. Transactional analysis then focuses on the communication between people. A transaction or communication between two people can be complementary, crossed, or ulterior. In a **complementary transaction** (Fig. 4-6), the arrows in the ego state diagram are parallel, and the communication flows smoothly.

COMPLEMENTARY TRANSACTION

PATIENT: **I know that when I get mad at my boss, I take it out on my wife and kids.**
NURSE: **Are you ready to think about some other ways you can handle your anger?**

If the arrows in the ego state diagram **cross,** however, communication breaks down (Fig. 4-7).

CROSSED TRANSACTION

PATIENT: **I know that when I get mad at my boss, I take it out on my wife and kids.**
NURSE: **Men always think that's okay, but the women have to suffer for it.**

The third type of transaction is **ulterior** transaction (Fig. 4-8). It takes place on two levels: the social, or overt, level and the psychological, or covert, level. These transactions tend to be destructive, because the communicators conceal their true motivations. One of the best known examples of this is the "Why Don't You . . . Yes But" (WDYYB) game. This game involves one person asking for a solution to a problem; however, every suggested solution is negated, until the

helper is silenced. On the surface, the interaction is two adults problem solving; in reality, one person is using his child to show what a bad parent the other person is.

ULTERIOR TRANSACTION

PATIENT: **I know that when I get mad at my boss, I take it out on my wife and kids, but I don't know what else to do.**

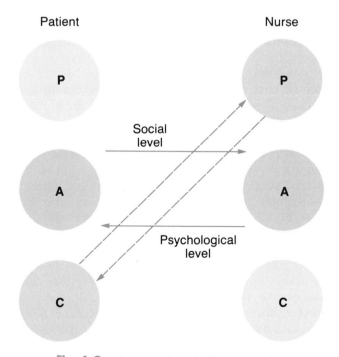

Fig. 4-8. Diagram of an ulterior transaction.

NURSE: **Do you think you could let your boss know how you're feeling?**
PATIENT: **He'll fire me for sure.**
NURSE: **Perhaps you could talk it over with someone you work with.**
PATIENT: **I don't have time to chat on the job like that. Besides, no one cares about someone else's beefs.**
NURSE: **Sometimes physical exercise helps people get rid of their anger. Have you ever tried it?**
PATIENT: **Sure. I work out a lot, but it doesn't help.**
NURSE: **Perhaps you can explain all this to your family.**
PATIENT: **My wife's tired of "all my talk" as she puts it. She says she wants some action.**

The value of the transactional analysis model of communication is that it provides a framework for the nurse to use in exploring the patient's recurrent behaviors, identifying patterns, postulating causes, and planning alternative ways to respond. Thus nonproductive communication patterns can be stopped and new, healthier, ones learned.

■ Therapeutic communication techniques

Ginott[23] believes that there are two basic requirements for effective communication:

1. that all communication be aimed at preserving the self-respect of both the helper and the helpee
2. that the communication of understanding precede any suggestions of information or advice giving

These requirements lay the groundwork for therapeutic communication. Such communication makes possible the formation of the nurse-patient relationship and the implementation of the nursing process. The collection of data and the planning, implementation, and evaluation activities are carried out *with* the patient, not *for* the patient, when the nurse uses therapeutic communication skills.

Some nurses reject the notion of therapeutic communication techniques because they view them as unnatural, ineffective, or stereotypical. Like all learned skills, these techniques can beabused, used too frequently, or incorrectly applied. Nor does knowledge of these skills ensure successful therapeutic communication. Although simple on the surface, these techniques are difficult and require practice and conscious thought to master. Because they are techniques, they are only as effective as the person using them. If they are worked into the nurse's existing interpersonal skills, they can enhance his or her effectiveness. If they are used as automatic responses and are inappropriate to

the nurse's manner of personal expression, they will negate both the nurse's and the patient's individuality and divest them of their dignity.

To ensure that the nurse is using these skills appropriately and effectively, the nurse needs to record interactions with the patient in some way and then analyze them. The nurse should also seek feedback from others. Many tools are available to help in this area. The nurse can benefit from maintaining a diary of his or her thoughts, feelings, and impressions in relation to clinical work. This can prove valuable in working through difficult aspects of termination or countertransference reactions.

The nurse may decide to tape record or videotape interactions with the patient. These are two of the most informative recording methods, and they also allow the nurse the freedom to concentrate on the patient. However, they do present problems: Sometimes another person is needed to operate the equipment; there is always the possibility of equipment failure; equipment can be expensive to obtain and operate and may be prohibited by the agency; and such equipment can raise questions about confidentiality.

Handwritten records are less expensive and do not require mechanical devices. They also allow the nurse to record his or her thoughts and feelings along with the verbal and nonverbal behavior. However, they require more time and energy. If such records are written in the patient's presence, they can be very distracting. If they are written afterward, some aspects of the interaction may be unconsciously forgotten or consciously ignored. Often these are most significant omissions.

The advantages and disadvantages of the various methods of recording nurse-patient interactions are summarized in Table 4-6. These must be considered, along with the nurse's and patient's preferences, before deciding on a particular method. Some form of recording that is as objective and comprehensive as possible is necessary. Only by analyzing the interaction can the nurse evaluate the degree of success in using therapeutic communication techniques.

Some of the more helpful techniques will now be described. Other sources present detailed information on the communication process and therapeutic and nontherapeutic communication techniques.[61,62] In addition, common errors in communication made by students in psychiatric nursing are analyzed in an article by Sayre listed in the annotated suggested readings at the end of this chapter. Nontherapeutic techniques are not discussed separately because basically they represent a failure to use an appropriate therapeutic skill. Rather, problems are discussed relative to some of the

TABLE 4-6

ADVANTAGES AND DISADVANTAGES OF VARIOUS METHODS OF RECORDING NURSE-PATIENT INTERACTIONS

Advantages	Disadvantages
Videotape	
Provides excellent opportunity to see, record, and analyze both nonverbal and verbal levels of communication	Mechanical devices are necessary
Participants are not distracted by writing	Mechanical failure can occur
Can be preserved for comparison with future interactions	At least one other person is necessary to operate equipment
Can provide participants with audiovisual feedback of their responses	Often distracting to participants, at least initially
Possible to see and hear entire interaction for review and supervision	Transcriptions are time consuming
Possible to replay segments for comparison, analysis, and supervision	Unless more than one monitor is available, comparison is time consuming
Tape recording	
Complete verbatim conversation is available	Mechanical devices are necessary
Participants are not distracted by writing	Mechanical failure can occur
Can be preserved for comparison with future interactions	Often distracting to participants, at least initially
Can provide participants with audio feedback of their responses	Transcriptions are time consuming
Possible to hear entire interaction for review and supervision	Unless more than one tape recorder is available, comparison is time consuming
Possible to replay segments for comparison, analysis, and supervision	Nonverbal communication is not available
	With cassette tape recorder, often necessary to disrupt interaction to turn tape over
Verbatim notes	
Possible to record thoughts and feelings during interaction	Difficult to concentrate on interaction until technique of writing without looking is mastered
Messages recorded as said rather than as what was intended	Often distracting to participants, at least initially
Possible to quickly review specific areas for comparison, analysis, and supervision	Requires greater skill in recording
Both verbal and nonverbal levels can be recorded	Segments of the interaction are usually missing or incomplete
No mechanical devices to distract participants	
General outline notes	
Possible to record thoughts and feelings during the interaction	Often distracting to participants, at least initially
Possible to quickly review specific areas for comparison, analysis, and supervision	Necessary to fill in general outline with specific data at a later time
Both verbal and nonverbal levels can be recorded	Often actual messages are distorted by intended messages
No mechanical devices to distract	
Requires less skill than verbatim notes	
Decreases amount of energy needed for writing during interaction, hence increases energy available for communication with client	
Postinteraction notes	
No distractions during interaction	Relies entirely on memory
Possible to focus attention entirely on communication process	Often actual messages are distorted by intended messages
Possible to record information at one's convenience	Often tends to be a more haphazard notation and analysis unless one is well organized

From Sundeen SJ et al: Nurse-client interaction: implementing the nursing process, ed 4, St Louis, 1989, The CV Mosby Co.

therapeutic techniques. The emphasis of learning is on a theoretical understanding of therapeutic communication and its appropriate application in a facilitative nurse-patient relationship.

■ **LISTENING.** Listening is essential if the nurse is to reach any understanding of the patient. Only the patient can tell the nurse how he feels, what he thinks, and how he sees himself and the world. Only by listening to the patient can the nurse enter his world and see things as he does. Therefore the first rule of a therapeutic relationship is to listen to the patient. It is the foundation on which all other therapeutic skills are built.

Obviously one cannot listen if one is talking, yet inexperienced nurses often find it difficult not to talk. This may be caused by their anxiety, the need to prove themselves, or a habitual manner of social interaction. It is helpful to remember that the patient should be talking more than the nurse during the interaction; the task of the nurse is to listen.

Real listening is difficult. It is an active, not a passive, process. The nurse should give complete attention to the patient and should not be preoccupied with himself or herself. The nurse should suspend his or her thinking of personal experiences and problems and personal judgments of the patient. Listening is a sign of respect for the patient and is a powerful reinforcer. It reinforces verbalization by the patient, without which the relationship could not progress.

■ **BROAD OPENINGS.** Broad openings such as "What are you thinking about?" "Can you tell me more about that?" and "What shall we discuss today?" confirm the presence of the patient and encourage him to select topics to discuss. They can also indicate that the nurse is there, listening to him and following him. Also serving in this way are acceptance responses such as "I understand," "And then what happened?" "Uh huh," or "I follow you."

■ **RESTATING.** Restating is the nurse's repeating to the patient the main thought he has expressed. It, too, indicates that the nurse is listening. Sometimes only a part of the patient's statement is repeated. This technique can serve as a reinforcer or bring attention to something important that might otherwise have been passed over.

■ **CLARIFICATION.** Clarification occurs when the nurse attempts to put into words vague ideas or thoughts that are implicit or explicit in the patient's talking. It is necessary, because statements about emotions and behaviors are rarely straightforward. The patient's verbalizations, especially when he is disturbed or feeling deeply, are not always clear and obvious. They may be confused, jumbled, hesitant, incomplete, disordered, or fragmentary. The nurse should not allow anything to go by that she does not hear or understand. Because of this uncertainty, clarification responses often are tentative or phrased as questions such as "I'm not sure what you mean. Are you saying that . . .?" or "Could you go over that again?" This technique is important because two functions of the nurse-patient relationship are to help clarify feelings, ideas, and perceptions and to provide an explicit correlation between them and the patient's actions.

■ **REFLECTION.** Reflection goes beyond simple acceptance or restating responses. *Reflection of content* is also called validation; it lets the patient know that the nurse has heard what he said and understands the content. It consists of repeating in fewer and fresher words the essential ideas of the patient and is like paraphrasing. Sometimes it helps to repeat a patient's statement, emphasizing a key word. Reflecting content is used to clarify the ideas that the patient is expressing and to validate that the nurse's understanding is consistent with the patient's meaning.

PATIENT: **When I walked into the room, I felt like I was going to faint. I knew I had tried to do too much too quickly, and I just wasn't ready for it.**
NURSE: **You thought you were ready to put yourself to the test, but when you got there, you realized it was too much too soon.**

Reflection of feelings consists of responses to the patient's feelings about the content. These responses let the patient know that the nurse is aware of what he is feeling. Broad openings, restatements, clarifications, and reflections of content need not represent empathic understanding. But reflection of feeling signifies understanding, empathy, interest, and respect for the patient. It increases the level of involvement between the nurse and patient.

The purpose of reflecting feelings is to focus on feeling rather than content to bring the patient's vaguely expressed feelings into clear awareness; it helps him accept or "own" those feelings as a part of himself. Skillful use of this technique depends on the nurse's ability to identify feelings and cues for feelings from the patient's nonverbal and verbal behaviors. The steps in reflection of feelings are to determine what feelings the patient is expressing, describe these feelings clearly, observe the effect, and judge by the patient's reaction whether the reflection was correct. Sometimes even inaccurate reflections can be useful, because the patient may correct the nurse and state his feeling more clearly.

Although reflecting techniques are some of the most useful, the nurse can also use them incorrectly.

One common error is stereotyping one's responses. This means that the nurse begins her reflections in the same monotonous way, such as "You think" or "You feel." A second error is in timing. Some nurses reflect back almost everything the patient says, which provokes feelings of irritation, anger, and frustration in the patient. The nurse appears to be insincere and in fact fails to be therapeutic with him. Other nurses may have trouble interrupting patients who continue talking in long monologues. Not only is it difficult to capture a feeling after it has passed, but in this case the nurse is failing to be a responsible, active partner in the relationship. Interruptions may at times be productive and necessary. Another error is inappropriate depth of feeling. The nurse fails by being either too superficial or too deep in assessing the patient's feelings. The final error is use of language that is inappropriate to the patient's cultural experience and educational level. Effective language is language that is natural to the nurse and readily understood by the patient.

■ **FOCUSING.** Focusing helps the patient expand on a topic of importance. It allows him to discuss central issues related to his problem and keeps the communication process goal directed. Intense focusing on an anxiety-producing topic can be detrimental to the relationship if it is not evaluated and balanced with other therapeutic techniques. Effectively used, it can help the patient become more specific, move from vagueness to clarity, and focus on reality.

By avoiding abstractions and generalizations, focusing helps the patient face his problems and analyze them in detail. It helps a patient talk about his situation or problem areas and accept the responsibility for improving them. If a patient is going to change his thoughts, feelings, or beliefs, he must first identify them as his own. If he fails to "own" them, he has lost control over a part of his life and becomes powerless to change it.

PATIENT: **Women always get put down. It's as if we don't count at all.**
NURSE: **Tell me how *you* feel as a woman.**

Encouraging a description of the patient's perceptions, encouraging comparisons, and placing events in time sequence are focusing techniques that promote specificity and problem analysis.

■ **SHARING PERCEPTIONS.** Sharing perceptions involves asking the patient to verify the nurse's understanding of what he is thinking or feeling. It is a way for the nurse to ask for feedback from the patient while also possibly providing him with new information. Perception checking can consist of paraphrasing what the patient is saying or doing, asking the patient to confirm the nurse's understanding, and allowing him to correct that perception if necessary. "You seem to be very irritated with me. Am I right about that?" Perception checking can also note the implied feelings of nonverbal language. When the technique is used in this way, it is best to describe the observed behavior first and then reflect on its meaning. "You say you really care about her, but every time you talk about her, you clench your fists. I wonder if you don't feel betrayed by her?" Perception checking is also a way to explore incongruent or double-blind communication. "You're smiling, but I sense that you're really angry with me." The value of perception checking as a therapeutic technique lies in the understanding it conveys to the patient and its potential for clearing up confusing communication.

■ **THEME IDENTIFICATION.** Themes are underlying issues or problems experienced by the patient that emerge repeatedly during the course of the nurse-patient relationship. Once the nurse has identified the patient's basic themes, he or she can better decide which of the patient's many feelings, thoughts, and beliefs to respond to and pursue. In this way the nurse can best promote the patient's exploration and understanding. Themes that are important tend to be repeated throughout the relationship. They can relate to feelings (depression or anxiety), behavior (rebelling against authority or withdrawal), experiences (being loved, hurt, or raped), or combinations of all three.

■ **SILENCE.** Silence on the part of the nurse has varying effects, depending on how the patient perceives it. To a vocal patient, silence on the part of the nurse may be welcome, as long as he knows the nurse is listening. When the patient pauses in his talk, he often expects and wants the nurse to respond. If the nurse does not, the patient may perceive this as rejection, hostility, or disinterest. With a depressed or withdrawn patient the nurse's silence may convey support, understanding, and acceptance. In this case verbalization by the nurse may be perceived as pressure or frustration. Sharing a patient's silence can be a most difficult task for the nurse but an essential one to furthering the therapeutic relationship.

Silence has several beneficial effects. It can prompt the patient to talk. Some introverted people find out that they can be quiet but still be liked. Silence allows the patient time to think and to gain insights. Finally, silence can slow the pace of the interaction. In general, the nurse should allow the patient to break a silence, particularly when the patient has introduced it. Obviously, sensitivity is called for in this regard, and silence should not develop into a contest. However, if the nurse is unsure how to respond to a patient's comments, a safe approach is to maintain silence. If the nurse's nonverbal behavior communicates interest and involvement, the patient often will elaborate on his statement or discuss a related issue.

An ineffective technique would be to begin questioning the patient. As a general technique, direct questioning has limited usefulness in the therapeutic relationship. Repetitive questioning takes on the tone of an interrogation and negates the element of mutuality. "Why" questions are particularly ineffective and are to be avoided, as are questions that can be answered simply by yes or no responses. Excessive questioning tends to be characteristic of inexperienced helpers. One consequence of it is that patients do not take the initiative and are discouraged or prevented from engaging in the process of exploration.

■ **HUMOR.** Humor is a basic part of the personality and has a place within the therapeutic relationship. It resolves paradoxes, tempers aggression, and is a socially acceptable form of sublimation. As a part of interpersonal relationships, it is a constructive coping behavior. By learning to express humor, a patient may be able to learn to express other feelings. Hutchinson[29] believes that humor can be used in three ways: (1) as an index to the developmental level of the patient, (2) as a planned approach for nursing intervention, and (3) as an indicator of change. As a planned approach to nursing intervention, humor can promote insight by making conscious repressed material. A change in the expression of humor and the quality of interpersonal relationships may be indicators of significant change in the patient.

Another important feature of humor as described by Heuscher[27] is that it can suddenly change or widen the patient's experiential horizon. Huescher believes that humor is an initial uncomplicated attempt at revealing new and wider visions of one's world; as such, it can further the growth of the person who is able to integrate some of the new vistas into his world design. "At worst, joking in psychotherapy is a 'playing at change' that allows the therapist and patient to retain their uneasy security in their unchanging individual existences. At best, it is a helpful revelation of new options."[27]

There are no rules for determining how, when, or where humor should be used in the therapeutic relationship. It depends on the nature and quality of the relationship, the patient's receptivity to such themes, and the relevance of the tale or witticism. Some occasions when the use of humor may be of therapuetic value include the following:

1. When the patient is experiencing mild to moderate levels of anxiety and humor serves as a tension reducer. It is inappropriate if a patient has severe or panic anxiety levels.
2. When it helps a patient cope more effectively, facilitates learning, puts life situations in perspective, decreases one's social distance, and is understood by the patient for its therapeutic value. It is inappropriate when it promotes maladaptive coping responses, masks feelings, increases social distance, and helps one avoid dealing with difficult situations.
3. When it is consistent with the social and cultural values of the patient and when it allows the patient to laugh at life, the human situation, or a particular set of stressors. It is inappropriate when it violates a patient's values, ridicules people, or belittles others.

Furthermore, the nurse must have insight into why he or she is using this technique. The nurse must also be aware of the dangerous ways it can be used to hide conflicts, ward off anxiety, manipulate the patient, and serve the nurse's own need to be liked and admired. Humor must be used cautiously. If it is indiscriminate, it meets only the nurse's needs and may be destructive to the relationship and frightening to the patient.

■ **INFORMING.** Informing, or the skill of information giving, needs little elaboration. It is an essential nursing technique in which the nurse shares simple facts with the patient. It is a skill used by nurses in health teaching or patient education, such as in teaching a patient when to take medication and informing him about necessary precautions and side effects. Giving information, however, must be distinguished from giving suggestions or advice.

■ **SUGGESTING.** Suggesting is the presentation of alternative ideas relative to problem solving. It is an appropriate therapeutic technique if used at the proper time and in a constructive way. As a therapeutic technique, it is a useful intervention in the working phase of the relationship when the patient has analyzed the problem area and is exploring alternative coping mechanisms. At that time, suggestions by the nurse will increase his perceived options and choices.

Suggesting, or giving advice, can also be nontherapeutic. Some patients who seek help do not really expect to work out their own problems; rather, they expect some pronouncement from the health care professional on what to do. So, too, nursing students often perceive their function as giving "common sense" advice. In these instances giving advice shifts responsibility to the nurse and reinforces the patient's dependence on her.

Another limitation is that the patient may take the

TABLE 4-7

THERAPEUTIC COMMUNICATION TECHNIQUES

Technique: **LISTENING**
Definition: An active process of receiving information and examining one's reaction to the messages received
Example: Maintaining eye contact and receptive nonverbal communication
Therapeutic value: Nonverbally communicates to the patient the nurse's interest and acceptance
Nontherapeutic threat: Failure to listen

Technique: **BROAD OPENINGS**
Definition: Encouraging the patient to select topics for discussion
Example: "What are you thinking about?"
Therapeutic value: Indicates acceptance by the nurse and the value of the patient's initiative
Nontherapeutic threat: Domination of the interaction by the nurse; rejecting responses

Technique: **RESTATING**
Definition: Repeating to the patient the main thought he has expressed
Example: "You say that your mother left you when you were 5 years old."
Therapeutic value: Indicates that the nurse is listening and validates, reinforces, or calls attention to something important that has been said
Nontherapeutic threat: Lack of validation of the nurse's interpretation of the message; being judgmental; reassuring; defending

Technique: **CLARIFICATION**
Definition: Attempting to put into words vague ideas or unclear thoughts of the patient to enhance the nurse's understanding or asking the patient to explain what he means
Example: "I'm not sure what you mean. Could you tell me about that again?"
Therapeutic value: Helps to clarify feelings, ideas, and perceptions of the patient and provide an explicit correlation between them and the patient's actions
Nontherapeutic threat: Failure to probe; assumed understanding

Technique: **REFLECTION**
Definition: Directing back to the patient his ideas, feelings, questions, and content
Example: "You're feeling tense and anxious and it's related to a conversation you had with your husband last night?"
Therapeutic value: Validates the nurse's understanding of what the patient is saying and signifies empathy, interest, and respect for the patient
Nontherapeutic threat: Stereotyping the patient's responses; inappropriate timing of reflections; inappropriate depth of feeling of the reflections; inappropriate to the cultural experience and educational level of the patient

Technique: **FOCUSING**
Definition: Questions or statements that help the patient expand on a topic of importance
Example: "I think that we should talk more about your relationship with your father."
Therapeutic value: Allows the patient to discuss central issues related to his problem and keeps the communication process goal-directed
Nontherapeutic threat: Allowing abstractions and generalizations; changing topics

Technique: **SHARING PERCEPTIONS**
Definition: Asking the patient to verify the nurse's understanding of what he is thinking or feeling
Example: "You're smiling but I sense that you are really very angry with me."
Therapeutic value: Conveys the nurse's understanding to the patient and has the potential for clearing up confusing communication
Nontherapeutic threat: Challenging the patient; accepting literal responses; reassuring; testing; defending

Technique: **THEME IDENTIFICATION**
Definition: Underlying issues or problems experienced by the patient that emerge repeatedly during the course of the nurse-patient relationship
Example: "I've noticed that in all of the relationships that you have described, you've been hurt or rejected by the man. Do you think this is an underlying issue?"
Therapeutic value: Allows the nurse to best promote the patient's exploration and understanding of important problems
Nontherapeutic threat: Giving advice; reassuring; disapproving

Technique: **SILENCE**
Definition: Lack of verbal communication for a therapeutic reason
Example: Sitting with a patient and nonverbally communicating interest and involvement
Therapeutic value: Allows the patient time to think and gain insights, slows the pace of the interaction and encourages the patient to initiate conversation, while conveying the nurse's support, understanding, and acceptance
Therapeutic threat: Questioning the patient; asking for "why" responses; failure to break a nontherapeutic silence

Continued.

TABLE 4-7—CONT'D

THERAPEUTIC COMMUNICATION TECHNIQUES

Technique: **HUMOR**
Definition: The discharge of energy through the comic enjoyment of the imperfect
Example: "That gives a whole new meaning to the word 'nervous,'" said with shared kidding between the nurse and patient
Therapeutic value: Can promote insight by making conscious repressed material, resolve paradoxes, temper aggression, reveal new options, and is a socially acceptable form of sublimation
Nontherapeutic threat: Indiscrimate use; belittling patient; screen to avoid therapeutic intimacy

Technique: **INFORMING**
Definition: The skill of information giving
Example: "I think you need to know more about how your medication works."
Therapeutic value: Helpful in health teaching or patient education about relevant aspects of patient's well-being and self-care
Nontherapeutic threat: Giving advice

Technique: **SUGGESTING**
Definition: Presentation of alternative ideas for the patient's consideration relative to his problem solving
Example: "Have you thought about responding to your boss in a different way when he raises that issue with you? For example, you could ask him if a specific problem has occurred."
Therapeutic value: Increases the patient's perceived options or choices
Nontherapeutic threat: Giving advice; inappropriate timing; being judgmental

nurse's advice and still not have things work out. The patient then returns to blame the nurse for failure. Most commonly, though, patients do not follow the advice offered by others, as in the transactional analysis model. The request for advice is often a child's expression of dependency, and the patient really knows what to do. The nurse who falls into the trap and responds with advice incurs the patient's wrath and contempt. A more productive strategy is for the nurse to deal with the patient's feelings first—feelings of indecision, dependence, and perhaps fear. Then the request for advice can be looked at and responded to in its proper perspective.

Suggesting is also nontherapeutic if it occurs early in the relationship before the patient has analyzed his conflicts or if it is a technique the nurse uses frequently. Then it negates the possibility of mutuality and implies that the patient is incapable of assuming responsibility for his own thoughts and actions. This assumption is also present when suggestion by the nurse is really covert coercion, as the nurse tells the patient how he *ought* to live his life.

The nurse's intent in using the suggesting technique should be to provide feasible alternatives and allow the patient to explore their potential value for himself. The nurse can then focus on helping the patient explore the advantages and disadvantages and the meaning and implications of the alternatives. In this way suggestions can be offered in a nonauthoritarian manner with such phrases as "Some people have tried. . . . Do you think that would work for you?" When using the technique of suggesting, nurses must be careful about both the timing of their intervention and their underlying motivation.

The therapeutic communication techniques presented in this chapter are summarized in Table 4-7.

Responsive dimensions

The nurse must achieve certain skills or qualities to initiate and continue a therapeutic relationship. These skills or qualities incorporate verbal and nonverbal behavior and the attitudes and feelings behind communication. Truax, Carkhoff, and Berenson[14-16] have identified specific core conditions for facilitative interpersonal relationships. They broadly divided these conditions into responsive dimensions and action dimensions. The responsive dimensions include genuineness, respect, empathic understanding, and concreteness.

Many nurses believe that they already demonstrate these qualities with their patients. However, a number of studies have reported that nurses are low in the

Some Illness-Maintaining Responses of Nurses with Patients

1. The nurse using a patient (who was similarly exploited at home) to do errands (bring coffee, clean office, carry messages).
2. The nurse burdening the patient with tales of his or her exciting social life—putting the patient in the position of "audience" and at the same time having little interest, if any, in his concerns; to cheer him up by "one-upping" him!
3. The nurse making "pets" of a few patients and thereby reinforcing previous "pet" status for those patients and reinforcing "unfavorable comparison" for other patients. Giving gifts to some but not all patients.
4. Arbitrating siblinglike disputes between two patients, so that one loses and one wins, as in sibling disputes at home.
5. Responding to dependency bids in ways that confirm and reconfirm the patient's self-view: "I am helpless, dependent, etc."
6. Responding to patient bids for derogation or punishment by giving it, thereby confirming and reconfirming these patient self-views.

7. Permitting, inviting, and responding to "tale bearing" in which one patient "tattles" on another, thereby reinforcing the patient's "informer role," which further isolates the patient from constructive interaction with other patients as peers.
8. Allowing or permitting "coalitions across generations"; that is, participating in nurse/patient discussion to the detriment of some other staff member. This replicates the patient's previous pattern of "pitting one against another," which may have effectively disunited mother and father, who are then reunited in concern for the now "identified patient."
9. Entering into pseudochum relationships with patients.
10. Nonuseful channeling of anxiety into overmedication, seclusion, EST, or work rather than into investigation of circumstances that evoked the anxiety in a given situation.
11. Using various problematic verbal inputs such as "mixed messages," "double-binds," etc.

From Peplau H: Int Nurs Rev 25(2):44, 1978.

qualities traditionally associated with therapeutic effectiveness in counseling—genuineness, nonpossessive warmth, and empathy.[49] A recent study is even more specific and suggests that nurses are most skilled in the authoritative interventions of prescribing, informing, and confronting patients and less skilled in the facilitative interventions of drawing out patient's emotions, encouraging their self-exploration, and confirming their self-worth.[47] Furthermore, the helping process can impede the patient's growth rather than enhance it, depending on the level of the nurse's responsive and facilitative skills. Some of the ways in which nurses may consciously or unconsciously hinder progress are given in the box on illness-maintaining responses.

The responsive dimensions are crucial in the orientation phase of a relationship to establish trust and open communication between the nurse and the patient. The nurse's goal at this time is to gain an understanding of the patient and to help him understand himself or gain insight. These responsive conditions then continue to be useful throughout the working and termination phases. All of the conditions are interrelated and contribute to each other in the therapeutic process, and some degree of all the responsive dimensions is necessary when initiating a relationship.

■ Genuineness

Genuineness implies that the nurse is an open, honest, sincere person who is actively involved in the relationship. He or she is a "real" person in a "real" encounter who is self-congruent, authentic, or "transparent."[32] Genuineness is the opposite of self-alienation, which occurs when many of one's real, spontaneous reactions to life are repressed or suppressed. Genuineness means that the nurse's response is sincere rather than phony, that the nurse is not thinking and feeling one thing and saying something different. It is an essential quality, because the nurse cannot expect openness, self-acceptance, and personal freedom in the patient if he or she lacks these qualities in the relationship.

Genuineness does not mean that the nurse must disclose his or her total self; but whatever the nurse does show must be a real aspect of himself or herself and not merely a "professional" response that has been learned and repeated. Genuineness also does not imply that the nurse will behave in the same way as with family, friends, or colleagues. In focusing on the patient, much of the nurse's personal need system is put aside, as well as some of his or her usual ways of relating to others. Genuineness does not require that the nurse always express all personal feelings, only that whatever he or she does express be congruent. Neither does genuineness imply impulsiveness or "anything goes." Carried to this extreme, genuineness can be destructive and work against the goals of a therapeutic relationship.

Following is an example of genuineness.

PATIENT: **I'd like my parents to give me my freedom and let me do my own thing. If I need them or want their advice, I'll ask them. Why don't they trust what they taught me? Why do parents have to make it so hard—like it's all or nothing?**

NURSE: **I know what you mean. My parents acted the same way. They offered advice, but what they expected was obedience. When they saw I could handle things on my own and used good judgment, they began to accept me as an individual. There are still times when they slip back into their old ways, but we understand each other better now. Do you think you and your parents need to share more openly and honestly your feelings and ideas?**

■ **Respect**

The quality of respect has also been called "non-possessive warmth" or "unconditional positive regard."[15] Positive regard is unconditional in that it does not depend on the patient's behavior. Caring, liking, and valuing are other terms for respect. The patient is regarded as a person of worth; he is respected. The nurse's attitude is nonjudgmental; it is without criticism, ridicule, depreciation, or reservation. This does not mean that the nurse condones or accepts all aspects of the patient's behavior as desirable or likeable. Yet the patient is accepted for what he is, as he is. The nurse does not demand that he change to be accepted or that he be perfect. Imperfections are accepted along with mistakes and weaknesses as part of the human condition. The inexperienced nurse may have difficulty accepting the patient without transferring his or her feelings about his thoughts or actions. However, acceptance means viewing his actions as coping behaviors that will change as he becomes less threatened and learns more adaptive mechanisms. It involves viewing his behavior as natural, normal, and expected, given his circumstances and perceptions.

Although there should be a basic respect for the patient simply as a person, respect is increased with understanding of his uniqueness. Respect can be com-

municated in many different ways: by sitting silently with a patient who is crying; by genuine laughter with the patient over a particular event; by accepting the patient's request not to share a certain experience; by apologizing for the hurt unintentionally caused by a particular phrase; by being open enough to communicate one's own anger or hurt caused by the patient. Being genuine with the patient and listening to him are also manifestations of respect for him. The nurse's ability to experience warmth for the patient depends in part on the ability to feel an unconditional positive regard for self and an acceptance of his or her own strengths and liabilities.

When the nurse communicates conditional warmth, he or she fosters feelings of dependency in the patient because the nurse becomes the evaluator and superior in the relationship, making mutuality impossible. This might occur because of the nurse's need to be in control and dominant, or it might be fostered by the dependent, clinging patient. If dependency feelings should arise in the patient, the nurse can effectively deal with them by acknowledging them and exploring them with him.

■ **Empathic understanding**

Empathy has been defined by Kalisch as "the ability to enter into the life of another person, to accurately perceive his current feelings and their meanings. It is an essential element of the interpersonal process. When communicated, it forms the basis for a helping relationship between nurse and patient."[33:1548] Without empathy there is no basis for practice; it is understanding the patient's world from his internal frame of reference rather than from the nurse's own external frame of reference. Rogers described it as "to sense the client's private world as if it were your own, but without losing the 'as if' quality."[51:284] Rogers believes that a high degree of empathy is one of the most potent factors in bringing about change and learning—"one of the most delicate and powerful ways we have of using ourselves."[52:2]

Accurate empathy involves more than knowing what the patient means. It also involves the nurse's sensitivity to the patient's current feelings and the verbal ability to communicate this understanding in a language attuned to the patient. It means frequently confirming with the patient the accuracy of one's perceptions and being guided by the patient's responses. It requires that the nurse lay aside personal views and values to enter another's world without prejudice. This can be done only by a nurse secure enough in the self to know that he or she will not get lost in what may possibly be the strange or bizarre world of the patient and who can comfortably return to his or her own world at will.

■ **DEVELOPMENT OF EMPATHY.** Empathic understanding consists of a number of stages. If the patient allows the nurse to enter his private world and attempts to communicate his perceptions and feelings, the nurse must be receptive to this communication. Next, the nurse must understand the patient's communication. To do this the nurse must be able to put himself or herself in the patient's place and assume his role. The nurse must then be able to step back into his or her own role and communicate understanding to the patient. It is not necessary or desirable for the nurse to feel the same emotion as the patient. Empathy should not be confused with sympathy. It is, instead, an appreciation and awareness of the patient's feelings. At deeper levels, empathy also involves enough understanding of human feelings and experiences to sense feelings that the patient only partially reveals.

A good deal of research has been conducted on empathy. The following discussion of the findings underscores its importance in counseling:

- Empathy is clearly related to positive outcome.
- Low empathy is related to a worsening in adjustment or pathological conditions.
- The ideal therapist is first of all empathic.
- Empathy is correlated with self-exploration and process movement.
- Empathy early in the relationship predicts later success.
- The patient comes to perceive more empathy in successful cases.
- Understanding is provided by the therapist, not drawn from him or her.
- The more experienced the therapist, the more likely he or she is to be empathic.
- Empathy is a special quality in a relationship, and therapists offer definitely more of it than even helpful friends.
- The better integrated the therapist is within himself or herself, the higher the degree of empathy he or she will be able to exhibit.
- Experienced therapists often fall far short of being empathic.Brilliance and diagnostic perceptiveness are unrelated to empathy.
- An empathic way of being can be learned from empathic persons.

The findings highlighted with solid blocks are particularly relevant to improving nursing practice. The last statement indicates that the ability to be accurately empathic is something that can be learned. This is especially likely to occur if one's nursing educators and supervisors are themselves individuals of sensitive understanding who establish an empathic climate for learning.

The first two findings indicate that, depending on the therapist's empathic level, therapeutic relationships can be "for better or worse." This is also true among nurses, shown by Williams' study,[67] which found that high and low levels of empathic communication were factors in changing the self-concept of institutionalized aged patients during group therapy.

Rogers[52] expands on the profound consequences empathy can have in promoting constructive learning and change. In the first place, it dissolves the patient's sense of alienation by connecting him on some level to a part of the human race. He can perceive that "I make sense to another human being . . . so I must not be so strange or alien. . . . And if I am in touch with someone else, I am not so all alone." On the other hand, if the patient is not responded to empathically, he may believe, "If no one understands me, if no one can see what I'm experiencing, then I must be very bad off. . . . I'm sicker than even I thought." Another benefit of empathy for the patient is that he can see that someone values him, cares for him, and accepts him for the person he is. Then perhaps he can come to think, "If this other person thinks I'm worthwhile, maybe I could value and care for myself. . . . Maybe I am worthwhile after all."

■ **EMPATHIC RESPONSES.** It is essential that the nurse first provide the contextual base for the relationship through genuineness and unconditional positive regard for the patient. Then, the understanding conveyed to the patient through empathy gives him his personhood or identity. Each person has the need to have his existence confirmed by another. Empathy gives the needed confirmation that one exists as a separate, valued, and unique person. The patient, as he perceives these new aspects of himself, incorporates them into his changing self-concept. And once his self-concept changes, his behavior changes, thus producing the positive outcome of therapy.

Gazda and co-workers[22] have described the following guidelines for responding with empathy:

1. Verbal and nonverbal behavior should be focused on by the helper.
2. The helper should formulate responses of empathy in a language and a manner that are most easily understood by the patient.
3. The tone of the helper's response should be similar to that of the patient.
4. In addition to concentrating on what the patient is expressing, the helper should also be aware of what is not being expressed.

5. The helper must accurately interpret responses to the patient and use them as a guide in developing future responses.

A nursing study conducted by Mansfield[42] identified specific verbal and nonverbal behaviors that conveyed high levels of empathy to the patient:

- Having the nurse introduce himself or herself to the patient
- Head and body positions turned toward the patient and occasionally leaning forward
- Verbal responses to the patient's previous comments, responses that focus on his strengths and resources
- Consistent eye contact and response to the patient's nonverbal cues such as sighs, tone of voice, restlessness, and facial expressions
- Conveyance of interest, concern, and warmth by the nurse's own facial expressions
- A tone of voice consistent with facial expression and verbal response
- Mirror imaging of body position and gestures between the nurse and patient

Another study of nonverbal communication and empathy of patients and nurses showed that, in comparison with patients, nurses spent approximately twice as much interview time with direct eye gaze; three times longer with head nodding; and virtually the entire interview with legs crossed. Although nurses tended to smile more and laugh less than patients, these findings were not significant. The researchers then compared the behaviors of high- and low-empathy nurses. They reported that high-empathy nurses kept their legs still and in a crossed position, whereas low-empathy nurses had more extraneous leg movements and laughed twice as much as high-empathy nurses.[26]

Additional studies are needed in nursing to identify more specifically the behavioral indicators and outcomes of this important dimension of nursing care.

- **EMPATHIC FUNCTIONING SCALE.** Kalisch[33] devised a "Nurse-Patient Empathic Functioning Scale," which describes five categories of empathy (Table 4-8). High levels of empathy (categories 3 and 4) communicate "I am with you"; the nurse's responses fit perfectly with the patient's conspicuous current feelings and content. The nurse's responses also serve to expand the patient's awareness of his hidden feelings through the use of clarification and reflection. Such empathy is communicated by the language used, voice qualities, and nonverbal behavior, all of which reflect the nurse's seriousness and depth of feeling.

At low levels of empathy (categories 0 and 1), the nurse ignores the patient's feelings, goes off on a tangent, or misinterprets what the patient is feeling. The nurse at this level may be uninterested in the patient or concentrating on the "facts" of what the patient says

TABLE 4-8

NURSE-PATIENT EMPATHIC FUNCTIONING SCALE

Categories of nurse empathic functioning	Level of patient's feelings	
	Conspicuous current feelings	Hidden current feelings
Category 0	Ignores	Ignores
Category 1	Communicates awareness that is accurate at times and inaccurate at other times	Ignores
Category 2	Communicates complete and accurate awareness of essence and strength of feelings	Communicates an awareness of presence of hidden feelings but is not accurate in defining their essence or strength; effort being made to understand
Category 3	Same as category 2	Communicates an accurate awareness of hidden feelings slightly beyond what patient expresses himself
Category 4	Same as category 2	Communicates without uncertainty an accurate awareness of deepest, most hidden feelings

From Kalisch B: Am J Nurs 73:1548, 1973. Copyright © 1973, American Journal of Nursing Company. Reproduced, with permission, from American Journal of Nursing, September, vol 73, no 9.

rather than his current feelings and experiences. The nurse is doing something other than listening; he or she may be evaluating the patient, giving advice, sermonizing, or thinking about personal problems or needs.

Empathic responses need to be properly timed within the nurse-patient relationship. Category 4 responses in the orientation phase may be viewed as too intense and intrusive. Usually a number of category 2 responses are required initially to build an atmosphere of trust and openness. In the later stages of the orientation phase and most particularly in the working phase, categories 3 and 4 responses are appropriate and most effective. Responses from categories 0 and 1 are nontherapeutic at all times and block the development of the relationship.

The various levels of empathy are evident in the following example:

PATIENT: **I'm really jittery today, and I hope I can get things out right. It started when I saw Bob on Friday, and it's been building up since then.**
NURSE: **You're feeling tense and anxious, and it's related to a talk you had with Bob on Friday. (Category 2.)**
PATIENT: **Yes. He began putting pressure on me to have sex with him again.**
NURSE: **It sounds like you resent it when he pressures you for sex. (Category 3.)**
PATIENT: **I do. Why does he think things always have to be his way? I guess he knows I'm a pushover.**
NURSE: **It makes you angry when he wants his way even though he knows you feel differently. But you usually give in and then you wind up disappointed in yourself and feeling like a failure. (Category 4.)**
PATIENT: **It happens just like that over and over. It's as if I never learn.**
NURSE: **So when the incident's all over, you're left blaming yourself and wallowing in self-pity. (Category 4.)**
PATIENT: **I guess that's right.**

Differences between nurses and patients are barriers to empathy. Differences in sex, age, religion, socioeconomic status, education, and culture can block the development of empathic understanding. Because everyone is unique, no one can completely understand another person. However, the wider a person's background and the more varied one's experiences, the greater will be the potential for understanding people.

Identical or similar experiences are not essential for empathy. No man can really experience what it is like to be a woman; no white can experience what it is like to be black. It is not necessary to be exactly like another, but it is desirable for nurses to prepare themselves in any way they can to understand potential patients. It is also important for nurses to realize that empathy can be learned and enhanced in a variety of ways, including staff development programs.

■ Concreteness

Concreteness involves using specific terminology rather than abstractions when discussing the patient's feelings, experiences, and behavior. It avoids vagueness and ambiguity and is the opposite of generalizing, categorizing, classifying, and labeling the patient's experiences. It has three functions: (1) to keep the nurse's responses close to the patient's feelings and experiences, (2) to foster accuracy of understanding by the nurse, and (3) to encourage the patient to attend to specific problem areas.[12] By focusing the patient in specific and concrete terms to his vague ramblings, the nurse helps the patient identify significant aspects of his problems.

The level of concreteness should vary during the various phases of the nurse-patient relationship. In the orientation phase, concreteness should be high; at this time, it can contribute to empathic understanding. It is essential for the formulation of specific goals and plans. As the patient explores various feelings and perceptions related to his problems in the working phase of the relationship, concreteness should be at a relatively low level to facilitate a thorough self-exploration. At the end of the working phase when the patient is engaging in action and during the termination phase, high levels of concreteness are again desirable.

Concreteness is evident in the following examples:

EXAMPLE 1

PATIENT: **I wouldn't have any problems if people would quit bothering me. They like to upset me because they know I'm high strung.**
NURSE: **What people try to upset you?**
PATIENT: **My family. People think being from a large family is a blessing. I think it's a curse.**
NURSE: **Could you give me an example of something someone in your family did that upset you?**

EXAMPLE 2

PATIENT: **I don't know what the problem is between us. My wife and I just don't get along anymore. We seem to disagree about everything. I think I love her, but she isn't affectionate or caring—hasn't been for a long time.**
NURSE: **You say you're not sure what the problem is, and you think you love your wife. But the two of you argue often and she hasn't given you any sign of love or affection. Have you felt affectionate toward her, and when was the last time you let her know how you felt?**

These four responsive dimensions or conditions—genuineness, respect, empathic understanding, and concreteness—facilitate the formation of a therapeutic relationship. However, few research instruments have been developed to evaluate nurse-patient interactions objectively. Aiken and Aiken[1] have adapted the scales developed by Carkhoff and Truax relative to the core dimensions of empathic understanding, positive regard, genuineness, concreteness, and self-exploration. Aiken and Aiken divided each dimension into facilitative levels that would allow a practitioner to score himself or herself on them. Methven and Schlotfeldt[45] developed an instrument designed to determine the nature of verbal responses nurses tend to give in emotion-laden situations typically encountered in nursing practice. The therapeutic level at which nurses function is unknown at present. Additional research is greatly needed on nurse-patient interactions, because there is little empirical evidence on which to base scientific practice in this area.

Action dimensions

Carkhoff[11] identified the action-oriented or initiative conditions for facilitative interpersonal relationships as confrontation, immediacy, and therapist self-disclosure. To these will be added the dimensions of catharsis and role playing. The separation of these therapeutic conditions into two groups—the understanding or responsive conditions, and the initiating or action conditions—is not a distinct separation. To some extent all the dimensions are present throughout the therapeutic relationship. The action dimensions must have a context of warmth and understanding. This is important for the inexperienced nurse to remember; he or she may be tempted to move into high levels of action dimensions without having established adequate understanding, empathy, warmth, or respect. The responsive dimensions allow the patient to achieve insight, but this is not enough. With the action dimensions, the nurse moves the therapeutic relationship upward and outward by identifying obstacles to the patient's progress and the need for both internal understanding and external action.

■ Confrontation

Confrontation usually implies venting anger and aggressive behavior. This has the effect of belittling, blaming, and embarrassing the receiver—all of which are harmful and destructive in both social and therapeutic relationships. However, confrontation as a therapeutic action dimension is an assertive rather than aggressive action. Confrontation is an expression by the nurse of perceived discrepancies in the patient's behavior. Carkhoff[11] identifies three categories of confrontation:

1. Discrepancy between the patient's expression of what he is (self-concept) and what he wants to be (self-ideal)
2. Discrepancies between the patient's verbal expressions about himself and his behavior
3. Discrepancies between the patient's expressed experience of himself and the nurse's experience of him

Confrontation is an attempt by the nurse to make the patient aware of incongruence in his feelings, attitudes, beliefs, and behaviors. It may also lead to the discovery of ambivalent feelings in the patient. Confrontation is not limited to negative aspects of the patient. It includes pointing out discrepancies involving his resources and strengths that are unrecognized and unused. It requires that the nurse collect sufficient data about the patient's history and accumulate sufficient perceptions and observations of his verbal and nonverbal communication so that validation of reality is possible. It also requires that the nurse take some risks, avoid venting his or her own feelings, and help the patient bring his discrepancies into his awareness.

The nurse must have developed an understanding of the patient to perceive discrepancies, inconsistencies in word and deed, distortions, defenses, and evasions. The relationship must also contain a bond that will weather the mild or severe crises that confrontation precipitates. The nurse must be willing and capable of working through the crisis after confronting the patient. Without this commitment the confrontation lacks therapeutic potential and can be quite damaging to both nurse and patient. Without question the effects of confrontation are challenge, exposure, risk, and the possibility for growth. The nurse who uses confrontation is modeling an active role to the patient; the nurse is using insight and understanding to remove ambiguity and inconsistency and thus seek deeper understanding.

■ **TIMING IN RELATIONSHIPS.** Bromley[6] suggests that before confrontation, the nurse assess the following factors: the trust level in the relationship, the timing, the patient's stress level, the strength of his defense mechanisms, his perceived need for personal space or closeness, and his level of rage and tolerance for hearing another perception. The patient has the capacity to deny or accept the nurse's observations, and his response to the confrontation can serve as a measure of its success or failure. Acceptance indicates appropriate timing and patient readiness. Denial by the patient serves to allay any threat that the confrontation posed to the patient. It provides the nurse with additional information; it tells her that the patient is resisting change and is unwilling to enlarge his view of reality at this time.

Confrontation must be appropriately timed to be effective. In the orientation phase of the relationship, the nurse should use confrontation infrequently and pose it as an observation of incongruent behavior. A simple "mirroring" of the discrepancy between a patient's actions and words is the most nonthreatening type of confrontation. The nurse might say, "You seem to be saying two different things." This type of confrontation closely resembles clarification at this time. The nurse might also identify discrepancies between how he or she and the patient are experiencing their relationship, point out unnoticed strengths or untapped resources of the patient, or provide the patient with objective but perhaps different information about his world. According to Carkhoff, "Premature direct confrontations may have a demoralizing and demobilizing effect upon an inadequately prepared helpee."[11:93] To be effective, confrontation requires high levels of empathy and respect.

In the working phase of the relationship, more direct confrontations may focus on specific patient discrepancies. The nurse may confront the patient with areas of weakness or shortcomings or may focus on the discrepancy between the nurse's experience of the patient and his own. This expands the patient's awareness and helps him move to higher levels of functioning. As Carkhoff says, "Confrontation of self and others is prerequisite to the healthy individual's encounter with life."[11:93] Confrontation is especially important in pointing out when the patient has developed insight but has not changed his behavior. This type of confrontation encourages the patient to act on his world in a reasonable and constructive manner, rather than assuming a dependent and passive stance toward life.

Research indicates that effective counselors use confrontation frequently, confronting patients with their assets more often in earlier interviews and with their limitations in later interviews.[2] Furthermore, Mitchell and Berenson[46] found that therapists who rated significantly higher on empathy, genuineness, respect, and concreteness confronted their patients significantly more often than those therapists who were less facilitative. In the initial interview, these confrontations were based on attempts to clarify the relationship, eliminate misconceptions, give the patient more objective information about himself and his world, and emphasize the patient's strengths and resources.

Inexperienced nurses frequently avoid confrontation. Certainly it does involve a risk. It can be nonther-apeutic when it is not associated with empathy or warmth or when it is used to vent the nurse's negative feelings of anger, frustration, and aggressiveness. However, carefully monitored confrontation can be viewed as an extension of genuineness and concreteness. It is a useful therapeutic intervention that can further the patient's growth and progress.

Following are seven examples of confrontation:

EXAMPLE 1

NURSE: **I see you as someone who has a lot of strength. You've been able to give a tremendous amount of emotional support to your children at a time when they needed it very much.**

EXAMPLE 2

NURSE: **It was my understanding that we were meeting together to talk about the problems that brought you to the hospital. But every time I come, you ask me to play cards with you, share a game of table tennis, or toss around a basketball. It seems to me that we're not in agreement on what these meetings are all about.**

EXAMPLE 3

NURSE: **The fact that Sue didn't accept your date for Friday night doesn't necessarily mean she never wants to go out with you. She could have had another date or other plans with her family or girlfriends. But if you don't ask her, you'll never find out why she refused you or if she'll accept in the future.**

EXAMPLE 4

NURSE: **We've talked three different times now and you've told me that you don't really have a problem or that other people make trouble for you. But I've noticed that on the ward you seldom talk to the other patients and little accidents like the spilled coffee at lunch really seem to upset you.**

EXAMPLE 5

NURSE: **You tell me that your parents don't trust you and never give you any responsibility, but each week you also tell me how you stayed out beyond your curfew or had friends over when your parents weren't home. Do you see a connection between the two?**

EXAMPLE 6

NURSE: **You say you want to feel better and go back to work, but you're not taking your medicine, which will help you to do that.**

EXAMPLE 7

NURSE: **We've been talking for 3 weeks now about your need to get out and try to meet some people. We even talked of different ways to do that. But so far you haven't made any effort to join aerobics, take a class, or do any of the other ideas we had.**

■ Immediacy

Immediacy involves focusing on the current interaction of the nurse and the patient in the relationship. It is a significant dimension, because the patient's behavior and functioning in the relationship are indicative of functioning in other interpersonal relationships. Most patients experience difficulty in interpersonal relationships; thus the patient's functioning in the nurse-patient relationship must be evaluated. As Carkhoff states, "The way he relates to the counselor is a snapshot of the way he relates to others. . . . If the counselor does not focus on trying to understand these things, growth possibilities for clients can be missed."[11:192] The nurse has the opportunity to intervene directly with the patient's problem behavior, and the patient has the opportunity to learn and change his behavior. Immediacy may be viewed as empathy, genuineness, or confrontation that involves a particular content—the relationship between the nurse and the patient.

Immediacy connotes sensitivity by the nurse to the patient's feelings and a willingness to deal with these feelings rather than ignore them. This is particularly difficult when the nurse must recognize and respond to negative feelings the patient expresses toward him or her. The difficulty is compounded by the fact that patients often express these messages indirectly and conceal them in references to other people.

It is not possible or appropriate for the nurse to focus continually on the immediacy of the relationship. It is most appropriate to do so when the relationship seems to be stalled or is not progressing. Frequently this is caused by factors in the immediate nurse-patient relationship, and focusing on them may help. It is also helpful to look at immediacy when the relationship is progressing particularly well. In both instances the patient is actively involved in describing what he feels is helping or hindering the relationship.

As with the other dimensions, high-level immediacy responses should not be suddenly presented to the patient. The nurse must first know and understand him and have developed a good, open relationship with him. The nurse's initial expressions of immediacy should be tentatively phrased; for example, "Are you trying to tell me how you feel about our relationship?" As the relationship progresses, observations related to immediacy can be made more directly, and as communication improves, the need for immediacy responses may decrease.

Following are two examples of immediacy:

EXAMPLE 1

PATIENT: **I've been thinking about our meetings, and I'm really pretty busy now to keep coming. Besides, I don't see the point in them, and we don't seem to be getting anywhere.**

NURSE: **Are you trying to say you're feeling discouraged and you feel our meetings aren't helping you?**

EXAMPLE 2

PATIENT: **The staff here couldn't care less about us patients. They treat us like children instead of adults.**

NURSE: **I'm wondering if you feel that I don't care about you or perhaps I don't value your opinion?**

■ Nurse self-disclosure

Self-disclosures have three characteristics. They are (1) subjectively true, (2) personal statements about the self, and (3) intentionally revealed to another person. In self-disclosure the nurse reveals information about himself or herself such as ideas, values, feelings, and attitudes. The nurse may share that he or she has had experiences or feelings similar to those of the patient and may emphasize both the similarities and differences. This kind of self-disclosure is an index of the closeness of the relationship and involves a particular kind of respect for the patient. It is an expression of genuineness and honesty by the nurse and is an aspect of empathy.

The rationale for nurse self-disclosure comes from the theoretical and research literature; it provides significant evidence that therapist self-disclosure increases the likelihood of patient self-disclosure. Patient self-disclosure is necessary for a successful therapeutic outcome. However, the nurse must use self-disclosure judiciously, and this is determined by the quality, quantity, and appropriateness of the disclosures.

The number of self-disclosures appears to be crucial to the success of the therapy. Although too few nurse self-disclosures may fail to produce patient self-disclosures, too many may decrease the time available for patient disclosure or may alienate the patient. Thus there appears to be a nonlinear relationship between nurse genuineness and patient disclosure. The problem for the nurse is knowing where the middle ground is. Clinical experience is necessary to determine the optimum therapeutic level.

The appropriateness or relevance of the nurse's self-disclosure is also important. The nurse should self-disclose in response to statements made by the patient. If the nurse's disclosure is far from what the patient is experiencing, it can serve to distract the patient from his problem or make him feel alienated from the nurse. A patient who is experiencing severe or panic levels of anxiety may feel threatened or frightened by the nurse's self-disclosure. In these cases the nurse must be careful, not to burden a patient with his or her own self-disclosures. Above all, disclosure by the nurse is always for the patient's benefit. The nurse does not disclose himself or herself to meet personal needs or to feel better. The nurse does not impose himself or herself on the patient. When self-disclosing, the nurse should have a particular therapeutic goal in mind.

Weiner has proposed guidelines that nurses can use to evaluate the potential usefulness of their self-disclosure.[65] These include:

1. Cooperation—Will the disclosure enhance the patient's cooperation, which is necessary to the development of a therapeutic alliance?
2. Learning—Will the disclosure assist the patient's ability to learn about himself, to set short- and long-term goals, and to deal more effectively with life's problems?
3. Catharsis—Will the disclosure assist the patient to express formerly held or suppressed feelings, important to the relief of emotional symptoms?
4. Support—Will the disclosure provide the patient with support or reinforcement for the goals that he is trying to accomplish in his life?

If all of these criteria are met, the nurse needs to consider the judicious use of self-disclosure. The nurse should take into account the type and goal of treatment, the context of the nurse-patient relationship, the patient's ego strength, the patient's feelings about the nurse, and the nurse's feelings about the patient. These guidelines govern the "dosage and timing" of self-disclosures and help the nurse assess the appropriateness, effectiveness, and anticipated response of the patient to the disclosure.

Self-disclosure by the nurse is evident in the following example:

PATIENT: **When he told me he didn't want to see me again, I felt like slapping him and hugging him at the same time. But then I knew the problem was really me and no one could ever love me.**

NURSE: **When I broke off with a man I had been seeing, I felt the anger, hurt, and bitterness you just described. I remember thinking I would never date another man.**

In this example the nurse self-disclosed to emphasize that the patient's feelings were natural. She also reinforced the external cause for the separation (boyfriend's decision to leave versus the patient's inadequacy) and implied that, with time, the patient will be able to resolve the loss.

Even though research has indicated the importance of this dimension for patient growth, it appears to be an area of some discomfort for nurses. Johnson[30,31] studied the level of reciprocal disclosure occurring between nurses and patients on four clinical units—med-

ical, surgical, psychiatric, and critical care. She found that anxiety levels tended to decrease among nurses and patients as their levels of self-disclosure increased. In addition, she reported low reciprocal self-disclosure in the psychiatric unit despite the verbal nature of psychiatric therapy and the lack of restrictions on talking about oneself. She concluded from her study that nurses and patients need to be assisted in learning to be open and authentic in their interactions with each other.

■ Emotional catharsis

Emotional catharsis occurs when the patient is encouraged to talk about things that bother him most. Catharsis brings fears, feelings, and experiences out into the open so that they can be examined and discussed with the nurse. The expression of feelings can be very therapeutic in itself, even if behavioral change does not ensue. The previously described responsive dimensions create an atmosphere within the nurse-patient relationship in which emotional catharsis is possible. The patient's responsiveness depends on the confidence and trust he has in the nurse.

The nurse must be able to recognize cues from the patient that he is ready to discuss his problems. It is important that the nurse proceed with the patient at the rate he chooses and support him as he discusses difficult areas. Forcing emotional catharsis on the patient could precipitate a panic episode, since the patient's defenses are attacked without sufficient alternative coping mechanisms available to him.

Patients are often uncomfortable about expressing feelings because of prohibitive social norms. Nurses may be equally uncomfortable with expressing feelings, particularly sadness or anger. Frequently nurses assume they know the patient's feelings and do not attempt to specifically validate them. The dimensions of empathy and immediacy require the nurse to notice and express emotions. Unresolved feelings and feelings that are avoided can cause stalls or barriers in the nurse-patient relationship. Specific examples are transference and countertransference phenomena, which are discussed later in the chapter.

If the patient is having difficulty expressing feelings, the nurse may help by suggesting how he or she might feel in the patient's place or how others might feel in that situation. The nurse might validate with the patient the feeling he seems to be describing in a general way. Some patients respond directly to the question "How did that make you feel?" Others intellectualize and avoid the emotional element in their answer. When patients realize they can express their feelings within an accepting relationship, they expand their awareness and potential acceptance of themselves.

The following example illustrates emotional catharsis:

NURSE: **How did you feel when your boss corrected you in front of all those customers?**

PATIENT: **Well, I understood that he needed to set me straight, and he's the type that flies off the handle pretty easily anyhow.**

NURSE: **It sounds like you're defending his behavior. I was wondering how you felt at that moment.**

PATIENT: **Awkward . . . uh . . . upset, I guess (pause).**

NURSE: **That would have made me pretty angry if it had happened to me.**

PATIENT: **Well, I was. But you can't let it show, you know. You have to keep it all in because of the customers. But he can let it out. Oh *sure* (emphatically)! He can tell *me* anything he wants. Just *once* I'd like him to know how *I* feel.**

■ Role playing

Role playing involves acting out a particular situation. It increases the patient's insight into human relations and can deepen his ability to see the situation from another person's point of view. Sedgwick[58] identifies the intent of role playing as being to represent closely real life behavior that involves the individual holistically, to focus attention on a problem, and to permit the individual to see himself in action in a neutral situation. It provides a bridge between thought and action in a "safe" environment in which the patient can feel free to experiment with new behavior. It is a method of learning that makes actual behavior the focus of study; it is action oriented and provides immediately available information. Role playing consists of the following steps:

1. Defining the problem
2. Creating a readiness for role playing
3. Establishing the situation
4. Casting the characters
5. Briefing and warming up
6. Considering the training design
7. Acting
8. Stopping
9. Involving the audience
10. Analyzing and discussing
11. Evaluation

When role playing is used for attitude change, it relies heavily on role reversal. The patient may be asked to play the role of a certain person in a specific situation or to play the role of someone with opposing beliefs. Research indicates that role reversal can help a person reevaluate the other person's intentions and become more understanding of the other person's posi-

tion.[5] After role reversal, patients may be more receptive to modifying their own attitudes.

As a method of promoting self-awareness and conflict resolution, role playing may help the patient "experience" a situation rather than just "talk about it." Role playing can elicit feelings in the patient that are similar to those experienced in the actual situation. It provides an opportunity for insight and for the expression of affect. For these reasons it is a useful method for heightening a patient's awareness of his feelings about a situation.

One of the specific ways in which role playing can be used to resolve conflicts and increase self-awareness is through a "dialogue" that requires the patient to take the part of each person or each side of an argument. He is then asked to "play out" the conflict through an imaginary dialogue. If the conflict is internal, the dialogue occurs in the present tense between his conflicting selves until one part of the conflict outweighs the other. If the conflict involves a second person, the patient is instructed to "imagine that the other person is sitting in the chair across from you." The patient is told to begin the dialogue by expressing wants and resentments about the other person. Then the patient changes chairs, assumes the role of the other person, and responds to what was just said. The patient assumes the first role again and responds to the other person. Using dialogue in this way not only serves as practice for the patient in expressing feelings and opinions but also gives a reality base for the probable response from the other party involved in the conflict. This can often remove the barrier that is keeping the patient from making a decision and acting on it.

Role playing is included as an action dimension because it can help the patient develop insight. Nurses need a variety of intervention skills. Role playing can be effective when an impasse has been reached in the patient's progress or when he is having difficulty translating insight into action. In these instances it can reduce tension and allow the patient the opportunity to practice or test new behaviors for future use.

Table 4-9 summarizes the responsive and action dimensions for therapeutic nurse-patient relationships. In concluding this section on therapeutic dimensions, we emphasize that the nurse's effectiveness is based on openness to learning what works best with particular kinds of patients. Both the use of communication techniques and the therapeutic conditions must be individualized to the nurse's personality and the patient's needs. Rote application can be destructive. The nurse must be willing to try other approaches and techniques that seem potentially helpful when the current approach seems ineffective at a given time.

TABLE 4-9

RESPONSIVE AND ACTION DIMENSIONS FOR THERAPEUTIC NURSE-PATIENT RELATIONSHIPS

Dimension	Characteristics
Responsive dimensions	
Genuineness	Implies that the nurse is an open person who is self-congruent, authentic, and transparent
Respect	Suggests that the patient is regarded as a person of worth who is valued and accepted without qualification
Empathic understanding	Viewing the patient's world from his internal frame of reference, with sensitivity to the patient's current feelings and the verbal ability to communicate this understanding in a language attuned to the patient
Concreteness	Involves the use of specific terminology rather than abstractions in the discussion of the patient's feelings, experiences, and behavior
Action dimensions	
Confrontation	The expression by the nurse of perceived discrepancies in the patient's behavior to expand his self-awareness
Immediacy	Occurs when the current interaction of the nurse and patient is focused on and is used to learn about the patient's functioning in other interpersonal relationships
Nurse self-disclosure	Evident when the nurse reveals information about himself or herself and personal ideas, values, feelings, and attitudes to facilitate the patient's cooperation, learning, catharsis, or support
Emotional catharsis	Takes place when the patient is encouraged to talk about things that bother him most
Role playing	The acting-out of a particular situation to increase the patient's insight into human relations and deepen his ability to see a situation from another point of view. It also allows the patient to experiment with new behavior in a safe environment

Therapeutic impasses

Therapeutic impasses are blocks in the progress of the nurse-patient relationship. They arise for a variety of reasons and may take many different forms, but they all create stalls in the therapeutic relationship. Impasses provoke intense feelings in both the nurse and the patient that may range from anxiety and apprehension to frustration, love, or intense anger. Four specific therapeutic impasses and ways to overcome them are discussed here: resistance, transference, countertransference, and gift giving.

■ **Resistance**

Resistance is the patient's attempt to remain unaware of anxiety-producing aspects within himself. It is a natural reluctance or learned avoidance of verbalizing or even experiencing troubled aspects of self. The term *resistance* was initially introduced by Freud to mean the patient's unconscious opposition to exploring or recognizing unconscious or even preconscious material. The patient's ambivalent attitudes toward self-exploration, in which he both appreciates and avoids anxiety-producing experiences, are a normal part of the therapeutic process. Primary resistance is often caused by the patient's unwillingness to change when the need for change is recognized. Patients usually display resistance behaviors during the working phase of the relationship, because this phase encompasses the greater part of the problem-solving process.

Resistance may also be a reaction by the patient to the nurse who has moved too rapidly or too deeply into the patient's feelings or who has intentionally or unintentionally communicated a lack of respect. It may also simply be the result of a patient who has a nurse working with him who is an inappropriate role model for therapeutic behavior.

Secondary gain is another cause of resistance. Favorable environmental, interpersonal, and situational changes occur, and material advantages may be secured as a result of the illness. Types of secondary gain include financial compensation, avoiding unpleasant situations, increased sympathy or attention, escape from responsibility, attempted control of people, and lessening of social pressures. Secondary gain can become a

Forms of Resistance Displayed by Patients

- Suppression and repression of pertinent information
- Intensification of symptoms
- Self-devaluation and a hopeless outlook on the future
- Forced flight into health where there is a sudden, but short-lived recovery by the patient
- Intellectual inhibitions, which may be evident when the patient says he has "nothing on his mind" or that he is "unable to think about his problems" or when he breaks appointments, is late for sessions, or is forgetful, silent, or sleepy
- Acting out or irrational behavior
- Superficial talk
- Intellectual insight in which the patient verbalizes self-understanding with correct use of terminology yet continues destructive behavior, or use of the defense of intellectualization where there is no insight
- Contempt for normality, which is evident when the patient has developed insight but refuses to assume the responsibility for change on the grounds that normality "isn't so great"
- Transference reactions

powerful force in the perpetuation and propagation of an illness, since it makes the environment more comfortable.

Resistance may take many forms. The accompanying box lists some of the forms of resistance that patients display as identified by Wolberg.[68]

■ Transference

Transference is an unconscious response of the patient in which he experiences feelings and attitudes toward the nurse that were originally associated with significant figures in his early life. Such responses utilize the defense mechanism of displacement. They may be triggered by some superficial similarity, such as a facial feature or manner of speech, or by the patient's perceived similarity of the relationship. The term transference refers to a group of reactions that attempt to reduce or alleviate anxiety. The outstanding trait defining transference is the inappropriateness of the patient's response in terms of intensity.

Transference reduces the patient's self-awareness by helping him maintain a generalized view of the world in which all people are seen in similar terms. Thus the nurse may be viewed as an authority figure from the past, such as a parent figure, or as a lost loved object, such as a former spouse. Transference reactions are harmful to the therapeutic process only if they remain ignored and unexamined.

Two types of transference present particular resistances in the nurse-patient relationship. The first is the **hostile transference.** If the patient internalizes his anger and hostility, he may express this resistance as depression and discouragement. He may ask to terminate the relationship on the grounds that he has no chance of getting well. If the patient externalizes his hostility, he may become critical, defiant, and irritable. He may express doubts about the nurse's training, experience, or personal adjustment. He may attempt to compete with the nurse by reading books on psychology and challenging him or her.

Hostility may also be expressed by the patient in detachment, forgetfulness, irrelevant chatter, or preoccupation with childhood experiences. An extreme form of uncooperativeness and negativism is evident in prolonged silences. Some of the most frustrating moments for the nurse are those spent in total silence with a patient. This is not the therapeutic silence that communicates mutuality and understanding. Rather, it is the silence that seems to be hostile, oppressive, and eternal. It is particularly disturbing for the nurse in the orientation phase, before a relationship has been established. Generally, silences are more uncomfortable for the patient than they are for the nurse, but in this case the reverse may be true. The nurse's task is to understand the meaning of the patient's silence and decide how to deal with it despite feeling somewhat awkward and useless.

A second difficult type of transference is the **dependent reaction transference.** This resistance is characterized by patients who are submissive, subordinate, and ingratiating and who regard the nurse as a "godlike" figure. The patient overvalues the nurse's characteristics and qualities, and their relationship is in jeopardy because the patient views it as magical. In this reaction the nurse must live up to the patient's overwhelming expectations, which is impossible because these expectations are completely unrealistic. The patient continues to demand more of the nurse, and when he or she does not meet his needs, he is filled with hostility and contempt.

Overcoming resistance and transference

Resistances and transferences can pose difficult problems for the nurse. The psychiatric nurse must be prepared to be exposed to powerful negative and positive emotional feelings coming from the patient, often on a highly irrational basis. The relationship can become stalled and nonbeneficial if the nurse is not prepared for the patient's expression of feelings, is not prepared to deal with them, or is so preoccupied by personal needs and problems that he or she cannot clearly perceive what is happening.

Sometimes resistances occur because the nurse and patient have not arrived at mutually acceptable goals or plans of action. Perhaps the patient expected the nurse to give him advice or solve his problems for him. This may occur if the contract was not clearly defined in the orientation stage of the relationship. The appropriate action here is to return to the goals, purpose, and roles of the nurse and patient in the relationship.

Whatever the patient's motivations, the analysis of the resistance or transference is geared toward his gaining awareness of these motivations and learning that he controls his behavior and ultimately is responsible for all he does and experiences. The first thing the nurse must do in handling resistance or transference is to listen. When she recognizes the resistance, she then uses clarification and reflection of feeling. Clarification helps give the nurse a more focused idea of what is happening. Reflection of content may help the patient become aware of what has been going on in his own mind. Reflection of feeling acknowledges the resistance and mirrors it to the patient. The nurse may say, "I sense that you're struggling with yourself. Part of you wants to explore the issue of your marriage and another part says 'No—I'm not ready yet.' "

It is not sufficient, however, to merely identify that resistance is occurring. The behavior must be explored and possible reasons for its occurrence analyzed. The depth of exploration and analysis engaged in by nurse and patient is related to the nurse's experience and knowledge base. The nurse prepared on the master's degree level has the background to review the resistance and work through the transference reaction with the patient. Supervision aids the nurse in this endeavor and minimizes the effect of any negative reactions the nurse may experience personally.

Countertransference

Countertransference is a therapeutic impasse created by the nurse. It refers to the nurse's specific emotional response generated by the qualities of the patient. This response is inappropriate to the content and context of the therapeutic relationship or inappropriate in the degree of intensity of emotion. It is transference applied to the nurse. Inappropriateness is the crucial element, as it is with transference, because it is natural that the nurse will have a warmth toward or liking for some patients more than others. The nurse will also be genuinely angry with the actions of certain patients. But in countertransference the nurse's responses are not justified by reality. In this case the nurse identifies the patient with individuals from his or her past, and personal needs will interfere with therapeutic effectiveness. The nurse's unresolved conflicts about authority, sex, assertiveness, and independence tend to create problems, rather than solve them.

Countertransference reactions are usually of three types: (1) reactions of intense love or caring, (2) reactions of intense hostility or hatred, and (3) reactions of intense anxiety often in response to resistance by the patient. Through the use of immediacy the nurse can identify countertransference in one of its various forms. The accompanying box lists some forms of countertransference displayed by nurses as described by Langs and Menninger.[38,44]

Forms of countertransference occur because the nurse is involved with the patient as a participant observer and is not a detached bystander. These reactions can be powerful tools in exploration and potent instruments for uncovering inner states. They are destructive only if they are brushed aside, ignored, or not taken seriously.

If studied objectively, these reactions can lead to further information about the patient. Analysis of countertransference can bring to light new material. The ability to remain objective does not mean that the nurse may not at times dislike what the patient says or may not become irritated. The patient's resistance to acquiring insight and transforming it into action and his refusal to change maladaptive and destructive coping mechanisms can be frustrating. But the nurse's capacity to understand his or her own feelings helps to maintain a working relationship with the patient.

Countertransference may also be manifested as a group phenomenon. Psychiatric staff members can become involved in countertransference reactions when they overreact to a patient's aggressive behavior, ignore available patient data that would promote understanding, or become locked in a power struggle with a patient. Other types of countertransference might in-

---

Forms of Countertransference Displayed by Nurses

- Inability to empathize with the patient in certain problem areas
- Depressed feelings during or after the session
- Carelessness about implementing the contract by being late, running overtime, etc.
- Drowsiness during the sessions
- Feelings of anger or impatience because of the patient's unwillingness to change
- Encouragement of the patient's dependency, praise, or affection
- Arguing with the patient or a tendency to push the patient before he is ready
- Trying to help the patient in matters not related to the identified nursing goals

- Involvement with the patient on a personal or social level
- Dreaming about or preoccupation with the patient
- Sexual or aggressive fantasies toward the patient
- Recurrent anxiety, unease, or guilt feelings about the patient
- A tendency to focus repetitively on only one aspect or way of looking at the information presented by the patient
- A need to defend nursing interventions with the patient to others

---

clude ignoring patient behavior that does not fit the staff's diagnosis, minimizing a patient's behavior, joking about or criticizing a patient, or becoming caught up in intimidation. Although these have been reported as phenomena of group countertransference, they can also illustrate individual countertransference reactions.

One difference between an inexperienced and an experienced psychiatric nurse is that the experienced nurse is constantly on the lookout for countertransference. He or she becomes aware of it when it occurs and holds it in abeyance or utilizes it to promote the therapeutic goals. In attempting to identify a countertransference, the nurse must apply the same standards of honest self-appraisal personally that he or she expects of the patient. The nurse should employ self-examination throughout the course of the relationship, particularly when the patient attacks or criticizes. The following questions may be helpful:

- How do I feel about the patient?
- Do I look forward to seeing him?
- Do I feel sorry for or sympathetic toward him?
- Am I bored with him and believe that we are not progressing?
- Am I afraid of him?
- Do I get extreme pleasure out of seeing him?
- Do I want to protect, reject, or punish him?
- Do I dread meeting him and feel nervous during the sessions?

- Am I impressed by him or do I try to impress him?
- Does he make me very angry or frustrated?

If any of these questions suggests a problem, the nurse should pursue it. What is the patient doing to provoke these feelings? Who does the patient remind me of? The nurse must discover the source of the problem. Because countertransference can be detrimental to the relationship, it should be dealt with as soon as possible. When it is recognized, the nurse can exercise control over it. Frequently the nurse needs help in dealing with countertransference. Individual or group supervision can be most beneficial. Weekly clinical seminars, peer consultation, and professional meetings can also offer emotional support.

■ **PROBLEM PATIENTS.** Countertransference problems are most clearly evident when a patient is labeled a "problem patient." Usually such a patient develops strong negative feelings such as anger, fear, and helplessness and is often described by nurses as "manipulative, a pain, dependent, inappropriate, and demanding." The label "problem patient" implies that the patient should change his behavior for the sake of the helper rather than for his own benefit. This labeling often causes the patient and nurse to become adversaries, and the nurse avoids contact with him.

A study of the treatment records of "difficult patients" revealed some interesting findings. Compared with controls, difficult patients were simultaneously involved in or referred to two or more treatment programs, had no one person primarily responsible for coordinating their treatment programs, had incomplete documentation of treatment contacts, and lacked a comprehensive diagnosis and treatment plan.[48] Another study of therapists' actions that address initially poor therapeutic alliances between the patient and therapist found that improved alliances and good outcomes were associated with (1) addressing the patient's defenses, (2) addressing the patient's guilt and expectations of punishment, (3) addressing the patient's problematic feelings in relation to the therapist, and (4) linking the problematic feelings in relation to the therapist with the patient's defenses.[19]

Rather than viewing the patient as a "problem patient," therefore, it is more productive for a nurse to view him as a patient who poses problems for the nurse. This turns the responsibility for action away from the patient and back onto the nurse. It forces the nurse to explore his or her responses to the patient and the behavior the nurse displays that reinforces the patient's unproductive behavior. In this way the nurse also makes the patient responsible for his own behavior. By stepping back and reviewing again the patient's needs and problems, the nurse becomes aware that he or she is failing to use the responsive dimensions of genuineness, respect, empathic understanding, and concreteness. Without this therapeutic groundwork, a therapeutic outcome is impossible.

■ **Gift giving**

Gift giving is included in this discussion of therapeutic impasses not because it necessarily precipitates an impasse, but because many nurses perceive it this way. This is partly because there has been a long-accepted taboo in nursing on accepting gifts from patients. Like many traditional taboos, it lacks a sound theoretical rationale, inhibits the nurse's independent decision making, and creates a feeling of anxiety or guilt.

Gifts can take many forms. They can be tangible or intangible, lasting or temporary. Tangible gifts may include such items as a box of candy, a bouquet of flowers, a hand-knit scarf, or a hand-painted picture. Intangible gifts can be the expression of thanks to a nurse by a patient who is about to be discharged or a family member's sense of relief and gratitude at being able to share an emotional burden with another caring person. The underlying element of all of these gifts is that something of value is voluntarily offered to another person, usually to convey gratitude.

Because gifts can be so varied, it is inappropriate to lump them all together and uniformly arrive at an appropriate nursing action. Rather, the nurse's response to gift giving and the role it plays in the therapeutic relationship depends on the timing of the particular situation, the intent of the giver, and the contextual meaning of the giving of the gift. Occasionally it may be most appropriate and therapeutic for the nurse to accept a patient's gift; on other occasions it may be quite inappropriate and detrimental to the relationship.

■ **TIMING IN THE RELATIONSHIP.** The timing of the gift giving is an important consideration. In the introductory, or orientation, phase of the relationship, nurses may be asked, "Do you have a cigarette I can borrow?" or "Will you buy me a cup of coffee?" These seemingly minor requests may make the nurse feel uncomfortable refusing them. The nurse may even rationalize compliance by thinking that it indicates interest in the patient and may help win his trust. But these responses indicate the nurse's failure to examine the patient's covert, or underlying, need and the nurse's own needs in complying with it. Also, in this early phase of the relationship, the nurse may be the one to initiate gift giving by giving the patient a book, plant, or some other item that he or she believes expresses her interest.

In the orientation phase of the relationship, gift giving can be detrimental because it often meets personal needs rather than therapeutic goals. For example, the patient may be trying to manipulate the nurse as his way of controlling the relationship and setting interpersonal limits on the level of intimacy he will allow. As such it can be a form of resistance and act as a therapeutic impasse. The nurse as the gift giver may also be distorting the nature and purpose of the therapeutic relationship. By giving gifts to the patient, the nurse is attempting to relate through objects instead of the therapeutic use of self. He or she is avoiding exploring possible feelings of inadequacy or frustration. If the patient accepts the gifts, the nurse may worry that he is relating to him or her out of a sense of obligation, and this aura of doubt may overshadow the course of the relationship. On the other hand, it may enhance the patient's sense of self to bring to his attention a magazine that has been on the ward and has an article on a topic of interest to him. The distinction lies in the meaning behind the gift and the sense of obligation it implies.

As the relationship progresses, gift giving may take on a different significance. In the working phase, for example, the patient may one day offer to buy the nurse a cup of coffee. This can be an indication of the patient's respect for the nurse and his belief in the mutuality of their work together. As an isolated incident, the nurse's acceptance of it can enhance the patient's confidence, self-esteem, and sense of responsibility.

Gift giving most often arises in the termination phase of the relationship, and it is in this phase that the meaning behind it can be the most complex and difficult to determine. At this time gift giving can be tangible or intangible and can reflect a patient's need to make the nurse feel guilty, delay the termination process, compensate for feelings of inadequacy, or attempt to transform the therapeutic nurse-patient relationship into a social one that can possibly go on indefinitely. The nurse can initiate gift giving for similar reasons. The feelings evoked during the termination process can be very powerful, and they must be acknowledged and explored if termination is to be a learning experience for both participants. If feelings are identified and clarified, then a small gift that reflects gratitude and remembrance can be exchanged, accepted, and valued. In this case it becomes not a therapeutic impasse but a memento of a treasured growth experience.

Effectiveness of the nurse

The nurse's effectiveness in working with psychiatric patients is related to his or her knowledge base, clinical skills, and capacity for introspection and self-evaluation. The nurse and patient, as participants in an interpersonal relationship, are entwined in a pattern of reciprocal emotions that directly affect the therapeutic outcome. The nurse conveys feelings to the patient. Some of these are in response to the patient; others arise from the nurse's personal life and are not necessarily associated with the patient. For example, a nurse is feeling angry because of an administrative problem involving the nursing service. The patient may sense these feelings and misconstrue their source as being himself. If he does not have the confidence to discuss this with the nurse, he or she may be unaware of the misconception.

Many painful feelings arise within the nurse because of the nature of the therapeutic process, which can be stressful. These "normal" stresses are caused by a variety of factors. Although the nurse must be a skilled listener, it is inappropriate for him or her to discuss personal conflicts or responses, except when they may help the patient. This bottling up of emotions can be painful. The nurse is expected to empathize with the patient's emotions and feelings. At the same time, however, the nurse is expected to retain objectivity and not be caught up in a sympathetic response. This can create a kind of double bind.

Termination poses another stress when the nurse must separate from a patient he or she has come to know well and care for deeply. It is common to experience a grief reaction in response to the loss. Many nurses find it emotionally draining when a patient communicates a prolonged and intense expression of emotion, such as sadness, despair, or anger. Discomfort also arises when the nurse feels unable to help a patient who is in great distress. Suicide dramatizes this situation. Treating suicidal individuals can arouse intense and prolonged anxiety in the nurse.

The painful nature of these emotional responses makes the practice of psychiatric nursing challenging and stressful. The therapeutic use of self involves the nurse's total personality, and total involvement is not an easy task. It is essential that the nurse be aware of his or her feelings and responses and receive guidance and support.

■ Supervision

According to Haller, supervision is a "process whereby a therapist, frequently but not always a relative beginner, is helped to become a more effective clinician. The goals of supervision are not only to guide the therapist in the successful handling of the supervised case, but to catalyze the therapist's creative and therapeutic use of self."[25:36] The supervisor serves as a provider of theoretical knowledge and therapeutic techniques, validates the use of the nursing process, and supports the working through of transference and countertransference reactions. Consultation is different from supervision in that it denotes a peer or collegial relationship; it is discussed in detail in Chapter 26.

Supervision also functions as a support system for those providing care and is an essential element in therapeutic relationships. One must care about oneself and experience being cared for before one can give care to others. All practicing psychiatric nurses experience some degree of clinical stress. There are stresses associated with such patient behaviors as hopelessness, self-destruction, and manipulation, as well as the stress inherent in the intimacy, openness, and responsiveness required of the nurse who has established a therapeutic relationship. Supervision provides the nurse with a system of clinical support and contributes greatly if indirectly to the quality of nursing care.

In many ways the process of supervision parallels the nurse-patient relationship. Both involve a learning process that takes place in the context of a deep and meaningful relationship that facilitates positive change. Self-exploration is a critical element of both. The supervisor should provide the same responsive and action dimensions present in the nurse-patient relationship to help the supervised nurse become a person who can live effectively with himself or herself and others.

Hughes advocates using a nursing model to provide the foundation for clinical teaching and supervision. Its purposes would be to:

- Improve the nurse's therapeutic relationships with patients
- Improve therapeutic nursing interventions
- Increase knowledge of the theories of human behavior
- Increase the nurse's self-awareness of the motivation of personal behavior
- Further the development of the nurse's personal endowments[28]

Hughes further identified three phases of supervision that parallel those of the nurse-patient relationship—the contracting, or beginning, phase; the working phase; and the termination phase.

There are three common forms of supervision: (1) the dyadic, or one-to-one, relationship, in which the supervisor meets the supervisee in a face-to-face encounter; (2) the triadic relationship, in which a supervisor and two nurses of similar experience and training meet for supervision; and (3) group supervision, in which several supervised nurses meet for a shared session with the supervisory nurse. All three forms have a similar purpose—exploring the problem areas and maximizing the strengths of the supervisees.

■ **THE PROCESS OF SUPERVISION.** The process of supervision requires the nurse to record the interactions with the patient. Both written processed recordings and audio recordings have been used for this purpose, but neither yields as accurate and complete information as that provided by videotape recordings. Videotaped sessions minimize distortion of data. The supervised nurse then analyzes the data, extracts themes, and identifies problems relevant to the nursing care. He or she reviews the literature, draws inferences, evaluates his or her effectiveness, and formulates plans for the next session. In the supervision conference the nurse shares this analysis and receives feedback from the supervisor and peers, if it is a group conference.

Supervision can be viewed in two ways. It can be a didactic process in which the theory, concepts, and practice of the individual therapeutic relationship are enunciated. Or it can be a quasitherapeutic process that explores countertransference problems, attitudes, values, and the nurse's emotional needs and personal biases. The more widely accepted view recognizes that the supervisor-therapist relationship is more important than a simple didactic adjunct to the treatment process; it has a major, if somewhat intangible, bearing on the therapist-patient relationship and the therapeutic process.

Three methods of supervision have been described. The first is **patient centered,** in which the therapist brings the technical problems with the patient to the supervisor and is given advice. The second type is **therapist centered,** in which the focus is on the therapist's blind spots and countertransference reactions. This helps the therapist see his or her influence on the therapeutic process. The danger with this method is that when it is used to the extreme, the patient is lost from sight and the supervision evolves into personal therapy for the supervisee. The third approach is **process centered,** in which the emphasis is on what is happening between the therapist, patient, and supervisor. The supervisor makes use of the analogy between the therapist-patient relationship and the therapist-supervisor relationship to help the supervisee use personal experience of emotional difficulties in receiving help from the supervisor to facilitate understanding of the patient's situation.

Ekstein and Wallerstein[17] have developed a process-centered model of supervision that is neither personal therapy nor simply a didactic process of conveying information on theory and technique. In their model the supervisor is an active participant in an affectively charged learning process, the focus of which is learning and personal growth rather than psychotherapy for the supervisee. The author's describe how and in what ways the problems between the therapist and the supervisor can shed light on and in fact often stand for problems that exist between the therapist and patient. The very problems experienced in the one relationship affect and are reflected in the other relationship; thus a parallel process exists between the supervisor-therapist relationship and therapist-patient relationship.

The goal of supervision, however, is not to eliminate these problems; it is to use them to achieve greater understanding of the ongoing dynamic processes at work in therapy. The problems become the vehicles through which therapeutic progress may be made. Ekstein and Wallerstein propose that the most effective supervision depends on active insight into the interplay of forces in the parallel processes of therapy and supervision.

Little research on the supervisory process is reported in the literature. One of the few studies to explore the nature of the process was conducted by Doehrman.[16] The results of this study highlight an important aspect of supervision—tension in the supervisory relationship is inevitable, but when understood and handled skillfully, it is instrumental to the therapist's growth. Learning to be therapeutic inspires fear and resistance in the learner. These feelings are expressed in the supervisee's characteristic way of resisting authority. The therapist's ways of resisting help in supervision are intimately related to his or her difficulties in helping patients. Insight into these resistances provides the supervisee with insight into his or her problems as a therapist and particular problems in the nurse-patient relationship. Deprived of these insights, the supervisee cannot grow as a therapist. There will be no learning, no change, and the status quo will be preserved.

Doehrman's study supports Ekstein and Wallerstein's model of supervision. This model entails the supervisor's addressing the problems of the supervisee that block the latter's functioning as an effective therapist. Doehrman concludes that the supervisor should deal with the supervisee's feelings toward her and toward the supervisory process when these feelings interfere with the therapist's effectiveness with patients or ability to learn from the supervisor. Clarifying these problems requires the supervisor to use certain therapeutic skills such as the exploration and expression of feelings and encouraging insight, and this may be intensely therapeutic for the supervisee.

■ **PURPOSE AND GOALS.** Despite the intensity involved, supervision is not therapy. The essential difference between the two is a difference of purpose. The aim of supervision is to teach psychotherapeutic skills, whereas the goal of therapy is to alter the patient's characteristic patterns of coping to function more effectively in all areas of life. In contrast, the supervisee's problems in the supervisory and therapeutic relationships are dealt with only to the extent that they affect the nurse's ability to learn from the supervisor and be effective with patients. Therefore the problems are limited in scope and depth; they do not include all other aspects of the supervisee's life situation. With the resolution of the particular problem, the focus of supervision returns to the teaching of psychotherapeutic skills and their implementation by the nurse with the patients. The therapeutic implications for the supervisee are therefore related to the primary goal of supervision—the teaching of psychotherapeutic skills.

Supervision or consultation is necessary for the practicing psychiatric nurse. Although it is crucial for novices, it is equally as important for experienced practitioners. Personal limitations create a need for assistance in remaining objective throughout the therapeutic process and the "normal" stresses it presents. Obviously supervision is only as helpful as the skill of the

---

DIRECTIONS FOR FUTURE RESEARCH

The following are some of the nursing research problems raised in Chapter 4 that merit further study by psychiatric nurses:

1. The extent to which psychiatric nurses possess the personal qualities associated with being able to help others
2. The levels of openness, authenticity, and empathic understanding in student-teacher relationships in nursing
3. The validity of Burgess and Burns' description of reasons why patients seek psychiatric care and which nursing approaches would be effective with each
4. The affective and behavioral patient outcomes associated with the nurse's use of personal space and spatial parameters
5. Valid and reliable instruments to measure the responsive and action dimensions of a therapeutic nurse-patient relationship
6. The extent to which psychiatric nurses demonstrate the responsive dimensions of genuineness, respect, empathic understanding, and concreteness and resulting therapeutic outcomes
7. The extent to which psychiatric nurses demonstrate the action dimensions of confrontation, immediacy, nurse self-disclosure, catharsis, and role playing and resulting therapeutic outcomes
8. An exploration of the role of gift giving within the context of a nurse-patient relationship
9. The process, methods, and outcomes of supervision used with and by psychiatric nurses
10. Different levels of therapeutic relationship skills possessed by psychiatric nurses with varying educational and experiential preparation

---

supervisor, the openness of the supervised nurse, and the motivation of both to learn and grow.

■ **SUGGESTED CROSS-REFERENCES** ■

This chapter serves as a foundation for formulating principles of psychiatric nursing and implementing psychiatric nursing practice. As such it is related to all other chapters of this text.

■ **SUMMARY** ■

1. The therapeutic nurse-patient relationship is a mutual learning experience and a corrective emotional experi-

ence for the patient. In this relationship the nurse uses personal attributes and specified clinical techniques in working with the patient to bring about behavioral change. General goals of the relationship were identified.

2. Self-awareness was described as the first step in providing quality nursing care through the therapeutic use of self. The following qualities needed by nurses to be effective helpers were analyzed: the awareness of self, the clarification of values, the exploration of feelings, the ability to serve as a role model, altruism, and a sense of ethics and responsibility.

3. The four phases of the relationship process were described and the tasks of the nurse in each of the phases were identified.

4. Communication incorporates the ideas of interpersonal influence and behavioral change. The structural and transactional analysis models were used to examine components of the communication process and to identify common breakdowns or problems. Helpful therapeutic communication techniques were also discussed.

5. The responsive dimensions of genuineness, respect, empathic understanding, and concreteness were presented. They interrelate with and contribute to each other in the therapeutic process, and some degree of each of them is necessary when initiating a relationship.

6. The action dimensions of confrontation, immediacy, nurse self-disclosure, catharsis, and role playing stimulate and contribute to patient insight.

7. Therapeutic impasses are roadblocks in the progress of the nurse-patient relationship. Resistance is the patient's attempt to remain unaware of anxiety-producing aspects within himself. Transference is an unconscious response of the patient in which he experiences feelings and attitudes toward the nurse that were originally associated with significant figures in his early life. Countertransference is the specific emotional response of the nurse, generated by the qualities of the patient, that is inappropriate to the content and context of the therapeutic relationship or inappropriate in the degree of intensity of emotion. It is transference applied to the nurse.

8. Supervision is a process in which the supervised nurse is helped to become a more effective clinician. It may occur individually or in groups and is distinct from consultation, which implies a peer relationship. Supervision is crucial for novices, but it is equally important for experienced practitioners.

■ **REFERENCES** ■

1. Aiken L and Aiken J: A systematic approach to the evaluation of interpersonal relationships, Am J Nurs 73:863, 1973.
2. Anderson S: Effects of confrontation by high- and low-functioning therapists on high- and low-functioning clients, J Counsel Psychol 16:299, 1969.
3. Argyle M: Bodily communication, New York, 1975, International Universities Press, Inc.
4. Berne E: Games people play: the psychology of human relationships, New York, 1964, Grove Press, Inc.
5. Bohart A: Role playing and interpersonal conflict reduction, J Counsel Psych 24:15, 1977.
6. Bromley G: Confrontation in individual psychotherapy, J Psychiatr Nurs 19(5):15, 1981.
7. Bugenthal J: The search for existential identity, San Francisco, 1976, Jossey-Bass, Inc, Publishers.
8. Burgess A and Burns J: Why patients seek care, Am J Nurs 73:314, 1973.
9. Campaniello J: The process of termination, J Psychiatr Nurs 18(2):29, 1980.
10. Campbell J: The relationship of nursing and self-awareness, Adv Nurs Sci 2(4):15, 1980.
11. Carkhoff R: Helping and human relations, vols 1 and 2, New York, 1969, Holt, Rinehart & Winston, Inc.
12. Carkhoff R and Berenson B: Beyond counseling and therapy, New York, 1967, Holt, Rinehart & Winston, Inc.
13. Carkhoff R and Truax C: Toward effective counseling and psychotherapy, Chicago, 1967, Aldine Publishing Co.
14. Coad-Denton A: Therapeutic superficiality and intimacy. In Longo D and Williams R, editors: Psychosocial nursing: assessment and intervention, New York, 1978, Appleton-Century-Crofts.
15. Cooper K: Territorial behavior among the institutionalized, J Psychosoc Nurs Ment Health Serv 22(12):6, 1984.
16. Doehrman M: Parallel process in supervision and psychotherapy, Bull Menninger Clin 40:9, 1976.
17. Ekstein R and Wallerstein R: The teaching and learning of psychotherapy, New York, 1958, Basic Books, Inc, Publishers.
18. Forchuk C and Brown B: Establishing a nurse-client relationship, J Psychosoc Nurs 27(2):30, 1989.
19. Foreman S and Marmar C: Therapist actions that address initially poor therapeutic alliances in psychotherapy, Am J Psychiatry 142(8):922, 1985.
20. Fox E, Nelson M, and Bolman W: The termination process: a neglected dimension in social work, Soc Work 14:53, Oct 1969.
21. Gaylin W: Feelings, New York, 1979, Harper & Row Publishers, Inc.
22. Gazda G, et al: Human relations development: a manual for educators, Boston, 1971, Allyn & Bacon, Inc.
23. Ginott H: Between parent and child, New York, 1965, Macmillan Co, Publishers.
24. Hall E: The silent language, Garden City, NY, 1959, Doubleday & Co, Inc.
25. Haller L: Clinical psychiatric supervision. In Kneisl, CR and Wilson HS, editors: Current perspectives in psychiatric nursing, vol 1, St Louis, 1976, The CV Mosby Co.
26. Hardin S and Halaris A: Nonverbal communication of patients and high and low empathy nurses, J Psychosoc Nurs Ment Health Serv 21(1):14, 1983.
27. Heuscher J: The role of humor and folklore themes in psychotherapy, Am J Psychiatry 137(12):1546, 1980.
28. Hughes C: Supervising clinical practice in psychosocial

nursing, J Psychosoc Nurs Ment Health Serv 23(2):27, 1985.

29. Hutchinson S: Humor: a link to life. In Kneisl CR and Wilson HS, editors: Current perspectives in psychiatric nursing, vol 1, St Louis, 1976, The CV Mosby Co.

30. Johnson M: Self-disclosure and anxiety in nurses and patients, Issues Ment Health Nurs 2(1):41, 1979.

31. Johnson M: Self-disclosure: a variable in the nurse-client relationship, J Psychiatr Nurs 18(1):17, 1980.

32. Jourard S: The transparent self, New York, 1971, Litton Educational Publishing, Inc.

33. Kalisch B: What is empathy? Am J Nurs 73:1548, 1973.

34. Kirschenbaum H and Simon S, editors: Readings in values clarification, Minneapolis, 1973, Winston Press, Inc.

35. Krieger D: The therapeutic touch: how to use your hands to help or to heal, New York, 1979, Prentice-Hall, Inc.

36. La Crosse M: Nonverbal behavior and perceived counselor attractiveness and persuasiveness, J Counsel Psychol 22:563, 1975.

37. Lane P: Nurse-client perceptions: the double standard of touch, Issues Mental Health Nurs 10:1, 1989.

38. Langs R: The technique of psychoanalytic psychotherapy, vol 2, New York, 1974, Jason Aronson, Inc.

39. Levinson H: Termination of psychotherapy: some salient issues. Paper presented at a meeting of the Illinois Society for Clinical Social Work, Chicago, Oct 1975.

40. Loomis M: Levels of contracting, J Psychosoc Nurs Ment Health Serv 23(3):9, 1985.

41. Luft J: Of human interaction, Palo Alto, Calif, 1969, National Press Books.

42. Mansfield E: Empathy: concept and identified psychiatric nursing behavior, Nurs Res 22(6):525, 1973.

43. Mehrabian A: Nonverbal communication, Chicago, 1972, Aldine Publishing Co.

44. Menninger K: Theory of psychoanalytic techniques, New York, 1958, Basic Books, Inc.

45. Methven D and Schlotfeldt R: The social interaction inventory, Nurs Res 11:83, 1962.

46. Mitchell K and Berenson B: Differential use of confrontation by high and low facilitative therapists, J Nerv Ment Dis 151(5):303, 1970.

47. Morrison P and Burnard P: Student's and trained nurse's perceptions of their own interpersonal skills: a report and comparison, J Adv Nurs 14:321, 1989.

48. Neill J: The difficult patient: identification and response, J Clin Psychiatry 40(5):209, 1979.

49. Peitchinis J: Therapeutic effectiveness of counseling by nursing personnel, Nurs Res 21(2):138, 1972.

50. Raths L, Harmin M, and Simon S: Values and teaching, Columbus, Ohio, 1966, Charles E Merrill Publishing Co.

51. Rogers C: On becoming a person, Boston, 1961, Houghton Mifflin Co.

52. Rogers C: Empathic: an unappreciated way of being, J Counsel Psychol 5(2):2, 1975.

53. Ruesch J: Communication and human relations: an interdisciplinary approach. In Ruesch J and Bateson G: Communication: the social matrix of psychiatry, New York, 1968, WW Norton & Co, Inc.

54. Ruesch J: Disturbed communication, New York, 1972, WW Norton & Co, Inc.

55. Schiff S: Termination of therapy, Arch Gen Psychiatry 6(1):77, 1962.

56. Schoffstall C: Concerns of student nurses prior to psychiatric nursing experience: an assessment and intervention technique, J Psychosoc Nurs Ment Health Serv 19(11):11, 1981.

57. Schultz F: The mourning phase of relationships, J Psychiatr Nurs 2(1):37, 1964.

58. Sedgwick R: Role playing: a bridge between talk and action, J Psychiatr Nurs 14(11):16, 1976.

59. Sigman P: Ethical choice in nursing, Adv Nurs Sci 1(3):37, 1979.

60. Stacklum M: New student in psychology, Am J Nurs 81:762, 1981.

61. Sundeen S et al: Nurse-client interaction: implementing the nursing process, ed 4, St Louis, 1989, The CV Mosby Co.

62. Travelbee J: Intervention in psychiatric nursing, Philadelphia, 1969, FA Davis Co.

63. Uustal D: Values clarification in nursing: application to practice, Am J Nurs 78:2058, 1978.

64. Watzlawick P, Beavin J, and Jackson D: Pragmatics of human communication: a study of interactional patterns, pathologies, and paradoxes, New York, 1967, WW Norton & Co, Inc.

65. Weiner M: Therapist disclosure: the use of self in psychotherapy, Boston, Mass, Butterworths, 1978.

66. Weiss S: Touch, Ann Rev Nurs Res 6:3,1988.

67. Williams C: Empathic communication and its effect on client outcome, Issues Ment Health Nurs 2(1):16, 1979.

68. Wolberg L: The technique of psychotherapy, ed 4, Orlando, 1988, Grune & Stratton, Inc.

■ ANNOTATED SUGGESTED READINGS ■

*Abraham I: Support groups for nursing students in psychiatric rotation, Issues Ment Health Nurs 4:159, 1982.

Presents and analyzes the content and process of a support group for undergraduate nursing students in clinical rotation in an inpatient psychiatric setting. Faculty might find this helpful reading.

*Albiez Sr A: Reflecting on the development of a relationship, J Psychiatr Nurs 9(6):25, 1970.

A nursing student describes her first experience in psychiatric nursing. She shares her feelings, fears, and problems in a way that other beginners can relate to. Can reassure the inexperienced nurse.

Berne E: Games people play, New York, 1967, Grove Press, Inc.

The founder of transactional analysis uses that technique to

---

*Asterisk indicates nursing reference.

explore a number of specific "games." A thought-provoking book that gives a different slant on relationships and challenges the reader to find ways to terminate destructive "games."

*Burnard P: Self-awareness for nurses, Gaithersburg, Md, 1986, Aspen Publishers, Inc.

Contains practical exercises, charts and diagrams, and concise, clear information in a step-by-step guide to developing self-awareness.

*Campbell J: The relationship of nursing and self-awareness, Adv Nurs Sci 2(4):15, 1980.

Reviews four theorists' contributions to self theory, then describes a holistic model of self-awareness that is related to nursing care. Presents a theoretical and conceptual discussion useful both to practice and research endeavors.

Carkhoff R: Helping and human relations, vols 1 and 2, New York, 1969, Holt, Rinehart & Winston.

Explores elements of research and practice in helping relationships. Presents scales used to rate the "core therapeutic dimensions."

*Claud E: The plateau in therapist-patient relationships, Perspect Psychiatr Care 10:112, 1972.

Presents the theoretical basis for resistance. Describes the author's approach in overcoming resistance in a patient she had been working with. Clinical experiences are clearly related.

*Cooper K: Territorial behavior among the institutionalized: a nursing perspective, J Psychosoc Nurs Ment Health Serv 22(12):6, 1984.

The crux of this paper is that nurses are an important part of the ward milieu and should attempt, whenever possible, to allow the institutionalized individual control and enjoyment of personal possessions and private living space. Draws attention to the needs of an often overlooked group of patients.

*Ferguson S and Campinha-Bacote J: Humor in nursing, J Psychosoc Nurs 27(4):29, 1989.

Presents an excellent overview of and reveiw of literature concerning the use of humor as a therapeutic intervention. Defining attributes and case examples included.

*Geach B and White J: Empathic resonance: a countertransference phenomenon, Am J Nurs 74:128, 1974.

The authors document a unique countertransference event—presenting characteristics, antecedents, and consequences. They identify a need for nurses to record similar experiences.

*Hayes M, Drake N, and Lindy J: The evening shift: an occasion for acting out transference phenomena, J Psychosoc Nurs Ment Health Serv 23(10):24, 1985.

Focuses on an underexplored aspect of nursing—issues on the evening shift. Views nurse-patient contacts in light of transference reactions and suggests that the disruptive, anxiety-producing behavior of patients, if viewed in this way, might have diagnostic and therapeutic value rather than being the occasion for professional self-doubt.

*Hughes C: Supervising clinical practice in psychosocial nursing, J Psychosoc Nurs Ment Health Serv 23(2):27, 1985.

Advocates a nursing model of clinical supervision and reviews phases of supervision, supervisory functions, relationship, and teaching methods.

Jourard S: The transparent self, New York, 1971, Litton Educational Publishing, Inc.

Proposes that a person can attain health only as he gains courage to be himself with others and finds goals that have meaning for him. Develops the concept of self-disclosure and the implications of it for the therapeutic relationship. Three chapters specifically addressed to nurses are highly recommended.

*Kalisch B: Strategies for developing nurse empathy, Nurs Outlook 19:714, 1971.

The author describes her experiment in developing empathic functioning in nursing students. The training includes discussion of the concept, discrimination training, communication practice, role playing, role model of empathy, and an experimental component.

*Krieger D: The therapeutic touch: how to use your hands to help or to heal, New York, 1979, Prentice Hall, Inc.

Presents the techniques of therapeutic touch, with detailed directions for the nurse who wants to expand her healing abilities in this way.

*La Monica E and Karshmer J: Empathy: educating nurses in professional practice, J Nurs Educ 17(2):3, 1978.

Describes in detail a staff development program that was effective in raising nurses' abilities to perceive and respond with empathy. Valuable reading for nurse educators and administrators who wish to design or use programs in behavioral empathy.

*McCann J: Termination of the psychotherapeutic relationship, J Psychiatr Nurs 17(10):37, 1979.

Discusses the psychodynamics and theories of termination. Also has a good bibliography.

Mueller W and Kell B: Coping with conflict—supervising counselors and psychotherapists, New York, 1972, Appleton-Century-Crofts.

Explores the goals, relationships, and processes that define supervision. Reviews conflict as the core of supervision and discusses in depth the concepts, principles, and guidelines that characterize supervision. Valuable reading for both supervisors and practitioners.

*Sayre J: Common errors in communication made by students in psychiatric nursing, Perspect Psychiatr Care 16(4):175, 1978.

Should be required reading for all students in psychiatric nursing. Identifies many of the communication errors made in each phase of the nurse-patient relationship and gives a clinical example of each. A useful article for enhancing student learning.

*Schoffstall C: Concerns of student nurses prior to psychiatric nursing experience: an assessment and intervention technique, J Psychosoc Nurs Ment Health Serv 19(11):11, 1981.

The authors describe a study they conducted to assess and reduce the anxiety of students about to begin their clinical experience in psychiatric nursing. Educators may find this useful.

*Schroder P: Transference and countertransference, J Psychosoc Nurs Ment Health Serv 23(2):21, 1985.

Clarifies and elaborates on the phenomena of transference and countertransference. Good supplementary reading on these topics.

*Sedgwick R: Role playing: a bridge between talk and action, J Psychiatr Nurs 14(11):16, 1976.

Describes the uses and steps of role playing. Techniques are included, with a brief description of how they are accomplished.

*Sundeen S et al: Nurse-client interaction: implementing the nursing process, ed 4, 1989, St Louis, The CV Mosby Co.

Describes the nursing process, including concepts related to self, communication, phases of the nurse-client relationship, and stress and adaptation. A useful reference for normative elements of relationship skills.

*Taylor S: Rights and responsibilities: nurse-patient relationship, Image 17(1):9, 1985.

Examines nurse-patient relationships in terms of rights and responsibility models of moral judgment, leading to a definition and description of maternalism.

*Uustal D: Values clarification in nursing: application to practice, Am J Nurs 78:2058, 1978.

Focuses on value clarification applied to nursing. Describes 10 strategies in applying the process that are helpful in identifying the nurse's own values.

*Vidoni C: The development of intense positive countertransference feelings in the therapist toward a patient, Am J Nurs 75:407, 1975.

Describes transference and countertransference feelings that influence the nurse-patient relationship. An excellent article that explores this important aspect of therapeutic work.

*Wheeler K: A nursing science approach to understanding empathy, Arch Psych Nurs 2(2):95, 1988.

Examines the nature of empathy in nursing and current conceptual frameworks used in empathy research. Proposes a unifying conceptual model of empathy based on Roger's paradigm of nursing science.

*Young J: Rationale for clinician self-disclosure and research agenda, Image: J Nurs Scholarship 20(4):196, 1988.

Reviews current knowledge on self-disclosure as a therapeutic intervention. Explores its role within the helping relationship and identifies directions for future research in this area.

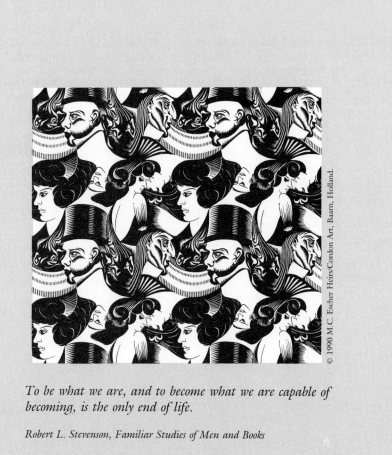

To be what we are, and to become what we are capable of becoming, is the only end of life.

Robert L. Stevenson, *Familiar Studies of Men and Books*

C H A P T E R   5

IMPLEMENTING THE NURSING PROCESS

LEARNING OBJECTIVES

After studying this chapter, the student should be able to:

- define nursing and its four characteristics as identified by the American Nurses' Association.

- define the nursing process and describe some of the unique challenges it presents when used with psychiatric patients.

- explain the need for a theoretical basis and conceptual framework for psychiatric nursing practice and its implications for the development and refinement of nursing theory.

- evaluate the role of culture, spirituality, and family in psychiatric care.

- describe the various psychiatric nursing activities in the phases of data collection, nursing diagnosis, planning, implementation, and evaluation.

- analyze the ways in which psychiatric nurses can participate in organizational evaluation of patterns of care through quality assessment measures.

- discuss the ways in which psychiatric nurses demonstrate professional accountability.

- explain why participation in research is an essential part of psychiatric nursing practice.

- assess the need for documentation related to each phase of the nursing process and describe various tools that nurses use for this purpose.

- describe the three elements of the problem-oriented medical record and the format used for each.

- incorporate elements of the nursing therapeutic process into the student's work with psychiatric patients.

- identify directions for future nursing research.

- select appropriate readings for further study.

Nursing defined

The nurse-patient relationship is the vehicle for applying the nursing process. The goal of nursing care is to maximize the patient's positive interactions with his environment, promote his level of wellness, and enhance his degree of self-actualization. By establishing a therapeutic nurse-patient relationship and using the nursing process, the nurse strives to promote and maintain patient behavior that contributes to integrated functioning. This is the essence of the nursing therapeutic process. It is also the framework on which this text is based.

Although it sounds simple, this concept actually involves a complex process with many related components and requires a skilled nursing practitioner. **The American Nurses' Association defines nursing as "the diagnosis and treatment of human responses to actual or potential health problems."[1:9]** This def-

inition suggests four defining characteristics of nursing*:

1. **Phenomena.** Nursing addresses a wide range of health-related responses observed in both sick and well people. The practice of medicine focuses on the actual health problem, whereas nursing centers on the patient's response to actual or potential problems.
2. **Theory.** Nurses use concepts, principles, and processes to guide their observations and to understand the phenomena that are the focus of their interventions. This use of theory precedes and serves as a basis for determining nursing actions to be taken.

---

*American Nurses' Association: Nursing a social policy statement, Kansas City, Mo, 1980. Reprinted with permission.

3. **Actions.** Nursing actions attempt to prevent illness and promote health. They are theoretically related to the observed phenomena and anticipated outcome of care.
4. **Effects.** The aim of nursing actions is to produce beneficial effects in relation to identified responses. By evaluating the results, nurses determine whether those actions have improved or resolved the conditions to which they were directed.

These characteristics describe nursing as an applied science that involves theory, investigation, and action. They also suggest some essential components of the nursing therapeutic process that merit further exploration. The characteristic of *phenomena* suggests that psychiatric nurses need a model of health and illness so that they may more fully understand the range of actual and potential health problems and possible responses to them. *Theory* maintains that nurses need a theoretical basis and conceptual framework for psychiatric–mental health nursing practice. *Action* requires that the nursing process be a problem-solving process, and the characteristic of *effects* demonstrates the need for standards of nursing practice to evaluate the quality of care. This chapter discusses each of these components of the nursing therapeutic process. It also relates them to the 1982 revised Standards of Psychiatric and Mental Health Nursing Practice* and the process criteria provided with each standard.

The nursing process

The nursing process is an interactive, problem-solving process, a systematic and individualized way to fulfill the goal of nursing care. It is a deliberate and organized approach requiring thought, knowledge, and experience. The nursing process acknowledges the au-

---

*Reprinted with permission from the American Nurses' Association, Kansas City, Mo 1982.

tonomy of the individual and his freedom to make decisions and be involved in his own care. Thus the nurse and patient emerge as partners in a relationship built on trust and directed toward maximizing the patient's strengths, maintaining his integrity, and promoting his adaptive response to stress.

Problem solving is a scientific way of thinking about and dealing with problems, and its principles are part of the nursing process. Table 5-1 compares the steps in problem solving with the phases of the nursing process.

In dealing with psychiatric patients, the nursing process presents unique challenges. Emotional problems are often vague and elusive, not tangible or visible like many physiological disruptions. Emotional problems also can show different symptoms and arise from a number of causes. Similar past events may lead to very different forms of behavior. Many psychiatric patients are initially unable to describe their problems. They may be severely withdrawn, highly anxious, or out of touch with reality. Their ability to participate in the problem-solving process may be limited because they see themselves as powerless victims who deny responsibility for their own behavior.

These factors make it more difficult to use the nursing process with psychiatric patients, but they do not negate its use. Geach has identified the following three hallmarks of clinically valid problem solving for psychiatric patients:

1. The nurse involves the patient in the process.
2. The problem that the nurse and patient address has immediate relevance to what is happening between them, at least initially.
3. The nurse and patient form some sort of relationship so that they can solve problems within a relationship rather than in isolation.[7]

It is essential that the nurse and the patient become partners in the problem-solving process. The

---

TABLE 5-1

COMPARISON OF THE STEPS IN PROBLEM SOLVING WITH THE PHASES OF THE NURSING PROCESS

Problem-solving steps	Phases of the nursing process
Observation and recognition of the problem	Data collection or assessment
Definition of the problem	Formulation of the nursing diagnosis
Formulation of the hypotheses or possible solutions	Planning nursing care
Implementation of the hypotheses or possible solutions	Implementation of nursing interventions
Formulation of conclusions	Evaluation of the nursing assessment, care plan, and actions

nurse may be tempted to exclude the patient, particularly if he resists becoming involved, but this should be avoided for two reasons. First, learning is most effective when the patient directly participates in the learning experience. Second, the patient's isolation from others and self-alienation is part of his unhealthy life-style that needs to be modified. By including the patient as an active participant in the nursing process, the nurse helps restore his sense of control over life and responsibility for action. It reinforces the message that the patient has been making decisions and currently continues to make them. He can choose either adaptive or maladaptive coping responses. Jourard states:

If a person believes himself to be weak, helpless or doomed to some fate or other, he will tend to behave or suffer in the way expected. If, on the other hand, he has a concept of himself as a being with much untapped potential to cope with problems and contradictions in his life, then when these arise, he will persist in efforts to cope with them long after someone who sees himself as ineffective and impotent has given up.[12:34]

The phases of the nursing process as described by the *Standards of Psychiatric and Mental Health Nursing Practice* include data collection, formulation of the nursing diagnosis, planning, implementation, and evaluation (Fig. 5-1). Sometimes data collection is also called the assessment phase of the nursing process. Validation is part of each step, and all phases may overlap or occur simultaneously.

Theoretical basis for practice

STANDARD I—THEORY
The nurse applies appropriate theory that is scientifically sound as a basis for decisions regarding nursing practice.
Process criteria
The nurse:

1. Examines basic assumptions on the nature of persons
2. Corrects erroneous beliefs
3. Uses theory and critical thinking to:
   a. Formulate generalizations (e.g., opinion, speculation, and assumption)
   b. Generate and test hypotheses
4. Uses inferences, principles, and operational concepts
5. Applies relevant theories

All actions of the psychiatric nurse should be based on an understanding of health-illness phenomena and a means for evaluating nursing care. This theoretical basis is drawn both from the nurse's own knowledge and from other sciences. The range of the-

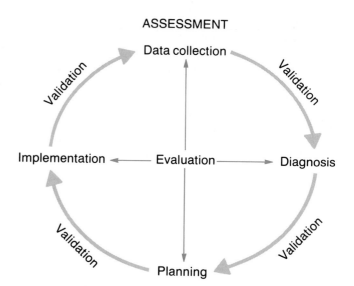

Fig. 5-1. Interrelated phases of the nursing process.

ories used by nurses includes intrapersonal, interpersonal, and systems theories. Intrapersonal theories explain within-person phenomena and focus on the individual level of care. Interpersonal theories elaborate on interactions between two or more people. Systems theories aid the nurse in understanding both complex networks or organizations and how their processes interact. They deal with the family, group, or community levels of care. Nursing requires using a range of theories because of the great variety in patients and patient responses, philosophical backgrounds of psychiatric nurses, and settings in which nurses work. No one theory is universally applicable; the appropriate theory should be selected for its relevance to the tasks at hand.

A conceptual framework is then formulated from relevant theoretical bases. It should integrate theory and nursing process and lead to a distinct body of nursing science by generating hypotheses, propositions, and relationships that can be empirically tested. In this way conceptual frameworks provide a basis for the direction of nursing practice, research, and education and contribute to the development of nursing theory.

Nursing theory

A number of nursing theories are being developed at this time. Prominent theorists who are developing conceptual models as a base for nursing practice include Roy,[26] Rogers,[25] Johnson,[11] Orem,[23] Neuman,[21] and King.[13] Flaskerud and Halloran have identified areas of agreement in nursing theory development. These include the concepts of man-person, society-environ-

TABLE 5-2

DEFINITION OF NURSING CONCEPTS BY NURSE THEORISTS

Nurse-theorist	Person	Environment	Health	Nursing
Roy and Roberts[26]	"An adaptive system with cognator and regulator acting to maintain adaptation in regard to the four adaptive modes"	Conditions, circumstances, and influences surrounding and affecting the development of an organism or group of organisms	The implied definition is that health exists if that person has adaptive responses that "promote the integrity of the person in terms of the goals of survival, growth, reproduction, and self-mastery"	Manipulating stimuli so that a person's coping mechanism can bring about adaptation
Rogers[25]	"Unitary man—a four-dimensional, negentropic energy field identified by pattern and organization and manifesting characteristics and behaviors that are different from those of the parts and which cannot be predicted from knowledge of the parts"	"A four-dimensional, negentropic energy field identified by pattern and organization and encompassing all that is outside any given human field"	Health not specifically defined; however, she does state that disease and pathology are value terms and since values change, phenomena perceived as disease, such as hyperactivity, may change over time and not be perceived as disease	Goal of nursing is that individuals achieve their maximum health potential through maintenance and promotion of health, prevention of disease, nursing diagnosis, intervention, and rehabilitation
Johnson[11]	Behavioral system composed of patterned, repetitive, and purposeful ways of behaving	Malfunctions in the behavioral systems are frequently caused by "sudden internal or external environmental change"	It seems reasonable to assume that health would be considered behavior that is orderly, purposeful, predictable, and functionally efficient and effective	"External regulatory force that acts to preserve the organization and integration of the patient's behavior at an optimum level under those conditions in which the behavior constitutes a threat to physical or social health, or in which illness is found"
Orem[23]	"A unity that can be viewed as functioning biologically, symbolically, and socially"	Although not explicitly defined, the role of the nurse in providing a developmental environment is discussed	"A term that has considerable general utility in describing the state of wholeness or integrity of human beings"	"A service, a mode of helping human beings" (Orem, 1980, p. 5); "nursing is contributed effort toward designing, providing, and managing systems of therapeutic self-care for individuals or multi-person units within their daily living environments"

From Stanhope M and Lancaster J: Community health nursing, St Louis, 1988, Mosby–Year Book, Inc.

Continued.

TABLE 5-2—cont'd

DEFINITION OF NURSING CONCEPTS BY NURSE THEORISTS

Nurse-theorist	Person	Environment	Health	Nursing
Neuman[21]	"Man is a system capable of intake of extrapersonal and interpersonal factors from the external environment. He interacts with this environment by adjusting it to himself"	"Environment consists of the internal and external forces surrounding man at a point in time"	"Health or wellness is the condition in which all parts and subparts (variables) are in harmony with the whole man"	"Nursing can . . . assist individuals, families, groups to attain and maintain a maximum level of total wellness by purposeful interventions . . . aimed at reduction of stress factors and adverse conditions which affect optimal functioning"
King[13]	A social, sentient, rational, reacting, perceiving, controlling, purposeful, action-oriented, and time-oriented being	Refers to human being interacting with the environment but does not define it	Dynamic life experiences of a human being, which implies continuous adjustment to stressors in the internal and external environment through optimum use of one's resources to achieve maximum potential for daily living	"Nursing is perceiving, thinking, relating, judging, and acting vis-a-vis the behavior of individuals who come to a nursing situation"

ment, health-illness, and nursing.[5] As the nurse interacts with people in society to facilitate health, the nursing process occurs. Table 5-2 describes how various nurse theorists define these common concepts.

Some believe that psychiatric nursing has not applied nursing models to its phenomena of concern. A notable exception to this is the work of Fitzpatrick, Whall, Johnson, and Floyd, which brings a unique perspective to psychiatric nursing theory.[4] Their text selects concepts and propositions from the behavioral sciences (such as Freudian, systems, and crisis theory) and relates them to the concepts of human beings, society, health-illness, and nursing. They believe it is necessary to adopt existing theories to make them reflect the unique perspective of psychiatric nursing practice. In doing this psychiatric nurses would contribute both to theory refinement and to the creation of clinically useful theory on which to base their practice.

 ## Data collection

STANDARD II—DATA COLLECTION

The nurse continuously collects data that are comprehensive, accurate, and systematic.

Process criteria
The nurse:

1. Informs the patient of their mutual roles and responsibilities in the data-gathering process
2. Determines what information is needed. Health data undergirding the nursing process for psychiatric and mental health patients are obtained through assessing the following:
   a. Biophysical, developmental, mental, and emotional status
   b. Spiritual or philosophical beliefs
   c. Family, social, cultural, and community systems
   d. Daily activities, interactions, and coping patterns
   e. Economic, environmental, and political factors affecting the patient's health
   f. Personally significant support systems and unutilized but available support systems
   g. Knowledge, satisfaction, and change motivation regarding current health status
   h. Strengths that can be used in reaching health goals
   i. Knowledge of pertinent legal rights
   j. Contributory data from the family, significant others, the health care team, and pertinent individuals in the community

Implementing the nursing process **151**

Data collection may be part of a formal admission procedure outside an established nurse-patient relationship. In this case the information is obtained from the patient in a direct and structured manner through observations, interviews, and examinations. An assessment tool or nursing history form can provide a systematic format that becomes part of the patient's written record. This format provides the facts on which the nurse can assess the patient's level of functioning and serves as a basis for diagnosis, planning, implementation, and evaluation of nursing care. Using a specified data collection format helps ensure that the necessary information is obtained. It also reduces the patient's repetition of his history and provides a source of information available to all health team members. The mental status examination, as described in Chapter 6, may be part of the psychiatric nurse's evaluation.

The assessment tool the nurse uses to collect data ideally should be derived from a conceptual framework of psychiatric nursing. More frequently, however, it is determined by the setting or program in which the nurse works. Regardless of the format, the nurse must obtain as complete a picture as possible of the patient's life situation.

The process criteria of standard II identify comprehensive areas in which data need to be collected. Each item listed (a-j) is important for a thorough and complete psychiatric nursing assessment. This list includes data relative to specific components of the nursing model of health-illness phenomena (see Chapter 3) used in this text—predisposing factors, precipitating stressors, primary appraisal of stressor, secondary appraisal of coping resources, and coping mechanisms as represented in Fig. 5-2. Together these components represent the data needed to complete the **nursing assessment** phase of the nursing process. The process criteria also identify from whom the data are to be collected and represent various levels of the model of social hierarchy—individual, family, group, and community.

The baseline data should reflect both content and process, and the patient is the ideal source of validation. The nurse should select a private place, free from noise and distraction, in which to interview the patient. Interviewing is a goal-directed method of communication that is required in a formal admission procedure. It should be focused but as open ended as possible, progressing from general to specific and allowing the patient to express himself spontaneously. The nurse's role is to maintain the flow of the interview, to listen to the verbal and nonverbal messages being conveyed by the patient, and to be aware of his or her own responses to the patient.

In an ongoing nurse-patient relationship, data collection may begin in the orientation phase. Gathering information is only one of many goals the nurse is pursuing at this time. Other tasks include establishing trust, acceptance, and open communication; creating a contract; and exploring the patient's feelings and actions. The nurse's approach therefore should be unstructured, flexible, and responsive to the patient's cues. Rather than working from a formalized data collection tool, the nurse may focus the patient on observing and describing his present thoughts, feelings, and experiences. To supplement his or her knowledge of the patient, the nurse can use a variety of secondary information sources, including the patient's medical record, nursing rounds, change-of-shift reports, nursing care plan, and the evaluation of other health professionals such as psychologists, social workers, or psychiatrists. In using secondary sources, nurses should not simply accept the assessment of another health team member. Rather, they should apply the information they obtain to their nursing framework for data collection and formulate their own impressions and diagnoses. This brings another perspective to the work of the health care team and an unbiased receptivity to the patient and his problems.

■ Cultural considerations

Some aspects of the data collection phase merit additional discussion. One is the assessment of the patient's cultural and socioeconomic background. Frequently these factors do not receive much attention. Yet they exert a powerful influence on the success of the nursing process for two important reasons. First, these factors contribute to a patient's belief system of health and illness. Sex, race, culture, family ties, and economic status, for example, all influence each component of the model of health-illness phenomena. Any one sociocultural factor may play a dominant role in an individual's life. Therefore any attempt to promote the patient's well-being must understand him as a unique individual who lives in a larger social, cultural, and economic community.

The second reason why sociocultural factors are important is that the response of the health care team is also influenced by the culture to which its members belong. The dominant psychotherapeutic approach of a society reflects the cultural attitudes of its time and place. This helps explain why there are differences in observed symptoms, frequency, distribution, and outcome of psychiatric illness among countries and cultures throughout the world. For instance, in developing nations such as Nigeria and India, the odds favor a fast and complete recovery from major psychoses. In

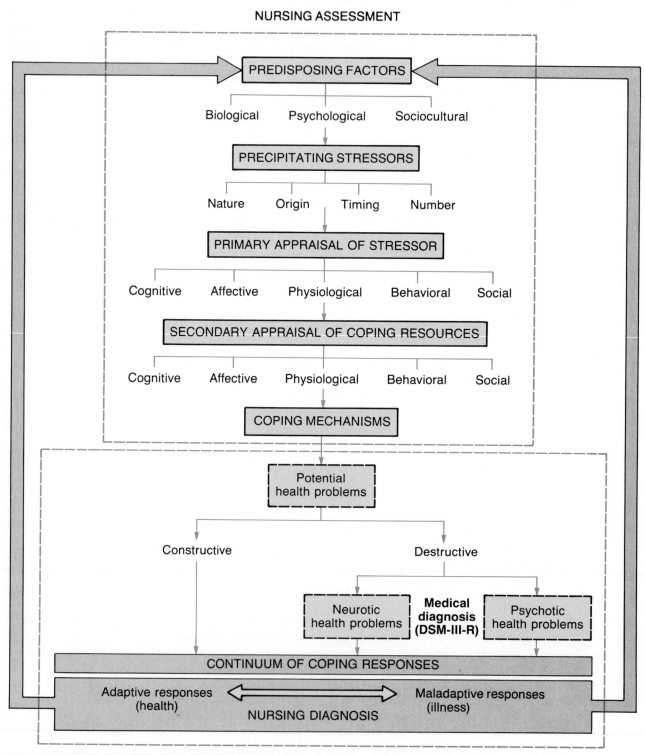

Fig. 5-2. Nursing model of health-illness phenomena and its relationship to nursing assessment and nursing diagnosis.

the more technologically advanced countries such as the United States, the prognosis is worse. This is the result, in part, of the cultural stigma against mental illness that is prevalent in the West.

Stigma, in its old definition, is referred to as a "scar left by a hot iron on the face of an evil doer." As such it has come to be seen as a mark of disgrace used to identify and separate out those people who society sees as deviant, sinful, or dangerous. For the psychiatrically ill, stigma is a barrier that separates them from society and keeps them apart from others. Patients and their families often report that the diagnosis of a mental illness is followed by increasing isolation and loneliness as family and friends retreat and withdraw. Patients feel rejected and feared by others and their families are met by blame. Stigma against mental illness is clearly a reflection of the cultural biases of contemporary American society; biases that are shared by consumers and health care providers alike.

Overcoming stigma and cultural bias is an important consideration for the psychiatric nurse. Two guiding principles that help the nurse make an assessment that incorporates culturological factors are: (1) to maintain a broad objective and open attitude toward people and their culture and (2) to avoid seeing all people as alike. Given this basis, the nurse can then explore various aspects of the patient's world view in the nursing assessment. Leininger has identified the following cultural components that should be part of a nursing assessment:

- patterns of life style
- specific cultural values and norms
- cultural taboos and myths
- world view and ethnocentric tendencies
- general things that the patient perceives as different or similar to other cultures
- health and life care rituals and health-related rites of passage
- folk and professional health-illness systems that are used
- degree of cultural change and acculturation
- self-care behavior[18]

By including these elements in one's nursing assessment, the nurse can better understand the content and context of a person's coping response.

Cultural bias can also affect the process of psychotherapy. One study reported that minority group patients received the least intensive psychotherapy. They were discharged more often or seen for minimum supportive psychotherapy.[37] A study among public health nurses found that they judged patients differently as a function of the patient's social class.[14] Consequently, some patients rather than being reviewed as culturally

different, are seen as disadvantaged, deprived, or underprivileged. Such prejudices do not form on the basis of race alone. They can also be based on a person's sex, religion, age, sexual preference, or ethnic background. However, the result is the same—prejudices influence the nurse's evaluation of the patient and limit the potential effectiveness of care.

Psychiatry needs to embrace the idea of intercultural psychotherapy. Schlesinger[28] believes this occurs when the patient and therapist acknowledge their different cultural backgrounds, and interaction of cultural variables results. This has implications for self-awareness, communications, diagnosis, nurse-patient relations, therapeutic models, and treatment goals. It requires that the nurse be aware of his or her own sociocultural identity and values, understand how social systems influence behavior, and remain willing to learn from a patient with another cultural set.

■ Spirituality

The holistic nature of nursing practice implies care for the body, mind, and spirit. Understanding a patient's spiritual beliefs allows the nurse to identify areas of potential problems for the patient and to suggest adaptive coping strategies that can be supported by the nurse. The interrelationship among the body, mind, and spirit are evident in one's response to stress. A biological stressor may influence a person's emotional reaction and lead to a questioning of philosophical or religious views. In the same way, emotional or spiritual stress may result in changes in a person's physical health and well-being. Spirituality, in a nursing assessment, should not be limited to a patient's membership in an organized religion but should include one's philosophical orientation to values, beliefs, and the meaning of life. It is an aspect of the total person that influences all other parts of life. Nursing questions on life, death, meaning, and values refer to this domain. Spiritual integrity is evident when a person experiences a sense of oneness in oneself, a sense of relatedness with other human beings, and a sense of transcendent relatedness with another realm. It is demonstrated through acts of love, hope, trust, and forgiveness.

Spiritual integrity can be altered in many ways, including experiences of pain, alienation, anxiety, guilt, anger, loss, and despair. Examples of altered spiritual integrity and their associated behaviors have been elaborated on by O'Brien[22] and Labun[17] and are summarized in Table 5-3. A profound feeling of demoralization or despiritization that is associated with spiritual distress may account for states of depression and anxiety and may give rise to thoughts of suicide.

Spiritual care involves helping the patient to rec-

TABLE 5-3

EXAMPLES OF ALTERED SPIRITUAL INTEGRITY AND THEIR ASSOCIATED BEHAVIOURS[17,22]

Experiences of altered spiritual integrity	Behaviours or expressions of altered spiritual integrity
Spiritual pain Experiences of discomfort or suffering related to one's human and/or transcendent relationships as well as one's values and beliefs.	Behaviours conveying discomfort or suffering relative to one's relationship with God, fellow human beings, and/or transcendent values and beliefs. Expression of feelings related to lacking of spiritual fulfillment or of feeling empty in relation to fulfillment and meaning. Inability to come to terms with one's reason for being or one's relationship with the source of creation.
Spiritual alienation Experiences of loneliness not filled by other human relationships.	Feelings of estrangement and remoteness between the events in a person's life and personal meaning and purpose for being. Feeling that no one can come to 'the core of one's being' and understand the person; that there is no 'connectedness' between one's self and other beings. A negative attitude toward receiving help or comfort from another spiritual being.
Spiritual anxiety Fear of the unknown and/or of impending doom for one's self or one's loved ones. Maybe based on specific events, on the unknown, or on possible events.	Worry about, or fear of, a God that is displeased, full of anger, or threatening punishment to one's self. Worry that those sources of ultimate strength or stability such as God, or the order of the Universe might not take care of one, either immediately or in the future. General fear of the future or of annihilation without a purpose or meaning.
Spiritual guilt Concern about one's life style, values, and beliefs.	Doubt or remorse about the life one has lived. Expressions suggesting that one has failed to live up to an idealized value or norm.
Spiritual anger Feeling about the injustice of a situation, blaming an undefinable transcendent source, God, or experiencing diffuse anger.	Expressions of outrage or feelings of powerlessness toward transcendent powers such as God or other undefinable sources for having allowed illness or other trials. Negative criticism or blaming of institutionalized religion and those who represent it.
Spiritual loss Feeling of having lost hold of those aspects of life which give ultimate and transcendent meaning and purpose.	Feelings of having lost or terminated the love of God or other deeply meaningful transcendent relationships. Expressions of fear that one has lost contact with God or that one's faith in a spiritual belief has been misplaced. Listlessness or 'drifting' with regard to things of ultimate or transcendent meaning which were meaningful in the past.
Spiritual despair Feeling that the person's hope in ultimate values, beliefs and transcendent experiences that were previously meaningful are no longer possible or that they will never be possible. A feeling that life makes no sense and that it is not possible to make sense of it.	Feelings that God no longer can or does care for one. No hope of ever experiencing fulfillment in a relationship with God or through transcendent experiences. No hope in past beliefs, or values, with a total feeling that life has become meaningless and purposeless. No hope of finding a philosophical explanation for life or of finding meaning or purpose.

ognize a personal unique meaning to life, strengthening one's relationship to a higher realm or deity, and helping to bring an appreciation of spiritual values into the patient's awareness. It requires that the nurse understand the patient's unique philosophical or religious views and respect his beliefs and practices even though they may be different from those of the nurse. In order to attain this level of understanding the nurse must establish trust and rapport that allow the patient to fully describe his spiritual beliefs. To do this, the nurse must be willing to recognize limitations and seek help from others when it is indicated.

■ Family systems

A final important aspect of data collection is the patient's role as a family member. If the patient is an active member of a family unit, it is necessary to include his view of the functional state of his family, as well as family resources and strengths. Sedgwick[29] describes the family as both a social organization and an emotional environment. As a social organization the family develops within its members sets of skills necessary for productive membership in a larger social system. It is a focal point of interaction for the individual as he relates to other family members, other families, the community, and the larger social network. So, too, the broader social system makes demands and places expectations on the family and requires it to process information, make decisions, attain financial and social productivity, and provide for the personal growth and development of its members.

The larger social context also influences the family's emotional environment. The family must create an atmosphere that promotes both group living and cooperation, and individual development and disagreement. Although the family's emotional environment is constantly changing, it must create a climate that is trusting, warm, concerned, accepting of differences in opinions and abilities, and adaptable to changes in individual members.

TABLE 5-4

DIMENSIONS OF THE FAMILY APGAR

Component	What is measured	Relevant open-ended questions
Adaptation	How resources are shared, or the degree to which a member is satisfied with the assistance received when family resources are needed	How have family members aided each other in time of need? In what way have family members received help or assistance from friends and community agencies?
Partnership	How decisions are shared, or the member's satisfaction with mutuality in family communication and problem solving	How do family members communicate with each other about such matters as vacations, finances, medical care, large purchases, and personal problems?
Growth	How nurturing is shared, or the member's satisfaction with the freedom available within the family to change roles and attain physical and emotional growth or maturation	How have family members changed during the past years? How has this change been accepted by family members? In what ways have family members aided each other in growing or developing independent life-styles? How have family members reacted to your desires for change?
Affection	How emotional experiences are shared, or the member's satisfaction with the intimacy and emotional interaction that exists in a family	How have members of your family responded to emotional expressions such as affection, love, sorrow, or anger?
Resolve	How time (and space and money) is shared, or the member's satisfaction with the time commitment that has been made to the family by its members	How do members of your family share time, space, and money?

Modified from Smilkstein G: J Fam Pract 6:1231, 1978.

Smilkstein[32] considers a healthy family to be a nurturing unit that demonstrates integrity in five components: *a*daptability, *p*artnership, *g*rowth, *a*ffection, and *r*esolve. He designed the acronym APGAR to refer to these components. To test these areas of family functioning, Smilkstein developed a brief screening questionnaire called the Family APGAR. Table 5-4 presents the functional components of the Family APGAR and relevant open-ended questions for family function information. This tool is useful in suggesting areas to be assessed relative to family functioning and potential areas of family strengths and resources.

Various types of family strengths may be noted. These include the ability to acquire resources, such as money or social support, and the productive use of them; the ability to communicate in depth with each other with openness and shared decision making; the presence of encouragement, ego support, praise, recognition, respect for individuality, and flexibility of family functions and roles; and family unity, loyalty, and cooperation. All of these strengths serve as potential family resources. Other resources may be present in the family's cultural pride, religious affiliation, community ties, economic status, and educational background. Including this information in the data collection phase of the nursing process not only gives depth to the nurse's assessment, it also suggests resources that will help the patient adapt.

 # Nursing diagnosis

STANDARD III—DIAGNOSIS

The nurse uses *nursing diagnoses* and standard classification of mental disorders to express conclusions supported by recorded assessment data and current scientific premises.

Process criteria
The nurse:

1. Identifies actual or potential health problems in regard to:
   a. Self-care limitation or impaired functioning whose general cause is mental and emotional distress, deficits in the ways significant systems are functioning, and internal psychic and/or developmental issues
   b. Emotional stress or crisis components of illness, pain, self-concept changes, and life process changes
   c. Emotional problems related to daily experiences such as anxiety, aggression, loss, loneliness, and grief
   d. Physical symptoms that occur simultaneously with altered psychic functioning, such as altered intestinal functioning or anorexia

   e. Alterations in thinking, perceiving, symbolizing, communicating, and decision-making abilities
   f. Impaired abilities to relate to others
   g. Behavior and mental states that indicate that the patient is a danger to self or others or is gravely disabled
2. Analyzes available information according to accepted theoretical frameworks
3. Makes inferences regarding data from phenomena
4. Formulates a nursing diagnosis subject to revision with subsequent data

After collecting all data, the nurse compares the information to documented norms of health and wellness. The psychosocial aspects of a patient's life present some special concerns for the nurse. It is important for the nurse to remember that what is acceptable and appropriate behavior in one social group may be considered deviant and bizarre in another. Since standards of behavior are culturally determined, the nurse should allow for both the patient's individual characteristics and the larger social group to which he belongs.

The nurse then analyzes the data and derives a nursing diagnosis. **A nursing diagnosis is a statement of the patient's nursing problem that includes both the adaptive or maladaptive health response and contributing stressors.** These nursing problems concern aspects of the patient's health that may need to be promoted or with which the patient needs help in adapting to stress. The subject of nursing diagnoses therefore is the patient's behavioral response to stress. This response, as represented in Fig. 5-2, may lie anywhere on the coping continuum from adaptive, healthy, to maladaptive, ill. Nursing diagnoses identify problems that may be overt, covert, existing, or potential. The professional nurse assumes the responsibility for therapeutic decisions regarding these patients' health responses.

Currently the classification of nursing diagnoses is in its infancy. However, nurses must define and clarify what they do in the psychiatric setting, and this requires the use of nursing diagnoses. McClosky believes:

In today's world, unless nurses can name the health problems they treat, they are speechless before legislators, third party payors, administrators, other health professionals, and perhaps even nurses themselves. Nursing diagnosis pinpoints what nursing is and what it does.[20]

The North American Nursing Diagnoses Association has been working on identifying, defining, and describing a classification system of nursing diagnoses. Additional work is needed both in defining the phenomena of concern to psychiatric nurses and in testing the identified diagnoses. If nurses diagnose problems, record their observations and conclusions, and describe the health responses they treat, the body of nursing knowledge will increase, as will the credibility of and value placed on nursing care.

■ **RELATIONSHIP TO MEDICAL DIAGNOSES.** Nursing does not exist in a vacuum. Although nurses are the largest group of health care professionals, they must work with other groups, such as physicians. Each group of health care providers serves as a resource to the others as they cooperate to improve the patient's health.

The interrelationship between medicine and nursing includes sharing information, ideas, and analyses and developing appropriate care plans for the patient. Interventions are based on the nursing assessment as well as the medical evaluation and ensure a thorough and coordinated plan of treatment for the psychiatric patient. Therefore, while formulating nursing diagnoses and using the nursing process, nurses should also be familiar with medical diagnoses and treatment plans.

Medical diagnosis refers to the health problem or disease states of the patient. In the medical model of psychiatry, the health problems are mental disorders or mental illnesses. These are classified in the DSM-III-R,[2] which comprehensively describes the symptoms of various mental disorders but does not attempt to discuss cause or how the disturbances come about. However specific diagnostic criteria are provided for each mental disorder. Chapters 2 and 3 of this text discuss the medical model and the DSM-III-R in greater detail.

Nursing and medical diagnoses may complement each other, but one is not a component of another. A patient with one specific medical diagnosis may have a number of complementary nursing diagnoses related to his range of health responses. On the other hand, a patient may have a specific nursing diagnosis without any identified medical diagnosis.

Coler conducted a small study correlating identified nursing diagnoses specific to psychiatric-mental health nursing with the diagnostic categories of DSM-III.[3] The study is significant because it demonstrated the overlap between the diagnostic labels of nursing and psychiatry. For instance, the nursing diagnosis of ineffective individual coping was identified 37 out of 56 times and in all the DSM-III categories. The second most common nursing diagnosis, potential for injury, appeared in all but two of the DSM-III categories. Additional research is needed to validate these nursing diagnoses and to examine their interaction with medical diagnostic categories. Table 5-5 lists the 17 diagnostic classes identified by the DSM-III-R along with the 11 psychiatric nursing diagnostic classes that are explored in this text.

Nursing diagnoses are usually formed in the orientation phase of the relationship. Inexperienced nurses often feel pressured to identify nursing problems quickly and are confused and frustrated by a withdrawn patient who does not share his feelings. In this case the primary nursing problem may be the patient's social isolation related to feelings of inadequacy or fear of interpersonal closeness. Nursing diagnoses describe the patient's current health responses. It is important for the nurse to begin with the patient's current behavior and to work from there. This requires both accepting the patient and setting nursing priorities.

TABLE 5-5

MEDICAL DIAGNOSTIC CLASSES DESCRIBED IN DSM-III-R*

Medical diagnostic classes described in Draft of DSM-III-R in Development*	Psychiatric nursing diagnostic classes
Disorders usually first evident in infancy, childhood, or adolescence	Anxiety
Organic mental syndromes and disorders	Psychophysiological illness
Psychoactive substance use disorders	Alterations in self-concept
Sleep and arousal disorders	Disturbances of mood
Schizophrenic disorders	Self-destructive behavior
Delusional (paranoid) disorders	Disruptions in relatedness
Psychotic disorders not elsewhere classified	Problems with expression of anger
Mood (affective) disorders	Impaired cognition
Anxiety disorders	Substance abuse
Somatoform disorders	Variations in sexual response
Dissociative disorders	Psychological responses to physical illness
Gender and sexual disorders	
Factitious disorders	
Impulse control disorders not elsewhere classified	
Adjustment disorder	
Other disorders associated with physical condition	
Personality disorders	

*American Psychiatric Association: Diagnostic and statistical manual of mental disorders, third edition revised, Washington DC, 1987, The Association.

❧ Planning

STANDARD IV—PLANNING

The nurse develops a nursing care plan with specific goals and interventions delineating nursing actions unique to each patient's needs.

Process criteria

1. The nurse collaborates with patients, their significant others, and team members in establishing nursing care plans
2. In the care plan the nurse:
   a. Identifies priorities of care
   b. States realistic goals in measurable terms with an expected date of accomplishment
   c. Uses identifiable psychotherapeutic principles
   d. Indicates which patient needs will be a primary responsibility of the psychiatric and mental health nurse and which will be referred to others with the appropriate expertise
   e. Stresses mutual goal setting and shared responsibility for goal attainment at the level of the patient's abilities
   f. Provides guidance for the patient care activities performed by others under the nurse's supervision
3. The nurse revises the care plan as goals are achieved, changed, or updated

Careful planning builds on the data collection and nursing diagnosis phases of the nursing process. It increases the chance of successful implementation and evaluation. The first step in planning is to develop clear objectives, or goals, for nursing care.

■ **CLARIFYING GOALS.** There are four important aspects of goal setting: mutuality, congruency, realism, and timing. However, before defining goals the nurse must recognize that the patient frequently comes to therapy with goals of his own. Generally they express his discomfort and relate to curing his symptoms. Often the patient's goals are not directly stated and may be difficult to clarify. Translating nonspecific concerns into specific goal statements is no easy task for the nurse. He or she must understand the patient's coping responses and the factors that influence them. Krumboltz and Thorensen[16] describe some of the difficulties in defining goals as follows:

1. The patient may view his problem as someone else's behavior. This may be the case of a parent who brings his adolescent son in for counseling. The parent may view the son as the problem, whereas the adolescent may feel his only problem is his father. One approach to this situation is to help the person who brings the problem into treatment, since he "owns" the problem at that moment. The nurse might sug-

gest, "Let's talk about how I could help you deal with your son. A change in your response might lead to a change in his behavior also."
2. The patient may express his problem as a feeling, such as, "I'm lonely," or "I'm so unhappy." Besides trying to help the patient clarify what he is feeling, the nurse might ask, "What could you do to make yourself feel less alone and more loved by others?" This helps the patient see the connection between actions and feelings and increases his sense of responsibility for himself.
3. The patient's problem may be that he lacks a goal or an idea of exactly what he desires out of life. In this case it might be helpful for the nurse to point out that values and goals are not magically discovered but must be created by people for themselves. The patient can then actively explore ways to construct his own goals or adopt the objectives of a social, service, religious, or political group with whom he identifies.
4. The patient's goals may be inappropriate, undesirable, or unclear. However, the solution here is not for the nurse to impose goals on the patient. Even if the patient's desires seem to be against his best interests, the most the nurse can do is reflect the patient's behavior and its consequences back to him. If he then asks for help in setting new goals, the nurse can help him do so.
5. The patient's problem may be a choice conflict. This is especially common if all the choices are unpleasant, unacceptable, or unrealistic. An example is a couple who wishes to divorce but do not want to see their child hurt or suffer the financial hardship that would result. Although the nurse cannot make undesirable choices desirable, he or she can help patients use the problem-solving process to identify the full range of alternatives available to them.
6. The patient may have no real problem but may just want to talk. Nurses must then decide what role to play and carefully distinguish between a social and a therapeutic relationship.

It becomes obvious that clarifying goals is an essential step in the therapeutic process. Out of this clarification and the nursing diagnoses emerges the mutually agreed on goals on which the patient-nurse relationship is based. A well-intentioned nurse often overlooks the patient's goals and devises a care plan leading to an outcome he or she feels is better. However, this approach may be one of the conflict-producing situations that the patient has experienced in the past. Therefore the experience of working cooperatively with the nurse to evolve mutually acceptable goals is extremely valuable. If the patient does not share one of the nurse's goals, it may be best to defer it until he agrees on its importance.

■ **SPECIFYING GOALS.** Once goals are agreed on, the nurse must state them explicitly for himself or herself and the patient. The more specifically one can state the goals of treatment, the more likely one is to achieve them. These goals also serve to guide later nursing actions and enhance the evaluation of care. Objectives should be written in behavioral terms. This means that the verb used to state the objective should represent a behavior that may be observed and should have as few interpretations as possible. Table 5-6 lists verbs with many and few interpretations. Goals should realistically describe what the nurse wishes to accomplish and within what time span. Often nurses err by using general statements that apply to all patients, such as the goals of forming a relationship or relieving depression. Although valid in general terms, they are not adequate in and of themselves.

Long- and short-term goals should be developed, with short-term objectives contributing to the long-term goals. Following are sample goals:

Long-term

> The patient will travel about the community independently within 2 months.

TABLE 5-6

INTERPRETATION OF VERBS

Appropriate verbs with few interpretations	Inappropriate verbs with many interpretations
To identify	To know
To list	To understand
To compare and contrast	To value
To describe	To appreciate
To discuss	To realize
To evaluate	To feel
To recall	To believe
To apply	To be familiar with
To demonstrate	To be aware of
To differentiate	To think
To state	To be interested in
To predict	To trust

Short-term

> 1. At the end of 1 week the patient will sit on his front steps.
> 2. At the end of 2 weeks the patient will walk to the corner and back to his house.
> 3. At the end of 3 weeks the patient, accompanied by the nurse, will walk around the block.
> 4. At the end of 4 weeks the patient will walk around the block alone.

The hierarchy would continue until the desired goal is achieved. Each goal is stated in terms of observable behavior and includes a period of time in which it is to be accomplished. It also includes any other relevant conditions, such as whether the patient is to be alone or accompanied by the nurse.

Most patients exhibit a number of nursing problems, each of which must be incorporated into the plan of care. Several goals may need to be written relative to each nursing diagnosis. As the nurse and patient work together to meet patient needs, new needs often arise. For this reason it is necessary to determine the relative priority of the various nurse-patient goals. Otherwise care would become haphazard and fragmented, with the focus first on one objective and then on the next, based only on what happened to come up at the time. Important and immediate needs could get lost in the general chaos.

■ **PRIORITIZING GOALS.** One of the most important tasks facing the nurse and patient is to assign priorities to goals. Frequently, several goals can be pursued simultaneously. Those related to protecting the patient from self-destructive impulses always receive top priority. Always, when identifying both long- and short-term goals, the nurse must keep the proposed time sequence firmly in mind.

Since the nursing care plan is dynamic and should adapt to the patient's coping responses throughout his contact with the health care system, priorities are constantly changing. If the focus is always on the patient's behavioral responses, priorities can be set and modified as the patient changes. This personalizes nursing care, and the patient participates in its planning and implementation.

■ **ACHIEVING GOALS.** Once the goals are decided, the next task is to outline the plan for achieving them. The nursing care plan applies theory from nursing and related biological and behavioral sciences to the unique responses of the individual patient. This assumes that as the nurse identifies patient needs, appropriate resources will be consulted. Failure to approach nursing care in this scientific manner can result in illogical decisions and a plan based on tradition, intuition, or trial and error. Although these decision-making methods may result in a valid plan, consistency of depth and accuracy over time will suffer, as will the overall care of the patient. Skilled nursing requires a commitment to the ongoing pursuit of knowledge that will enhance professional growth.

The patient's active involvement leads to more successful care plans. If the nurse collects data, returns to the nurse's station, consults textbooks, and then writes up a plan of care, an important step has been missed. After writing a tentative care plan, the nurse must validate this plan with the patient. This saves time and effort for them both as they continue to work together. It also communicates to the patient his responsibility in getting well. The patient can tell the nurse that a proposed plan is unrealistic regarding financial status, life-style, value system or, perhaps, personal preference. Usually there are several possible approaches to a patient's problem. Choosing the one most acceptable to the patient improves the chances for success.

If a goal answers the question of "what," the plan of care answers the questions "how" and "why." The plan chosen obviously will depend on the nursing diagnosis, the nurse's theoretical orientation, and the nature of the goals pursued. In general, the goals will influence the selection of therapeutic techniques. Failure to reach a goal through one's plan can lead to the decision to adopt a new approach or reevaluate the goal. These activities commonly occur in the working phase of the relationship.

 Implementation

STANDARD V—INTERVENTION

The nurse intervenes as guided by the nursing care plan to implement nursing actions that promote, maintain, or restore physical and mental health, prevent illness, and effect rehabilitation.
Process criteria
The nurse:

1. Acts to ensure that health care needs are met either by using nursing skills or by obtaining assistance from other health care providers when indicated
2. Acts as the patient's advocate when necessary to facilitate the achievement of health
3. Reviews and modifies interventions based on the patient's progress

Implementation refers to the actual delivery of nursing care to the patient and his response to that care. Good planning increases the chances of successful implementation. Such factors as available people, equipment, resources, time, and money must be con-

sidered as nursing actions are planned. Well-planned nursing care also takes into account the personalities and experiences of the nurse and the patient and their interaction.

The most valid basis for nursing action applies the scientific method to nursing practice. It is also acceptable to use theory selectively from the biological and behavioral sciences. In most situations there is more than one way to accomplish the stated objectives. It is helpful when planning care to identify alternative nursing actions that are also appropriate to the goal. If this is done, the nurse is not left floundering should the first approach fail. Considering several alternatives makes the implementation phase of the nursing process highly flexible.

STANDARD V-A—PSYCHOTHERAPEUTIC INTERVENTIONS

The nurse (generalist) uses psychotherapeutic interventions to help patients to regain or improve their previous coping abilities and prevent further disability.
Process criteria
The nurse:

1. Identifies the patient's responses to health problems
2. Reinforces functional responses to health problems and helps the patient modify or eliminate dysfunctional responses
3. Employs principles of communication, interviewing techniques, problem solving, and crisis intervention when performing psychotherapeutic interventions
4. Uses knowledge of behavioral concepts such as anxiety, loss, conflict, grief, and anger to help the patient cope with, adapt to, and constructively deal with feelings
5. Demonstrates knowledge of and skill in the use of psychotherapeutic interventions specifically useful in the modification of thought, perception, affect, behavior, and motivation
6. Uses health team members to help evaluate the outcome of interventions and to formulate modification of psychotherapeutic techniques
7. Reinforces useful patterns and themes in the patient's interactions with others
8. Uses crisis intervention to promote growth and to aid the personal and social integration of patients in developmental, situational, or suicidal crisis

In implementing psychotherapeutic interventions, the nurse helps the psychiatric patient do two things: **develop insight** and resolve problems through **carrying out a plan of positive action.** These two areas for nursing intervention correspond with the responsive and action dimensions of the nurse-patient relationship described in Chapter 4. Insight refers to the patient's development of new emotional and cognitive organizations. Often the patient becomes more anxious as his defense mechanisms are broken down. This is the time when resistance commonly occurs. But knowing something on an intellectual level does *not* inevitably lead to a change in behavior. Nurses who terminate their interventions at this point are not fully carrying out the therapeutic process to the patient's benefit. An additional step is needed. The patient must decide if he will revert to maladaptive coping mechanisms, remain in a resisting, immobilized state, or adopt new, adaptive, and constructive approaches to life.

The first step in helping a patient translate insight into action is to build adequate incentives to abandoning old patterns of behavior. The nurse should help the patient see that his old patterns do him more harm than good and inflict much suffering and pain. The patient will not learn new patterns until the motivation to acquire them is greater than his motivation to retain old ones. The nurse therefore should encourage any desires the patient expresses for mental health, emotional growth, and freedom from suffering. The nurse also should continue to motivate and support the patient as he tests new behaviors and coping mechanisms. The individual's social support system is vital in this regard. This is relevant to all levels of nursing intervention—primary, secondary, and tertiary—and all patient populations.

STANDARD V-B—HEALTH TEACHING
The nurse helps patients, families, and groups achieve satisfying and productive patterns of living through health teaching.
Process criteria
The nurse:

1. Identifies patients' health education needs
2. Employs principles of learning and appropriate teaching methods
3. Teaches the basic principles of physical and mental health
4. Teaches communication, interpersonal, and social skills
5. Provides opportunities for patients to learn experientially

Health education is an important nursing activity to help patients change maladaptive coping responses. The four-step process is included in primary, secondary, and tertiary prevention activities:

1. Increasing a patient's awareness of issues and events related to mental health
2. Helping a patient understand potential stressors, possible outcomes, and alternative coping responses

3. Increasing a patient's knowledge of where and how to acquire the needed resources
4. Increasing the patient's actual abilities

Therapeutic education can take place anywhere and with any group of individuals. For example, a classroom course for psychiatric patients that focuses on how to cope with and regain control over their lives can be effective. Similarly, patient education groups can have a positive effect on patient compliance with medication regimens.

There is also a trend toward using education for families with mentally ill relatives. Such psychoeducational approaches—plus training in communication, problem solving, information giving, and behavioral management—help families understand mental illness.

Health teaching is one of nursing's oldest and most important functions. But too often it is given a low priority by nurses who are overwhelmed with other tasks. In a psychiatric setting, the need for patient and family education is great and many opportunities arise for formal and informal health teaching by the nurse. Chapters 8 and 10 discuss strategies and areas for health education that both promote mental health and assist in the rehabilitation of patients who have experienced mental illness.

STANDARD V-C—SELF-CARE ACTIVITIES
The nurse uses the activities of daily living in a goal-directed way to foster adequate self-care and the physical and mental well-being of patients.
Process criteria
The nurse:

1. Respects and protects the patient's rights
2. Encourages the patient to collaborate in developing a self-care plan
3. Sets limits in a manner that is humane and the least restrictive necessary to assure safety of the patient and others

STANDARD V-D—SOMATIC THERAPIES
The nurse uses knowledge of somatic therapies and applies related clinical skills in working with patients.
Process criteria
The nurse:

1. Uses knowledge of current psychopharmacology to guide nursing actions
2. Observes and interprets pertinent responses to somatic therapies in terms of the underlying principles of each therapy
3. Evaluates effectiveness of somatic therapies and recommends changes in the treatment plan as appropriate

4. Collaborates with other team members to provide for safe administration of therapies
5. Supervises the patient's chemotherapeutic regimen in collaboration with the physician
6. Provides opportunities for patients and families to discuss, question, and explore their feelings and concerns about past, current, or projected use of somatic therapies
7. Reviews expected actions and side effects of somatic therapies with patients and their families
8. Uses prescribing authority for medications as congruent with the state nursing practice act

STANDARD V-E—THERAPEUTIC ENVIRONMENT

The nurse provides, structures, and maintains a therapeutic environment in collaboration with the patient and other health care providers.

Process criteria

The nurse:

1. Assures that patients are adequately oriented to the milieu and are familiar with scheduled activities and rules that govern behavior and daily living
2. Observes, analyzes, interprets, and records the effects of environmental forces upon the patient
3. Assesses and develops the therapeutic potential of the practice setting on behalf of patients through consideration of the physical environment, the social structure, and the culture of the setting
4. Fosters communications in the environment that are congruent with therapeutic goals
5. Collaborates with others in the development and institution of milieu activities specific to the patient's physical and mental health needs
6. Articulates to the patient and staff the justification for use of limit setting, restraint, or seclusion and the conditions necessary for release from restriction
7. Participates in ongoing evaluation of the effectiveness of the therapeutic milieu
8. Helps patients living at home to achieve and maintain an environment that supports and maintains health

STANDARD V-F—PSYCHOTHERAPY

The nurse (specialist) uses advanced clinical expertise in individual, group, and family *psychotherapy*, child psychotherapy, and other treatment modalities to function as a psychotherapist and recognizes professional accountability for nursing practice.

Process criteria

The nurse:

1. Structures the therapeutic contract with the patient in the beginning phase of the relationship, including such elements as purpose, time, place, fees, participants, confidentiality, available means of contact, and responsibilities of both patient and therapist

2. Engages in interdisciplinary and intradisciplinary collaboration to achieve treatment goals
3. Engages patients in the process of determining the appropriate form of psychotherapy
4. Identifies the goals of psychotherapy
5. Uses knowledge of growth and development, psychopathology, psychosocial systems, small group and family dynamics, and knowledge of selected treatment modalities as indicated
6. Articulates a rationale for the goals chosen and interventions used
7. Fosters increasing personal and therapeutic responsibility on the part of the patient
8. Provides for continuity of care for the patient in the therapist's absence
9. Determines with the patient, when possible, that goals have been achieved and facilitates the termination process
10. Refers patients to other professionals when indicated
11. Respects and protects the patient's legal rights
12. Avails self of appropriate opportunities to increase knowledge and skill in the therapies utilized in nursing practice
13. Obtains recognized educational preparation and ongoing supervision for types of psychotherapy used, (e.g., individual psychotherapy, group and family psychotherapy, child psychotherapy, psychoanalysis, or other forms of therapy)
14. Uses clinical judgment in determining whether providing physical care (especially procedures prone to misinterpretation, e.g., injections, enemas) will enhance or impair the therapist-patient relationship and delegates such care as needed

The standards of practice and related process criteria for implementing nursing care are detailed and explicit. The standards clearly identify the range of activities psychiatric nurses employ: psychotherapeutic interventions, health teaching, self-care activities, somatic therapies, therapeutic milieu, and, if the nurse has advanced training, psychotherapy. The process criteria detail the many specific activities involved.

Within the nurse-patient relationship the patient can actively work toward adaptive goals. It is important to allow sufficient time for change. Many of the patient's maladaptive patterns have been building up over years; he cannot be expected to change them in a matter of days or weeks. Finally, the nurse must help the patient evaluate these new patterns, integrate them into his life experiences, and practice problem solving to prepare for future experiences. In this way secondary prevention nursing interventions also fulfill primary and tertiary prevention goals. Chapters 8 and 10 describe primary and tertiary prevention nursing interventions in greater detail.

Evaluation

STANDARD VI—EVALUATION

The nurse evaluates the patients' responses to nursing actions in order to revise the data base, nursing diagnoses, and nursing care plan.

Process criteria

The nurse:

1. Pursues validation, suggestions, and new information
2. Discusses observations, insights, and data with colleagues
3. Documents the results of evaluation of nursing care
4. Conducts a nursing audit

When evaluating care, the nurse should review all previous phases of the nursing process and determine whether the patient has met his goals. Fig. 5-3 illustrates the overall flow of the nursing process. Clearly the nurse makes many decisions throughout the process. He or she must first consider if the conceptual framework was appropriate to the particular patient situation. Next, was the data collection adequate, and were all relevant coping responses, objective signs, and subjective symptoms identified? Was the nursing diagnosis accurate, considering the normal parameters used, the analysis and synthesis of data, the application of theory, and its appropriateness for nursing therapy? Were the nursing goals and plan of care relevant and mutual? Did they show appropriate priorities, and were all realistic alternatives considered? The nurse should also evaluate whether the nursing interventions were appropriate, efficient in use of time and energy and, most important, effective. The timing, relevance, communication, and outcome of the nursing interventions must all be critically analyzed. It is worthwhile to note explicitly the achievement of goals. Often progress with psychiatric patients is slow and occurs in tiny steps rather than dramatic leaps. Realizing that progress has been made can produce growth in itself and inspire new enthusiasm in both the patient and the nurse.

One approach to evaluating psychiatric nursing is goal attainment scaling as described by Stanley.[34] This method assesses preestablished individual goals by constructing a review plan. The steps involved in creating a review plan include

1. Identifying specific patient goals
2. Weighting the relative importance of each goal
3. Deciding on a way of measuring progress for each goal that is useful, relevant, and easily rated

4. Determining the expected patient outcome for each goal
5. Creating a scale of levels of goal attainment
6. Setting a date to review a patient's overall progress toward the goals
7. Calculating a goal attainment score to summarize the patient's overall progress

Such an approach links evaluation to planning, thereby strengthening the scientific basis of nursing practice by developing empirical methods. Nurse administrators can use the same method to assess the effectiveness of a nursing service area.

The nurse must remain flexible to modify interventions according to the patient's changing needs and the nurse's continuing evaluation. Modifying a care plan does not necessarily mean nursing care has failed. Failure can occur if the plan of care is not relevant to the patient's needs or is not revised as his needs change or become clearer. Thus reassessment, reordering priorities, setting new goals, and revising the care plan are all essential evaluation activities.

Evaluation is a mutual process based on the patient's previously identified goals and level of satisfaction. Rather than a cumbersome task left for the termination phase of the relationship, it is a continuous, active process that begins early in the relationship and continues throughout. Key words for the evaluation phase of the nursing process are mutual, continuous, adequate, effective, appropriate, efficient, and flexible.

■ Organizational evaluation

Nurses need to actively participate in yet another level of evaluation: the formal organizational evaluation of overall patterns of care through *quality assessment measures*. In these activities the focus is not on the nurse practitioner but on the patient and the overall program of care. The current growth and commitment to critically reviewing health care stems from several sources: consumer demand for quality but reasonable health care; third-party payors for controlled health care costs; increased professional accountability; and regulatory and federal groups that monitor the quality of care. At this higher level of analysis a comprehensive evaluation should include:[31]

- Systems evaluation of treatment and allocation of resources
- Consumer evaluation of patient needs and satisfaction
- Clinical evaluation of treatment outcome and process

Of these three types of evaluation, clinical evaluation is the oldest and most common. It is gaining at-

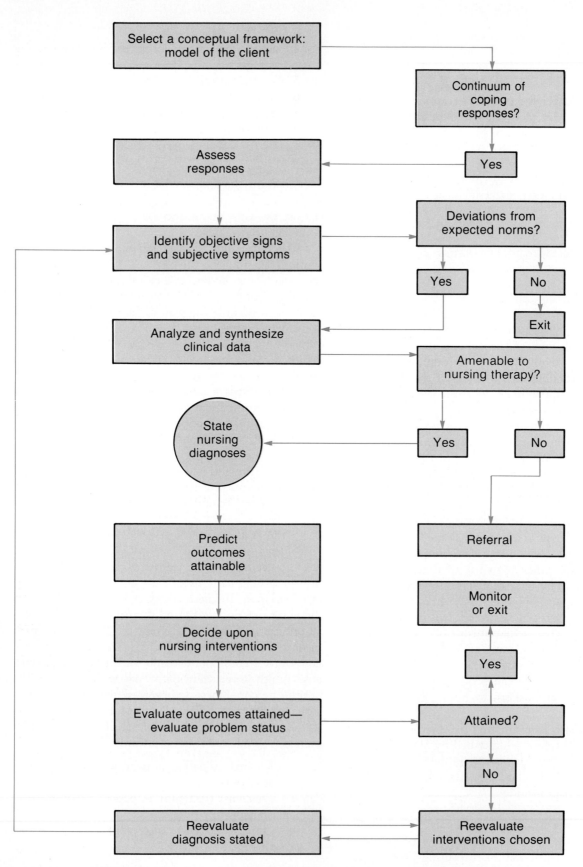

Fig. 5-3. Flowchart of the nursing process. (Modified from Gordon M: Nurs Clin North Am 14:492, 1979.)

tention and acceptance as the public becomes better educated and more assertive. Systems evaluation has primarily been limited to improving operations in private industry; only recently has it been applied to health care.

■ **SYSTEMS EVALUATION.** Systems evaluation assesses the organization of the delivery system, including patient flow, paperwork, procedures for scheduling patients, staff-patient ratio, disciplinary mix, and use of resources. It supplements clinical evaluation and has three components: (1) systems analysis, (2) economic analysis, and (3) operations research. Systems analysis attempts to simplify and improve the organization. Economic analysis emphasizes money spent and what, in turn, it produces. Operations research helps hospital management allocate available resources most effectively. Together these analyses, by evaluating the actual organization of treatment, have the potential to improve the performance of the clinical operation.

■ **CONSUMER EVALUATION.** Consumer evaluation has not received as much attention in the psychiatric literature as it has in other areas of health care. One of the few studies to examine consumer satisfaction with nurse psychotherapy was reported by Hardin and Durham,[10] who found that 90% of the patients expressed satisfaction and 70% were extremely satisfied. Assessing consumer satisfaction with nursing care is difficult, because the health care team works together and numerous variables can explain the findings. Nevertheless, additional studies are needed to both evaluate nursing services and document their cost-effectiveness.

■ **CLINICAL EVALUATION.** Clinical evaluation of ongoing programs takes place through various quality assurance activities that include both evaluation and corrective action. Some of the functions of quality assurance are listed in the accompanying box. Zimmer[38] defines quality assurance as estimating the degree of excellence in three areas: (1) patient health outcomes, (2) process or activity, and (3) resource cost outcomes. A common method reflecting two of these areas is the patient care audit, which, when restricted to nursing care, is also called the **nursing audit.** An audit may target a disease, nursing diagnosis, patient behavior, therapeutic measure, or nursing procedure. An audit that focuses on nursing actions is called a **process audit.** In a process audit, data are collected relative to a specific nursing activity and compared to a preset standard of nursing care, such as the American Nurses' Association *Standards of Nursing Practice.* If the audit focuses on the patient's response to care, it is an **outcome audit.** This type of audit parallels the evaluation

---

Functions of Quality Assurance

1. Tied to the philosophy of the hospital
2. Improves the performance of all professionals and protects the patients
3. Focuses on the quality of patient care
4. Sets the quality of care delivered against standards and measurable criteria
5. Prevents future losses or patient injuries by continuous monitoring of problem resolution areas
6. Searches for patterns of noncompliance with goals, objectives, and standards. The following steps of the quality assurance process are applied: problem identification, problem assessment, implementation of corrective action, follow-up, and reporting of findings.

From Orlikoff J and Lanham G: Hospitals 55(15):55, 1981.

---

phase of the nursing process. Specific examples of nursing audits conducted in the psychiatric setting are described in some of the annotated suggested readings at the end of this chapter.

Both process and outcome audits have advantages, depending on the information desired. Zimmer[38] believes that in quality assurance efforts, nurses should first start by determining the desired patient health outcomes and the degree to which they are attained. Next, they identify the most powerful and cost-effective activities that cause these results. Finally, when activities are identified and their relationship to specific outcomes is clear, nurses should proceed to the third step, determining the cost of the nursing activities and related resources.

Two important components of quality assurance should be emphasized. The first is the necessity for peer review, which should consist of expert nurse peers who are all involved in delivering care. They are the only people with the needed nursing knowledge to judge desired patient health outcomes, how patients should progress toward those outcomes, and which nursing activities cause the changes. They are also the ones who will be most involved with the second component of quality assurance—correcting the deficiencies or problems that the audit reveals. This concept of corrective action, actually making improvements, differentiates quality assurance from simple program evaluation or evaluation research. The reports of quality assurance should reach the highest level of the organization, so that steps are taken to improve the situation. These steps may include administrative changes in policies or procedures, continuing education programs, reallocation of personnel, changes in activities or procedures, or further research.

All nurses must be involved in this level of clinical program evaluation, because through such activities they demonstrate professional accountability. As Zimmer has stated:

Members of the nursing profession will be able to take their place among the disciplines that function in patient health review when and only when they can identify the specific alterations in patient health status secured through nursing activities. The development and the use of nurses' capability to function in quality assurance thus deserves the highest priority in the nursing profession.[38:93]

Nurse accountability

STANDARD VII—PEER REVIEW

The nurse participates in peer review and other means of evaluation to assure quality of nursing care provided for patients.
Process criteria
The nurse:

1. Assumes responsibility for review of clinical practice with peers, supervisors, and/or consultants
2. Considers recommendations for change that may arise from review

STANDARD VIII—CONTINUING EDUCATION

The nurse assumes responsibility for continuing education and professional development and contributes to the professional growth of others.
Process criteria
The nurse:

1. Initiates independent learning activities to increase understanding and update skills
2. Participates in inservice meetings and educational programs either as an attendee or as a teacher
3. Attends conventions, institutes workshops, symposia, and other professional meetings
4. Systematically increases understanding of theories related to psychiatric and mental health nursing
5. Helps others identify areas of educational needs
6. Formally and informally communicates to professional colleagues and others new knowledge regarding clinical observations and interpretations

Implementing the nursing process is the ongoing professional responsibility of every nurse. Inherent in this responsibility is the need for professional accountability requiring both peer review and continuing education on the part of each psychiatric nurse. Supervision by a peer, a group of peers, or a more experienced person is an important part of professional practice. Whether formal or informal, peer review helps the nurse examine care planning and serves as an ongoing learning experience.

Continued education is a valuable tool that also helps nurses to grow professionally. This includes a variety of professional activities from reading journals to attending workshops to participating in psychiatric nursing organizations. Another important aspect of continued education is sharing new knowledge with colleagues.

STANDARD IX—INTERDISCIPLINARY COLLABORATION

The nurse collaborates with interdisciplinary teams in assessing, planning, implementing, and evaluating programs and other mental health activities.
Process criteria
The nurse:

1. Participates in the formulation of overall goals, plans, and decisions
2. Includes the patient in the collaboration of the mental health team whenever possible and appropriate
3. Recognizes, respects, accepts, and demonstrates trust in colleagues and their contributions
4. Consults with colleagues as needed and is available to be consulted by them
5. Articulates knowledge and skills so that these may be coordinated with the contributions of others working with a patient or program
6. Collaborates with other disciplines in teaching, supervision, and research

Planning and implementation of accountable nursing care do not take place in isolation from the patient's other experiences with the health care team and the health care system. The nurse has a responsibility to be sure that the nursing care plan is consistent with the plans of other health care professionals who are involved with the patient. Sometimes conflict can be avoided by discussing roles and responsibilities with other professionals. Knowing how responsibility is distributed within the health team, the nurse can consult colleagues appropriately as indicated by the patient's needs. Although the nurse may have information about these needs, it is much more efficient and appropriate to refer the patient to team members who specialize in dealing with the patient's needs in those areas. Adequate background information should accompany the referral to avoid duplicating the assessment process.

STANDARD X—UTILIZATION OF COMMUNITY HEALTH SYSTEMS

The nurse (specialist) participates with other members of the community in assessing, planning, implementing, and evaluating mental health services and community systems that include the promotion of the broad continuum of primary, secondary, and tertiary prevention of mental illness.

Process criteria

The nurse:

1. Uses knowledge of community and group dynamics and systems theory to understand the structure and function of the community system
2. Recognizes current social and political issues that influence the nature of mental health problems in the community
3. Encourages active consumer participation in assessing and planning programs to meet the community's mental health needs
4. Brings the community's needs to the attention of appropriate individuals and groups, including legislative bodies and regional and state planning groups
5. Plans and participates in didactic and experiential educational programs related to the community's mental health
6. Uses consultative skills to facilitate the development and implementation of mental health services
7. Interprets mental health services to others in the community
8. Participates with other health care professionals and members of the community in the planning, implementation, and evaluation of mental health services
9. Participates in the delineation of high-risk population groups in the community and identifies gaps in community services
10. Assesses strengths and coping capacities of individuals, families, and the community in order to promote and increase their mental health
11. Uses knowledge of community resources to assist consumers' referral to and appropriate use of health care resources.
12. Collaborates with staff members at other agencies to facilitate continuity of service for individuals and families

Even when dealing with an individual patient, the nurse must not overlook the impact of the family and community. Interventions related to these other levels should be part of each phase of the nursing process. The psychiatric nurse generalist, in working with the family and community, aims to enhance the patient's resources and to maximize adaptive health responses. The psychiatric nurse specialist can also implement the nursing process with community health systems. At this level the nurse uses consulting skills to affect the health care needs of the larger community system.

Nursing research
STANDARD XI—RESEARCH

The nurse contributes to nursing and the mental health field through innovations in theory and practice and participation in research.

Process criteria

The nurse:

1. Approaches nursing practice with an inquiring and open mind
2. Uses research findings in practice
3. Develops, implements, and evaluates research studies as appropriate to level of education
4. Uses responsible standards of research in investigative endeavors
5. Ensures that a mechanism for the protection of human subjects exists
6. Obtains expert consultation and/or supervision as required

The relationship between theory, practice, and research is interactive and reciprocal. For theory to be useful, it must have implications for practice, and for practice to be tested and validated, it must be based in theory. Theory that arises out of practice is validated by research, which returns to direct practice and has implications for clinical care. This cyclical relationship, as diagrammed by O'Toole,[24] is represented in Fig. 5-4. It shows how the casual, nonsystematic observation of a problem in practice leads to a more systematic observation and definition of terms, including the nature of the problem and influencing factors. Descriptive, observational, and exploratory research can further define a problem. Hypotheses may be developed concerning relationships between identified variables, which may be tested in correlational or survey research designs. One might then test cause-and-effect relationships between the variables in various experiments with natural or controlled settings. Only after establishing cause-and-effect can one prescribe and test specific interventions aimed at changing the clinical problem. In this way prescriptive studies feed knowledge back into practice to improve health care.

This progression of observing from practice, theorizing, testing in research, and subsequently modifying practice must become an essential part of psychiatric nursing if it is to survive as a practice discipline. The gap between research and practice must be bridged.

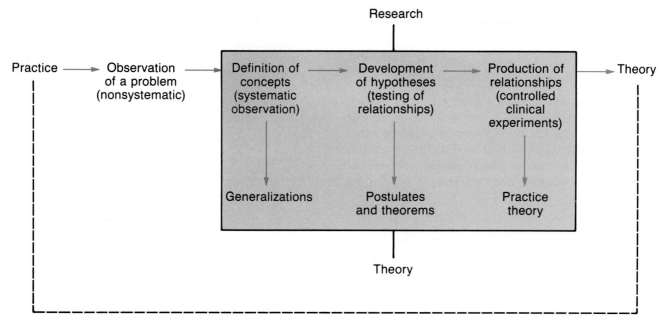

Fig. 5-4. Relationship between theory, practice, and research. (From O'Toole A: J Psych Nurs Ment Health Serv 19(2):11, 1981.)

One solution is to encourage closer collaboration between nurse researchers and nurse clinicians to ensure that the right questions are asked and the right variables are tested.

It has been noted that clinical practice in psychiatry is "more intuitive than it is scientific."[33:9] Research in this area is difficult for many reasons. Problems such as sample size, outcome measurements, and the complexity of human behavior all compound the difficulties. It is also hard to balance the rights of the individual against the desire to accomplish sound research. For example, consent to psychiatric research is complex. First, one needs to consider whether the subject is able to consent and the degree to which it is an informed choice. Next is the issue of the treatment itself and whether it alters the subject's ability by changing his affect, perceptions, or ability to process information. The risks involved in psychiatric research must be carefully studied and ethics must be maintained.

Research is sorely needed on the outcomes of nursing intervention to determine its effectiveness and how psychiatric nurses compare to other mental health care providers. Important data are being accumulated regarding the cost-effectiveness of nursing interventions in acute care, chronic care, primary care, and health promotion. One controlled investigation conducted in England demonstrated that community psychiatric nurses' clinical and social care of neurotic patients was comparable with that provided by outpatient psychiatrists.[19] In addition, the patients assigned to the nurses reported greater consumer satisfaction and had higher rates of discharge. Finally, over the whole study period, the care provided by the psychiatric nurses was less expensive. Psychiatric nurses need to undertake and report similar research studies if this speciality area of practice is to survive and remain viable.

Research on psychiatric nursing has increased in the past decade, and it is obvious that nurses can construct sophisticated designs with both theoretical and practical importance. The clinical problems are numerous, and as nurses gain the skills and experience to validate their work scientifically, they can make a significant contribution to psychiatric theory and practice.

Clinical case analysis

Clinical example 5-1 is a case study of a long-term relationship that demonstrates the use of the nursing process with a patient. It illustrates the interrelationship of the phases of the nurse-patient relationship, the therapeutic dimensions, and the various activities as the nurse works with the patient to foster adaptive coping behavior and more integrated functioning.

Documentation

Each phase of the nursing process should be documented in writing. This is essential to the successful planning and implementation of nursing care.

CLINICAL EXAMPLE 5-1

Ms. G came to the psychiatric outpatient department of the local hospital requesting treatment with a female therapist. After consultation with a psychiatrist, the psychiatric nurse specialist agreed to perform the initial screening and evaluation and consider serving as her primary therapist.

ASSESSMENT

To collect the initial data, the nurse followed the admission format required by the department. A description of the presenting problem revealed that Ms. G was a 29-year-old single woman who was neat in appearance and markedly overweight. She reported feelings of "confusion and depression" and said that superficially she appeared "outgoing and friendly and played the role of a clown." In reality, however, she said she had few close friends, felt insecure about herself, felt unsuccessful in her job, and believed she "overanalyzed her problems."

Additional information was obtained in other significant areas of her life. Her psychosocial history revealed a disrupted family situation. Her mother died of tuberculosis when she was 11 years of age. Her father, age 73, was alive but had been an alcoholic "for as long as Ms. G could remember." She had one sister, age 20, who married at age 16 and was now divorced. She also had one stepsister, age 45, who was married, had two adopted sons, and lived out of state. In exploring this family information, Ms. G revealed that her stepsister was her natural mother, but she had continued to call her father's wife "mother." After her "mother" died, her stepsister took over the house. Two years later, however, this stepsister married and moved out of state. Ms. G reported feeling closest to this stepsister and felt abandoned when she left. Ms. G then took charge of the house until age 14, when her father placed her and her sister in a group home where she had difficulty making friends.

She completed high school and college. In college she had four good friends who were all married now. Her only close heterosexual relationship was in high school, and this boyfriend eventually married her best friend. Since that time she had never dated and stated she had no desire to marry.

After college she obtained a job as a "girl Friday" for a law firm and expressed much pleasure with it. She then saw the opportunity to make more money as a waitress and switched jobs. She currently worked at a restaurant and her schedule involved day and night rotations as well as weekend shifts. She expressed dissatisfaction with many aspects of her job but was unable to identify alternatives. Her goal in life was to have a fulfilling career.

She lived alone. Her best friend was her immediate supervisor at work. She currently had no male friends and only two other female acquaintances.

Pertinent medical history revealed a major weight problem. She was 36 kg (80 pounds) overweight and extremely conscious of it. She viewed her body negatively and believed others were also "repulsed" by her weight. She was also recently recovered from infectious hepatitis. She drank an occasional beer when out with friends (once or twice a month), denied any drug use, and smoked three fourths of a pack of cigarettes a day.

NURSING DIAGNOSIS

After consultation the psychiatric nurse agreed to work with Ms. G as primary therapist. In the following session they established a contract for working together, and a fee was set by the agency's financial secretary. At this time they explored her expressed guilt over seeking help, the reason for her request for a female therapist, their mutual roles, and the confidential nature of the relationship. The nurse also shared with Ms. G. the maladaptive coping responses she had noted and the inferences she had made. They discussed these areas, and the following nursing diagnoses were identified from the psychiatric nursing diagnostic classes:

1. Self-concept, disturbance in self-esteem, related to childhood rejection and unrealistic self-ideals
2. Social isolation, related to ambivalence regarding male-female relationships and lack of socialization skills
3. Self-concept, disturbance in role performance, related to job dissatisfaction with working hours and nature of the work
4. Self-concept, disturbance in body-image, related to weight control problem
5. Anxiety, related to the possibility of change and the therapy process

PLANNING

In discussing these areas they agreed that problem 1 was a central one and problems 3 and 4 directly contributed to it. Her coping mechanisms included intellectualization and denial, and she compensated for her self-doubts by an outward appearance that was social, joking, and

Continued.

CLINICAL EXAMPLE 5-1—cont'd

friendly, yet superficial. Problem 5 presented an immediate demand on the therapeutic relationship. The strengths Ms. G brought to the therapy process included her introspective nature and ability to analyze events, her openness to new ideas, the resource people available to her in her immediate environment, and a genuine sense of humor. They mutually agreed to work on her problem areas in weekly therapy sessions. After 5 months they would evaluate the achievement of the following long-term goals:

1. Ms. G will describe her expectations of the therapeutic process and her commitment to it.
2. Aspects of Ms. G's self-ideal will be identified.
3. Factors influencing her self-concept and negative, stereotyped self-perceptions will be evaluated.
4. Interpersonal relationships will be analyzed to include her patterns of relating, her expectations of others, and specific areas of difficulty.
5. Alternative employment opportunities will be identified.
6. The advantages and disadvantages of a job change will be compared.

IMPLEMENTATION

Since they were in the introductory phase of the relationship, many of the goals involved areas needing further assessment. During this phase of treatment Ms. G displayed much anxiety, testing behavior, and ambivalence, and the nursing actions were focused on promoting respect, openness, and acceptance and minimizing her anxiety. Through the nurse's use of empathic understanding, Ms. G became less jovial and superficial and began to attain some intellectual insight into her behavior. With guidance she began to appraise her own abilities and became more open in expressing feelings.

She feared intimate personal involvement and could not tolerate physical closeness. The nurse incorporated this into nursing actions by initially minimizing confrontation, setting limits on anxiety-producing topics, and arranging the office seating to allow the patient to select her proximity to the nurse.

As they discussed the patient's relationships, the nurse confronted her with the dependent role Ms. G played and the unrealistic expectations she placed on others in the exclusiveness and amount of time she demanded from them. Her pattern of relating was also manipulative in that she elicited a sympathetic response and then used it to meet her own needs. She had great difficulty with mutuality and autonomy in relating to others. She was inexperienced in heterosexual relationships and missed many of the normal adolescent growth experiences in this area. Finally, she had much emotion and fear vested in her family of origin. The only trusting relationship Ms. G could recall was with her step-sister-mother. When this stepsister abruptly left home to marry, Ms. G perceived this as a personal rejection. She had since isolated herself from her family and continued to blame herself for her rejection by others, thus lowering her self-esteem and ability to trust others.

At the end of 4 months Ms. G was being considered for a promotion at work to hostess but on the basis of an evaluation by her best friend and supervisor was rejected for it. This precipitated a suicide attempt, which Ms. G revealed at her next regular session. At this point the issue of trust within the relationship became critical, as well as her inability to express anger because she feared rejection. The nurse now began more actively confronting Ms. G in her areas of ambivalence and inconsistency, setting limits on her self-destructive behavior, and suggesting alternatives. Ms. G then revealed that her relationship with her friend-supervisor was also a sexual one, and she expressed fears of homosexuality and loss of identity.

In later sessions Ms. G's relationship with this friend would become a critical therapeutic issue because many of her conflicts were acted out in it. The therapy process presented a threat to the pathological nature of this relationship, and during the course of therapy Ms. G would need to choose between maladaptive behaviors and more growth-producing options.

The relationship had now moved into the working phase where focus was placed on specifics, and problem-solving activities began. After 5 months the nursing diagnoses were reevaluated to include the following:

1. Violence, potential for self-directed, related to perceived rejection by friend
2. Self-concept, disturbance in personal identity, related to childhood rejection and unrealistic self-ideals
3. Social isolation, related to inability to trust, lack of socialization skills, and feelings of inadequacy
4. Powerlessness, related to fear of rejection by others

CLINICAL EXAMPLE 5-1—cont'd

5. Self-concept, disturbance in role performance, related to job dissatisfaction with working hours and nature of the work
6. Coping, ineffective individual, related to work and social stressors and lack of coping resources

At this time the nurse sought consultation as she further evolved her plan of care. Neither medication nor hospitalization were indicated. These formulations were shared with Ms. G, and together they collaborated about her future progress. They agreed to focus on changing Ms. G's maladaptive behavior by exploring past events and conflicts, and helping her learn more productive patterns of living. Ms. G was now ready to commit herself to the work of therapy and interpersonal change, and she began to assume increased responsibility for this therapeutic work.

Because her self-ideal was unrealistically high, specific short-term goals became essential. The nurse's theoretical orientation incorporated the dynamics of Sullivan's and Peplau's interpersonal theories, Beck's cognitive framework, and Glasser's reality therapy. The relationship was focused on frequently through the use of immediacy and became a model for examining many of her conflicts. This proved to be an excellent learning opportunity as Ms. G and the nurse dealt with resistance, transference, and countertransference reactions. During the next year Ms. G made much progress, including the following changes:

1. She moved into an apartment with another girlfriend.
2. She left her previous job and resumed working in an office where she received more personal satisfaction and a work schedule that would allow her to increase her social activities.
3. She began a diet regimen.
4. She participated in additional activities, such as a dancing class and a health spa.
5. She learned to verbalize her anger more freely with the nurse, friends, and others at work. This included discussing the many relationships in her past that were terminated without her agreement and in which she had internalized her anger.
6. She contacted her step sister-mother and visited her. This was an important therapeutic goal, because it allowed her to review her early experiences and provided her with actual feedback from those involved.

Consequently, many of her misperceptions became evident and open to exploration in therapy.
7. She was able to admit her ambivalent feeling about her friend-supervisor and discuss the negative aspects of the relationship. She stopped further sexual contact with her because she felt exploited. Over time, the nature of this relationship changed, and it eventually became a casual acquaintance.
8. She learned about the variety of sexual feelings and responses and saw her needs in this area as appropriate developmental tasks.
9. Her perception of personal space changed, and her tolerance for physical closeness increased.
10. She developed new male and female friends and socialized frequently with them.

EVALUATION

The terminating phase of the relationship began after about 18 months. At this time Ms. G was independently solving problems and, in therapy, the nurse primarily validated and supported her thinking. She was now receiving and accepting much positive feedback from others, had lost 15 kg (40 pounds), was continuing to diet, was planning future career goals, and had achieved more satisfactory interpersonal relationships with both men and women. The mutual goals for therapy had been met.

Terminating was difficult because of the close, trusting bond that had developed between them. The nurse had feelings of pleasure in Ms. G's growth, as well as personal satisfaction in her effectiveness as therapist. Ms. G openly described her feelings about terminating and raised the question of a possible social relationship between them. Over the course of 6 months she came to realize that the premise of the relationship was therapy and changing individual perceptions or patterns of relating would not be feasible or desirable. Most important, she had control for terminating this relationship and the opportunity to work it through in a positive way. The sessions were spaced to monthly intervals and considerable time was spent reviewing initial problem areas and the progress she had made in them. After 6 months, or 2 years of therapy, the nurse and patient mutually agreed to terminate regular sessions.

■ Assessment tools

Documentation begins with collecting data. If the nurse's data are not recorded, other mental health clinicians may attempt to obtain the same information. This repetition for the patient is unnecessary and inappropriate. By entering all collected data on the patient's record, omissions and areas of confusion can be easily identified and clarified with the patient.

To gather information the nurse should use an organized and systematic format. This tool may be called a data collection tool, nursing assessment form, or nursing history. It may include elements of the psychiatric evaluation, as described in Chapter 6 and outlined in the tool in Appendix A, but goes beyond this evaluation to include subjective and objective data relative to a nursing diagnosis. A variety of such nursing assessment tools have appeared in the psychiatric nursing literature.* In addition, agencies, nursing departments, psychiatric units, educational programs, and individual nurse clinicians often use a format that they have developed themselves. These tools may be adapted to the needs of a particular patient or institution.

Currently these tools need to be tested empirically for validity, reliability, and usefulness in nursing practice. One of the most complete sociopsychologic assessment forms is the one developed by Francis and Munjas,[6] which consists of 315 questions divided into 10 areas of assessment. The thoroughness of this tool makes it a valuable basis for decisions on data collection. (See the box on page 173, which lists these and other areas to include in a complete nursing assessment.)

Four critical areas that also need to be included in a nursing assessment are the patient's social support network, medication and drug history, physiological health status, and family information. Although a reliable method for measuring social support has not yet been developed, some elements that should be included in a clinical assessment of social support are listed in the box on nursing assessment.

The psychiatric nursing assessment should also explore the patient's medication and drug history, since it can affect the effectiveness of treatment and the patient's response to psychopharmocological agents. Appendix B presents a detailed assessment form for medications and drugs, and the assessment should include the pharmacological aspects outlined in the box on nursing assessment.

Nurses should also assess the patient's past and current physical health, since maladaptive coping responses have physiological as well as psychosocial effects. Furthermore, physiological imbalances can cause or intensify symptoms of emotional dysfunction. Other tools can be used to judge physiological functioning (Appendix C), and they should include the appropriate areas listed in the box on nursing assessment.

Finally, the nurse may wish to focus less on the individual and more on the quality of the family functioning—the degree to which the family can deal with problems successfully. To do this the nurse may need to use a family analysis tool that examines the family as a unit, including its structure, relationships, and coping potential.[29,36] Helm, at Yale University School of Nursing, developed a useful guide to family analysis (Appendix D), which evaluates factors listed in the box on areas to include in a complete nursing assessment.

A complete biopsychosocial assessment of the patient, based on these tools, would take hours to complete. Sometimes this might be necessary, but in other cases, based on the patient's situation and a team approach to care, the nurse may need to collect data relevant to only a few of these areas. A skilled psychiatric nurse, although familiar with all areas of assessment, must use his or her own judgment to determine what information is needed.

More recently another approach to data collection forms has been suggested. Guzzetta et al,[8] created a psychiatric assessment tool that is organized around the nine human response patterns of NANDA's taxonomy of nursing diagnoses—communicating, knowing, exchanging, moving, perceiving, relating, feeling, choosing, and valuing. The tool identifies areas to assess on the left side of the form and a column for related nursing diagnoses on the right side of the form (see Appendix E). The value of a nursing assessment tool such as this is that it organizes the nurse's approach around a nursing, rather than medical, model of practice and readily suggests appropriate nursing diagnoses as the outcome of the nursing assessment. Table 5-7 summarizes the areas a nurse would emphasize in a psychiatric nursing assessment that is organized around the NANDA human response patterns.

■ Nursing care plans

The next type of documentation is the nursing care plan, which should reflect all of the remaining stages of the nursing process—nursing diagnosis, planning, implementation, and evaluation. The format of the care plan may differ from agency to agency, because it is based on the nursing process, but the differences tend to be minor. A complete nursing care plan includes relevant demographic data on the patient, objective and subjective behaviors, nursing diagnoses,

---

*References 7, 9, 15, 42, 44.

Areas to Include in a Complete Nursing Assessment

Psychosocial

Demographic and vital data
  Name
  Address
  Birth
  Marital status
  Sex
  Race
Presenting data
  Nature of the problem
  Time of occurrence
  Reason for seeking care at this time
Family information
  Family system
  Communication patterns
  Interaction patterns
  Crisis response
Socioeconomic status
  Occupation
  Education
  Leisure time
  Residence
  Income
Life values
  Ethnicity/culture
  Religious behavior/spirituality
  Beliefs about illness
  Attitudes toward life
  Living standards and self-care behavior
Social habits
  Eating
  Drinking
  Drug use
  Hygiene
Sexual behavior
  Preference
  Sex role
  Sex activity
Cognition
  Consciousness
  Orientation
  Attention
  Perception
  Apperception
  Thought content
  Thought form
  Thought progress
  Memory
  Self-concept
  Body image
Affect
  Depersonalization

  Continuum of despair to ecstasy
  Affective ambivalence
  Inadequate affect
  Inappropriate affect
  Anxiety
Conation (observed)
  Appearance
  Motor activity
  Communication

Social support

Size of social network
Intensity, durability, multidimensionality, dispersion, and frequency of social linkages
Normative context of the relationships
Social roles
Support available to meet role obligations during illness
Patterns of social affiliation
Need for social affiliation

Medications and Drugs

Psychiatric medications
Prescription (nonpsychiatric) medications
Over-the-counter (nonprescribed) medications
Alcohol and street drugs

Physiological

Medical history
  Development
  Past illnesses and injuries
  Hospitalizations
  Family history
Physiological status
  Body systems
  Present illnesses
  Medications and ongoing treatments
Health maintenance
  Health goals

Family

Family's generational structure
Home environment
Physical and mental health
Financial status
Developmental stage in family life cycle
Family structure
Intrafamily relationships
Sociocultural family context
Strengths and weaknesses
Identified problem

TABLE 5-7

AREAS OF NURSING ASSESSMENT BY NANDA HUMAN RESPONSE PATTERNS[8]

NANDA Patterns	Emphasis areas to determine
Communicating	Verbal communication
	Nonverbal communication
	Grooming and appearance
Knowing	Orientation
	Perception or knowledge of planned therapy
	Readiness to learn
Exchanging	Physical integrity
	Toxicology screen
Moving	Leisure or social activities
	Acccess to firearms and weapons
	Self-care
Perceiving	Sensory perception
	Self-concept
	Meaningfulness
Relating	Role (home or occupation)
	Quality of relationships with others
Feeling	Emotional or integrity states
	Recent stressful life events
	Cognitive manifestations
	Coping with anxiety, fear, anger, guilt, envy, shame, and sadness
Choosing	Patient and family coping methods
	Patient's usual defense methods
	Compliance with health care regimen
	Judgment or decision-making ability
Valuing	Important religious practices
	Important life values

priority of the diagnoses, nurse-patient goals, nursing actions, rationale, and evaluation with modifications of the plan.

There are many advantages to keeping a written record of the nursing care plan as it evolves. The nurse who writes the plan must think through the whole nursing process in a logical and structured manner, so the plan is more likely to be based on sound rationale. This is helpful since others often scrutinize nursing care plans and may question specific components. It also helps the nurse evaluate himself or herself. An up-to-date working care plan requires that the nursing process be consistently reviewed and revised.

Many agencies are aware that well-written nursing care plans reflect the course of the patient's contact with nursing personnel, so it is often included in the patient's permanent agency record. This can greatly improve nursing care if the patient contacts the agency again in the future. Much data from the original assessment need not be collected again, thereby freeing both the patient and nurse to work on current concerns.

Detailed nursing care plans are useful learning tools. However, daily use of a care plan by the nursing staff and other personnel may require an abbreviated format. Recording information in a concise manner can save both time and energy, but the dangers of vague generalities and routine analysis are great. Many institutions use shortened care plans, such as Kardex forms. A sample format for a psychiatric nursing Kardex form is presented in Fig. 5-5. Nurses using such formats must ensure that patients receive clearly defined and individualized nursing care.

Writing documentation can be difficult, since it is hard to crystallize one's thinking and be specific. Krall* suggests the following five questions she found helpful in formulating written mental health treatment plans:

1. What is the exact behavior keeping the patient in the hospital?
2. Is the treatment plan written in behavioral terminology?
3. Is the stated behavior written in such a way that the patient can understand it?
4. Are the stated behaviors written in such a way that all nursing personnel can readily understand them?
5. How is the written treatment plan to be used? 15:236

■ **Charting**

Santora and Willer[27] examined the frequency, length, and content of staff member's discussions and written reports about 90 hospitalized psychiatric patients. They found that nursing staff members were more likely than psychiatrists to record patient progress but usually limited this to behavioral descrip-

---

*From Krall ML: Am J Nurs 76:236, 1976. Copyright by the American Journal of Nursing Co.

PSYCHIATRIC NURSING CARE PLAN

Precautions: _____   Special nursing needs: _____
_____   _____
_____   _____

Visitors: { } No restrictions   Telephone: { } Limited
{ } Family only   { } Unlimited
{ } Restricted to:
_____
{ } No visitors

Privileges: { } Restricted to unit
{ } Off unit accompanied by staff
{ } Off unit accompanied by family/visitor
{ } Off unit unaccompanied
{ } Out of hospital leave (dates) _____

Assessment data summary: _____
_____
_____
_____

Nursing diagnoses: _____
_____
_____
_____

Treatment goal: _____
_____

Date	Problem/need	Expected outcome (objective)	Target Date	Nursing Intervention

Room	Patient's name	Age	Doctor	Primary nurse	Admit date

Date	Medications	Date	P.R.N. Medications	Diagnostic & psychiatric tests	Req.	Done
		Date	Treatments	Special orders and concerns		

Allergies: Medical diagnosis: Diet:
(axis I-III)

Fig. 5-5. Psychiatric nursing Kardex form.

tions, whereas psychiatrists were more likely to focus on treatment goals or plans. Overall, the quality of the records and reporting habits was low.

Partly as a response to such problems, Weed[35] developed the **problem-oriented medical record.** Traditional medical records have often been repetitive, confusing, and disorganized. Separating nursing notes from the rest of the chart tended to block communication among various health team members. Nurses often were less motivated to write good notes, especially in settings where it was the practice to destroy nursing records after the patient's discharge. Frequently, incidents that nurses thought were significant enough to

record in detail were also documented by other health team members. The problem-oriented medical record avoids this duplication, because all notes are written chronologically, allowing each person to concentrate on adding new observations. It is also more convenient to read, which improves communication.

Many mental health facilities use the problem-oriented medical record. It consists of three basic elements: (1) the data base, (2) the problem list and treatment plan, and (3) progress notes.[35] The data base is the sum total of information from which the patient's problems can be identified. Many mental health professionals, including nurses, psychiatrists,

---

TABLE 5-8

SAMPLE PROBLEM-ORIENTED MEDICAL RECORD

Problem list and treatment plan

Date	Problem list	Treatment plan	Resolved
3-24-86	1. Agitated depression—loss of appetite, loss of interest in housework, difficulty sleeping	1. Amitriptyline (Elavil), 50 mg t.i.d. 2. Group therapy, Tuesdays 3. Explore patient's self-concept and perception of role performance 4. Encourage expression of emotion, particularly feelings of guilt, sadness, and hostility	
3-24-86	2. Marital conflict—states she and her husband are not compatible sexually and feels that he is not interested in her	1. Conjoint marital therapy, Fridays 2. Explore nature of sexual incompatibility 3. Confront patient with her inability to communicate her feelings and thoughts to her husband	

Treatment team progress notes

Date and time	Problem list		Progress notes
3-29-86 4 PM	4. Marital difficulty	S	Patient attended group therapy session today. Talked about difficulties with her husband, feels he doesn't love her.
		O	Appears nervous in group, feigns eye contact, but does participate somewhat.
		A	Still not comfortable with group members. Blames herself for problems at home, feels guilty.
		P	Support her in group, encourage her to express her emotions freely. *F. Hawkins, R.N.*
	5. Depression	S	Patient stated she was feeling better and liked participating in ward activities.
4-20-86 2 PM		O	Appears more enthusiastic and motivated. Increase in appetite and better sleeping habits.
		A	Adjusting to ward well. Appears antidepressants have taken effect.
		P	Continue medication and encourage patient to become even more involved on the unit. *L. Wilson, M.D.*

psychologists, and social workers, may contribute to it. The problem list and treatment plan are drawn up as soon after the patient is admitted as possible. Every significant problem and related treatment should be included. Problems should be dated and labeled active or inactive, and a note should be made when they are resolved.

Progress notes usually are written in SOAP format, preceded by a date, problem number, and problem name. A SOAP note includes the following:

S **Subjective data,** which include verbal comments, complaints, or information obtained from the patient or from a source other than the patient, such as the family

O **Objective data,** which may be a factual observation of a patient's behavior, such as his appearance or nonverbal behavior; a physiological measurement, such as height, weight, or blood pressure; or a test result, such as an x-ray examination or laboratory data

A **Assessment,** the interpretation of the subjective and objective data

P **Plan,** which is the specific plan of action for the problem, including diagnostic studies, treatment approaches, and patient education plans.

Here is a sample SOAP note:

S "I'm scared to go for a job interview . . . scared of all the strange people looking at me."

O Patient's hand rubbed forehead, biting on fingernails, frequent changes in sitting positions, no eye contact. Patient smoked rapidly and continuously while discussing his employment status.

A Patient experiencing moderate anxiety over the thought of going for a job interview. Strangers continue to make him feel self-conscious and inferior.

P Encourage patient to verbalize his fears and anxiety. He must be approached by staff members in a firm but caring manner, since he will not initiate social contacts. He requires persistent encouragement to verbalize feelings.

Table 5-8 shows a sample of the two basic elements of the problem-oriented medical record, the problem list and treatment plan, and related progress notes.

A recent approach to documentation is the use of a computerized system that writes, retrieves, and analyzes psychiatric treatment plans.[9] Such software can provide rapid entry and retrieval of required treatment plans and produces a document that is clinically expressive and readable. It stores clinical data that may

DIRECTIONS FOR FUTURE RESEARCH

The following are some of the nursing research issues raised in Chapter 5 that merit further study by psychiatric nurses:
1. The identification, classification, and validation of phenomena of concern to psychiatric nurses
2. The degree of mutuality in the nurse-patient relationship at the various phases of the nursing process, particularly in a psychiatric care context
3. The impact of cultural biases on the nursing care given to patients of different ethnic groups and social classes
4. Nursing diagnoses used by psychiatric nurses, including the extent and consistency of use, the format, their validity and reliability, and their usefulness in suggesting nursing actions that will promote adaptive coping responses.
5. The correlation and individuation of nursing and medical diagnoses
6. The content, process, and structure of health teaching conducted by psychiatric nurses and related outcomes
7. Outcomes of psychiatric nursing care, including levels of patient satisfaction
8. The cost-effectiveness of psychiatric nurses relative to other mental health care providers
9. The quality assurance activities engaged in by psychiatric nurses and resulting patient outcomes, nursing activities, and costs
10. Models of interdisciplinary collaboration in psychiatric practice, research, and education

also be useful for research, quality assurance, and management.

The specific format may vary, but the important issue is that information about the plan of care must be communicated so that staff members can treat the psychiatric patient consistently. Written records are subject to review by professional colleagues and in some states by the patient himself. In one study,[30] patients in a psychiatric unit of a general hospital read their complete medical records daily, and the practice was evaluated to determine its effect on patients and staff members. Both medical and nursing staff members along with patients found this an effective way to educate patients, help them become more actively involved in their treatment, correct inaccuracies in the medical record, and promote thoughtful charting by the staff. Committing oneself in writing is a necessary part of implementing the nursing process. Its implications should be seriously considered by all psychiatric nurses.

■ SUGGESTED CROSS-REFERENCES ■

This chapter serves as a foundation for formulating principles of psychiatric nursing and implementing its practice. As such it relates to all other chapters of this text.

■ SUMMARY ■

1. The American Nurses' Association defines nursing as "the diagnosis and treatment of human responses to actual or potential health problems." Nursing has four characteristics: phenomena, theory, actions, and effects. The need for a theoretical basis and conceptual framework for psychiatric nursing practice was presented.

2. The nursing process is an interactive, problem-solving process used by the nurse as a systematic and individualized way to fulfill the goal of nursing care. It is essential that the nurse and patient become partners in this process. The five phases of the nursing process were described, with the American Nurses' Association's *Standards of Nursing Practice* used as the organizing framework.

   a. Data collection is based on observation and may be facilitated by a systematic assessment tool. Data should reflect both content and process, and information relative to the patient's biopsychosocial world. The patient is the ideal source of validation. Cultural, religious, and socioeconomic data are crucial. The data base should also include the patient's view of the functional state of his family, as well as family strengths and resources.

   b. A nursing diagnosis is the independent judgment of a nurse through which the patient's nursing problems are identified. These problems may be overt, covert, existing, or potential. The subject of nursing diagnosis is the patient's behavioral response to stress. The statement of a nursing diagnosis should include both the adaptive or maladaptive health response and contributing stressors.

   c. Planning involves setting goals that are mutual, congruent, realistic, and appropriately timed. The plan of nursing care also includes priorities and prescribed nursing approaches to achieve the goals derived from the nursing diagnoses.

   d. Implementation refers to the actual delivery of nursing care to the patient. With psychiatric patients, nursing interventions should be directed toward helping the patient develop insight and resolve problems through carrying out a plan of positive action.

   e. Evaluation involves reviewing all previous phases and determining the degree of goal achievement by the patient. It is a mutual, continuous process that incorporates reassessment and modification of the care plan. Organizational evaluation of overall patterns of care through quality assessment measures also was discussed.

3. The need for nurse accountability was described in relation to peer review, continuing education, interdisciplinary collaboration, and utilization of community health systems.

4. The progressive process of observing from practice, theorizing, testing in research, and subsequently modifying practice must become an essential part of psychiatric nursing if the specialty is to survive as a practice discipline. Research is also needed on the outcomes of psychiatric nursing care.

5. A case analysis of a long-term relationship with a patient illustrated the use of the nursing process, phases of the relationship, and various therapeutic dimensions.

6. Activities of each phase of the nursing process should be documented in writing. The problem-oriented medical record was described.

■ REFERENCES ■

1. American Psychiatric Association: Nursing: a social policy statement, Kansas City, Mo, 1980, The Association.
2. American Psychological Association: Diagnostic and statistical manual of mental disorders, third edition, revised, Washington DC, 1987, The Association.
3. Coler M: I am nursing diagnosis: color me DSM-III green. In Kim M, McFarland G, and McLane A, editors: Classification of nursing diagnoses, St Louis, 1984, Mosby–Year Book, Inc.
4. Fitzpatrick J, Whall A, Johnson R, and Floyd J: Nursing models and their psychiatric mental health applications, Bowie, Md, 1982, Robert J Brady Co.
5. Flaskerud J and Halloran E: Areas of agreement in nursing theory development, Adv Nurs Sci 4:1, 1980.
6. Francis G and Munjas B: Manual of social psychologic assessment, New York, 1976, Appleton-Century-Crofts.
7. Geach B: The problem-solving technique: as taught to psychiatric students, Perspect Psychiatr Care 12:9, 1974.
8. Guzzetta C et al: Clinical assessment tools for use with

nursing diagnoses, St Louis, 1989, Mosby—Year Book, Inc.

9. Hammond K and Munnecke T: A computerized psychiatric treatment planning system, Hosp Community Psychiatry 35(2):160, 1984.

10. Hardin S and Durham J: First rate: exploring the structure, process, and effectiveness of nurse psychotherapy, J Psychosoc Nurs Ment Health Serv 23(5):8, 1985.

11. Johnson D: The behavioral system model for nursing. In Riehl J and Roy SC, editors: Conceptual models for nursing practice, ed 2, New York, 1980, Appleton-Century-Crofts.

12. Jourard S: Toward a psychology of transcendent behavior in explorations. In Otto H, editor: Human potentialities, Springfield, Ill, 1966, Charles C Thomas, Publisher.

13. King I: A theory for nursing: systems, concepts, process, New York, 1981, John Wiley & Sons.

14. Kini J: The effects of patient social class on the judgments of public health nurses, Nurs Res 17(3):261, 1968.

15. Krall ML: Guidelines for writing mental health treatment plans, Am J Nurs 76:236, 1976.

16. Krumboltz J and Thorensen C: Behavioral counseling, cases and techniques, New York, 1969, Holt, Rinehart & Winston.

17. Labun E: Spiritual care: an element in nursing care planning, J Adv Nurs 13:314, 1988.

18. Leininger M: Transcultural nursing: concepts, theories and practice, New York, 1978, John Wiley & Sons.

19. Mangen S et al: Cost-effectiveness of community psychiatric nurse or out-patient psychiatrist care of neurotic patients, Psychol Med 13:407, 1983.

20. McClosky J: Nurses' orders: the next professional breakthrough, RN 431(2):99, 1980.

21. Neuman B: The Neuman systems model: application to nursing education and practice, Norwalk, Conn, 1982, Appleton-Century-Crofts.

22. O'Brien ME: The need for spiritual integrity. In Yura H and Walsh B, editors: Human needs and the nursing process, Norwalk, 1982, Appleton-Century-Crofts.

23. Orem D: Nursing: concepts of practice, ed 2, New York, 1980, McGraw-Hill Book Co.

24. O'Toole A: When the practical becomes theoretical, J Psychosoc Nurs Ment Health Serv 19(2):11, 1981.

25. Rogers M: An introduction to the theoretical basis of nursing, Philadelphia, 1970, FA Davis Co.

26. Roy SC and Roberts S: Theory construction in nursing: an adaptation model, Englewood Cliffs, NJ, 1976, Prentice-Hall.

27. Santora E and Willer B: The reporting habits of staff in a psychiatric hospital, Hosp Community Psychiatry 26:362, 1975.

28. Schlesinger R: Cross-cultural psychiatry: the applicability of Western Anglo psychiatry to Asian-Americans of Chinese and Japanese ethnicity, J Psychosoc Nurs Ment Health Serv 19(9):26, 1981.

29. Sedgwick R: Family mental health: theory and practice, St Louis, 1981, Mosby—Year Book, Inc.

30. Simonton M, et al: The open medical record: an educational tool, J Psychiatr Nurs 15:25, 1977.

31. Singh A, May P, and Messick J: The role of operations research and systems analysis in holding down the cost of hospitals and clinics, J Psychiatr Nurs 16(9):24, 1978.

32. Smilkstein G: The family APGAR: a proposal for a family function test and its use by physicians, J Fam Pract 6:1231, 1978.

33. Smoyak S: Clinical practice: intuitive or based on research? J. Psychosoc Nurs Ment Health Serv 20(4):9, 1982.

34. Stanley B: Evaluation of treatment goals: the use of goal attainment scaling, J Adv Nurs 9:351, 1984.

35. Weed L: Medical records, medical education and patient care, Cleveland, 1969, The Press of Case Western Reserve University.

36. Whall A: Nursing theory and the assessment of families, J Psychiatr Nurs 19(1):30, 1981.

37. Yamamoto J, James Q, and Palley N: Cultural problems in psychiatric therapy, Arch Gen Psychiatry 19:45, 1968.

38. Zimmer M: Quality assurance in the provision of hospital care. A model for evaluating nursing care, Hospitals 48:91, 1974.

■ ANNOTATED SUGGESTED READINGS* ■

*Apostoles F, Little M, and Murphy H: Developing a psychiatric nursing audit, J Psychiatr Nurs 15:9, 1977.

Describes the experience of developing the first nursing audit, primarily a process one, in one clinical division of a large psychiatric hospital. Eight specific steps are described in a way that makes this useful reading for nurses involved in a similar process.

*Bevilacqua J: Voodoo—myth or mental illness? J Psychiatr Nurs 18(2):17, 1980.

A fascinating clinical study of a 14-year-old Haitian girl's experience with what has been diagnosed as mental illness. The author raises many questions on etiology, interventions, and the influence of voodoo and makes the reader consider how the system we work in perpetuates rather than relieves mental illness.

*Boettcher E: Nurse-client collaboration: dynamic equilibrium in the nursing care system, J Psychiatr Nurs 16:7, 1978.

Explores the process of nurse-patient collaboration, which parallels the nursing process. Highly recommended for the clinical example it includes that describes a nursing care plan, including behaviors, nursing diagnosis, mutual goals, specific interventions, rationale, and evaluation.

Comas-Diaz L and Griffith E: Clinical guidelines in cross-cultural mental health, New York, 1988, John Wiley & Sons.

Focuses on the clinical implications of assessment, evaluation for treatment, and mental health care for ethnoculturally different populations. A resource book for all practitioners.

*Erickson H, Tomlin E, and Swain M: Modeling and role-modeling, Englewood Cliffs, NJ, 1983, Prentice Hall.

An easy-to-read text that presents a practical approach to the study of a theory-based model for nursing. Based on the idea that the nurse should understand the patient's model of his world and then role model that world so that the patient can grow healthier. Clinical examples are provided.

*Evans C and Lewis S: Nursing administration of psychiatric-mental health nursing, Rockville, Md, 1985, Aspen Publishers, Inc.

The only text that addresses psychiatric nursing administration. Relevant chapters discuss evaluation, continuing education, documentation, and research implementation.

*Fitzpatrick J, Whall A, Johnson R, and Floyd J: Nursing models and their psychiatric mental health applications, Bowie, Md, 1982, Robert J Brady Co.

An important text that examines borrowed theories that psychiatric nurses frequently use and explores their congruence with nursing models. Highly recommended reading.

*Foreman M: Building a better nursing care plan, Am J Nurs 79(6):1086, 1979.

Presents a general semantics approach to formulating a nursing care plan. The author believes that by asking oneself a series of questions, a more specific and more useful plan of care can be developed. A well-written article that presents a concise, unique approach to care plan writing.

*Francis G and Munjas B: Manual of social psychologic assessment, New York, 1976, Appleton-Century-Crofts.

Presents a systematic method for nurses to assess the sociological and psychological aspects of patients. A comprehensive analysis of variables is presented along with suggested questions. A valuable resource for nurse practitioners.

*Hauser M and Feinberg D: Problem solving revisited, J Psychiatr Nurs 15:13, 1977.

The authors present a framework consisting of a combination of the problem-solving process and the creative thinking process. The processes directed in a complementary manner are suggested as a means of solving problems creatively in situations that call for unique and novel solutions.

*Kibbee P: Methods of monitoring quality in a psychiatric setting, J Nurs Quality Assurance 1(3):64, 1987.

Detailed discussion of volume and quality indicators, nursing monitors, and outcome-oriented systems as they apply to psychiatric nursing.

*Labun E: Spiritual care: an element in nursing care planning, J Adv Nurs 13:314, 1988.

Discusses basic aspects of spirituality as an aspect of holistic nursing care. The nursing process is used to show how spirituality can be incorporated into the patient's plan of care.

Lefley HP: Culture and chronic mental illness, Hosp Comm Psychiatry 41(3):277, 1990.

Extremely thorough review of the relationship of culture to chronic mental illness. Issues related to etiology, service delivery, diagnosis, and treatment are all explored. Highly recommended in both scope and depth of analysis.

*Lucas M and Folstein M: Nursing assessment of mental disorders on a general medical unit, J Psychiatr Nurs 18(5):31, 1980.

The authors of this study found that current nursing assessments on general medical units failed to identify cognitive disorders and symptoms of emotional distress. To correct this omission, the authors suggest the use of two brief tools to measure psychiatric disorders quantitatively.

Mager RF: Preparing instructional objectives, ed 2, Palo Alto, Calif, 1984, Fearon Publishers.

This is a classic text on the art of writing behavioral objectives. It is written in a programmed learning format and is easy to read and informative. This is highly recommended for inexperienced objective writers.

*Marriner-Tomey A: Nursing theorists and their work, St Louis, 1989, Mosby–Year Book, Inc.

Describes the work of the major nursing theorists in a thorough, referenced, and easily understood manner. Highly recommended for both students and clinicians.

*Miller T and Lee L: Quality assurance: focus on environmental perceptions of psychiatric patients and nursing staff, J Psychiatr Nurs 18(2):9, 1980.

A unique application of quality assurance is described in this study, which assessed the ward atmosphere of an inpatient psychiatric service. This information was used for staff education and enrichment.

Olson D and McCubbin H: Families: what makes them work, Beverly Hills, Calif, 1983, Sage Publications.

"Normal" family life is described in this book, which is based on a study of more than 1000 families. Types of families, the stresses they encounter, and their coping resources are all explored.

*O'Toole A: When the practical becomes theoretical, J Psychosoc Nurs Ment Health Serv 19(12):11, 1981.

Explores the relationship between practice, theory, and research and reviews studies in psychiatric nursing, with an assessment of the progress of the field in developing practice theory. Implications and suggestions for future direction highlight important areas that psychiatric nursing needs to address to survive.

*Rowan F: The chronically distressed client, St Louis, 1980, Mosby–Year Book, Inc.

Uses eight in-depth psychiatric case studies to illustrate the application of nursing process methodology. Highly recommended for its consistent, thorough analysis in a case-specific presentation.

*Singh A, May P, and Messick J: The role of operations research and systems analysis in holding down the costs of hospitals and clinics, J Psychiatr Nurs 16(9):24, 1978.

Explores the applications of operations research and systems analysis techniques to find ways to improve clinical operations and contain costs within medical care facilities.

*Stanley B: Evaluation of treatment goals: the use of goal attainment scaling, J Adv Nurs 9:351, 1984.

Describes goal attainment scaling in detail. The authors argue that the key to successful evaluation lies in evaluation planning, which strengthens the scientific basis of nursing practice by empirical methods.

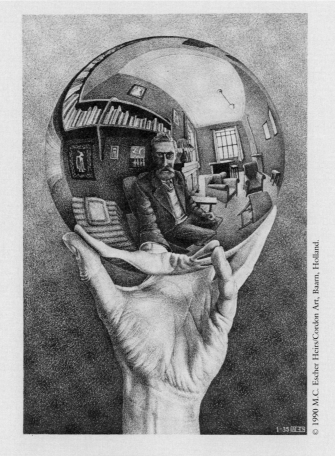

Information is of no value for its own sake, but only because of its personal significance.

Eric Berne

C H A P T E R   6

PSYCHIATRIC EVALUATION

E. Susan Batzer
Michele T. Laraia

LEARNING OBJECTIVES

After studying this chapter, the student should be able to:

- state the role of the nurse in a psychiatric evaluation of patients and the knowledge and skills needed.

- identify the two basic elements of a psychiatric interview and interviewing skills.

- describe the stages of psychiatric evaluation related to collecting data on the presenting problem, patient's history, mental status examination, formulation of a diagnostic impression, and case disposition.

- identify the major categories of data the nurse should collect regarding the patient's presenting problem, history, and mental status.

- analyze the behavior to be assessed in the six major categories of a mental status examination.

- discuss additional resources for completing patient assessment, including psychological and physiological measurements.

- identify the usefulness of brain visual imaging for psychiatric practice.

- relate the formulation of a medical diagnosis to that of a nursing diagnosis.

- consider the factors in deciding a case disposition.

- discuss future trends in the psychiatric evaluation of patients.

- identify directions for future nursing research.

- select appropriate readings for further study.

Clinical examples 6-1 and 6-2 provide cases of unusual behavior. The vignette in Clinical example 6-1 is somewhat typical of a person with a manic episode, but it might also represent other conditions such as substance-induced organic disorder or schizophrenic disorder. What information does the nurse need to assess this woman's mental functioning and to determine whom to ask for assistance?

In Clinical example 6-2, was the man's depression so well masked that no clinical symptoms were evident during his hospital stay? Were there any clues recorded in the initial interview and assessment? Was a psychiatric evaluation done along with evaluation of the gastrointestinal, genitourinary, cardiopulmonary, and other systems?

These clinical examples demonstrate the importance of a psychiatric evaluation. They have several things in common: behaviors that are viewed as a psychiatric problem, nurse-patient interaction, and a lack of sufficient data to effectively assess and plan a treatment program. As vital members of the health care team, nurses must assume a role in the psychiatric evaluation of patients.

Role of the nurse

At one time psychiatric evaluation was the job of the physician, usually a psychiatrist. However, Imboden[7] has pointed out the need for psychiatric evaluation as part of the routine physical examination of patients. If the patient's problem is psychologically based, a psychiatric evaluation might save him costly tests and procedures. The holistic approach implies assessment of psychological needs and potential. Nurses trained in caring for the patient as a total being will include the psychiatric evaluation as part of the assessment skills they acquired in nursing school.

A psychiatric evaluation is not something totally new to be learned. It is primarily a reorganization of knowledge and skills acquired by nurses. Basic knowledge of human behavior and psychodynamics, psychopathology, and psychotherapy, combined with interviewing and assessment skills, are the tools nurses need to perform a psychiatric evaluation. Like most things it is a skill easily learned with practice. What might often impede nurses in their performance is not a lack of knowledge but an uneasiness with psychiatric problems. It is important therefore that nurses be aware of their own negative or uncomfortable feelings toward patients with psychiatric symptoms.

As in other areas of nursing, the role assumed by the nurse depends on his or her level of preparation and the health care setting. The general practitioner should include the psychiatric evaluation as part of the nursing history. Clinical example 6-3 illustrates the need for such an assessment.

This illustration presents the roles of two nurses. The staff nurse assessed the patient, including a brief psychiatric evaluation, and then called on the liaison nurse. This nurse consultant has advanced knowledge of psychiatric nursing that will enable her to determine the patient's problem and to help the staff nurse design a care plan.

Nurses in a community mental health center may have advanced knowledge in psychiatric nursing through education at the master's degree level or through experience and in-service education in mental health. They often perform the initial evaluation of patients and assign them to the appropriate health team members, such as the psychiatrist and psychologist, for further evaluation or treatment. Nurses in this setting may also arrange for hospitalization or may engage the

patient in a form of psychotherapy, including crisis intervention and insight-oriented therapy.

Nurses working in a psychiatric inpatient setting can perform a variety of functions based on the philosophy of the unit. Whether these functions include primary nursing, patient advocate, or other conceptually defined roles, nurses need to review mental functioning continuously. This provides a focus on the patient's problems and ongoing evaluation of patient needs as well as assessment of treatment.

The psychiatric interview

The basic elements of a psychiatric assessment are the psychiatric history and the mental status examination. For clarity these are addressed separately in this chapter. The psychiatric interview provides the structure for assessing the patient. Assessment denotes systematic collection of patient data. A data base on which nursing judgments can be made is assembled through history taking and the mental status examination.

The nurse's approach and line of inquiry during the psychiatric evaluation will vary, depending on the presenting problem and the patient. There are many formats for performing and recording the psychiatric evaluation.[1,7,8,10] This chapter presents one framework for organizing and recording data.

The purpose of the psychiatric interview is to establish rapport with the patient, describe his symptoms, gain knowledge of his living patterns and coping behaviors, and assess how his mind is working. The interview is goal-directed communication to experience who the patient is and how he has developed. This attempt at fully acknowledging and understanding the patient enables the nurse to determine needs and a plan of care more effectively. The plan of care is most successful when it reflects concern for the patient as an individual. Consider the case of a man with high blood pressure who is told to relax. The nurse does not know he has six children, debts, and is the only working member of his family. It is not surprising to find that the plan was ineffective and that the patient has uncontrolled blood pressure and depression when he next visits the hospital. Loss of appetite and an inability to sleep, characteristic of an affective disorder, have compounded the original problem of high blood pressure.

Establishing a rapport with a patient is often taken for granted or viewed as an intuitive skill. However, it should be thought about and planned for as any other nursing goal. A basic factor is respect for and awareness of the patient's sense of security. A threat to the individual's security produces anxiety, which in turn influences data obtained in the interview. The nurse conveys sensitivity by demonstrating a genuinely warm, concerned, and competent approach. This atmosphere of acceptance makes it easier for the patient to express his feelings and concerns.

The nurse can convey respect for the patient by addressing him by name and by introducing himself or herself by name and title. Following this identification, a definition of purpose should be established so that a framework for the interview is set. This provides an opportunity for sharing expectations and allaying anxiety, since both nurse and patient are clear about what is to follow. As interviewer, the nurse is governed by the purpose of the interview, which is distinct and specific for each situation encountered. For example, consider a patient who has had a thoracotomy as part of the treatment for Hodgkin's disease and is struggling with acceptance of this chronic condition. The psychiatric liaison nurse will help secure psychiatric treatment elsewhere. A second type of interview is the initial meeting in brief psychotherapy or in continued treatment. The nurse's purpose here is to establish both a diagnosis and a professional acquaintance, with the intent of carrying on treatment himself or herself. A third type of interview with a different purpose would involve the parents of a child who is handicapped or has a chronic disease. Although the focus of the interview might be a problem the child is having, the parent's particular difficulties and needs must be considered in planning for the child's treatment.

Whenever the nurse conducts an interview, the environment should be private. Ideally, this would mean a comfortable room used solely by the interviewer and the person being interviewed. More often than not this occurs only in settings where there are private offices in which the patient and nurse can meet. The nurse must often overcome environmental constraints, and his or her creativity is called on to convey an atmosphere of privacy to the patient. This can be accomplished by turning chairs in a crowded room away from others or by leaving a message with other personnel that the interview should be interrupted only for specified reasons.

■ Interviewing skills

Thus far, understanding the patient through demonstrating respect, acceptance, and concern has been described. However, setting the stage for self-disclosure is not enough. The nurse must actively participate in the process by being what Sullivan[13] refers to as a participant observer. This implies participation with and observation of the patient to collect relevant data on which nursing care can be based.

Communication skill is a valuable tool of the participant observer. Maintaining eye contact and using open-ended questions and reflection are familiar techniques in promoting communication. It should be noted, however, that active participation in the interview is not synonymous with increased verbalization by the nurse. A facial expression that reflects interest and concern is just as effective as a verbal message in denoting participation with the patient.

Two skills of utmost importance in conducting a psychiatric interview are listening and observation. Here they are specifically addressed, because they are perhaps the most difficult skills to acquire. Listening attentively to and observing another person involves transcending oneself, and this is a difficult task. Being sure that what is said is heard as the sender of the message intended, and not as the receiver of the message had expected or hoped for, requires introspection on the part of the nurse. Biases, stereotypes, and cultural differences can also interfere with this communication.

The nurse must listen both to what is being said and to what is not being said. For example a patient may describe his mother as "kind, loving, helpful, someone (he) could always turn to." However, as more information is shared, the patient describes her as "having been out of the house a lot working and leaving him with various baby-sitters throughout his childhood." From these limited data the nurse might wonder how the mother was able to communicate the kind, helpful, loving attitude her son describes. Or the nurse might question if this is more a description of what the patient needed and wanted but did not receive from his mother. As a result of conflict, the defense mechanisms of denial and fantasizing may be operating to protect the patient as he tells of his early childhood. Much more information is needed before an assumption such as this one can be made. What is implied in this description is that the nurse must strive to understand what the patient is trying to communicate. Does the nurse know what he means by his statements? Could it mean something other than what immediately occurs to the nurse?

Throughout the interview the nurse must also listen for the themes that develop as the patient describes himself and his current and past history. In describing his life, a 22-year-old patient pointed out that his parents taught him at an early age to please other people. It also became evident that his parents were consulted on most of the decisions he made throughout his life, such as the friends he had, the schools he attended, what his major was to be in college, and where he lived with his wife. He expressed trouble in placing limits on co-workers who constantly asked him to do favors for them and to join clubs, which he was not able to refuse. One of the themes inherent in this description is the patient's inability to assert himself. It is important to focus on this, since it may be one of the stressors related to his depression.

CLINICAL EXAMPLE 6-4

Although Mrs. S is only 31 years of age, her torn clothing that fits loosely and her slumped posture and furrowed brow give an appearance of someone much older who has weathered many storms. She continuously wrings her hands as she talks about the death of her husband 6 years ago when her children were still infants. At one point tears come to her eyes as she talks about her inability to give her children the things she would like them to have.

Observation also requires a special attentiveness in the nurse. It is important to observe the patient's verbal content and the nonverbal communication represented in the body language he uses. Does he look older or younger than his stated age? Is there a message in his style of dress or the gestures he uses in the interview? Does his manner of communicating reflect his educational level? Is his affective response to a particular topic congruent with the content he presents? Clinical example 6-4 contains many nonverbal cues that the nurse should note.

These observations, along with others obtained in the mental status examination, form the data base on which the nursing diagnosis and a treatment plan are made. Other observations are addressed in more depth in the discussion of the mental status examination.

If the nurse uses the skills described, an open atmosphere that encourages self-disclosure by the patient will be created. A tense, hurried, and anxious approach should be avoided. The nurse's awareness of his or her feelings, subjectivity, and misperceptions before meeting the patient should help to avoid communicating anxiety to the patient. If immobilized by insecurity and anxiety, the nurse will be unable to provide the open atmosphere that allows participation in the other individual's experience.

A vital concern of the beginning clinician is where to begin with the patient. Simply stated, it is best to start where the patient is. Yet few patients spontaneously begin on their own; rather, they wait for the nurse to open the interview. A brief statement of what the nurse has learned about the patient, either from observation or from a referral, usually gives the patient the opportunity to tell his story in his own way. The patient with Hodgkin's disease described earlier was approached by the nurse in the following way.

MS. J: **Good afternoon, Ms. X. My name is Ms. J, and I am a psychiatric nurse.**

MS. X: **(Looks up) Hello.**

MS. J: **The head nurse, Ms. K, asked me to come and talk with you today. She is concerned about you, because she noticed that you had been crying on several occasions when she entered your room.**

MS. X: **(Beginning to tear) I'm tired of talking, I'm tired of tests, I just want to be left alone.**

MS. J: **It sounds like you are feeling frustrated.**

MS. X: **(Looking directly at the nurse) What would you know? All of this, and for what? Most people with cancer end up dead, so what's the use?**

The nurse had provided the patient a chance to disclose some of her feelings about her illness and her fear of death. From this point, considering the patient's emotional status and readiness, the nurse can proceed with psychiatric evaluation.

With the hospitalized patient an account of the presenting problem and events leading up to the hospitalization, as well as historical data, may have previously been obtained and recorded in the chart by other health care professionals. If so, the nurse would modify his or her approach and discuss particular areas not included in the original evaluation or areas believed to be important to the patient's current mental functioning. The nurse can rely on collateral sources such as the medical history or social history and select the focus for the interview.

■ Presenting problem

A clear account of the presenting problem must be obtained, consisting of a chronological reconstruction of the current illness. If this account is not spontaneously offered by the patient or identified elsewhere, the nurse uses his or her skills in obtaining this information. How does the patient perceive the problem? Is it interpersonal, somatic, or sociological? When was the problem first noticed (onset)? How long has it lasted (duration)? Does the patient know possible causes of the problem? Has it become worse (progressed) or changed in degree? If so, when did the change occur? Has the patient found any solution or obtained any relief?

In eliciting this information the nurse looks for other factors of which the patient may not be aware, such as a change in personal relationships, job, financial condition, and other circumstances surrounding the initial occurrence. In the preceding dialogue it was assumed, perhaps because of the nurse's own conflicts, that the patient's crying spells were related to her present condition—the thoracotomy for Hodgkin's disease. When asked about the onset of her crying, the patient told the nurse about her husband's recent job loss and his inability to find another job. Just that information could change the entire assessment of this patient's needs. She may have already worked through acceptance of the chronic illness and currently be concerned with medical insurance for future treatment. Although the original statement she makes about death might reflect an ongoing conflict, without more specific inquiry by the nurse her immediate concerns could go unnoticed.

It is therefore necessary to strive for specificity. The patient must be encouraged to describe actual incidents and to record these in his own words rather than in a general statement. Skill in discouraging trivia and repetition helps the patient focus on the current problem.

After a description is obtained about the presenting problem and the incidents that led to its occurrence, the patient's view of responsibility needs to be assessed. Does he see the problem as something he needs to change, something someone else is responsible for, or something that no one can control, such as a patient who believes the devil has entered his body?

Whom the patient views as responsible for the problem directly relates to what changes are desired. The 22-year-old man previously described felt depressed and questioned what he could do to overcome these feelings. Although the relationship with his parents may have been causative in his depression and a conflict he could work through in therapy, it was not his current focus. However, placing limits on expectations he had of himself and that others at work had of him was something he consciously desired to do. This focused on an identified problem and a definition of goals. Agreement between the nurse and patient on problem identification is essential if resolution is to occur. Whether the nurse's task is to refer the patient for treatment or to undertake therapy personally, a mutually agreed on diagnosis is essential.

In the initial stage of the psychiatric interview, the nurse has created an open atmosphere with a concerned approach to the patient and has gathered information about his current illness. The patient has described the symptoms in behavioral terms, (such as a desire to be alone or frequent fighting with spouse), and in body disturbances (such as an inability to sleep, loss of weight, or heart palpitations). How the nurse views the presenting problem depends on whether there were previous episodes and if the problem is an exaggeration of long-term trends or something new. To make an assumption about patterns of living and coping behaviors, further data collection is necessary.

■ History taking

A brief survey of the patient's life in the second stage of the interview provides the nurse with a rough social sketch. Of particular significance are events contributing to a psychological disruption, which may be secondary to maladaptive coping behaviors or indicate resources and strengths to consider in treatment planning. To help the patient see the relevance of questions about the past, the nurse can summarize briefly what he has said about his problems and then move to the history. For example, the nurse might say "For me to understand you better and the events of your present situation, I will need to learn something about your life."

There are various sources used to obtain historical information.[7,8,10] They include medical, psychiatric, family, personal, sexual, and drug histories (see Appendixes A-E). The latter two areas are usually not spontaneously offered by the patient because of anxiety-laden material. Starting with a survey of the patient's life is usually less threatening. The nurse guides the patient by progressing from topics that promote the least anxiety to those that promote the most. The interview will have a smoother progression if the nurse asks questions in a logical sequence, without abrupt changes from one topic to another.

■ **MEDICAL HISTORY.** The depth of information included in the medical history depends on the patient's age, the problems encountered in his life, and the resources available to the nurse. If a young woman reports good physical health throughout her life, the detail required would be less than from the middle-aged man who has had some physical ailment since childhood. Other family members or significant others in the patient's life, such as the mother or family physician, can be vital sources of data. This is especially true if the patient is uncertain about events surrounding a particular illness or hospitalization.

Following are areas addressed in the patient's general medical history:

1. Illnesses and operations, when they occurred, the outcome, and the chronicity of the condition
2. Congenital, biological, chemical, or physical injury to the nervous system, specifically any head injuries
3. Current medical treatments or medication being taken

When an account of these experiences is given, it is important to note the patient's reaction to illnesses, operations, or accidents he has had.

■ **PSYCHIATRIC HISTORY.** After the medical history, the nurse should inquire about any previous psychiatric illnesses or encounters with mental health professionals. Have there been any psychiatric problems in the past? Is the current episode similar to those or different? What were the frequency and duration of the past episodes? If the patient was involved in treatment, what kind was it and how did he feel about it?

The psychiatric history includes data about the patient's family. Relatives who have had psychiatric illnesses and the prevalence of suicide in the family should be identified. The significance of this to the patient's current illness is twofold. In certain psychiatric disorders, such as affective ones, heredity is considered one of the predisposing factors. Psychiatric illness or suicide in the family may also show how individuals in the patient's life coped with stress and whether this has

influenced his repertoire of coping behaviors. It is essential to point out, however, that the patient's *reaction* to mental illness in his family is more significant than the illness itself.

■ **FAMILY HISTORY.** Assessment of the patient's capacity to form relationships begins with the family history. It is through the relationship the infant has with the significant adults in his life, usually the parents, that the basis of his security is formed. Sullivan[11] believes the goal of life is interpersonal security. By assessing the patient's relationships throughout his life, data can be obtained about his interpersonal needs and level of self-esteem. The family provides the first learning situation for the individual. Areas of dysfunction and support need to be determined, since the family can be considered one of the support systems available to the patient throughout his life.

Although the patient may not remember a lot about his early childhood, he has often been told of significant events. These events may include when and where he was born, his place in the family structure, what the family circumstances were, including any financial stresses, and whether the patient's birth was planned. He may know of problems his mother experienced during the pregnancy or labor and delivery, who besides the parents was frequently in the home, what the discipline was like, and what his parents' attitudes toward his development seemed to be. Interactions with parents, siblings, and other family members during childhood, with specific reference to violence, rejection, deaths, or separation, are important factors influencing the patient's sense of self as "good" or "bad."

■ **PERSONAL HISTORY.** These data tell the nurse what the emotional climate was for this individual's personality development from his point of view. Obviously, the nurse determines content areas by the purpose of the interview and the length of time the patient can participate in the interview. When and how early developmental tasks were achieved, such as entering school, leads into the personal history. A continuation of the chronological approach includes schooling, vocational pursuits, sexual experiences, and drug experimentation. These experiences are more easily addressed if they are described as they first occurred.

Starting school is a big event in childhood. It is also the individual's first opportunity to compare himself to others. Socialization patterns have begun to develop. The relationships with teachers and fellow students, friendships formed, and special interests and activities such as Scouts portray early social values. Conflicts during the early primary years are expressed as nail biting, nightmares, sleepwalking, enuresis, truancy, and poor academic achievement. Although most children exhibit some of these behaviors, the parents' response and what the individual remembers are important to elicit.

As the individual approaches adolescence—a time of rapid physical development and emotional turmoil—he begins the task of self-identification and the formation of intimate relationships. People outside the family become important sources for comparisons of values, attitudes, and experiences. Experimentation with drugs, including alcohol, and sex are likely to occur and should be addressed.

On entering high school, what was the extent and type of participation in sports, parties, church, and political activities? What was the individual's experience with groups and leadership, especially during school? Was he a member of the "in group"? Did his level of academic performance change? What were his age and status on leaving school? Did he graduate or leave school to work? Did he have any special interests or hobbies? Were they solitary or group activities? When did he first drink alcohol, smoke marijuana, and experiment with other drugs such as LSD, amphetamines, or barbiturates? What pattern was established at the time, and how has it changed? Questions about drug use can be intimidating to the individual. It is important to phrase the questions so he feels free to answer without having a value judgment placed on him. Phrases such as "when" or "how often," rather than "did you" assume that the behavior occurred and make it easier for the individual to answer.

With the onset of puberty, sexual attitudes become important. How and from whom did the patient learn about sexual matters? With a woman, information about the time of menarche is elicited. Did the individual experience an early or delayed onset of body development, and what was the reaction to this in relation to peers? What were the experiences with necking, petting, and intercourse? How were these experiences viewed by family and friends? Friendship, dating, and early sexual experiences, including autosexual, homosexual, and heterosexual activities, are usually important issues for the adolescent. Were these experiences comfortable and pleasurable or associated with guilt?

An individual's sex life can be viewed as a barometer of emotional health. It is therefore important to learn his current sexual behaviors, and if there have been any changes in sexual habits. The nurse must feel comfortable discussing sexual matters to talk about the patient's sexual habits in each stage of his life. This is a sensitive area to most people. Further information on

discussing sexual material with patients appears in the publication *Assessment of Sexual Function.*[6]

Occupational and marriage history are included in assessing the period of maturity. What are the patient's goals and ambitions, positions held, promotions, and relationships with bosses and peers? Are there any discrepancies between stated goals and the individual's efforts to achieve them? Continuing education and military experiences can be discussed when applicable.

The marriage history should include dating and courtship, circumstances of the marriage, sexual adjustment, frequency of sexual intercourse, living conditions, financial difficulties, and previous marriages. If there are children, what were reactions to the pregnancies and births, and are there any prominent problems in the family now? What is the patient's relationship with his parents? If they are deceased, what was the patient's reaction to the loss?

To complete the social sketch of the patient, it is essential to determine his talents, strengths, and assets. Asking him to describe his daily activities can give a clue as to what the patient is trying to achieve. The richness or poverty of activities may indicate the meaning of life for him. Church, community, and leisure activities often are sources of emotional support, especially in times of stress.

The second stage of the evaluation has simply been an attempt to understand how the patient comes to be there. It depicts the development of a patient's self-concept. As with any assessment that the nurse performs, the amount of detail depends on the patient, his presenting complaint, and the environmental constraints such as time. Hopefully, the areas just addressed will be included in some detail in each psychiatric evaluation. Clinical example 6-5 illustrates the type of data obtained in the first two stages.

Mental status examination

The historical information obtained gives the nurse a perspective on areas with which the patient may have difficulty, such as forming relationships, consistent job performance, and other significant areas. Further assessment of limitations and strengths is obtained in the mental status examination, the third stage of the psychiatric evaluation. Appendix A provides a detailed format of the mental status examination.

The mental status examination is a way of organizing observational data about all aspects of a patient's mental functioning. While obtaining information about the presenting problem and taking a history, the nurse is informally and indirectly accumulating information. However, formal questioning usually is

CLINICAL EXAMPLE 6-5

Ms. T is a 22-year-old single, white, unemployed clerical worker who comes to the mental health clinic stating she does not socialize any more and is becoming increasingly self-conscious about going out of the house for fear of "making a fool" of herself. She is currently living with her father, three siblings, and an aunt in the aunt's home. She states she would like to "make something" of herself but is afraid that people won't accept her.

Ms. T relates the onset of her feelings to the problems that occurred at work 18 months ago. She states she felt a lot of pressure at work, felt "extremely nervous" around her boss, was denied two promotions for "trivial reasons," and began to feel inferior to other workers, which made her depressed and led to her resignation.

During the time that problems were occurring at work, several incidents happened at home that also affected how Ms. T was feeling. She broke up with her steady boyfriend of 2 years, her younger sister was using drugs, and the police had been called to the home several times. Ms. T was concerned about the effect this had on her aunt, for whom she has a great deal of affection and gratitude. Her paternal grandmother had died in February, and her twin brother had married and left the home in June. Both these individuals were a source of support to Ms. T. She wishes that her siblings and father would move out of the house, leaving only herself and the aunt, because "none of them are decent people anyway and they only cause trouble for my aunt."

Her medical history includes hospitalization at age 6 for a tonsillectomy. Ms. T says she enjoyed being in the hospital and remembers playing in the play area. She had no major illnesses during childhood or adolescence that she could recall. She believes that she had the usual childhood illnesses, measles and mumps.

Ms. T's psychiatric history was negative for herself and her family. She was seen by Dr. X at the Community Health Facility 6 months ago for a questionable somatoform disorder. Her father has been seen by Dr. X for 10 years for multiple physical complaints.

Ms. T was born and raised in Baltimore. She is the eldest, along with a twin brother, of five children. She has two sisters, age 21 and 19, by her father's first marriage and one sister, age 15, by his second. Ms. T states she has little recollection of her biological mother. She remembers going to the movies with her at about age 4 and has heard from other family members that she was a "nice lady." Her father was described as a "very emotional" person who gets "very upset" easily. He drank heavily when the children were young and was taken out of the house several times by the police for disorderly conduct. Ms. T and her siblings were basically raised by her paternal aunt and grandmother. Even after the father's second marriage, she and her siblings lived with the aunt and the grandmother. Her father remarried when Ms. T was 6 years old and lived with his second wife in an apartment close to her aunt's home. She states that the family would celebrate holidays together and go on picnics but that she never felt close to any of her siblings or to her father.

Ms. T started school at age 5 and achieved "above average" grades. She was a safety guard in grade school and a cheerleader for 3 years in high school. She graduated from high school at age 17 without any failures. Ms. T says she was a "shy kid" most of her life but had several girl friends. However, she rarely brought them home because of her father's drinking.

Her sexual experiences include kissing and petting. Ms. T states she wants to be a virgin when and if she marries. She learned about menstruation from girl friends and a movie at school and her first period was at age 13. She states that she has never talked with family members about sexual matters.

Ms. T feels she has cut herself off from friends during the past 2 years. Several of them still call or drop by, but she never goes out to socialize with them. She spends most of her day cleaning the house, making the meals, and listening to music in her room.

The only position Ms. T held was as a clerical worker at the bank. She acquired the job after graduation and believes that she did okay until 18 months ago. She gives a vague description of her boss, stating he just "didn't like me" and was "always on my back about something."

Ms. T denies any experimentation with drugs. She used to drink wine on social occasions when dating but stopped after she broke up with her boyfriend.

needed to complete an accurate and comprehensive mental status examination. Verbatim samples of the patient's speech and thought present a precise picture. For clarity the mental status examination should be recorded in a certain order and organized according to certain categories: general observations, sensorium and intelligence, thought processes, affect, mood, and insight. Each item is addressed here with clinical examples, followed by a continuation of the case history presented earlier.

■ General observations

Specific aspects of the patient's behavior are included in the remainder of the mental status examination. It is useful, however, to record in the beginning general observations, especially those characteristics of the patient that appear outstanding to the interviewer.

■ **APPEARANCE.** The patient's appearance should be described in terms of consistency with his age and station in life, his manner of dress (conservative, tasteful, meticulous, inappropriate), his personal habits (clean, unkempt, disorderly), his characteristic facial expression (alert, vacant, sad, bewildered, hostile, masklike), and his state of health and nutrition.

■ **REACTION TO INTERVIEW.** The patient's reaction to the interview, with the circumstances surrounding it taken into account, is addressed. Has he been cooperative, friendly, evasive, ingratiating, indifferent, passive, dependent, or hostile in his responses to the interviewer? If he has been observed in various situations, does he respond differently to people (physicians, nurses, other patients)? Each patient reacts to the situation whether he is hospitalized, referred for psychiatric evaluation by the court, or voluntarily seeking counseling.

■ **CONSISTENCY OF BEHAVIOR.** As previously discussed, communication is expressed both verbally and nonverbally. Examples of the patient's verbal and nonverbal behavior are included and the consistency of both is noted. Characteristics of speech such as speed, vocabulary, and goal directedness are observed. Any overt behaviors such as finger tapping, hair twirling, hand wringing, pacing, posturing, gait, and bizarre movements are described.

■ **RESPONSE TO PATIENT.** It is important that the nurse also become aware of the response he or she has to each of the patients interviewed. The response can contain diagnostic information about the patient. A depressed patient may elicit a sense of sadness and hopelessness in the nurse. In contrast, the nurse might feel anger toward a patient who is hostile. The principal feeling elicited should be identified with the behaviors observed, as in Clinical example 6-6.

■ Sensorium and intelligence

This section describes the patient's state of consciousness and his ability to accurately perceive the environment. His orientation, memory, intellectual function, judgment, and comprehension are assessed. Impairment in more than one area may relate to diagnosis of an organic mental disorder.[11] Since the disorder can vary from mild transient alterations to a permanent disruption of all areas, it is important to carefully document each area.

■ **LEVEL OF CONSCIOUSNESS.** A variety of terms can identify the patient's level of consciousness. Is he alert and awake or stuporous and sleepy? Is he easily distracted or hyperalert? Can he sustain attention to both external and internal stimuli? A clouded state of consciousness is an essential feature in delirium.

■ **ORIENTATION.** The patient is questioned regarding his orientation to time, place, person, and situation. Does he know who he is, where he is, who the people around him are, and the date? Does he seem to understand the rationale for the interview and his role in it? Patients with organic disruptions may give grossly inaccurate answers, especially for time relationships. In contrast, the schizophrenic disorders may cause the patient to say he is someone else or somewhere else or to reveal his personalized orientation to the world.

■ **MEMORY.** Memory impairment is a prominent behavior observed in dementia, ranging from forgetfulness to a total lack of understanding of significant people and events. Three areas must be tested under memory: immediate recall, recent memory, and remote memory. Immediate recall involves attention, concentration, and ability to retain material just learned. The digits-span test requires that the patient repeat digits either forward or backward within a 10-second interval. The nurse recites a series of randomly selected digits, beginning with three digits and progressing until the patient is unable to repeat the digits in proper sequence. The procedure is then repeated, but the patient is asked to say the numbers with the order reversed. The patient may need to be given an example to ensure that he understands the procedure. An approximate comparison to educational level can be made: five digits forward and four digits backward equals an eighth-grade education; seven digits forward and five digits backward indicates a twelfth-grade education. However, high anxiety or some psychotropic medicines may interfere with the patient's ability to concentrate and should be considered if the performance is poor.

Recent memory can be tested by asking the patient when he came to the hospital and by having him recall the events of the past 24 hours. A reliable informant may be needed to verify the statements made. A test of recent memory can be performed by asking the patient to remember three words (an object, a color, an address) and then having him repeat them 15 minutes later in the interview.

The patient's ability to give a consistent account of his history requires an intact remote memory. Available records or reliable informants are needed to verify information such as date of birth, age, when started and finished school, date of marriage, birth dates of children, and other significant events.

■ **INTELLECTUAL FUNCTION.** A patient's intellectual function is assessed in relation to his educational, occupational, and attainment levels. Testing vocabulary, counting and calculating ability, abstract ability, and fund of general knowledge provides some information about the patient's intelligence. Vocabulary can be assessed by asking for word definitions or synonyms. Counting and calculating involve simple arithmetic (9×6, $21 + 7$) and asking the patient to serially subtract 7 from 100. If he has difficulty subtracting 7 from 100, he can be asked to subtract 3 from 20 in the same manner. This task also involves the ability to concentrate and complete a task.

The ability to conceptualize and abstract can be tested by having the patient explain a series of proverbs. He is given an example of a proverb with its interpretation and then asked to tell what several proverbs mean to him. Following are frequently used proverbs: "When it rains, it pours," "A stitch in time saves nine," "A rolling stone gathers no moss," and "The proof of the pudding is in the eating." Most adults are able to interpret proverbs as a representation or symbolization of human behavior or events. Cultural background is a set factor that should be considered when

the patient is not able to complete the task. If the patient's educational level is less than ninth grade, asking him to list similarities between a series of paired objects will assess his ability to abstract. The following series of paired objects are frequently used: bicycle, bus; apple, pear; television, newspaper. A good reply would be in terms of function, whereas a reply in terms of structure may indicate a tendency toward concrete thinking.

To determine the patient's fund of general knowledge, he can be asked to name the last five presidents, the mayor, five large cities, the capital of France, or other similar questions congruent with his education. With all these tests the patient's background should be kept in mind so that he is given tasks he can perform. If the patient cannot read or does not work, he may not be able to describe recent events or local news but could relate plots of television shows or local neighborhood information. If, after the patient completes some general tests of intelligence, the nurse has doubts or suspects deterioration from a history of changes at work, home, or school, a referral for psychological testing should be considered.[4]

■ **JUDGMENT.** The patient's judgment can best be assessed from an account of past decisions and how they were reached and from responses in the interview. Judgment involves the ability to understand facts and draw conclusions from relationships. In discussing recent events does the patient appear to exercise sound judgment? A teenage boy referred for counseling after repeated arrests for car theft exhibits poor judgment. It is useful to determine if the judgments are deliberate, impulsive, or inappropriate. Several hypothetical situations can be presented for the patient to evaluate: What would he do if he found a stamped, addressed envelope lying on the ground? How would he find his way out of a forest in the daytime? What would he do if he entered his house and smelled gas?

■ **COMPREHENSION.** Throughout the interview the patient's ability to understand the meaning of the questions is assessed, as well as his ability to comprehend incidents in his environment such as local, political, and personal events. Does he understand his role as a patient and, if hospitalized, does he understand the hospital routine? An organic brain syndrome could interfere with the patient's level of comprehension.[11]

The assessment data obtained in the area of sensorium and intelligence are particularly important in determining disorders classified as organic mental disorders. The acute picture presented to the clinician often is easy to identify, whereas the more subtle changes that can occur as a result of a degenerative disease or brain lesion require attentive observation by

CLINICAL EXAMPLE 6-7

It was apparent that the patient was alert and awake but almost totally distracted by something within himself. Questions and directions were repeated frequently so that they were understood. He was oriented to person, place, and situation. He performed six digits forward and three digits backward and remembered two of three objects after 15 minutes. He remembered the third with help. He listed presidents to Truman and performed serial sevens with relative ease, making two mistakes. He could not identify any recent events or discuss television shows and seemed limited in his fund of general knowledge. This may relate to his social isolation since quitting school at age 16, as described by his mother.

the nurse, who should carefully document behavior, as shown in Clinical example 6-7.

■ Thought processes

■ **FORM OF THOUGHT.** The patient's thought process is observed through his speech. The patterns or forms of verbalization, rather than the content of speech, are assessed. What is the rate or flow of speech? Is it overly fast or retarded? Does the patient proceed in a clear, logical, goal-directed manner? As he talks about topics relating to himself, the nurse should note if the patient is able to express himself in an understandable manner or if his ideas are vague, leaving the nurse uncertain about their meaning. Can the patient move freely from one topic to another with relative ease and flexibility? Is there continuity of thought, or are his associations disconnected (loose), constantly changing (flight of ideas), wide of the point (tangential), interrupted suddenly (blocked), or distorted and bizarre, as when new words are made up to express ideas symbolically (neologisms)?

■ **CONTENT OF THOUGHT.** Recurring patterns of content such as delusions, hallucinations, or illusions may be observed and may reflect a disruption in perception. Misperceptions include a variety of thoughts, feelings, or fears the patient may have that interfere in some way with his reality testing.

Hallucinations refer to sensory perceptions that have no external stimuli. Sometimes the patient's behavior indicates that he is hallucinating; he may adopt a listening attitude, mumble, pick at unseen objects, or stop suddenly as if guarding himself. Asking if he has heard noises or voices when no one was around or had

any unusual experiences leads the patient to describe any such experiences. Characteristics such as the source, manner of reception, content, and time of the experience should be described.

Delusions are recurring false beliefs not congruent with the patient's culture or background. Again, tactful questioning helps the patient focus on delusional material. Does he misinterpret what happens to him, giving it special or false meaning? Does he feel that he has been singled out or watched? Does he experience his thoughts or actions as being controlled by an external force? Can people read his mind, or does he have psychic powers? These concerns may be complicated, are concealed by the patient, and require extensive questioning.

Illusions refer to misperceptions with an external stimulus. The hospitalized patient may believe his room is a jail cell and the staff members are security guards. A schoolteacher with an organic mental disorder may perceive her family as pupils and the bedside table as her desk.

The patient's thoughts can be focused on obsessions, compulsions, or phobias that also interrupt the normal thought process. Repetitive thoughts, impulses, or behaviors unwanted by the individual are defined as obsessions or compulsions. These can be assessed by asking the patient if he has any intrusive recurring thoughts or actions that he feels unable to control and that occupy an extensive amount of his time. Objects and/or situations irrationally and persistently feared by the patient are identified as phobias. The individual can exert great energy avoiding certain situations or thinking about the feared object.

Disruptions in both the form and content of thought are seen in schizophrenia, affective disorders, anxiety disorders, organic mental disorders, and paranoid disorders in varying degrees of intensity and varying combinations. In the following example, the nurse includes a detailed description of the patient's thought processes:

The patient's speech was rapid, and he acknowledged feeling as if his thoughts were coming too fast, "My mind is racing ahead." The rapidity of his speech compounded the difficulty understanding him as he quickly moved from one topic to another in what appeared to be an unrelated manner. He denied any visual or auditory hallucinations; however, he believed that he could talk with God if he needed a consultant on his life situation. He felt this was a special blessing given to him over other men.

■ Affect

Observations of the range, appropriateness, and intensity of the patient's emotional expressions (affect)

CLINICAL EXAMPLE 6-8

Ms. T was a stylishly dressed, neatly groomed, slender female, in apparent good physical health who appeared her stated 22 years of age. She was cooperative during the interview but had difficulty expressing herself in specific terms. Her vague responses at times left the interviewer feeling perplexed about the difficulties she was describing.

The patient was alert and awake and oriented to person, place, and situation. Immediate recall and recent memory were intact, demonstrated in her ability to recall three unrelated objects immediately and again in 15 minutes. Some of the historical information given was inconsistent with historical factors reported by her father. Although the vocabulary used by Ms. T and her knowledge of general information was congruent with her twelfth-grade education and past employment, she had difficulty completing the serial sevens but performed serial threes with relative ease. She stated she was "nervous," which may be a factor related to performance. She was able to abstract two of three proverbs presented.

Proverb	Interpretation
Don't cry over spilled milk.	"If something happens, then forget about it. Maybe things will get better."
A rolling stone gathers no moss.	"A good person gathers no enemies. If a person stays active, he won't get depressed."
People who live in glass houses shouldn't throw stones.	"The glass will break."

Her responses to hypothetical situations were appropriate; however, the manner in which she coped with difficulties at work and home showed impaired judgment about personal issues.

Ms. T's speech was clear, coherent, and of normal rate and tone. Except for the vague tangential manner in which she discussed her concern for her aunt, her communication was goal directed. There were no apparent delusions, hallucinations, or illusions. She denied any obsessions, compulsions, or phobias.

The central theme during the interview was her fear of being irresponsible and hurting her aunt. Her sadness and concern about her behavior in relation to the aunt pervaded the interview. She appeared nervous (looking away, fidgeting) and cried whenever she talked about her aunt. She described her mood as "low" and rated it as a four. She denied any suicidal or homicidal ideas or plan previously or at the present time.

Her insight is questionable, since she questioned her need for treatment, although she agreed to return. She knew a problem existed but was unaware of the causative factors related to her behavior.

in relation to the circumstances of the interview and the ideas expressed are documented. Does the patient demonstrate variability in the expression of feeling, or does his affectual response appear blunted or restricted in some way? Does he report significant life events without any emotional component (flat)? Is the patient's affectual response congruent with the content of his speech? (For example does he report that he is being persecuted by the police and then laugh?) Does he rapidly shift from one affectual response to another (labile)? The patient's statements of emotion and the nurse's empathic responses may provide clues to the appropriateness of the affect or character of the prevailing mood.

■ Mood

The pervasive, relatively enduring emotional state of the patient reflects his mood and can influence his perception of his life situation. Does his appearance reflect his mood? Does he look "down in the dumps"? How would he describe his mood? Does it remain the same or change during the day or from day to day? Asking the patient to rate his mood on a scale of 0 to 10 can be useful for an immediate rating and valuable for comparison of changes that occur during treatment. When the clinical picture is highlighted by a continuous intensification or change in the patient's mood, an affective disorder is suspected.

If the nurse perceives a potential for suicide, he or she should attempt to bring out the patient's thoughts about self-destruction. Suicidal or homicidal thoughts should be addressed directly. Has the patient had the desire to harm himself or someone else? Has he made any previous attempts, and if so, what events surrounded the attempts? To judge suicidal or homicidal risk, the nurse assesses the patient's plans, ability for implementation (availability of guns), attitude about death, and support systems available, as in the following example:

The patient responded to most of the questions in a flat, dull manner. Although he stated he felt sad about the recent changes in his life, his lifeless posture and tone of voice did not convey any emotional response. He denied any current suicidal or homicidal plans. He related having made two suicidal gestures in the past year by "taking pills."

■ Insight

The degree of insight the patient has about the nature of his problem and how it affects his feelings, thoughts, and behavior may be assessed informally as he talks. It is important to determine if he sees the problem as something brought on by external factors

Elements of Psychiatric Evaluation

A. Data collection
1. Presenting problem
   a. Onset, duration, symptoms noted, and progression
   b. Solutions attempted
   c. Significant changes in the patient's life
   d. How responsibility for the problem is viewed
2. Characteristic patterns of living and coping behaviors
   a. Medical history and current problems
   b. Psychiatric history for self and family
   c. Family history and personal history: Chronological approach with emphasis on interpersonal relationships and major areas of life experiences
3. Mental status examination
   a. General observations: Appearance, reaction to the interview, consistency of behavior, and response to the patient
   b. Sensorium and intelligence: Level of consciousness, orientation, memory, intellectual functioning, judgment, and comprehension
   c. Thought processes: Characteristics of speech, patterns of verbalizations, manner of communication of thoughts, organization of ideas, coherence of associations, recurring patterns of thoughts, and misperceptions described
   d. Affect: Range, appropriateness, and intensity of affect
   e. Mood: behavioral manifestations and description of mood; suicidal/homicidal idea or plan
   f. Insight: Understanding of current situation and solutions
B. Organization and interpretation of data
1. Problem identification: Medical and nursing diagnoses
2. Identification of patient resources
C. Treatment plan

or stemming from within himself. Whether he can see his treatment needs realistically affects the treatment plan and the setting of mutual goals. Several questions may be helpful to ascertain the patient's degree of insight. What does he think about all he has told the nurse? What does he want to do about it? What does he want others, including the nurse, to do about it? The following example illustrates a patient's level of insight:

The patient enumerated several problems he encountered at work. He reluctantly stated that he might have to change, but really thought his difficulties were because of his wife's drinking. He believed he could do nothing until she changed.

This third stage of the psychiatric interview completes the assessment of the patient. The mental status examination describes comprehensive data about the patient's mental functioning in an organized manner. Clinical example 6-8 finishes the clinical portrayal of Ms. T.

The nurse has assembled a comprehensive data base through history taking and the mental status examination. She has collected objective facts based on observation of the patient's behavior during the interview. In the final stage of the psychiatric evaluation, the nurse critically examines the information she has organized in the preceding stages and interprets these data to formulate a treatment plan. The elements of a psychiatric evaluation are summarized in the accompanying box.

Additional resources

The psychiatric interview provides the structure for obtaining pertinent information about the patient. Additional resources are often used to complete a comprehensive assessment. The medical chart is one resource the nurse can use to collect information about medical and social histories. This information is recorded in designated sections of the patient's chart by various members of the health team.

Significant others in the patient's life, including family, friends, a minister, or the family physician, can participate in the interview and share valuable perceptions about the patient and his situation. Family theorists stress the importance of the patient's social system in both diagnosis and treatment of psychiatric problems.

The expressive therapies are essential resources for assessing and treating children. Children often are brought for psychiatric evaluation by the family or referred by the school system for behavioral disruptions. Art, dance, or play therapy can provide the means for establishing an initial relationship with the child. These therapies are especially important when the child is unable to express his ideas or does not want to talk. Again the family is a vital resource to the clinician working with children.

■ Psychological measurements

Research in recent years has provided a variety of formalized questionnaires and standardized tests as adjunctive methods for assessment. Computers are now used to collect and collate data, to diagnose symptom clusters, and to evaluate specific treatment modalities. Rating scales can be used to gather information from the patient and significant others. The common rating scales given in the box at right list those most fre-

---

Common Rating Scales

Beck Depression Inventory
Hamilton Depression Scale (HAM-D)
Manic-State Scale
Nurses' Observation Scale (NOSIE)
Brief Psychiatric Rating Scale (BPRS)
Clinical Global Impressions Scale (CGI)
Hamilton Anxiety Scale (HAM-A)
Self-Report Symptom Check List (SCL-90)

Situations Where Testing Is Frequently Indicated

Children

1. *Presence of a learning disorder*
   Psychological testing can help delineate the etiology and treatment in learning disabilities, which may involve central nervous system dysfunction, intellectual deficiency, and/or personality and emotional factors. Tests often provide clues to family and/or school influences.
2. *Emotional-social disturbances*
   Psychological testing can be useful in understanding such problems as hyperactivity; antisocial behavior; excessive withdrawal; difficulty adapting to peers, home, and/or school; and language disorders.
3. *Developmental deviations*
   Testing gives information about age-appropriateness of the child's functioning (intellectual, personal-social, perceptual-motor coordination).

Adults

4. *Mental retardation/intellectual deficiency*
   Testing can throw light on the factors interfering with an adult's use of intelligence, as well as assess mental retardation. State laws may require an IQ score as part of the diagnosis of mental deficiency in certain situations, such as for custodial care and support for children with learning disabilities.
5. *Psychotherapy*
   A psychological evaluation can help determine the therapeutic mode and goals. It often is useful in deciding when to terminate therapy or in understanding changes during therapy.
6. *Differential diagnosis*
   Psychological evaluations measure function ranging from perceptual-cognitive and ego level factors to personality structure, dynamics, and the unconscious. The analysis of strength and weakness contributes to an understanding of the whole person. For adults, testing is often helpful in detecting borderline psychosis, early signs of organicity, and early signs of schizophrenia.
7. *Forensic psychiatry*
   Psychological evaluation is often a helpful adjunct in cases involving mental illness or central nervous system impairment following injury. Psychological testing also has many applications in the criminal justice system.

From DeCato CM and Wicks RJ: J Psychiatr Nurs 14:25, June 1976.

TABLE 6-1

COMMONLY USED PSYCHOLOGICAL TESTS

Name	General classification	Description	Special features
Bellak Children's Apperception Test	Projective technique	Drawings of animals for children	Designed specifically for children
Bender (Visual-Motor) Gestalt Test	Graphomotor technique; may be used as projective technique	Geometric designs that the patient is asked to draw or copy, with design in view	Useful for detecting psychomotor difficulties correlated with brain damage
California Personality Inventory	Objective personality test	Seventeen scales developed presumably for normal populations for use in guidance and selection	Less emphasis on mental illness than MMPI scales, such as dominance, responsibility, socialization
Cattell 16 Personality Factor Questionnaire (16 PF)	Objective personality test	Questionnaire covering 16 personality factors derived from factor-analytical studies	Bipolar variables allow for interpretation of scores varying either above or below the norm, such as reserved vs. outgoing; trusting vs. suspicious, timid vs. venturesome
Draw-a-Person Test	Graphomotor projective technique	Patient asked to draw a person and then one of the sex opposite to the first drawing	Projects body image, how the body is conceived and perceived; sometimes useful for detecting brain damage; modifications include: draw an animal; draw a house, a tree, and a person (H-T-P); draw your family; draw the most unpleasant concept you can think of
Minnesota Multiphasic Personality Inventory (MMPI) (Forms: Individual, Group, and Shortened R)	Objective personality test	Questionnaire yielding scores for 9 clinical scales in addition to other scales	Includes scales related to test-taking attitudes; empirically constructed on basis of clinical criteria; computer interpretation services available
Rorschach Technique	Projective technique	Ten inkblots used as basis for eliciting associations	Especially revealing of personality structure; most widely used projective technique
Rosenzweig Picture Frustration Test	Projective technique	Cartoon situations, dialogue to be completed by subject	Designed specifically to assess patterns of reaction to typical stress situations; child, adolescent, and adult forms
Sentence Completion Test (SCT)	Varies from direct-response questionnaire to projective technique	Incomplete sentence stems that vary as to their ambiguity	Highly flexible; may be used to tap specific conflict areas; reveals generally more conscious, overt attitudes and feelings
Symonds Picture Story Test	Projective technique	Pictures of adolescents	Designed specifically for adolescents
Thematic Apperception Test (TAT)	Projective technique	Ambiguous pictures used as stimuli for making up a story	Especially useful for revealing personality dynamics; some pictures are designed specifically for women, men, adolescent girls, and adolescent boys
Wechsler Adult Intelligence Scale (WAIS)	Intelligence test	Eleven subtests: vocabulary, comprehension, information, similarities, digit span, arithmetic, picture arrangement, picture completion, object assembly, block design, and digit symbol	Most commonly used intelligence scale that yields a measure of intelligence expressed as IQ scores; differences in subtests can also be useful clinically

Modified from Freedman AM, Kaplan HI, and Sadock BJ, editors: Comprehensive textbook of psychiatry, ed 3, Baltimore, 1980, The Williams & Wilkins Co.

TABLE 6-1—cont'd

COMMONLY USED PSYCHOLOGICAL TESTS

Name	General classification	Description	Special features
Wechsler Intelligence Scale for Children (WISC)	Intelligence test	Similar to the WAIS	Standardized for children ages 5 to 15
Wechsler Preschool and Primary Scale of Intelligence (WPPSI)	Intelligence test	Similar to the WAIS and WISC	Standardized for children ages 4 to 6½
Word-Association Technique	Projective technique	Stimulus words to which patient responds with first association that comes to mind	Flexible; may be used to tap associations to different conflict areas; generally not as revealing as SCT responses

quently used (also see Appendix G). Self-report questionnaires filled out by the patient give an account of subjective distress. This description can be a more accurate account of the patient's emotional state than that inferred or elicited in the interview. Questionnaires directed to family members or friends can relate specific characteristics of the patient's social or family life. Some of the circumstances in which psychological testing may be useful are given in the situations testing box on page 195.

Psychological tests are of two types: those designed to evaluate intellectual and cognitive abilities and those designed to describe personality functioning. Some of these tests are described briefly in Table 6-1. Commonly used intelligence tests are the Wechsler Adult Intelligence Scale (WAIS) and the Wechsler Intelligence Scale for Children (WISC). Although intelligence tests often are criticized as culturally biased, their ability to determine an individual's strengths and weaknesses within the culture provides essential therapeutic information.

Material obtained from projective tests reflects aspects of an individual's personality function, including reality testing ability, impulse control, major defenses, interpersonal conflicts, and self-concept. A battery of tests is usually administered to provide comprehensive information. The Rorschach Test, Thematic Apperception Test (TAT), Bender Gestalt Test, and Minnesota Multiphasic Personality Inventory (MMPI) are commonly used by the clinical psychologist.

A more detailed discussion of the psychological tests available and their clinical applicability can be found elsewhere.[4,5] It is important for the clinician to be aware of the resources available and of the general information that can be obtained from standardized scales and tests. Some of these tests may be administered by a nurse, and others require the training and skill of a psychologist. Collaboration with the psychologist to review assessment data and to plan treatment is a responsibility of the nurse as a member of the health team.

■ Physiological measurements

Special diagnostic procedures are especially important when the patient or his family describes abrupt changes in his behavior or losses of consciousness for even brief periods of time. These procedures are the electroencephalogram (EEG), computed tomography (CT) scan, lumbar puncture, and blood chemistry values. A listing of normal laboratory values is presented in Table 6-2. Electroencephalography records any changes in the electrical activity in various areas of the brain. The test is useful in diagnosing epilepsy, brain lesions, and other diseases of or injury to the brain. According to the area of the lesion, specific symptoms would be demonstrated. The symptom complex would reflect the disruption in function of the brain area involved. Distortion of taste, smell, sight, or hearing could occur. The patient's ability to speak clearly or understand what is being said could affect his pattern of communication. Changes in his personality or mental ability could be displayed in lapses of memory, absentmindedness, or loss of initiative. All these behaviors would be ascertained in the mental status examination. However, if the symptoms are treated psychopathologically, a brain tumor or seizure disorder could be overlooked and the right treatment denied. The EEG, CT scan, and lumbar puncture can be essential procedures for detecting specific brain dysfunctions.

Chemical analysis of various substances in the

TABLE 6-2

BOEHRINGER MANNGEIM 8700
*Normal values for blood chemistry.**

BUN	6-22	mg/dl	Creatinine	0.5-1.5	mg/dl	Alkaline phosphatase	29-74	μ/l
Na	131-146	mEq/l	Ldh	112-217	μ/l	Bilirubin	0.1-1.2	mg/dl
K	3.5-5.0	mEq/l	SGOT	6-36	μ/l	Uric acid	2.5-7.7	mg/dl
Cl	95-108	mEq/l	SGPT	9-54	μ/l	Total protein	5.8-7.7	gm/dl
CO_2	23-31	mEq/l	Ca	8.5-10.5	mg/dl	Albumin	3.0-4.5	gm/dl
Glucose	70-110	mg/dl	Phosphorus	2.4-4.2	mg/dl	Cholesterol	0-170	mg/dl

*The range may vary slightly depending on the laboratory where the analysis was done.

blood can give the clinician diagnostic information. This is especially valuable when a drug-induced delirium is suspected. Many drugs and poisons can cause organic mental disorder. The most commonly implicated drugs are the opiates, barbiturates, amphetamines, and hallucinogens. The patient may display behaviors ranging from mild confusion and drowsiness to overwhelming anxiety and hallucinations. The blood level and toxic level of the drug involved would be important, possibly life-saving, information.

Symptoms of cerebral dysfunction, including mental confusion, hallucinations, and convulsions, might also occur in certain hypoglycemic states. In this instance the patient's behavior reflects a variation in the normal amount of glucose in the blood. The factors that might be involved are numerous. It is particularly important to differentiate these factors so the appropriate treatment can be instituted.

■ Brain visual imaging in psychiatry

Brain visual imaging has not yet affected the clinical practice of psychiatry in a profound way. However, it shows great promise for increasing knowledge of the pathophysiology of mental illness, enhancing diagnostic assessment, and choosing more specific treatments. Psychiatric research using these five new imaging techniques attempts to identify brain abnormalities underlying psychiatric illnesses. The following descriptions provide a brief explanation of each technique:[3,9]

1. Computed tomography (**CT scan**) is a radiological technique that takes cross-sectional x-ray films (coupled with radiation detectors and computers) of the brain. Structural changes such as ventricular enlargement can be identified. These changes have been found in psychi-

atric patients with a variety of diagnoses and after chronic ingestion of substances such as alcohol, but the research concentration to date has been focused on schizophrenia because of its unknown origin and devastating effects. CT scanning is an expensive procedure with some risk of x-ray overexposure to the patient. It is not indicated if a patient does not show gross neurological deficits on careful mental status or physical examination or on an EEG. Newer imaging techniques are likely to yield more information with less risk.

2. Brain electrical activity mapping (**BEAM**) uses computer analysis to topographically display EEG (electroencephalography) rhythms and evoked response (external electrical and sensory stimulation, i.e., flashes of light, noise, muscle stimulation, etc.) data. The BEAM uses color maps of condensed and summarized data on electrophysiological activity in the brain. It involves easy and relatively inexpensive modifications of equipment that is familiar and accessible. It seems likely that this technique will be useful for patients who do not fit the diagnostic categories listed in the DSM-III-R[2] and who may be suspected of having subtle organic impairments that are not fully characterized after initial neurological screening.

3. Regional cerebral blood flow techniques (**RCBF**) use probes applied to the scalp to measure decreasing activity of a chemically inert and diffusable gas that emits gamma activity. RCBF provides information on blood flow in gray matter and white matter and on relative tissue weights. The gas inhalation technique is used more often than injection into the internal

carotid artery. RCBF techniques have been used for research purposes to study a variety of psychiatric disorders; they are less expensive than positron emission tomography (PET scanning), and may prove useful in the study of transient mental states. Single photon emission computed tomography **(SPECT)** is one method used to study RCBF, and offers a means of assessing presumed neuronal activity in resting states and with tasks and pharmacological challenges.

4. Positron emission tomography **(PET scan)** quantitatively measures physiological and biochemical brain function rather than structure. A compound tagged with a positron-emitting nuclide is given to the patient either by inhalation or by injection. As the positrons are annihilated, these events are measured and a computer generates color-coded displays. The PET scanner has provided measures of cerebral glucose use that are directly related to functional activity in regions of the brain. These results have shown glucose use to be abnormal in a variety of psychiatric disorders. PET scanning is an extremely expensive procedure requiring sophisticated equipment, and it entails exposing a patient to a dose of radiation. Although PET scanning is in an early stage of development, it is already having a major effect on theory and knowledge of the pathophysiology of mental illness. It allows a look at the sites of action of drugs by imaging the drug receptor molecules on the surface of cells in living humans.

5. Magnetic resonance imaging **(MRI)** is a technique for obtaining cross-sectional pictures of the entire body. It can provide information on the metabolic and biochemical status of live organs. Simply stated, MRI permits detection of the frequencies at which chemical elements in body tissue resonate. Computer-coded visual displays create detailed pictures of brain structures from the characteristic frequencies of various brain tissues. MRI can detect lesions resulting from tumors, metastases, strokes, and abscesses and can detect abnormalities in some psychiatric disorders, as well as drug effects. This technique does not expose the patient to x-rays or to any apparent health risks, thereby allowing for studies of children and repeated studies of patients over many years. Potential uses include studying cell energy metabolism and determining specific sites of action of drugs in the brain.

Diagnostic impression

At this point in the psychiatric evaluation, a diagnostic impression is formulated. Diagnosis implies identified problems—overt, covert, existing, or potential. It is important to validate these problems with the patient.

The presenting problem has been identified in terms of onset, duration, and course. The nurse has identified stressors or the precipitating factors that prompted the patient to seek help. These behaviors, along with those assembled in the interview, are compared to documented norms to identify deviations. The nurse's base may include personality development, behavior, or systems theories. Each provides a framework for comparing behaviors and identifying deviations. Personality development involves the completion of identified tasks and incorporation of certain skills at various points in an individual's life. Behavior theory encompasses the broad spectrum of human behavior and incorporates individual set factors, such as culture and nationality, in determining the function of certain behavior. Systems theory can also provide a framework for evaluating the patient's environment (family, community, nation).

The patient's behavior is the critical evidence used in formulating a diagnostic impression, regardless of the observer's theoretical framework. The difficulty that arises in psychiatric diagnosis is in part caused by the lack of specificity and simple, valid criteria for classifying human behavior. Thus psychiatric diagnosis can be a complex and controversial issue.

DSM-III-R has attempted to increase reliability through specific criteria to define each diagnosis. These criteria were used in clinical facilities throughout the United States during the development of this system to identify and solve problems in classifying disorders. The predecessors to the DSM-III-R, DSM-I and DSM-II, lacked sufficient detail in the classification for either clinical or research purposes.

In the DSM-III-R, clinically significant behavioral or psychological syndromes that include symptom clusters of patient behaviors are classified as mental disorders (Chapters 2 and 3). A descriptive approach is used in the discussion of each disorder and in the division into diagnostic classes. This results in the grouping of syndromes with common clinical features.

The DSM-III-R points out that the classification categorizes disorders, not individuals, and that each disorder is not an entity unto itself. Thus the need for an individualized approach to diagnosis is warranted. The approach of the DSM-III-R is atheoretical in relation to cause unless a specific pathophysiological process is known to be causative. Then the cause is included in the definition of the disorder.

The nurse should have a working knowledge of the DSM-III-R so that effective communication can occur through sharing a common terminology. The nurse's knowledge can also help him or her to ascertain other behavioral characteristics that suggest a particular syndrome. With certain disorders, especially schizophrenic and affective disorders, treatments can be considered according to the similarity of problems within each category.

Although the DSM-III-R follows a medical model, identification of specific clinical syndromes makes correlation with the nursing process model possible. The nurse, knowledgeable about the clinical syndrome involved, would focus on the nursing diagnosis. The nursing diagnosis reflects a discrepancy between the patient's behavior and the expected behaviors for a person with similar set factors related to stressors. For example, alteration in self-concept might be inferred from certain patient behaviors: shabby clothing, unkempt hair, preoccupation with physical concerns, refusal to participate in social activities. Specific nursing actions are then correlated with the nursing problem identified. The patient exhibiting an alteration in self-concept might benefit from information on grooming and self-care.

The organization and interpretation of assessment data depend on the purpose of the interview and the interviewer's background. As previously discussed, the nurse is guided by the purpose of the interview. A complete psychiatric evaluation is not always warranted, as in an emergency situation, and can be conducted over several interviews with the patient. The nurse may perform the mental status examination along with clarification of the presenting problem and rely on other resources such as the medical chart for historical data.

The woman described in Clinical example 6-1 may not be able to give an accurate account of historical factors when seen by the nurse. However, her mental status should be assessed to determine the degree of incapacitation and the immediate ramifications, if any. She was disturbing the peace, but should she be kept in jail overnight or allowed to leave the hospital in her current state? These are examples of judgment a nurse will need when assessing patients in an emergency room or crisis clinic.

The nurse's educational background and experience also help determine the comprehensiveness of the psychiatric evaluation. Nurses employed in mental health facilities have more opportunity to practice psychiatric evaluation. However, all nurses need to be knowledgeable about psychiatric evaluation and must be able to identify deviations from the norm. The nurse may need to call on someone more knowledgeable, such as the clinical specialist, to identify particular disorders and help determine care. It is important to assess the patient as a total being. This involves knowledge of psychological, sociological, and biological behaviors.

■ Case disposition

A brief summary of considerations about case disposition is presented here. The three general areas are the identified problem, the limitations and strengths of the individual, and the treatment resources available. Each area is discussed separately and followed by a continuation of the case study of Ms. T.

The problem areas in the psychiatric evaluation are addressed in order of priority. The symptoms described by the patient in the presenting problem should be addressed first, since they are usually causing the most discomfort. However, as in other areas, the patient may not always be aware of or admit to important problems. Priority is always given to problems that will threaten the life of the individual or of another if not treated. Suicidal or homicidal potential must be considered first and a treatment plan provided. Another factor is whether the behavior expresses a failure of coping mechanisms, as in a crisis, or lifelong maladjustment. The individual's limitations in coping with problems, especially in self-protection, are considered. In certain instances of psychotic behavior the individual may not be aware of his inability to care for himself and therefore may need brief hospitalization. The depressed person is also a candidate for hospitalization, and his suicidal risk must be evaluated at all times. A number of factors should be considered in determining whether the patient should be hospitalized or referred for outpatient treatment. These factors include the family and significant others available to the patient; his strengths, including past coping abilities; the values and beliefs he has; and his ability to meet the demands of the situation.

The nature of the problem indicates treatment and related goals. For example, the patient who complains that he cannot form intimate relationships may benefit from individual and group therapy. The man who complains of impotence with his spouse may do best in couples therapy. If the nurse is involved in therapy, the problem should be defined in measurable terms so that he or she and the patient can evaluate any changes. It is useful to know what change the patient wants, since this focuses on a particular issue and the goals for therapy.

Whatever the nurse's goal, on completing the psychiatric evaluation he or she should be able to make a

---

CLINICAL EXAMPLE 6-9

Ms. T stated she does not socialize any more, as evidenced by her leaving her job and withdrawal from family and friends. She spends her day at home cleaning, cooking, and listening to the radio alone in her room, which are solitary activities. She stated she felt inferior to her peers at work and was denied two promotions. She feels fearful about going out because she might make a fool of herself.

Ms. T's history reveals a lack of consistent nurturing in the home and an unstable family structure. The grandmother seemed to be a source of support and nurturance to Ms. T and has recently died. There was no evidence of role models for the development of intimate relationships in the home. Ms. T described herself as a "shy kid" who had few friends in childhood. She expressed feelings of hatred for most of her siblings. The aunt has provided for her, and the overwhelming concern Ms. T has about hurting the aunt may relate to fear of rejection, thereby losing the one stable relationship she believes she has left.

Ms. T presented an attractive appearance. She appeared to have difficulty relating to the interviewer, which was evidenced in her vague responses. She seemed to hide behind the sunglasses that she wore throughout the interview. She stated a concern about her decreasing ability to relate to others and a fear of attempting to do so.

The developmental tasks of the young adult include an increase in socialization and intimacy. It is a time when an individual's involvement in relationships and special interests provide for a sense of self-satisfaction. A pursuit of career goals occurs. The relationships formed and goals attained related to work or school become a source of positive feelings about oneself. In comparing the data obtained in the interview with developmental norms, a discrepancy exists. Two problem areas are evident: a decrease in socialization and a decrease in self-esteem.

The related nursing diagnoses would include (1) social isolation related to increased stress at work and home evidenced in withdrawal and (2) disturbance in self-concept related to feelings of guilt evidenced by statements of self-blame.

The treatment modality selected is long-term individual psychotherapy with the following goals. The patient will (1) establish a relationship with the therapist, (2) reestablish contact with friends, (3) resume vocational activities (school or work), and (4) experience activities within her capabilities to increase self-esteem. Conjunctive therapies considered are group and family therapy. Group therapy would provide the patient with the opportunity to develop and test socialization skills. Family therapy would focus on the interrelationship of the patient's problem with the family process. The selection of the type of therapy depends on the framework of the therapist and the availability of other modalities.

---

recommendation to the patient. The nurse should know what community agencies are available and what services they provide.

Clinical example 6-9 (above) illustrates how the data obtained in a psychiatric evaluation are used in a final disposition and a formulated treatment plan. Interviewing, differentiating symptoms, establishing a diagnosis, and formulating a treatment plan are skills the nurse develops with experience and a sound theoretical base. As in other areas of nursing, it is essential that the nurse be aware of the health team working with the patient. The treatment must be congruent with their plans. Communication among the physician, social worker, and psychologist should occur throughout all stages.

The psychiatric evaluation is similar to the nursing process model in that it is a systematic problem-solving approach. Assessment data are obtained during the initial stages, and a treatment plan with identified goals is formalized in the final stage. Whether the nurse is involved only in the initial contact with the patient or participates in the treatment plan, he or she has been involved in implementing the nursing process. The nurse has been involved in assessment, planning, intervention, and evaluation, even though the time spent in the last two stages may be minimal if a referral is made.

Future trends

It is difficult to project what might occur in the future. Experience, wisdom, and technology developed in the past century have brought changes no one could have foreseen. The study of the psyche has historically perplexed human beings. Various schools of thought have emerged in an attempt to understand the development of the human species. Theories of personality were developed by Freud, Sullivan, Erikson, and others as they observed and recorded the behavior of their patients. Objective evaluation of behavior as an expression of the inner self remains a difficult task. Psychiatric evaluation still takes place in a subjective relationship. As advancement in technology has influenced the effectiveness of health care, in the future evaluation of the subjective side of humans will become increasingly objective.

Psychological testing is being used more to expand or validate objective impressions, as described earlier in the discussion of resources available to the practitioner. Research has produced a variety of assessment tools, such as questionnaires, that aim to elicit certain information for comparison to standardized results. Methods for computerized psychiatric evaluation have been developed.

The nurse's role is being redefined as nurses con-

tinue to increase their independent functions and identify their unique contributions. Nurses with advanced knowledge and experience in psychiatry are becoming private practitioners. In private practice, they often use other nurses and psychiatrists as consultants.

In considering future trends in psychiatric evaluations, legal implications increase as the population becomes more health oriented and adept at pursuing care. Diagnosis and treatment of health problems are scrutinized by the population and by the courts. Cases of negligence and malpractice are on the rise. This trend makes objective evaluation essential for the future practitioner. Integration of research and clinical practice is crucial for optimum care of human psychosocial needs. Care implies prevention and maintenance and should complement the established goal, cure.

■ **SUGGESTED CROSS-REFERENCES** ■

The DSM-III-R and the medical model are discussed in Chapters 2 and 3. Therapeutic relationship skills are discussed in Chapter 4. Implementing the nursing process is discussed in Chapter 5. Impaired cognition is discussed in Chapter 19.

■ **SUMMARY** ■

1. Basic knowledge of psychodynamics, psychopathology, and psychotherapy, combined with interviewing and assessment skills, is needed to perform a psychiatric evaluation. The nurse's role depends on his or her level of preparation and the health care system.

2. The basic elements of a psychiatric evaluation are the psychiatric interview and the mental status examination. Through the interview the nurse establishes rapport with the patient, gains knowledge of his living patterns and coping behaviors, and assesses his mental functioning.

3. A clear account of the presenting problem and the events that led up to it are obtained in the initial stage of a psychiatric evaluation.

4. Data collection through history taking involves the patient's medical, psychiatric, family, personal, sexual, and drug histories. These data are collected in the second stage of the psychiatric evaluation.

5. The mental status examination organizes data in six categories: general observations, sensorium and intelligence, thought processes, affect, mood, and insight. These data represent the third stage of a psychiatric evaluation.

6. Additional resources for data collection include the medical chart, significant others in the patient's life, formalized questionnaires, and standardized tests.

7. Brain imaging techniques may be helpful in completing a thorough assessment.

8. A diagnostic impression is formulated from integration of historical data, the mental status examination, and special tests and diagnostic procedures. Formulating a diag-

---

DIRECTIONS FOR FUTURE RESEARCH

Following are some of the nursing research issues raised in Chapter 6 that merit further study:
1. Effectiveness of the psychiatric nurse as the primary patient evaluator for the multidisciplinary treatment team
2. Validity and reliability of the psychiatric nursing assessment and the formation of nursing diagnoses
3. Effects of cultural diversity on patient presentation of symptoms and interviewer interpretation
4. The relationship between DSM-III-R diagnoses and NANDA nursing diagnoses
5. Characteristics of the interview process that effect the accurate collection of data
6. Responsive and active dimensions used by the interviewer that influence the self-disclosure of the patient
7. Effects of the availability of technology on the quality, costs, and outcomes of the psychiatric evaluation
8. Early identification of suicidal ideation in patients at risk for self-destructive behavior
9. The role of nurse-patient rapport during the interview process on the formulation of the treatment plan
10. Comparisons between patient and interviewer perceptions of the presenting problem and its effect on patient compliance with the treatment plan

nostic impression entails identifying the clinical syndrome and the nursing diagnoses.

9. Organization and interpretation of the collected data and identification of a case disposition complete the final stage of a psychiatric evaluation. Making a case disposition involves awareness of the identified problems and nursing diagnoses, the individual's limitations and strengths, and the treatment resources available.

10. Psychiatric evaluation is similar to the nursing process model in that it is a systematic, problem-solving approach to patient care. The assessment data obtained and their organization and interpretation depend on the purpose of the interview and the background of the interviewer, the nurse.

11. Future trends in the psychiatric evaluation of patients include the development of more objective tests and measurements in computerized form. A practical consideration for obtaining skill in psychiatric evaluation is the legal implication of an undiagnosed psychiatric problem.

■ **REFERENCES** ■

1. Alston JF and Levet JM: What's happening: practical application of the mental status exam, Nurs Pract 2:37, 1977.
2. American Psychiatric Association: Diagnostic and statistical manual of mental disorder, third edition, revised, Washington, DC, 1987, The Association.
3. Andreasen NC: Brain imaging: applications in psychiatry, Science 239:1381, 1988.
4. DeCato CM and Wicks RJ: Psychological testing referrals: a guide for psychiatrists, psychiatric nurses, physicians in general practice, and allied health personnel, J Psychiatr Nurs 14:24, 1976.
5. Freedman AM, Kaplan HI, and Sadock BJ, editors: Comprehensive textbook of psychiatry, ed 3, Baltimore, 1980, Williams & Wilkins.
6. Group for the Advancement of Psychiatry: Assessment of sexual function: a guide to interviewing, New York, 1973, Mental Health Materials Center, Inc.
7. Imboden JB: Practical psychiatry in medicine. Part 16. Psychiatric evaluation of the medical patient, J Fam Pract 10:4, 1980.
8. Nyman G: The mental status examination. In Balis GU, Wurmser L, and Grenell R, editors: Psychiatric foundations of medicine, Woburn, Mass, 1978, Butterworth Publishers, Inc.
9. Sargent M: Update on brain imaging, Hosp Comm Psych 39(9):933, 1988.
10. Snyder JC and Wilson MF: Elements of a psychological assessment, Am J Nurs 77:235, 1977.
11. Sullivan HS: The psychiatric interview, New York, 1954, WW Norton & Co, Inc.

■ **ANNOTATED SUGGESTED READINGS** ■

Baker FM: Screening tests for cognitive impairment, Hosp Comm Psych 40(4):339, 1989.

Five tests to screen for cognitive impairment are reviewed. The tests are easily administered tools that help the non-psychiatric clinician determine whether an individual's cognitive function is normal or impaired.

Bates B: Mental Status. In A guide to physical examination and history taking, Philadelphia, 1987, JB Lippincott Co.

Provides a basic but thorough guide for beginning interviewer or experienced clinician wanting a comprehensive review. Definitions of terms are clear, developmental changes are reviewed, techniques of the examination are described, and abnormal findings are discussed.

*Cihlar CR: Mental status assessment for the ET nurse: psychologic impact of physical trauma, J Enterostomal Ther 13(2):49, 1986.

Discusses characteristic reactions to physical trauma in the emergency trauma patient and the specific assessment of mental status, particularly in reference to nursing care approaches.

*Critchley DL: Mental status examination with children and adolescents: a developmental approach, Nurs Clin North Am 14:3, 1979.

The author describes the developmental framework she uses for organization of the mental status examination with children and adolescents. Suggestions for age-appropriate activities, such as play and art, are included in a discussion of the structure of the interview.

Freedman AM, Kaplan HI, and Sadock BJ, editors: Comprehensive textbook of psychiatry, ed 5, Baltimore, 1989, Williams & Wilkins.

An in-depth discussion of the diagnosis and classification of symptoms observed in the psychiatric patient is presented in the chapters that address psychiatric evaluation. Specific guidelines are provided in a well organized, easily understood format for obtaining pertinent information in the psychiatric interview, taking a history, and performing the mental status examination.

Group for the Advancement of Psychiatry: Assessment of sexual function: a guide to interviewing, New York, 1973, Mental Health Materials Center, Inc.

Gives a straightforward approach to the assessment of sexual function. Specific questions are included with the discussion of various age groups and particular problems that might occur at the stages of development.

Hankoff LD et al: A program of crisis intervention in the medical setting, Am J Psychiatry 131(1):47, 1974.

Deals with interventions associated with the assessment of problems affecting general medical patients.

*Hundley J, Sullivan CH, and Coburn KL: Computerized EEG: forming a mental image, J Psychosoc Nurs 28(2):19, 1990.

Effects of technological advances on the expanding role of the psychiatric nurse are explored, including the greater opportunities for patient education, patient preparation, family education, and nursing subspecialization.

Imboden JB: Practical psychiatry in medicine. Part 16. Psy-

---

*Asterisk indicates nursing reference.

chiatric evaluation of the medical patient, J Fam Pract 10:4, 1980.

The importance of a psychiatric evaluation of the medical patient is conveyed in the discussion of the relationships between biological and psychosocial factors in illness. A general review of the broad classification of psychiatric illness, elements of a psychiatric diagnosis, factors to consider in a psychiatric interview, and the format for a psychiatric evaluation are described clearly and concisely.

Lesser AL: Problem-based interviewing in general practice: a model, Med Educ 19(4):299, 1985.

Integrates mental health and evaluation principles into the general assessment of medical patients, presenting to the general practitioner a systems approach to diagnosis.

*Ninns M and Makohon R: Alzheimer's disease: functional assessment of the patient, Geriatric Nursing 6(3):139, 1985.

A timely article about early detection of Alzheimer's disease related to observations of behavioral levels of function.

Nyman G: The mental status examination. In Balis GU, Wurmser, L, McDaniel E, and Grenell R, editors: Psychiatric foundations of medicine, Woburn, Mass, 1978, Butterworth Publishers, Inc.

A comprehensive discussion of the mental status examination. Case histories are included and compared as each section of the mental status examination is discussed. An excellent reference for a more thorough examination of the psychiatric patient.

Rapp MS: Re-examination of the clinical mental status examination, Can J Psychiatry 24:8, 1979.

The author questions the objectivity of the data obtained in the mental status examination, especially in the areas of insight, memory, judgment, and intelligence. He implies that individual differences in the examiner and patient could distort the judgments made.

*Rector CS and Foster ME: Assessment and care of the patient experiencing alcohol withdrawal syndrome, Crit Care Nurse 4(4):64, 1984.

Defines characteristics of alcohol withdrawal syndrome and the subsequent nursing care involved as a result of individual assessment techniques.

*Robitaille-Tremblay M: A data collection tool for the psychiatric nurse, Can Nurse 81(7):26, 1984.

The author has developed a structured brief assessment tool for systematic collection and analysis of psychiatric patient data.

Shea SC: Psychiatric interviewing, Orlando, Florida, 1990, WB Saunders Co.

Reviews interviewing skills in a humanistic way. Includes case studies, sample interviews and commonly made mistakes.

Spitzer RL, Skodol AE, Gibbon M, and Williams JBW: DSM-III case book, Washington, DC, 1981, The American Psychiatric Association.

A collection of case vignettes that is helpful in its descriptive correlation of clinical material to the principles of the DSM-III. The discussion following each vignette includes the rationale for the diagnosis according to the diagnostic criteria outlined in the DSM-III.

Sullivan HS: The psychiatric interview, New York, 1954, WW Norton & Co, Inc.

Sullivan describes both the patient and therapist as they interact during the psychiatric interview. He stresses the importance of the patient-therapist relationship in understanding the patient as a unique person. Assessment of the patient is incorporated throughout the book as the stages of the interview are presented.

Taylor M: The neuropsychiatric mental status examination, New York, 1982, Spectrum.

A review of the mental status examination that includes the exploration of organicity factors in cognitive function.

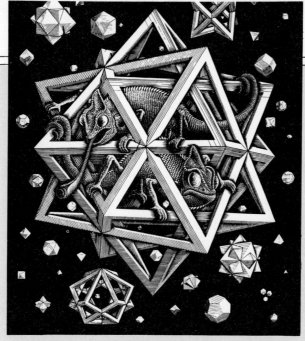

Pinel immediately led Couthon to the section for the deranged, where the sight of the cells made a painful impression on him. Couthon asked to interrogate all the patients. From most, he received only insults and obscene apostrophes. It was useless to prolong the interview. Turning to Pinel, Couthan said: "Now, citizen, are you mad yourself to seek to unchain such beasts?" Pinel replied calmly: "Citizen, I am convinced that these madmen are so intractable only because they have been deprived of air and liberty."

Philippe Pinel, *Traite Complet du Regime Sanitaire des Alienes* 56 (1836)

CHAPTER 7

LEGAL AND ETHICAL ASPECTS OF PSYCHIATRIC CARE

LEARNING OBJECTIVES

After studying this chapter, the student should be able to:

- state the admission, discharge, and status of civil rights as they pertain to informal, voluntary, and involuntary admission of a patient to a psychiatric hospital.

- describe the legal justification for a patient's commitment, the commitment process, and the three types of resulting hospitalization.

- analyze the moral, legal, and psychiatric implications of involuntary commitment, including the issues of assessing a patient's dangerousness and freedom of choice.

- identify the common civil and personal rights retained by psychiatric patients.

- define the following terms: testamentary capacity, incompetency, confidentiality, privileged communication, and malpractice.

- evaluate the potential benefits and problems that may arise from the right to treatment, the right to refuse treatment, and the right to treatment in the least restrictive setting.

- discuss the rights, responsibilities, and potential conflict of interest attendant in the three legal roles of the nurse: provider, employee, and citizen.

- compare and contrast the four sets of criteria commonly used in the United States to determine the criminal responsibility of a person believed to be mentally ill.

- assess the role of ethics in psychiatric nursing.

- define an ethical dilemma and relate one that arises in psychiatric nursing practice.

- apply the model for ethical decision making to a personally encountered ethical dilemma.

- critique the five forces currently affecting the mental health delivery system and the mechanisms and resources needed to improve the quality of mental health care in the United States.

- identify directions for future nursing research.

- select appropriate readings for further study.

To assess psychiatric professionals' knowledge of their patients' legal rights, Trancredi and Clark[40] conducted a study that included psychiatrists, psychiatric residents, nurses, and social workers. The results indicated that these professionals were generally unaware of a patient's legal rights at the time of admission and during hospitalization. Yet the relationship between psychiatry and law reflects the tension between individual rights and social needs, and the two areas have many similarities. Both psychiatry and law deal with human behavior, interrelationships between people, and responsibilities people assume based on these relationships. Both also play a role in controlling socially undesirable behavior. Together they analyze whether psychiatric treatment should be therapy, custodial care, or incarceration.

There are also differences between the two disciplines. Psychiatry is concerned with the meaning of behavior and personal life satisfaction, whereas law addresses the outcome of behavior and a system of rules to encourage orderly social functioning. These differences are evident in terminology. For example, "insane" and "legal commitment" are predominantly legal, not psychiatric, terms. Lawyers, judges, and juries decide whether a person was insane when he acted and whether a psychotic person should be legally committed for treatment.

The law impacts psychiatric nursing, particularly in concern for the rights of patients and the quality of care they receive. In the past 20 years, civil, criminal, and consumer rights have been established and expanded through judicial decision. Previously powerless and neglected groups such as the mentally ill are now using the legal system both to express legitimate grievances and to fight for social change. Many of the laws vary from state to state, and professionals must become familiar with the legal provisions of their own states. This knowledge enhances the freedom of both nurse and patient.

Hospitalizing the patient

One out of every eight Americans needs some form of mental health services, and a fourth of the people receiving psychiatric care are hospitalized. Not everyone who requires psychiatric care receives it, but the population statistics of mental hospitals are still impressive. Ten of every 10,000 Americans are patients in public mental hospitals, and state hospitals provide a major portion of long-term care for the chronically ill. Psychiatric patients occupy more than 25% of all hospital beds in the United States, and there are three times as many patients on record at psychiatric hospitals as there are criminals in prison.[29] Hospitalization can be traumatic or supportive for the individual, depending on the institution, attitude of family and friends, response of the staff, and type of admission. There are three major types of admission: informal, voluntary, and involuntary. Table 7-1 summarizes their distinguishing characteristics.

■ Informal admission

Informal admission to a psychiatric hospital resembles admission to a general medical hospital, that is, without formal or written application. The client is free to leave at any time. If he leaves before treatment is completed, he is often requested to sign himself out

"against medical advice," but he is not required to do so.

■ Voluntary admission

Under this procedure any citizen of lawful age may apply in writing (usually on a standard admission form) for admission to a public or private psychiatric hospital. He agrees to receive treatment and abide by hospital rules. He may seek help based on his own personal decision or the advice of family or a health professional. If someone is too ill to apply but voluntarily seeks help, a parent or legal guardian may request admission for him. In most states a child under the age of 16 years may be admitted if his parents sign the required application form.

Voluntary admission is preferred because it is similar to a medical hospitalization. It indicates that the individual acknowledges problems in living, seeks help in coping with them, and will probably actively participate in finding solutions. Most patients who enter private psychiatric units of general hospitals are voluntary.

When admitted in this manner, the patient retains all his civil rights, including the right to vote, possess a driver's license, buy and sell property, manage personal affairs, hold office, practice a profession, and engage in a business. It is a common public misconception that all admissions to a mental hospital involve the loss of civil rights.

If the voluntary patient wishes to be discharged, most states require that he give written notice to the hospital. In some states he can be released immedi-

---

TABLE 7-1

DISTINGUISHING CHARACTERISTICS OF THE THREE TYPES OF ADMISSION TO PSYCHIATRIC HOSPITALS

	Informal admission	Voluntary admission	Involuntary admission
Admission	No formal application needed	Formal application must be completed by patient	Application did not originate with patient
Discharge	Initiated by patient	Initiated by patient	Initiated by hospital or court but not by patient
Status of civil rights	Retained in full by patient	Retained in full by patient	Patient may retain none, some, or all, depending on state law
Justification	Voluntarily seeks help	Voluntarily seeks help	Mentally ill and one or more of the following: 1. Dangerous to others 2. Dangerous to self 3. Need for treatment

ately; in others he can be detained from 48 hours to 15 days before being discharged. This allows the hospital staff time to confer with the patient and family members and decide if additional inpatient treatment is necessary. If it is and the patient will not withdraw his request for discharge, the family may begin involuntary commitment proceedings, thereby changing the patient's status.

Although voluntary admission is the most desirable, it is not always possible. Sometimes a patient may be acutely disturbed, suicidal, or dangerous to himself or others, yet rejects any therapeutic intervention. In these cases involuntary commitments are necessary.

■ Involuntary admission (commitment)

In the late 1940s the World Health Organization reported that almost 90% of admissions to state mental hospitals in the United States were involuntary and approximately 10% were voluntary. The trend has shifted to more voluntary admissions. In 1963, 30% were voluntary, and by 1980 nearly half of all admissions to psychiatric hospitals were voluntary.[17] This trend has resulted from the greater variety of admission statuses and stricter rules regarding involuntary commitment. This is still a striking contrast to England, however, where more than 80% of patients are admitted voluntarily.

Although involuntary commitment has come under intense scrutiny, the United States Supreme Court continues to recognize it based on two legal theories. First, under its "police power," the state has the authority to protect the community from the dangerous acts of the mentally ill; and second, under its *parens patriae* powers, the state can provide care for citizens who cannot care for themselves, such as some mentally ill persons. In the past 20 years, the police power rationale for civil commitment has been supplanting the *parens patriae* doctrine through statutory changes. There has also been a trend toward increasing the requirements for standards of proof and procedural due process for such commitments.

Involuntary commitment does not always imply compulsion. It means that the patient did not originate the request for hospitalization and may have opposed it or was indecisive and did not resist. The standards for commitment vary among states and reflect the confusion present in the medical, social, and legal arenas of society. Most laws permit commitment of the mentally ill on three grounds: (1) dangerous to others, (2) dangerous to self, or (3) need for treatment. The deciding factor is whether the person can function in a reasonable manner without becoming an undue burden on his family or the community. The patients who are committed to psychiatric hospitals reflect the vagueness of these criteria.

■ THE COMMITMENT PROCESS.

State laws vary, but they try to protect the individual who is not mentally ill from being detained in a psychiatric hospital against his will for political, economic, family, or other nonmedical reasons. Certain procedures are standard. The process begins with a sworn petition by a relative, friend, public official, physician, or any interested citizen stating the person is mentally ill and needs treatment. Some states allow only specific individuals to file such a petition. One or two physicians examine the patient's mental status. Some states require that at least one of the physicians be a psychiatrist.

The decision whether to hospitalize the patient is then made. Precisely who makes this decision determines the nature of the commitment. **Medical** certification means a specified number of appointed physicians make the decision. This power to certify is given to all physicians, not just psychiatrists. A judge or jury decides on **court or judicial** commitment in a formal hearing. In this case the court is required to notify the patient so that he can retain legal counsel if he desires to contest commitment. A jury trial is not mandatory in most states but can be requested by the patient. Most states recognize the patient's right to legal counsel, but only about half actually appoint a lawyer for the patient if he does not have one. **Administrative**

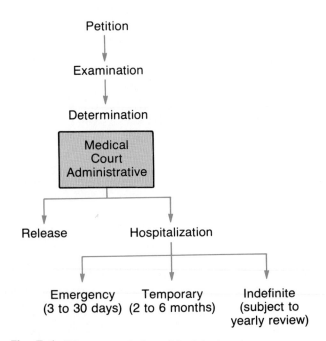

Fig. 7-1. Diagrammatical model of the involuntary commitment process.

commitment is determined by a special tribunal of hearing officers. The Fourteenth Amendment to the U.S. Constitution protects citizens against infringements on liberty without "due process of the law." Because of this, medical certification is used rarely, primarily in emergencies, and administrative commitment is subject to judicial review.

If the individual is determined to need treatment, he is hospitalized. The length of hospital stay varies, depending on the patient's needs. Fig. 7-1 diagrams the involuntary commitment process. It identifies three types of hospitalization: emergency, temporary, and indefinite. Table 7-2 describes characteristics of these types of hospitalization.

Emergency hospitalization. Almost all states permit emergency commitment for patients who are acutely ill. The goals for the commitment are short term, and they are primarily intended to control an immediate threat to self or others. In those states lacking such a law, police often detain the acutely ill individual in jail on a disorderly conduct charge, which is a criminal charge. Such a practice is inappropriate and often harmful to the patient's mental status.

To obtain an emergency commitment, the patient's family, a physician, or someone designated by the state must file a petition that includes a supporting report by a psychiatrist. It is reviewed by a judge or hospital official, and hospitalization is provided. Most state laws limit the length of emergency commitment to 3 to 30 days. Emergency hospitalization allows detainment in a psychiatric hospital only until proper legal steps are taken to provide for additional hospitalization.

Temporary or observational hospitalization. This type of commitment is primarily used for diagnosis and short-term therapy and does not require an emergency situation. Again, the commitment is for a specified time, but in this case it ranges from 2 to 6 months. The commitment process is similar to that for emergency hospitalization. Some states require a court order for all temporary commitments, whereas others require one only if the person protests. If at the end of the stipulated period the patient is still not ready for discharge, a petition can be filed for an indefinite commitment.

Indefinite hospitalization (formal commitment). A formal commitment provides for hospitalization for an indefinite time or until the patient is ready for discharge. The process is usually a court commitment. Patients in public or state hospitals more frequently have indefinite commitments than patients in private hospitals. Even when committed, these patients maintain their right to consult a lawyer at any time and to request a court hearing to determine if additional hospitalization is necessary. The hospital ultimately discharges the patient, however, and a court order is not necessary to do this.

■ Commitment dilemma

In nine states involuntary commitment assumes incompetency and the patient loses his civil rights. He is restricted in his ability to make contracts, vote, drive, obtain a professional license, serve on a jury, marry, or enter into civil litigation. In addition, the patient must suffer the stigma attached to the label "committed" in all his future activities. Because of the many people affected by involuntary commitment and the loss of personal rights that it entails, it becomes a matter of great legal, moral, social, and psychiatric significance. In general medicine there is no equivalent loss of individual rights, except for rare cases requiring quarantine for carriers of potentially epidemic diseases.

The question may be asked, "How ill does one need to be to merit commitment as being insane?" It is not necessary to be psychotic, as shown by the number of elderly, addicted, and neurotic patients hospitalized, as well as by the many psychotic individuals who remain free. Perhaps a person's dangerousness to himself or others is a more pertinent consideration. Certainly psychiatric professionals consider hospitalization in

TABLE 7-2

DISTINGUISHING CHARACTERISTICS OF THE THREE TYPES OF INVOLUNTARY HOSPITALIZATION

	Emergency	Temporary	Indefinite
Goals	Controlling an immediate threat to self or others	Diagnosis and short-term therapy	Treatment until determined ready for discharge
Time limit	3 to 30 days	2 to 6 months	Indeterminate

this instance as a humanitarian gesture that protects both the individual and society. "Dangerousness," however, is a vague term.

Dangerousness. Interestingly, courts guard the freedom of people who are mentally healthy but dangerous. After a prison sentence is served, the individual is automatically released and can no longer be retained. However, someone who is mentally ill and dangerous can be confined indefinitely. Ennis observes:

> Of all the identifiably dangerous groups in society, only the mentally ill are singled out for preventive detention and . . . they are probably the least dangerous as a group. Why should society confine a person if he is dangerous and mentally ill but not if he is dangerous and sane?[12.101]

To support his suggestion that the mentally ill are less dangerous than the mentally healthy, Ennis cites a 5-year study of 5,000 patients discharged from a state mental hospital in New York. The results showed that their arrest rate was one-twelfth that of the general population.

Similar findings were reported in a major study by Templin who observed over 2,000 police-citizen encounters in an urban area.[43] She found that police contact with people exhibiting signs of serious mental disorder was a relatively rare event. In addition, there were no differences found between the mentally disordered suspects and the non-mentally disordered suspects regarding the type of crimes that were committed. Research studies such as this one help to dispel the myth that the mentally ill are a more dangerous group who are also more prone to violent crime. Yet the idea of preventive detention does not exist in most areas of the law, since the ability to predict an action does not confer the right to control it in advance. Only illegal acts result in a prolonged confinement for most citizens—except the mentally ill.

Another issue is that there are no reliable indicators of dangerousness. Even if some mentally ill individuals are potentially dangerous, psychiatrists cannot necessarily predict future violence. Frequently psychiatrists overpredict the patient's potential for dangerous acts and the extent of his illness.

Oran[26] believes this results from psychiatrists' medical training, which cautions that underdiagnosis is more harmful than overdiagnosis. It is compounded by their conflicting roles as an agent of both the patient and the community, which require them to be therapist, warden, and judge. If psychiatrists underpredict a psychiatric illness and the patient later causes harm, the community holds them responsible. If they overpredict illness, however, a patient is subjected to treatment against his will. Thus multidisciplinary

teams rather than psychiatrists alone should be involved in determining dangerousness. Input from those familiar with the patient's home setting and sociocultural background might also improve evaluations.

Szasz[39] states that the real issue is not whether a person is dangerous, but who he is and how he is dangerous. He believes society condones danger in some ways but not others. For example, drunken drivers are very dangerous and kill many more people than do people with paranoid ideation. Drunken drivers are not committed, however, and people labeled paranoid are. In fact, some kinds of dangerous behaviors required in certain roles, such as race car driver, trapeze artist, and astronaut, are admired and valued. Some suggest that the assessment of danger involves four separate questions[9]:

1. What type of harmful act is to be considered dangerous: physical or psychological harm, harm to persons, or harm to property?
2. What degree of injury constitutes harm: verbal abuse, assault, or assault with a weapon?
3. How likely is it that the harmful act will occur? Do actuarial tables or clinical judgments allow us to predict it?
4. How frequently will the harmful act recur? Do the compulsively repeated acts of the exhibitionist make him more dangerous than a man whose only violent act was to murder both his parents?

The answers to these questions can be very subjective, which suggests that the underlying issue is noncomformity in ways that offend others. In this context, social role becomes important.

Before the law all men and women are equal, but it is also true that most committed patients are members of the lower classes. Scheff has observed the following:

> There is a large portion of the patient population, 43 percent, whose presence in the hospital cannot readily be explained in terms of their psychiatric condition. Their presence suggests the punitive character of the societal reaction to deviance.[35:168]

The behavioral standard of dangerousness can be said to change the function of the psychiatric hospital from a place of therapy for mental illness to a place of confinement for offensive behavior. This suggests that the psychiatric hospital's covert function is social control. This idea is supported by the various behavioral disorders that justify commitment, including drug addiction, alcoholism, and sexual offenses. In addition, epileptics may be committed in many states despite the fact that epilepsy is not a mental illness but a controllable physical condition.

Freedom of choice. The legal and psychiatric question thus raised is freedom of choice. Some professionals believe that at certain times the individual cannot be responsible for himself. To protect both the patient and society, it is necessary to confine him and make decisions for him. An example is the suicidal patient. In most states it is against the law to kill oneself, so law and psychiatry join to protect the person and help him resolve his conflict.

How does this compare with the cancer or cardiac patient who may reject medical advice and his identified therapeutic regimen? Should society, through law and medicine, attempt to cure him by involuntary methods? Some physicians, such as Chodoff,[7] view civil commitment as basically a benevolent system that makes bona fide treatment available. He disagrees with the assumption that mentally ill persons are competent to exercise free will and make decisions in their own best interest, such as whether to take medications or remain outside a hospital. He contends that there are mentally ill people who may not be physically dangerous but nevertheless endanger their own prospects for a normal life. Chodoff believes institutions can at least protect them and in many cases help them. Thus he thinks it would be immoral to abolish involuntary civil commitment.

Other people, such as Szasz, oppose intervention. Szasz favors responsibility for self and the right to choose or reject treatment. If one's actions violate criminal law, he suggests the individual be punished through the penal system:

> For some time now I have maintained that commitment—that is, the detention of persons in mental institutions against their will—is a form of imprisonment; that such deprivation of liberty is contrary to the moral principles embodied in the Declaration of Independence and the Constitution of the United States; and that it is a gross violation of contemporary concepts of fundamental human rights. The practice of "sane" men incarcerating their "insane" fellow men in "mental hospitals" can be compared to that of white men enslaving black men. In short, I consider commitment a crime against humanity.[39:113]*

There is currently a trend toward due process and legal procedures that approach the rigor of those used in the criminal process. The Massachusetts Mental Health Act of 1970, for example, recoded the statutes

governing the admission, treatment, and discharge of the mentally ill and mentally retarded. It involved changes in both content and procedure. Significantly, it eliminated very broad criteria for commitment and replaced them with guidelines that required proving the likelihood of serious harm to self or others before involuntary hospitalization.

This act also involved two important procedural changes. One was the abolition of an indefinite period of involuntary hospitalization; the commitment was for limited periods only. The second important change was the requirement of factual evidence, not just expert opinion, proving the prospective patient met the legal criteria for commitment. Nine other states (Maine, Nebraska, New Mexico, Ohio, Rhode Island, South Carolina, Tennessee, Washington, and Wisconsin) have since drafted similar laws.

In 1986 another important development occurred. The National Center for State Courts through its Institute on Mental Disability and Law formulated guidelines for involuntary civil commitment that contain practical solutions to problems associated with the process.[24] These guidelines are very comprehensive. They include the essential elements for an equitable, efficient, and effective commitment process, as well as measures for screening individuals before they are involuntarily detained. They call for greater cooperation and communication among the mental health, social service, public safety, and justice systems, and outline the roles of law enforcement officers, lawyers, mental health professionals, and judges in maintaining the continuity of the commitment process.

■ **ETHICAL CONSIDERATIONS.** Each nurse must resolve for herself whether she favors commitment. What should be done if the nonconformist does not wish to change his behavior? Does he maintain his freedom to choose even if his thinking appears to be irrational or abnormal? Is coercion fair? Can social interests be served by less restrictive methods such as outpatient therapy? Every nurse is responsible for reviewing commitment procedures in her state and working for necessary legal reforms.

Thus the commitment dilemma exposes present practices and opens areas of controversy for the future. The present mental hospital has been described as a jail, hospital, poorhouse, and home for the elderly. It protects, treats, feeds, maintains, and houses socially incompetent individuals who are often feared by society. When discharged, they often lack alternatives and come to the attention of law enforcement agencies or welfare offices.

Approximately one third of the total population of homeless adults are seriously mentally ill. Another

---

*Excerpt from *Ideology and Insanity* by Thomas Szasz. Copyright © 1970 by Thomas S. Szasz. Used by Permission of Doubleday & Co., Inc.

third are alcoholics and drug addicts, and the remaining third are homeless for economic reasons, including the lack of low income housing.[44] Robert Jones, president of the Philadelphia Committee for the Homeless, blamed deinstitutionalization as the major cause of homelessness, but also mentioned economic recession, high unemployment rates, and cutbacks in federal programs.[14] In addition to blaming cutbacks in aid to individuals, he noted the cutbacks in programs for medical care, aging studies, alcoholism and drug abuse, families and children, and employment training. Finally, Jones cited urban renewal for severely reducing low-cost housing units and increasing the number of evictions.

Local communities deny the problem by resisting the establishment of halfway houses or sheltered homes in their neighborhoods. Third-party insurance seldom covers extended outpatient psychiatric care. In today's mobile and impersonal society, family and friends are often unwilling or unable to care for the newly released patient, who may end up in a dismal run-down hotel or boarding house with nothing to do but watch television and wander the streets.

These issues must be addressed by psychiatric nurses, patients, and citizens across the United States. The value of commitment, goals of hospitalization, quality of life, and rights of patients must be preserved through the judicial, legislative, and health care systems.

Discharge

A patient who voluntarily admits himself into the hospital can be discharged by the staff when he has received "maximum benefit" from the treatment. He may also request discharge. Most states require written notice of his desire for discharge, and some hospitals will also request he sign a form that states he is leaving "against medical advice." These forms become part of his permanent record. He is usually released 24 to 72 hours after submitting a discharge request. If a voluntarily admitted patient elopes from the hospital, he can be brought back only if he again agrees. Staffs frequently attempt to contact such patients and discuss alternatives. If he refuses to return, either he must be discharged or involuntary commitment procedures must begin.

An involuntarily committed patient has lost the right to leave the hospital when he wishes. Temporary and emergency commitments specify the maximum length of detainment. Indefinite commitments do not, although the patient's status should be reviewed periodically. The patient may also apply for another commitment hearing. If a committed patient leaves secretly, the staff has the legal obligation to notify the police and committing courts. Frequently these patients return home or visit family or friends and can be easily located. The legal authorities then return the patient to the hospital. Additional steps are not necessary, since the original commitment is still effective.

There are three kinds of discharges: conditional, absolute, and judicial.

■ Conditional discharge

Specified leaves of absence or liberties help many committed patients make the transition from hospital to community. These are known as conditional discharges because certain things are expected of the patient. Most frequently he is required to attend outpatient therapy through the hospital or community mental health center. If he is progressing well, his leaves may be extended for 30 to 90 days or more. During this time the commitment order is still in effect, and, should he relapse while in the community, he can be brought back to the hospital.

This type of discharge planning allows a gradual integration into the community, and many patients have benefited from it. If at the end of the conditional period the patient has adjusted well, the hospital can issue an absolute discharge.

■ Absolute discharge

As the name implies, an absolute discharge terminates the patient's relationship with the hospital. It is a final discharge, and if the patient needs to return to the hospital at some future time, new admission proceedings must begin. Usually the hospital is required to notify the court when a committed patient receives an absolute discharge.

This type of discharge occurs most often when the patient has made substantial progress and can function well in the community. However, there are also cases when patients who have not improved and are unlikely to do so in the future are granted absolute discharges. In these instances, families or guardians are contacted to arrange satisfactory care for the patient. In addition, some laws require that the hospital notify other state officials.

■ Judicial discharge

Nearly 40 states have laws allowing a patient or his family the right to appeal for a discharge even though the hospital does not agree with the discharge request. The process and requirements for such cases vary from state to state, but they give the patient another option if he believes hospitalization is no longer appropriate. Such laws may be important for further defining patients' rights in future years.

Patients' rights

In 1973 the American Hospital Association issued a Patient's Bill of Rights, which many general hospitals throughout the United States have adopted. Psychiatric hospitals, however, continue to struggle with the issue of individual civil rights. Recent legislation throughout the United States supports the civil and personal rights of the mentally ill. The new laws also reflect the past restrictions and discriminations suffered by the mentally ill. Some states now allow the committed patient to retain all civil rights, similar to the voluntary patient, except the right to leave the hospital and to terminate treatment.

It has been estimated that one third of the states do make some provision to ensure that notice of rights is given to patients.[32] Frequently, a document is posted for reading in a location that is easily accessible to patients. In some hospitals, the patient's are given a list of rights on admission.

Allowing for great variation among states, patients presently have the following rights:

- Right to communicate with people outside the hospital through correspondence, telephone, and personal visits
- Right to keep clothing and personal effects with them in the hospital
- Right to religious freedom
- Right to be employed if possible
- Right to manage and dispose of property
- Right to execute wills
- Right to enter into contractual relationships
- Right to make purchases
- Right to education
- Right to habeas corpus
- Right to independent psychiatric examination
- Right to civil service status
- Right to retain licenses, privileges, or permits established by law, such as a driver's or professional license
- Right to sue or be sued
- Right to marry and divorce
- Right not to be subject to unnecessary mechanical restraints
- Right to periodic review of status
- Right to legal representation
- Right to privacy
- Right to informed consent
- Right to treatment
- Right to refuse treatment
- Right to treatment in the least restrictive setting

Some of these deserve more discussion.

■ Right to communicate with people outside the hospital

This right allows the patient to visit and hold telephone conversations in privacy and send unopened letters to anyone of his choice, including judges, lawyers, families, and staff. Although the patient has the right to communicate in an uncensored manner, the staff may limit his access to the telephone or visitors when such access could harm the patient or be a source of harrassment for the staff. The hospital can also limit the times when telephone calls are made and received and when visitors can enter the facility. On occasions hospital staff have intercepted and destroyed letters presumed to be threatening or abusive. In states where this is not illegal, such activity raises the moral question of individual freedom vs. the good of the community.

■ Right to keep personal effects

The patient may bring clothing and personal items to the hospital, taking into consideration the amount of storage space available. The hospital is not responsible for their safety, and valuable items should be left at home. If the patient brings something of value to the hospital, the staff should place it in the hospital safe or otherwise provide for safekeeping. The hospital staff is also responsible for maintaining a safe environment and should take dangerous objects away from the patient if necessary.

■ Right to be employed if possible

This includes the right to work whenever possible and the right to be compensated for it, including payment for work-therapy programs within the hospital. Involuntary servitude or work without pay within institutions is on the decline because courts have held that the Thirteenth Amendment, which abolished slavery, also applies to psychiatric patients. This means that mental institutions cannot force patients to work, either by punishing them or by making privileges or discharge depend on work. If patients choose to work, they must be assigned jobs on documented therapeutic grounds and be paid the minimum wage.

The U.S. Department of Labor is notifying all institutions that if they fail to pay patient workers, they are breaking the law. The ultimate effect of this move is not yet known. Some professionals fear that the money to pay patients will come out of treatment funds and that the patients will fare worse in the end. Others fear that hospitals will hire regular labor and leave the patients with nothing to do. Some argue that institutions will charge patients for room and board to recover the money. A further concern is that if the Department of Labor enforces the law, institutions may be forced to close because of lack of funds.

■ Right to execute wills

A person's competency to make a will is known as *testamentary capacity*. He can make a valid will if he (1) knows that he is making a will, (2) knows the nature and extent of his property, and (3) knows who his friends and relatives are and what the relationships mean. Each of these criteria must be documented for the will to be considered valid. This means the patient must not be mentally confused at the time he signs his will. It does not imply that he must know exact details of his property holdings or specific bank account figures, but he cannot attempt to give away more than he possesses. Furthermore, the law requires that he know who his relatives are but does not require him to bequeath anything to them.

A patient's commitment or diagnosis as being psychotic does not immediately invalidate his will. It is still valid if it was made during a lucid period and the patient met the three criteria. The problem most debated in determining testamentary capacity involves the delusional patient, particularly if the delusional thinking could alter the outcome of the will. The important question is whether the false belief or delusion caused the person to dispose of his property differently than he would have otherwise.

Two or three people must witness the will by watching the patient sign it and watching each other as they sign it. Later a nurse may be summoned to testify to the patient's condition at the time he drew up his will. Her testimony should relate to the three criteria just listed. It is important for the nurse to report pertinent observations, recall information as accurately as possible, and express herself concisely and objectively. Hospital charts and the nurse's notes may also be used in the court proceedings.

■ Right to enter into contractual relationships

The court considers contracts valid if the person understands the circumstances involved in the contract and its consequences. Once again, a psychiatric illness does not invalidate a contract, although the nature of the contract and degree of judgment needed to understand it would be influencing factors.

■ **INCOMPETENCY.** Related to this right is the issue of mental incompetency. Every adult is assumed to be mentally competent, mentally able to carry out his affairs. To prove otherwise requires a special court hearing to declare him "incompetent." This is a legal term without a precise medical meaning. To prove that an individual is incompetent, it must be shown that

(1) he has a mental disorder, (2) this disorder causes a defect in judgment, and (3) this defect makes him incapable of handling his own affairs. All three elements must be present, and the exact diagnostic label is not as important in this case. If a person is declared incompetent, the court will appoint a legal guardian to manage his estate. This frequently is a family member, friend, or bank executive. Incompetency rulings are most often filed for persons with senile dementia, cerebral arteriosclerosis, chronic schizophrenia, and mental retardation.

The legislative trend is to separate the concepts of incompetency and involuntary commitment, since the reasons for each are essentially different. Incompetency arises from society's desire to guard a person's assets from his own inability to understand and transact business. Involuntary commitments are intended to protect the patient from himself (in the case of suicide), protect others from the patient (as in homicide), and administer treatment. However, many states still consider the two equivalent. Hospital policies and procedures may impose incompetent status on the patient.

If ruled incompetent, one cannot vote, marry, drive, or make contracts. A release from the hospital does not necessarily restore competency. Another court hearing is required to reverse the previous ruling before the individual can once again manage his own affairs.

■ Right to education

Many parents exercise this right on behalf of their emotionally ill or mentally retarded children. The U.S. constitution guarantees this right to everyone, although many states have not provided adequate education to all citizens and are now required to do so.

■ Right to habeas corpus

Habeas corpus is an important right the patient retains in all states even if he has been involuntarily hospitalized. It originated in English Common Law and is included in the U.S. Constitution. Its goal is the speedy release of any individual who claims he is being detained illegally. A committed patient may file a writ at any time on the grounds that he is sane and eligible for release. The hearing takes place in court, where those who wish to restrain the patient must defend their actions. A jury is sometimes impaneled to determine the patient's sanity. If he is judged sane, he is discharged.

■ Right to independent psychiatric examination

Under the Emergency Admission Statute, the patient has the right to demand a psychiatric examination by a physician of his own choice. If this physician determines that he is not mentally ill, the patient must be released.

Right to marry and divorce

Since marriage is a formal contract, the same general criteria apply. The marriage is considered valid if the individual understands the nature of the marriage relationship and the duties and obligations it brings. The crucial factor is his mental capacity at the time of the marriage, not before or after. In general, courts are reluctant to declare a marriage void. Many states have laws forbidding the marriage of mentally ill persons, since mental illness, whether caused by genetics or environment, often runs in families. Thus the primary objective of such laws is to prevent the birth of children who might be mentally ill. These laws are not based on any scientific evidence that mental illness can be inherited.

In most states psychiatric illness is not in itself grounds for divorce. However, some states will grant divorces if the mentally ill spouse has been hospitalized for a certain number of years (usually 3 to 5). Sometimes it is also necessary to specify that the spouse is "incurably insane." Understandably, many psychiatric professionals hesitate to make such a diagnosis.

Right to privacy

The right to privacy implies the individual's right to keep some information about himself completely secret. *Confidentiality* involves the disclosure of certain information to another person, but this is limited to authorized individuals. Every psychiatric professional is responsible for protecting a patient's right to confidentiality, including even the knowledge that he is in therapy or in a hospital. Revealing such information might damage the patient's reputation or hamper his ability to obtain a job. The protection of the law applies to all patients. This can create ethical and professional dilemmas, such as the one experienced by the nurse in the following true case,[18] Clinical example 7-1.

The issue of confidentiality is becoming increasingly important, since various agencies demand information about a patient's history, diagnosis, treatment, and prognosis and sophisticated methods for obtaining information (e.g., wiretapping and computer banks) have developed. These threaten the individual's right to privacy. Clinicians are free from legal responsibility if they release information with the patient's written and signed request. As a rule, it is best to reveal as little information as possible and discuss with the patient what will be released.

Little research has been done on how patients feel about this important issue. One study found that psy-

---

CLINICAL EXAMPLE 7-1

On a Wednesday morning in 1981 in Springfield, Illinois, a man walked into Lauterbach's Cottage Hardware Store, grabbed an ax, and began swinging. When he left, one person was dead and two others were critically injured. Ten days later, police received a call from Mr. K, who was a patient in the 49-bed psychiatric unit at St. John's Hospital. Mr. K told the police that his roommate at the hospital confessed the crime. However, he didn't know his roommate's name. He asked Nurse M to identify him but she refused to do so, since she believed his name was shielded by a state law guaranteeing the privacy of mental health records. Hospital administrators supported her decision even after she was fined $250 by a county judge for refusing to give the man's name to a grand jury. Nurse M did tell the police that the suspect was not a patient in St. John's at the time of the murder and that he resembled their composite sketch.

---

chiatric inpatients valued confidentiality highly and worried about the possibility of unauthorized disclosures, particularly to employers.[36] They were unfamiliar, however, with their legal rights or options should breaches in confidentiality occur. This study emphasizes the importance of confidentiality and the need for additional research and patient education in this area.

Confidentiality builds on the element of trust necessary in a patient-therapist relationship. The patient places himself in the care of others and reveals vulnerable aspects of his personal life. In return he expects high-quality care and the protection of his interests. Thus the patient-therapist relationship is an intimate one that demands trust, loyalty, and privacy.

■ **PRIVILEGED COMMUNICATION.** The legal phrase *privileged communication* applies only in court-related proceedings. It includes communications between husband and wife, attorney and client, and clergy and church member. The right to reveal information belongs to the person who spoke, and the listener cannot disclose the information unless the speaker gives permission. This protects the patient, who could sue the listener for disclosing privileged information. It also gives the patient the confidence necessary to make a full account of symptoms and conditions so that he can be treated.

Privileged communication between health professionals and patients exists only if established by law. Thirty-three states currently recognize privileged communication between physicians and patients; twelve do not. Five states have laws providing for privileged communication between nurses and patients, including Arkansas, New York, Oregon, Vermont, and Wisconsin.[27] In these states the nurse is exempt from giving information obtained in a professional capacity if the information was necessary to provide nursing care. In all other states, a nurse would be required to reveal this information in court. In general, however, a nurse rarely is called into court to divulge information of this kind.

In 1975 the Federal Rules of Evidence were revised to extend physician-patient privilege only to psychotherapist-patient privilege. Acknowledging, however, that sometimes it was necessary to obtain information for the public good or to avoid fraud, the following exceptions were noted[45]:

1. Communications *not* made for purposes of diagnosis and treatment
2. Commitment and restoration proceedings
3. Issues as to wills or other contracts between parties and the patient
4. Actions on insurance policies
5. Required reports (venereal diseases, gunshot wounds, child abuse)
6. Communications in furtherance of the crime of fraud; mental or physical condition put in issue by the patient (personal injury cases)
7. Malpractice actions
8. Some or all criminal prosecutions, depending on the state

■ **PATIENT RECORDS.** Most hospitals keep psychiatric records separately so that they are less accessible than medical records. The law and psychiatric profession view them as more sensitive than medical records. Generally, psychiatrists retain the right to decide if they should release medical information to the patient, and some states bar patients from viewing them at all. A hospital chart can be brought into court, however, and its contents can be used in a lawsuit. Privileged communication does not apply to hospital charts, so nursing notes should be written carefully. Furthermore, as a general rule only those involved in a patient's care may read his chart. This includes physicians, nurses, aides, students, and others directly involved in treatment.

■ **PROTECTING A THIRD PARTY.** Another dimension to the concepts of confidentiality and privileged communication stems from the case of *Tarasoff v. Regents of the University of California et al.*[41] In this case the psychotherapist did not warn Tatiana Tarasoff or her parents that his client had stated he intended to kill her when she returned from summer vacation. In the lawsuit that followed Tatiana's death, California's Supreme Court decided that the treating therapist has a duty to warn the intended victim of a patient's violence. When a therapist is reasonably certain that a patient is going to harm someone, the therapist has the responsibility to breach the confidentiality of the relationship and warn or protect the potential victim. This can be done in several ways, including alerting the proper authorities or hospitalizing the patient. Four states (Massachusetts, Maryland, Michigan, and Arizona) have passed legislation outlining the specific options available to mental health professionals for how and when a potential victim should be warned.

■ **Right to informed consent**

Informed consent means a physician must give the patient a certain amount of information about the proposed treatment and must attain the patient's consent, which must be competent, understanding, and voluntary. The physician should explain the special treatment and possible complications and risks. The patient must be able to consent and not be a minor or judged legally incompetent or insane. Failure to obtain consent may lead to lawsuits of "assault and battery" or negligence.

Psychiatric outpatients usually express consent by their willingness to come for treatment. Only unusual treatments, such as experimental drugs or electroconvulsive therapy (ECT), require specific written consent. Informally admitted and voluntary patients usually sign a paper on admission consenting to psychiatric treatment, which includes milieu therapy, chemotherapy, psychotherapy, and occupational therapy. Again, unusual treatments need special permission. For the involuntarily admitted patient, the commitment procedure gives the hospital the right to treat the patient.

Consent forms usually require the signatures of the patient, a family member, and two witnesses. Nurses are often called on to be witnesses. The form then becomes part of the patient's permanent hospital record.

■ **Right to treatment**

The concept of the right to treatment is relatively recent. In 1960 Birnbaum, a graduate student in both medicine and law, wrote, "there does not appear to have been any significant and realistic consideration given, from a legal viewpoint, to the problem of whether or not the institutionalized mentally ill person receives adequate medical treatment so that he may regain his health, and therefore his liberty, as soon as possible."[5] In a 1966 case in the District of Columbia

(Rouse v. Cameron), the court held that mental patients committed by criminal courts had the right to adequate treatment. Furthermore, confinement without treatment was imprisonment and transformed the hospital into a penitentiary. The case affirmed that the purpose of involuntary hospitalization was treatment, not punishment. If treatment was not provided, the patient could be transferred, released, or even awarded damages. The hospital did not need to show that the treatment would improve or cure the patient, only that there was a true attempt to do so.

A 1972 case *(Wyatt v. Stickney)* extended the right to treatment to all mentally ill and mentally retarded persons who were involuntarily hospitalized. The court stated:

> To deprive any citizen of his or her liberty upon the altruistic theory that the confinement is for humane therapeutic reasons and then fail to provide adequate treatment violates the very fundamentals of due process.[48]

The court defined three criteria for adequate treatment:

1. A humane psychological and physical environment
2. A qualified staff with a sufficient number of members to administer adequate treatment
3. Individualized treatment plans

The keystone of the Wyatt decision is the requirement for an individualized treatment plan. Failure to provide it means the patient must be discharged unless he agrees to remain voluntarily.

This decision was upheld again in 1986. It is important because it goes beyond the earlier right-to-treatment case to require judicially enforceable standards of care in mental hospitals. It will also have economic implications, since meeting the three criteria will clearly cost more money. This may force states to reconsider the budgets presently allotted to mental health.

The Supreme Court made a landmark decision in 1975 in the case of *Donaldson v. O'Connor,* which freed a Florida State psychiatric patient after 15 years of confinement. The court ruled that he was not dangerous and was not receiving treatment. Therefore continuing to confine him would violate his right to liberty.

The right to treatment is based on the Eighth and Fourteenth Amendments to the Constitution. The Eighth Amendment deals with the issue of cruel and unusual punishment and the Fourteenth with due process and equal protection under the law. Various right-to-treatment cases have been introduced in state courts throughout the country, and their outcome will greatly affect the care of the mentally ill.

This new right, however, also poses several questions. One involves the appropriateness of treatment and whether confinement itself can be therapeutic. A second question deals with the untreatable patient. Should he be released after a certain time? Another problem is the unwilling patient. Might a person refuse treatment and then seek release, claiming he was denied his right to adequate treatment? A more pressing question is whether the public is willing to pay the costs required to provide adequate treatment to the mentally ill in public institutions. In current times of high inflation and reduced government funds, programs often struggle to survive at existing funding levels, let alone expansion. Thus budget constraints may play an even greater role than judicial decisions in affecting the care of the mentally ill.

■ Right to refuse treatment

The relationship between the right to treatment and the right to refuse treatment is complex. The right to refuse treatment includes the right to refuse involuntary hospitalization. It has been called the "right to be left alone." Some people believe therapy can control a person's mind, regulate his thoughts, and change his personality, and the right to refuse treatment protects the patient against this. This argument states that involuntary therapy conflicts with two basic legal rights: freedom of thought and the right to control one's own life and actions as long as they do not interfere with the rights of others.

In recent years, there has been an increase in the number of lawsuits concerning the right to refuse treatment, especially treatment involving psychotropic drugs. Many states have guidelines for the administration of electroconvulsive therapy and psychosurgery; however, the controversy over refusal of medication is a more recent one. Related to this is the right to refuse experimentation. Any experimental treatment requires the written consent of the patient. However, evidence exists that certain institutions obtained only inadequate consent, whereas others made no attempt at all to obtain it.[38]

The 1979 landmark case that established this right for psychiatric patients was *Rogers v. Okin.* This upheld the rights of hospitalized psychiatric patients to refuse medication. It emphasized that restraint may be used only in cases of emergency, such as the occurrence or serious threat of extreme violence, personal injury, or attempted suicide. Judge Tauro held that:

> The committed patient has a right to be wrong in his analysis of that information (regarding a particular treatment

program)—as long as the consequences of such error do not pose a danger of physical harm to himself, fellow patients or hospital staff. And so, while the state may have an obligation to make treatment available, and a legitimate interest in providing such treatment, a competent patient has a fundamental right to decide to be left alone, absent an emergency.[34]

The court's decision meant that committed psychiatric patients were presumed competent to make decisions regarding treatment in nonemergencies.

On the other hand, the 1982 Supreme Court decision in *Youngberg v. Romeo* supported the exercise of professional judgment in using seclusion or restraint.[49] The standard to be applied is that of usual and customary professional practice.

The right-to-refuse-treatment concept raises many questions. Does the right apply to all treatments, including medications, or only to those that are hazardous, intrusive, or severe, such as psychosurgery? How can staff meet their obligation for the right to treatment when a patient refuses to be treated? How does one differentiate between refusal, resisting treatment, and noncompliance, and does each of these require a different response? No solutions exist to these complex issues, but they concern nurses, who are frequently responsible for delivering prescribed treatments such as medications.

A recent review of the literature on the refusal of medication shows that while short-term refusal is common, continuing long-term refusal is rare.[21] Symptomatology such as delusions and denial may cause the refusal, and refusing patients are generally sicker than compliant ones. A study of patient's attitudes after involuntary medication suggests that for most patients, the decision to refuse medication is a sign of the patient's illness and does not reflect autonomous functioning or consistent beliefs about mental illness or its treatment.[37]

Rhoden provides an additional perspective. She suggests that staff members who overrule a patient because they believe they are doing "what is best for the patient" may sacrifice increased patient-staff communication and cooperation.[31] Although drug treatment may help a patient, taking his views seriously by not forcing the medication shows respect for him and may, in itself, be therapeutic.

Staff members faced with the patient who is refusing medication have several options. First, they can offer the patient a lower dosage—or no medication at all. A second option would be to discharge the patient against medical advice if no other staff action can relieve his symptoms and the patient does not meet the criteria for commitment. Another approach would be

to have the patient declared incompetent and seek a court order permitting the medication. Similarly, a guardian can consent to medication when the patient's refusal can be shown to result from incompetence and resultant inability to make a rational decision.

Nurses should judge each situation on a case-by-case basis. The Task Force on Behavior Therapy has examined the issue of coerced treatment and suggested three criteria that may justify it[3]:

1. The patient must be judged to be dangerous to himself or others.
2. It must be believed by those administering treatment that it has a reasonable chance to benefit the patient and those related to him.
3. The patient must be judged to be incompetent to evaluate the necessity of the treatment.

Even if these three conditions are met, the patient should not be deceived. He should be informed regarding what will be done, the reasons for it, and its probable effects.

Future court decisions will certainly explore the many aspects of this issue. Peck indicates possible outcomes:

The right-to-treatment movement . . . will undoubtedly do away with some of the injustices and deplorable conditions that have resulted in support for the right to refuse treatment and involuntary hospitalization. The end result might be more humane hospitals and treatment, which would lessen the impact of this movement. On the other hand, the right to treatment will probably also tend to make hospitals force their treatment, out of fear of being sued, on persons who were previously ignored. This in turn might result in an increase in cases maintaining the right to refuse treatment.[28:315]

Nurses are frequently on the front line in dealing with patients who refuse treatments and medications. It is clear that voluntary patients have the right to refuse any and all treatments and should not be forcibly medicated except in exceptional situations when the patient is actively violent to himself and others and when all less restrictive means have been unsuccessful. The behavior of the patient should be clearly documented and all interventions recorded.

Nurses must know the guidelines identified by the courts in the state in which they practice in administering medication properly to involuntarily committed patients. Some questions that can help guide the nurse's decision are[30]:

1. Has the patient been given a psychiatric diagnosis?
2. Is the treatment consistent with the diagnosis?

3. Is there a set of defined "target symptoms?"
4. Has the patient been informed about the treatment outcome and side effects?
5. Have medical and nursing assessments been completed prior to introducing drug therapy?
6. Are the therapeutic effects of treatment being monitored?
7. Are side effects being monitored?
8. Is the patient over or under medicated?
9. Is drug therapy being changed too quickly?
10. Are PRNs and stat doses being used too often?
11. Is drug therapy being prescribed for an indefinite period of time?

Finally it is important for the nurse to remember that a therapeutic nurse-patient relationship is critical in working with a patient who refuses to take medication. A positive, caring relationship between the nurse and patient can play a vital role in reversing treatment refusal.

TABLE 7-3

SIX CLINICAL DIMENSIONS OF THE CONCEPT OF RESTRICTIVENESS IN PSYCHOSOCIAL NURSING

Dimension	Component
Structural	Type of treatment setting and objective means of physical restraint or limitations on physical freedoms
Institutional policy	Rules, procedures, routines, and regulations for operating the institution and degree of patient involvement in planning
Enforcement	Staff-determined consequences of rule breaking or inability of the patient to leave the setting
Treatment	Use and level of antipsychotic medications and the use of other somatic treatments such as electroconvulsive therapy or psychosurgery
Psychosocial atmosphere	Status difference between patients and staff and degrees of staff authoritarianism
Patient characteristics	Patient's ability to manage his own care and level of functioning as influenced by the severity of his disorder

From Garritson S: J Psychosoc Nurs 21(12):9, 1983.

Right to treatment in the least restrictive setting

The right to treatment in the least restrictive setting is closely related to the right to adequate treatment. Its goal is evaluating the specific needs of each patient and maintaining the greatest amount of personal freedom, autonomy, dignity, and integrity in determining his treatment. Table 7-3 presents six clinical dimensions of the concept of restrictiveness in psychosocial nursing. This right applies to both community- and noncommunity-based programs. Greater consideration of this right might limit some of the controversy surrounding commitment and the right to refuse treatment.

The cases behind this right assert that if patients can function in some setting other than a mental hospital, the court has the responsibility of placing them in that setting. In the 1973 case *Dixon v. Weinberger,* the judge ruled that patients in Washington, D.C., have a statutory right to confinement in the least restrictive facility.[11] Washington, D.C., and the federal government are responsible for developing a plan to identify those who should be transferred to community-based facilities and the means for achieving this transfer, including creating new facilities if necessary.

The right to the least restrictive alternative tends to support patients' needs for normalization more effectively than do right-to-treatment cases. However, they are complicated by the need for new models, more facilities, and larger budgets for aftercare, so that discharged and chronically ill patients can be supported in the community.

Mental health laws regarding involuntary commitment are under pressure for reform in many states and one alternative proposed is the greater use of direct involuntary commitment to outpatient treatment. Despite more emphasis on treatment in the least restrictive setting, states are reticent to use outpatient treatment as an alternative to involuntary hospitalization. One study examined the effects of changes in North Carolina commitment laws designed to foster appropriate outpatient commitment.[22] Although the new laws increased outpatient commitment, hospital clinicians doubted its effectiveness and remained reluctant to use it. Problems associated with involuntary outpatient treatment include issues of legal liability and control over patients, costs of implementation, right treatment litigation, staff resistance to coerce patients, and need for close coordination with the criminal justice system.[47]

This right to treatment in the least restrictive setting raises a number of difficult questions. How do mental health professionals balance human rights versus the human needs of patients? Will sufficient funds be available to provide adequate supportive care in the community? What will happen to the other chronically ill patients who are not discharged into less restrictive settings? Will the community centers be able to provide better care than institutions? How can one counter community resistance to local placement of mentally ill patients? And most important, given present economic constraints, will the limited resources allotted to mental health go to community centers at the expense of large hospitals?

A final consideration in the right to the least restrictive alternative is that it applies not only to when a person should be hospitalized, but also to how a person is cared for within the hospital setting. It requires that a patient's progress be carefully monitored so that treatment plans can be changed based on the patient's current condition.

Issues related to the use of seclusion and restraints are of particular concern in this regard. There must be adequate rationale for the use of these practices and appropriate documentation should include a description of the precipitating event that warranted seclusion or restraints, alternatives attempted or considered, the patient's behavior while secluded or restrained, nursing interventions implemented, and ongoing evaluation of the patient. It is important to remember that seclusion and restraint must be therapeutically indicated and justified. Nurses may find it helpful to refer to the guidelines developed on them by a task force of the American Psychiatric Association.

■ Nursing's role in patients' rights

The National League for Nursing in 1977 issued a statement on the nurse's role in patients' rights.[25] It identified respect and concern for patients and assurance of competent care as basic rights, along with patients receiving the necessary information to understand their illness and make decisions about their care. The League urged nurses to get involved in assuring patients' human and legal rights.

The League identified many of the previously mentioned rights, plus the following:*

- Right to health care that is accessible and that meets professional standards, regardless of the setting
- Right to courteous and individualized health care that is equitable, humane, and given without discrimination as to race, color, creed, sex,

---

*National League for Nursing: Nursing's role in patients' rights, New York, 1977, The League. Used with permission.

national origin, source of payment, or ethical or political beliefs
- Right to information about their diagnosis, prognosis, and treatment, including alternatives to care and risks involved
- Right to information about the qualifications, names, and titles of personnel responsible for providing their health care
- Right to refuse observation by those not directly involved in their care
- Right to coordination and continuity of health care
- Right to information on the charges for services, including the right to challenge these
- Above all, the right to be fully informed as to all their rights in all health care settings

Perhaps the single most important factor is the attitude of psychiatric professionals. Sensitivity to patients' rights cannot be imposed by the court, the legislature, administrative agencies, or professional groups. If nurses ignore them, implement them casually, or are outwardly hostile about honoring them, patients' rights remain an empty legal concept. But if professionals are sensitive to patients' needs in all aspects of their relationships with them, they will secure these human and legal rights.

■ Summary

The 1978 report from the President's Commission on Mental Health[30] recommends that each state have a "Bill of Rights" for all mentally disabled people. This should be included in educational programs directed to patients, staff, families, and the general public. It proposes that a copy of the rights be prominently displayed in all mental health settings, given to each patient, and explained in an understandable manner.

The Mental Health Systems Act of 1980 supported the recommendations of the President's Commission on Mental Health. Included within the act itself is a Bill of Mental Health Rights.[22] (See the box on the 1980 Mental Health Systems Act's Rights and Advocacy.) The act recommended, but did not mandate, that the bill of rights be included in state legislation. This was unfortunate since a survey found that only 22 states complied with at least one third of the act's major recommendations and only five states complied with one half of them. Another survey in 1985 found that only thirteen states had amended their laws based on the recommendations and only Hawaii provided for most of the recommended rights.[19] Subsequently, in 1986, Congress passed the Protection and Advocacy for Mentally Ill Individuals Act, which au-

---

1980 Mental Health Systems Act's Rights and Advocacy

1. Right to appropriate treatment supportive of a person's personal liberty
2. Right to an individualized, written treatment plan and its appropriate periodic review and reassessment
3. Right to ongoing participation in the treatment plan and a reasonable explanation of it
4. Right not to receive treatment, except in an emergency situation
5. Right not to participate in experimentation without informed, voluntary, written consent
6. Right to freedom from restraint or seclusion
7. Right to a humane treatment environment
8. Right to confidentiality of records
9. Right to access of one's mental health care records
10. Right to access of telephone, mail, and visitors
11. Right to be informed of these rights
12. Right to assert grievances based on the infringement of these rights
13. Right of access to a qualified advocate to protect these rights
14. Right to exercise these rights without reprisal
15. Right to referral to other mental health services on discharge

---

thorized the establishment of systems in each state to protect and advocate for the rights of the mentally ill. However, presidential commissions, mental health legislation, and litigation have usually brought only abstract victories. Efforts to implement these decisions have been slowed by confusing requirements, inadequate resources, and insufficient knowledge.

Clearly the reforms mandated by law will cost money, yet public willingness to pay for more and better psychiatric care is questionable. Limited resources continue to be a major factor, regardless of how well organized, numerous, and well intentioned are the advocates of better mental health care. Protecting the rights of the mentally ill will depend on the effectiveness of any new programs arising from executive, judicial, or legislative orders.

Legal role of the nurse

Professional nursing practice is not determined by simply following patients' rights. Rather, it is an interplay between the rights of patients, the legal role of the nurse, and concern for quality psychiatric care (Fig. 7-2). There are three roles that the psychiatric nurse moves in and out of while completing professional and personal responsibilities: provider of services, employee or contractor of services, and private citizen. These roles are simultaneous, and each carries certain rights and responsibilities.

■ Nurse as provider

■ **MALPRACTICE.** All psychiatric professionals have legally defined duties of care and are responsible for their own work. If these duties are violated, malpractice exists. Malpractice involves the failure of professionals to provide the proper and competent care that is given by members of their profession in the community, resulting in harm to the patient. Most malpractice claims are filed under the law of negligent tort. A *tort* is a civil wrong for which the injured party is entitled to compensation. Because, under the law, everyone is responsible for his own torts, each nurse can be held responsible in malpractice claims. Under the law of negligent tort the plaintiff must prove the following:

1. A legal duty of care existed.
2. The nurse performed the duty negligently.
3. Damages were suffered by the plaintiff as a result.
4. The damages were substantial.

When patients are admitted to a psychiatric hospital, the problems of litigation in connection with their care are many and varied. The Bill of Rights in the Mental Health Systems Act helps clarify the sometimes conflicting roles of mental health professionals. It asserts that a health professional is not obligated to: administer treatment contrary to her clinical judgment, prevent the discharge of any person for whom appropriate treatment is impossible as a result of the person's refusal to consent, admit any person who has repeatedly frustrated treatments in the past by withholding consent, or provide treatment to anyone admitted solely for diagnostic or evaluative purposes.[20] Such legislation helps to shed some light on the role of

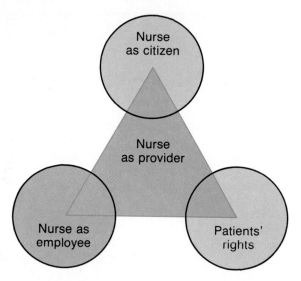

Fig. 7-2. Model of interactive influences of psychiatric nursing practices.

health providers in such issues as right to treatment and right to refuse treatment.

Litigation. Lawsuits alleging malpractice in psychiatric diagnosis or treatment, once rare, are now increasing. The American Psychiatric Association has identified most frequent sources of claims, in order of decreasing frequency:

- Patient suicide
- Improper treatment
- Ineffective or improper medication
- Breach of confidentiality
- Wrongful commitment
- Injuries resulting from electroshock therapy
- Sexual abuse of patients
- Failure to obtain informed consent[42]

Similarly, lawsuits against nurses were relatively uncommon. However, they can occur when the nurse errs while acting either dependently or independently. The box on page 223 describes three recent cases involving psychiatric nurses. A study of nursing malpractice litigation between 1967 and 1977 indicated that approximately 14 cases occurred in psychiatric hospitals.[6] Most incidents involved administration of treatments or medications, communications, and supervision of patients.

The most common causes of malpractice suits against psychiatric nurses are negligence in suicide precautions and assisting in ECT. When a patient is believed to be suicidal, the psychiatrist writes an order for suicide precautions. The nurse then has the responsibility to follow that order in a way that ensures the patient's safety. The exact procedure varies from hospital to hospital, but it should include close observation, limiting his activity to the ward only, and removing any potentially harmful objects. Another potential problem area concerns the patient receiving ECT. The nurse must take proper precautions to prepare him before the treatment and to monitor his status afterward until he is fully conscious and alert.

■ **LEGAL RESPONSIBILITIES.** Creighton[8] stresses that the nurse is responsible for reporting pertinent information about the patient to co-workers involved in caring for him. The degree of nursing care must depend on the patient's condition, with the seriously ill demanding a higher degree of care to protect them from injury and self-destruction.

Reporting information includes written as well as oral communication, and accurate records are crucial. Clear, concise nursing notes can avoid many problems. For example, notes that record specific suicidal precautions clarify the nurse's actions. The nurse should also record the occasion when she explained to a patient and his family the food precautions he needed to observe when taking his monoamine oxidase (MAO) inhibitor medication. Such a note would prevent a possible lawsuit should the patient violate his dietary restrictions and become ill. Accurate reporting is an element of good nursing care that should be completed promptly and thoroughly.

The legal responsibilities of nonphysician therapists have not yet been well defined. The nurse can follow these preventive measures to avoid possible lawsuits:

1. Implement nursing care that meets the *Standards of Psychiatric–Mental Health Nursing Practice* as described by the American Nurses' Association.
2. Know the laws of one's state, including the rights and duties of the nurse as well as the rights of the patients.
3. Keep accurate and concise nursing records.
4. Maintain the confidentiality of patient information.
5. Consult a lawyer should any questions arise.

■ **Nurse as employee**

The role of employee, or contractor of service, is less frequently scrutinized but also very important. This mandates the practitioner's rights and responsibilities in relation to one's employers, partners, consultants, and other professional colleagues. Professionals often do not know the rights and responsibilities of employees and contractors of service. However these

Selected Litigation Involving Psychiatric Nurses

Case 1: Valentine v. Strange (597 F. Supp. 1316 VA)

Problem: Nurses sued when psychiatric patient set self on fire

Facts: Despite two previous attempts to burn herself, the health care providers permitted the patient to keep her cigarettes and lighter. Patient subsequently set fire to her clothing and suffered third-degree burns.

Legal Lesson: The failure of health care professionals to take precaution in the face of imminent danger to the life of an involuntarily committed patient constitutes a violation of liberty interests protected by the due process clause of the Fourteenth Amendment.

Case 2: Vattimo v. Lower Bucks Hospital (428 A. 2nd 765—Pa.)

Problem: Need for restraint and supervision of patients by psychiatric nurses

Facts: A patient with a psychotic fascination with fire set fire to his hospital room, resulting in the death of the other occupant. The patient had been diagnosed as a paranoid schizophrenic, and staff had been warned of his preoccupation with fire.

Legal Lesson: The hospital was required to exercise reasonable care under the circumstances to restrain, supervise, and protect mentally deficient patients.

Case 3: Delicata v. Bourlesses (404 N.E. 2nd 667—Mass.)

Problem: Nursing psychiatric assessment vs. the psychologist's

Facts: A nursing assessment indicated that a depressed patient should be closely supervised as potentially suicidal. An evaluation by the staff psychologist advised that suicidal precautions were *not* necessary. The patient subsequently killed herself in a locked bathroom.

Legal Lesson: Medical orders by a staff psychiatrist or an evaluation by a staff psychologist must be questioned when there is a change or deterioration in a patient's condition. Nursing assessments should include the evaluation of such changes in the patient's apparent physical and psychological condition. The responsibility of assessment includes the necessity for making appropriate nursing judgments and implementing nursing actions based on these assessments.

---

are the basis of one's economic security, professional future, and peer relationships.

As an employee, a nurse has the responsibility to supervise and evaluate those under her authority for the quality of care given. She must also observe her employer's rights and responsibilities to clients and other employees, fulfill the obligations of the contracted service adequately, inform the employer of circumstances and conditions that impair the quality of care, and report negligent care by others when and where appropriate. This includes the legal duty to communicate any concerns about other mental health professionals.

In return, a nurse can expect certain rights from her employer. These include consideration for service, adequate working conditions, adequate and qualified assistance where necessary, and the right to respect all of her other rights and responsibilities.

■ Nurse as citizen

The third role that the nurse plays is that of citizen. This is particularly significant because all other roles, rights, responsibilities, and privileges are awarded because of the inherent rights of citizenship. The U.S. government grants these as inherent: civil rights, property rights, right to protection from harm,

Maryland Nurses' Association
The Bill of Rights for Registered Nurses

We, the Council on Human Rights of the Maryland Nurses' Association, in order to promote increased knowledge and understanding of the rights and responsibilities of all registered nurses, have developed The Bill of Rights for Registered Nurses. We propose that this Bill will aid in educating consumers and health care professionals about the rights of registered nurses, as well as their corresponding responsibilities. Therefore, we submit the Bill of Rights for Registered Nurses as a position statement of the Maryland Nurses' Association.

The nurse has a right:

Individual

to practice according to the Maryland Nurse Practice Act.

to make independent nursing judgments.

to question any delegated medical order or any plan of care that may cause possible harm to the patient/client or others.

to refuse to carry out any delegated medical order or any plan of care that may cause possible harm to the patient/client or others.

to pursue quality continuing education.

to teach individuals and groups health care practices that facilitate treatment, prevent illness, and provide optimal wellness.

Employment

to competitive hiring and promotion which is based on knowledge and experience and which is unrestricted by consideration of sex, race, age, creed, or national origin.

to realistic assignments that can assure the patient/client quality care that includes safety, dignity, and comfort.

to negotiate salary and individual conditions of employment.

to work in a safe and adequately equipped environment.

to work with qualified, competent nursing personnel.

to periodic, fair, objective evaluations by peers.

to pay increases based on demonstrated performance.

to due process whenever accused of unethical, incompetent, illegal, or unqualified practice or of prejudicial or inappropriate conduct.

to be an advocate for the patient/client and the public when health care and safety may be affected by incompetent, unethical, or illegal practices.

to representation by a negotiator in labor matters.

The nurse has a responsibility:

to assume personal accountability for individual nursing judgments and actions which consider the individual value systems and the uniqueness of each patient/client.

to implement the nursing process in providing individualized nursing care.

to safeguard the patient/client and the public from incompetent, unethical, or illegal health care practices.

to refuse to perform any nursing action which will jeopardize the patient/client or the public, and the obligation to communicate the rationale to the proper authority.

to avail one's self of opportunities which will broaden knowledge and refine and increase skills.

to educate the patient/client and the public.

to maintain competence and prepare one's self adequately for promotion.

to evaluate one's own work environment and to communicate and document unrealistic work loads through appropriate channels.

to make known individual convictions and preferences prior to hiring.

to assess, evaluate, document, and correct unsafe conditions and to communicate such information to the appropriate authority promptly.

to objectively document and report to appropriate authority evidence of competent, as well as incompetent performance and to evaluate, inform, counsel, and teach nursing personnel when indicated.

to participate in the development of reliable and valid evaluation criteria for peer review.

to maintain competence, incorporate new techniques and knowledge, and continuously upgrade the quality of health care.

to participate in the planning, establishment, and implementation of procedures to ensure due process.

to be alert to any instances of incompetent, unethical, or illegal practices by any member of the health care system and to take appropriate action regarding these practices.

to select and utilize a knowledgeable and impartial negotiator.

Maryland Nurses' Association
The Bill of Rights for Registered Nurses—cont'd

The nurse has a right:	The nurse has a responsibility:
Professional to receive support from the nursing profession at all levels. to belong to an autonomous nursing organization. to have expert testimony supplied by the nursing organization for both legal and legislative issues. to full and equal representation on all decision-making bodies concerned with health care. to be involved actively in the political decision-making process at all levels of the government.	to participate in activities that contribute to the ongoing development of the profession's body of knowledge. to be an active member and to participate in the nursing organization's effort to implement and improve standards of nursing. to provide knowledgeable, objective, articulate expert testimony. to provide knowledgeable, active, and effective collaborating with members of the health professions. to be knowledgeable, active, and effective in the legislative process by direct involvement, effective education and selection of representative legislators, lobbying, and creating citizen awareness in promoting local, state, and national efforts to meet the health needs of the public.

---

right to a good name, and right to due process. These form the foundation for the nurse's other legal relationships.

■ **CONFLICT OF INTEREST.** Unfortunately, the best interests of the patient, nurse, and employer do not always merge. Conflict can occur when, for example, the nurse's right to live and work without threat to personal security is violated by a patient who harms her. Take the case of a psychotic patient who has hallucinations that are adequately controlled with psychotropic medications but who refuses to take them. Intervention with this patient must consider the following possibilities:

- Failing to medicate the patient may deny his right to treatment.
- Failing to medicate the patient could have harmful side effects, such as the unnecessary and possibly irreversible continuation of his illness.
- Failing to medicate the patient may lead to a psychotic episode and result in injury to himself, other patients, or the staff.
- Failing to medicate the patient may lead to a psychotic episode but no violence.

- Medicating the patient in the absence of an emergency situation and without a clear threat of violence violates his right to refuse treatment.

In the following case the staff decided not to medicate the patient. When the night nurse checked on the patient in his room that evening, he struck the nurse in the face, resulting in severe bruises and the loss of some teeth. This development leads to new questions.

- Was the patient competent and legally liable for his actions?
- What were the circumstances of the incident?
- Was the nurse sufficiently aware of the potential hazard and, if so, was she responsible for assuming the risk?
- Was staffing adequate to discourage, respond to, and control a potentially violent situation?
- Was there a provision in the unit for potentially violent patients and, if so, why wasn't it used for this patient?

Obviously, there are no simple or perhaps even equitable solutions to such dilemmas; yet they are real and ever present. All mental health professionals must focus on prevention. This requires a knowledge of legislation, rights, responsibilities, and potential conflicts.

Nurses in Maryland have developed the bill of rights for registered nurses shown in the box on pages 224 and 225. This commendable document educates nurses and the public and also clarifies rights and responsibilities. In addition, professional nursing judgment requires examining the context of nursing care, the possible consequences of one's actions, and practical alternatives. Only then do rights and responsibilities become meaningful.

Psychiatry and criminal responsibility

The determination of criminal responsibility concerns the accused person's condition when he committed the offense. It has received much public attention as the "insanity defense." This proposes that a person who has committed an act usually considered criminal is not guilty by reason of "insanity." This is a difficult decision to make. Usually defense attorneys and prosecutors offer many arguments pro and con and frequently call on psychiatrists to testify. Nurses are seldom directly involved, but they should understand the law in this area as both citizens and psychiatric professionals.

This defense is based on the humanitarian rationale that a person should not be blamed if he "did not know what he was doing" or "could not help himself." With the complexity of today's society and judicial system, however, many believe this defense is being abused, and it is highly controversial. Much of this controversy stems from John Hinckley's shooting of President Reagan in 1981, from which he was acquitted by the verdict of "not guilty by reason of insanity." One recent change is the movement away from using the defense "not guilty by reason of insanity" (NGBI) to the more recent "guilty but mentally ill" (GBMI). This has been adopted by Michigan, Indiana, Illinois, and Georgia.

At present four sets of criteria are used in the United States to determine the criminal responsibility of an offender who is mentally ill: the M'Naghten Rule; the Irresistible Impulse Test; the Durham Test or "Product Rule"; and the American Law Institute's, or ALI, Test, the one most frequently used (see Table 7-4).

■ M'Naghten Rule

This law originated with the 1832 London trial of Daniel M'Naghten when he was tried for the murder of Edward Drummond, private secretary of Sir Robert Peele. M'Naghten had suffered from delusions of persecution and had complained to public authorities many times. Receiving no help, however, he decided to resolve the situation himself. He began watching the house of Sir Robert Peele and one evening, under the belief he was shooting Peele, shot Edward Drummond as he emerged from the house. His attorney entered an appeal of "partial insanity," and M'Naghten was declared of unsound mind and committed to an institution for the criminally insane. In deciding the case, the judges identified two rules to determine the criminal responsibility of a person who pleads insanity. The first rule states that the individual at the time of the crime did not "know the nature and quality of the act." The second states that if he did know what he was doing, he did not know that it "was wrong." These two rules are called the "nature and quality" rule and "right from wrong" test. This case was the first major test of criminal responsibility, and it is still used in most states and criminal courts.

TABLE 7-4

FOUR SETS OF CRITERIA COMMONLY USED TO DETERMINE THE CRIMINAL RESPONSIBILITY OF A MENTALLY ILL OFFENDER

Name of test	Criteria
M'Naghten Rule	1. The individual did not know the nature and quality of the act. 2. The individual did not know that what he was doing was wrong.
Irresistible Impulse Test	An individual is impulsively driven to commit the criminal act with lack of premeditation and a strong urge to do so. This test is seldom used in isolation.
Durham Test, or Product Rule	An individual's act was the "product of mental disease." This test is seldom used.
American Law Institute's Test	An individual lacks the capacity to "appreciate" the wrongfulness of his act or to "conform" his conduct to the requirements of the law. It excludes the psychopath and is a popular criterion for determining criminal responsibility.

■ Irresistible Impulse Test

A number of states have adopted the Irresistible Impulse Test along with the M'Naghten Rule. It is never used in isolation. According to this test, a person may know the difference between right and wrong but finds himself impulsively driven to commit the criminal act. It is usually necessary to show a lack of premeditation and that the urge was so strong that it would have been followed regardless of the circumstances. This test is a frequent defense for sudden, violent behavior displayed under stress.

■ Durham Test, or "Product Rule"

The Durham Test is based on a 1954 decision in the District of Columbia. The rule states that the accused is not criminally responsible if his act was the "product of mental disease." Thus it is sometimes called the "Product Rule," although this phrase and "mental disease" have been difficult to define. Many people object to this test because it greatly expands the number of individuals who may plead insanity. It is seldom used at this time.

■ American Law Institute's Test

The ALI test is similar to the combination of the M'Naghten Rule and Irresistible Impulse Test. It states that a person is not responsible for his criminal act if he lacks the capacity to "appreciate" its wrongfulness or to "conform" his conduct to the law. It also excludes "an abnormality manifested only by repeated criminal or otherwise antisocial conduct," which excludes the psychopath who has repeated criminal conduct. This popular test is now used by all the federal circuit courts and a number of states' courts.

■ Disposition of mentally ill offenders

If a person is found not guilty by reason of insanity (NGBI), he is rarely set free. In some states he may be committed at the court's discretion, and in almost a third of the states he is automatically hospitalized. Some offenders are treated in special hospitals, others are sent to state mental hospitals, and still others go to prison treatment facilities. If an offender is found guilty but mentally ill (GBMI), he is never freed. Since the insanity defense is used most frequently in capital offenses, it is usually better to have good security, and penal institutions are the best option.

After hospitalization and recovery, the patient may be discharged by the court that ordered his commitment. In other states the governor may discharge him. Still others allow the mental institution to make that decision. The major criteria for discharge are that he is not likely to repeat his offense and that it is relatively safe to release him to the community.

Ethics in psychiatric nursing

Ethical considerations combine with legal issues to impact on all the elements of the psychiatric nursing process. The concept of ethics means something diferent to each individual. It implies what is right and wrong and reflects one's ideas on values and morality.

■ Ethical standards

An ethic is a standard of behavior or a belief valued by an individual or group. It describes what ought to be, rather than what is—a goal to which one aspires. These standards are learned through socialization, growth, and experience. As such, they are not static but evolve to reflect social change.

Groups, such as professions, can also hold a code of ethics. Such a code guides the profession in serving and protecting consumers. It also provides a framework for decision making for members of the profession. Moore[23] has defined two major purposes for a code of ethics as "structuring" and "sensitizing." Structuring is preventive and aims to restrain impulsive and unethical behavior. The second purpose, sensitizing, is educative, with the goal of raising members' ethical consciousness.

The American Nurses' Association published a code of ethics for nurses (see the box on page 228).[1] It emphasizes the nurse's accountability for the quality of care and his or her duty to act as a patient advocate in ensuring the quality of care given by others.

Nurses should follow these professional standards as they deliver health care. Knowing one's own values and implementing them within the framework of the code can increase both the quality of the care one gives and the satisfaction the nurse receives from her practice.

■ Power and paternalism

A discussion of ethics and nursing must also consider the crucial element of power. In the psychiatric setting, the nurse can function in many roles, from a custodial keeper of the keys to a skilled therapist. Each of these roles includes a certain amount of power, since all nurses have the ability to influence the patient's treatment and serve as the major source of information regarding his behavior. This is particularly true in inpatient settings, where a nurse and patient spend more time together and the nursing staff is the only group to work a 24-hour day. Nurses also participate in team meetings, individual and group psychotherapy, and behavior modification programs. Finally,

---

American Nurses' Association Code for Nurses

1. The nurse provides services with respect for human dignity and the uniqueness of the client unrestricted by considerations of social or economic status, personal attributes, or the nature of health problems.
2. The nurse safeguards the client's right to privacy by judiciously protecting information of a confidential nature.
3. The nurse acts to safeguard the client and the public when health care and safety are affected by the incompetent, unethical, or illegal practice of any person.
4. The nurse assumes responsibility and accountability for individual nursing judgments and actions.
5. The nurse maintains competence in nursing.

6. The nurse exercises informed judgment and uses individual competence and qualification as criteria in seeking consultation, accepting responsibilities, and delegating nursing activities to others.
7. The nurse participates in activities that contribute to the ongoing development of the profession's body of knowledge.
8. The nurse participates in the profession's efforts to implement and improve standards of nursing.
9. The nurse participates in the profession's efforts to establish and maintain conditions of employment conducive to high-quality nursing care.
10. The nurse participates in the profession's effort to protect the public from misinformation and misrepresentation and to maintain the integrity of nursing.
11. The nurse collaborates with members of the health professions and other citizens in promoting community and national efforts to meet public health needs.

From American Nurses' Association: Code for nurses with interpretive statements, Kansas City, Mo, 1976, The Association. Reprinted with permission.

---

nurses can greatly influence decisions about patient medications, such as type, dosage, and frequency.

The literature describes the ethical dilemmas that arise from health care professionals' "paternalistic" attitude toward their patients. Paternalism can be defined as acting on one's own idea of what is best for another person, without asking that individual. It occurs when something is done "for the patient's own good" even though the patient would likely disagree with the action. This attitude reduces the adult patient to the status of a child and interferes with his freedom of action.

Gert and Culver present five criteria to evaluate whether a particular action is paternalistic.[13] They suggest that a nurse is acting paternalistically if, and only if, her behavior indicates that she believes:

1. One's action is for the patient's good
2. One is qualified to act on the patient's behalf
3. One's action involves violating a moral rule (e.g., deceiving, breaking a promise, causing pain)
4. One is justified in acting on the patient's behalf whether or not the patient has ever given or will ever give consent
5. The patient thinks (perhaps falsely) that he knows what is for his own good

Thus paternalism involves acting on one's own beliefs, as well as breaking a commonly held moral rule.

To avoid this potential danger, the nurse should realize that her ethical obligations span a wide range of individuals, including the patient, the patient's family or support system, herself, her own family, other health care professionals, the health care institution or organization in which she works, and the larger social community. Furthermore, her ethical obligations arise within a context of laws and government regulations that may, at times, create dilemmas. By remaining aware of these laws, she can examine these problems from both clinical and ethical perspectives.

■ Ethical dilemmas

An ethical dilemma exists when moral claims conflict with one another. It can be defined as (1) a difficult problem that seems to have no satisfactory solution or (2) a choice between equally unsatisfactory alternatives. Ethical dilemmas pose such questions as "What should I do?" and "What is the right thing to do?" They can occur both at the nurse-patient-family level of daily nursing care and at the policy-making level of institutions and communities. Although ethical dilemmas arise in all areas of nursing practice, some are unique to psychiatric and mental health nursing. Many of these dilemmas fall under the umbrella issue of behavior control.

At first glance, behavior control may seem a simple issue—behavior is a personal choice, and any behavior that does not impose on the rights of others is acceptable. Unfortunately, this does not help one address complex situations. For example, a severely depressed person may choose suicide as an alternative to an intolerable existence. This is, on one level, an individual choice not directly harming others, yet suicide is strongly forbidden in American society. In many states, it is a crime that can be prosecuted. As another example, in some states it is illegal for consenting adults of the same sex to have sexual relations, although it is not illegal for a man to rape his wife. These examples raise difficult questions: When is it appropriate for society to regulate personal behavior? Who will make this decision? Is its goal personal adjustment, personal growth, or adaptation to social norms? And finally, how do we measure the costs and benefits of attempting to control personal freedom in a free society?

One of the most fundamental problems is that psychiatry lacks definitions for mental health, normalcy, mental illness, and insanity. These terms have been debated for centuries, yet there are no universally accepted definitions. This demonstrates the blurry line between science and ethics in the field of psychiatry. Theoretically, science and ethics are separate entities. Science is descriptive, deals with "what is," and rests on validation; ethics is predictive, deals with "what ought to be," and relies on judgment. However, psychiatry is neither purely scientific nor value free.

The fact that psychiatry is not a predictable science is reflected in the existence of more than 100 schools of psychotherapy. Each has its own theory of causation, treatment goals, and therapeutic practices, which include screaming cures (Janov's primal therapy), reasoning cures (Ellis' rational therapy), realism cures (Glasser's reality therapy), orgasm cures (Reich's orgone therapy), profound-rest cures (transcendental meditation), and even chemical cures (megavitamin therapy). Thus psychiatry represents neither pure science nor pure ethics, but a branch of the healing professions that resides somewhere in between and that often may be affected by culture, chance, and faith.

Despite these ambiguities, each mental health professional must identify his own professional commitment. Is he committed to the happiness of the individual or the smooth functioning of society? Ideally, these values should not conflict, but in reality they sometimes do. The patient's rights to treatment, to refuse treatment, and to informed consent highlight this conflict-of-interest question. As a nurse, one must consider if one is forcing a patient to be socially or politically acceptable at the expense of his personal happiness. The nurse may not be working for either the patient's best interests or her own; she may be acting as an agent of society and not be aware of it.

All nurses participate in some therapeutic psychiatric regimens whose scientific and ethical bases are ambiguous. The American health care system continues to apply a medical model of wellness and illness to human behavior. Wellness is socially acceptable behavior, and illness is socially unacceptable. It becomes critically important for each nurse to analyze such ethical dilemmas as freedom of choice versus coercion, helping versus imposing values, and focusing on cure versus prevention. She must also become active in defining adequate treatment and deciding resource allocations.

■ Ethical decision making

Ethical decision making involves trying to determine right from wrong in situations without clear guidelines.

Everything is neither right nor wrong. The right or wrong is the choosing, the keeping, the losing. All paths are light and shadow, and every path is a different thing to each man. The right and the wrong, the good and the evil lie not upon the silent pathway, but in the man that walks it.[33:198]

There are three dimensions to ethical decision making, each of which influences one's analysis of the dilemma and related decisions:

1. The existence of a code of value judgments or ethics that one knows about
2. The awareness of one's personal moral beliefs and values
3. A complex social and legal context

The nurse should relate the code of nursing ethics to his or her own personal value system and identify areas of similarity and difference. This will allow the nurse to base ethical decisions on behavior that involves responsibility, accountability, risk, and commitment. Responsibility requires the capacity for rational, moral decision making. Accountability signifies action. Risk involves taking the chance of peril, jeopardy, or loss, and commitment implies loyalty, trust, and a pledge of self. In addition, the nurse's ethical choice must consider the circumstances, social customs, and any legal ramifications.

■ MODEL FOR ETHICAL DECISION MAKING.

A decision-making model can help identify factors and principles that affect a decision. Curtin[10] proposed

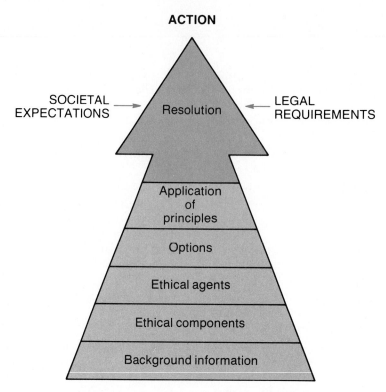

Fig. 7-3. Model for ethical decision making. Societal expectations and legal requirements may sway the resolution of the conflict one way or another. However, one must not confuse the notions of what is legal (or expected) with what is good, right, or proper—they may or may not coincide. (From Curtin L: Nurs Forum 17:12, 1978.)

a model for critical ethical analysis (Fig. 7-3), which describes steps or factors that the nurse should consider in resolving an ethical dilemma. The first step is **gathering background information** to obtain a clear picture of the problem. This includes finding available information to clarify the underlying issues. The next factor is **identifying the ethical components** or the nature of the dilemma, such as freedom versus coercion or treating versus accepting the right to refuse treatment. The next step is the **clarification of the rights and responsibilities of all ethical agents,** or those involved in the decision making. This can include the patient, the nurse, and possibly many others, including the patient's family, physician, health care institution, clergy, social worker, and perhaps even the courts. Those involved may not agree on how to handle the situation, but their rights and duties can be clarified. **All possible options must then be explored** in light of everyone's responsibilities, as well as the purpose and potential result of each option. This step eliminates those alternatives that violate rights or seem harmful. The nurse then engages in the **application of**

principles, which stem from her philosophy of life and nursing, her scientific knowledge, and her ethical theory. Ethical theories suggest ways to structure ethical dilemmas and judge potential solutions. Here are four possible approaches[4]:

1. **Utilitarianism** focuses on the consequences of actions. It seeks the greatest amount of happiness or the least amount of harm for the greatest number: "the greatest good for the greatest number."

2. **Egoism** is a position in which one seeks the solution that is best for oneself. The self is most important, and others are secondary.

3. **Formalism** considers the nature of the act itself and the principles involved. It involves the universal application of a basic rule, such as "do unto others as you would have them do unto you."

4. **Fairness** is based on the concept of justice, and benefit to the least advantaged in society becomes the norm for decision making.

The final step is **resolution into action.** Within the context of social expectations and legal requirements, the nurse decides on the goals and methods of implementation. Table 7-5 summarizes these steps and suggests questions nurses can ask themselves in making complex ethical choices in psychiatric nursing practice.

TABLE 7-5

STEPS AND QUESTIONS IN ETHICAL DECISION MAKING

Steps	Relevant questions
Gathering background information	Does an ethical dilemma exist? What information is known? What information is needed? What is the context of the dilemma?
Identifying ethical components	What is the underlying issue? Who is affected by this dilemma?
Clarification of agents	What are the rights of each involved party? What are the obligations of each involved party? Who should be involved in the decision making? For whom is the decision being made? What degree of consent is needed by the patient?
Exploration of options	What alternatives exist? What is the purpose or intent of each alternative? What are the potential consequences of each alternative?
Application of principles	What criteria should be used? What ethical theories are subscribed to? What scientific facts are relevant? What is one's philosophy of life and nursing?
Resolution into action	What are the social and legal constraints and ramifications? What is the goal of one's decision? How can the resulting ethical choice be implemented? How can the resulting ethical choice be evaluated?

Future challenges

The interface between psychiatry and the law is becoming increasingly complex. Historically, the mental health delivery system had only two components—mental health professionals and patients. Now, however, the system has grown to include five forces, each of which must be taken into account when dealing with any mental health problem. Kopolow[15] describes this five-sided relationship (Fig. 7-4) as consumers, providers of services, governmental regulators and lawmakers, the judiciary, and third-party insurers. These groups have related, but slightly different, interests. The consumer is concerned that services be available when and where he wishes them, that they are appropriate, and that he is involved in establishing their priorities. The provider has clinical and professional biases. If outside controls must exist, the provider wants them applied fairly, with responsibilities and liabilities clearly defined. The government wants citizens to have quality care at the lowest cost and wants providers to be accountable for their care. The courts, after years of neglect, are focusing on patients' constitutional rights and have begun to scrutinize patient care and treatment. Finally, insurance companies are concerned with making a profit by paying for covered services by appropriately licensed and credentialed professionals. The changing priorities and interactions of these five forces affect the quality, availability, and responsiveness of mental health services in the United States.

At present there are simultaneous trends toward adequate treatment of the psychiatrically ill and protection of their constitutional rights. Both trends are emerging at a time of fiscal restraint. It would appear as if one's choice is between abandoning former pa-

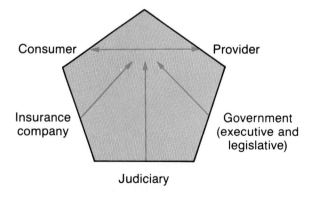

Fig. 7-4. Pentagonal relationship that characterizes the mental health delivery system. (From Kopolow L: Patient's rights and psychiatric practice. In Barton W and Sanborn C, editors: Law and the mental health professions, New York, 1978, International Universities Press, Inc.)

tients to their rights in the community or warehousing them in large institutions, whether these be hospitals or jails.[46]

Mental health professionals are concerned about the quantity and quality of psychiatric care. Legal reformers are indignant about patients' rights and object to a law that justifies commitment based on a single professional's prediction of some unproven harm. Criminal court judges are angry that in the day-to-day implementation of the commitment law, their only option is to prosecute the mentally ill defendant. Psychiatric hospitals are understaffed, underfunded, and attacked on all sides for their inability to "care for" and "cure" psychiatric patients. Community programs are few and poorly supported, often resulting in deinstitutionalized patients living without treatment in urban ghettos or being treated as criminals. The public is frightened at the thought of psychiatric patients in their neighborhoods. Concerned citizens demand that mental health programs exercise greater control over this population, whom they perceive as dangerous.

Clearly, mechanisms are needed by which patients, mental health professionals, attorneys, and concerned citizens can work together to advance mental health care and the rights of all patients. The mentally ill need not only protection of their legal rights, but also protection of their clinical needs and general welfare. No one profession can fulfill all these needs, but increased cooperation among the various mental health advocates can achieve this goal.

■ **Advocacy and patient education**

Mental health advocacy is evolving into one effective method for protecting the rights of all citizens to high-quality mental health care that is clinically and constitutionally appropriate. New Jersey, for example, has a Division of Mental Health Advocacy mandated by the state legislature that works to improve the delivery of mental health care. It is staffed by lawyers, psychologists, psychiatric nurses, social workers, and others who work as advocates for those caught in the psychiatric system. Minnesota, New York, Michigan, and California have adopted similar programs. The purpose of mental health advocacy is to ensure that both clinical and legal concerns are properly weighed. More and more it is considered a service to which patients are entitled.

Under the Protection and Advocacy for Mentally Ill Individuals Act of 1986, all states must designate an agency that is responsible for protecting the rights of the mentally ill. There are three areas of advocacy that would help to maximize the fulfillment of patients'

rights: (1) to educate the mental health staff and to implement policies and procedures that recognize and protect patients' rights; (2) to establish an additional procedure to permit the speedy resolution of problems, questions, or disagreements that occur based on legal rights; and (3) to provide access to legal services when a patients' rights have been denied.

While the advocacy movement has helped to bring about many positive changes in the health care system, it has also been criticized for inadequate definition of terms and irresponsibility. "Advocate," "legal representative," and "ombudsman" are often defined differently in different programs. "Legal advocacy" and "legal services" are also confused, and "information and advice" are often equated with "advocacy." Lamb has also noted that the patients' rights activist has power without clinical responsibility.[16] He cautions that major problems can result when power is wielded by people

DIRECTIONS FOR FUTURE RESEARCH

The following are some of the nursing research problems raised in Chapter 7 that merit further study.

1. Psychiatric nurses' knowledge of a patient's legal rights at the time of admission and during psychiatric hospitalization.
2. Psychiatric nurses' ability to evaluate the potential dangerousness of psychiatric patients.
3. Patients' rights most commonly violated in psychiatric settings.
4. Nursing interventions implemented with patients who refuse medication.
5. Litigation involving psychiatric nurses, including the number of cases, basis of the lawsuit, other persons named in the suit, and outcome.
6. Resolution of conflict of interest relative to the legal roles of the psychiatric nurse as provider, employee, and citizen.
7. The ethical dilemmas arising from psychiatric nurses' paternalistic attitude toward their patients.
8. The dimensions of the ethical decision-making process used by psychiatric nurses in critically analyzing ethical issues.
9. Psychiatric nurses' participation in formal and informal mental health advocacy programs.
10. Mechanisms used by psychiatric nurses to impact on mental health issues at the local, state, and national levels and identification of issues in which they are involved.

who do not understand the complex clinical needs of the severely mentally ill. Mental health professionals, therefore, must distinguish responsible advocacy from irresponsible lobbying. He suggests that advocates be required to have in-depth experience with severely disturbed patients for 6 months to a year and that advocates be rigorously screened.

It has been noted that the ratio of patients to prisoners is three to one. Does this mean that for every public defender there should be three mental health lawyers? Whether this becomes a reality, it is still possible to safeguard the rights of patients by (1) periodically reviewing those involuntarily committed, (2) considering the least restrictive setting when determining treatment, and (3) using more alternatives to hospitalization, including foster home and day treatment programs. States are being required to reorder their priorities at a time when many have been forced to cut their mental health budgets. One can only speculate on what the result will be.

In the Sixteenth Century the deranged were expelled, shipped off, or executed; in the Seventeenth Century the insane were locked up in jails and houses of correction; in the Eighteenth Century madmen were confined in madhouses; in the Nineteenth Century lunatics were sent to asylums; in the Twentieth Century the mentally ill are committed to hospitals; in the Twenty-first Century . . . .
K. Jones, *Lunacy, Law, and Conscience*

■ SUGGESTED CROSS-REFERENCES ■

This chapter serves as a foundation for formulating principles of psychiatric nursing and implementing psychiatric nursing practice. As such, it is related to all other chapters of this text.

■ SUMMARY ■

1. Informal admission to a psychiatric hospital occurs without formal or written application. The patient admitted in this way is free to leave at any time.

2. Voluntary admission requires the individual to make written application to a psychiatric hospital and agree to receive treatment and abide by hospital rules. If he wishes to be discharged, it is usually required that he give written notice to the hospital.

3. Involuntary admission means that the request for hospitalization did not originate with the patient, and when he is committed, he loses the right to leave the hospital when he wishes. It is usually justified on the grounds of (1) dangerous to others, (2) dangerous to self, or (3) need for treatment. The procedure for commitment includes filing a petition, completing a mental status examination, and determining the need for hospitalization, which can be a medical, court, or administrative decision.

4. The civil and personal rights of psychiatric patients are presently being supported in legislative acts throughout the United States. The nature of these rights varies greatly from state to state.

   a. The person's competency to execute wills is called the testamentary capacity. To make a valid will, it is required that he (1) know he is making a will, (2) know the nature and extent of his property, and (3) know who his friends and relatives are and how he is related to them.

   b. "Incompetency" is a legal term that must be proved in a special court hearing. To determine incompetency, it must be shown that the person has a mental disorder that causes a defect in judgment, and this defect makes him incapable of handling his own affairs. As a result of this ruling, he loses many of his civil rights. This can be reversed only in another court hearing that declares him competent.

   c. Habeas corpus is an important right all patients retain. It provides for the speedy release of any individual who can show he is being deprived of his liberty and detained illegally.

   d. The right to privacy implies the right to keep some information about oneself completely secret from others. "Confidentiality" involves disclosure of certain information to another specifically authorized person. "Privileged communication" applies only in court-related proceedings and must be established by law. At present, most states do not provide for privileged communication between nurses and patients.

   e. The right to informed consent requires that a physician explain the treatment to the patient, including its possible complications and risks. The patient's consent to it must imply competency, understanding, and volition. All unusual and experimental treatments require special permission.

   f. The rights to treatment, refuse treatment, and receive treatment in the least restrictive setting are recent developments that are being delineated in various court decisions.

5. The psychiatric nurse has rights and responsibilities attendant to each of three legal roles: nurse as provider, nurse as employee, and nurse as citizen. As a provider, every nurse is responsible for the quality of care she gives and can be held responsible in malpractice claims. For a nurse to be proved negligent, it must be shown that (1) a legal duty of care existed, (2) the nurse performed the duty negligently, (3) the patient suffered damages, and (4) the damages were substantial.

6. Criminal responsibility concerns the accused person's condition at the time of the alleged crime. At present, three tests are commonly used in the United States to determine criminal responsibility. These are the M'Naghten Rule, the Irresistible Impulse Test, and the American Law Institute's Test. A fourth test, the Durham Test, or "Product Rule," is seldom used.

7. An ethic is a standard of valued behavior or beliefs adhered to by an individual or group. It describes a goal to which one aspires. An ethical dilemma exists when moral claims conflict with one another. Ethical decision making involves trying to determine right from wrong in situations where clear guidelines are not evident. A model for critical ethical analysis was presented and discussed.

8. Five forces currently affect the mental health delivery system—the consumer, the provider, the government, the judiciary, and the insurance companies. The future must provide for independent, responsible, and collaborative approaches to advocacy so that it can become an effective mechanism for creating a more responsive mental health system.

■ **REFERENCES** ■

1. American Nurses' Association: Code for nurses with interpretive statements, Kansas City, Mo, 1976, The Association.
2. APA task force issues guidelines for use of selection and restraint in inpatient settings, Hosp Community Psych 36(6):677, 1985.
3. Arkin A et al: Behavior modification, NY State J Med 76:190, 1976.
4. Aroskar M: Anatomy of an ethical dilemma: the theory, Am J Nurs 80:658, 1980.
5. Birnbaum M: The right to treatment, Am Bar Assoc J, p 499, 1960.
6. Campazzi B: Nurses, nursing and malpractice litigation: 1967-1977, Adv Nurs Sci 4(1):1, 1980.
7. Chodoff P: The case for involuntary hospitalization of the mentally ill, Am J Psychiatry 133:496, 1976.
8. Creighton H: Law every nurse should know, Philadelphia, 1975, WB Saunders Co.
9. *Cross v Harris,* 418 F 2d (DC Cir 1969).
10. Curtin L: A proposed model for critical ethical analysis, Nurs Forum 17(1):12, 1978.
11. *Dixon v Weinberger,* No 74285 (CDDC Feb 14, 1974).
12. Ennis BJ: Civil liberties and mental illness, Criminal Law Bull, p 101, 1971.
13. Gert B and Culver M: Paternalistic behavior, Philos Pub Affairs 6:45, 1976.
14. Jones R: Street people and psychiatry: an introduction, Hosp Community Psychiatry 34(9):807, 1983 Suppl.
15. Kopolow L: Patients' rights and psychiatric practice. In Barton W and Sanborn C, editors: Law and the mental health professions, New York, 1978, International Universities Press, Inc.
16. Lamb R: Securing patients' rights—responsibly, Hosp Community Psychiatry 32(6):393, 1981.
17. Lambert R and Heston A, editors: The annals of the American Acadamy of Political and Social Science: the law and mental health, Beverly Hills, 1986, Sage Publications.
18. Law briefs, Time, p 44, July 6, 1981.
19. Lyons-Levine M, Levine M, and Susman J: Patient bill of rights: a survey of state statutes, Mental Dis Law Report 6(3):178, 1982.
20. Mental Health Systems Act, Report No 96-980, Amendment to Senate Bill 1177, Sept 23, 1980.
21. Miller R: Involuntary civil commitment of the mentally ill in the post-reform era, Springfield, Ill, 1987, Charles C Thomas.
22. Miller R and Fiddleman P: Outpatient commitment: treatment in the least restrictive environment? Hosp Community Psychiatry 35(2):147, 1984.
23. Moore R: Ethics in the practice of psychiatry: origins, functions, models and enforcement, Am J Psychiatry 135:157, 1978.
24. National Center for State Courts' guidelines for involuntary civil commitment, Mental Physical Dis Law Report 10(5), 1986.
25. National League for Nursing: Nursing's role in patient's rights, Pub No 11-1671, New York, 1977, The League.
26. Oran D: Judges and psychiatrists lock up too many people, Psychol Today 7:27, Aug 1973.
27. O'Sullivan A: Privileged communication, Am J Nurs 80:947, 1980.
28. Peck C: Current legislative issues concerning the right to refuse versus the right to choose hospitalization and treatment, Psychiatry 38:303, Nov 1975.
29. President's Commission on Mental Health: report to the president, vol I, Washington, DC, 1978.
30. Rapoport D and Parry J, editor: The right to refuse antipsychotic medication, Washington DC, The American Bar Association's Commission on the Mentally Disabled, 1986.
31. Rhoden N: The presumption for treatment: has it been justified? Law Med Health Care 13(2):65, 1985.
32. Rights of disabled persons in residential facilities, Mental Dis Law Report 3(5):348, 1979.
33. Rogers C: Nakao: Blackfoot philosophy, New York, 1972, Warner Books, Inc.
34. *Rogers v Okin,* 478, Fed Supp 1342, 1979.
35. Scheff T: Being mentally ill: a sociological theory, Chicago, 1966, Aldine Publishing Co.
36. Schmid D, Applebaum P, Roth L, and Lidz C: Confidentiality in psychiatry: a study of the patient's view, Hosp Community Psychiatry 34(4):353, 1983.
37. Schwartz H, Vingiano W, and Perez C: Autonomy and the right to refuse treatment: patient's attitudes after involuntary medication, Hosp Community Psychiatry 39(10):1049, 1988.
38. Spece R: Conditioning and other techniques used to 'treat'? 'rehabilitate'? 'demolish'? prisoners and mental patients, South Calif Law Rev, p 616, 1972.
39. Szasz T: Ideology and insanity, New York, 1970, Doubleday & Co, Inc.
40. Tancredi L and Clark D: Psychiatry and the legal rights of patients, Am J Psychiatry 129:328, 1972.
41. *Tarasoff v Regents of the University of California et al,* 529 p 2d 553.

42. Taub S: Psychiatric malpractice in the 1980s: a look at some areas of concern, Law Med Health Care 11(3):97, 1983.
43. Teplin L: The criminality of the mentally ill: a dangerous misconception, Am J Psych 142(5):593, 1985.
44. Torrey EF: Thirty years of shame, Policy Review 15:10, 1989.
45. 28 USCS Appendix 476, 1975.
46. Whitmer G: From hospitals to jails: the fate of California's deinstitutionalized mentally ill, Am J Orthopsychiatry 50(1):65, 1980.
47. Wilk R: Implications of involuntary outpatient commitment for community mental health agencies, Am J Orthopsych 58(4):580, 1988.
48. *Wyatt v Stickney*, 344, Fed Supp 373, 375, 1972.
49. *Youngberg v Romeo*, 102 Supreme Ct 2452, 1982.

■ ANNOTATED SUGGESTED READINGS ■

*Aroskar M: Anatomy of an ethical dilemma: the theory, the practice, Am J Nurs 80:658, 1980.

First describes the theory related to ethical dilemmas and decision making and then uses the theory to analyze a specific clinical dilemma. Application to practice particularly useful.

Chodoff P: The case for involuntary hospitalization of the mentally ill, Am J Psychiatry 133:496, 1976.

Examines three points of view on the question of involuntary hospitalization. Discusses an overreliance on the dangerousness standard and favors a return to use of medical criteria by psychiatrists.

Cournos F: Involuntary medication and the case of Joyce Brown, Hosp Community Psychiatry 40(7):736, 1989.

Describes the highly publicized case of a homeless woman who was hospitalized and contested her forced medication.

*Ethical guidelines for the Colorado Society of Clinical Specialists in Psychiatric Nursing, J Psychosoc Nurs 28(2,3,4,5),1990.

A series of four articles describing the work of psychiatric nurses in Colorado on patient's rights, confidentiality, accountability, and competence. Recommended reference for professional practice.

*Fromer M: Paternalism in health care, Nurs Outlook 29(5):284, 1981.

Contends that nurses, physicians, and administrators exhibit paternalism—the tendency to limit the patient's autonomy. One reason for this is the socialization process of nurses. Studious, analytical discussion of an important problem in psychiatric practice.

*Garritson S and Davis A: Least restrictive alternative: ethical considerations, J Psychosoc Nurs 21(12):17, 1983.

Critically evaluates how the principles and assumptions underlying the least restrictive alternative concept relate to the human rights versus human needs dilemma that confronts practitioners. Addresses rights, paternalism, autonomy, and needs.

*Gonzalez H: The consumer movement: the implications for psychiatric care, Perspect Psychiatr Care 14:186, 1976.

Briefly examines the consumer movement and its two major components: the consumer as consumer and the consumer as a provider of health care. Analyzes the implications of the consumer movement for health care providers in the delivery of psychiatric care. Thought-provoking article.

Kittrie N: The right to be different, Baltimore, 1971, Johns Hopkins University Press.

Describes the conflict between the humanitarian ideals of the therapeutic state and the practical results of the administration of criminal law. Examines the problems of mental illness, commitment, and due process and the future implications of implementing a therapeutic state. Particular attention devoted to delinquent youths, psychopaths, addicts, alcoholics, and methods of dealing with the population explosion. Provides advanced reading in this controversial area.

Kopolow L and Bloom H, editors: Mental health advocacy: an emerging force in consumers' rights, Rockville, Md, 1977, US Department of Health, Education and Welfare.

Seeks to stimulate interest in patient advocacy. Reviews major concepts in advocacy and describes statewide mental health–advocacy programs and unique judicial decision.Appendix includes a model state advocacy statute and an excellent bibliography.

*Laben J and MacLean C: Legal issues and guidelines for nurses who care for the mentally ill, ed 2, Thorofare, NJ, 1989, Charles B Slack.

Explores basic legal concepts in clear, concise language. Well-researched, authoritative reference discusses both issues and case decisions with application to nurses.

Means H: Criminal case number 16836: the State of Maryland vs Sherry Windt, The Washingtonian 38:102, 1978.

Describes the interplay between psychiatry and the law in a true case presentation of 16-year-old Sherry Windt, who killed her mother. Presents both legal and psychiatric records of the complex trial and psychiatric assessment. Invokes numerous questions regarding psychiatry and the law.

Plum K: Moving forward with deinstitutionalization: lessons of an ethical policy analysis, Am J Orthopsych 57(4):508, 1987.

Explores deinstitutionalization from an ethical viewpoint and applies moral principles to public policy. Excellent but advanced reading.

*Rabinow J: Where you stand in the eyes of the law, Nursing 89 15:34,1989.

Brief overview of important nursing and legal issues. Clearly presented.

*Saunders J and Du Plessis D: An historical view of right to treatment, J Psychosoc Nurs 23(9):12, 1985.

Analyzes the professional nurse's responsibilities in the right-to-treatment issue. Describesproviding active, individualized psychiatric treatment and monitoring the patient's environment, thus safeguarding the legal rights of the mentally ill.

Szasz T: Law, liberty, and psychiatry, New York, 1963, The Macmillan Co, Publishers.

Classic inquiry into the social and legal uses of psychiatry

*Asterisk indicates nursing reference.

attempts to show that psychiatry in the United States is often used to subvert traditional political guarantees of individual liberty. Describes many faults committed in the name of mental illness and proposes solutions for them. Considered a classic in its field.

Szasz T: Insanity: the idea and its consequences, New York, 1988, John Wiley & Sons.

Most recent work by this psychiatrist explores the social dimensions of mental illness and its consequences for the individual.

*Thorner N: Nurses violate their patients' rights, J Psychiatr Nurs 14:7, 1976.

Reports on a study conducted on the refusal of medication by patients. Reveales that medication refusals do not occur often in the psychiatric setting and that nurses deal with refusals by first using psychological methods. Also reports on nurses' inadequate knowledge of the patients' right to refuse medication and of the legal responsibility in medication administration.

*Veatch R and Fry S: Case studies in nursing ethics, Philadelphia, 1987, JB Lippincott.

Basic text reviewing ethical issues in nursing using a case study format. One chapter addresses the concerns of psychiatry.

*Winkler L and Fennell K: Values and nursing ethics: a bibliography, J Psychiatr Nurs 19(4):19, 1981.

Presents a complete bibliography of journal articles on values and nursing ethics.

*Witt P: Notes of a whistleblower, Am J Nurs 83:1649, 1983.

Personal story of a psychiatric nurse who saw abuse in her work setting and tried to resolve a legal and ethical dilemma.

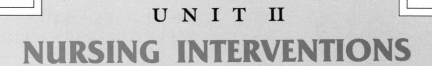

UNIT II
NURSING INTERVENTIONS

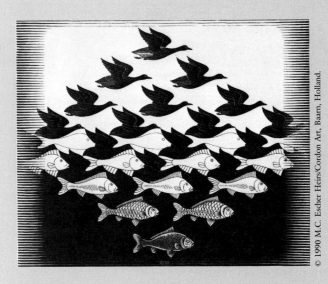

What is this thing called health?
Simply a state inwhich the individual
happens transiently to be perfectly
adapted to his environment. Obviously,
such states cannot be common, for the
environment is in constant flux.

H.L. Mencken, in the American Mercury, March 1930*

C H A P T E R 8

PREVENTIVE MENTAL HEALTH NURSING

© 1990 M.C. Escher Heirs/Cordon Art, Baarn, Holland.

LEARNING OBJECTIVES

After studying this chapter, the student should be able to:

- define primary, secondary, and tertiary prevention.

- compare and contrast the epidemiological, behavioral, and nursing paradigms of primary prevention.

- assess the vulnerability of the following groups to developing maladaptive coping responses: children and adolescents, new families, established families, women, mature adults, and the elderly.

- describe the levels of intervention and activities related to the following primary prevention nursing interventions: health education, environmental change, and supporting social systems.

- compare and contrast group psychotherapy, therapeutic groups, and self-help groups in relation to group goals, desired outcomes, and role of the nurse.

- assess the importance of evaluation of the nursing process when applied to primary prevention.

- identify directions for future research.

- select appropriate readings for further study.

Many people regard prevention of mental disorders as a desirable goal that should be actively pursued. Although this may seem obvious, in fact, the issues of prevention are complex and controversial. Caplan discussed basic concepts underlying preventive mental health endeavors in his classic work, *Principles of Preventive Psychiatry.*[9] He applies the three levels of preventive intervention from the public health model to mental illness and emotional disturbance. He defined **primary prevention** as lowering the *incidence* of mental disorders or reducing the rate at which new cases of a disorder develop. **Secondary prevention** involves reducing the *prevalence* of a disorder by reducing its duration. Secondary prevention activities for control of a disorder include early case finding, screening, and prompt effective treatment. **Tertiary prevention** activities attempt to reduce the *severity* of a disorder and associated disability.

Currently the major thrust in the United States is in secondary prevention activities or the treatment of mental disorders. This is evident in the allocation of economic resources, the nature of caregiving organizations and institutions, and the characteristic activities of psychiatric professionals. Specifically, in 1985 the National Institute of Mental Health (NIMH) was re-organized and established biomedical research of serious mental illnesses as the institute's highest priority. Part of the reorganization included the elimination of the Office of Prevention. One result of this change was a decrease in NIMH's emphasis on primary prevention activities in its funded research initiatives.

Tertiary prevention is evident in rehabilitative activities that often reflect a chronically ill patient group. This group is underserved and undervalued. Although it represents a substantial number of the mentally ill, this group and their needs appear to have a low priority within American society. Chapter 10 examines the area of tertiary prevention in more depth.

Although primary prevention is often espoused with such slogans as "An ounce of prevention is worth a pound of cure" or "Curing is costly—prevention, priceless," it has yet to evolve as a substantial force in the mental health movement. This is partly because of the fuzziness of the concepts and definitions underlying the issues. For example, primary prevention programs may be aimed at an entire population or only at persons believed to be at high risk for developing a disorder. This depends on how one views primary prevention in general—is it disease prevention or health promotion? There also needs to be agreement on what one is promoting or preventing to best determine what action should be taken.

Conceptualizing primary prevention

The idea of promoting mental health in general is an attractive one. Promotion sounds optimistic and positive. It is consistent with the idea of self-help and taking responsibility for one's own health. It implies changing human behavior and draws on a holistic approach to health. A continuing problem, however, with the strategy of promoting mental health is the vastness and vagueness of its goals. Theoretically, everything has implications for primary prevention, for reducing emotional disorders, and for strengthening and fostering mental health. Thus goals are often ill defined, and evaluation of promotion activities is difficult. Even if goals of a project can be identified and measured, their relation to long-term goals and behavior is questionable. For example, successfully teaching coping skills to schoolchildren may attain one's short-term goals, but what this precisely means for their mental health as adults is unclear and unsupported by empirical evidence.

■ Epidemiological prevention paradigm

Another problem is that there is basic disagreement on what is important in understanding and preventing mental disorders. One group of mental health professionals favors the genetic-biochemical explanation that each mental disease has a separate physical cause. The prevention model they favor focuses narrowly on genetic counseling and on biochemical and brain research to discover the specific causes of mental illness. They argue that there is no real proof that social stresses cause mental illness, and that the high rate of mental illness among the poor may be because disturbed people tend to "drift downward" from the upper and middle classes into poverty.

Lamb and Zusman, in a critique of primary prevention, state this view boldly:

> The cause and effect relationship between social conditions and mental illness is extremely questionable. In the area of mental health, most—if not all—successful primary preventive activities have been aimed at specific diseases. In contrast to the situation in large areas of physical illness, there is no evidence that it is possible to strengthen "mental health" and thereby increase resistance to mental illness by general preventive activities. Despite massive efforts to combat poverty (at least partly in the name of mental health), to increase social welfare and Social Security benefits, and to change the educational systems and methods of child rearing, there is no indication of a decrease in frequency of any of the functional

mental illnesses. Nor is there obvious evidence that other countries with stronger social welfare systems and different child-rearing practices have different rates of mental illness. Thus, as far as we can see, the major functional mental illnesses (as well as the very frequent diagnosable minor illnesses) remain untouched by primary prevention in the sense of trying to strengthen mental health.[35:13]

This suggests that primary prevention activities are perhaps best focused on illness prevention. Viewing mental illness as a disease in the medical model perspective allows one to use the classic, epidemiological paradigm in primary prevention. This paradigm consists of the following steps:

1. Identify a disease of sufficient importance to justify the development of a preventive intervention program. Develop reliable methods for its diagnosis so that people can be divided into groups according to whether they do or do not have the disease.
2. By a series of epidemiological and laboratory studies identify the most likely theory of that disease's path of development.
3. Launch and evaluate an experimental preventive intervention program based on the results of those research studies.[2:182]

This paradigm has been effective for a broad array of communicable diseases, such as smallpox, typhus, malaria, diphtheria, tuberculosis, rubella, and polio, and nutritional diseases, such as scurvy, pellagra, rickets, kwashiorkor, and endemic goiter. It has also proved useful in a variety of mental disorders caused by poisons, chemicals, licit or illicit drugs, electrolyte imbalances, and nutritional deficiencies. All these diseases have one thing in common. For each, there is a known necessary, although not always sufficient, causative agent.

■ Behavioral prevention paradigm

A contrasting view of the causes and prevention of mental illness is presented by mental health professionals who support a social-learning model. In this model mental disorders are believed to result from faulty early learning of social coping skills, from low levels of competence, from low self-esteem, and from poor support systems interacting with high levels of stress. This viewpoint stresses that mental disorders do not appear to have a single identified precondition and may have causative factors that are multiple, interactive, situational, and sociocultural in nature. They thus require that prevention of mental illness be conceptualized in a more behavioral way as the prevention of problems or maladaptive responses. This view calls for prevention of the following:

1. **Specific behaviors** that are self-defeating or harmful to others, such as poor or unhealthy habits, overeating, procrastinating, evasiveness, blaming others, and "setting the stage" to fail
2. **Role failures,** as a student, a parent, or an employee
3. **Relationship breakdowns** between husband and wife, parent and child, boss and employee, including detection and control of interpersonal "games" that are destructive
4. **Feeling overreactions,** such as panics, new situation anxiety, flights, and temper tantrums
5. **Psychological disabilities,** such as the social deterioration of a confined ill person, decompensation, "going to pieces," or falling into melancholia instead of experiencing normal grieving

With such a conceptualization, many of the services already given in the community by mental health and other helping agencies can be identified and publicly acknowledged as prevention efforts.[28:41-48]

By defining problems in this way they can include both single-episode events, such as a divorce, or a long-standing condition, such as marital conflict. They can also reflect either an acute health problem or a chronic health problem. For example, Room[52] has identified the following categories of problems that can arise from the abuse of alcohol:

1. Acute health problems, such as overdose or delirium tremens
2. Chronic health problems, such as cirrhosis or head or neck cancer
3. Casualties, such as accidents on the road, in the home or elsewhere, and suicide
4. Violent crime and family abuse
5. Problems of demeanor, such as public drunkenness and use of alcohol by teenagers
6. Default of major social roles—work or school and family roles
7. Problems of feeling state—demoralization and depression and experienced loss of control

This conceptualization requires the use of a new paradigm for primary prevention, which has been developed by Bloom.[5] It assumes that problems are multicausal, that everyone is vulnerable to stressful life events, and that any disability or problem may arise as a consequence of them. For example, four vulnerable persons can face a stressful life event—perhaps the collapse of their marriage or the loss of their job. One person may become severely depressed, the second may be involved in an automobile accident, the third may head down the road to alcoholism, and the fourth may develop a psychotic thought disorder or coronary artery disease. This behavioral paradigm does not search for a cause for each problem. Rather, it attempts to reduce the incidence of stressful life events as outlined in the following steps:

1. Identify a stressful life event that appears to have undesirable consequences in a significant proportion of the population. Develop procedures for reliably identifying persons who have undergone or who are undergoing that stressful experience.
2. By traditional epidemiological and laboratory methods, study the consequences of that event and develop hypotheses related to how one might reduce or eliminate the negative consequences of the event.
3. Launch and evaluate experimental preventive intervention programs based on these hypotheses.[5:183]

This paradigm shifts attention from nonspecific predisposing factors of mental illness to more discrete and identifiable precipitating stressors. These factors may be single-episode life events, such as loss of a job, or more long-term life event stressors, such as job dissatisfaction. Narrowing the focus of the study in this way allows one to limit the population at risk and use financial and program resources more wisely.

■ **Nursing prevention paradigm**

It is possible to identify the specific dimensions needed for nurses to engage in primary prevention activities based on the nursing model of health-illness phenomena used in this text. It would involve the systematic application of the nursing process with a focus on the primary prevention of maladaptive health responses associated with an identified stressor. This would incorporate the following aspects:

1. *Assessment.* **Identification of a stressor that precipitates maladaptive responses and a target or vulnerable population group that is at high risk in relationship to it.**
2. *Planning.* **Elaboration of specific strategies of prevention and relevant social institutions and situations through which the strategies may be applied.**
3. *Implementation.* **Application of selected nursing interventions aimed at decreasing maladaptive responses to the identified stressor and enhancing adaptation.**
4. *Evaluation.* **Determining the effectiveness of the nursing interventions with regard to short- and long-term outcomes, use of re-**

sources, and comparison with other prevention strategies.

The nursing process can thereby be used in a goal-directed way to decrease the incidence of mental illness and promote mental health among individuals, families, groups, and communities.

Assessment

Three types of primary prevention programs have been identified by Bloom: community-wide, milestone, and high-risk.[6] In a community-wide program, the target group is all people living within a specified geographic area. The people receiving intervention are not selected on a case-by-case basis but rather are included based on geographic considerations. In a milestone program, residents of a community become the target of an intervention at a particular point in the life cycle. Examples of such programs include those aimed at women who are pregnant for the first time and preschool screening programs whose goals are to identify and provide effective intervention for children who may be at risk for emotional or learning problems in later years. The third type of primary prevention program is a high-risk program in which specific individuals or groups are identified as being at increased risk for certain conditions and become the target of an intervention program.

While all people and all families face similar developmental tasks, not everyone adapts to them or copes with them positively. Individuals or groups in our society have additional stressors placed on them, inadequate coping resources, and fewer positive experiences to balance out their perceived stress. These people and groups are thus particularly vulnerable or at high risk for developing maladaptive responses. It is extremely helpful if the nurse has an awareness of these vulnerable people. The increased sensitivity that results from this awareness will affect the nurse's assessment of both existing and potential problems and actual work with people from these high-risk groups. Nurses, as the largest group of health care providers, can make a significant impact in promoting mental health if they would anticipate problems and commit their time and skill to preventing their occurrence.

Assessment in primary prevention therefore involves identifying groups of people who are vulnerable to developing mental disorders or maladaptive coping responses to specific stressors or risk factors. To complete such an assessment, the nurse needs to draw on information generated from theory, research, and clinical practice. Some of these vulnerable groups will now be briefly described. Each group could merit, in itself, a separate chapter or perhaps a textbook. The intent of this discussion, however, is to highlight the unique ways in which some people are particularly vulnerable to maladaptive responses.

It should also be noted that these are not the only high-risk groups for developing mental disorders. The actual identification of vulnerable groups depends on one's geography and life experiences. And not all individuals within these groups are at equal risk. What these groups do share, however, is the experience of a life event, stressor, or risk factor that represents a loss of some kind or places an excessive demand on the ability to cope. These broad categories are intended to help one conceptualize common stressful experiences. Using them in clinical research or practice would require further specification of a particular subgroup within these broad categories based on a particular stressor or risk factor. The more clearly the subgroup can be defined, the more specifically the prevention strategies can be researched, identified, and implemented.

■ Children and adolescents

The mental health needs of children are noteworthy. Recent studies suggest that between 17% and 22% (11 to 14 million children) suffer from some type of diagnosable mental disorder. The most conservative estimate is that 12% of the 63 million children and adolescents in the United States suffer from clinical maladjustment. Of the nearly 7.5 million youngsters, nearly half are presumed to be severely handicapped by their mental disorder.[29] In less severe cases, the young person may have difficulty coping with the demands of school, family, and community life.

Many adult problems have their origins in childhood. Childhood and adolescence are periods for learning coping skills, and the success in achieving such skills can have profound effects throughout life. Childhood conditions that merit a primary prevention effort are presented in the box on page 242. Some of these problems probably result from a dysfunction in the biological development and organization of the brain. Others may result from major stressors beyond the child's control. Regardless, they must be viewed from the most holistic nursing perspective because they occur in the context of the fragile relationships of a child's genetic makeup, mental development, physical health, and family and social environment.

The identification of children at risk for developing a mental disorder is very important for both the implementation of preventive intervention programs and the adequate distribution of clinical resources. Among children who are at risk are those whose par-

Childhood Conditions Meriting Primary Prevention Intervention

1. Antisocial behavior
   a. Physical aggressiveness (e.g., fighting, wanton destructiveness, robbery)
   b. Other antisocial behaviors (e.g., truancy, running away, petty theft)
2. Learning disorders
3. Mental retardation
4. Childhood schizophrenia
5. Suicide
6. School failure
7. Child abuse and neglect (including sexual abuse)
8. Severe neurotic disorders
9. Psychiatric sequelae of chronic medical illness

ents are mentally ill or substance abusing, children with chronic medical illnesses, children living in foster care, Native American children from certain tribes, children in families living on welfare, and homeless children. Each of these high-risk groups have rates of mental disorders far exceeding those of the general population.

Other risk factors include prolonged parent-child separation and lack of consistent caretakers, living in crowded, inner-city neighborhoods, physical or sexual abuse, catastrophic events, bereavement, and marital discord or instability in the family environment. Internal factors leading to increased risk of childhood mental disorders include low birth weight, developmental delay, brain damage, epilepsy, early difficulties with temperment, and mental retardation. Each of these factors increases the risk of developing a mental disorder, and many of them tend to occur in combination.

Less is known about factors that protect children and make them more resilient even when exposed to adversity. Potential protective factors include good problem-solving abilities, good social skills, a warm, caring relationship with an adult, and positive experiences outside the home.

Adolescence poses its own set of challenges and stressors. It is an accepted time of great biological, psychological, and social change. Many demands are placed on the young person, and not all adolescents have sufficient resources to cope with them. One usual resource of the adolescent, the peer group, can actually become a stressor by pressuring the young person to participate in experiences, such as drugs or sex, not in his or her best interests. Concerns about sex typing and homosexuality may develop at this time, as do questions about contraception, pregnancy, abortion, and sexually transmitted disease.

Late adolescence may be a time of moving away from home, making an initial career choice, or becoming involved in advanced schooling. All of these events may lead to questions about independence, motivation, competence, control, and capacity for intimacy. The need to develop intimate psychosocial relationships with others may be a major source of stress even though it is considered a normal developmental task. Many questions and insecurities may surround the issues of marriage, selecting a mate, conjoint living, and shared decision making. Each of these demands may combine and compound adolescents' level of stress. If this occurs and their coping resources are not adequate, this group will be highly vulnerable to the development of maladaptive responses.

Reporting the many studies and statistics pertaining to this high-risk group is beyond the scope of this chapter. However, the problems are self-evident in the large numbers of adolescent suicides, runaways, drug abusers, and school failures, and the tremendous problems posed by juvenile prostitution, unwanted pregnancies, delinquency, and crime. These problems are discussed in Chapter 31.

■ New families

The family poses opportunities for primary prevention. In a society beset with stress and rapid change, the stability and smooth functioning of the family cannot be taken for granted. Issues such as working mothers, divorce, and single-parent families have ramifications for nursing as does the broader area of parenting.

The stress involved in decisions regarding children, conception, birth, and the parental role has been well documented in both the professional literature and popular press. The decision whether or not to have children has become increasingly complex with recent changes in American society. Women now may have more extensive career options, less geographical proximity to their own families of origin, more earning potential, greater medical technology available, changing sex-role perceptions, and a more frequently used option to have children later in adulthood. However, these changes may be at odds with the cultural norms or personal beliefs of the couple. Rather than serving to increase one's options, they may instead create conflict and dissonance. How the couple copes with this stress has far-reaching implications for their health and that of their children.

Clearly new parents are at high risk for developing maladaptive responses. Bieber and Bieber[4] describe a psychiatric syndrome that often appears in both men and women in the first year after the birth of a child. Signs and symptoms include combinations of acute anxiety, depression, psychosomatic disorders, changes in affectional responses toward the spouse, changes in sexual behavior, the onset of various types of frigidity in the woman, potency difficulties in the man, an apparent loss of interest in the marriage, and the first involvement in extramarital relations, often leading to divorce. Pregnancy thus sets in motion a series of changes and stressors that challenge the coping resources of the man and woman and can result in either adaptive or maladaptive responses.

■ **MOTHERS.** The transition to motherhood is a stressful period for women of all ages. Pregnancy and the postpartum period are generally regarded as maturational crises for women equal in importance to those of adolescence and midlife. Stressors undergone during this period include the following:

1. Endocrine changes
2. Changes in body image
3. Activation of psychological conflicts pertaining to pregnancy
4. Intrapsychic reorganization of becoming a mother

The result of these stressors is often depression of varying intensity during pregnancy and after delivery. In some cases postpartum psychosis may develop. Studies indicate that approximately 10% of pregnant women describe being depressed during pregnancy and 20% to 40% report feeling depressed or have other signs of emotional distress. Psychotic disorders occur less often but are associated with greater impairment.

It is possible to identify women who may be at risk for developing depression during pregnancy or in the postpartum period.[18] Nurses should be aware that recent research suggests that depression appears to be as prevalent during pregnancy as it is in the postpartum period. In addition, pregnant women who are relatively young, who are not well-educated, who already have children at home, and who are not employed outside the home are at increased risk for developing depression. Understanding these risk factors will allow the nurse an opportunity to assess and plan early interventions to promote the expectant mother's mental and physical health.

■ **FATHERS.** The response of men to pregnancy and fatherhood has most often been described in the literature in terms of the benefits of parental involvement to father, mother, and infant. Little attention has been given to their more problematic responses, despite the fact that both minor emotional reactions and severe reactions are common. For example, Lacoursiere[34] reported that about 2% of hospitalized patients with a diagnosis of paranoid psychosis developed symptoms in relation to fatherhood. Another interesting study found that one of the most important factors in female maladjustment to pregnancy was rejection of the pregnancy by the husband or father of the child.[26]

Yet, if one views childbirth as a maturational crisis, it must serve as a stressor for the man as well as the woman. For both, it is a time to recapitulate some of the developmental problems of earlier phases. The following variables have been suggested as significant instigators of psychopathological reactions in men: increased financial responsibility, triggering of latent homosexual conflicts by restriction of heterosexual opportunities during the prenatal period, rearousal of unacceptable childhood anger toward parents or siblings, reactivation of unresolved oedipal conflict, and frustration of dependency demands as the wife's attention is diverted to the baby's needs.

■ **INFANTS.** The mental health of parents directly affects the health of the infant. This is demonstrated in a study by Nuckolls, Cassel, and Kaplan,[48] which found that the proportion of women having pregnancy and birth complications was significantly higher among those women who had experienced a high frequency of life changes accompanied by a low degree of social-emotional support during their pregnancies. When social support was high, there was no increase in complications. Conflict over the acceptance of pregnancy has been associated with increased length of the labor process, as well as increased levels of maternal anxiety. The degree of wantedness of the pregnancy has been associated with increased risk of low birth weight. Cobb[11] cites several studies showing that wanted children tend to adapt to or cope with the stresses of growing up better than do those who began life under circumstances where parental preference had been abortion. Wanted children fared better in terms of the decreased incidence of juvenile delinquency and need for psychiatric treatment and were better able to adapt to the school socialization and educational achievement processes.

Another dimension of stress in this high-risk group is related to the bonding and attachment process and the development of parent-child relationships. Stressors related to childbirth can place the family at risk for child maltreatment. A number of circumstances, including a medically abnormal pregnancy, difficult labor or delivery, neonatal separation, other separations in the first 6 months, illnesses in the infant during the first year of life, and maternal illness during the first year of life all place a family at risk for child maltreatment. Threats to the parent-infant bond are particularly dangerous. In one study,[40] 66% of abused children experienced 48-hour separations from their parents in the first week of life, whereas only 3% of those same children's siblings had been separated. Medically high-risk infants are particularly in danger. In a study[33] of 146 infants who had been in an intensive care nursery, a lack of parental visits was associated with the likelihood of later maltreatment.

Although these results are not definitive, when combined with other research findings they are persuasive. Disruption in parent-infant bonding predicts greater risk for maltreatment. Where the mother has an active role and high status in the childbirth process, there are fewer medical complications, less resort to medications that suppress infant functioning, fewer cesarean section deliveries, and fewer induced labors. These, in turn, positively influence the child and may serve to reduce the risk of child maltreatment.

■ **ROLE TRANSITIONS.** The abuse and neglect of children are evidence of parental difficulty in assuming the maternal or paternal role. Both roles are assumed through a complex social and cognitive learning process. They are not intuitive, nor are they universally present in couples who have given birth. Many variables have been identified as affecting the maternal role. Mercer[42] identifies these as age, perceptions of the birth experience, early maternal-infant separation, support system, self-concept and personality traits, maternal illness, child-rearing attitudes, infant temperament, infant illness, and socioeconomic status. Although all of these variables have been described in the literature, there is no evidence that one variable is most predictive or how they interact to account for variance in the maternal role. The nursing framework proposed by Mercer for studying these variables is necessary to guide research projects that can identify stressors and suggest prevention strategies.

A similar nursing research paradigm has been developed by Cronenwett and Kunst-Wilson[14] for the transition to fatherhood. They believe that a separate paradigm for fathers is necessary because the experience of becoming a parent differs for men and women, and the stress associated with becoming a father is least understood. The framework they propose for understanding the processes involved in a man's transition to fatherhood includes many variables and can help stim-

ulate further research. More precise knowledge of the nature of the stress and the intervening variables that promote adaptation will be necessary for the nurse to actively work to prevent potential problems.

Three other subgroups of new parents may also be particularly vulnerable in their role transitions: teenage parents, unwed parents, and the parents of adopted children. Pregnancy in adolescence brings together two maturational crises, each of which compounds the problems of the other. At this time, the adolescent has not yet achieved his or her own sense of identity and independence and yet must assume the role of parent for an infant who is totally dependent. The unwed mother experiences to some degree a lack of coping resources that may include social support, financial assistance, and shared care-taking responsibilities. The stressor of parenthood thus makes excessive demands on one's coping ability.

Stress is also experienced by parents throughout the process of adoption. The parents who are not able to conceive their own child have undergone an extensive period of testing, waiting, hoping, and accepting one's physiological limitations. Once the decision to adopt has been made, a long waiting period usually follows. The actual arrival of an adopted child requires a readjustment of roles and family dynamics. In addition, the relatively recent phenomena of surrogate mothers may initiate changes and problems that are new to the couple and society at large.

■ **Established families**

The family unit is of critical importance. It continues to be a primary personal and cultural institution that has undergone major and minor structural changes in response to the larger social environment. The majority of Americans continue to seek and contract marriages, desire and have children, and live in households independent of the nuclear family. Important changes have also occurred. Because of increased longevity and fertility control, the "shape" of the family life cycle has changed, so that parenting no longer dominates most of the family's life cycle. Raising a family may occupy only half or a third of a couple's married life. In addition, today over 50% of American mothers work outside the home. Of married women with school-age children, two thirds are employed. The employment of married women thus appears to be an accepted and perhaps even expected social pattern because of economic and personal fulfillment needs. A final important change is the increasing divorce rate, which has given rise to single-parent families. It is estimated that one out of four children lives in a single-parent home. Although maternal custody has been the predominant pattern in separation and divorce, paternal custody is becoming more common, and joint custody of children has emerged as an alternative. Remarriage is also increasing, with the result that families may have stepparents, stepchildren, and multiple sets of grandparents.

Although these changes may not necessarily be destructive in themselves, they do place demands on the family's functioning and create a more complex set of needs. For example, all parents need some relief from their child and home care responsibilities. Often these needs can be met through an evening out or an informal arrangement with families and friends. However, in families in which both parents work, child care that is consistent, dependable, and high quality becomes a necessity.

Another type of family at high risk for developing problems is the one in which there is lack of knowledge of effective parenting. Because parenting is not an established course in educational curriculum and families are more geographically mobile, it is not surprising that this need has emerged. Yet one's child-rearing practices do have a significant effect on one's children and even future generations.

Pratt[50] has observed that the use of the developmental style of child rearing (reasons, information, rewards, and autonomy) tends to be more effective than disciplinary methods in assisting children to develop resources and capacities for coping, learning, and self-care. Maladaptive behaviors associated with the strongly disciplinary style of child rearing have been identified as social aggressiveness, hostility, and dependency in boys and regressiveness, fearfulness, and social withdrawal in girls. Studies have shown that, when parents have tended to be lax or inconsistent in the use of appropriate rules or controls, their children's failure to develop adequate coping mechanisms in early life can cause subsequent maladjustment in their neurophysical development and lead to lifelong patterns of psychosomatic and social complications.[31]

Numerous subgroups of families are under stress. Many of these high-risk family groups have been researched, analyzed, and reported on in both the popular literature and that of the psychiatric community. Although the potential problems are significant, there is a major deficit in programs to either prevent or alleviate them.

■ **DIVORCE.** The divorce rate in the United States has risen sharply in the past few years, provoking a crisis situation in many families and necessitating immediate intervention directed toward stress reduction. Although the increasing divorce rate is startling, attention is also directed toward the number of marriages that do not dissolve but rather maintain themselves in a constant state of disequilibrium. Of the 49 million married couples in the United States, nearly 80% of them are in their first marriage.

In contrast, about 1 million divorces have occurred annually in the United States. Between 1966 and 1976 the divorce rate doubled. Since then it has leveled off and even begun to decrease slightly.[1] There are many reasons for the increase in divorce, including changing social norms, new divorce laws, improved social and economic status of women, and improved methods of contraception. However, the recent high rates cannot be taken as a sign that marriage as an institution is dying. Rather, these rates reflect a new assertion of independence from unhappy or unsuccessful marriages. Such marriages have always existed, and in earlier years they were protected by stringent divorce laws, social stigma, financial pressures, large family size, and lack of equal opportunity for women. In light of the women's movement and other social changes, an outbreak of divorces occurred, revealing long-suppressed marital grievances and new expectations. The high divorce rate may decrease if couples start marriages later and on better foundation. It may be too soon to predict, but many of the social changes that led to high divorce rates may now contribute to stronger marriages and families in the future.

Divorce, one of the most traumatic crises a family faces, confronts each member with the task of examining and often changing his or her role in the family system. Although divorce is often a healthy step toward reestablishing family homeostasis, stress is involved. A body of knowledge is being accumulated regarding the reactions of both spouses and children to the experience. The first year after the divorce is particularly difficult. During this time, money constitutes a major source of stress as one household divides into two, each needing financial support. Women complain of feeling helpless and physically unattractive and of experiencing an acute loss of identity. On the other hand, men describe not knowing who they are, feeling as though they have no roots, structure, or predictable home life. Many divorced men buy sports cars and flashy clothes and plunge into a wide range of social activities to offset the loneliness.

Divorce therapy is gaining attention as a tool for primary prevention. The ultimate goal of divorce counseling or therapy is to help the couple disengage from their former relationship with a minimum amount of destructive and malicious behavior toward each other or their children. Divorce is dealt with as a family systems problem, which includes not only the immediate family but also the extended family. Each person in the family has an opinion about the situation and may need to lay blame on someone; each is affected by the family disruption.

One framework for understanding divorce moves through the stages of grief to explain reactions to the separation and loss. Regardless of how fraught a marriage is with frustration and conflict, it is never easy to terminate. Even painful relationships have meaning for the participants. Denial serves to shield the marriage partners from the reality of the separation and their subsequent loss, since it "buys" time for individuals to reconstruct coping abilities. In nursing intervention, denial is supported by listening to and helping the person describe his fear and dismay. Denial is transitory and is not supported when it becomes disproportionate to the actual situation.

Anger often follows denial and may be directed outwardly toward the ex-spouse or inwardly when it is manifested as depression. As the former partners are forced into new roles, they may feel helpless. Since helplessness causes a person to feel vulnerable, a common coping mechanism is to become angry and attempt to impose control on the situation.

Just as in the stages of grief, bargaining often follows anger. One or both spouses wonder if the marriage could have been saved "if I had just. . . ." Depression often occurs when one or both parties realize that the emotional investment they once had in a marriage no longer exists.

In the final stage, acceptance, the individual can move beyond regret and begin to make plans. Throughout the counseling, but particularly once acceptance begins, the primary nursing approach is problem solving, or application of the nursing process to assess, plan, and implement coping strategies.

A major issue in relation to divorce counseling is that of family roles. Traditional family roles are often disrupted as each spouse assumes responsibilities previously carried out or shared with the other partner. Men may assume responsibility for household maintenance when previously their wives handled this task. Women may be forced to support themselves and their children; for some, employment may constitute a major alteration in role.

Specific interventions are either child centered, relationship focused, or adult centered. Child-centered interventions assist the parents to understand and deal with their child's responses to divorce. Children are particularly at risk for mental health disruption during a divorce in that they are often caught in the middle of bitter parental battles, and visitation rights, custody, and child support can become bargaining issues. Children from divorced families also tend to constitute a

significant portion of the case loads in psychiatric facilities with common problems being depression, aggressive outbursts, or behavioral problems at school or in social groups. Some frequently observed age-specific responses to divorce and pertinent nursing interventions are given in Table 8-1.[32]

Relationship-centered interventions are used when knowledge of the child's growth and development is less an issue than is the ability of the parent to cope with the stress of divorce. Many parents become immobilized with their increased responsibility and the pressing need to make decisions and deal with the daily reactions of family members to the divorce. Children often get caught up in the parental conflict. Nursing intervention helps family members remain open and honest with one another and not use each other for harmful purposes.

Adult-centered counseling focuses on helping the partner who seeks counseling adapt to the new role and cope with the stresses implicit in a major life change. Even the most desperate marriage provides some security and division of labor. Women particularly need to examine their alternatives in advance of major decisions to make the best choice as they assume expanded roles, which often include financial support of self or family.

■ **ILLNESS.** Another major source of stress for all families is illness. The illness of one family member affects all other members and can result in maladaptive responses and a variety of pathological states. The premature birth of a child, the child born with a genetic defect, and the handicapped child all place great and unanticipated demands on the family. Parents of such children, and the children themselves, have special needs. Studies show that parental attitudes about having produced handicapped children vary widely (regret, denial, anger, and rejection), since these children may represent parental incompetence both to the parents themselves and to others. Parental coping patterns include the projection of false reports of progress, statements of grief, and the development of cynical acceptance of the disabilities.

Nurses are particularly aware that major and minor illnesses of family members take a significant toll. Illnesses requiring hospitalization and surgery precipitate multiple threats to the family unit. Adapting to a hyperactive child, an alcoholic parent, a psychotic sibling, or an arthritic spouse may be impossible without the extended use of outside resources.

A final well-documented stressor for the individual and family is the death of a family member. Bereavement and its sequelae have been studied in various forms—widows, widowers, stillborn death, death of a

TABLE 8-1

RESPONSES TO DIVORCE AND RELATED NURSING INTERVENTIONS

Behavior observed	Nursing intervention
Preschool Regression, confusion, irritability Difficulty understanding what is happening Repeatedly asks same questions (e.g., "Where is Daddy?" "When is Daddy coming home?")	Provide guidance to custodial parent who serves as child's best support person Teach communication skills related to interpreting meaning of divorce Examine alternatives for intervening in the child's regressive behavior
Early latency Often immobilized by parental separation Developmentally denial does not serve these children well, yet open confrontation with reality is traumatic Nearly insatiable need to maintain contact with both parents Anger (common reaction)	Open discussion may be too threatening; nurse might use a "divorce monologue" to talk about how other children react to divorce Focus on helping both parents support child's need for contact "Divorce monologue" may give child permission to express anger
Later latency Torn in loyalty toward parents Worries a great deal Can both express their feelings verbally and channel them into organized activities Superego controls may be threatened as external controls decrease because of stress	Encourage child to express fears and worries to parents Support child as he deals with pain and anger Encourage parents to be consistent and firm in approach
Adolescence Intense feelings of pain (anger, sadness, loss, and betrayal) Strong feelings of shame and embarrassment Concern about their own future as a marital partner Concern about adequacy as a sexual partner in their current dating, as well as for future married life Often unrealistic concern about finances Shortened disengagement from and shift in perceptions of parents Accelerated individuation from parents Heightened awareness of parents as sexual objects Loyalty conflicts Strategic withdrawal as a defense against pain	Provide an opportunity for open discussion of feelings, including helping them plan ways to express feelings directly and constructively Discuss feelings of shame, embarrassment, and fear of the future Use communication strategies, such as role playing or psychodrama to help adolescents learn to deal with feelings Practice improved, honest, open communication

Modified from Kelley J and Wallerstein J: Am J Orthopsychiatry 47:23, 1977.

parent, death of a child, sudden death, sudden infant death, and death after a protracted illness. Research in this area has led to the elaboration of the normal mourning or grieving process and the identification of strategies for anticipatory guidance, support systems, and preventive intervention (Chapter 14). Perhaps of all the vulnerable groups discussed in this chapter, the bereaved have been the focus of the most research and the most concrete prevention strategies. The task of adequately implementing these strategies remains to be done.

■ Women

In a descriptive nursing research study, Griffith analyzed broad areas of stress, common stress responses, and usual coping patterns of women according to age.[21,22] The stress categories and factors included in the study are presented in Table 8-2. One

TABLE 8-2

CATEGORIES AND FACTORS OF POTENTIAL STRESSORS EXPERIENCED BY WOMEN

Category	Factors
Love relationships	Being in love
	Satisfactory sex life
	Relationship with loved one
Personal success	Success in life
	Success in occupation/role
	Degree of recognition
	Personal growth and development
Physical health	Nutrition and eating patterns
	Physical attractiveness
	General health and physical condition
	Exercise and physical activity
Parent-child relationships	Being a parent
	Relationship with children
Personal time	Time to oneself
	Balance between work, family, leisure, home, and self
Social relationships	Relationships with close friends
	Relationships with co-workers
	Social life with significant others

From Griffith J: Women's stressors according to age group: part I, Issues in Health Care of Women, 6:311, 1983.

fourth of all women in the study reported that their physical health was a major stressor. Women between 25 and 34 years old indicated that personal time and personal success were also major stressors. For women over 35, physical health was the primary stressor, followed by personal time. Younger women were more likely to report physical and emotional symptoms of stress than older women. The physical symptoms most frequently reported included restlessness, sinus problems, frequent backaches and headaches, and trouble sleeping. Emotional responses to stress included feeling overweight, depression, nervousness, anxiety, sudden mood shifts, and irritability.

Women's usual coping patterns also vary with age. Younger women were more likely to talk with friends or associates about their problems, whereas older women relied on work or religion. Almost one third of the women in the study used consumption of food as a means of coping with their problems. These are significant findings because they document current physical and mental health care needs. Additional research is needed to identify effective ways to assist women in reducing their stress symptoms and developing more adaptive coping responses.

■ **MENTAL HEALTH NEEDS.** The mental health of women is intimately connected to the idea of equal-ity. Unfortunately our society is one of structured social inequality based on gender, race, and class differences. Women have a disadvantaged status in this society, which increases their vulnerability to stress and their potential for developing maladaptive responses. The status of women is summarized in the 1978 President's Commission on Mental Health:

1. **Salary.** More than half of all women are now employed outside of the home, but they are clustered in the lowest paying occupations and at the bottom of the achievement ladder. One woman in four compared to one man in 18 lives on an annual income of less than $4000.

2. **Dual roles.** Whether or not a woman is employed outside the home, housework remains largely "women's work." Thus many American women have two full workdays in every 24 hours.

3. **Politics.** Only about 3.5% of the House and 2% of the Senate of the United States and about 9% of the state legislators are women. This greatly reduces the political capacity of women to improve their status.

4. **Business.** It is still unusual to see women in the bastions of financial power and in high corporate echelons.

5. **Law.** In many states when a woman marries, she trades the rights of a person for the duties of a wife. A husband who deserts his wife and takes a temporary job in another state can seriously affect his wife's credit rating and her right to vote, serve on juries, run for office, and so on.[51:1027]

The Subpanel on the Mental Health of Women of this commission reported that circumstances and conditions that society accepts as normal and ordinary often lead to despair, anguish, and mental illness in women.[51] The subpanel documented the ways in which inequality creates dilemmas and conflicts for women in the contexts of marriage, family relationships, reproduction, child rearing, divorce, aging, education, and work. These same conditions encourage the frequency of incest, rape, and marital violence, which also heighten women's vulnerability to mental illness. Finally, the epidemiological data that establish conditions associated with mental illness are particularly relevant to women. These include poverty, alienation, and powerlessness. The convergence, therefore of multiple stressful events with the chronic stressful conditions in which women frequently live places women at high risk for mental disorders.

This risk is substantiated by a high incidence and prevalence of mental illness among women. One of the most consistent findings is that depression is closely associated with being female. The ratio of depressed women to men is about two to one. Data also show that young poor women who head single-parent families and young married women who work at dead-end jobs have shown the greatest rise in the rate of both treated and untreated depression. The most recent research data suggest, however, that the excess of psychological symptoms in women is not intrinsic to femaleness but to the conditions of subordination, stress, and powerlessness that characterize traditional female roles.

■ **POWERLESSNESS.** Families are usually viewed as providing support networks for people, yet Carmen, Russo, and Miller[10] believe that it is in the traditional construct of marriage that the subjugation of women is the most apparent and destructive. For example, in rigidly traditional families, female adults and children are at highest risk for violence and sexual abuse.[74] Violence is said to occur in 50% of American families,[42] and it has been estimated that 30% of all girls have been sexually abused before age 18, most often by family or household members (Chapter 32).

These destructive patterns of family roles and relationships are reinforced by society's pervasive pattern of sex discrimination. Women who leave unhappy or violent homes are denied equal educational, vocational, and economic opportunities; quality and supportive child care facilities; and a legitimate self-supporting role in society. Women are clustered in "female" jobs that are characterized by low pay; they earn less than men in the same occupation; and they are not equally compensated with men for work involving similar education or experience. In 1979 the median annual income of women who worked full time was 60% that of men. By 1986 that figure fell to 57% of what men earn. The earnings gap is greatest for minority women. Of divorced women, only 14% are awarded alimony and only 44% are awarded child support. Less than half of these, or only 21% of divorced mothers, collect child support regularly, and even then the payments are generally insufficient.[57] It would appear then, that the alternative to depression in an unhappy marriage can be a life of poverty with a dead-end job and great difficulty in attempting to provide adequate care for one's children.

The idea of powerlessness in the development of psychological distress and mental disorders among women is evident in one study, which reported that women who became depressed had previously made many attempts to cope. Those with the highest rates of depression were continuously faced with multiple and chronic stresses affecting themselves and their children. Efforts to deal with these stresses led to repeated frustration in employment possibilities, housing conditions, protection against violence and crime, child care assistance, and the unhelpful responses of social service and mental health agencies.[20]

■ **RESPONSE OF THE MENTAL HEALTH SYSTEM.** The responsiveness of the health community is critical to illness prevention and health promotion. New knowledge about women, men, and sex roles has not generally been incorporated into mental health education or clinical practice. This is evident in the following criticisms:

1. A double standard exists for mental health based on sex-role stereotyping and adjustment to one's environment. Broverman's now classic study[7] of mental health clinicians' attitudes indicates that healthy women are viewed differently from men and adults of unspecified gender in being more submissive, less independent, less adventurous, more suggestible, less competitive, more excitable in minor crises, more likely to have their feelings hurt, more emotional, more conceited about appearance, less objective, and more illogical. Although this study was conducted in 1970, Sherman[56] in 1980 concluded that sex-role stereotyping is still present in mental health standards

and that sex role–discrepant behaviors are viewed as more of a maladjustment. Although nurses were not included in Broverman's study, Davis[15] believes that, as a group, they are not very different from others practicing in the mental health field. She notes that despite nurses' perceptions to the contrary, research seems to indicate that as an occupational group, nurses have a traditional view of sex roles.

2. Sexual abuse and exploitation in the male therapist–female patient relationship is more common than has previously been realized. This includes such erotic activities as kissing, hugging, touching, and therapist-patient sex. Some studies have indicated that as many as 10% of men psychiatrists and psychologists in practice report having sexual contact with women patients.

3. A related danger in the male-female therapeutic relationship is that it may replicate rather than remedy the oppressed position in which women frequently find themselves in life. This may encourage the woman to fantasize that an idealized relationship with a more powerful male is a better solution to life problems than is taking autonomous control of one's own life. This possibility is strengthened by the predominance of male therapists.

4. Therapeutic theories in psychiatry have often supported stereotypes about sex roles, including the assumption that dependency, masochism, and passivity are normal for women, and that assertiveness and aggression are male traits and should not be encouraged in women. Women are also subjected to theories of psychopathology that "blame-the-mother," particularly in reference to schizophrenic children and the general "antifeminine" nature of Freudian psychology.

5. A pervasive sex bias has been documented in the therapeutic relationship. Evidence reveals that therapists' knowledge about issues affecting the lives of women is inadequate.[56] Adjustment to traditional female roles is stressed, yet realistic appraisals of the occupational hazards of the housewife role have been lacking. Anger in women is often labeled pathological and inappropriate. Thus many women experience conflict about anger and have difficulty expressing it adaptively.

The consequences of these practices affect both the quality and quantity of mental health care available to women. Carmen notes:

Women can be considered *both* overserved and underserved by mental health delivery systems. For disorders congruent with sex-role stereotypes, such as depression, conversion hysteria, and phobias, women show higher rates of service utilization than do men. In contrast, problems of women that are congruent with societal views of male au-

thority and female devaluation, such as rape, incest, and wife beating, have been ignored. Thus, services for female victims of male aggression have been provided largely through the coordinated efforts of women themselves at a time when mental health professionals were often either blaming the victims or not noticing them. Similarly, for disorders that are incongruent with society's idealized view of women, such as alcoholism and illicit drug abuse, women's service needs have usually been hidden and ignored.[10:1327]

Yet the incidence of alcoholism among women is high, and in the United States more than two thirds of all tranquilizers, stimulants, and antidepressants are used by women. Homemakers over age 35 have been identified as the largest single group of tranquilizer users.[13] In summary, women at high risk for psychiatric illness are often separated or divorced, nonwhite, poorly educated, of low socioeconomic status, and coping with the stress of raising small children and being a breadwinner on a low income.

■ **WORKING MOTHERS.** An increasing number of women are in the labor force because of personal career choice or financial need. In the United States, because of the increasing divorce rate, more women are becoming the primary financial support for themselves and their children. It is often difficult to juggle three roles—wife, mother, employee. Employment outside the home can create positive, growth-producing feelings, resulting in increased self-esteem and a heightened sense of independence. Working can also cause negative, often immobilizing feelings of guilt and anxiety about "abandoning" one's family. It is common for a working mother to assume responsibility for everything that goes wrong with the family in her absence. Many women are socialized to accept the belief that a woman's place is in the home; hence, when a woman seeks employment, she thinks she is defying societal norms.

Although feminism has expanded some opportunities for women, it has also created new dilemmas. Four syndromes have been identified: (1) reentry anxiety when a long homebound woman returns to work in the outer world, (2) performance anxiety and fear that career success may be viewed as social failure, (3) conflict between social expectations of accommodation and compliance and the need to assert herself and fight for her rights when they have been imposed on, and (4) conflict between a woman's sense of personal identity and her professional identity, in which marriage or family may be viewed as a threat to independence.[43]

Three defense mechanisms seem symptomatic of underlying guilt: rationalization, projection, and overcompensation. In rationalization the mother thinks up a socially approved reason for her behavior, such as "I would just play bridge or do volunteer work if I stayed at home." Projection involves blaming someone or something else for one's need to work, and overcompensation is evidenced by trying to repay the child with gifts.

Nurses can help the working mother cope with her many roles. First, they can encourage and provide a medium in which the mother can come to grips with her conflicting feelings. The mother needs to be aware that it is the quality rather than the quantity of mother-child interactions that has the greatest impact on growth and development. Moreover, children often benefit from their mother's feelings of self-satisfaction related to job success.

The nurse can also support working mothers as they make or change child care arrangements. Few situations have as profound an effect on the working mother as disruptions in child care. Essentially, selecting the best arrangement for each family is a problem-solving strategy whereby the family examines each available alternative and selects the one that seemingly will bring more comfort.

Another problem-solving area relates to assigning responsibility for household chores. It takes 105 hours a week to carry out full-time employment and meet the domestic responsibilities of the family. Recent studies show that working women still do the majority of the housework, with child care taking priority over other chores. Many sacrifice leisure time and sleep to manage. A variety of household management alternatives exist, and the nurse can help the mother select the one that suits the needs of her family. Five guidelines have been developed for nurses working with mothers who are experiencing role conflict[36]:

1. Help the mother examine and accept her reasons for working.
2. Encourage the woman to choose a job carefully. Working mothers cannot afford to transfer hostility from the job to the family.
3. Communicate honestly with family members to determine their response to employment. Discussion of differences cannot occur without honest expression.
4. Assist the mother in finding a suitable surrogate whose attitudes are consistent with hers.
5. Explore ways in which help can be provided by others, the family, or the housekeeper.

■ Mature adults

The issues of midlife and advancing age are problematic for some adults. As people approach midlife they reflect on the choices they have made and their progress in attaining the goals they had set. Marriage, life-style, children, career, and quality of life all are subject to scrutiny. Certain types of stressors, including career changes (promotion, change of job, demotion, or being fired), changes in the family unit (death, divorce, or departure of the last child), and the aging process, may precipitate anxiety, depression, or psychosomatic illnesses. Midlife combines the sense of "another chance" with that of a "final chance."

Midlife has traditionally been given very little attention in theory, research, or practice. Recently, it has been explored as a time of development and change, rather than a period merely focused on impending aging and death.[44] The middle years range in the 30s to the 40s, although defining it by chronological age has been more recently criticized. Neither can it any longer be defined as the time of menopause for the woman. Rather, it relates to a combination of biological, psychological, and sociological events. Notman compares it to the period of adolescence:

This importance of separation, the change in relationship to family, and the potential for further development of one's own interests, are common to both periods. However, the differences are highly significant. At adolescence the separation is from parents, who are incestuous object choices. At midlife the separation is from children, and the experience often revives some sense of loss. The adolescent perspective of infinite time and choices to be made differs from the midlife sense of the finite and the reassessment of choices that have been made. The reality is that time is limited and that although choices do exist or even increase, there is also a limited range and variety of careers, new physical pursuits, and new relationships.[47:1273]

Important in a discussion of midlife is the fact that it is viewed differently by men and women. According to Levenson's work,[37] men give central importance to the role of work in establishing oneself in the world. Thus, at midlife, men focus heavily on evaluating their work and their career goals. Women, on the other hand, focus on the world in relation to their family or potential to have one, as well as their work or career goals. Women who have not had children feel a last chance to consider motherhood. Women with children experience a decrease in their focus on the burdens of child care. Children may either be sent into the world or function independently at home. Consequently, these women may feel relieved, renewed, and ready to return to the work world.

Although this can be an exciting time, it can also be viewed negatively if one feels displaced, unprepared, or unaccepted. Extramarital affairs, divorces, and major life changes can result from a midlife crisis and can pose problems for the individual, as well as the family.

■ The elderly

Later adulthood and old age is another time of increased stress. In the past, it has been largely ignored by researchers and clinicians in the mental health field who focus heavily on the early developmental stages. One of the most obvious reasons for this may be evident in the changing distribution of the population. Between 1960 and 1980, the percentage of persons aged 60 years or older throughout the world grew by 50%. Experts have projected a 57% growth between 1980 and 2000 and a 65% increase between 2000 and 2020.

In the United States today, approximately 34 million people, or 12% of the population is 65 years of age or older. Since 1900 the percentage of Americans over age 56 has tripled, and the number has increased nine times from 3.1 million to 30 million in 1988. By the year 2000, it is anticipated that the very elderly (80 years or older) will be the largest single federal entitlement group, consuming $82.8 billion in benefits. By 2030, these numbers are anticipated to increase to 64.6 million elderly persons, comprising 21.2% of the United States' population.

Elderly people are at high risk for mental illness for several reasons, including their susceptibility to the effects of rapid social and environmental change. Since the 1950s social and technological changes have occurred at an unprecedented pace. This poses problems for elderly people who are physiologically less able to adapt to rapidly changing events in their lives.

A number of barriers exist for the elderly that interfere with their ability to meet their mental health needs. First, more national resources are devoted to children than to the elderly. Also, elderly people who live on fixed incomes are especially susceptible to the effects of inflation. People are at high risk for lowered self-esteem during inflationary periods when their expectations for either social mobility or maintenance of at least an adequate standard of living are destroyed by the high cost of living. Elderly people are susceptible to lowered self-esteem and resignation when they have spent a lifetime of saving for retirement only to find that they are not able to make ends meet. In addition, transportation often presents a major barrier for the elderly who do not have ready access to services. Retirement also can deal a serious blow to self-esteem, since so much of contemporary society revolves around what people do for a living.

Although the majority of the elderly population is not poor and 95% of those over 65 remain commu-nity, rather than institutional, residents, certain noticeable changes impose constraints on the aging adult. In reviewing the literature, Hefferin[25] identified three life stages of people living beyond age 65. The first stage is between ages 65 and 75, in which most people continue with normal activities unless a specific illness exists. In the second stage, from age 75 to 85, normal activities can also be carried out, although the effects of aging are evident. The final stage occurs after 85, in which most people need some help to maintain normal activities, and some may even require institutionalization.

As these stages reflect, the period extending from middle age into early old age is often characterized at the outset by the height of social and economic success and physical well-being. But slowly changes occur that for most people are simply a somewhat lower level of physical and psychological energy, accompanied by society's subtle and open pressures to make room for the next generation. The evidence is strong that individual differences in the maintenance of behavioral competence are related primarily to the person's state of health and the opportunities and tendencies to be fully involved in a stimulating environment.

Despite this evidence, society still holds many myths and stereotypes about the elderly that decrease feelings of worth. Language and humor are full of negative clichés. Phrases like the "old goat," "silly old biddy," or "dirty old man" do not reflect a positive image of the elderly. The very word *elderly* tends to call forth a set of images, including graying and thinning hair, a slow stooped gait, and a tendency toward forgetfulness. In a major study by the National Council on Aging[3] it was found that older people were almost as negative in their attitudes about aging as were their younger counterparts. Few people in a sample of 4000 chose the years between 60 and 80 as "the best of my life," and about one third considered this period as the least desirable time of their life.[8]

■ **LIFE STRESSORS.** As people live longer, new life stressors create the possibility of maladaptive responses. For example, certain life events, such as forced retirement and loss of friends and family, become more likely with increasing age, and loss of a spouse is often perceived as the single greatest loss that an individual can experience in the life cycle. The combined physical, social, financial, and psychological changes that result from the loss of a spouse severely tax the coping ability of the bereaved.

Although death of a spouse may be perceived as the greatest stressor, multiple other social, psychological, and biological stressors overlap, interact, and enhance the vulnerability of aging adults. These are de-

TABLE 8-3

SUMMARY OF STRESSES FACING THE ELDERLY

Category of stress	Influencing factors	Outcomes
Social Stresses		
Family-cultural	Smaller family size Increased mobility One fourth of elderly have no children One half of elderly have only distant relatives	Weakened traditional nuclear family unit Less opportunity for role modeling by elderly Shift from family to public responsibility for care of the aged
Employment	Security not based on ability to work but on government and union pensions Elderly capable of work function beyond age 65 In 1900, 66% of those over 65 still worked Now less than 33% work Retirement age is now 70 by new federal law	Retirement represents a major change that may be responded to adaptively or maladaptively Some models of part-time work have been developed
Commercial	Society values youth and views older people and objects as obsolescent Commercial advertising is aimed at youth and deplores aging in principle	Aging is devalued
Logistical	Physical disabilities, costs, fears, access, distances, and weather are all problems affecting the mobility of the elderly	Transportation is difficult for many of the elderly Access to activities and health care is often limited The elderly are easy targets for robbery and assault
Financial	Pensions are outstripped by the cost of living Health insurance is often inadequate with rising premiums and poor psychiatric coverage Statistics for physical and psychiatric illness demonstrate the elderly's great need for services	Inflation has a severe impact on the elderly
Discriminatory	Negative stereotypes of the elderly are commonly accepted Providing health care to the elderly lacks prestige and is often avoided by caregivers Courses in aging and care of the aged are seldom part of the educational curricula of health care professionals	Ageism, or prejudice toward the elderly, exists in American society Health problems of the elderly often receive inadequate treatment
Psychological Stresses		
Mastery	The elderly experience decreasing influence over their outer life and preoccupation with their inner life	Through denial and projection the elderly evolve a "magical mastery" of their external environment
Coping style	The elderly tend to use coping styles that were effective earlier in life Denial, somatization, projection, and constructed affect may occur	If previously used and trusted coping styles fail, the elderly may display maladaptive responses
Generation gap	At the time of the elderly's need, younger relatives may be at crucial points in their own lives and lack the time and insight to help	Younger relatives have difficulty understanding the aging process
Fears	Common fears include the following: 1. Maintaining control over their lives and environment 2. Maintaining physical functioning 3. Retaining a sense of purpose and productivity	

Continued.

TABLE 8-3, cont'd

SUMMARY OF STRESSES FACING THE ELDERLY

Category of stress	Influencing factors	Outcomes
	4. Maintaining independence while acknowledging the possible need of a dependent status for survival 5. Failing cognition and senility 6. Death 7. Losing the interest of others	Predictable fears are common among the elderly and may cause significant psychological stress
Love cues	The elderly have acquired skills in interpreting nonverbal communication They easily detect and respond to cues of lack of interest or respect	If the elderly perceive lack of interest or honesty, they believe they are unliked and respond by withdrawing
Self-image	The elderly may dislike their dependent status or interpret it as a sign of their own failures	The elderly may have an aversion to youth or an acceptance of the stereotypes of the aged
Loss	Losses are predictable, steady, numerous, and often arrive in bunches	Losses for the elderly represent the most basic psychological stress
Death of family and friends	Loss of family and friends suggests impending loss of self	Results in loss of security and companionship and depletion of the pool of caregivers
Relocation	Relocation can involve loss of privacy, accustomed diet, favorite belongings, and familiar faces It may be accompanied by a feeling of aloneness or abandonment	Stress is a function of losing the familiar and facing the unsure new environment
Money	Loss of money affects the availability of goods, care, identity, and status	This compounds any other stressor experienced by the elderly
Retirement	Some external sources of gratification may be lost, and the couple may have to deal with changes in privacy and daily routine	Results in changes in income, identity, and life-style
Deteriorating body function	This decreases a person's skills	Loss of body functioning may affect one's identity and sense of productivity and usefulness
Attractiveness	Aging produces physical changes The effect of aging on one's physical appearance is subject to personal evaluation	One potential outcome is negative self-image and withdrawal from others
Visual and auditory acuity	Acuity in sensory cues is important for orientation, processing information, and maintaining daily activities	Diminution in sight or hearing can create inaccurate interpretation of the environment and may lead to paranoid or avoiding behavior
Prestige	The elderly often are retired from membership in decision-making bodies or are given an "honorary" membership without voting privileges	They perceive that their opinions are not valued and that their experience does not count
Sex	Sexual ability is determined by availability of a partner, past sexual activity, physical health, and support from family and health professionals The elderly may be embarrassed to discuss their sexual needs or experience side effects from medications One's ability to enjoy sex can be maintained throughout the life cycle	Natural physiological changes, if explained to the elderly and understood by them, can result in increased closeness, satisfaction, and communication
Cognition	Subtle changes in cognitive ability are detected first by the elderly Cognitive changes can be compounded by other life stresses	Resulting changes and perceptions can affect practical coping abilities and be psychologically disturbing

Continued.

TABLE 8-3, cont'd

SUMMARY OF STRESSES FACING THE ELDERLY

Category of stress	Influencing factors	Outcomes
Biological Stresses		
Illness and accidents	Result in decreased function and pain	Can erode activity, appearance, finances, employability, and self-esteem
Physiological aging	Aging inevitably occurs in body organs, biochemical and metabolic pathways, musculoskeletal systems, and central nervous system	Requires specific and sensitive guidelines for treatments, medications, education, and compliance
	It occurs at different rates in different people and among different organs in the same person	
Medications	The elderly tend to collect large numbers of medications from multiple sources, using an average of 13 prescriptions a year	Prescribing medications must be accompanied by proper discussion, written instructions, and careful monitoring
	They often take higher than prescribed doses and for longer periods of time	
	Of psychogeriatric admissions, 20% are precipitated by adverse effects of psychotropic drugs	
Other ingested substances	Changes in appetite, decreased activity, and poor physical function interfere with proper food intake among the elderly	Nutrition is often a problem for the elderly
		Drugs and alcohol may be used as tranquilizers or to allay loneliness
	Assessment of caffeine, nicotine, and alcohol is often overlooked in the elderly	
Iatrogenic biological stresses	The negative stereotypes of aging may block the reality of medication side effects and infection sequelae	Major iatrogenic problems arise from failing to diagnose and treat the causes of illness because of stereotyped thinking and an inappropriate prescription of medications to "keep the patient happy"

Modified from Goodstein R: Am J Orthopsychiatry 51(2):219, 1981.

scribed in detail by Goodstein.[17] He notes that the social sphere presents a major source of stress, including family-cultural, employment, commercial, logistical, financial, and discriminatory stresses as described in Table 8-3. He observes that the elderly's social status and physical function have decreased at the same time this population has increased.

The elderly also have a bombardment of emotional pressures as they struggle with the issues of integrity and independence. Stressors involving mastery, coping style, generation gap, fears, love cues, self-image, loss, death of family and friends, relocation, money, retirement, deteriorating body functions, attractiveness, visual and auditory acuity, prestige, sex, and cognition (Table 8-3) all pose emotional hardship to the elderly. Goodstein believes that no matter what the specific psychological stress, the commonalities of sequelae to loss are reduced self-esteem and dignity, plus the implication that life and personal usefulness are slipping away.

Finally, without question, biological stress takes a toll on the elderly. Consider these statistics:

The elderly represent one third of the nation's health bill, one third of the family physician's practice time, two times the number of outpatient visits of other age populations, twice the number of days in the hospital of other age populations, three and a half times the cost of health care in other age populations, and 45% of the elderly have some physical limitations.[17:226]

Major sources of biological stress for the elderly include illness and accidents, physiological aging, medications, other ingested substances, and iatrogenic biological stresses (Table 8-3).

Despite these multiple stresses, most elderly persons are able to live in the community reasonably secure financially and in social contact with family and friends. However, older persons experiencing multiple stresses and inadequate coping resources are at greater risk to require institutional support. Access to and use of social support systems are important determinants of an older person's response to stress, along with previous life experiences, premorbid coping styles, physical and emotional status, and the approach health professionals provide to the elderly from both a practical and an attitudinal standpoint.

■ **BARRIERS TO MENTAL HEALTH CARE.** Attitude barriers on the part of both the elderly and health care providers interfere with effective service utilization. Hagebak and Hagebak[23] described psychological barriers held by both therapists and the elderly. They found six major attitude barriers commonly held by therapists: (1) the "you can't teach an old dog new tricks" attitude, which discounts the elderly person's ability to learn, adapt, or change; (2) the "my God, I'm mortal too" syndrome, which forces therapists to acknowledge their own aging process; (3) the "why bother?" attitude, which holds that since elderly people have a shortened life span it is hardly worth the effort to work with them; (4) the "I'm a child" belief, which is seen when role reversal occurs and the therapist responds to the older person as though to a parent; (5) the "patient is a child" approach, which discounts the elderly people's abilities by treating them like children; or (6) "senility is natural," an attitude that labels the elderly person as forgetful or slow. Often the elderly respond to these attitudes like a self-fulfilling prophecy and thus behave accordingly.

Nurses can overcome these attitude hurdles by first recognizing that the older person is a person who just happened to grow older but is not basically different from other people. The next step is introspection or conscious examination of one's feelings toward aging and death. Attitudes, beliefs, and feelings are generally clearly transmitted to others, hence personal awareness is extremely important.

Like nurses and other health care providers, elderly people often hold attitudes that are barriers to obtaining mental health services. They often believe that "senility is natural" and expect to evidence psychological changes. Thus they view any mental health changes as inevitable and often fail to seek assistance for problems that could be treated or reversed. Elderly people often question their value by asking "who/why am I?" They believe that since they no longer work and their children are grown, they have lost their value to society. A third attitude held by the elderly is one of fierce independence, or "do for yourself," whereby they hesitate to seek the aid of others. The counterpart

to this attitude is "I'm distrustful and afraid," in which the elderly fear the services provided by anyone associated with the mental health system. Last, elderly people may evidence a "doing what's expected" syndrome in which they support stereotypes or their perceptions of what others expect of them.[35] These barriers tend to arise because both nurses and the elderly are unfamiliar with the aging process.

Severe psychological decline is not an inevitable part of aging. Although some physiological changes do occur with aging, many others can be prevented by modification of the environment, such as overcoming attitudes that expect the elderly to respond in less than functional ways, reducing stress, and using simple techniques, such as speaking clearly and audibly. As with all age groups, stress interferes with accurate perception of environmental cues, as well as with problem-solving ability. Stimuli that tend to set off a stress response are ones that are novel, rapidly changing, or unexpected.

The most common psychiatric problem among the elderly is depression. Old age is a time of numerous losses. For many, retirement, while eagerly anticipated, reflects a loss of meaningful involvement with the larger society. Also, friends and family members begin to die, skills and abilities may diminish, and even homes and familiar possessions are lost. The effects of several drugs commonly consumed by elderly people contribute to depression, including digitalis; antihypertensives, especially reserpine; antiparkinsonism drugs; corticosteroids; antianxiety drugs; and even some antidepressants.

The interaction of drugs is a particular problem for the elderly who often mix medications. Comfort[12] says that the first operation in geriatric psychiatry is the "plastic bag test," which means to collect all the medication the patient is taking. Often some were prescribed, others were purchased over the counter, and still other medication was provided by friends or family. Not only do the elderly inadvertently mix medications, but many use drugs and alcohol to cope with stress, or loneliness, or feelings of fear, anxiety, or loss.

The elderly are not a homogeneous group. Each one is a unique person with needs, desires, assets, and support networks. In providing mental health services it is important to remember that most elderly people do not live in institutions but rather are able to maintain their own home or live with friends or family members. Often a primary mental health goal is that of helping the family identify and use its own strengths to support and respond effectively to elderly members.

Hamrick and Blazer[24] describe a program that helps family members identify and use their own strengths to help elderly relatives. They assess areas such as recent events that may have been stressful, the developmental history of both the patient and the family, impairments in the older adult, family conflicts, and support (both tangible and intangible). Once the assessment is completed, one or more of five major approaches is generally used: (1) explain the patient's impairment and capabilities to the family, (2) inform the family about community resources and how to use them, (3) evaluate respite activities of the family, (4) allow members to express and work through their feelings, and (5) provide opportunities for the family to make decisions about care of the older adult.

To respond effectively to the mental health needs of the elderly, nurses must use an integrated approach that takes into account the multiple stressors and the resources available for effective coping. Schaie believes that "the quality of life in developed societies can be readily sensed from the manner in which transition from midlife to old age is accomplished with a minimum of stress and the preservation of maximum personal freedom and opportunities."[55:216] If this is true, primary prevention activities directed toward the elderly must command the attention of psychiatric nurses and other health professionals.

♦ Planning and implementation

Under the sponsorship of the Public Health Service, a national incentive has been undertaken to promote health and prevent disease in this country. A number of potential measures have been identified to meet one of the 1990 objectives for the control of stress and violent behavior. These include education, service, and technological and legislative measures as identified in the box on page 258.[58] This list provides the nurse with a good overview of the many areas appropriate for nursing intervention.

In addition, the nursing model of health-illness phenomena presented in Chapter 3 and represented in Fig. 8-1 is useful for the nurse in planning strategies for primary prevention. It suggests both target areas and types of activities that might be useful. If the overall nursing goal is to promote constructive coping mechanisms and maximize adaptive coping responses, then the model suggests that prevention strategies should be directed toward influencing predisposing factors, precipitating stressors, appraisal of stressors, and coping resources and mechanisms through the following interventions: (1) health education, (2) environmental change, and (3) supporting social systems. Because the process depicted in the model is a dynamic one, it is not possible to discretely link a particular strategy with a particular component of the model.

Rather, the strategies can affect multiple aspects of a person's life. For example, an environmental change, such as changing jobs, can affect one's predisposition to stress, decrease the amount of stress, change one's appraisal of the threat, and perhaps increase one's financial or social coping resources. This interactive effect can thus serve to justify the use of these prevention strategies for vulnerable groups.

■ Health education

This strategy of primary prevention in mental health involves the strengthening of individuals and groups through **competence building.** It is based on the assumption that many maladaptive responses are the result of a lack of competence, that is, a lack of perceived control over one's own life, of effective coping strategies, and the lowered self-esteem that results. Bloom[5] believes that competence building is perhaps the single most persuasive preventive strategy for dealing with individual and social issues in most communities. A competent community is one that is aware of resources and alternatives, can make reasoned decisions about issues facing them, and can cope adaptively with problems. In this sense the concept of a competent community parallels the concept of positive mental health.[30]

■ LEVELS OF INTERVENTION. Health education or competence building can be viewed as having four aspects. The first is increasing the individual's or group's awareness of issues and events related to health and illness. Awareness of normal developmental tasks and potential problems is fundamental. The second aspect is increasing one's understanding of the dimensions of potential stressors, possible outcomes (both adaptive and maladaptive), and alternative coping responses. A third element is increasing one's knowledge of where and how to acquire the needed resources. Many health professionals assume this is common knowledge, although for many individuals it is not. The fourth and final aspect of health education focuses on increasing the actual abilities of the individual or group. This means improving or maximizing one's coping skills, such as problem-solving skills or interpersonal skills, tolerance of stress and frustration, motivation, hope, self-esteem, and power. Ryan contends the following:

Self-esteem is to some extent an essential requirement to the very survival of the human organism . . . and is partially dependent on the inclusion of a sense of power within the self-concept. . . . A mentally healthy person must be able to perceive himself as at least minimally powerful, capable of influencing his environment to his own benefit, and

Potential Primary Prevention Measures

Education and information measures

- Increasing the public's awareness, through planned campaigns using the appropriate media, that stress can be an antecedent of illness and that stress management can be an important component of health
- Creating new educational pathways for developing enhanced professional skills in bio-behavioral fields of medicine and public health
- Developing the capacities of health care professionals in stress diagnosis and management
- Helping parents recognize and deal with stress
- Training secondary, elementary, and preschool teachers to include discussion of stress recognition and management in school health curricula
- Training of police in handling calls involving domestic and interpersonal disputes which would potentially lead to violent behavior
- Public education, especially for high-risk groups, on steps to take to reduce risks of rape
- Training all "helping" professionals regarding signs which indicate high risk for suicide
- Helping the public be aware of indicators of possible suicide

Service measures

- Hotlines for people under acute stress (suicide, child abuse prevention)
- Stress management programs in work places
- Stress management programs targeted to adolescents, parents, and the elderly
- Stress appraisal analysis (self-administered or performed by a legitimate objective outside source)
- Professional and social support systems to assist in resolution of stressful life events, including mutual aid and self-help groups such as Reach for Recov-

ery, child abusing parents, bereavement groups, single parent groups
- Information and counseling with regard to individually appropriate leisure and stress-reducing activities including exercise
- A variety of self-help relaxation and biofeedback techniques, which can be individualized in concert with a diversity of life-styles and work requirements
- Psychophysiologic tests to aid in assisting employees who are having difficulty adjusting to their work and to their coworkers
- Support services for inevitable or necessary life change events—especially in relation to death, separation, job changes, and geographic relocation
- Domestic crisis teams to defuse domestic disputes
- Targeting the above measures to high risk populations and individuals with low coping abilities
- Evaluating intervention efforts
- Follow-up services for persons who have attempted suicide
- Shelters for abused wives (and husbands)
- Training all health (and other human services—including educational) personnel to be alert to evidence of child abuse

Technological measures

- Actions by employers, labor, and government to reduce stress-creating work environments
- Reducing stressful aspects of the environment such as noise pollution and overcrowding

Legislative and regulatory measures

- Activities to create employment opportunities for youth
- Action to limit the availability of handguns, to reduce homicides and suicides that occur during stressful periods
- Strengthening mandatory child abuse reporting laws

Modified from US Department of Health and Human Services: Promoting health, preventing disease: objectives for the nation, Washington, DC, 1984, Public Health Service.

further . . . this sense of minimal power has to be based on the actual experience and exercise of power.[54:50]

■ **PROGRAMS AND ACTIVITIES.** Health education has long been regarded by nurses as an essential part of nursing practice. However, it is difficult to quantify the degree or quality of mental health education actually implemented by nurses. It can take place in any setting, can assume a formal or informal structure, can be directed toward individuals or groups, and can be related to predisposing factors or potential stressors. Health education directed toward strengthening an individual's predisposition to stress can take various forms. Growth groups may be formed for parents that focus on parent-child relations, normal

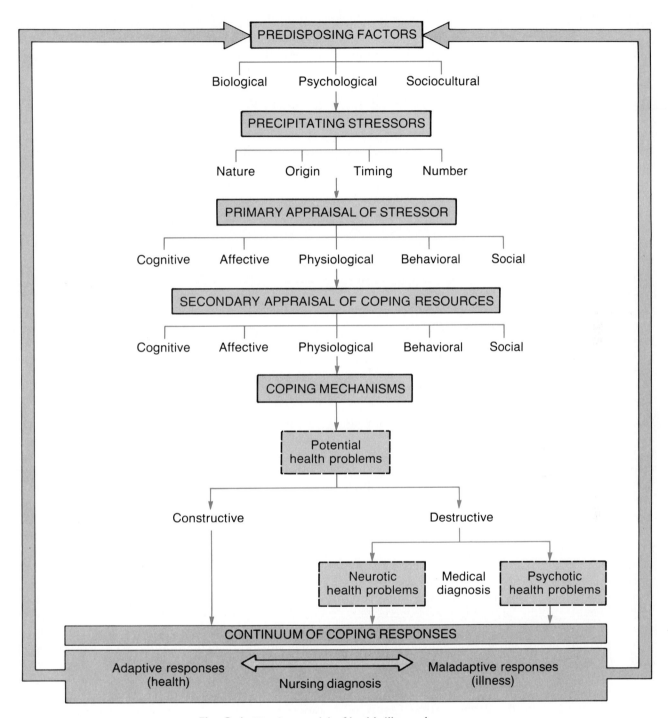

Fig. 8-1. Nursing model of health-illness phenomena.

growth and development, or effective methods of child rearing. Groups of children or adolescents can discuss peer relationships, sexuality, or potential problem areas, such as drug abuse or promiscuity. Employee groups can form to discuss career burnout and related issues. Or a more activity-centered educational pro-

gram can be initiated, such as Outward Bound, which helps the individual discover that step by step one can expand competence in mastering new, unexpected, and potentially stressful situations in an adaptive way.

Probably the most common type of health education program implemented at present is one that aids the individual in coping with a specific potential stressor. Consider, for example, the impending stressor or risk factor of marital separation. Families about to experience marital separation are vulnerable to emotional problems, physical complaints, and increased use of health care facilities. Children and adults about to experience stressful events may be offered educational and supportive group intervention aimed at enhancing their ability to cope. Education groups can similarly be offered to those experiencing retirement, bereavement, or any other stressful event.

Parent education classes are a well-known example of the type of anticipatory guidance that can be offered to high-risk groups. Although raising children is considered a serious aspect of life, until recently little attention has been directed to the belief that effective parenting is not an innate ability. Whether nurses subscribe to a specific set of beliefs and strategies for parenting or choose an eclectic approach, the opportunities for promoting mental health abound. Possibly one of the most beneficial results of parent education is the acknowledgment that all parents become frustrated, angry, and ambivalent toward their children. Parent education goes beyond acknowledging feelings and includes learning and practicing alternative ways of interacting with children. During these classes, situations are anticipated and discussions focus on identifying potential crisis situations and dealing with them through simulated encounters such as role playing. Education for mental health can thus address the needs of both children and parents as family roles shift and respond to societal change.

Finally, health education activities can be directed to the larger community. One way to do this is by changing the attitudes and behavior of health care providers and consumers. This may involve activities related to dispelling myths and stereotypes associated with vulnerable groups, providing knowledge of normal parameters, increasing sensitivity to psychosocial factors affecting health and illness, and enhancing the ability to give sensitive, supportive, and humanistic health care.

An example of one such activity is an educational pamphlet published by the Parental Stress Center of Pittsburgh.[2] The Center serves families in which one or both parents abuse or neglect their children, many of whom are infants when the pattern of abuse begins. The pamphlet was developed as a resource for new mothers to help them understand and prepare for the special stresses during the first 3 months of life. In providing this mental health information, the Center considered the issues of the social stigma of mental illness, the cognitive ability of the patient, educational

background, legitimacy of popular psychotherapy fads, and the use of pamphlets, films, etc.

Another community-level strategy requires public education on mental health issues and community resources. Misconceptions regarding vulnerable subgroups of the population need to be corrected. The stigma, misunderstanding, and fear surrounding mental illness are related to both the agencies providing mental health services and the people receiving these services who are often elderly or poor, or members of social minority groups. Unlike physical illness, which tends to evoke sympathy and the desire to help, mental disorders tend to disturb and repel people. Yet everyone encounters stress, and all people are subject to maladaptive coping responses. Mental health professionals can educate the public that health is a continuum and illness is caused by a complex combination of factors. In doing so, consumers "may begin to understand that none of us is immune from mental illness or emotional problems, and that the fear, anxiety, and even anger we feel about people who suffer these problems may merely reflect some of our own deepest fears and anxieties."[51:57]

■ Environmental change

Activities in primary prevention involving environmental change have a social setting focus. They require the modification of an individual's or group's immediate environment or the larger social system. They are particularly appropriate actions when the environment has placed new demands on the person, when it is not responding to his developmental needs, and when it provides a diminished level of positive reinforcement for the individual. The nursing literature gives evidence that this is not an area of primary prevention in which nurses have been actively involved.

For the individual, various types of environmental changes may prove to promote one's mental health, including changes in one's economic, work, housing, or family situations. **Economically,** there may be the location of resources for financial aid or assistance obtained in budgeting and managing of income. **Work** changes may include vocational testing, guidance, education, or retraining that can result in a change of jobs or careers. It may also mean that an adolescent, a homemaker, or an older adult may be placed in a new career. Changes in one's **housing** can involve moving to new quarters, which may mean leaving family and friends or returning to them, improvements in existing housing, or the addition or subtraction of coinhabitants, whether they are family, friends, or roommates. Environmental changes that may benefit the **family** include attaining child care facilities, enrollment in a nursery school, grade school, or camp, or obtaining access to recreational, social, religious, or community facilities.

The potential benefit of all of these changes should not be minimized or overlooked by mental health practitioners. They can promote mental health by increasing one's coping resources, modifying the nature of one's stressors, and possibly increasing one's positive, rewarding, and self-enhancing experiences.

■ **ORGANIZATIONS AND POLITICS.** Nurses can also effect environmental changes at a larger organizational and political level. One way is by influencing health care structures and procedures. Given the vulnerability of new parents, for example, nurses can work to implement birthing rooms and family suites in obstetrical settings. They might also become involved in training community, nonprofessional caregivers to increase the social supports available to vulnerable groups. Another approach would be to stimulate support for women's issues related to mental health, such as through studying the psychology of women; dispelling sex-role stereotypes; promoting feminist therapy; sponsoring programs, conferences, and workshops on women's issues; and recruiting more women professionals into the mental health field.

Obviously, if nurses believe that their profession makes a valuable contribution to health promotion, they should document the cost-effectiveness and quality of nursing care, lobby for greater patient access by nurses, and seek adequate compensation and reimbursement for nursing services. Many of these goals can be obtained if nursing has greater participation in the decision-making structures of health care institutions, such as hospital boards, advisory groups, health system agencies, and legislative bodies.

Within organizations, environmental change can be achieved through program consultation. Such consultation with a large corporation, for example, may lead to the formulation of more flexible retirement plans or a preretirement counseling program. Involvement in community planning and development can have an impact in many different areas. For instance, a community may be helped to meet the needs of the elderly for educational opportunities, recreational programs, and access to social support networks through telephone tielines or special transportation services. So too, the stress associated with environmental pollutants, such as chemicals and radiation, can be addressed.

Some environmental changes require involvement at the national level which may be directed toward the media's portrayal of violence, laws on drunk driving, gun control legislation, access to family planning services, federal funding of abortion, the advocation of changes in child-rearing practices, including the provision of day-care centers, flex time and paternity leave, or the passage of equal rights legislation.

Of course, many attitudes in and areas of the social system are in need of change, including racism, sexism, ageism, inadequate housing, poverty, and problems with the educational system. The dilemma is that global problems such as these are too broad, too pervasive, and too diffuse to be adequately addressed, let alone resolved. Furthermore, the changes under the Republican administration mean that fewer governmental resources are available to aid such primary prevention efforts. For any prevention strategies to be successful in the future, it will be necessary to document the ways in which a particular group is vulnerable to a specific stressor, how the proposed prevention program will be beneficial and cost-effective, and the degree to which it succeeded or failed.

■ **Supporting social systems**

As a primary prevention strategy, supporting social systems is not an approach that attempts to remove or minimize the stressor or risk factor. Rather, its rationale is that of strengthening social supports as a way of buffering or cushioning the effects of a potentially stressful event. It is such an important concept for all levels of prevention—primary, secondary, and tertiary—that an entire section of the President's Commission on Mental Health was devoted to exploring ways to expand personal and social networks of families, neighbors, and community organizations to which people naturally turn to help them cope. It has implications for promoting health, helping people seek assistance earlier, supporting them in times of stress, and aiding the situation of the chronically mentally ill. Social support systems can be helpful in emphasizing the strengths of individuals and families and focusing on health rather than illness. For these reasons the commission recommended that "a major effort be developed in the area of personal and community supports which will":

1. Recognize and strengthen the natural networks to which people belong and on which they depend
2. Identify the potential social support that formal institutions within communities can provide
3. Improve the linkages between community support networks and formal mental health services
4. Initiate research to increase our knowledge of informal and formal community support systems and networks[51:15]

Given the goal that social support systems should be maximized, how does one go about achieving it?

First, one needs to determine how much social support a high-risk group will need and then compare it to the amount of social support that is available. Although the question is straightforward, it is complicated by the fact that there are multiple determinants of each element. One's need for social support will be influenced by predisposing factors, the nature of the stressors, and the availability of other coping resources such as economic assets, individual abilities and skills, and defensive techniques. The availability of social supports will similarly be influenced by predisposing factors such as age, sex, socioeconomic status, the nature of the stressor, and the characteristics of the environment. Acute episodic stressors tend to elicit more intense support, whereas in chronic problems, support resources tend to not persist. So too, changes or stressors viewed in a positive way by one's social network, such as the birth of a baby or a promotion, may elicit a great deal of support, whereas a negative event, such as a sudden death, may generate little support.

In addition, the quantity and type of social support that meets one need may not meet another. Research suggests that different characteristics of social support may be needed for different stresses. For example, in one study, family cohesiveness, family expressiveness, and spouse support were significant sources of support for the patient receiving dialysis, but the presence of a confidant was not.[16] However, Brown's study[8] found that an important factor in preventing depression in women was an intimate confiding relationship with a husband or boyfriend. Support from other relationships was not shown to be a specific factor. Thus the match between the type and level of social support and the nature of the stressor is an important, but not entirely understood, one.

■ **TYPES OF INTERVENTIONS.** Even though many variables related to social support need further study, one can still use social support in designing and implementing interventions in primary prevention. Four particular types of interventions are possible. First, social support patterns can be used to assess communities and neighborhoods to identify problem areas and high-risk groups. Not only will information about the quality of life be gained, but also the social isolation of a particular group might become apparent as well as central individuals whose aid may then be enlisted in developing community-based programs.

A second preventive intervention would be to improve linkages between community support systems and formal mental health services. Often mental health professionals are not aware of or comfortable with the existence or functioning of community support systems. To correct this, they should be taught the skills involved in using and mobilizing community resources and social support systems. All health care providers need to recognize when patients need social support and to provide them with access to appropriate community support systems.

The third type of intervention is to strengthen natural, existing caregiving networks. Health professionals can provide information and support to the variety of informal caregivers in the community who serve a very important and somewhat different function than more formalized and organized support systems. Gottlieb[19] notes that informal support systems provide (1) a natural training ground for the development of problem-solving skills, (2) a medium in which personal growth and development is based on repeated episodes of people learning to direct the process of change for themselves, and (3) a supportive milieu that capitalizes on the strength of existing ties among people in our communities, rather than fragmenting intact social units on the basis of diagnosed needs or specialized services.

Numerous informal support groups exist. They may include church groups, civic organizations, clubs, women's groups, or work and neighborhood supports. Self-help groups are becoming more common as members organize themselves to solve their own problems. The members all share a common experience, work together toward a common goal, and use their own strengths to gain control over their lives. The processes involved in self-help groups are social affiliation, learning self-control, modeling methods to cope with stress, and acting to change the social environment.[38]

Self-help groups are familiar to the public through such groups as Alcoholics Anonymous, Weight Watchers, Parents Without Partners, and Parents Anonymous. They have also demonstrated their ability to help those people experiencing grief reactions, such as widows and parents of children who died from sudden infant death syndrome. Since self-help groups use a variety of methods and membership criteria, each group should be assessed individually for its general effectiveness and appropriateness for particular individuals and families. Newton has identified some areas for the nurse to assess before recommending involvement in a self-help group.[45] These are presented in Table 8-4.

Working with natural, informal support systems should be done cautiously, however, to minimize undesirable consequences. One should attempt to create the least amount of disruption possible. Gottlieb[19]

TABLE 8-4

ASSESSMENT GUIDELINES FOR SELF-HELP GROUPS

Questions for the group	Questions for the potential member
1. What is its purpose?	7. How does the person feel about attending a self-help group?
2. Who are the group members and leaders?	8. How compatible is the group and the individual's approach to the problem?
3. What are the beneficial aspects of the group?	9. How accessible is the group to the potential member?
4. For whom would the group not be suitable?	
5. What problems are inherent in the group?	
6. Is the group effective in preventing further emotional distress?	

From Newton G: J Psychosoc Nurs Ment Health Serv 22(7):27, 1984.

---

warns against the potentially damaging effects of well-intentioned consultation with informal caregivers by inadvertently suppressing their natural repertoire of helping behaviors. This might be an important point to remember in relation to all primary prevention strategies.

Finally, if an individual's social support is inadequate, interventions may need to be more direct. To determine what interventions are possible, Norbeck suggests that the following questions be asked:

1. What is the capacity of the network to change?
   a. *Network structure.* Are there persons who can be brought into (or back into) the network?
   b. *Network functioning.* Can existing network members be assisted to provide the kind of support that is needed (e.g., allow talk about the pregnancy or about a loss)?
   c. *Network disruption.* Can policies be changed or resources employed to minimize network disruption (e.g., due to hospitalization at a distant tertiary care facility)?
2. Does the individual have the interpersonal skills and attitudes required to establish and maintain contact with network members?
3. Is the individual receptive to using existing self-help or support groups or to having contact with a person who has coped with a similar experience?
4. If help from the indigenous social support system cannot be made available or acceptable, exactly what support does this individual require to cope with the current stressors or illness?
5. What long-term help would be required to assist the individual to establish and maintain an adequate social support network?[46:54]

A fourth possible intervention may be to help the person or group develop, maintain, and use a network. The person may also be encouraged to consider expanding his network. This might require health education strategies with the goal of competence building. Alternatively, one can influence the network more directly. Network therapy involves assembling and mobilizing all the important members of the family's kin and friendship network. The focus is then on tightening social bonds within the network and breaking dysfunctional patterns. For families who are isolated and whose networks are depleted, network members may not be available for such a strategy. In this case, arranging for the use of mutual support groups may be effective.

Finally, it should be noted that although supporting social supports is an effective intervention, it is not one that is limited to primary prevention activities. Rather, all nurses in all settings can use this strategy as a way of providing holistic care to maximize the health of individuals, families, and groups.

■ Working with groups

The nurse who is working in the area of primary prevention in mental health may be working with any level of the social hierarchy—individuals, families, communities, or even the larger society (Fig. 8-2). At this time she is likely to be working with groups of people as a way of maximizing the impact she can make and mobilizing the environment's potential to be supportive. A group approach, however, may not always be the most effective or efficient one. To decide if a group approach is indicated for a particular intervention, Loomis suggests that the nurse ask herself the following questions:

1. What are the client needs I am attempting to meet?
2. Can these needs be met in a group?
3. What are my own objectives for the proposed group?
4. What are the expectations of the system relative to the proposed group?
5. Is there any discrepancy or conflict between the answers to questions 1 through 4?[39:18-20]

Assuming that a group approach has been decided on, the next task of the nurse is to decide what type of group would be most appropriate. This may be ac-

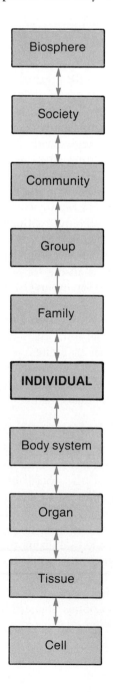

Fig. 8-2. Levels of organization that make up the social hierarchy.

The diagram (top to bottom) reads:
Biosphere — Society — Community — Group — Family — **INDIVIDUAL** — Body system — Organ — Tissue — Cell

complished by considering one's group goals, desired outcomes, and role of the nurse. It is particularly important to examine the role of the nurse, because different types of groups often have similar goals and outcomes. For example, providing emotional support to members is usually a function of many groups—formal, informal, natural, and professional. So too, giving new information to members can be a common outcome. A distinguishing characteristic, however, can be found in how the nurse functions in the group.

■ **TYPES OF GROUPS.** Marram describes three types of groups in which the psychiatric nurse is particularly likely to be involved.[41] The first is **group psychotherapy,** which uses the group process to treat people with existing mental disorders. They may vary in intensity and in the underlying theoretical framework used by the leaders. These groups can be distinguished by their overall emphasis on (1) personality reconstruction, (2) insight without reconstruction, (3) remotivation, (4) problem solving, (5) reeducation, or (6) support.[41] Nurses who lead such groups actively and formally engage patients in a therapeutic endeavor. However, the context is changed from that of a one-to-one relationship to that of a group relationship. Regardless, the responsibility for group psychotherapy resides with the nurse, and, for her to function in this role, she needs to have advanced education or extensive supervised experience. This type of group is associated with secondary and tertiary levels of prevention. Examples include inpatient groups, outpatient groups, special problem groups, family groups, therapy groups, and married couples groups.

The second type of group is commonly implemented in primary prevention strategies. This is the **therapeutic group,** which may be differentiated from group psychotherapy according to (1) how large a role emotional stress has played in the person's current level of health and (2) the primary goal or central objective of the group experience.[41] In group psychotherapy the emotional stress of the patient is of primary importance, and the group goal is treatment. In therapeutic groups, stress is the result of some change or life event that has the potential of producing a maladaptive response. One's goal, therefore, is prevention, education, and providing support. The individual in this group is on the healthy end of the health-illness continuum, although he may be experiencing a situational crisis of some type. The nurse still maintains responsibility for these groups, although her role may now be that of a health educator and facilitator. Examples of these groups can be found in general hospitals, clinics, nursing homes, industrial settings, business, schools, and penal institutions.

The third type of group is the **self-help, or mu-**

tual support, group, which has been described under the strategy of supporting social systems. Their primary aims are to (1) control member behavior, (2) ameliorate stress due to common problems, and (3) maintain member self-esteem and social integration.[41] They do not focus on personality reconstruction or insight analysis. Although the goals of these groups may not necessarily differentiate them from other types of groups, they do differ in one very important criterion: they are led by the group members themselves. If a nurse is the leader with primary responsibility for the group, then it is not a self-help, or mutual support, group. In these groups, if professionals participate at all, they do so by invitation and usually only in an ancillary role.

Finally, the nurse who uses a group approach should have an understanding of the development and processes that occur in groups to increase the therapeutic potential of the group for its members. These are described in Chapter 28.

 Evaluation

Throughout this chapter on primary prevention in mental health, mention has been made of the lack of clarity of concepts and assumptions, the lack of empirical studies identifying causal or predictive relationships, and the lack of understanding of the essential processes underlying preventive interventions. All of these problems are serious, and perhaps they all contribute to the lack of support for primary prevention as a public priority. Until we know more about an optimum fit between an individual and his social environment, it will be difficult to be able to help people define, select, create, and use environments that are growth producing for them.

When talking about primary prevention, one tends to think in terms of the total elimination of mental illness and stress. Yet these are not realistic goals, and maintaining them can only discourage any possible action. Perhaps it is possible to set goals of the reduction in suffering and the enhancement of the capacity to cope. But even these may be unattainable, given that the environment is constantly changing and adaptation is an ongoing challenge. Rather, if one focuses on the specific problems of a vulnerable group in our society, one's activity becomes more directed and the chance of success increases.

Clearly a need exists for the evaluation of programs in primary prevention. In a world of shrinking resources, only those programs with proven effectiveness are likely to be supported in the future. It needs to be demonstrated that the prevention strategy used had both short-term and long-term effects that benefited the individual and society. One also needs to de-termine whether the specific strategy implemented was the most effective, appropriate, and efficient one. Considering alternative approaches and comparing outcomes is an essential part of the evaluation process.

Offord believes that in the initial evaluation of primary prevention programs, close attention must be given to two points: (1) the program or intervention must be described in reproducible terms, and (2) the target of the intervention program must be stated.[49] Given these two prerequisites, he has identified the following points that should then be considered in evaluating particular primary prevention interventions or programs.

1. *Efficacy.* Does the program or intervention do more good than harm among those who agree to it?
2. *Effectiveness.* Does the intervention do more good than harm to those to whom it is offered?
3. *Efficiency.* Is the intervention being made available to those who could benefit from it with optimal use of resources?
4. *Length and timing of intervention.* Is there any evidence about the optimal length or timing of an intervention program?
5. *Harmful effects.* Are there data to suggest that the interventions may have harmful effects perhaps resulting from the unfavorable consequences of labeling?
6. *Screening programs.* Is there any evidence about the sensitivity, specificity, and predictive accuracy of the screening program?
7. *Possible high-risk groups.* Is there any evidence that the program would be more efficient if it were applied to those at increased risk for the disorder to be prevented?
8. *Economic analysis.* What are the results of the cost-benefit and cost-effectiveness analyses?

Finally, when evaluating certain aspects of the interventions, Offord suggests that the quality of the evidence supporting the conclusion should be rated systematically in the following way:

Grade I: If evidence is obtained from at least one properly randomized control trial
Grade II-1: If evidence is obtained from well-designed cohort or case-controlled analytic studies
Grade II-2: If evidence is obtained from comparisons between times and places with or without the intervention
Grade III: If support is derived from the opinions of respected authorities, based on clinical experience, descriptive studies, or reports of expert committees

He believes that when this grading system is applied to a particular primary prevention intervention or program, it will make explicit the strength of the scientific evidence supporting its possible implementation and provide a framework from which research priorities can be readily identified.[49]

Although preventing all illness is not possible, preventing some particular problems is. But a number of barriers exist that make expansion of primary prevention activities difficult. When faced with a choice, the needs of the presently ill consistently take precedence over preventing problems in the future. This holds true for nurses, as well as for the larger society. Yet by being more farsighted, both groups could benefit greatly. Nursing has long maintained its role in health education and supportive care. If it can document these actions and their effectiveness, it will demonstrate its value as a profession and its importance in promoting the well-being of society.

DIRECTIONS FOR FUTURE RESEARCH

The following are some of the nursing research problems raised in Chapter 8 that merit further study by psychiatric nurses:

1. Mental health services available to women on a regional basis in relation to rape, family violence, and substance abuse
2. Study of psychiatric nurses' attitudes toward sex roles
3. Specific preventive strategies and relevant social institutions and situations through which the strategies may be applied
4. The degree, level, and type of environmental change implemented by psychiatric nurses
5. The extent of participation of nurses in mutual support groups
6. The degree, domain, and type of mental health education implemented by psychiatric nurses
7. The effectiveness of preventive nursing interventions with regard to short- and long-term outcomes, use of resources, and comparison with other prevention strategies
8. The degree and type of intervention used by psychiatric nurses in supporting social systems
9. Preventive programs implemented by nurses who work with the mental health needs of women
10. The extent to which nurses engage in the primary prevention measures identified to meet the national 1990 objectives for the control of stress and violent behavior

■ SUGGESTED CROSS-REFERENCES ■

The model of health-illness phenomena, including stressors, coping resources, social support systems, and family assessment, are discussed in Chapter 3. Chapter 25 describes prevention in relation to community mental health. Therapeutic aspects of groups are discussed in Chapter 28. Problems experienced by children are discussed in Chapter 30 and adolescents are discussed in Chapter 31. Problems of family violence and abuse are discussed in Chapter 32. Problems experienced by the elderly are discussed in Chapter 35.

■ SUMMARY ■

1. Caplan's three levels of preventive intervention were described. The major thrust in present psychiatric care is in secondary prevention, and primary prevention has yet to evolve as a major force in the mental health movement.

2. The idea of promoting mental health was critiqued, and it was suggested that primary prevention activities focus on illness prevention to be effective. A paradigm for primary prevention was presented that attempts to reduce the incidence of particular stressful life events for vulnerable groups, and it was applied to the nursing process.

3. Assessment in primary prevention was presented as the identification of groups of people who are vulnerable to developing mental disorders or maladaptive coping responses to specific stressors or risk factors. The following vulnerable groups were described: children and adolescents, new families, established families, women, mature adults, and the elderly.

4. Prevention strategies should be directed toward influencing predisposing factors, precipitating stressors, appraisal of stressors, and coping resources through the following interventions: health education, environmental change, and supporting social systems.

   a. Health education involves the strengthening of individuals and groups through competence building.
   b. Environmental change involves the modification of an individual's or group's immediate environment or the larger social system.
   c. Supporting social systems is a way of buffering or cushioning the effects of a potentially stressful event. Four strategies for supporting social systems were described.

5. Working with groups is useful to maximize the preventive impact of the nurse's actions and the environment's potential to be supportive. Three types of groups—group psychotherapy, therapeutic groups, and self-help groups—were described in relation to group goals, desired outcomes, and role of the nurse.

6. Evaluation of primary prevention activities is impeded by the lack of clarity of assumptions, empirical studies in the area, and essential processes underlying preventive interventions. In evaluating preventive strategies, one needs to consider specific criteria and use a systematic rating scale of scientific evidence.

REFERENCES

1. American Psychiatric Association: Changing family patterns in the United States, Washington DC, 1986, The Association.
2. Angier J: Issues in consumer mental health information, Bull Med Libr Assoc 72(3):262, 1984.
3. Beverly E: The beginning of wisdom about aging, Geriatrics 30(7):117, 1975.
4. Bieber T and Bieber T: Postpartum reactions in men and women, J Am Acad Psychoan 6(4):511, 1978.
5. Bloom B: Prevention of mental disorders: recent advances in theory and practice, Community Ment Health J 15(3):179, 1979.
6. Bloom B: The evaluation of primary prevention programs. In Roberts L, Greenfield N, and Miller N, editors: Comprehensive Mental Health, Madison, 1968, University of Wisconsin Press.
7. Broverman I, Broverman D, and Clarkson F: Sex-role stereotypes and clinical judgments of mental health, J Consult Clin Psychol 34:1, 1970.
8. Brown F and Harris T: Social origins of depression, London, 1978, Tavistock Publications, Ltd.
9. Caplan G: Principles of preventive psychiatry, New York, 1964, Basic Books, Inc, Publishers.
10. Carmen E, Russo N, and Miller J: Inequality and women's mental health: an overview, Am J Psychiatry, 138:1319, 1981.
11. Cobb S: Social support as a moderator of life stress, Psychosom Med 38(5):306, 1976.
12. Comfort A: Geriatric psychiatry: mental symptoms in old age, Ala J Med Sci 18(2):177, 1981.
13. Cooperstock R: Sex differences in psychotropic drug use, Soc Sci Med 12B:179, 1978.
14. Cronenwett L and Kunst-Wilson W: Stress, social support and the transition to fatherhood, Nurs Res 30(4):196, 1981.
15. Davis A: The woman as therapist and client, Nurs Forum 16(34):250, 1977.
16. Diamond M: Social support and adaptation to chronic illness: the case of maintenance hemodialysis, Res Nurs Health 2:101, 1979.
17. Goodstein R: Inextricable interaction: social, psychologic, and biologic stresses facing the elderly, Am J Orthopsychiatry 51(2):219, 1981.
18. Gotlib I et al: Prevalence rates and demographic characteristics associated with depression in pregnancy and postpartum, J Consult Clinical Psychol 57(2):269, 1989.
19. Gottlieb B: The primary group as supportive milieu: application to community psychology, Am J Community Psychol 7(5):469, 1979.
20. Greywold E, Reese M, and Belle D: Stressed mothers syndrome: how to short circuit the stress depression cycle, Behav Med 7(11):12, 1980.
21. Griffith J: Women's stressors according to age groups: part I, Issues in Health Care of Women 6:311, 1983.
22. Griffith J: Women's stress responses and coping patterns according to age groups: part II, Issues in Health Care of Women 6:327, 1983.
23. Hagebak J and Hagebak B: Serving the mental health needs of the elderly: the case for removing barriers and improving service integration, Community Ment Health J 16:263, 1980.
24. Hamrick K and Blazer D: Older adults and their families in a community mental health center: strategies for intervention, Hosp Community Psychiatry 31:332, 1980.
25. Hefferin E: Life-cycle stressors: an overview of research, Fam Community Health 2(4):71, 1980.
26. Helper M et al: Life-events and acceptance of pregnancy, J Psychosom Res 12:183, 1968.
27. Hilberman E: Overview: the "wife-beater's wife" reconsidered, Am J Psychiatry 137:1336, 1980.
28. Hollister W: Basic strategies in designing primary prevention programs. In Klein D and Goldston S, editors: Primary prevention: an idea whose time has come, Department of Health, Education, and Welfare No (ADM)77-447, Rockville, Md, 1977, National Institute of Mental Health.
29. Institute of Medicine: Research on children and adolescents with mental, behavioral, and developmental disorders: mobilizing a national incentive, Washington DC, 1989, National Academy Press.
30. Iscoe I: Community psychology and the competent community, Am Psychol 29:607, 1974.
31. Jonas AD and Jonas DF: The influence of early training on the varieties of stress responses: an ethological approach, J Psychosom Res 19(5-6):325, 1975.
32. Kelley J and Wallerstein J: Brief interventions with children in divorcing families, Am J Orthopsychiatry, 47:23, 1977.
33. Kennell J, Voos D, and Klaus M: Parent-infant bonding. In Heffer R and Kempe C, editors: Child abuse and neglect: the family and the community, Cambridge, Mass, 1976, Ballinger Publishing Co.
34. Lacoursiere R: Fatherhood and mental illness: a review and new material, Psychiatr Q 46:109, 1972.
35. Lamb H and Zusman J: Primary prevention in perspective, Am J Psychiatry 136(1):12, 1979.
36. Lancaster J: Coping mechanisms of working mothers, Am J Nurs 75:1322, 1975.
37. Levenson D, Darrow C, and Kelin E: The seasons of a man's life, New York, 1978, Alfred A Knopf, Inc.
38. Levy L: Self-help groups: types and psychological processes, J Appl Behav Sci 12:310, 1976.
39. Loomis ME: Group process for nurses, St Louis, 1979, The CV Mosby Co.
40. Lynch M: Ill-health and child-abuse, Lancet, vol 2, Aug 16, 1975.
41. Marram GD: The group approach in nursing practice, ed 2, St Louis, 1978, The CV Mosby Co.
42. Mercer R: A theoretical framework for studying factors that impact on the maternal role, Nurs Res 30(2):73, 1981.

43. Moulton R: Some effects of the new feminism, Am J Psychiatry 134(1):1, 1977.
44. Neugarten B, editor: Middle age and aging, Chicago, 1968, University of Chicago Press.
45. Newton G: Self-help groups: can they help? J Psychosoc Nurs Ment Health Serv 22(7):27, July 1984.
46. Norbeck J: Social support: a model for clinical research and application, Adv Nurs Sci 3(4):42, 1981.
47. Notman M: Midlife concerns of women: implications of the menopause, Am J Psychiatry 136:1270, 1979.
48. Nuckolls KB, Cassel J, and Kaplan BH: Psychosocial assets, life crisis and the prognosis of pregnancy, Am J Epidemiol 95:431, 1972.
49. Offord D: Primary prevention: aspects of program design and evaluation, J Am Acad Child Psychiatry 21(1):225, 1982.
50. Pratt L: Child-rearing methods and children's health behavior, J Health Soc Behav 14(3):61, 1973.
51. President's Commission on Mental Health, vols 1 to 4, Washington, DC, 1978, US Government Printing Office.
52. Room R: The case for a problem prevention approach to alcohol, drug and mental problems, Public Health Rep 96(1):26, 1981.
53. Russell D: Incidence and prevalence of intrafamilial sexual abuse of female children, Child Abuse Neglect 7:133, 1983.
54. Ryan W: Preventive services in the social context: power, pathology and prevention. In Bloom B and Buch D, editors: Preventive services in mental health programs, Boulder, Colo, 1967, Western Interstate Commission for Higher Education.
55. Schaie K: Psychological changes from midlife to early old age: implications for the maintenance of mental health, Am J Orthopsychiatry 51(2):199, 1981.
56. Sherman J: Therapist attitudes and sex-role stereotyping. In Brodsky A and Hare-Merstin R, editors: Women and psychotherapy, New York, 1980, The Guilford Press.
57. "To . . . form a more perfect union . . .": Justice for American Women: Report of the National Commission of the Observance of International Women's Year, Washington, DC, 1976, US Government Printing Office.
58. US Department of Health and Human Services: Promoting health, preventing disease: objectives for the nation, Washington DC, 1984, Public Health Service.
59. United States Senate Committee on Aging: Aging America: trends and projections, Washington DC, 1987.

■ ANNOTATED SUGGESTED READINGS ■

Belsky J: Here tomorrow: making the most of life after fifty, Baltimore, 1988, Johns Hopkins University Press.
Excellent reference for a positive perspective on how growing older is yet another phase of human growth and development. Reviews health aspects of aging.

*Boettcher E: Linking the aged to support systems, J Gerontological Nurs 11(3):27, 1985.
Presents a conceptual framework based on socioeconomic factors, social exchange, power, and linkages that can help nurses formulate and implement more effective care plans for the elderly.

Bond L and Wagner B: Families in transition: primary prevention programs that work, Beverly Hills, Calif, 1988, Sage Publications.
Reviews normative transitions, the mystique of the traditional family, family crises, and principles that characterize effective prevention program.

*Bushy A and Smith T: Lobbying: the hows and wherefores, Nurs Manage 21(4):39, 1990.
Describes how, by becoming politically active, nurses can prepare for the future by influencing change in the health care system. Reviews the process of lobbying that nurses can use.

Eisenberg L: A research framework for evaluating the promotion of mental health and prevention of mental illness, Public Health Rep 96(1):3, 1981.
Excellent review article addressing specific topics and ways in which health may be promoted. Broad in scope and important in content.

*Ellison E: Social networks and the mental health caregiving system: implications for psychiatric nursing practice, J Psychosoc Nurs Ment Health Serv 21(2):18, 1983.
Examines the social network perspective as it relates to the design and delivery of mental health services for the chronically mentally ill. Assessment, diagnoses, and intervention strategies are described.

*Gallo J, Reichel W and Anderson L: Handbook of geriatric assessment, Rockville, Maryland, 1988, Aspen Publishers.
A thorough and clear manner, this text describes a multidimensional approach to assessing the elderly patient, including mental, functional, social, values, economic and physical components.

*Gammonley J: New directions for mental health education, J Psychiatr Nurs 16(12):40, 1978.
One of the few articles in the psychiatric nursing literature that focuses on mental health education, which is described in relation to both preventive and therapeutic programs.

Hefferin E: Life-cycle stressors: an overview of research, Fam Community Health 2(4):71, 1980.
An extensive, thorough, and well-organized review of research on life-cycle stressors. A valuable reference article.

*Jacobson A: Melancholy in the 20th century: causes and prevention, J Psychiatr Nurs 18(7):11, 1980.
Explores depression among women with a particular focus on primary prevention using support networks and anticipatory guidance for this high-risk population during critical developmental stages.

Journal of Family Issues
This quarterly journal focuses on the family in contemporary society. It includes theoretical and applied research writing with special issues focusing on a particular topic in depth.

---

*Asterisk indicates nursing reference.

*Newton G: Self-help groups: can they help? J Psychosoc Nurs Ment Health Serv 22(7):27, 1984.

Detailed description of assessment guidelines for evaluating self-help groups. Will help nurses determine therapeutic potential of such groups since not all of them are effective for all people.

*Nix H: Why parents anonymous? J Psychiatr Nurs 18(10):23, 1980.

Describes the formation of Parents Anonymous, the self-help group aimed at preventing child abuse. Includes the group's definition, structure, roles, and processes.

Price R, Cowen E, Lorion R, and Ramos-McKay J: The search for effective prevention programs: what we learned along the way, Am J Orthopsych 59(1):49, 1989.

Summarizes model prevention programs for high-risk groups throughout the life span. Program content is described and implications for planning, implementing, and evaluating effective programs are discussed.

*Roberts F: A model for parent education, Image 13:86, 1981.

Looks at why parent education is often ineffective and presents a new model for reconceptualizing its planning and delivery. The model has application for preventive health education in other areas.

*Robinson K: Working with a community action group, J Psychiatr Nurs 16(8):38, 1978.

Describes the role of nurses working with a community action group. Analyzes stages of group development and related problems.

Satir V: Peoplemaking, Palo Alto, Calif, ed 2, 1987, Science & Behavior Books.

Written for families about family process. Analyzes self-worth, communication systems, and family rules in an enjoyable way.

*Sedgwick R: Family mental health: theory and practice, St Louis, 1981, The CV Mosby Co.

Divided into three sections: an overview of concepts and principles, a discussion of the clinical process, and clinical application through case illustrations. Should be read by all nurses.

*Social Support, Adv Nurs Sci 10(2), 1988.

This entire journal issue is devoted to the theoretical and clinical application of social support to nursing practice. Excellent overview of the topic.

*Welch M, Boyd M, and Bell D: Education in primary prevention in psychiatric-mental health nursing for the baccalaureate student, International Nurs Rev 34(5):128, 1987.

Discusses how the concept of primary prevention can be taught to students of psychiatric nursing.

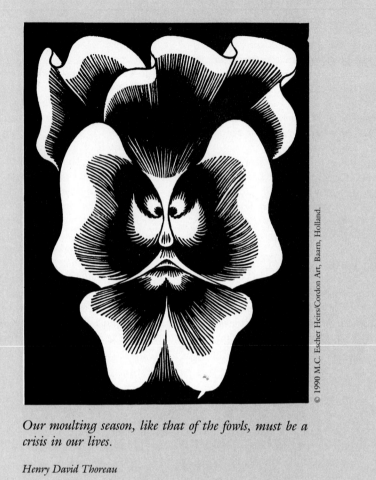

Our moulting season, like that of the fowls, must be a crisis in our lives.

Henry David Thoreau

C H A P T E R   9

CRISIS INTERVENTION

Sandra E. Benter

LEARNING OBJECTIVES

After studying this chapter, the student should be able to:

- describe the history of crisis theory, including the contributions of Lindemann and Caplan.

- define crisis and explain its potential for disorganization or personal growth.

- relate Caplan's four phases of a crisis and impinging "balancing factors."

- discuss the three types of crises: maturational, situational, and adventitious.

- analyze the goal, scope, and phases of crisis intervention.

- assess the relationship between nursing diagnoses and medical diagnoses appropriate to crisis intervention.

- describe four levels of crisis intervention and eight therapeutic techniques.

- evaluate the various modalities of crisis intervention and the settings in which they may be used.

- apply crisis intervention principles in the care of a patient.

- discuss future trends in crisis therapy.

- identify directions for future nursing research.

- select appropriate readings for further study.

Historical perspective

Historically, crisis theory comes from psychoanalytical theory. Analytical theory proposes that there are unconscious links to behavior and that psychological interpretations can be made to explain the causes of behavior. The causes are found in one's early experiences of infancy and childhood and affect one throughout life. There are many areas of conflict within the person. If conflicts are to be resolved constructively, they must be adapted to the environment; for example, to be socially acceptable, one's aggressive impulses can be channeled into competitive business practices rather than the physical harm of a rival.

Those who studied and practiced preventive psychiatry used psychoanalytical concepts to develop crisis theory. They explored the possibility of intervening briefly during stressful periods to resolve the problem in a healthy way. They observed a sequence of phases that people experienced during stressful situations and studied the outcomes of the crises. Crisis intervention techniques were then identified for promoting favorable outcomes.

In 1944, Eric Lindemann[25] studied 101 patients in crisis. He included psychoneurotic patients who lost a relative during the course of treatment, relatives of patients who died in the hospital, bereaved disaster victims (Coconut Grove fire) and their relatives, and relatives of members of the armed forces. Lindemann observed the course of normal grief and the symptoms of morbid grief reactions. Those persons undergoing normal grief showed signs of somatic distress, preoccupation with the image of the deceased, hostile reactions, guilt, changes in patterns of activity, and sometimes the taking on of characteristics of the deceased. Those persons undergoing morbid grief reactions showed either delayed or distorted reactions. Distorted reactions included overactivity without a sense of loss, the acquisition of symptoms belonging to the last illness of the deceased, the development of a medical disease, an alteration in relationships with friends and relatives, the development of furious hostility against specific persons, and the development of a clinical agitated depression.

Lindemann saw the role of mental health workers to be that of helping the patient free himself from his ties to the deceased and find new patterns of rewarding interaction. He believed the concept of intervention during bereavement could be applied to other stressful situations such as marriage and the birth of a child. Thus the prevention of psychiatric disorders could be accomplished. He thought this could take place in the community and be patterned after a public health model so that many people could be reached. Lindemann, along with Gerald Caplan, actually set up a community mental health clinic in Massachussets where crisis intervention was practiced.

In 1964 Caplan published the concepts of community mental health practice, including primary, secondary, and tertiary prevention.[6] He defined crisis theory and described crisis intervention as a separate form of therapy. He viewed **primary prevention** as the social and interpersonal actions that help meet the basic needs of a community and allow it to deal constructively with its crises. Its aim is the prevention of mental disorder. Social action involves working with political and social policies to help people cope with crises. Interpersonal action involves helping individuals with their specific stresses.

Secondary prevention aims to decrease the number of existing cases through early diagnosis and effective treatment. Early referral, screening programs, and improvement in diagnostic tools are examples of secondary prevention. This type of prevention is the more traditional treatment-oriented method of approaching mental illness. Caplan emphasizes that attention must be paid to effective use of mental health workers so that the numbers treated successfully will be large enough to make a difference in community rates.

Tertiary prevention aims to reduce the rate of disability caused by one's lowered ability to contribute to the community after recovering from mental disorder. Rehabilitation programs therefore focus on tertiary prevention. Secondary prevention includes primary prevention, and tertiary prevention includes both primary and secondary prevention. Crisis therapy is a primary prevention concept and is one of the most effective ways of preventing mental disorder.

In 1963 President Kennedy issued a message on community treatment of mental illness and mental retardation in the introduction of the Community Mental Health Centers Act. Communities then began to assume more responsibility for their own mental health needs. Although many clinicians thought that long-term psychotherapy was still the preferred treatment, it was impractical because it was expensive, required a long-term commitment, and did not meet the needs of all socioeconomic groups. Therefore a treatment method that was brief, direct, and here-and-now—oriented was necessary. Crisis therapy then became more widely used.

Definition of crisis

A crisis is an internal disturbance caused by a stressful event or a perceived threat to self. The person's usual way of coping becomes ineffective in dealing with the threat, causing a rise in anxiety. The threat, or precipitating event, can usually be identified. It may have occurred weeks or days ago, and its significance may or may not be linked (in the individual's eyes) to the crisis state. Precipitating events are perceived losses, threats of losses, or challenges. Losses may include the death of a spouse, divorce, or loss of a job. Threats of losses may include illness of a family member or an increase in arguments with a spouse. Challenges may include a change in responsibilities at work or a change to a different line of work. Additional threats or stresses are identified in the Social Readjustment Rating Scale (Chapter 3).

Following the precipitating event the person's anxiety rises and Caplan's four phases of a crisis[6] emerge. In the first phase the anxiety activates one's usual methods of coping. If these do not bring relief and there is inadequate situational support, the person progresses to the second phase. He becomes even more anxious because his coping mechanisms have failed. In the third phase he tries out new coping mechanisms or redefines the threat so that old ones can work. Resolution of the problem therefore can occur in this phase. However, if resolution does not occur, the person goes on to the fourth phase in which the continuation of severe or panic levels of anxiety may lead to psychological disorganization.

In describing the phases of a crisis, it is important to consider the following balancing factors[1]: one's perception of the event, situational supports, and coping mechanisms. Successful resolution of the crisis is more likely if the person has a realistic view of the event, if he has situational supports that can help him solve the problem, and if he has effective coping mechanisms. These balancing factors are shown in the paradigm developed by Aguilera and Messick (Fig. 9-1).

The phases of a crisis and the impact of balancing factors are similar to the components of the nursing model of health-illness phenomena described in Chapter 3. However, by definition, crises are self-limiting. People in crisis are too emotionally upset to continue such a high level of anxiety indefinitely. A period of 6 weeks has classically been considered the time span needed for resolution, whether it be a positive solution or a state of disorganization. However, some researchers consider it unlikely that any specific time can be applicable to all people undergoing all crises.[2]

People in crisis experience many symptoms, including helplessness, anxiety, confusion, depression, anger, withdrawal, psychosomatic symptoms, inefficiency, and hopelessness. Suicidal and homicidal thoughts may be present. Feelings of alienation from others often occur. Sometimes these symptoms can cause further problems; for example, inefficiency at work may lead to the loss of a job, financial problems, and lowered self-esteem. Crises can also be complicated by old internal conflicts. Previous conflicts can be brought out by the present conflict and make crisis resolution more difficult.

Periods of intense conflict can cause increased vulnerability but can also produce increased growth. How one handles the crises determines whether growth or disorganization results. Growth comes from experiencing and learning in new situations. People in crisis feel uncomfortable and often reach out for help. They are in turmoil and are ready to accept help from others until they feel psychological equilibrium has returned. The fact that crises can lead to personal growth is an important one for the nurse to remember when working with patients in crisis situations.

Types of crises

There are three types of crises: maturational, situational, and adventitious. Sometimes more than one type of crisis can occur at the same time. Thus an individual undergoing a maturational crisis can simultaneously have a situational stress that adds to his anxiety. For example, an adolescent who is having difficulty adjusting to his change of role and body image may, at the same time, undergo the stresses related to the death of a parent.

■ Maturational crises

Developmental psychology describes a series of steps one must take in growing toward maturity. As a person passes from one stage to another, he goes through transitional periods during which his psychological equilibrium can be upset. These periods are developmental, or maturational, crises.

Erik Erikson[13,14] described eight stages of development from infancy to old age and the relationship of each stage to the ones before and after. Each stage presents a problem or task that the person must complete before moving on to the next stage. Erikson emphasizes that development is a continuum in which each stage has a part. The tasks of each stage must be completed for the individual to grow and move toward maturity. The person learns to cope with the stresses of life as his personality matures. Erikson points out that this mastery of tasks leads to successful solutions of maturational crises.

Havighurst[18] also identified specific tasks for each major developmental period from infancy through death. Table 9-1 compares Erikson's and Havighurst's developmental stages and tasks.[35] Together they pre-

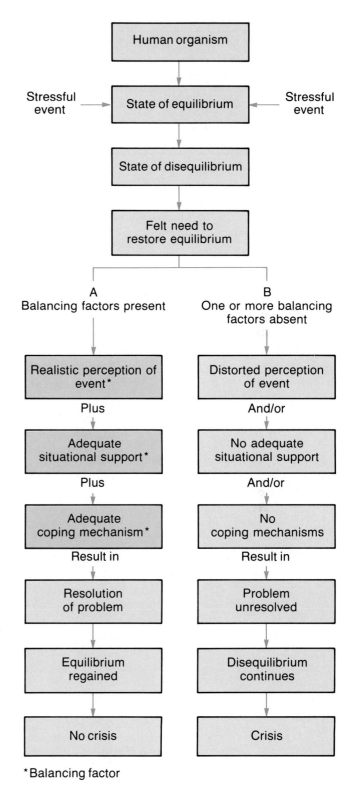

Fig. 9-1. Effect of balancing factors in a stressful event. (From Aguilera DC: Crisis intervention: theory and methodology, ed 6, St Louis, 1990, Mosby–Year Book, Inc.)

TABLE 9-1

COMPARISON OF ERIKSON'S AND HAVIGHURST'S DEVELOPMENTAL STAGES AND TASKS

Developmental stage	Erikson	Havighurst
	Trust versus mistrust 1. Oral needs of primary importance 2. Adequate mothering necessary to meet infant's needs 3. Acquisition of hope	1. Learning to walk 2. Learning to take solid foods 3. Learning to talk 4. Learning to control elimination of body wastes 5. Learning sex differences and sexual modesty 6. Achieving physiological stability 7. Forming simple concepts of social and physical reality 8. Learning to relate oneself emotionally to parents, siblings, and other people 9. Learning to distinguish right and wrong and developing a conscience
Toddler years	*Autonomy vs. shame* 1. Anal needs of primary importance 2. Father emerges as important figure 3. Acquisition of will	
Early childhood	*Initiative vs. guilt* 1. Genital needs of primary importance 2. Family relationships contribute to early sense of responsibility and conscience 3. Acquisition of purpose	
Middle childhood	*Industry vs. inferiority* 1. Active period of socialization for child as he moves from family into society 2. Acquisition of competence	1. Learning physical skills necessary for ordinary games 2. Building wholesome attitudes toward oneself as a growing organism 3. Learning to get along with age mates 4. Learning an appropriate sex role 5. Developing fundamental skills in reading, writing, and calculating 6. Developing concepts necessary for everyday living 7. Developing conscience, morality, and scale of values 8. Developing attitudes toward social groups and institutions
Adolescence	*Identity vs. identity diffusion* 1. Search for self in which peers play important part 2. Psychosocial moratorium is provided by society 3. Acquisition of fidelity	1. Accepting one's physique and accepting a masculine or feminine role 2. New relations with age mates of both sexes 3. Emotional independence of parents and other adults 4. Achieving assurance of economic independence 5. Selecting and preparing for an occupation 6. Developing intellectual skills and concepts necessary for civic competence 7. Desiring and achieving socially responsible behavior 8. Preparing for marriage and family life 9. Building conscious values in harmony with adequate scientific world picture
Adulthood	*Intimacy vs. isolation* 1. Characterized by increasing importance of human closeness and sexual fulfillment 2. Acquisition of love	1. Selecting a mate 2. Learning to live with marriage partner 3. Starting family 4. Rearing children 5. Managing home 6. Getting started in occupation 7. Taking on civic responsibility 8. Finding congenial social group

From Sundeen SJ et al: Nurse-client interaction: implementing the nursing process, ed 4, St Louis, 1989, The CV Mosby Co.

TABLE 9-1, cont'd

COMPARISON OF ERIKSON'S AND HAVIGHURST'S DEVELOPMENTAL STAGES AND TASKS

Developmental stage	Erikson	Havighurst
Middle age	*Generativity vs. self-absorption* 1. Characterized by productivity, creativity, parental responsibility, and concern for new generation 2. Acquisition of care	1. Achieving adult civic and social responsibility 2. Establishing and maintaining economic standard of living 3. Assisting teenage children to become responsible and happy adults 4. Developing adult leisure activities 5. Relating oneself to one's spouse as a person 6. Accepting and adjusting to physiological changes of middle age 7. Adjusting to aging parents
Old age	*Integrity vs. despair* 1. Characterized by a unifying philosophy of life and a more profound love for mankind 2. Acquisition of wisdom	1. Adjusting to decreasing physical strength and health 2. Adjusting to retirement and reduced income 3. Adjusting to death of spouse 4. Establishing explicit affiliation with age group 5. Meeting social and civic obligations 6. Establishing satisfactory physical living arrangements

sent a comprehensive view of human development and its crises.

Maturational crises are periods requiring role changes. For example, when a person grows from early childhood to middle childhood, he is expected to become socially involved with people outside the family. When he moves from adolescence to adulthood, he is expected to be financially responsible for himself. Both social and biological pressures to change can precipitate a crisis. The nature and extent of the maturational crisis can be influenced by the adequacy of role models, interpersonal resources, and the ease of others in accepting the new role. Adequate role models show the person how to act in the new role. Interpersonal resources allow him to try out many new interpersonal behaviors in his attempt to achieve role changes. The use of others in accepting the new role determines the strength or resistances one comes up against in making role changes. The greater the resistance of others, the more stress the person faces in making the changes.

Transitional periods during adolescence, parenthood, marriage, midlife, and retirement are key times for maturational crises to occur. Some conflicts related to parenthood are in Clinical example 9-1.

Some of the conflicts related to retirement are presented in Clinical example 9-2.

CLINICAL EXAMPLE 9-1

Ms. J was a 19-year-old black, single, unemployed woman who came to the mental health clinic a month after the birth of her first child. Ms. J complained of feeling depressed. Her symptoms included difficulty falling asleep, early morning awakening, crying spells, a poor appetite, difficulty in caring for the baby because of fatigue and apathy, and thoughts of wanting to hurt the baby. The patient lived with her parents and siblings and had never lived on her own. She had always been dependent on her mother to take care of her and relieve her stresses. Her mother, however, worked and the patient was totally responsible for her daughter's care each day. Also, Ms. J's mother was angry that she had had a child and usually refused to care for the baby. The patient's boyfriend, who was the baby's father, had promised to marry her, but he had recently decided he was too young to handle the responsibility of a wife and child. In summary, a young woman who had unmet dependency needs of her own was now in a position of parenthood and had to meet the dependency needs of an infant. This precipitated a crisis for her.

> ## CLINICAL EXAMPLE 9-2
>
> Mr. R was a 67-year-old white, married pharmacist who came to the mental health clinic complaining of anxiety, depression, and insomnia. His symptoms had begun 2 weeks ago when the patient's wife decided that they should move to a retirement community in Florida. The patient described his wife as a strong, willful woman who was also outgoing and charming and made friends easily. He considered himself a quiet, nervous person who was comfortable only with old friends and his two sons and their families. Mr. R, although of retirement age, had continued to work as a pharmacist, doing relief work for a drugstore chain when the regular pharmacists were absent. In moving to Florida, the patient would lose his pharmacist's license, which was valid only for his present state of residence. He expressed difficulty in making the transition from a working person to a retired person. He had fears of becoming directionless and useless. He was anxious about leaving his sons and his friends. The possibility of both complete retirement and moving to another state precipitated his present distress.

> ## CLINICAL EXAMPLE 9-3
>
> Mrs. H is a 55-year-old white, married woman whose husband was hospitalized for mitral stenosis. Heart surgery was scheduled for the following week. Mr. H appeared appropriately concerned, but the nursing staff noticed that the patient's wife was becoming increasingly anxious. She spent each day running from her husband's bedside to the nurses' station demanding constant attention. She moved and spoke rapidly and continuously, and at times her thoughts seemed confused. Mrs. H stated that once in the past she had had a "nervous breakdown," and she hoped the stress of her husband's surgery would not result in another one.

Situational crises

Situational crises occur when an external event upsets an individual's or a group's psychological equilibrium. Examples of situational crises include loss of a job, loss of a loved one, an unwanted pregnancy, the onset or worsening of a medical illness, divorce, and school problems. The loss of a job can result in financial stress, feelings of inadequacy as a breadwinner, and marital conflict caused by a spouse's anger over the lost job. The loss of a loved one results in bereavement and can also cause financial stress, change of roles of family members, and loss of emotional support. The onset or worsening of a medical illness causes fear of the loss of a loved one. Again, financial stress and change of roles of family members often occur. Divorce is similar to the stress of the loss of a loved one, and there is the stress of dealing with the ex-spouse as well. An unwanted pregnancy is stressful because it requires decisions to be made about whether to complete the pregnancy or to abort it, and whether to keep the baby or place it for adoption. If the baby is to be kept, changes in life-style will be required. School problems are also stressful and can lead to serious feelings of inadequacy. Parents often blame themselves or each other, and total family disequilibrium can result.

Some of the stresses related to the course of a medical illness can be seen in the situational crisis presented in Clinical example 9-3.

Adventitious crises

Adventitious crises are accidental, uncommon, and unexpected. Multiple losses with gross environmental changes result. For example, fires, earthquakes, hurricanes, or floods, which disrupt entire communities, are adventitious crises. Recent mass tragedies, which have become all too common, are also examples of adventitious crises and include group kidnappings (the taking of hostages), nuclear accidents, group killings in communities, airplane crashes, volcanic eruptions, and floods complicated by the deposit of industrial waste material.

Unlike maturational and situational crises, adventitious crises do not occur in the lives of everyone. When they do occur, however, they challenge every coping mechanism because of the severity of the stress. During adventitious crises, mental health workers must reach larger numbers of people in crisis states. The multiple losses and gross environmental changes that result from adventitious crises can be seen in the following situation described in a Department of Health, Education and Welfare publication[9:5].

In West Virginia a river filled with coal sludge overflowed when a dam broke, and an entire community was damaged. There were many deaths and injuries, loss of homes and possessions, disruption or loss of employment, sudden relocation, and extreme demands on physical endurance. The solidarity of this isolated rural community was grossly dis-

TABLE 9-2

FIVE PHASES OF HUMAN DISASTER RESPONSE

Phase	Response
Impact phase	Includes the event itself and is characterized by shock, panic, or extreme fear; the person's judgment and assessment of reality factors are very poor, and self-destructive behavior may be seen.
Heroic phase	A cooperative spirit exists between friends, neighbors, and emergency teams; constructive activity at this time can help to overcome feelings of anxiety and depression but over-activity can lead to "burnout".
Honeymoon phase	Begins to appear 1 week to several months after the disaster; the need to help others is sustained, and the money, resources, and support received from various agencies causes life to begin again in the community; psychological and behavioral problems may be overlooked.
Disillusionment phase	Lasts from about 2 months to 1 year; a time of disappointment, resentment, frustration, and anger; victims often begin to compare their neighbors' plights with their own and may start to resent, envy, or show hostility toward others.
Reconstruction and reor-ganization phase	Individuals recognize that they must come to grips with their own problems; they begin to rebuild their homes, businesses, and lives in a constructive fashion; this period may last for years after the disaster.

Data from Frederick C and Garrison J: Behav Today 12:32, 1981.

turbed. The residents suffered a high incidence of mental illness as a result.

Disaster-precipitated emotional problems often surface weeks or even months after the disaster. The symptoms usually occur in roughly five phases, which are described in Table 9-2.[15] If the reconstruction phase does not begin within 6 months of the onset of the disaster, the likelihood of lasting psychological problems is greatly increased. The severe psychological stress resulting from adventitious crises can be further illustrated by the findings of Terr who studied 23 child kidnap victims[37:14]:

In the town of Chowchilla, California, a school bus containing 26 children and a bus driver was stopped by three masked men and taken over at gunpoint. The captured children were driven around in boarded-over vans for 11 hours and were then transferred to a buried truck trailer. After 16 additional hours, two of the oldest boys dug them out. The children suffered from initial misperceptions, fears of further trauma, and hallucinations. Later they experienced posttraumatic play reenactment, personality change, repeated dreams, fears of being kidnapped again, and a fear of common mundane experiences.

Crisis intervention

Aguilera and Messick state[1:1]:

Crisis intervention can offer the immediate help that a person in crisis needs to reestablish equilibrium. This is an inexpensive, short-term therapy that focuses on solving the immediate problem.

Crisis intervention is frequently limited to a period of 6 weeks. The goal of crisis intervention is for the patient to return to his precrisis level of functioning. Often the patient advances to a level of functioning that is higher than the precrisis level, because he has learned new ways of problem solving. There are four phases of crisis intervention that are similar to those of the nursing process: assessment, planning, implementation, and evaluation.

■ Assessment

The first step of crisis intervention is assessment. During this phase, data regarding the nature of the crisis and its effect on the patient must be collected. It is from these data that a plan for intervention will be developed. During this phase the nurse begins to establish a positive working relationship with the patient. A number of specific areas should be assessed by the nurse. These are the balancing factors that are important in the development and resolution of a crisis:

1. Identifying the precipitating event
2. Identifying the patient's perception of the event
3. Identifying the nature and strength of the patient's support systems
4. Identifying the patient's previous strengths and coping mechanisms

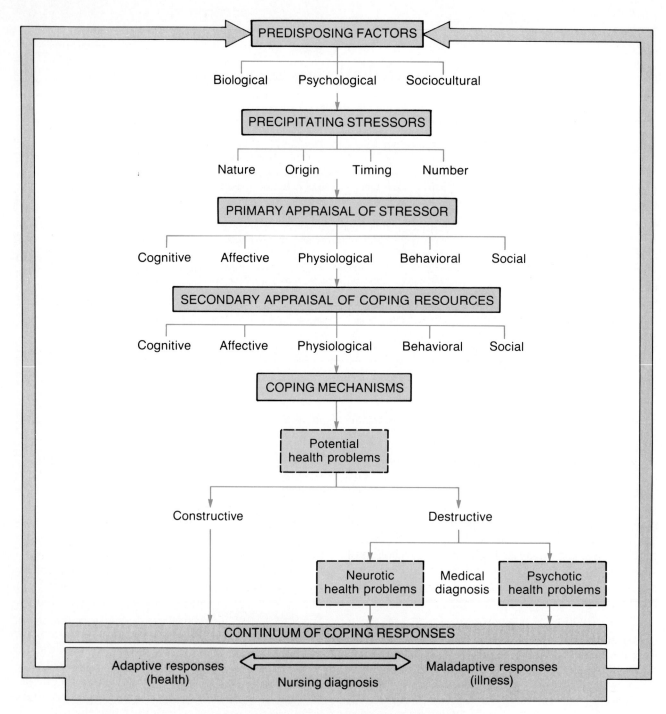

Fig. 9-2. Nursing model of health-illness phenomena.

The components of the nursing model of health-illness phenomena that parallel the balancing factors in crisis intervention are highlighted in Fig. 9-2.

■ **PRECIPITATING EVENT.** To help identify the precipitating event, the nurse should explore three areas: the patient's needs and the events that threaten those needs, the point at which symptoms appear, and the themes or memories that the patient talks about. Four kinds of needs that have been identified are related to self-esteem, sexual role mastery, dependency, and biological function.[33] Self-esteem is achieved when the person attains successful social role experience. Sexual role mastery is achieved when the person attains vocational, sexual, and parental role successes. Dependency is achieved when a satisfying interdependent relationship with others is attained. Biological function is achieved when a person is safe and his life is not threatened.

The nurse determines which needs are not being met by asking the patient how he feels about himself, what areas of his life he thinks successful, what kinds of relationships he has with others, and how safe and secure he feels in life. The nurse looks for obstacles that might interfere with meeting the patient's needs. What recent experiences have been upsetting? What areas of life have had changes?

■ **PERCEPTION OF THE EVENT.** The patient's perception of the precipitating event is very important. What may seem trivial to the nurse may have great meaning to the patient. An overweight adolescent girl may have been the only girl in the class not invited to a dance. This may have threatened her self-esteem. A man with two unsuccessful marriages may have just been told by a girlfriend that she wants to end their relationship; this may have threatened his need for sexual role mastery. An emotionally isolated, friendless woman may have had car trouble and been unable to find someone to give her a ride to work. This may have threatened her dependency needs. A chronically ill man who has had a recent relapse of his illness may have had his need for biological function threatened.

Coping patterns become ineffective and symptoms appear usually after the stressful incident. When did the patient begin to feel anxious? When did his sleep disturbance begin? At what point in time did his suicidal thoughts start? If symptoms began last Tuesday, ask what took place in the patient's life on Tuesday or Monday. As the patient connects life events with the breakdown in coping mechanisms, an understanding of the precipitating event can emerge.

Themes and surfacing memories of the patient give further clues to the precipitating event. Present issues of concern are symbolically connected to past issues of concern. For example, a female patient who talks about the death of her father, which occurred 3 years ago, may, on questioning, reveal a recent loss of a relationship with a male. A patient who talks about feelings of inadequacy he had as a child because of poor school performance may, on questioning, reveal a recent experience in which his feelings of adequacy on his job were threatened. Since most crises involve losses or threats of losses, the theme of losses is a common one expressed. In assessment the nurse therefore looks for a recent occurrence that may be connected to an underlying theme.

■ **SUPPORT SYSTEMS.** The patient's living situation and his supports in the environment must be assessed. Information is sought concerning present and potential sources of support. Does the patient live alone or with family or friends? With whom is he close? Who does he think understands him and offers him strength? Is there a supportive clergyman or church friend? Assessing the patient's support system is important in determining who should come for the crisis therapy sessions. It may be decided that certain family members should come with the patient so that the family members' support can be strengthened. If the patient has few supports in his life, he may need to be involved in a crisis therapy group so that the support of other group members can be elicited. Assessing the patient's support system is also vital in determining whether hospitalization would be more appropriate than outpatient crisis therapy. If there is a high degree of suicidal and homicidal risk along with a weak outside support system, hospitalization may be a safer and more effective treatment.

■ **COPING MECHANISMS.** Next, the nurse assesses the patient's strengths and previous coping mechanisms. How has the patient handled other crises in his life? To whom has he turned? How did he relieve anxieties? Did the patient talk out problems with a relative? Did he leave his environment for a period of time to think things out from another perspective? Did he participate in physical activity to relieve tension? Did he find relief in crying? Besides exploring previous coping mechanisms, the nurse should also note the absence of other possible successful mechanisms.

■ **NURSING DIAGNOSES.** The final step in the assessment phase of crisis intervention is the formulation of nursing diagnoses. These diagnoses may be related to any aspect of the patient's life and can reflect the variety of nursing problems described in Chapters 11 to 21. The box on page 280 presents the primary NANDA nursing diagnoses appropriate to crisis intervention and examples of complete nursing diagnoses. Nursing diagnoses related to the range of possible maladaptive responses of the patient are identified along with related medical diagnoses in Table 9-3.

■ **RELATED MEDICAL DIAGNOSES.** Related medical diagnoses may include a variety of psychiatric disorders. However, many patients who require crisis intervention fall under the category of adjustment disorder. Posttraumatic stress disorder (PTSD)[21] is one type of anxiety disorder that is often treated by crisis intervention therapy. If not treated early, this disorder can become chronic.[5,10,16] Two populations that often experience PTSD are rape victims and war veterans. For example, it is estimated that 20% to 60% of the

---

Nursing Diagnoses Related to Crisis Intervention

Primary NANDA Nursing Diagnoses

Coping, ineffective individual
Coping, ineffective family: compromised
Family processes, altered

Examples of Complete Nursing Diagnoses

Ineffective individual coping related to child's illness evidenced by limited ability to concentrate and psychomotor agitation

Ineffective individual coping related to daughter's death evidenced by inability to recall events pertaining to the car accident

Ineffective family coping, compromised, related to separation from husband evidenced by excessive dependency on friends and preoccupation with having husband return home

Ineffective family coping, compromised, related to wife's cancer diagnosis evidenced by feelings of grief, fear, and guilt

Altered family process related to move to a new town evidenced by social withdrawal and rejection of help from others

Altered family process related to marriage of daughter evidenced by unclear family boundaries and distorted communication patterns

---

stressor that occurs within 3 months of the onset of the stressor but has not persisted for more than 6 months. Behaviors include impairment in social or occupational functioning or symptoms of an excessive reaction to the stressor. There are various types of adjustment disorders, such as the following:

Adjustment disorder with depressed mood: The other essential feature is tearfulness or hopelessness.

Adjustment disorder with anxious mood: The other essential features are nervousness, worry, and jitteriness.

Adjustment disorder with mixed emotional features: The other essential feature is a combination of depression and anxiety and other disorders.

Adjustment disorder with disturbances of conduct: The other essential feature is the violation of the rights of others or of major age-appropriate societal norms and rules.

Adjustment disorder with mixed disturbance of emotions and conduct: The other essential features are both emotional features and a disturbance of conduct.

Adjustment disorder with work or academic inhibition: The other essential feature is a decrease in work or academic functioning.

Adjustment disorder with withdrawal: The other essential feature is social withdrawal without significant depressed or anxious mood.

Adjustment disorder with physical complaints: The other essential feature is the presence of physical symptoms such as headache, backache, or fatigue.

Adjustment disorder NOS: This is a residual category for disorders involving maladaptive reactions to psychosocial stressors that are not classifiable as specific types of adjustment disorder.

Posttraumatic stress disorder. The essential feature of posttraumatic stress disorder is the development of characteristic symptoms after a psychologically traumatic event. The characteristic symptoms involve reexperiencing the traumatic event; a numbing of responsiveness or reduced involvement with the external world; recurrent, distressing dreams of the event; and a variety of autonomic, depressed, or anxious symptoms.

■ Planning

The second step of crisis intervention is planning. During this phase the previously collected data are analyzed and specific interventions are proposed. Dynamics underlying the present crisis are formulated from the information about the precipitating event. Alternative solutions to the problem are explored, and steps for achieving the solutions are identified. The nurse decides which environmental supports to engage or strengthen and how to do this. She also decides

---

2.5 million Vietnam war veterans who saw combat have had or continue to have psychological adjustment problems at home. Their long-term adjustment should ideally follow four stages identified by Figley: (1) recovery, (2) avoidance, (3) reconsideration, and (4) adjustment.[5] In recovery, the veteran realizes that he is safe. In avoidance, he tries not to think about his experiences so that he does not have to face overwhelming feelings. In reconsideration, the veteran reflects on his experiences and begins to deal with his thoughts and feelings. Finally, having successfully reflected, he enters the stage of adjustment. Immediate psychological help in following through these stages may prevent chronic disorder. The medical diagnoses of adjustment disorder and posttraumatic stress disorder will now be briefly described.

Adjustment disorder. Adjustment disorder is a maladaptive reaction to an identifiable psychosocial

TABLE 9-3

MEDICAL AND NURSING DIAGNOSES RELATED TO CRISIS INTERVENTION

Related Medical Diagnoses (DSM-III-R)*	Related Nursing Diagnoses (NANDA)
Adjustment disorder with depressed mood	Adjustment, impaired
Adjustment disorder with anxious mood	Anxiety
Adjustment disorder with mixed emotional features	†Coping, ineffective family: compromised
Adjustment disorder with disturbances of conduct	†Coping, ineffective individual
Adjustment disorder with mixed disturbance of emotions and conduct	†Family process, altered
Adjustment disorder with work or academic inhibition	Fear
Adjustment disorder with withdrawal	Grieving, anticipatory
Adjustment disorder with physical complaints	Growth and development, altered
Adjustment disorder NOS	Health maintenance, altered
Posttraumatic stress disorder	Knowledge deficit
	Parenting, altered
	Post-trauma response
	Rape trauma syndrome
	Self-esteem disturbance
	Social isolation
	Spiritual distress

*From American Psychiatric Association: Diagnostic and Statistical Manual of Mental Disorders (Third Edition—Revised). American Psychiatric Association, October 1987.
†Indicates primary nursing diagnoses for crisis intervention.

which of the patient's coping mechanisms to develop and which ones to strengthen.

■ Intervention

The third step of crisis intervention is implementing the intervention itself. The intervention can take place on many levels using a variety of techniques. Shields[31] has described four specific levels of crisis intervention, which represent a hierarchy from the most superficial to the most in-depth:

1. Environmental manipulation
2. General support
3. Generic approach
4. Individual approach

Each step includes the lower levels of intervention. The progressive order of the steps also indicates the degree of knowledge and skill needed by the nurse for application.

■ **ENVIRONMENTAL MANIPULATION.** Environmental manipulation includes interventions that directly change the patient's physical or interpersonal situation. These interventions provide situational support or remove stress. For example, a patient who is having trouble coping with her six children may temporarily send several of the children to their grandparents'

house. In this situation some stress is alleviated. Similarly, a patient having difficulty on his job may take a week of sick leave so he can be removed temporarily from that stress. A patient who lives alone may move in with his closest sibling for several days. In this situation some support is provided. Likewise, involving the patient in family or group crisis therapy provides environmental manipulation for the purpose of providing support.

■ **GENERAL SUPPORT.** General support includes interventions that provide the patient with the feeling that the nurse is on his side and will be a helping person. The nurse uses warmth, acceptance, empathy, caring, and reassurance to provide this type of support.

■ **GENERIC APPROACH.** The generic approach is a type of crisis intervention that is similar to the public health model. It is designed to reach high-risk individuals and large groups as quickly as possible. It applies a specific method to all individuals faced with a similar type of crisis. The course of the particular type of crisis is previously studied and mapped out. The intervention is then set up to ensure that the course of the crisis results in an adaptive resolution.

As described earlier in this chapter, grief is an example of a type of crisis with a known pattern that can be influenced toward a positive outcome. Lindemann's study[25] described the pattern of grief. He believed that helping the patient free himself from his ties to the deceased and find new patterns of rewarding interaction would help the patient effectively resolve his grief. Applying this specific intervention to people experiencing grief, especially when a high-risk group is evident (e.g., families of local disaster victims), is an example of providing a generic approach. Use of the generic approach does not require the nurse to have a thorough understanding of the unique psychodynamics of the patient.[22]

■ **INDIVIDUAL APPROACH.** The individual approach is a type of crisis intervention similar to the model of diagnosis and treatment of a specific problem in a specific patient. The nurse must understand the patient's psychodynamics that led to the present crisis and must use the intervention that is most likely to help the patient to a healthy resolution to his crisis. This type of crisis intervention can be effective with all types of crisis. It is particularly useful in combined situational and maturational crises. The individual approach is also beneficial when symptoms include homicidal and suicidal risk. The individual approach should be applied if the course of the crisis cannot be determined. It also should be applied to crises that have not responded to the generic approach. It is often helpful to consult with others when deciding which approach to use for a specific patient.

■ **TECHNIQUES.** The nurse uses techniques that are active, focal, and explorative to carry out the interventions. The intervention must be aimed at achieving quick resolution. The nurse also must be active in guiding the crisis intervention through its various steps. A more passive approach is inappropriate for this type of psychotherapy because of the time limitations of the crisis situation.

The nurse is creative and flexible, trying many different techniques. Some of these include abreaction, clarification, suggestion, manipulation, reinforcement of behavior, support of defenses, raising self-esteem, and exploration of solutions.[30] A brief description of these techniques will now be presented.

Abreaction is the release of feelings that takes place as the patient talks about emotionally charged areas. As he becomes aware of his feelings about the events, he experiences tension reduction. Abreaction is often used in crisis intervention. The nurse encourages abreaction by asking the patient how he feels about his situation, recent events, and significant people involved in his crisis. The nurse asks open-ended questions and reflects the patient's words back to him so that he will further ventilate his feelings. The nurse does not discourage crying or angry outbursts but rather sees them as a positive release of feelings. Only when feelings seem out of control, such as in extreme rage or despondency, should the nurse discourage abreaction and help the patient concentrate on thinking rather than feeling. For example, if a patient angrily talks of wanting to kill a specific person, it is better to help him focus on thinking through the consequences of carrying out the act rather than encouraging free expression of the angry feelings.

Clarification is used when the nurse helps the patient to identify the relationship between certain events in his life. For example, helping a patient see that it was after he was passed over for a promotion that he began feeling too sick to go to work is clarification. Clarification helps the patient gain a better understanding of his feelings and how they led to the development of a crisis. In crisis intervention the clarification of unconscious processes is minimal.

Suggestion is the process of influencing a person so that he accepts an idea or belief. In crisis intervention the nurse influences the patient to see him or her as a confident, calm, hopeful, empathic leader who can help. By believing the nurse can help, the patient feels optimistic and in turn will feel less anxious. He also may want to please the nurse by fulfilling his or her expectations of getting better.

Manipulation is a technique in which the nurse uses the patient's emotions, wishes, or values to his benefit in the therapeutic process. Like suggestion, manipulation is a way of influencing the patient. For example, the nurse may want to point out to the patient who prides himself on his independence that he is responsible for much of the work of solving his problem.

Reinforcement behavior occurs when healthy, adaptive behavior of the patient is reinforced by the nurse. He or she strengthens positive responses made by the patient by agreeing with or complimenting those responses. For example, when a patient who has passively allowed himself to be criticized by his boss states that he asserted himself in an interaction with his boss, the nurse can tell him she is pleased with his assertiveness.

Support of defenses occurs when the nurse encourages the use of healthy defenses and discourages those that are unhealthy. Defense mechanisms are indirect behaviors used to cope with stressful situations. The purpose of defense mechanisms is to maintain self-esteem and ego integrity. When defenses deny, falsify, or distort reality to the point that the person cannot deal effectively with reality, they are maladaptive. The nurse should encourage the patient to use adaptive defenses and discourage those that are maladaptive. For example, when a patient denies the fact that her husband wants a separation despite the fact that he has told her what he wishes, the nurse can point out to her that she is not facing facts and dealing realistically with the problem. This is an example of discouraging the use of the defense mechanism of denial. If a patient who is furious with his boss writes a letter to his boss's supervisor rather than assaulting his boss, the nurse should encourage his adaptive use of the defense mechanism of sublimation.

In crisis intervention, defenses are not attacked but rather are more gently encouraged or discouraged. When defenses are attacked, the patient cannot maintain his self-esteem and ego integrity. There is not enough time in crisis intervention to help replace the attacked defenses with new healthier defenses. Returning the patient to his previous level of functioning is the goal of crisis intervention, not the restructuring of defenses.

Raising self-esteem is a particularly important technique. The patient in a crisis feels helpless and may be overwhelmed with feelings of inadequacy. The fact that he has found it necessary to seek outside help for his problem may further increase his feelings of inadequacy. The nurse should help the patient regain his feelings of self-worth. She does this by communicating her confidence that the patient can participate actively in finding solutions to his problems. The nurse also communicates to the patient that he is a worthwhile person by listening to him, accepting his feelings, and relating to him with respect.

Exploration of solutions is essential because crisis intervention is geared toward solving the immediate crisis. The nurse and patient actively explore solutions to the crisis. Answers that the patient had not thought of before may become apparent as he talks to the nurse and his anxiety decreases. For example, a patient who has lost his job and has not been able to find a new one may become aware of the fact that he knows many people in his field of work whom he could contact to get information regarding the job market and possible openings.

These crisis intervention techniques are summarized in the box below. In addition to using these

Techniques of Crisis Intervention

Technique: **Abreaction**
Definition: The release of feelings that takes place as the patient talks about emotionally charged areas
Example: "Tell me about how you have been feeling since you lost your job."

Technique: **Clarification**
Definition: Encouraging the patient to express more clearly the relationship between certain events in his life
Example: "I've noticed that after you have an argument with your husband you become sick and can't leave your bed."

Technique: **Suggestion**
Definition: Influencing an individual so that he accepts an idea or belief, particularly the belief that the nurse can help and that he will feel better
Example: "Many other people have found it helpful to talk about this and I think you will too."

Technique: **Manipulation**
Definition: Using the patient's emotions, wishes, or values to his benefit in the therapeutic process
Example: "You seem to be very committed to your marriage and I think that you will work through these issues and have a stronger relationship in the end."

Technique: **Reinforcement of behavior**
Definition: Giving the patient positive responses to adaptive behavior
Example: "That's the first time you were able to defend yourself with your boss and it went very well. I'm so pleased that you were able to do it."

Technique: **Support of defenses**
Definition: Encouraging the use of healthy, adaptive defenses and discouraging those that are unhealthy or maladaptive
Example: "Going for a bicycle ride when you were so angry was very helpful, since when you returned you and your wife were able to talk things through."

Technique: **Raising self-esteem**
Definition: Helping the patient to regain feelings of self-worth
Example: "You are a very strong person to be able to manage the family all this time. I think you will be able to handle this situation too."

Technique: **Exploration of solutions**
Definition: Examining alternative ways of solving the immediate problem
Example: "You seem to know many people in the computer field. Couldn't you contact some of them to see if they might know of available jobs?"

techniques, Morley, Messick, and Aguilera[28] listed attitudes that are essential for the crisis worker to have. The crisis worker should see this work as the treatment of choice with persons in crisis rather than as a second-best treatment. Assessment of the present problem should be viewed as necessary for treatment, but complete diagnostic assessment should be viewed as unnecessary. The goal and time limitations of crisis intervention should be kept in mind constantly, and unrelated material should not be explored. An active directive role must be taken, and flexibility of approach is essential.

■ **Evaluation**

The fourth step of crisis intervention is evaluation. During this phase the nurse and patient evaluate whether the intervention resulted in the desired effect—a positive resolution of the crisis. Has the patient returned to his precrisis level of functioning? Have the patient's original needs, which were threatened by the precipitating or stressful event, been met? Have the patient's symptoms, which demonstrated ineffective use of coping mechanisms, subsided? Have the patient's useful coping mechanisms begun to function again? Does the patient have a strong support system to rely on now? The nurse and patient review the changes that have occurred. The nurse credits these changes to the patient so that he can see his own effectiveness and discusses how what he learned from the experience of crisis intervention may help in coping with future crises. As in any evaluation process, if goals have not been met the patient and nurse can go back to the first step, assessment, and continue through the four phases again. At the end of the evaluation process, if the nurse and patient believe referral for another type of professional help would be useful, the referral is made.

Clinical case analysis

The phases of crisis intervention just described can be seen in Clinical example 9-4.

Modalities and settings for crisis therapy

Nurses work in many settings in which they see individuals in crisis. Medical hospitalizations are stressful for patients and their families and are often precipitating causes of crises. The patient who becomes demanding or withdrawn or the wife who becomes known as a "pest" to the nursing staff is a possible candidate for crisis therapy. The diagnosis of an illness, the limitations imposed on one's activities, and the changes in body image because of surgery can all be viewed as losses or threats that may precipitate situa-

tional crisis. Simply the stress of being dependent on nurses for care can precipitate a crisis for the hospitalized patient. Strain and Grossman[32] identified the following categories of psychological stress in hospitalized patients:

1. Threat to narcissistic integrity
2. Fear of strangers
3. Separation anxiety
4. Fear of loss of love and approval
5. Fear of loss of control of developmentally achieved functions
6. Fear of loss or injury to body parts
7. Reactivation of feelings of guilt and shame and fear of retaliation

Nurses who work in obstetric, pediatric, geriatric, or adolescent settings can readily observe patients or family members undergoing maturational crises. The anxious new mother, the acting-out adolescent, and the newly retired depressed patient are all possible candidates for crisis therapy. If physical illness is an added stress during maturational turning points, the patient is at an even greater risk. Emergency room settings are also flooded with crisis cases. People who attempt suicide, psychosomatic patients, and crime and accident victims are all possible candidates for crisis therapy. If the nurse is not in a position to work with the patient on an ongoing basis, a referral for crisis therapy can be made.

Community health nurses can observe patients in their own environments and can often spot and intervene in family crises. The child who refuses to go to school, the man who refuses to learn how to give himself an insulin injection, and the family with a member dying at home are possible candidates for crisis therapy. Community health nurses are in a position to evaluate high-risk families for their need of crisis therapy. Families with new babies, ill members, recent deaths, and a history of difficulty coping are all possible high-risk families.

Recently, new community-oriented crisis intervention modalities have been developed. These are based on the philosophy that the health care team must be aggressive and go out to the patients rather than wait for the patients to come to them. Two such modalities are mobile outreach services and psychiatric home care services. Nurses working in these modalities intervene in a variety of settings, ranging from patients' homes to street corners.

■ **Family work**

The family concept of crisis defines the crisis as a family problem, regardless of who the patient is or who is exhibiting symptoms.[7] Because the crisis is seen

CLINICAL EXAMPLE 9-4

ASSESSMENT

Mr. A was a 29-year-old, medium-built, casually dressed black man who was referred to the crisis clinic by another agency. The patient came to the clinic alone. The nurse working with Mr. A collected the following data.

The patient worked in a large steel-making company. The company was laying off many workers and reassigning others. One month earlier Mr. A was temporarily assigned to an area where he had had difficulty 2 years ago. The foreman, the patient believed, was now harrassing him as he had previously. Two weeks ago the patient got angry at the foreman and had thoughts of wanting to kill him. Instead of taking violent action, Mr. A became dizzy, and his head ached. He requested medical attention but was refused. He then "passed out" and was taken by ambulance to the dispensary.

Since that time Mr. A had a comprehensive physical examination and was found to be in excellent health. His physician prescribed diazepam (Valium) on an as-needed basis, but this was only slightly helpful. The patient returned to work for 2 days this week but felt "sick" again. The agency to which Mr. A registered a complaint against his foreman was the agency that referred him to the clinic.

Mr. A complained of being depressed, nervous, and tense. He was not sleeping well, was irritable with his wife and children, and was preoccupied with angry feelings toward his foreman. He had paranoid feelings about his foreman harassing him. Mr. A denied suicidal thoughts while admitting to homicidal thoughts. He felt the homicidal thoughts were under control. At one point during the initial interview the patient was tearful despite strong attempts at control. He demonstrated adequate comprehension, above-average intelligence, a good capacity for introspection, an adequate memory, an affect more of anxiety than depression, and paranoid ideation in regard to the foreman at work. His thought processes were organized, and there was no evidence of a perceptual disorder. Ego boundary disturbance was evident in the patient's paranoid thoughts. It seemed that the foreman was, in fact, a difficult man to get along with. However, the description of personal harassment seemed distorted. There were no depressive symptoms.

Mr. A was raised by his parents. His father was "boss" and beat him and his siblings often.

His mother was quiet and always agreed with his father. Mr. A's parents were Jehovah's Witnesses, and he was Baptist. The patient has a younger brother, a younger sister, and an older sister. The patient and his brother had always been close. The two of them had stopped their father's beatings by ganging up on him and "psyching him out." As a child Mr. A hung around with a "tough crowd" and fought frequently. He stated he believed that he can physically overpower others, but tries to keep out of trouble by talking to people rather than fighting and by working hard.

Mr. A had never before sought aid from a mental health facility. His physical health, as stated, was excellent. He was taking no medication at the time of his first interview. Mr. A had a tenth-grade education and had always achieved above-average grades. His work record up until this time was good. His interests included bowling and other sports. He also periodically took courses at a local community college for his own personal growth rather than in preparation for a degree.

Mr. A had been married for 9 years. His wife was 2 years younger than he. They had three daughters ages 9, 7, and 9 months. Mr. A stated that his relationships with his wife and daughters were satisfactory. Both his wife and his brother were strong supports at this time.

Mr. A's usual means of coping were talking calmly with the threatening party and working hard on his job, in school, and in leisure activities. These coping mechanisms failed to work for him at this time but had been successful in the past. Other strengths the patient exhibited were a good work record under the other foreman and only mild impairment in spheres of his life outside work. He had no arrest record and showed the ability of not acting impulsively but rather of thinking through his actions. Mr. A showed strong motivation for working on his problem. He was reaching out for help, and the beginning of a therapeutic relationship was developing.

Environmental supports seemed strong. Although the patient's wife and brother were supportive, the patient saw his problem as not involving them. It was therefore decided that the patient would be seen alone for the sessions. The patient felt no supports at work.

PLANNING

Mr. A was in a situational crisis, an internal disturbance that resulted from a perceived threat. The

Continued.

CLINICAL EXAMPLE 9-4—cont'd

threat or precipitating stress in this case was the transfer to a new boss. The patient's need for sexual role mastery was not being met, since he wasnot attaining vocational role success. Soon after the transfer Mr. A's usual means of coping became ineffective and he experienced increased anxiety. Symptoms that appeared included attacks of dizziness, headache, passing out, and paranoid thinking. There was no suicidal intent, but feelings toward the foreman contained some homicidal ideation. The patient demonstrated enough control over his impulses that hospitalization was believed to be unnecessary. The patient's memories and themes emphasized his feelings of being harassed. Difficulty with his boss could be related to an earlier conflict, that is, the patient's feelings toward his father, another harassing boss.

The overall goal of treatment would be for the patient to return to at least his precrisis level of functioning. If possible, he could reach a level above, having learned new methods of problem solving. A crisis intervention approach was decided on that considered the patient's needs and desires, the presenting problem, and the limitations of the clinic. The patient demonstrated a good potential for problem solving and the nurse made a contract with him for crisis intervention on a weekly basis.

Possible solutions were mutually explored:

1. It was believed that the patient should remain away from work temporarily so that his rage would not be likely to explode.
2. The patient's intellectual understanding of the crisis would be sought. By understanding what had happened to cause his anxiety, the patient would be able to see more clearly ways of solving the problem. Intellectual understanding rather than affective understanding is sought because of the time limitations and goals of crisis intervention. Affective understanding involves long-term treatment with much emphasis on unconscious processes.
3. Old constructive ways of handling anger would be reinforced. These included submitting a formal complaint at work and ventilating his feelings both to the nurse during the sessions and to his family and friends at other appropriate times.
4. New ways of coping would be taught. These included seeking support at work and following several official avenues of protest.
5. Because of the strength of the patient's feelings toward his boss, it was possible that new ways of handling anger would not suffice and that a transfer to another department might be a better solution.

INTERVENTION

The level of intervention used by the nurse was the **individual approach,** which is the most sophisticated approach and includes the generic approach, general support, and environmental manipulation. The individual approach was chosen because Mr. A's crisis was not one for which a known course could be mapped. Also, since there was a homicidal component to the patient's symptoms, it was believed to be the safest approach. With a clear understanding of psychodynamics, the nurse geared the intervention to aid the patient to achieve an adaptive resolution to his crisis.

Environmental manipulation was achieved by having the patient remain home from work temporarily. Letters were written by the nurse to his employer explaining his absence in general terms. The patient was encouraged to talk to his wife about his difficulties so that she could understand his anxiety and be emotionally supportive.

General support was given by the nurse, who provided an atmosphere of reassurance, nonjudgmental caring, warmth, empathy, and optimism. Mr. A was encouraged to talk freely about the problem without having his feelings judged as good or bad. The nurse offered reassurance that the problem was one that could be solved and that the patient would be feeling better. The nurse let the patient know that she understood his feelings and would help him overcome his crisis.

The **generic approach** was used to decrease the patient's anxiety and guide him through the various steps of problem solving common to all crises. Levels of anxiety were assessed and means of reducing anxiety or helping the patient tolerate moderate anxiety were employed. The patient was encouraged to use his anxiety consciously and constructively to solve his problem and develop new coping mechanisms.

The **individual approach** was used in assessing the specific problems of Mr. A and treating those specific problems. An understanding of the patient's individual psychodynamics was sought and dealt with by the nurse and patient. The patient was reexperiencing harassment from a male authority figure as he had experienced with his father during his youth. Because of the repetition of harassing experiences, Mr. A perceived his treatment by his boss in a personal and paranoid way. In other words, he was strongly sensitive to unfair

CLINICAL EXAMPLE 9-4—cont'd

treatment and overreacted as a result of early repetitive childhood experiences. His emotional response was to strike out physically, as his father had struck out at him. Intellectually, Mr. A knew this would be a disastrous action, and his conflict was solved by becoming sick and passing out so that he could not assault his boss. Mr. A's intense anger was recognized and a high priority was placed on channeling the anger in a positive direction.

The first two interviews were used for data gathering and establishing a positive therapeutic relationship. Through the use of **abreaction** the patient ventilated angry feelings but did not concentrate on wanting to kill his boss. The nurse used **clarification** to help the patient begin to attain an intellectual understanding of the precipitating event and its effect on him. **Suggestion** was used by influencing the patient to see the nurse as one who can help. The nurse told the patient the problem could be worked out by the two of them and that he would soon be feeling better. Mr. A decided to contact several people at work to obtain information about transferring to another department or being laid off. The patient and nurse therefore were **exploring solutions.** The nurse **reinforced** the patient's use of problem solving by telling him his ideas about alternative solutions were good ones well worth his looking into. Throughout these and other sessions the nurse **raised his self-esteem** by communicating her confidence that he could participate actively in finding solutions to his problems. She also listened to and accepted his feelings and treated him with respect. By contacting others at work in his pursuits, the patient found some supportive individuals at work.

During the third session the patient described an incident in which he became furious at a worker at an automobile repair shop. The repairs on the patient's car were never right, and the patient kept returning the car there. The patient shoved the worker but limited his physical assault to that. He then felt nervous and jittery. The patient had previously expressed pride in his ability to control his angry feelings and not physically strike out at others. **Manipulation** was used by telling the patient he showed control in stopping the assault before it had become a full-blown fight and it seemed apparent he could continue to exhibit this ability. During this session, also, the patient spoke of old angry feelings toward his father. Some of this ventilation was allowed, but soon thereafter the focus was guided back to the present crisis.

In the fourth session the patient reported no episode of uncontrollable anger. He still put much emphasis, however, on being harassed by others. The nurse questioned the fact that others were out to intentionally harass the patient. Mr. A's defenses were not attacked, but his gross use of projection was discouraged. In the fifth session the patient reported that a car tried to run him off the road. At a red traffic light the patient spoke calmly to the driver and the driver apologized. The nurse **reinforced this behavior** and **supported his use of sublimation as a defense.** Discussion of termination of the therapy was begun.

In the sixth session Mr. A told of his plans to return to work the following week. He would be going to a different department even though it seemed he would soon be laid off. He also talked about a course he had begun at a community college. He showed no evidence of anxiety or paranoia. Termination of the therapeutic relationship was further discussed. Only a few of the techniques of crisis intervention are described here. It should be kept in mind that the techniques, in actuality, are repetitively used in all sessions to be effective.

EVALUATION

The interventions resulted in the desired effect, an adaptive resolution of the crisis. The changes that occurred were discussed with the patient. The patient's need for sexual role mastery was being met. He was returning to work in a department in which he felt comfortable and successful. His symptoms of anxiety, paranoia, dizziness, headaches, passing out, and homicidal thoughts had ended. He no longer felt harassed. His original coping mechanisms were again effective. He was talking calmly to people he was having difficulty with, and he was again working hard in a goal-oriented way (i.e., a college course). He had learned new methods of coping, which included talking about his feelings to significant others, following administrative or official avenues of protest, and seeking support. The patient and nurse discussed how Mr. A could use the methods of problem solving he had learned from the experience to help cope with future problems. The goal, return to the precrisis level of functioning, had been attained.

It was also recommended to the patient that he engage in psychotherapy so that he could deal with the old angers that interfered with his present life. Mr. A refused the recommendation at this time and stated he would contact the clinic if he changed his mind.

as a family problem, responsibility for the patient's symptoms is placed on the family. It is assumed that a series of family events led to the present problems. The family is viewed as a system so that each member affects and is affected by each other member. For example, when a child refuses to go to school, it is believed not only that the child fears school and wishes to remain with mother but also that the mother is afraid to be alone and wants the child home with her. The crisis is a family one, not just the child's crisis. It is also assumed that role problems cause disequilibrium in families, and new role assignments may be helpful. For example, if a mother appears to be the leader of the family and the father is discounted as ineffective, the nurse can assign certain tasks to the father, such as deciding on proper bedtimes for the children, so that the father will assume some leadership. At other times, tasks are given to the entire family so that emphasis is removed from the symptoms and conflicts. The family is given the responsibility of meeting each member's needs and of changing so that the present problem can be solved.[23]

One family crisis model developed by Hill[19] is based on family systems theory. It was formulated as a result of his research on forced separation and reunion during World War II. In the model, known as the ABCX model, the event (A) interacts with the family's coping resources (B) in combination with the family's definition of the event (C) and produces the crisis (X). If the crisis is not quickly resolved, the family eventually reorganizes into either an adaptive or maladaptive family structure. Another model adds postcrisis adaptation to Hill's model and is called the double ABCX model.[26] This model suggests that if the change in the family system continues over time, the family experiences further hardships. However, new ways of perceiving the situation and new ways of coping can occur and result in new family organization.

Crisis intervention programs have been implemented for families with special problems such as for families of servicemen missing in action,[36] families going through perinatal bereavement,[29] and families with children in the intensive care nursery.[11] One innovative program was started to help patients with chronic renal failure and their families adjust to the unique demands of home dialysis.[24]

Finally, nurses in community mental health centers or departments of psychiatry see many patients in crisis. Patients and families have varied major complaints: depression, anxiety, marital conflict, suicidal thoughts, illicit drug taking, and psychotic symptoms. Crisis therapy modalities available in mental health centers include individual, family, and crisis groups.

■ Group work

Crisis groups function along the same sequential phases of resolution that individual intervention follows. The nurse and group help the patient to solve his problem. Thereafter the group reinforces the patient's new problem-solving behavior. The nurse's role in the group is active, focal, and present oriented. The group follows the nurse's example and uses similar therapeutic techniques. The group acts as a support system for the patient and is therefore of particular benefit to socially isolated individuals. Often the way the patient functions in the group will highlight the faulty coping pattern that is responsible for his present problem. For example, it may become apparent from a patient's interaction with group members that he does not appear to listen to anything said by others but continues talking as though nothing were said. This same patient may be in a crisis because his girlfriend left him because she thought he did not care about her thoughts and feelings. The nurse can comment on the faulty coping behavior seen in the group and encourage group discussion about it.

Crisis groups can be open ended or time limited and can be geared toward a homogeneous or heterogeneous population. Donovan, Bennett, and McElroy[12] describe a limited crisis group in a health maintenance organization. They suggest that the group's success results from the cohesiveness of the group culture, the supportive and accepting attitude of the group, and the group's expectation that the patients will work out their problems. Chen[8] describes a successful open-ended crisis group in a community mental health center. In her group, Chen uses an individual interpersonal focus and a mass group focus to help patients resolve their present crises. Homogeneous crisis groups have been initiated for groups with specific problems. For example, groups have been implemented for men accompanying women seeking abortion[17] and families in the waiting room for intensive care patients.[4]

There is a trend for psychiatric hospitalizations to be short term. Nurses practicing on these units can use crisis therapy in working with the patient and his family either individually or in groups so that the patient can return to the community as soon as possible. This can also prevent rehospitalization. The hospitalization itself may be viewed as an environmental manipulation and thus as part of the crisis intervention.

Crisis intervention is sometimes practiced by telephone rather than in face-to-face contacts. Nurses working for hot-lines or nurses who become involved in answering emergency telephone calls may find themselves practicing crisis intervention without the use of visual cues. Referrals for face-to-face contact should be made, but often, because of the patient's unwillingness or inability to cooperate, the telephone remains the only contact. Listening skills must therefore be emphasized in the nurse's role. Most emergency telephone services have extensive training programs to teach this specialized type of crisis intervention. Manuals written for the crisis worker include content such as suicide-potential rating scales, community resources, drug information, guidelines for helping the caller discuss his concerns, and advice on understanding the limitations of one's role.[27]

■ Disaster work

As part of the community, nurses are called on when adventitious crises strike the community. Floods, earthquakes, airplane crashes, fires, nuclear accidents, and other natural and unnatural disasters precipitate large numbers of crises. Frederick and Garrison[15] have described a "service model" in which mental health workers in the immediate postdisaster period should go to places where victims are likely to gather, such as morgues, hospitals, and shelters. Later, if Federal Disaster Assistance Centers are established, mental health workers may assist in the centers. Rather than waiting for people to publicly identify themselves as persons who are unable to cope with stress, it is suggested that the mental health workers work with the Red Cross, talk to people waiting in lines to apply for assistance, go door-to-door, or, at a relocation site, ask people how they are managing their affairs and explore their reactions to stress.

Nurses providing crisis therapy during large disasters would use the public health or generic approach so that as many individuals as possible can receive help in a short amount of time. Tragedies such as group kidnappings and group killings in communities may affect fewer people and may at times require the individual approach. The nurse may choose to work with families or groups rather than individuals during adventitious crises so that individuals can gain support from others in their family or community who are undergoing stresses similar to theirs.

A good example of mental health professionals helping victims of an adventitious crisis occurred in Kansas City, Missouri, in the days and weeks following the crash of the overhead walkways at the Hyatt Hotel in July 1981. Eight mental health centers in the Kansas City metropolitan area joined to help care for the emotional sufferings of the individuals involved. The centers formed an unofficial coalition and prepared a joint press release describing the many aspects of the grieving process and publicizing the services that they would offer to the survivors of those killed at the hotel—the injured, the observers, and the rescue workers. The services were of three kinds. First, all the centers offered phone counseling and support groups free of charge. Second, special services were planned, such as a grief workshop that was attended by about 200 people who had been at the crash scene. Other related seminars were also held. Third, the centers and media worked together to let the general public know about other resources and services as these became available and to reassure people that their strong reactions to the tragedy were normal.

■ Preventive work

Crisis therapy is a major technique of preventive psychiatry. Maladaptive behavior can be prevented by identifying a crisis and intervening immediately. Crisis can actually be avoided by determining factors that can lead to a crisis and taking action to stop the process. When the nurse sees a potentially stressful situation, he or she should watch the individual's level of anxiety. The nurse should talk and listen to persons under stress so that anxiety levels can be lessened before they reach severe or crisis proportions.

For example, an elderly patient with a known psychiatric illness was being seen in supportive psychotherapy with his wife. The wife telephoned the nurse who was working with them to state that her husband had died 2 weeks ago and they therefore would not be coming back to the clinic. The nurse believed that the patient's death was most definitely a stress for his wife and that there was a potential for a crisis. The nurse asked the patient's wife to come into the clinic one more time so that they could evaluate how she was getting along. The wife was seen and the nurse encouraged her to talk about her husband's death and her future plans. The nurse assessed that the wife was going through the grieving process in a normal adaptive way and that as long as the wife continued talking about her feelings to family and friends, a crisis would be avoided.

Prevention of crises can be directed toward high-risk groups as well as individuals. These groups include children of divorce, care givers of the elderly, victims of violence, and families of AIDS patients. Thus nurses working in primary, secondary, and tertiary care settings can contribute greatly to prevention by early case finding and treatment.

■ Patient education

Educating patients about crisis prevention and early adaptive response to stressful situations is important. This education can be provided by the nurse to individual patients and to society at large. Although patient education takes place during the entire crisis intervention process, it is emphasized during the evaluation phase. At this time the patient's anxiety has decreased, and he can better use his cognitive abilities. The nurse and patient summarize the course of the crisis and the intervention to teach the patient how to avoid other similar crises. For example, the nurse identifies with the patient the feelings, thoughts, and behaviors he experienced as his anxiety rose following the stressful event. He or she explains that if these feelings, thoughts, and behaviors are again experienced, the patient should immediately consider that he is stressed and needs to take action to stop the anxiety from increasing. The nurse then teaches the patient ways in which he can use his newly learned coping mechanisms in future situations.

Nurses are also involved in identifying patients who are at high risk for developing crises and teaching coping strategies to avoid the development of the crises. For example, coping strategies that can be taught to potential patients (e.g., all hospitalized patients) are (1) how to obtain information, (2) how to elicit support with accomplishing tasks and meeting physical needs, and (3) how to elicit emotional support.

The general public is also in need of education so that they can identify those in need of crisis services, be aware of available services, change their attitudes so that people will feel free to seek services, and obtain information about how others deal with potential crisis-producing problems. For example, a mother who learns about reactions to rape may identify her daughter as a rape victim. She then takes her daughter to the nearest crisis center that services rape victims. The mother, in encouraging her daughter to go to the crisis center, tells her daughter that rape is not the fault of the victim, thus enabling her daughter to change her attitude about the rape and feel positive about obtaining outside help. At the center the mother is given a pamphlet that describes how to help rape victims and shares this pamphlet with friends so that they can cope quickly and effectively if their loved ones are raped.

The nurse provides education to society at large by participating in programs in the media (both publicly and privately funded), by leading or participating in educational groups in the community, and by taking every possible opportunity to advertise crisis services. For instance, if a nurse is a member of a church group that has developed crisis services, she should share the availability of these services with her child's parent-teacher association. Thus the information is disseminated to the school's families, the teachers' families, and to other groups to which the parents and teachers belong. Crisis prevention and crisis therapy are necessary for improving the mental health of society. Nurses, as health care professionals, are in a position to provide much patient education about crisis on both a small and large scale.

Future trends

Crisis therapy is popular as the treatment of choice for many patient populations such as victims of violence, disaster victims, and individuals who are newly diagnosed with AIDS. It is considered both practical and effective by mental health workers and patients. Because it is a short-term therapy, it is inexpensive in terms of time and money for patients and caregivers. In our mobile and fast-moving society crisis therapy is also practical, because it requires a short-term commitment from the patient and caregiver. Many people can be reached in a limited period.

Some crisis services are finding a need to change the nature and scope of the treatment they offer because of a change in the populations that use them. Seriously mentally ill persons and their families living in the community often seek help when symptoms become severe. Because of the recurrent nature of many mental illnesses, these individuals are at high risk for periodic crises, and they often have fewer coping mechanisms and support resources. Research is just beginning to identify and measure the major sources of life stress facing people with psychiatric disabilities. However, the need for crisis services is clearly documented by increasing hospital readmission rates, emergency room visits, and the numbers of mentally ill persons who are placed in jail. Some early findings in the field suggest that crisis services can reduce state hospital admissions; that crisis intervention programs produce as good or better outcomes as inpatient treatment at a lower cost; and that a wide range of settings other than hospitals can be used effectively for crisis resolution.

Most recently some communities have established residential crisis services to provide persons in crisis with a protective and supportive setting in which to stay temporarily while they stabilize.[34] Although these services are relatively uncommon, interest in them is growing as a cost-effective and perhaps better alternative to acute psychiatric hospitalization.

Persons other than mental health professionals are being educated to do certain levels of crisis intervention. Neighborhood workers, police, clergy, bartenders, and lawyers are but a few of the many people who come in frequent contact with the target population. These persons who deal with people in crisis are being taught by professionals, including nurses, how to identify individuals in crisis, how to intervene on a generic level, and how to refer individuals needing professional treatment to mental health personnel.

Some people believe that there is not one systematic model of crisis therapy, but many. Conceptualization of crisis work is at present vague rather than detailed and refined. More research is needed so that crisis theory can be better defined operationally.[3] The choice of a crisis intervention modality for specific patients seems at times to be arbitrary and dependent on the practitioner's or agency's orientation rather than based on theory. Further research is needed to identify which crisis intervention modality—individual, group, or family—is most effective under which circumstances. At present the family modality is selected when the crisis directly involves other family members and when strong family support is essential for the individual. When the identified crisis patient is a child or adolescent, family crisis intervention is the preferred mode.[20]

At times, when family members are uncooperative and refuse to become involved in the treatment, an individual or group approach is selected. For individuals in crisis who are isolated and have little support from family or friends, a group is helpful because the other group members form a support system. The individual approach is selected when the crisis does not seem to directly involve the family or when the patient believes he can best handle the crisis on his own. A patient whose crisis stems from his asserting his independence from his family may also want to be seen individually. Most recently, much attention in individual and family development study is being focused on normative developmental changes. For example, a new mother is described as going through a natural transition rather than a developmental crisis. But the differentiation between transition and crisis has not yet been clearly defined.

Nurses are more frequently being placed in the role of primary therapist and therefore are becoming more involved in the direct practice of crisis therapy. This trend seems to be continuing and will grow as certification procedures for nurses further develop. Nurses are also involved in indirect services in the field of crisis therapy. The theory and practice of crisis intervention is taught by nurses to other nurses in various settings and also to paraprofessionals, and to members of the community whose work frequently brings them in contact with persons in crisis. Nurses frequently function in the role of consultant, advising others in their work with individuals in crisis.

Additional nursing research is needed in crisis therapy. What level of education and skill is needed to perform the different levels of crisis intervention?

DIRECTIONS FOR FUTURE RESEARCH

The following are some of the nursing research problems raised in Chapter 9 that merit further study by psychiatric nurses:

1. The conditions under which natural developmental transitions become crises
2. The relationship between length of time for crisis resolution and individual personality factors
3. Appropriate outcome measures to use in evaluating the effectiveness of crisis theory
4. The relationship between the length of time for crisis resolution and type of crisis
5. Empirical validation of the course of grief
6. Family functioning characteristics associated with family vulnerability to crisis
7. The relationship between characteristics of role models and the incidence of developmental crises
8. Empirical validation of Caplan's four phases of crisis
9. Ability of nurses to use the four levels of crisis intervention
10. The level of nursing education and skill needed to perform the different levels of crisis intervention

Which nursing interventions are most effective for whom? Follow-up studies are also needed so that the long-term effects of crisis therapy can be evaluated.

■ SUGGESTED CROSS-REFERENCES ■

Therapeutic relationship skills are discussed in Chapter 4. The phases of the nursing process are discussed in Chapter 5. Interventions in primary prevention are discussed in Chapter 8.

■ SUMMARY ■

1. A crisis is an internal disturbance that results from a perceived threat. Crises are a time of increased vulnerability and can stimulate personal growth.

2. Crises can be maturational, situational, or adventitious. Maturational crises develop from stress during transitional periods of the maturing process when psychological equilibrium is upset. Situational crises occur when a specific external event upsets one's psychological equilibrium. Adventitious crises are accidental, uncommon, and unexpected crises with multiple losses and gross environmental changes.

3. Crisis intervention is a brief, here-and-now-oriented, active mode of psychotherapy with the goal of reestablishing psychological equilibrium. On completion of the process of crisis intervention, the patient is returned to at least his pre-crisis level of functioning.

4. The methodology of crisis intervention includes the steps of assessment, planning, intervention, and evaluation. In completing an assessment, the nurse attempts to identify the precipitating event, the patient's previous strengths and coping mechanisms, and the nature and strength of the patient's support systems. The nurse further assesses the patient's needs and the events that threaten those needs, the point at which symptoms appear, and the themes or memories that are described by the patient.

5. Levels of crisis intervention are environmental manipulation, general support, generic approach, and individual approach. Environmental manipulation includes interventions that directly change the patient's physical or interpersonal situation to provide situational support or remove stress. General support includes interventions that provide the patient with the feeling that the nurse is on his side and will be a helping person. The generic approach includes interventions that guide patients through a particular known course of a crisis so that an adaptive solution will be the outcome. The individual approach includes interventions that aid a particular patient to achieve an adaptive resolution to this crisis and requires a clear understanding of the patient's specific psychodynamics.

6. Techniques of crisis intervention include abreaction, clarification, suggestion, manipulation, reinforcement of behavior, support of defenses, raising self-esteem, and exploration of solutions.

7. Nurses are frequently in a position to use crisis intervention techniques. Settings include all areas of general hospitals, communities, mental health centers, psychiatric hospitals or units, emergency telephone services, and disaster areas. Modalities of crisis intervention used include the individual, family, and group approaches.

8. Trends in crisis therapy seem to demonstrate continued use and increasing sophistication of techniques. Nurses are involved with crisis therapy in both their direct and indirect services. The use of specific techniques and modalities of crisis therapy needs further research.

■ **REFERENCES** ■

1. Aguilera DC and Messick JM: Crisis intervention: theory and methodology, ed 6, St Louis, 1990, Mosby–Year Book, Inc.

2. Auerbach SM: Crisis intervention research: methodological considerations and some recent findings. In Cohen W, Claiborn WL, and Specter GA, editors: Crisis intervention, New York, 1983, Human Sciences Press, Inc.

3. Auerbach S and Stolberg A: Crisis intervention with children and families, Washington DC, 1986, Hemisphere Publishing Corporation.

4. Bloom ND and Lynch JG: Group work in a hospital setting, Health Soc Work 4:48, 1979.

5. Burgess AW and Baldwin BA: Crisis intervention theory and practice, Englewood Cliffs, NJ, 1981, Prentice-Hall, Inc.

6. Caplan G: Principles of preventive psychiatry, New York, 1964, Basic Books, Inc.

7. Chandler HH: Family crisis intervention: point and counterpoint in the psychosocial revolution, J Natl Med Assoc 64:211, 1972.

8. Chen ME: Applying Yalom's principles to crisis work . . . some intriguing results, J Psychiatr Nurs 16:15, 1978.

9. Crisis intervention programs for disaster victims in smaller communities, Washington, DC, 1979, Department of Health, Education and Welfare Pub No (ADM) 79-675, US Government Printing Office.

10. Davidson J, et al: A diagnostic and family study of post-traumatic stress syndrome, Am J Psychiatry 142:1, 1985.

11. Dillard RG, Auerbach KG, and Showalter AH: A parents' program in the intensive care nursery: its relationship to maternal attitudes and expectations, Soc Work Health Care 5:245, 1980.

12. Donovan JM, Bennett MJ, and McElroy CM: The crisis group—an outcome study, Am J Psychiatry 13:906, 1979.

13. Erikson EH: Childhood and society, New York, 1963, WW Norton & Co, Inc, Publishers.

14. Erikson EH: Identity, youth and crisis, New York, 1968, WW Norton & Co, Inc, Publishers.

15. Frederick C and Garrison J: Disaster and mental health: an overview, Behav Today 12:32, 1981.

16. Friedman MJ: Post-Vietnam syndrome: recognition and management, Psychosomatics 22:54, 1981.

17. Gordon RH: Efficacy of a group crisis—counseling program for men who accompany women seeking abortions, Am J Community Psychol 6:239, 1978.

18. Havighurst RJ: Human development and education, New York, 1953, Longman, Inc.

19. Hill R: Families under stress, New York, 1949, Harper.

20. Hoff LA: People in crisis: understanding and helping, Menlo Park, Calif, 1989, Addison-Wesley.

21. Horowitz M: Stress-response syndromes: a review of posttraumatic and adjustment disorders, Hosp Community Psychiatry 37:241, 1986.

22. Jacobson G, Strickler M, and Morley WE: Generic and individual approaches to crisis intervention, Am J Public Health 58:339, 1968.

23. Langsley DG and Kaplan DM: The treatment of families in crisis, New York, 1968, Grune & Stratton, Inc.

24. Levenberg SB, Jenkins C, and Wendorf DJ: Studies in family-oriented crisis intervention with hemodialysis patients, Int J Psychiatry Med 9(1):83, 1978-1979.

25. Lindemann E: Symptomatology and management of acute grief, Am J Psychiatry 101:141, 1944.

26. McCubbin H and Patterson J: Family adaptation to crisis. In McCubbin H, Cauble A, and Patterson J, editors:

Family, stress, coping, and social support, Springfield, Ill, 1982, Charles C Thomas.

27. Mills P: Crisis intervention resource manual, Vermillion, SD, 1973, Educational Research and Service Center.
28. Morley WE, Messick JM, and Aguilera DC: Crisis paradigms of intervention, J Psychiatr Nurs 5:537, 1967.
29. Quirk TR, O'Donohue S, and Middleton J: The perinatal bereavement crisis, J Nurse Midwife 24:13, 1979.
30. Rusk TN: Opportunity and technique in crisis psychiatry, Compr Psychiatry 12:249, 1971.
31. Shields L: Crisis intervention: implications for the nurse, J Psychiatr Nurs 13:37, 1975.
32. Strain JJ and Grossman S: Psychological care of the mentally ill, New York, 1975, Appleton-Century-Crofts.
33. Strickler M and LaSor B: Concepts of loss in crisis intervention, Ment Hygiene 54:302, 1970.
34. Stroul B: Residential crisis services: a review, Hosp Community Psychiatry 39:1095, 1988.
35. Sundeen SJ et al: Nurse-client interaction: implementing the nursing process, ed 4, St Louis, 1989, Mosby–Year Book, Inc.
36. Teichman Y, Spiegel Y, and Teichman M: Crisis intervention with families of servicemen missing in action, Am J Community Psychol 6:315, 1978.
37. Terr LC: Psychic trauma in children: observations following the Chowchilla schoolbus kidnapping, Am J Psychiatry 138:14, 1981.

■ ANNOTATED SUGGESTED READINGS ■

*Aguilera DC: Crisis intervention: theory and methodology, ed 6, St Louis, 1990, Mosby–Year Book, Inc.

Detailed, comprehensive, and thorough presentation of crisis theory and method. Includes historical development, psychotherapeutic techniques, group therapy concepts, socioeconomic factors affecting intervention, the problem-solving approach, situational and maturational crises, and levels of prevention and trends as they relate to crisis intervention. Paradigms are included to facilitate understanding.

*Brownell MJ: The concept of crisis: its utility for nursing, Adv Nurs Sci 6:4, 1984.

Explores various definitions and uses of the concept of crisis and presents a crisis continuum for conceptualizing crisis states. The article is scholarly and provides implications for nursing practice and research.

Burgess AW and Baldwin BA: Crisis intervention theory and practice, Englewood Cliffs, NJ, 1981, Prentice-Hall, Inc.

Clinical handbook providing guidance for practice by specifying a typology of six types of crises, and formats for intervention in each type. Many contemporary crisis-producing issues, such as sexual abuse, incest, divorce, mothers going to work, and combat stress are addressed in the typology.

Caplan G: Principles of preventive psychiatry, New York, 1964, Basic Books, Inc.

Classic in psychiatry that places a historical perspective on the development of crisis intervention from preventive psychiatry. A public health model is used to explain the approaches of primary, secondary, and tertiary prevention of mental disorders.

*Chen ME: Applying Yalom's principles to crisis work: some intriguing results, J Psychiatr Nurs 16:15, 1978.

Written for the serious group therapist; translates some conventional group therapy principles into a crisis group theoretical framework. The literature on crisis groups is reviewed, followed by a description of an open-ended crisis group that uses Yalom's process-focused interventions. Theory is clearly defined and illustrated with clinical examples.

Cohen LH, Claiborn WL, and Specter JD, editors: Crisis intervention, New York, 1983, Human Sciences Press, Inc.

Written for the academician, researcher, or anyone interested in scientific information. Presents material about crisis theory, technique, training, and research. Written in a scholarly manner, presenting numerous citations on which its tenets are founded.

Gilliland B and James R: Crisis intervention strategies, Pacific Grove, Calif, 1988, Brooks Cole Publishing.

Crisis intervention text that includes definitions, techniques, and strategies for specific situations such as sexual assault, substance abuse, and personal loss. Useful for students because it includes case-centered learning exercises in most chapters.

*Hall J and Weaver B: Nursing of families in crisis, Philadelphia, 1974, JB Lippincott Co.

Compilation of articles written by nurses dealing with families in crisis. Text attempts to increase the reader's understanding of crisis theory as it applies to nursing situations; provides examples of strategies and tactics that may be useful in helping families resolve crises. A variety of nursing practice settings are presented.

*Harrison D: Nurses and disasters, J Psychosoc Nurs 19(2):34, 1981.

Brief paper reviewing some of the acute psychiatric problems that can result from disaster experiences. Effective use of nurses in these emergencies is also described.

Hoff LS: People in crisis: understanding and helping, Menlo Park, Calif, 1989, Addison-Wesley.

Presents theory and practice of crisis intervention and stresses the social and cultural contexts that influence that theory and practice. Crisis intervention approaches described include individual, group, family, and community networking.

Jacobson G, Strickler M, and Morley WE: Generic and individual approaches to crisis intervention, Am J Public Health 58:339, 1968.

The nature of crisis is described and two possible approaches in crisis intervention are presented—general and individual. Circumstances under which each approach is selected are identified, and clinical examples of each method are presented.

*Lancaster J and Berkovsky D: An ecological framework for crisis intervention, J Psychiatr Nurs 16:17, 1978.

Written for the nurse educator. Describes how to help bac-

---

*Asterisk indicates nursing reference.

calaureate nursing students use an ecological framework for crisis intervention with children placed in an institution for dependent and neglected children. Both theory and clinical examples are presented, making this article a useful one for students too.

Lindemann E: Symptomatology and management of acute grief, Am J Psychiatry 101:141, 1944.

Describes an early study of the grieving process. Stages of grief are identified, and normal and morbid grief reactions are differentiated. Use of crisis intervention to guide grief toward a favorable outcome is explored.

*Mitchell CE: Identifying the hazard: the key to crisis intervention, Am J Nurs 77:1194, 1977.

Concentrates on identifying the precipitating or stressful event from which a crisis develops; details what clues to look for and how to use the clues to intervene effectively.

*Narayan SM and Joslin DJ: Crisis theory and intervention: a critique of the medical model and proposal of a holistic nursing model, Adv Nurs Sci 2:27, 1980.

Provides an alternative to the disease prevention orientation of crisis intervention, describing a holistic model that emphasizes the alteration of health potential as one strives for a high level of wellness. Medical and holistic nursing models of crisis are compared both theoretically and in implications for intervention.

National Institute of Mental Health: Innovations in mental health services to disaster victims, Rockville, Md, 1985, US Department of Health and Human Services.

Monograph written for policymakers, administrators, and service providers that evaluates ways in which crisis intervention was used in specific disasters. Provides an update on research projects and a useful list of reference material for both child and adult disaster victims.

National Institute of Mental Health: Training manual for human service workers in major disasters, Rockville, Md, 1978, US Department of Health, Education and Welfare.

Highly recommended manual that uses crisis intervention theory and is a training instrument to help people cope after a disaster strikes. Excellent coverage includes phases of a disaster, key concepts, community relationships, selection and education of human service workers, special risk groups, self-awareness sessions, and identification of available resources.

Parad H, editor: Crisis intervention: selected readings, New York, 1965, Family Service Association of America.

Compilation of readings on a range of theoretical formulations of crisis theory; shows the way crisis intervention is used in practice. It applies crisis theory to various practice settings and a number of commonly encountered stressful situations affecting the individual, group, and family. A highly recommended reading.

Strickler M and Allgeyer J: The crisis group: a new application of crisis theory, Soc Work 12:28, 1967.

Describes a study in which individuals in crisis were treated in group therapy. The authors claim most patients made progress in the crisis group modality and explain theoretically how the progress occurred. A clinical example is given to further illustrate the concepts.

*Wallace MA and Morley WE: Teaching crisis intervention, Am J Nurs 70:1484, 1970.

Written for the nurse educator; describes problems that evolve in clinical supervision of graduate nursing students learning to practice crisis intervention. Both initial and advanced problem patterns are identified and solutions are described.

Woolsey S: Support after sudden infant death, Am J Nurs 88:1347, 1988.

Crisis intervention strategies described for working with families and staff following sudden infant death syndrome. Author describes the grieving process and the nurse's role in planning interventions appropriate to the family's stage of grief.

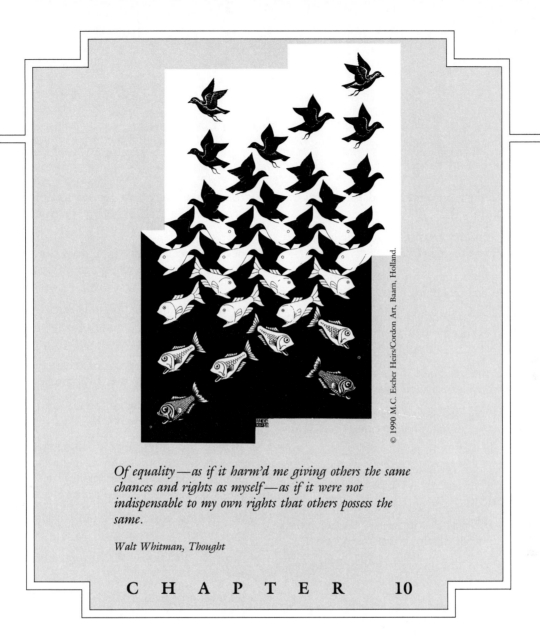

© 1990 M.C. Escher Heirs/Cordon Art, Baarn, Holland.

Of equality—as if it harm'd me giving others the same chances and rights as myself—as if it were not indispensable to my own rights that others possess the same.

Walt Whitman, Thought

C H A P T E R   10

REHABILITATIVE PSYCHIATRIC NURSING

LEARNING OBJECTIVES

After studying this chapter, the student should be able to:

- define tertiary prevention and psychiatric rehabilitation.

- discuss concepts relative to an individual's rehabilitative nursing needs.

- identify four trends in the development of psychosocial treatment.

- describe the concepts of primary and secondary gain as they pertain to psychiatric rehabilitation.

- analyze the readiness of a patient for discharge from a treatment program.

- identify and discuss five factors relative to assessment of the family's resources for assisting the patient.

- describe and evaluate community resources relative to the needs of the recovering psychiatric patient.

- discuss the role of the nurse in interaction with the needs of the recovering patient.

- identify and discuss eight principles of psychiatric rehabilitation.

- compare and contrast several models for the provision of rehabilitative psychiatric services.

- develop specific behavioral goals for rehabilitative psychiatric nursing care in conjunction with the patient and family.

- describe group interventions that are appropriate to tertiary prevention, including the nurse's role with self-help groups.

- discuss nursing interventions that are directed toward meeting the needs of families.

- develop a mental health education plan relevant to tertiary prevention.

- analyze the importance of nursing intervention at a community level, including mental health education, membership in advocacy groups, networking, and political action.

- describe the current status of tertiary prevention program evaluation.

- identify directions for future nursing research.

- select appropriate readings for further study.

The public health model of prevention includes three levels of preventive health care activity: primary, secondary, and tertiary. **Primary prevention,** as discussed in Chapter 8, focuses on decreasing the number of new cases (incidence) of a health problem by intervening before an illness occurs. **Secondary prevention** focuses on prompt intervention when illness occurs to limit the length and severity of an episode. This has been the major area of intervention for psychiatric nurses. It is the focus of much of this book. **Tertiary prevention** is the limitation of disability related to an episode of illness. It is the subject of this chapter.

Any episode of illness may involve lasting change in the individual's level of functioning. A person who has been more seriously ill is more likely to have serious problems living productively in the community. Hospitalization is especially disruptive to the person's life, and it is difficult to adjust after discharge. Nurses who work in institutional settings must be aware of the total range of present and potential patient care needs.

Tertiary prevention usually begins before discharge from the hospital. Caplan[15] says the goal of tertiary prevention is to reduce the rate of defective functioning related to mental disorder in a community. This definition includes the other levels of prevention, but adds that common usage usually limits the meaning to reduction of the rate of residual defect.[15] This is the sense in which it will be used in this chapter.

Rehabilitation

Tertiary prevention is carried out by the performance of activities identified as *rehabilitation*. Rehabilitation is the process of enabling the individual to return to his highest possible level of functioning. The goal is usually to match or exceed the pre-illness functional level. This may be achieved by capitalizing on strengths, relearning old skills, or learning new skills, depending on the effects of the health care problem and the person's response to it.

Like primary prevention, the tertiary level of prevention was largely ignored until the advent of community mental health programs in the 1960s. The development of effective treatments for psychosocial disorders allowed mental health care providers to begin to think about the future of patients who were able to reenter the community. Medication and psychotherapy, in particular, assisted patients to develop positive interpersonal relationships. Hospitalization was avoided for some patients who were able to function in the community with the help of intensive intervention.

A new interest in the civil rights of psychiatric patients led to increased importance of psychiatric rehabilitation. The right to treatment in the least restrictive setting was established in the courts. This resulted in reassessment of patients in hospitals. Some of them had been there for many years. It soon became obvious that many people who were returning to communities lacked the skills needed for daily life. Scandals occurred in many cities as discharged psychiatric patients were discovered in shabby boarding houses, soup kitchens, jails, and skid row. Many became victims of crime because they lacked the skills to protect themselves. Many returned to the hospital for brief admissions, creating a "revolving door" between the hospital and the community. Others became inmates of other kinds of institutions, especially jails and nursing homes, as they demonstrated their inability to cope.

The process of moving long-term hospital patients to the community is called **deinstitutionalization.** For this process to succeed, patients must be prepared to function at least minimally well in the community. This has become an important focus of psychiatric rehabilitation. However, *all* patients who have received treatment for a disruption in mental or emotional functioning are potentially in need of rehabilitation. This chapter focuses on the nursing process as applied to psychiatric rehabilitation for any degree of residual impairment. The care of the chronically mentally ill person is discussed in greater depth in Chapter 33.

Psychiatric rehabilitation approaches have also been termed *psychosocial treatments*. Heinrichs[23] has identified four trends in the development of psychosocial treatment: (1) psychoeducation and the medical model, (2) working with families, (3) group therapy, and (4) social skills–social learning theory.

■ Psychoeducation and the medical model

The traditional medical approach to a patient with a physical illness includes diagnosing the problem, telling the person what to expect from the illness, and discussing treatment alternatives. In the past, people with mental illnesses were discouraged from asking questions about their problems, which caused misconceptions and fear. As more has been learned about the probable biological origin of the major illnesses, mental health care providers have become more willing to teach patients and families. Heinrichs[23:126] states,

> An important function of psychoeducational work is to identify hitherto unspoken fears and to correct myths and prejudices by providing basic information in a context of respect and hope.

This is in contrast to the approach labeled "mystification" by Banes,[10] a former patient. She relates mystification to a lack of education of patients about their illnesses, treatments, and medications.

■ Working with families

The professional has taken the role of consultant to the family. This is in contrast to past attitudes of suspicion and blame directed from providers toward families. Families can now be partners in providing care.

■ Group therapy

For many severely mentally disabled people, group treatment is more effective than individual therapy. Positive aspects of group therapy include an opportunity for ongoing contact with others, consensual validation of perceptions, and an allowance for varying levels of activity and intensity of participation.

■ Social skills–social learning theory

This theoretical framework is based on a behavioral approach. It involves teaching specific living skills that the patient is expected to need to survive in a community setting. At the present time, research is needed to test the usefulness of this approach and to study whether or not skills that are learned in the hospital can be transferred to the community.

Bennett[13] discusses the conflict between the needs of society and the needs of the mentally ill person. Closing hospital wards leads to loss of jobs for hospital staff. Community living expenses must be met through tax revenues. Taxpayers may object to this use of their funds. Families may have been relieved by the decision to hospitalize a troubled member. They may not be eager to take him back. He recommends that the resolution to this dilemma may rest in study of the needs of patients and of the characteristics of hospital and community environments.[13] Therapeutic and damaging elements in both settings should be identified, and this information used to develop more helpful patient care settings.

Rehabilitative psychiatric nursing must be studied in the context of the patient and his social system. This requires the nurse to focus on three elements: the individual, the family, and the community. This chapter has been designed to discuss each of these elements relative to the nursing process. Relevant nursing interventions are identified at each phase.

 Assessment

■ The individual

Assessment of the need for rehabilitation begins at the time of the first contact between the nurse and the patient. A comprehensive psychiatric nursing assessment, as described in Chapters 5 and 6, is directed toward obtaining information that will enable the nurse to assist the patient to achieve his maximum possible level of functioning. This is the definition of rehabilitation. Nurses are expected to identify and reinforce the patient's strengths as one means of assisting him to cope with his weaknesses. This, too, is basic to the concept of rehabilitation. Thus good nursing care is really the same as rehabilitative nursing care.

The nursing model of health-illness phenomena (Fig. 10-1) may be applied within the context of rehabilitative nursing practice. It is particularly important for the nurse to identify stressors that may interfere with the patient's adjustment to a health-promoting life-style. The Holmes and Rahe approach[24] to rating life stressors was presented in Chapter 3. Baker and associates[9] have questioned whether this list of stressors is appropriate for subpopulations such as the chronically mentally ill. They conducted a study to identify life stressors that are relevant to this group. To evaluate the relative impact of stressors, they asked study participants to rate life events according to two sets of factors.

The first set of variables related to whether the event was *positive* and growth-enhancing or *negative* and psychologically distressing. The other set focused on whether the event was under the control of the individual. The life events that were evaluated included

changes in structured daily activities, residence, physical health, finances, family relationships, interpersonal relations with nonrelatives, relationship with spouse, and hospitalization.

It is possible to hypothesize potentially more distressing events as one moves from a positive/controlled combination to negative/uncontrolled. Although the investigators did not report this type of analysis, they did find that, if an event was viewed as positive, it was more likely that the patient had initiated it. Nurses need to be aware of patients' perceptions of their experiences. Research provides guidelines for this. It is also essential to validate each individual's response to significant changes in his life.

When conducting the initial assessment of the patient, the nurse needs to think beyond the limits of his or her own patient care setting and try to anticipate the nature of the patient's other contacts with the health care system. In hospitals this process is discharge planning, and the need is obvious. However, nurses in community settings should also expect patients to progress to other levels of care. Although some people will need long-term outpatient care, many will be discharged from psychiatric care.

■ PRIMARY AND SECONDARY GAIN.
To assess the patient's readiness to move from one level of care to another, the nurse must understand the concepts of primary and secondary gain. **Primary gain** refers to the individual's efforts to cope with the predisposing and precipitating stressors. For instance, a person who feels compelled to wash his hands repetitively experiences a reduction in anxiety as a result of the behavior. The decrease in anxiety is the primary gain. Nursing care at the secondary prevention level focuses on interventions to assist the patient to develop healthier ways of accomplishing the primary gain.

Secondary gain refers to the other advantages that are associated with the sick role. In the American culture, sick people are expected to have difficulty meeting their own needs. Therefore they expect to receive help and attention from others. In return, they are expected to show that they want to get well by cooperating with a plan of care. The extra attention and nurturing that is given to sick people can decrease the motivation to get better. Most people experience this even with a minor illness. A cold provides an excuse to stay home from school or work, sleep late, eat favorite foods, and indulge in relaxing activities. Even when one feels below par, there is pleasure associated with the release from daily responsibilities and a reluctance to resume them. The problem is greater for the person who has difficulty coping with the stresses of daily life. Being a patient can protect the person from the need

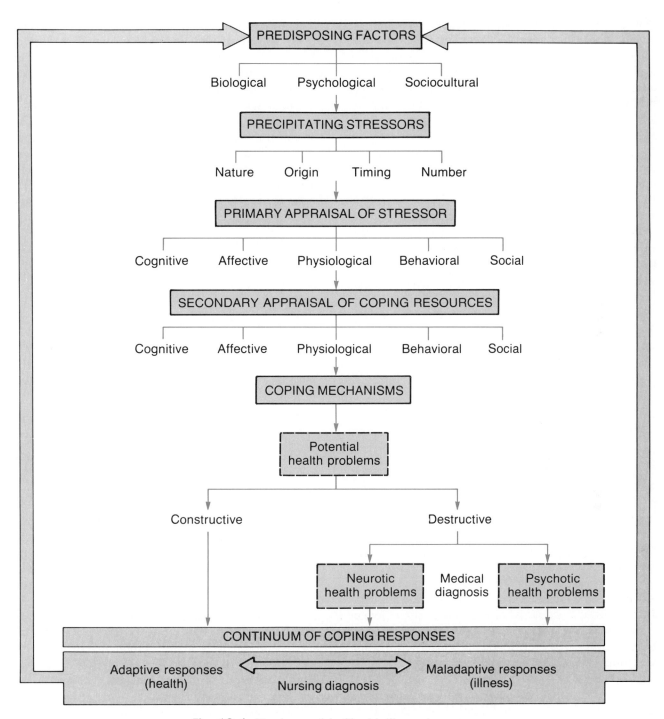

Fig. 10-1. Nursing model of health-illness phenomena.

to face situations that cause anxiety. The resistance that is associated with secondary gain is sometimes thought to be a purposeful manipulation to avoid assuming responsibility.

Even when more effective coping mechanisms have been developed, it can be frightening to test them in a situation has been intolerable in the past. Bachmann[6] has described her experience as an ex-patient reentering the community. She discovered that it was difficult to relate to her old friends because of their difficulty in understanding her experience. On the other hand, she lacked the self-confidence to reach out to new people. The greatest source of support for her was contact with other former patients. But she says that these significant relationships were discouraged by staff members who viewed them as a way of perpetuating illness. Bachmann also found the community boring compared to the hospital and began to develop a life pattern of working and sleeping. Nurses who are involved in busy community and family lives may fail to recognize the contrast that the patient experiences between the hospital and the community. Thus the nurse must try to understand the patient's world and respect his needs as he sees them.

A punitive attitude toward the patient who is reluctant to move ahead is not helpful. The person needs support and understanding. Helpful nursing interventions include the following:

1. Planning with the patient to resume activities one by one, starting with the least threatening
2. Role playing difficult situations before attempting to confront them
3. Accompanying the patient into the community to offer support if needed
4. Providing honest and timely feedback about the patient's attempts to become reengaged in his environment
5. Advocating for the patient's needs with family members and community agencies

Axelrod and Wetzler[5] studied a group of patients who were discharged from a general hospital psychiatric unit to identify the factors that were related to keeping outpatient appointments. They found that the first appointment must be scheduled as soon as possible after discharge. In addition, people who had been hospitalized several times were more likely to keep appointments. Patients who acknowledged their need for treatment and medication were also more compliant. In this group, people who were hospitalized longer were more likely to follow through with treatment after discharge. However, following longer-term hospitalizations, the reluctance to reenter the community tended to grow.

When a person is hospitalized for months or years, the handicap that Wing and Olsen[43] have called "institutionalism" develops. This is characterized by social withdrawal and resistance to leaving the hospital, even when the surroundings are barely adequate. The institutional environment becomes comfortable because it is predictable and few demands are made. Some patients become angry or have more symptoms when they are being encouraged to move to the community. Some experts think that this social withdrawal is caused by the lack of stimulation in the environment;

others believe that it is related to severe mental illness, usually chronic schizophrenia. Although it is important that the cause be identified through research, in any case the nurse must help the patient develop trusting and caring relationships.

Discharge from an inpatient or partial hospitalization program should be based on careful interdisciplinary assessment of the patient's level of functioning. Gallagher[20] defines patient discharge as a process of social negotiation. He has reviewed the literature and identified factors other than symptoms of illness that frequently appear to determine readiness for discharge:

1. **Age.** Young patients are more likely to be discharged.
2. **Length of stay.** Potential for discharge decreases as the length of stay in the program increases.
3. **Life circumstances.** Housing and employment in the community increase the likelihood of discharge. Employment is a more important factor for men. Marriage, implying available housing, is more significant for women.
4. **Family wishes.** Family request facilitates release.
5. **Patient request for release.**

Although the success of the negotiation process and the influence of life factors may in reality determine discharge, nurses should assess the patient's living skills and interpret this assessment to the patient, family, and interdisciplinary team. Anthony[2] has developed a matrix (Table 10-1) of the skills required for successful functioning in the community. He describes the physical, emotional, and intellectual components of the skills required for living, learning, and working. The nurse may use these examples in working with the patient to identify strengths, establish goals, and set priorities for skill development. Such a model provides a rational basis for assessing the patient's readiness to function productively in the community. It also provides objective information that can be shared with the mental health care providers who will work with the patient in the community agency.

Nurses who work in community settings must also be concerned about the relationship between the treatment that is given and the help that the patient wants. In a study of 99 long-term patients of a community mental health center, Spivack and associates[39] found that the patients' focus was on social interaction and health status. However, the treatment goals were directed toward work and task accomplishment. The investigators wondered if the treatment that the patients were receiving would help them succeed in living in

TABLE 10-1

POTENTIAL SKILLED ACTIVITIES NEEDED TO ACHIEVE THE GOAL OF PSYCHIATRIC REHABILITATION

Physical	Emotional	Intellectual
Living skills		
Personal hygiene	Human relations	Money management
Physical fitness	Self-control	Use of community resources
Use of public transportation	Selective reward	Goal setting
Cooking	Stigma reduction	Problem development
Shopping	Problem solving	
Cleaning	Conversational skills	
Sports participation		
Using recreational facilities		
Learning skills		
Being quiet	Speech making	Reading
Paying attention	Question asking	Writing
Staying seated	Volunteering answers	Arithmetic
Observing	Following directions	Study skills
Punctuality	Asking for directions	Hobby activities
	Listening	Typing
Working skills		
Punctuality	Job interviewing	Job qualifying
Use of job tools	Job decision making	Job seeking
Job strength	Human relations	Specific job tasks
Job transportation	Self-control	
Specific job tasks	Job keeping	
	Specific job tasks	

From Anthony WA: Principles of psychiatric rehabilitation, Baltimore, 1980, University Park Press.

the community. They recommended the adoption of a skills development model to prepare patients for vocational settings.

■ The family

The image of the isolated chronically mentally ill person who returns to a community where he has no connections has been widely publicized in recent years. However, most mentally ill people are involved with their families and will have frequent contact with family members while they are in the community.[29] Therefore family resources must be assessed when a rehabilitation plan is being developed. Unfortunately, health care providers and patients' families frequently become adversaries. The family may be viewed by the providers as the cause of the problem or as resistant to the treatment plan. Family members have a right to provide input to the treatment plan. They can identify

potential problem areas and help to enhance the patient's compliance with the plan.

The nurse who assesses the family as part of a rehabilitation plan should include the following areas:

1. Family structure, including developmental stage, roles, responsibilities, norms, and values
2. Family attitudes toward the mentally ill member
3. The emotional climate of the family
4. The social supports that are available to the family, including extended family, friends, financial support, religious involvement, and community contacts
5. The family's understanding of the patient's problem and the plan of care

Some of this information may be obtained from the social worker. However, it is the nurse's responsibility to be available to the family. This includes regular planned contacts with the family and inclusion of the family as part of the treatment team.

■ **The community**

The community greatly influences rehabilitation of its mentally ill members. Mental health professionals have a unique role in the community because they are community members and advocates of the mentally ill at the same time. It can be difficult for patients and their families to demand that the community provide adequate services. Care providers, including nurses, can and should assume a leadership role in assessing the adequacy and effectiveness of existing community resources and in recommending changes.

Nurses in all settings must be familiar with the community agencies that provide services to patients. Most communities have a social and medical services directory that can be consulted for basic information such as location, type, and cost of the services provided. Most agencies serve people who come from a particular geographical area such as one part of a city or, in a rural area, one or several counties. As the nurse works with patients, she will become more familiar with other agencies that provide services for the same people. Nurses should pay attention to patients' evaluations of the agencies from which they receive services. This information helps to identify agencies that are responsive and helpful as opposed to those that are difficult for patients to approach.

Personal contact with other community agencies can be very useful as part of a community assessment. This may be achieved by making an appointment with an agency staff member. However, a more realistic picture of an agency's services can be obtained by going to the agency with a patient who is requesting services. This allows the nurse to see how the agency responds to the patient and how the patient handles his affairs in the community. The nurse can also provide emotional support to the patient if he is insecure in a new situation. The nurse should identify himself or herself to the staff of the agency and explain that he or she and the patient would like to learn more about the services. Collaborative relationships between mental health care providers and community agencies are absolutely essential if rehabilitation is to succeed.

A wide range of services must be provided to patients in tertiary prevention. Those that are directed toward basic needs include provisions for shelter; food, clothing, and household management; income and financial support; meaningful activities; and mobility and transportation.[19] Other services provide for special needs that may differ from one patient to the next such as general medical services, mental health services, habilitation and rehabilitation programs, vocational services, and social services.[19] A third group of services are integrative, with the purpose of coordinating the system. These include patient identification and outreach, individual assessment and service planning, case service and resource management, advocacy and community organization, community information, and education and support.[19] This overview of a community service system was developed by the Steering Committee on the Chronically Mentally Ill of the United States Department of Health and Human Services. It is described in greater detail in Table 10-2. Although the plan focuses on the chronically mentally ill, it may be used to assess the services available to all mentally ill patients. These services may be provided in a variety of settings. Table 10-3 identifies the types of settings in which mental health care services might be provided according to the level of care that is needed.

⚜ Planning and implementation

■ **The individual**

Treatment planning and intervention in rehabilitative psychiatric nursing focuses on fostering independence by maximizing the person's strengths. This is directly parallel to the nurse's role in physical rehabilitation. It differs from nursing care that is given to patients when they are acutely ill. During acute illness, people require a nurturing approach. The nurse must provide for all of the basic life functions that the person is unable to manage. However, the relationship gradually becomes less dependent as the patient grows stronger and better able to care for himself. Residual functional deficits may remain. The nurse and patient must then work together to find ways for the patient to overcome any remaining impaired areas of functioning.

Peplau[35] described nursing roles relative to the patient's needs and ability to function. The unconditional mother–surrogate role is related to the acutely ill phase. This implies that the nurse would act in a maternal nurturing way. When the patient begins to feel better, the nurse would continue some of the mother-surrogate functions, but she would add counseling, leadership, and resource person activities. These additional activities are related to the shift of responsibility from the nurse to the patient. People who choose nursing as a profession often have strong needs to nurture. It is important to be aware of this and not to let it interfere with the patient's need to develop self-care skills.

The close relationship between physical and psy-

TABLE 10-2

COMPREHENSIVE ARRAY OF SERVICES AND OPPORTUNITIES FOR CHRONICALLY MENTALLY ILL PERSONS

Basic needs/opportunities	Special needs/opportunities

Shelter

Protected (with health, rehabilitative, or social services provided on site)
Hospital
Nursing Home
Intermediate-care facility
Crisis facility
Semi-independent (linked to services)
Family home
Group home
Cooperative apartment
Foster care home
Emergency housing facility
Other board and care home
Independent apartment/home (access to services)

Food, clothing, and household management

Fully provided meals
Food purchase/preparation assistance
Access to food stamps
Homemaker service

Income/financial support

Access to entitlements
Employment

Meaningful activities

Work opportunities
Recreation
Education
Religious/spiritual
Human/social interaction

Mobility/transportation

General medical services

Physician assessment and care
Nursing assessment and care
Dentist assessment and care
Physical/occupational therapy
Speech hearing therapy
Nutrition counseling
Medication counseling
Home health services

Mental health services

Acute treatment services
Crisis stabilization
Diagnosis and assessment
Medication monitoring (psychoactive)
Self-medication training
Psychotherapies
Hospitalization: acute and long-term care

Habilitation and rehabilitation

Social/recreational skills development
Life skills development
Leisure time activities

Vocational

Prevocational assessment counseling
Sheltered work opportunities
Transitional employment
Job development and placement

Social services

Family support
Community support assistance
Housing and milieu management
Legal services
Entitlement assistance

Integrative services

Client identification and outreach
Individual assessment and service planning
Case service and resource management
Advocacy and community organization
Community information
Education and support

From Department of Health and Human Services Steering Committee on the Chronically Mentally Ill: Toward a national plan for the chronically mentally ill, Pub No (ADM)81-1077, Washington, DC, 1981, US Government Printing Office.

TABLE 10-3

TYPICAL SETTINGS FOR PROVIDING SERVICE CLUSTERS

Acute treatment	Residential treatment	Rehabilitation	Psychosocial support
Housing setting			
Apartment/home (on site)	Public psychiatric hospital	Family	Family
Family (on site)	Nursing homes	Halfway house	Apartment
Foster family	Veterans hospital	Cooperative apartment	Congregate housing (long term)
Crisis hotel	Forensic unit at public	(transitional)	Board and care home
Respite care home	psychiatric hospital		Lodge
Emergency housing	Community forensic unit		Foster care home
General hospital			
Public psychiatric hospital			
Private psychiatric hospital			
Community mental health center inpatient unit			
Service setting			
Work		Social club	Social club
Telephone hotline		Psychosocial rehabilitation center	Psychosocial rehabilitation center
Other housing and hospital settings previously listed		Sheltered workshop	Sheltered workshop
		Industry setting	Community mental health center outpatient services
		Community college	Outpatient clinic
		Community mental health center outpatient services	Day treatment program
		Outpatient clinic	
		Day treatment program	

From Department of Health and Human Services Steering Committee on the Chronically Mentally Ill: Toward a national plan for the chronically mentally ill, Pub No (ADM)81-1077, Washington, DC, 1981, US Government Printing Office.

chiatric rehabilitation is demonstrated in the eight principles of psychiatric rehabilitation, as described by Anthony, Cohen, and Cohen.[3]

1. The primary focus of psychiatric rehabilitation is on improvement of capabilities and competencies.
2. The patient benefits by developing skills that will be useful in his own environment.
3. Psychiatric rehabilitation uses a variety of theories and therapeutic constructs. It is based on the philosophy and principles of rehabilitation.
4. Improvement of vocational outcome is a central focus.
5. Hope is essential for psychiatric rehabilitation.
6. Deliberately increasing independent behavior can ultimately lead to increased independent functioning.
7. The patient is encouraged to be actively involved in planning and implementing his own rehabilitation.
8. The fundamental psychiatric rehabilitation interventions are patient skill development and the development of environmental resources.

■ **ALTERNATIVE CARE SETTINGS.** It may be difficult to alter traditional nurse-patient roles in a hospital or clinic setting. In recent years efforts have been underway to develop alternative settings for the delivery of mental health care such as foster homes, halfway houses, and psychosocial rehabilitation centers. Malone[32] described Community Bound, a rehabilitation program for long-term mentally ill people in Austin, Texas. She identified several concepts that contributed to the rehabilitation of the patients. The dominant category was related to *"survival skills."* This referred to all of the activities that enabled the patient to remain in the community, including living skills such as housekeeping, money management, and shopping; socialization skills such as manners, assertiveness, and other interpersonal behaviors; and vocational skills. Another concept was *cooperation*. The patient had to be able to obey rules and participate in the program. The concept of *hanging out* was related to the importance of socializing with others in an informal setting. It allowed the patients to experience friendship. *Checking up* was the staff activity of ensuring that things were going well with a patient. Staff and patients often helped someone deal with community agencies. This was called *backing*. The final concept described was *supplementing*. This referred to providing material resources such as food or clothing to patients. Malone points out that many of the activities that she identified are traditionally performed by nurses.

Another alternative intervention program attempts to keep patients in their own homes in the community. This is the Training in Community Living program designed by Stein and Test.[40] In this model, when a person is referred for hospital admission, staff are assigned to be with him in the community. Nurses accompany patients as they perform their usual activities and provide support and assistance when needed. This real-world experience with the patient enables the nurse to accurately assess the skills that the person needs to learn. The nurse and patient mutually agree on realistic goals. Staff contact is decreased as the patient demonstrates the ability to function independently. When the person is living with his family, they may also receive counseling and assistance in dealing with the patient's behaviors.

A third nonhospital intervention model is the Southwest Denver Model developed by Polak and co-workers.[36] The author stresses the need to consider and manipulate the social forces that influence the patient. This model also uses direct intervention in the social environment as the treatment approach. The major difference between this model and Training in Community Living is the focus. The latter model helps the patient adjust to the environment. The Southwest Denver Model assists in adjusting the environment to the patient's needs. Intervention again takes place in the patient's social setting. If the patient must get away from his environment for a short time, foster care is arranged. Hospitalization is viewed as a last resort. If a patient is acutely psychotic or suicidal, an "intensive observation apartment" is available with close 24-hour supervision provided. A home day care program provides training in living skills in a home setting.

The programs described above generally maintain a clear distinction between the helpers and the helped. Chamberlin,[16] a former mental health services consumer, has described three other models that claim to decrease or eliminate this differentiation.

■ **Partnership model.** Patients in this type of program are told that they are partners. How-

ever, there is still a clear distinction between care givers and receivers. Chamberlin refers to these as "alternatives in name only." One example of a partnership model program is Fountain House. This program is described in detail in Chapter 33. It is run by professionals and, according to Chamberlin, looks and functions like an institution. She further criticizes the apparent assumption that all ex-patients are like the severely disabled people on whom the program focuses.

■ **Supportive model.** Membership is open to all who want mutual support. Ex-patients and those who have never been hospitalized are equal. It is believed that any person can sometimes be in need of help and can sometimes be able to provide help to others. Professionals are excluded, except to promote community support or funding.

■ **Separatist model.** Ex-patients support each other and run the service. All others are excluded. It is believed that anyone who has never experienced the psychiatric patient role will interfere with the consciousness-raising process and will have stereotyped attitudes.

Chamberlin believes very strongly that alternative treatment programs should be run by patients. Successful programs also include many other elements. They must address needs identified by the patients, and participation must be voluntary. There should be options to participate in all or part of the total program. Help is provided either by patients to patients or by others whom the patients select. The patients are responsible for the administrative direction of the program. Criteria for participation are determined by the patient group. Finally, the program is mainly accountable to the patient. Strict confidentiality is maintained, but all information related to his treatment is made available to the patient.

As experience with alternative treatment programs has grown, it has become apparent that there are groups of patients who need modified or special programs. For instance, Setze and Bond[37] conducted a study of hospital readmission for 400 admissions to a psychosocial rehabilitation program. They found that women, whites, those under 21 years old, and those who had been hospitalized three or more times were more likely to be readmitted. Bachrach's[8] recognition of the unique service needs of men and women support this viewpoint.

Foster home care is sometimes recommended for discharged people, particularly those who have been hospitalized for a long time and who have lost contact with relatives. There has been concern about foster home placement; lack of regulation in some foster homes has resulted in situations in which foster care givers exploit the resident. However, well-run foster care settings have been effective.[31] Foster homes must be supplemented by treatment programs and provision for other psychosocial needs.

These program examples are not the only approaches to psychiatric rehabilitation. They demonstrate the use of creativity to manage a complicated problem. Nurses have been involved in most of these programs. There is a risk involved for nurses who challenge traditional mental health care structures. There is also a potential reward as people who have been excluded from society are reintegrated as productive members. It should be noted that comprehensive psychosocial rehabilitation programs such as Fountain House are widely recommended for intervention with chronically mentally ill patients. These programs are discussed in Chapter 33.

Rehabilitative psychiatric nursing tries to maximize the person's strengths and minimize his weaknesses. The nursing care plan should be organized around very specific behavioral goals that are based on a comprehensive assessment of the patient's living skills. These goals should build on those that are developed as part of the secondary prevention process. Examples of such goals may be found in Chapters 11 to 21. This part of the nursing care plan may be labeled the *discharge plan* in an inpatient treatment setting. Discharge plans should also be developed in community settings. This will remind both the nurse and the patient that the ultimate goal is for independent functioning. Even patients who need long-term medication can usually receive maintenance prescriptions from their family physician as part of their general health care program. This helps to put the mental illness into perspective as a chronic health problem that is not so different from other chronic problems the patient might have.

The nurse and the patient must decide together on the desired level of functioning. If the patient is unwilling to take on activities that the nurse thinks would be helpful, it is important to discover why. Sometimes nurses try to push a patient ahead too rapidly. Patient behavior that has developed gradually over time cannot be changed quickly. Learning new behavior patterns and giving up old ones is frightening and causes anxiety.

Lamb[27] has suggested the following reasons that the homeless mentally ill may resist help:

1. Severe illness and disorganization
2. Low tolerance for intimacy and closeness
3. Rejection of the mentally ill identity
4. Desire to maintain an isolated lifestyle and anonymity
5. Fear of dependency

The nurse must be sure that the patient's coping skills are adequate to deal with the stress of growth. Feedback must be requested from the patient to be sure that the rehabilitation plan continues to address his needs. Sometimes the plan assumes greater importance than the patient. The nurse must prevent this.

■ **PATIENT EDUCATION.** Several theorists have suggested educational approaches to assist with rehabilitation. This type of intervention has also been called **psychoeducation.** Goldman[21] defines psychoeducation as "education or training of a person with a psychiatric disorder in subject areas that serve the goals of treatment and rehabilitation, for example, enhancing the person's acceptance of his illness, promoting active cooperation with treatment and rehabilitation, and strengthening the coping skills that compensate for deficiencies caused by the disorder."[21:667] He adds that patient education must be provided by a qualified person and should be part of the treatment plan.

Barter and associates[11] have described the Community Interaction Program in Sacramento, California. Three of the components of this program emphasize education. Transitional employment training teaches attitudes and behaviors required for success in the work force. Adult basic education is offered to meet needs for basic academic education. Local teachers present these classes, thereby providing involvement of community members in the program. There are also weekly seminars on medications. These sessions begin with a pretest, are followed by a lecture/discussion presentation, and end with a posttest. At times, other topics such as health and nutrition have been added. This practical type of education is very useful in helping people who have been hospitalized survive in the community.

Bellack and associates[12] reported on a social skills training program. This is a structured learning experience that prepares the patient to develop social relationships and decreases the stress of interpersonal conflict and failure. The content includes training in participating in brief conversations, assertiveness skills, and sharing positive feelings. Special topics related to patient need such as dating or job interviewing may be added. A role modeling, role playing, and feedback teaching method was used. The patients responded

TABLE 10-4

MODEL OF AN EDUCATION PLAN FOR PSYCHIATRIC PATIENTS IN REHABILITATION PROGRAMS

Content	Instructional activities	Evaluation
Identify and describe common psychiatric diagnoses	Provide handouts outlining behaviors Discuss coping behaviors Assign homework from lay literature Compare mental illness to physical illness	Patient recognizes characteristics of the diagnosis he has been given Patient distinguishes between cure and coping
Describe the role of stress in contributing to psychiatric disorders	Sensitize the patient to signs of increased stress Define stress as a test of coping skills Teach relaxation exercises	Patient verbalizes level of stress Patient performs relaxation exercises and describes a reduction in perceived stress
Assist to gain a sense of control by recognizing personal pattern of signs and symptoms	Provide feedback when symptomatic behavior occurs Instruct patient to keep a diary of behavior and to identify symptoms	Patient consistently labels symptoms and seeks professional help when necessary
Development of social skills to enable participation in vocational and recreational activities	Role play social interaction in a variety of situations Field trips to community activities Supervised vocational training in real work settings	Patient participates in progressively more independent social and work activities
Identify and describe community support systems	Provide a list of community support programs, including self-help groups, mental health care agencies and social agencies Invite representatives of programs to speak to patient group Escort to first agency contact	Patient selects community programs that offer resources needed by him Patient becomes able to access agency independently
Describe and discuss psychoactive medications	Instruct about actions, side effects, and contraindications to common psychoactive medications Distribute handouts describing the patient's medications Suggest systems to help patient remember when to take medication and how much	Patient describes characteristics of prescribed medications Patient reports effects of prescribed medications Patient takes medication as prescribed

Modified from Buckwalter KC and Kerfoot KM: J Psychosoc Nurs Ment Health Serv 20:(5):15, 1982.

well to the high structure and goal orientation of the program.

Patient education should be part of the nursing role. Buckwalter and Kerfoot[14] identified several topics that can help the patient avoid rehospitalization. These are presented in the format of a teaching plan in Table 10-4. A mental health education program such as this can be used in hospital or community settings. Specific content can be planned to meet the needs of a patient or a group. Consumers are growing to expect health teaching as a part of professional service. Nurses are the best equipped health care providers to provide this service.

Lamb et al.[30] identified several guiding principles for the care of long-term psychiatric patients in the community. First, the patient must feel control over internal drives, symptoms, and environmental demands. The second principle advises the care provider to work with the well part of the patient's ego. "The goal is to expand the remaining well part of the person rather than to remove or cure pathology."[30:10] Third, treatment should be located in a noninstitutional setting if possible. Another principle requires clear definition of goals. The fifth principle is that work therapy should be a cornerstone of the program. The next principle emphasizes the importance of the person's status change from mental patient to community resident. The final principle states that helping the person find a normal environment should always be a goal. The nurse can help the patient with the last two goals by encouraging social activities in the community.[29]

Sometimes it is assumed that community-based rehabilitation is the ideal model of care for all people with long-term mental illnesses. Lamb[28] has challenged this assumption. He points out that mentally ill people are a heterogeneous group. Some may be unable to tolerate the stress of living in the community. He recommends that high-quality long-term hospital or residential care be made available to this group of people. Nurses will then need to modify their expectations from patient improvement to maintaining stability.

■ **SOCIAL SUPPORT.** The role of nurses relative to social support groups has been described by Norbeck.[34] She relates the following assumptions about social support:

1. Supportive relationships are needed by people to manage everyday role demands and to cope with life changes and unusual stressors.
2. A network of social relationships forms the context for the giving and receiving of social support.
3. Social network relationships are relatively stable over time, especially those that are the individual's primary ties.
4. To be supportive, a relationship should be basically healthy, not pathological.
5. The quantity and type of support that is needed depends on the characteristics of the individual and the nature of the situation.
6. The quantity and type of support that is available also depends on the characteristics of the individual and the situation.

Norbeck states that many psychotic patients have inadequate social supports. Nursing interventions that she recommends for these patients are described in Table 10-5. The interventions focus on the type of problem being experienced. Situational problems are handled by using coping skills or environmental supports.

TABLE 10-5

TYPOLOGY OF DEFICIENCIES IN SOCIAL SUPPORT AND RECOMMENDED INTERVENTIONS

Deficiencies	Nursing interventions
I. Situational	
1. Losses of network members	1. a. Assist client to deal with losses and provide temporary support
	b. Assist client to "repeople" the network
2. Crisis or problem exceeds network's capacity or experience	2. a. Influence key network member to provide support
	b. Volunteer linking
	c. Mutual aid groups
	d. Professional support
II. Pathological	
A. *Person deficiencies*	
3. Inadequate social skills	3. a. Training in social skill development
	b. Environmental manipulation to facilitate interaction
4. Negative network orientation	4. a. Assist client to decrease over-generalization from pathological relationships to other relationships
B. *Network deficiencies*	
5. Pathological relationships	5. a. Decrease face-to-face contact with key person
	b. Change attitudes and behavior of key person
6. Maladaptive network structure	6. a. Encourage non-kin contact
	b. Network therapy

From Norbeck JS: J Psychosoc Nurs Ment Health Serv 20:(12):22, 1982.

Pathological problems require changing the patient's behavior or the network. The nurse may need to work with other members of the health care team to help the patient overcome serious problems.

Support may also be found through involvement in self-help groups. These are groups of patients who meet to offer peer support and encouragement. Self-help groups do not ask for and often discourage involvement by mental health care providers. Providers may be viewed as agents of an illness-focused system. Self-help groups emphasize the abilities of their members to serve as advocates for themselves and for others with similar problems. Knight and co-workers[26] reported that members have described social support as the most helpful aspect of self-help groups. Recovery, Inc., was the first self-help group formed by people with emotional problems. This group was modeled after Alcoholics Anonymous. More recently, other groups have organized to bring together chronically mentally ill people or those with a specific medical diagnosis such as schizophrenia. Some self-help groups draw their membership from the families of mentally ill people. Family members often feel caught between the demands of the patient and the health care providers. Nurses can make patients aware of these groups and encourage them to attend. They can also offer themselves as resources to the group. Membership in a self-help group can be an important step toward independence by a person recovering from a mental illness.

■ **The family**

Family support is very important to the successful rehabilitation of a mentally ill person. The mental illness of a member is often a shock and a source of great stress to the family. Nurses are in a favorable position to help families cope with the stress and adapt to changes in the family structure.

Walsh,[42] a parent of a schizophrenic, has suggested several common trouble spots in family life. The first is disrupted communications. Another problem area is the mechanics of everyday life, including the need for privacy and control over one's own space, keeping a regular schedule, nutrition, television usage, money management, and grooming. Families are concerned about responding to hallucinations, delusions, and odd behavior. They particularly need help to cope with violent or suicidal threats. Alcohol and drug use also cause disruptions in family life.

The last area of concern identified by Walsh is frequently ignored by family members and professionals alike. That is the need for relatives to remember to take care of themselves. She recommends the following ways to accomplish this:

1. Accept the fact of a mentally ill family member.
2. Plan a self-care program.
3. Continue to pursue personal activities and interests.
4. Get involved with organizations such as self-help groups or churches.
5. Avoid the advice and opinions of those who have not lived with a schizophrenic.
6. Remember that happiness is possible.
7. Stop blaming yourself.

Reviewing this list gives the nurse some understanding of the pain and stress that is experienced by the family of a mentally ill person. Nurses can help ease that pain by giving advice such as that listed above.

■ **NURSE-FAMILY ALLIANCE.** Wing and Olsen[43] identified helpful attitudes for professionals working with families of mentally ill patients. Instead of assuming the role of expert with the family, which can lead to feelings of powerlessness and hostility, they recommend establishing a relationship of mutual learning. The nurse can then concentrate on empathizing with the family and can work with them in problem solving.

Unfortunately, families and mental health care providers sometimes become engaged in power struggles related to the care of the mentally ill family member. Spaniol, Zipple, and FitzGerald[38] suggest the following ways that professionals can share power with families for the benefit of the patient:

1. Clarify mutual goals.
2. Learn about rehabilitative and educational methods.
3. Separate intervention from explanation of causation.
4. Acknowledge limitations.
5. Develop a team relationship with the family and the community.
6. Recognize and identify the family's strengths.
7. Learn to accept criticism of the system.
8. Encourage family members to recognize and meet their own needs.
9. Keep up with current information about psychiatric illnesses and medications and share this knowledge with families.
10. Incorporate practical advice from families into health-teaching plans.
11. Seek knowledge about the availability and quality of community resources.
12. Establish a positive relationship with family support groups and refer families to them.
13. Demonstrate personal commitment through advocacy.

14. Learn to accept diverse beliefs.
15. Cultivate a personal support system.

Several helpful approaches to families have been identified by Grunebaum and Friedman.[22] The first is to allow the family members to express their feelings about the patient's illness and how it relates to their lives. The next task is to provide the information that families need to participate in decision making. Families have feelings related to the member's illness. These may include relief that the member is receiving help, guilt over hospitalizing the member, fear about what will happen in the future, and depression if the member does not respond well to treatment. Another task is to assist them to deal with these feelings. Families may try to cope with the member's mental illness by denying the seriousness of the problem, by being over-controlling, or by withdrawing. A task of the nurse is to identify the coping method that is being used and assess its helpfulness. Finally, the nurse must help the family learn to balance their own needs with those of the patient. Because nurses are usually viewed as supportive and helpful, they are in a good position to be sensitive to the needs of families and to address them in their practice.

■ **FAMILY INTERVENTION PROCESS.** Anderson, Hogarty, and Reiss[1] have described a four-phase process for intervention with the families of schizophrenic patients. This model is summarized in Table 10-6. Phase I focuses on establishing a connection with the family. At first the therapist "joins" the family in social talk and shares information. This decreases anxiety by creating an atmosphere that is familiar to the family. Next the therapist assumes the role of "family ombudsman." This implies an alliance with the family and the avoidance of assigning blame for the patient's problems. The therapist shares information with the family and asks for their input for the treatment plan. The clinician's role is established as the family's representative and their link with other parts of the health care system. The family's reactions to the illness are sought, and their concern is put into action in the patient's behalf. Finally, a treatment contract is agreed on that includes the establishment of mutual goals.

Phase II focuses on teaching survival skills for liv-

TABLE 10-6

OVERVIEW OF THE FAMILY INTERVENTION PROCESS

Phases	Goals	Techniques
Phase I	Connection with the family and enlistment of cooperation with program	Joining
		Establishment of treatment contract
	Decrease of guilt, emotionality, and negative reactions to the illness	Discussion of crisis history and feelings about the patient and the illness
	Reduction of family stress	Empathy
		Specific practical suggestions that mobilize concerns into effective coping mechanisms
Phase II Survival skills workshop	Increased understanding of illness and patient's needs by family	Multiple family education and discussion
	Continued reduction of family stress	Concrete data on schizophrenia
	Deisolation—enhancement of social networks	Concrete management suggestions
		Basic communication skills
Phase III Reentry and application	Patient maintenance in community	Reinforcement of boundaries (generational and interpersonal)
	Strengthening of marital/parental coalition	
	Increased family tolerance for low-level dysfunctional behaviors	Task assignments
	Decreased and gradual resumption of responsibility by patient	Low-key problem solving
Phase IV Maintenance	Reintegration into normal roles in community systems (work, school)	Infrequent maintenance sessions
	Increased effectiveness of general family processes	Traditional or exploratory family therapy techniques

From Anderson CM, Hogarty GE, and Reiss DJ: Schizophr Bull 6:495, 1980.

ing with schizophrenia. This is done in a daylong workshop. It is also hoped that a support network will be formed among the families who attend. In Phase III the content from the workshop is discussed with the individual family. There are generally two main themes during this phase: reinforcing family boundaries and the gradual resumption of patient responsibility. Respect for boundaries is communicated by allowing members to speak for themselves and to engage in separate activities and by recognizing each member's vulnerabilities and limitations. The patient gradually assumes responsibility. He may first help with simple tasks, then gradually become more independent. This can be a long, slow process; thus the family will need much patience. Expectations must be realistic; one change should be made at a time. Phase IV begins when goals have been attained to the greatest possible extent. At this point, the family chooses between traditional family therapy or decreased involvement focusing on maintenance.[1] Although the model was developed for work with the families of schizophrenic patients, many of the principles apply to families of other mentally ill patients as well. Intervention using the model should not be attempted without advanced education at the graduate level. However, nurses can be very helpful if they try to understand family needs and reinforce family coping mechanisms.

■ The community

There are several ways that nurses can intervene in the community to encourage the establishment of tertiary prevention programs. Among these are health education, membership in advocacy groups, networking, and political action. It has been noted that stigma decreases with increased formal education. Cumming and Cumming[17] thought that community-based health education programs on the topic of mental health might have the same effect. They conducted a study based on this idea to try to change negative community attitudes toward the mentally ill. They failed in their efforts but made some interesting observations related to the study. They believed that they should have found a way to motivate the community members to want to learn. They also assumed that they were aware of community attitudes but later discovered that this was not so. They had used a psychiatrist as the educator in the project. They later decided that it might have been more effective to use community members who were well informed about the subject. The psychiatrist was a good teacher, but this was not the role expected of him by the community members. Finally, they decided that they should have promoted direct involvement between community members and

patients by encouraging volunteer activity as a part of the program.

Most nurses have a strong background and a firm belief in health education. Mental health education in the community provides a real opportunity to have an impact on the experience of patients as community members. Greater understanding of the behaviors and needs of the mentally ill could increase acceptance. This could lead to the development of better services. People who refuse to allow group homes in their neighborhoods usually have irrational fears that are fueled by the media's distorted portrayal of mentally ill people. Education combined with direct contact with members of rehabilitation programs can be helpful in overcoming negative attitudes. Nurses should take advantage of opportunities to speak to community groups about mental health.

Membership by nurses in community advocacy groups can also be helpful. Nurses can join forces with other professional and lay people who share concerns about the care of the mentally ill. The National Mental Health Association is the largest advocacy group that addresses mental health issues. Members of this organization have been useful in drawing attention to the needs of the mentally ill and in supporting positive legislation at the federal and state levels. They monitor the effectiveness of the mental health care system. Nurses can provide useful input to this part of their activities.

Nurses can also promote working relationships among advocacy groups, professional organizations, self-help groups, and concerned citizens. As fewer funds are available for the care of the mentally ill, the formation of coalitions is essential to lobby for the allocation of resources to mental health care. Coalition formation is also referred to as networking. Mitchell and Trickett[33] have identified functions served by social networks. They include (1) emotional support; (2) task-oriented assistance; (3) communication of expectations, evaluation, and a shared world view; and (4) access to new and diverse information and social contacts.[33:30] These functions are also the factors that capture members' commitment to united action.

The activities of community-wide networks are frequently directed toward the political system. Aside from allocation of money and other resources, the nature of mental health care in a community is strongly influenced by the political structure of that community. As has been seen in Chapter 7, legal issues have a great effect on mental health care delivery. Nurses need to be aware of and involved in the political process. They should communicate directly with their legislators at all levels, sharing their interests and concerns. Politicians are well aware of the need to respond to the priorities of their constituents. The number of nurses in the United States makes them a potentially powerful political force, but that power has seldom been exerted. If nurses are committed to positive health care, particularly at the primary and tertiary prevention levels, they must become visibly involved.

Nurses can also become more directly involved in the political system. They can run for office and support other nurses who are legislators. Nurses are often invaluable members of appointed boards and commissions having to do with health care. Their knowledge can be shared with others who are planning community health care systems. These voluntary activities are time consuming, but they can have great impact on the health care system. Community-level policies can either inhibit or facilitate direct care efforts. Active involvement in professional organizations often leads to productive and rewarding community activities. There is a great sense of satisfaction to be derived from selling a community on a new idea and seeing it become a reality.

 Evaluation

■ **Program evaluation**

Many of the approaches to tertiary prevention that have been described are relatively new. Because of the long-term nature of many types of mental illness, the evaluation of these programs is in its early stages. Longitudinal studies will provide more valid and reliable measures of success or failure. Bachrach[7] has reviewed the literature on model programs for the care of chronically mentally ill people. She analyzed these programs at four levels. The first level is an evaluation of the success or failure of the individual program. Externally determined criteria (e.g., cost-effectiveness or licensure standards), accomplishment of stated objectives, patient functioning, and patient or staff satisfaction are approaches to evaluation that have been used at the programmatic level. The second level is the assessment of commonalities among programs. Bachrach found the following eight common elements in successful programs[7]:

1. The targeting of a specific group of patients
2. Realistic linkages with other community resources
3. Provision of a full range of services
4. Individualized treatment
5. Conformity with the local cultural system
6. Specialized training for staff

7. Liaison with a hospital for access to inpatient beds when needed
8. Presence of an internal evaluation system

The third level of evaluation relates to whether or not the program can be duplicated in other settings. This is identified as a problem by Bachrach for several reasons. One is that each program is developed in a cultural context that differs from others. Another is that model programs often have the advantage of special funding and other resources that are not available for duplicates. The very fact that it is a model and therefore special can influence the outcome of a program. Another potential problem is the extent to which most successful programs depend on the leadership of one person or a small group of people who are extraordinarily committed to their program. There is frequently a charismatic leader associated with successful programs. Finally, the model programs are too new to tell whether they will stand the test of time.[7]

The fourth level of evaluation is that of relevance. This examines the relationship of the program to the mental health care system. Bachrach[7] has named this impact evaluation. She questions whether model programs can really provide the answers to broader social problems. The model must be considered in the context of the system within which it exists.

■ **Patient evaluation**

Others focus on evaluating the effectiveness of rehabilitation programs by assessing the impact on the individual patient. Kelly and co-workers[25] looked for predictors of success in aftercare programs. They identified two: involvement in occupational therapy and responsiveness to reinforcement in group therapy. Anthony and co-workers[4] also recommended patient evaluation criteria. They settled on decrease in rehospitalization rates and posthospital employment as the most useful measures of community adjustment. However, they also recommended that evaluation efforts be extended and that rehabilitation programs examine the results more closely.

Turkat and Buzzell[41] suggest an evaluation approach based on member movement within a psychosocial rehabilitation program. They found that, as patients move from one program component to another, progress toward increased independence is inconsistent. Patients tend to move back and forth, "alternating cycles of progression, regression, and maintenance." Therefore it is important not to base program evaluation on an expectation that most patients will progress in a stepwise fashion. A decrease in rehospitalization rates may be a more significant criterion of program success.

Cutler[18] identified clinical, programmatic, and administrative principles for psychosocial rehabilitation programs that may serve as evaluation guidelines. The clinical principles are continuity of care, availability of services, and the provision of services in the patient's natural environment. Programmatically, the services should be comprehensive. The administrative principles include integration of planning with all service providers and agencies, planned staff development, and a constant and ongoing evaluation program. Patients of the *Living in the Community* program in Oregon, on which these principles are based, experienced a 9% rehospitalization rate in 6½ years.

It is becoming obvious that, if tertiary prevention efforts are to be supported in the future, it is necessary to prove that they are effective in both human and economic terms. Therefore evaluation criteria must be developed and used.

■ SUGGESTED CROSS-REFERENCES ■

The nursing process is discussed in Chapter 5. Intervention in social support systems is discussed in Chapter 8. Family assessment is discussed in Chapter 5, and identification of vulnerable families is discussed in Chapters 8 and 29. The care of the chronically mentally ill patient is discussed in Chapter 33.

■ SUMMARY ■

1. Tertiary prevention was defined as reduction of the rate of residual defect related to an episode of mental illness.

2. Psychiatric rehabilitation was identified as the process by which tertiary prevention is carried out.

3. Four trends in the development of psychosocial treatment were identified as psychoeducation and the medical model, working with families, group therapy, and social skills–social learning theory.

4. Stressors were discussed in terms of the experience of the chronically mentally ill.

5. Concepts related to the assessment of the individual and rehabilitative nursing needs were described.

6. The concepts of primary and secondary gain were discussed as they relate to psychiatric rehabilitation.

7. Readiness for discharge from inpatient or partial hospitalization programs was analyzed in terms of patient characteristics and required skills.

8. Family assessment was discussed in the context of available resources for patient support. Important factors include family attitudes toward the patient, alterations in the roles of family members, the emotional climate of the family, the availability of social support, and the family's understanding of the patient's illness.

9. Community assessment was described in terms of the nurse's responsibility to identify and evaluate community resources.

10. The role of the nurse in planning and intervening in rehabilitative psychiatric care was related to responsiveness to the patient's readiness for increased independence.

11. Eight principles of psychiatric rehabilitation were presented to demonstrate similarities to physical rehabilitation concepts.

12. Several model community programs for the provision of tertiary prevention services were described.

13. The development of specific mutual nurse-patient goals that are stated in behavioral terms was discussed relative to tertiary prevention.

14. Group intervention, including fostering self-help groups, was suggested as an appropriate activity for the nurse.

DIRECTIONS FOR FUTURE RESEARCH

The following are some of the nursing research problems raised in Chapter 10 that merit further study by psychiatric nurses:

1. Nursing interventions that limit dependency by inpatients on the institution
2. Testing of the generalizability of social skills learned in a hospital or other institutional setting to a community environment
3. Exploration of various models of independent living skills training
4. Survey of the amount of classroom and clinical time allotted to content relative to rehabilitative psychiatric nursing in basic and graduate nursing programs
5. The relationship between contact with unrelated mentally ill people and attitudes toward mental illness
6. Constructive roles that nurses may perform relative to self-help groups
7. Evaluation of the helpfulness of self-help group membership as compared to participation in other types of treatment programs
8. Description of community support groups planned to address the unique needs of subpopulations of the chronically mentally ill: women, young adults, the elderly
9. Development of generalizable and reproducible evaluation criteria to be applied to tertiary prevention programs
10. The relationship of various tertiary prevention program elements to patient outcomes

15. Strategies were presented for the support of the families of psychiatric patients. These include involving the family in a team relationship, incorporating the family's strengths, educating the family, referring them to community resources including self-help groups, and advocating for appropriate services.

16. A model mental health education plan for consumers of tertiary rehabilitation services was presented.

17. Community interventions were proposed to encourage and support the development of tertiary prevention services. These include mental health education, membership in advocacy groups, networking, and political action.

18. Program evaluation was discussed in terms of the state of the art. Some criteria were identified, as were levels of evaluation. However, more work is needed in this area.

■ REFERENCES ■

1. Anderson CM, Hogarty GE, and Reiss DJ: Family treatment of adult schizophrenic patients: a psychoeducational approach, Schizophr Bull 6:490, 1980.
2. Anthony WA: The principles of psychiatric rehabilitation, Baltimore, 1980, University Park Press.
3. Anthony WA, Cohen MR, and Cohen BF: Psychiatric rehabilitation. In Talbott JA, editor: The chronic mental patient: five years later, New York, 1984, Grune & Stratton, Inc.
4. Anthony WA et al: Efficacy of psychiatric rehabilitation, Psychol Bull 78:447, 1972.
5. Axelrod S and Wetzler S: Factors associated with better compliance with psychiatric aftercare, Hosp Community Psychiatry 40:397, 1989.
6. Bachmann BJ: Reentering the community: a former patient's view, Hosp Community Psychiatry 22:19, 1971.
7. Bachrach LL: Overview: model programs for chronic mental patients, Am J Psychiatry 137:1023, 1980.
8. Bachrach LL: Chronic mentally ill women: emergence and legitimation of program issues, Hosp Community Psychiatry 36:1063, 1985.
9. Baker F et al: The impact of life events on chronic mental patients, Hosp Community Psychiatry 36:299, 1985.
10. Banes JS: An ex-patient's perspective of psychiatric treatment, J Psychosoc Nurs Ment Health Serv 21:(3):11, 1983.
11. Barter JT, Queirolo JF, and Ekstrom SP: A psychoeducational approach to educating chronic mental patients for community living, Hosp Community Psychiatry 35:793, 1984.
12. Bellack AS et al: An examination of the efficacy of social skills training for chronic schizophrenic patients, Hosp Community Psychiatry 35:1023, 1984.
13. Bennett D: Deinstitutionalization in two cultures, Health Society 57:516, 1979.
14. Buckwalter KC and Kerfoot KM: Teaching patients self care: a critical aspect of psychiatric discharge planning, J Psychosoc Nurs Ment Health Serv 20:(5):15, 1982.
15. Caplan G: Principles of preventive psychiatry, New York, 1964, Basic Books, Inc, Publishers.
16. Chamberlin J: On our own, New York, 1978, McGraw-Hill Book Co.
17. Cumming E and Cumming J: Closed ranks: an experiment in mental health education, Cambridge, Mass, 1957, Harvard University Press.
18. Cutler DL et al: Disseminating the principles of a community support program, Hosp Community Psychiatry 35:35, 1984.
19. Department of Health and Human Services Steering Committee on the Chronically Mentally Ill: Toward a national plan for the chronically mentally ill, Pub No (ADM)81-1077, Washington, DC, 1981, US Government Printing Office.
20. Gallagher BJ III: The sociology of mental illness, Englewood Cliffs, NJ, 1980, Prentice-Hall, Inc.
21. Goldman CR: Toward a definition of psychoeducation, Hosp Community Psychiatry 39:666, 1988.
22. Grunebaum J and Friedman H: Building collaborative relationships with families of the mentally ill, Hosp Community Psychiatry 39:1183, 1988.
23. Heinrichs DW: Recent developments in the psychosocial treatment of chronic psychotic illnesses. In Talbott JA: The chronic mental patient: five years later, New York, 1984, Grune & Stratton, Inc.
24. Holmes TH and Rahe RH: The social readjustment rating scale, J Psychosom Res 11:213, 1967.
25. Kelly JA et al: Objective evaluation and prediction of client improvement in mental health aftercare, Soc Work Health Care 5:187, 1979.
26. Knight B et al: Self-help groups: the members' perspectives, Am J Community Psychol 8:53, 1980.
27. Lamb HR: Deinstitutionalization and the homeless mentally ill, Hosp Community Psychiatry 35:899, 1984.
28. Lamb HR: Deinstitutionalization at the crossroads, Hosp Community Psychiatry 39:941, 1988.
29. Lamb HR and Goertzel V: The long-term patient in the era of community treatment, Arch Gen Psychiatry 34:679, 1977.
30. Lamb HR et al: Community survival for long-term patients, Washington, DC, 1976, Jossey-Bass, Inc, Publishers.
31. Linn MW et al: Hospital vs. community (foster) care for psychiatric patients, Arch Gen Psychiatry 34:78, 1977.
32. Malone J: Concepts for the rehabilitation of the long-term mentally ill in the community, Issues Ment Health Nurs 10:121, 1989.
33. Mitchell RE and Trickett EJ: Task force report: social networks as mediators of social support, Community Ment Health J 16:27, 1980.
34. Norbeck JS: The use of social support in clinical practice, J Psychosoc Nurs Ment Health Serv 20:(12):22, 1982.
35. Peplau HE: Interpersonal relations in nursing, New York, 1952, GP Putnam's Sons.

36. Polak PR: A comprehensive system of alternatives to psychiatric hospitalization. In Stein LI and Test MA, editors: Alternatives to mental hospital treatment, New York, 1978, Plenum Press.
37. Setze PJ and Bond GR: Psychiatric recidivism in a psychosocial rehabilitation setting: a survival analysis, 36:521, 1985.
38. Spaniol L, Zipple A, and FitzGerald S: How professionals can share power with families: practical approaches working with families of the mentally ill, Psychosoc Rehab J 8:77, 1984.
39. Spivack G et al: The long-term patient in the community: life-style patterns and treatment implications, Hosp Community Psychiatry 33:291, 1982.
40. Stein LI and Test MA: An alternative to mental hospital treatment. In Stein LI and Test MA, editors: Alternatives to mental hospital treatment, New York, 1978, Plenum Press.
41. Turkat D and Buzzell V: Psychosocial rehabilitation: a process evaluation, Hosp Community Psychiatry 33:848, 1982.
42. Walsh M: Schizophrenia: straight talk for families and friends, New York, 1985, William Morrow and Co, Inc.
43. Wing JK and Olsen R: Community care for the mentally disabled, New York, 1979, Oxford University Press.

■ ANNOTATED SUGGESTED READINGS ■

Anthony WA: The principles of psychiatric rehabilitation, Baltimore, 1980, University Park Press.

An excellent, clearly written book that describes a psychiatric rehabilitation program in great detail. Reflects the author's extensive experience in training mental health care providers to care for the seriously mentally ill.

Bachrach LL: Deinstitutionalization: an analytical review and sociological perspective, Department of Health, Education, and Welfare Pub No (ADM)79-351, Washington, DC, 1979.

Attempts to pull together the many theories and opinions related to deinstitutionalization. Provides a comprehensive overview of the issues and includes a sociological analysis by the author. Recommended for the advanced student or the nurse who is interested in performing research.

*Banes JS: An ex-patient's perspective of psychiatric treatment, J Psychosoc Nurs Ment Health Serv 21(3):11, 1983.

An eloquently written article about the mental health system that reflects the perspective of a mental health professional who was a mental patient. Contains observations about the effects of institutionalization and the dilemmas of deinstitutionalization that should be read by all nurses who work with troubled people.

Bogin DL et al: The effects of a referral coordinator on compliance with psychiatric discharge plans, Hosp Community Psychiatry 35:702, 1984.

Report of a research project that clearly demonstrates the importance of actively assisting patients to become involved in aftercare services. Intervention of a specific staff person who was responsible for discharge planning was found to enhance patient compliance with outpatient treatment.

*Buckwalter KC and Abraham IL: Alleviating the discharge crisis: the effects of a cognitive-behavioral nursing intervention for depressed patients and their families, Arch Psychiatric Nursing 1:350, 1987.

Describes a nursing intervention using the cognitive and behavioral models of treatment. Discharged depressed patients and their families were found to display better coping skills if they had been involved in the program.

Chamberlin J: On our own, New York, 1978, McGraw-Hill Book Co.

Presents the viewpoint of a woman who was a client of the mental health system. Describes experiences in a graphic manner and also discusses in detail alternative approaches to mental health care that she believes to be more humane and helpful than those that she experienced. Presents a strong case for greater patient involvement in planning and carrying out treatment and rehabilitation.

Gudeman JE and Shore MF: Beyond deinstitutionalization: a new class of facilities for the mentally ill, N Engl J Med 311:832, 1984.

Identifies five groups of patients who do not function adequately in the community: the elderly, demented, and behaviorally disturbed; the mentally retarded and psychotic; the brain-damaged and assaultive; the psychotic and assaultive; and the chronically schizophrenic, disruptive, and endangered. Suggests specialized inpatient units for these people to provide long-term treatment-oriented care.

*Hjorten MK: A volunteer support system for the chronically ill, Persp Psychiatr Care 20:17, 1982.

A personal account of the experience of a nursing student in planning and later directing a community support program for the chronically mentally ill. Provides several suggestions for the organization of such programs and demonstrates the value of volunteer services and community involvement.

Hospital and Community Psychiatry

Journal that is a rich resource of information about psychosocial rehabilitation and in which most current research in this field is reported. Multidisciplinary focus.

*Jack LW: Using play in psychiatric rehabilitation, J Psychosoc Nurs Ment Health Serv 25:13, 1987.

Proposes that play, which is a normal part of life, should be incorporated into outpatient treatment programs for chronic schizophrenic patients. Discusses appropriate incorporation of play into nursing intervention.

Langsley DG, Barter JT, and Yarvis RM: Deinstitutionalization—the Sacramento story, Compr Psychiatry 19:749, 1978.

Demonstrates the effect of legislation on the provision of mental health care. Describes the changes that took place in Sacramento, California in response to the passage of the Lanterman-Petris-Short Act, which reorganized the mental health care system in the state.

*Asterisk indicates nursing references.

*Leavitt M: The discharge crisis: the experience of families of psychiatric patients, Nurs Res 24:33, 1975.

Describes the results of interviews with the families of 16 psychiatric patients before discharge from the hospital. Concludes that the families were not prepared to deal with the patient at home and analyzes several reasons for this response.

*Norbeck JS: The use of social support in clinical practice, J Psychosoc Nurs Ment Health Serv 20(12):22, 1982.

An excellent discussion of the concept of social support. Presents relevant research findings. Develops a typology of social support–related problems and suggests nursing interventions.

Skirball BW and Pavelsky PL: The compeer program: volunteers as friends of the mentally ill, Hosp Community Psychiatry 35:938, 1984.

Describes a program in which trained volunteers, in coordination with the patient's therapist, provide support services to mentally ill patients and provides the patient with an added dimension of a normal friendship.

*Stokes F and Keen I: Developing self-care skills and reducing institutionalized behavior in a long-stay psychiatric population: the role of the nurse in behaviour modification, J Adv Nurs 12:35, 1987.

Use of case histories to demonstrate the value of using a behavior modification approach to the rehabilitation of patients who have been hospitalized for a long period of time. Emphasizes the role of the nurse as critical to the success of such a program.

*Sweeney D et al: Mapping urban hotels: life space of the chronic mental patient, J Psychosoc Nurs Ment Health Serv 20(5):9, 1982.

States that community care providers should seek out patients on their own turf such as urban hotels and enlist proprietors and/or staff as community caregivers. Emphasizes that the object is not to "professionalize" them, but to assist them to provide social support to the residents.

Talbott JA: The chronic mental patient: five years later, New York, 1984, Grune & Stratton, Inc.

An important anthology that includes chapters written by most of the recognized authorities in the care of the chronically mentally ill. Scope of topics covered and depth of presentation make this an invaluable resource to the psychiatric nurse.

Walsh M: Schizophrenia: straight talk for families and friends, New York, 1985, William Morrow and Co, Inc.

An excellent presentation of the impact of schizophrenia on the family. The author is very frank in describing experiences with the mental health care system and those of other families. Nurses should also recommend this book to families of patients. Contains much information and advice, including a list of rehabilitation resources.

Wong SE et al: Training chronic mental patients to independently practice personal grooming skills, Hosp Community Psychiatry 39:874, 1988.

Presents an example of a program that was very effective in assisting seriously mentally ill patients to learn good habits of grooming and dress. Designed to be implemented by various levels of nursing staff.

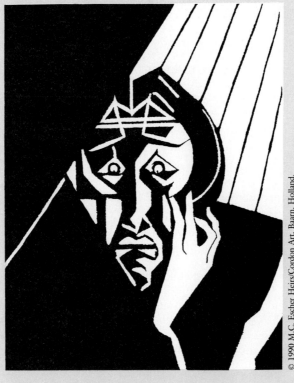

. . . . The fears we know
Are of not knowing . . . It is getting late.
Shall we ever be asked for? Are we simply
Not wanted at all?

W.H. Auden, The Age of Anxiety

C H A P T E R   11

ANXIETY

DIAGNOSTIC PREVIEW

MEDICAL DIAGNOSES RELATED TO ANXIETY

- Panic disorder
- Social phobia
- Obssessive-compulsive disorder
- Generalized anxiety disorder

- Agoraphobia without panic attacks
- Simple phobia
- Post-traumatic stress disorder

LEARNING OBJECTIVES

After studying this chapter, the student should be able to:

- describe the characteristics of the concept of anxiety.

- compare and contrast the four levels of anxiety with regard to perceptual field, potential for learning, and continuum of coping responses.

- discuss the predisposing factors that have been proposed for the origin of anxiety.

- analyze precipitating stressors that contribute to the development of anxiety.

- state the value of a unified multicausal model of anxiety.

- identify the physiological, behavioral, cognitive, and affective behaviors associated with anxiety.

- identify and describe the coping mechanisms associated with task-oriented and ego-oriented reactions.

- analyze the position of anxiety within the nursing model of health-illness phenomena.

- formulate individualized nursing diagnoses for patients with varying levels of anxiety.

- assess the relationship between nursing diagnoses and medical diagnoses associated with anxiety.

- develop long-term and short-term individualized nursing goals with patients experiencing anxiety.

- apply therapeutic nurse-patient relationship principles with appropriate rationale in planning the care of the patient experiencing anxiety.

- describe nursing interventions appropriate to the needs of the patient experiencing panic, severe, moderate, and mild levels of anxiety.

- analyze the indications for, techniques of, and problems associated with promoting the relaxation response.

- develop a mental health education plan to promote a patient's adaptive anxiety responses.

- assess the importance of the evaluation of the nursing process when working with patients who experience anxiety.

- identify directions for future nursing research.

- select appropriate readings for further study.

During the past 20 years, anxiety, a pervasive aspect of contemporary life, has been the subject of more than 500 articles or books. A recent study determined that between 10% and 25% of the population of the United States suffers from an anxiety disorder.[22] It is created within the environment by threats of war, monetary inflation, the energy crisis, and political kidnappings. Anxiety is also created within the individual by inner confusion, conflicting values, role diffusion, and personal disenchantment. The seventeenth century was known as the Age of Enlightenment, the eighteenth as the Age of Reason, and the nineteenth as the Age of Progress. The twentieth century is known as the Age of Anxiety. Anxiety has always existed, however, and belongs to no particular era or culture. It derives from the Greek root meaning "to press tight" or "to strangle." The Latin term for "anxious" means narrowness or constriction, usually with discomfort.

Although the concept of anxiety is timeless, its great impact on human life has been realized only recently. Every aspect of human endeavor is affected by anxiety. It resembles the term "anger," when defined as "grief or trouble." It is also related to "anguish," which is described as "acute pain, suffering, or distress." Anxiety is a multidimensional concept. It is manifested as a somatic, experiential, and interpersonal phenomenon. It therefore involves one's body, perceptions of self, and relationships with others. These elements make it a foundational concept in the study of psychiatric nursing and human behavior.

Continuum of anxiety responses

May defines anxiety as "diffuse apprehension that is vague in nature and associated with feelings of uncertainty and helplessness."[15:190] Feelings of isolation, alienation, and insecurity are also present. The person perceives that the core of his personality is being threatened. Experiences provoking anxiety begin in infancy and continue throughout life. They end with the fear of the greatest unknown, death.

■ Defining characteristics

The concept of anxiety can be better understood by exploring some of its characteristics. Anxiety is an emotion and a subjective individual experience. It is an energy and therefore cannot be observed directly. A nurse infers that a patient is anxious based on certain behaviors. As with all inferences, the nurse needs to validate this with the patient. Also, anxiety is an emotion without a specific object. It is provoked by the unknown and precedes all new experiences such as entering school, starting a new job, or giving birth to a child.

This characteristic of anxiety differentiates it from fear. Fear is an individual ideation that has a specific source or object. The person can identify and describe the source of fear. Fear involves the intellectual appraisal of a threatening stimulus; anxiety involves the emotional response to that appraisal. A person generally fears a set of circumstances that may occur at some point in the future. A fear is caused by physical or psychological exposure to a threatening situation. Fear produces anxiety. Thus, fear is the appraisal of danger; anxiety is the unpleasant emotion evoked by fear. The two emotions are differentiated in speech. One speaks of *having* a fear but of *being* anxious.

Another characteristic of anxiety is that it is communicated interpersonally. This is significant to the nurse. If a nurse is talking with a patient who is anxious, within a short time the nurse will also experience feelings of anxiety. Similarly, if a nurse is anxious in a particular situation, this will be readily communicated to the patient. The contagious nature of anxiety can therefore have positive and negative effects on the therapeutic relationship. The nurse must diligently monitor these effects. It is also important to remember that anxiety is part of everyday life. It is basic to the human condition and provides a valuable warning system to the individual. In fact, the capacity to be anxious is necessary for survival.

The crux of anxiety is preservation of self. Anxiety occurs as a result of a threat to a person's selfhood, self-esteem, or identity. Tillich describes it as "the state in which a being is aware of its possible non-being."[25] It results from a threat to something central to one's personality and essential to one's existence and security. It may be connected with the fear of punishment and disapproval or withdrawal of love. It may stem from the fear of disruption of a relationship, isolation, or loss of body functioning. Anxiety is experienced when the values a person identifies with his existence are threatened. Culture is related to anxiety because culture can influence the values the individual considers most important. These values include the physical, social, moral, and emotional elements of life. Underlying every fear is the anxiety of losing one's own being. This is the frightening element. However, a person can meet the anxiety and grow from it to the extent that his values are stronger than the threat.

All people therefore need a balance between courage and anxiety to preserve themselves, fulfill their beings, and affirm their existence. It is only by moving through anxiety-creating experiences that one achieves self-realization. Whenever a person moves through new possibilities, he enlarges his self-awareness, increases the scope of his activity, and expands his freedom. As May summarizes it, "the positive aspects of selfhood develop as the individual confronts, moves through and overcomes anxiety-creating experiences."[15:234]

■ Levels of anxiety

Peplau[20] identified four levels of anxiety and described the effects of each on the individual (Fig. 11-1). The first is **mild anxiety,** which is associated with the tension of day-to-day living. During this stage the person is alert and his perceptual field is increased. He sees, hears, and grasps more than previously. This kind of anxiety can motivate learning and can produce growth and creativity. The second level is **moderate anxiety,** in which the person focuses only on immedi-

ate concerns. His perceptual field is narrowed as he sees, hears, and grasps less. He blocks out selected areas but can attend to more if directed to do so. The third level is **severe anxiety,** in which the person's perceptual field is greatly reduced. He tends to focus on a specific detail and not think about anything else. All his behavior is aimed at relieving his anxiety, and he needs much direction to focus on another area. The final level is **panic,** which is associated with awe, dread, and terror. At this stage details are blown out of proportion. Because the individual has lost control, he is unable to do things even with direction. Panic involves the disorganization of the personality. A person can no longer function as an organized human being. There is increased motor activity, decreased ability to relate to others, distorted perceptions, and loss of rational thought.[18] Panic is a frightening and paralyzing experience for the individual. He is unable to communicate or function effectively. This level of anxiety cannot

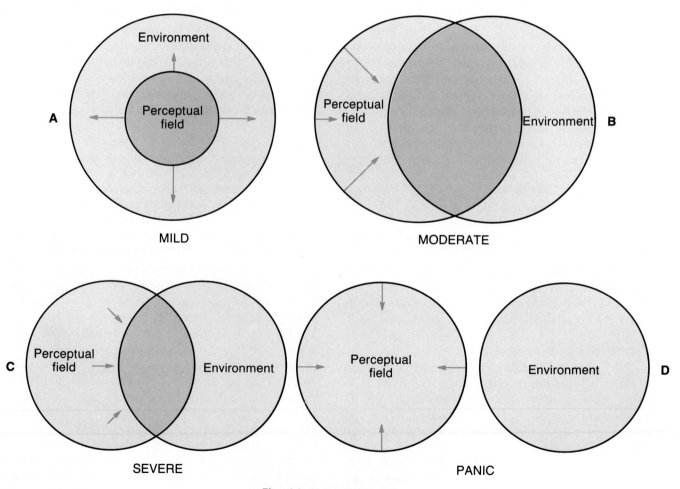

Fig. 11-1. Levels of anxiety.

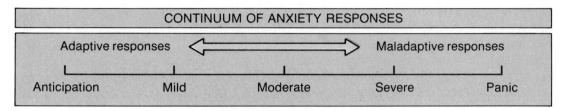

Fig. 11-2. Continuum of anxiety responses.

persist indefinitely because it is incompatible with life. A prolonged period of panic would result in exhaustion and death.

The nurse will be able to identify which level of anxiety a patient is experiencing by the behaviors she observes. The anxiety response may then be conceptualized on the continuum of coping responses described in the nursing model of health-illness phenomena (see Chapter 3). Fig. 11-2 shows the range of the anxiety response from the most adaptive response of anticipation to the most maladaptive response of panic. The patient's level of anxiety and its position on the continuum of coping responses will be relevant to the nursing diagnosis. The type of intervention the nurse implements will be based on these factors.

 ## Assessment

■ Predisposing factors

Anxiety is a prime factor in the development of the personality and formation of individual character traits. Because of this importance, various theories of the origin of anxiety have been developed. Very few facts, however, support these theories.

■ **PSYCHOANALYTIC VIEW.** Freud initiated the study of anxiety. In the beginning Freud regarded anxiety as a purely physiological reaction to a person's chronic inability to reach an orgasm in sexual relations. He believed that unexpressed sexual energy was converted into anxiety. Alleviation of anxiety therefore merely required improved sexual technique. Not until 30 years later did he see the importance of anxiety for a theory of personality development.[8,9]

His later viewpoint included two types of anxiety—primary and subsequent. The essence of primary anxiety is the "traumatic" state. This state begins in the infant as a result of the sudden stimulation and trauma of birth. Experiences of anxiety continue with the possibility that one's hunger and thirst might not be satisfied. Primary anxiety therefore is a state of tension or a drive produced by external causes. The environment is capable of threatening as well as satisfying. This im-

plicit threat predisposes the individual to anxiety in later life.

With increased age and ego development, a new kind of anxiety arises. Freud viewed this subsequent anxiety as the emotional conflict that takes place between two elements of the personality—the id and the superego. The id represents one's instinctual drives and primitive impulses. The superego reflects one's conscience and culturally acquired restrictions. The ego, or I, tries to mediate the demands of these two clashing elements. Freud therefore suggested that one major function of anxiety was to warn the person of impending danger. It was a signal to the ego that it was in danger of being overtaken.

■ **INTERPERSONAL VIEW.** Sullivan[24] disagreed with Freud. He believed that anxiety could not arise until the organism had some awareness of its environment. Sullivan viewed the fear of disapproval as central to his theory of anxiety. He believed that anxiety originated in the early bond between the infant and mother. Through this close emotional bond, anxiety is first conveyed by the mother to the infant. The infant responds as if he and his mother were one unit. As the child grows older, he sees this discomfort as a result of his own actions. He believes that his mother either approves or disapproves of his behavior. In addition, developmental traumas such as separations and losses can lead to specific vulnerabilities. Sullivan believed that anxiety in later life arises when a person perceives he will be viewed unfavorably or will lose the love of a person he values.

Sullivan identified two other aspects of anxiety that will be important in the nurse-patient relationship. The first is that a mild or moderate level of anxiety is frequently expressed as anger. The second is that areas in the personality marked by anxiety often become the areas of significant growth. This can result when the individual learns to deal with his anxiety constructively, as in a therapeutic relationship.

Will[27] believes that an individual's level of self-esteem is an important factor related to anxiety. A person who is easily threatened, has a low level of self-esteem, or has a poor opinion of himself is more susceptible to anxiety. This is evident in a person with test anxiety. His anxiety is high because he doubts he can succeed. This may have nothing to do with his actual abilities or how much he studied. The anxiety is caused only by his perception of his ability, which reflects his self-concept. He may, for instance, be well prepared for the examination. His severe level of anxiety, however, will reduce his perceptual field significantly, and he may omit, misinterpret, or distort the meaning of the test items. He may even block out all his previous studying. The result will be a poor grade, which will reinforce his poor perception of self. Research supports the theory that individuals with high anxiety have a greater discrepancy between their perceived self and ideal self.[23] Thus low self-esteem can result in predisposition to high anxiety.

■ **BEHAVIORAL VIEW.** Some behavioral theorists propose that anxiety is a product of frustration caused by anything that interferes with attaining a desired goal. The actual precipitating factor acts to block the individual's attempt to obtain satisfaction and security. An example of an external frustration for a young man might be the loss of his job. Many of his goals may be potentially blocked, such as financial security, pride in work, and perception of self as family provider. An internal frustration is evidenced by the young college graduate who sets unrealistically high career goals and is frustrated by job offers of a clerical or apprentice nature. In this case his view of self is being threatened by his unrealistic goals. He is likely to experience feelings of failure, insignificance, and mounting anxiety.

Other experimental psychologists regard anxiety as a drive that is learned because of an innate desire to avoid pain. They believe that anxiety begins with the attachment of pain to a particular stimulus. If the reaction is strong enough, it may become generalized to similar objects and situations. Learning theorists believe that individuals who have been exposed in early life to intense fears are more likely to be anxious in later life. In this respect, parental influences are important. The child who sees his parents respond with anxiety to every minor stress soon develops a similar pattern. Paradoxically, if the child's parents are completely unmoved by potentially stressful situations, the child feels alone and lacks emotional support from the family. The appropriate emotional response of parents gives the child security and helps him learn constructive coping methods of his own.

Anxiety is also theorized to arise through conflict, which is defined as the clashing of two opposing interests. The person experiences two competing drives and must choose between them. A reciprocal relationship exists between conflict and anxiety. Conflict produces anxiety, and anxiety increases one's perceived conflict by producing feelings of helplessness. Dollard and Miller[5] conceptualize conflict as deriving from two tendencies: approach and avoidance. Approach is the tendency to do something or move toward something. Avoidance is the opposite tendency—not to do something or not to move toward something. The authors identify four kinds of conflict (Fig. 11-3). The first is the **approach-approach** conflict in which the individual is motivated to pursue two equally desirable but incompatible goals. This type of conflict seldom produces anxiety. **Approach-avoidance** conflict occurs when the individual wishes to both pursue and avoid the same goal. The patient who wants to express his anger but feels great anxiety and fear in doing so experiences this type of conflict. Another example is the ambitious business executive who must compromise his values of honesty and loyalty to be promoted. **Avoidance-avoidance** is a third kind of conflict in which the person must choose between two undesirable goals. Since neither alternative seems beneficial, this is a difficult choice usually accompanied by much anxiety. The most common type of conflict situation is the **double approach-avoidance.** In this case the person can see both desirable and undesirable aspects of both alternatives. This is the kind of conflict experienced by a person living with the pain of his social and emotional life and destructive coping patterns. His alternative is to seek psychiatric help and expose himself to the threat and potential pain of the therapy process. Double approach-avoidance conflict feelings are frequently described as ambivalence. In summarizing their theory, Dollard and Miller stress the importance of conditioning early in life. However, they assert that little is known about how most complex learned drives are acquired. Also, little is known about what permits one person to easily resolve a conflict, whereas another is plunged into a tumultuous emotional state.

■ **FAMILY STUDIES.** Epidemiological and family studies show that anxiety disorders clearly run in families and that they are common and of different types.[26] Anxiety disorders can overlap, as do anxiety disorders and depression. A person with one anxiety disorder is more likely to develop another or to experience a major depression within his lifetime. It has been estimated that about a quarter of those with anxiety disorders receive treatment. However, these persons are high users of health care facilities for reasons other than emotional problems.[26]

■ **BIOLOGICAL BASIS.** Basic science advances in understanding anxiety have been considerable in recent years. Investigators have learned that the brain con-

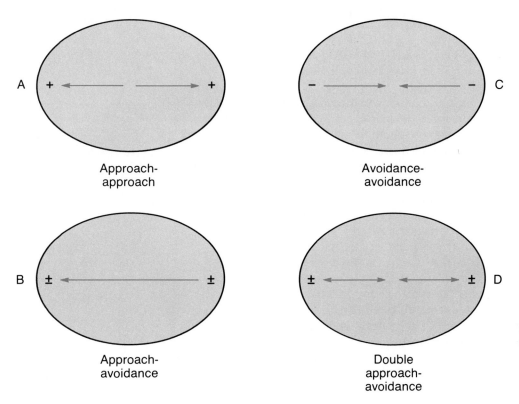

A
+ ←————————————→ +

Approach-
approach

B
± ←———————————— ±

Approach-
avoidance

C
– ———————→←———————— –

Avoidance-
avoidance

D
± ←————————→←————————— ±

Double
approach-
avoidance

Fig. 11-3. Types of conflict.

tains specific receptors for benzodiazepines and that these receptors probably help to regulate anxiety. The discovery of benzodiazepine receptors has prompted a search for naturally occurring brain substances that bond to them. The inhibitory neuroregulator gamma-aminobutyric acid (GABA) also may play a major role in biological mechanisms relating to anxiety, as may the endorphins. Although the theory is still controversial, some investigators believe that an area deep in the brain may have a key role in certain forms of anxiety. This area, called the locus ceruleus, is known to be important in several behaviors. Rigorous studies of drugs that relieve and produce anxiety should help provide additional information regarding the biological basis for anxiety disorders.

In addition, it has been shown that an individual's general health has a great effect on his predisposition to anxiety. Anxiety may accompany some physical disorders. Growing evidence suggests that it can worsen such dangerous illnesses as hypertension, heart disease, and peptic ulcer. Hyperthyroidism, hypoglycemia, and severe pulmonary disease are other illnesses associated with high levels of anxiety. One's coping mechanisms may be impaired by toxic influences, dietary deficiencies, reduced blood supply, hormonal changes, and

other physical causes. Input from somatic sources in the presence of physical illness may reduce one's capacity to cope with additional stressful inputs. One study examined the relationship between selected health-related stressful life events and anxiety levels. The researchers found that anxiety was strongly related to the number of days the individual had been sick during the last month. It was also related to the incidences of hospitalization, involvement in an accident, and four out of five medical conditions.[6] In addition, symptoms from some physical disorders, including hyperthyroidism, may mimic or exacerbate anxiety.

Similarly, fatigue increases irritability and feelings of anxiety. It appears that fatigue caused by nervous factors predisposes the individual to a greater degree of anxiety than does fatigue caused by purely physical causes. Thus fatigue may actually be an early symptom of anxiety. Patients complaining of nervous fatigue may already be suffering from a moderate anxiety state and be more susceptible to future stress situations.

■ **Precipitating stressors**

Given these numerous theories about the origin of anxiety, what kinds of events might precipitate feelings of anxiety? Precipitating stressors can be grouped into two categories: threats to one's physical integrity and threats to one's self-system.

■ **THREATS TO PHYSICAL INTEGRITY.** This category suggests impending physiological disability or decreased capacity to perform the activities of daily living. They may include both internal and external sources. External sources may include exposure to viral and bacterial infection or to environmental pollutants or safety hazards. Lack of adequate housing, food, or clothing, and traumatic injury are other examples of external sources. Internal sources may include the failure of physiological mechanisms such as the heart, immune system, or temperature regulation. The normal biological changes that can occur with pregnancy and failure to participate in preventive health practices are other internal sources that threaten physical integrity. Pain is often the first indication that physical integrity is being threatened. It creates anxiety that often motivates the person to seek health care. Thus some preventive health programs try to generate mild anxiety. Because threats to one's physical integrity do produce anxiety, many patients will experience these feelings.

■ **THREATS TO SELF-SYSTEM.** Threats in this second category are quite pervasive. Basically, they imply harm to one's identify, self-esteem, and integrated social functioning. Both external and internal sources can threaten self-esteem. External sources may include the loss of a valued person through death, divorce, or relocation. A change in job status, an ethical dilemma, and social or cultural group pressures are other examples of external sources. Internal sources may include interpersonal difficulties at home or at work or assuming a new role, such as parent, student, or employee. In addition, many of the threats to physical integrity previously mentioned also threaten self-esteem, since the mind-body relationship is an intimate and overlapping one.

This distinction of categories is only theoretical. The person responds to all stressors, whatever their nature and origin, as an integrated whole. Also, no specific event will be as equally stressful to all individuals or even to the same individual at different times.

■ **AN INTEGRATIVE MODEL.** A true understanding of anxiety requires integration of knowledge from all the various points of view (Fig. 11-4). Akiskal has proposed a model that integrates data from psychoanalytical, interpersonal, behavioral, genetic, and biological perspectives.[1] This multicausal model provides a useful frame of reference for the nurse. It is holistic in nature and encourages the assessment of behaviors and perceptions in developing appropriate nursing interventions. It also suggests a variety of causative factors and stresses the interrelationship among them in ex-

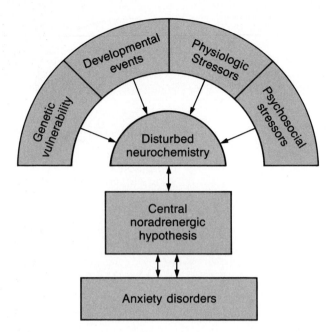

Fig. 11-4. Unified model of anxiety disorders.

plaining present behavior. It proposes that anxiety disorders can best be understood as an integration of the following factors:

1. There is a built-in neurobiological substance that prepares the individual to cope with danger.
2. Evolution has affected this substance in such a way that certain stimuli threatening to survival are selectively avoided.
3. Certain individuals may be born with a central autonomous nervous system that is overly sensitive to stimuli that are generally harmless.
4. Childhood and adult learning experiences may ultimately determine the extent, severity, and nature of the situations that will evoke anxiety.
5. Chronic inability to cope with dangerous situations adaptively could increase the tendency to respond with anxiety.
6. The cognitive functions might permit continual focusing on anxiety reactions, so that the mere anticipation of aversive stimuli would provoke anxiety.
7. Such a person would perhaps be more vulnerable to insecurities, especially if intelligent and introspective.

Thus the person's response will depend on the number and timing of the stressor and the predisposing factors previously described. It will also be affected by the person's perception of the event and the resources he has available. By observing specific behaviors, the nurse will be able to assess the individual's level of anxiety and identify his coping responses. An appropriate nursing diagnosis can then be formulated.

■ Behaviors

Anxiety can be expressed directly through physiological and behavioral changes. It can also be indirectly manifested through the formation of symptoms or coping mechanisms developed as a defense against anxiety. The nature of the behaviors displayed by the patient depends on his level of anxiety. The intensity of the behaviors will increase with increasing anxiety.

In describing anxiety's effects on **physiological responses,** one can see that mild and moderate anxiety heighten one's capacities. Conversely, severe and panic levels paralyze or overwork capacities and structures. The physiological responses associated with anxiety are primarily mediated through the autonomic nervous system. This involves the internal adjustment of the body without a conscious or voluntary effort. Two types of autonomic responses exist: the sympathetic, which activate body processes, and the parasympathetic, which conserve body responses.

Experimental studies support the predominance of the sympathetic reaction. This reaction prepares the body to deal with an emergency situation by either a "fight" or a "flight" reaction. When the cortex of the brain perceives a threat, it sends a stimulus down the sympathetic branch of the autonomic nervous system to the adrenal glands. Because of a release of epinephrine, respiration deepens, the heart beats more rapidly, and arterial pressure rises. Blood is shifted away from the stomach and intestines to the heart, central nervous system, and muscle. Glycogenolysis is accelerated, and the blood glucose level rises. For some individuals, however, the parasympathetic reaction may coexist or predominate and produce somewhat opposite effects. Other physiological reactions may also be evident. The variety of physiological responses to anxiety that the nurse may observe in patients are summarized in Table 11-1.

Psychomotor manifestations, or **behavioral responses,** will also be observed in the anxious patient. Its effects have both personal and interpersonal aspects. High levels of anxiety affect one's coordination, involuntary movements, and responsiveness. They also act as disjunctive forces in human relationships. In an interpersonal situation, anxiety can warn a person to withdraw from a situation where discomfort is anticipated. The anxious patient therefore typically withdraws and decreases interpersonal involvement. The

TABLE 11-1
PHYSIOLOGICAL RESPONSES TO ANXIETY*

Cardiovascular	**Gastrointestinal**
Palpitations	Loss of appetite
Heart racing	Revulsion toward
Increased blood pres-	food
sure	Abdominal discomfort
Faintness (p)	Abdominal pain (p)
Actual fainting (p)	Nausea (p)
Decreased blood	Heartburn (p)
pressure (p)	Diarrhea (p)
Decreased pulse rate	
(p)	**Urinary Tract**
	Pressure to urinate (p)
Respiratory	Frequency of urination
Rapid breathing	(p)
Shortness of breath	
Pressure on chest	**Skin**
Shallow breathing	Face flushed
Lump in throat	Localized sweating
Choking sensation	(palms)
Gasping	Itching
	Hot and cold spells
Neuromuscular	Face pale
Increased reflexes	Generalized sweating
Startle reaction	
Eyelid twitching	
Insomnia	
Tremors	
Rigidity	
Fidgeting	
Pacing	
Strained face	
Generalized weakness	
Wobbly legs	
Clumsy movement	

*(p) indicates parasympathetic response

possible behavioral responses the nurse might observe are presented in Table 11-2.

Mental, or intellectual, functioning is also affected by anxiety. **Cognitive responses** the patient might display when experiencing anxiety are described in Table 11-2.

Finally, the nurse will be able to assess a patient's emotional reactions, or **affective responses,** to anxiety by his subjective description of his personal experience. Frequently patients describe themselves as "tense, jittery, on edge, jumpy, worried, or restless." One patient attempted to describe his feelings in the follow-

TABLE 11-2

BEHAVIORAL, COGNITIVE, AND AFFECTIVE RESPONSES TO ANXIETY

Behavioral	Cognitive	Affective
Restlessness	Impaired attention	Edginess
Physical tension	Poor concentration	Impatience
Tremors	Forgetfulness	Uneasiness
Startle reaction	Errors in judgment	Tension
Rapid speech	Preoccupation	Nervousness
Lack of coordination	Blocking of thoughts	Fear
Accident proneness	Decreased perceptual field	Fright
Interpersonal withdrawal	Reduced creativity	Alarm
Inhibition	Diminished productivity	Terror
Flight	Confusion	Jitteriness
Avoidance	Hypervigilance	Jumpiness
Hyperventilation	Self-consciousness	
	Loss of objectivity	
	Fear of losing control	
	Frightening visual images	
	Fear of injury or death	

ing way: "I'm expecting something terribly bad to happen, but I don't know what. I'm afraid, but I don't know why. I guess you can call it a generalized bad feeling." All these phrases are expressions of a person's apprehension and overalertness. They convey the impression that all is not well. It seems clear that the person interprets his anxiety as a kind of warning sign. Additional affective responses are listed in Table 11-2.

Anxiety is an unpleasant and uncomfortable experience that most people will go to extremes to avoid. They frequently try to replace anxiety with a more tolerable feeling. Pure anxiety is rarely seen. Anxiety is usually observed in combination with other emotions. Patients might describe feelings of anger, boredom, contempt, depression, irritation, worthlessness, jealousy, self-depreciation, suspiciousness, sadness, or helplessness. These feelings may be viewed as defenses to shield them from the distress of anxiety. This makes it difficult for the nurse to discriminate between anxiety and depression, for instance, because the patient's descriptions may be similar.

Close ties exist between anxiety, depression, guilt, and hostility. These emotions often function reciprocally; one feeling acts to generate and reinforce the others. The relationship between anxiety and hostility is particularly close. The pain one experiences with anxiety frequently causes anger and resentment toward those thought to be responsible. These feelings of hostility in turn increase anxiety.

This cycle is evident in the case of a dependent and insecure wife who was very attached to her husband. She expressed numerous vague fears. In exploring her feelings, she also expressed great hostility toward him and their relationship. This symbolized her helplessness and increased her feelings of weakness. Verbalizing these angry feelings, however, further increased her anxiety and her unresolved conflict.

Thus anxiety is frequently expressed through anger, and a tense and anxious person is more likely to become angry.

■ Coping mechanisms

As the level of anxiety increases to the severe and panic levels, the behaviors displayed become more intense and injurious to the individual. These behaviors may be painful, uncomfortable, and unpleasant. Understandably, people seek to avoid anxiety and the circumstances that produce it. When experiencing anxiety, the individual uses various coping mechanisms to try to relieve it. The inability to cope with anxiety constructively is a primary cause of pathological behavior. To neutralize, deny, or counteract anxiety, the individual develops patterns of coping. The pattern used to cope with mild anxiety dominates when anxiety becomes more intense. Anxiety plays a major role in the psychogenesis of emotional illness, since many symptoms of illness develop as attempted defenses against anxiety. These symptoms also allow disguised symbolical expression of elements of the conflict.

It is helpful for the nurse to be familiar with the coping mechanisms people use when experiencing the various levels of anxiety. The **mild level of anxiety** is the anxiety caused by the tension of day-to-day living. Menninger and coworkers[17] identified several coping mechanisms people use to relieve this kind of tension. These include crying, sleeping, eating, yawning, laughing, cursing, physical exercise, and daydreaming. Oral behavior, such as smoking and drinking, is another means of coping with mild anxiety. When dealing with other people, the individual copes with low levels of anxiety through superficiality, lack of eye contact, use of clichés, and limited self-disclosure. The person can also protect himself from anxiety by assuming comfortable roles and limiting his close relationships to those with people having values similar to his own. Mild levels of anxiety are often handled without conscious thought, and their effects can be easily minimized.

Moderate, severe, and panic levels of anxiety, however, pose greater threats to the ego. They require more energy to cope with the threat. These coping mechanisms can be categorized as task-oriented reactions and ego-oriented reactions.

■ **TASK-ORIENTED REACTIONS.** Task-oriented reactions are thoughtful, deliberate attempts to solve problems, resolve conflicts, and gratify one's needs. They are aimed at realistically meeting the demands of a stress situation that has been objectively appraised. These are consciously directed and action oriented. These types of reactions can include attack, withdrawal, and compromise.

In **attack behavior** a person attempts to remove or overcome obstacles to satisfy a need. There are many possible ways of attacking problems, and this type of reaction may be destructive or constructive. Destructive patterns are usually accompanied by great feelings of anger and hostility. These feelings may be expressed by negative or aggressive behavior that violates the rights, property, and well-being of others. Constructive patterns reflect a problem-solving approach. They are evident in self-assertive behaviors that respect the rights of others.

Withdrawal behavior may be expressed physically or psychologically. Physically, withdrawal involves removing oneself from the source of the threat. This can apply to biological stressors, such as smoke-filled rooms, exposure to irradiation, or contact with contagious diseases. An individual can also withdraw in various psychological ways, such as by admitting defeat, becoming apathetic, or lowering aspirations. As with attack, this type of reaction may be constructive or destructive. When it isolates the individual from others and interferes with his ability to work, the reaction creates additional problems. It is often accompanied by fear, hostility, and guilt.

Compromise is necessary in situations that cannot be resolved through either attack or withdrawal. This involves changing one's usual way of operating, substituting goals, or sacrificing aspects of one's personal needs. Compromise reactions are usually constructive and are frequently employed in approach-approach and avoidance-avoidance situations. When the decision resolves the problem, the individual can then move on to other activities. Occasionally, however, the person realizes with time that the compromise is not acceptable. He must then renegotiate a solution or adopt a different coping mechanism.

A person's capacity for task-oriented reactions and effective problem solving is greatly influenced by his expectation of at least partial success. This in turn will depend on remembering past successes in similar situations. On this basis he can go forward and deal with the current stressful situation. Perseverance in problem solving also depends on the person's expectation of a certain level of pain and discomfort and his belief that he is capable of tolerating this. Here lies the balance between courage and anxiety.

■ **EGO-ORIENTED REACTIONS.** Task-oriented reactions are not always successful in coping with stressful situations. Consequently, ego-oriented reactions are often used to protect the self. These reactions, also called **ego defense mechanisms,** are the first line of psychic defense. Everyone uses defense mechanisms, and they frequently help one cope successfully with mild and moderate levels of anxiety. They protect the person from feelings of inadequacy and worthlessness and prevent awareness of anxiety. They can be used to such an extreme degree, however, that they distort reality, interfere with interpersonal relationships, and limit one's ability to work productively. This results in ego disintegration instead of self-integrity.

As coping mechanisms, they have certain drawbacks. First, ego-oriented reactions operate on relatively unconscious levels. The person has little awareness of what is happening and little control over events. Second, they involve a degree of self-deception and reality distortion. Therefore they usually do not

TABLE 11-3

EGO DEFENSE MECHANISMS

Defense mechanism	Example	Defense mechanism	Example
Compensation: Process by which a person makes up for a perceived deficiency by strongly emphasizing a feature that he regards as an asset.	A businessman perceives his small physical stature negatively. He tries to overcome this by being aggressive, forceful, and controlling in business dealings.	**Projection:** Attributing one's own thoughts or impulses to another person. Through this process one can attribute intolerable wishes, emotional feelings, or motivations to another person.	A young woman who denies she has sexual feelings about a coworker accuses him without basis of being a "flirt" and says he is trying to seduce her.
Denial: Avoidance of disagreeable realities by ignoring or refusing to recognize them; probably simplest and most primitive of all defense mechanisms.	Mrs. P has just been told that her breast biopsy indicates a malignancy. When her husband visits her that evening, she tells him that no one has discussed the laboratory results with her.	**Rationalization:** Offering a socially acceptable or apparently logical explanation to justify or make acceptable otherwise unacceptable impulses, feelings, behaviors, and motives.	John fails an examination and complains that the lectures were not well organized or clearly presented.
Displacement: Shift of emotion from a person or object to another usually neutral or less dangerous person or object.	A 4-year-old boy is angry because he has just been punished by his mother for drawing on his bedroom walls. He begins to play "war" with his soldier toys and has them battle and fight with each other.	**Reaction formation:** Development of conscious attitudes and behavior patterns that are opposite to what one really feels or would like to do.	A married woman who feels attracted to one of her husband's friends treats him rudely.
Dissociation: The separation of any group of mental or behavioral processes from the rest of the person's consciousness or identity.	A man is brought to the emergency room by the police and is unable to explain who he is and where he lives or works.	**Regression:** Retreat in face of stress to behavior characteristic of any earlier level of development.	Four-year-old Nicole, who has been toilet trained for over a year, begins to wet her pants again when her new baby brother is brought home from the hospital.
Identification: Process by which a person tries to become like someone he admires by taking on thoughts, mannerisms, or tastes of that individual.	Sally, 15 years old, has her hair styled similarly to her young English teacher whom she admires.	**Repression:** Involuntary exclusion of a painful or conflictual thought, impulse, or memory from awareness. It is the primary ego defense, and other mechanisms tend to reinforce it.	Mr. R does not recall hitting his wife when she was pregnant.
Intellectualization: Excessive reasoning or logic is used to avoid experiencing disturbing feelings.	A woman avoids dealing with her anxiety in shopping malls by explaining that she is saving the frivolous waste of time and money by not going into them.	**Splitting:** Viewing people and situations as either all good or all bad. Failure to integrate the positive and negative qualities of oneself.	A friend tells you that you are the most wonderful person in the world one day, and how much she hates you the next day.
Introjection: Intense type of identification in which a person incorporates qualities or values of another person or group into his own ego structure. It is one of the earliest mechanisms of the child; important in formation of conscience.	Eight-year-old Jimmy tells his 3-year-old sister, "Don't scribble in your book of nursery rhymes. Just look at the pretty pictures," thus expressing his parents' values to his little sister.	**Sublimation:** Acceptance of a socially approved substitute goal for a drive whose normal channel of expression is blocked.	Ed has an impulsive and physically aggressive nature. He tries out for the football team and becomes a star tackle.
		Suppression: A process often listed as a defense mechanism but really a conscious counterpart of repression. It is intentional exclusion of material from consciousness. At times, it may lead to subsequent repression.	A young man at work finds he is thinking so much about his date that evening that it is interfering with his work. He decides to put it out of his mind until he leaves the office for the day.
Isolation: Splitting off of emotional components of a thought, which may be temporary or long term.	A second-year medical student dissects a cadaver for her anatomy course without being disturbed by thoughts of death.	**Undoing:** Act or communication that partially negates a previous one; primitive defense mechanism.	Larry makes a passionate declaration of love to Sue on a date. On their next meeting he treats her formally and distantly.

help the individual to cope with the problem realistically. Many defense mechanisms have been identified in the literature; Table 11-3 lists some of the more common ones .

When discussing ego-oriented reactions, or defense mechanisms, it is important to note that individuals frequently monitor their own level of emotional tolerance and the resulting need to use ego defenses.

This idea is supported by Elliott,[7] who believes denial in particular may effectively allay anxiety immediately following a stressful event. She believes that if denial is gradually eliminated as the stress begins to subside, the person may better adapt to the new situation.

The evaluation of whether the patient's use of certain defense mechanisms is adaptive or maladaptive involves four issues:

1. The accurate recognition of the patient's use of the defense mechanism by the nurse.
2. The degree to which the defense mechanism is used. Does it imply a high degree of personality disorganization? Is the person unresponsive to facts about his life situation?
3. The degree to which use of the defense mechanism impedes the patient's progress toward regained health.
4. The reason the patient used the ego defense mechanism.

The nurse will better understand the patient and plan more effective nursing care after considering these areas.

If the ego defense mechanisms fail and the person's level of anxiety remains high, he must use exaggerated and inappropriate coping mechanisms. These coping patterns are maladaptive responses that may appear deviant or abnormal to others. They include the many hidden, unconscious, and devious pathways in which the effects of anxiety are converted psychologically.

Obviously, many coping mechanisms are available to the individual for minimizing anxiety. Some of these defense mechanisms appear to be essential for all human beings to maintain emotional stability. The exact nature and number of the defenses used by the individual strongly influence his personality pattern. When these defenses are overused or used unsuccessfully, they cause many physiological and psychological symptoms commonly associated with emotional illness. As Freud has said, "One thing is certain, that the problem of anxiety is a nodal point linking up all kinds of most important questions; a riddle, of which the solution must cast a flood of light upon our whole mental life."[14:118]

 # Nursing diagnosis

Formulating a nursing diagnosis depends on a clear understanding of the position of anxiety within the nursing model of health-illness phenomena (Fig. 11-5). First, it emerges as a "generalized anxiety reaction" when a person perceives a stressor to be threatening or harmful. Three aspects of anxiety are activated at this time:

1. The central nervous system is aroused.
2. Anxiety is felt and is evident in various cognitive, affective, physiological, behavioral, and social changes.
3. Ways of coping with anxiety are brought into play.

These coping mechanisms may be constructive or destructive in nature and may represent neurotic or psychotic health problems.

■ Differentiating anxiety responses

Most behaviors and coping mechanisms described in this chapter in relation to anxiety could be classified as neurotic disorders or health problems. A **neurosis** is a mental disorder characterized by anxiety that involves no distortion of reality. Neurotic disorders are maladaptive anxiety responses associated with moderate and severe levels of anxiety (Fig. 11-4).

Psychosis, however, can emerge with the panic level of anxiety as the individual feels he is "breaking into pieces." The anxiety of psychosis is not just fear of failure or fear of being unable to cope with the threatening situation. It is the fear that the failure will reveal defeat in the "process of living" and failure in the "process of being." This can be seen in the woman who has just given birth to a baby and experiences a postpartum psychosis. In this case the fear manifests itself in connection with being a mother. The woman identifies with her own mother and with the child. She experiences feelings of unfulfilled needs and personal inadequacies.

In addition to differentiating between neurotic and psychotic anxiety responses, the nurse will need to discriminate between anxiety and depression. These frequently overlap because anxious patients are often depressed and depressed patients are often anxious. For example, both anxious and depressed patients share the following symptoms: sleep disturbances, appetite changes, nonspecific cardiopulmonary and gastrointestinal complaints, difficulty concentrating, irritability, and fatigue or lack of energy. Yet there are often discrete, if subtle, differences between the two groups. These are described in Table 11-4.

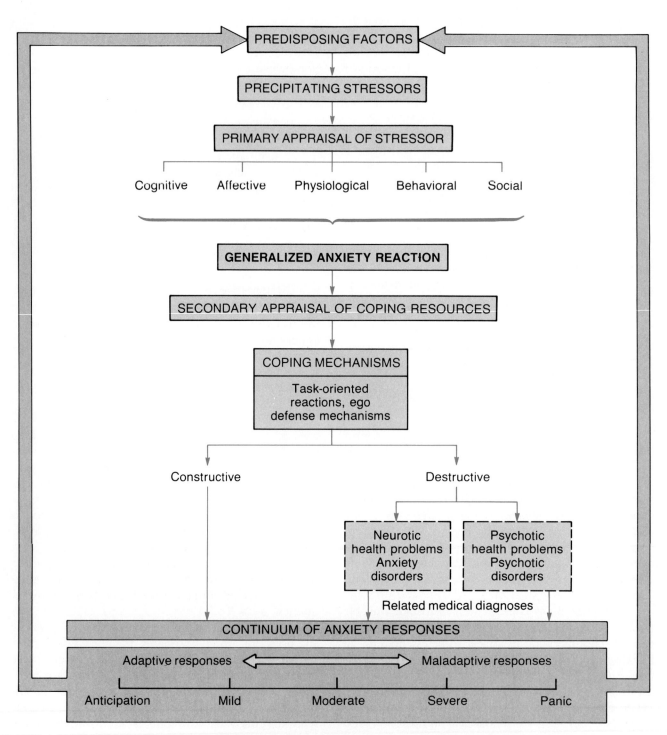

Fig. 11-5. Nursing model of health-illness phenomena related to anxiety.

TABLE 11-4

DIFFERENCES BETWEEN ANXIETY AND DEPRESSION

Anxiety	Depression
Predominantly fearful or apprehensive with feelings of dread	Predominantly sad or hopeless with feelings of despair
Difficulty falling asleep (initial insomnia)	Early morning awakening (late insomnia) or hypersomnia
Phobic avoidance behavior	Diurnal variation (feels worse in the morning)
Rapid pulse and psychomotor and autonomic hyperactivity	Slowed speech and thought processes
Breathing disturbances	Delayed response time
Tremors and palpitations	Psychomotor retardation (agitation may also occur)
Sweating and hot or cold spells	Loss of interest in usual activities
Faintness, light-headedness, dizziness	Inability to experience pleasure
Depersonalization (feelings of detachment from one's body)	Thoughts of death or suicide
Derealization (feeling that one's environment is strange, unreal or unfamiliar)	Negative appraisals are pervasive, global, and exclusive
Negative appraisals are selective and specific and do not include all areas of life	Sees the future as blank and has given up all hope
Sees some prospects for the future	Regards mistakes as beyond redemption
Does not regard defects or mistakes as irrevocable	Absolute in negative evaluations
Uncertain in negative evaluations	Global view that nothing will turn out right
Predicts that only certain events may go badly	

■ Identifying nursing problems

The nurse who has adequately assessed a patient and uses a conceptual model for understanding anxiety will be able to formulate a nursing diagnosis based on the patient's position on the continuum of anxiety responses. The nurse will review the objective data collected, as well as the subjective responses of the patient to questions and statements. The patient's history will be important. The nurse's personal response to the patient will also be important, since anxiety is readily communicated interpersonally.

In formulating the nursing diagnosis related to anxiety, the research of Lagina[12] shows that nurses tend to refer more frequently to subjective observations than to objective behaviors. They appear to rely heavily on the patient's medical diagnosis of health problems, prognosis, and the therapy indicated. Lagina stresses the need for nurses to go beyond the patient's medical diagnosis. Nurses need to identify the patient's behavior and his pattern of responding to anxiety. She also suggests that nurses, in diagnosing their patients' anxiety, may be projecting their own anxiety. She underscores the need to distinguish between the two.

To formulate a nursing diagnosis, the nurse must determine the quality and quantity of the anxiety experienced by the patient. The coping mechanism mobilized must also be categorized as constructive or destructive. In considering the quality of the anxiety, the nurse might question the appropriateness of the patient's response to the perceived threat. Is it warranted and adaptive, or absurd and irrational? A problem may exist if the response is out of proportion to the threat. This would indicate that the patient's cognitive appraisal of the threat is unrealistic. The quantity of the reaction is the next consideration in determining the degree or level of anxiety. When anxiety reaches the severe and panic levels, it indicates that the conflict is increasingly problematic and incapacitating for the patient.

The nurse also needs to explore how the anxiety is being met or coped with. Constructive coping mechanisms are protective responses that consciously confront the threat. Destructive coping mechanisms involve repression into the unconscious. They tend to be ineffective, inadequate, disorganized, inappropriate, and exaggerated. They may be evident in bizarre behavior or symptom formation.

Finally, the nurse needs to determine the overall effect of the anxiety on the individual. Is it stimulating growth? Or is it interfering with effective living and life satisfaction? Is it enhancing one's sense of self? Or is it depersonalizing and despiritizing? Whenever possible, the patient should be included in identifying problem areas. This may not always be feasible, however, particularly if the patient's anxiety level is at the severe or panic level.

An appropriate nursing diagnosis would reflect these criteria. It should include the nursing problem, the related stressor, and maladaptive health responses. Primary North American Nursing Diagnosis Association (NANDA) diagnoses and examples of complete nursing diagnoses related to anxiety are presented in

---

Nursing Diagnoses Related to Anxiety

Primary NANDA Nursing Diagnoses

Anxiety
Coping, ineffective individual
Fear

Examples of Complete Nursing Diagnoses

Panic level of anxiety related to family rejection evidenced by confusion and impaired judgment

Severe anxiety related to sexual conflict evidenced by repetitive handwashing and recurrent thoughts of dirt and germs

Severe anxiety related to marital conflict evidenced by inability to leave the house

Moderate anxiety related to financial pressures evidenced by recurring episodes of abdominal pain and heartburn

Moderate anxiety related to assumption of motherhood role evidenced by inhibition and avoidance

Moderate anxiety related to poor school performance evidenced by excessive use of denial and rationalization

Ineffective individual coping related to daughter's death evidenced by inability to recall events pertaining to the car accident

Ineffective individual coping related to child's illness evidenced by limited ability to concentrate and psychomotor agitation

Fear related to impending surgery evidenced by generalized hostility to staff and restlessness

---

the accompanying box. A complete nursing assessment would include all maladaptive responses of the patient. Many additional nursing problems would be identified from the way the patient's anxiety reciprocally influences his interpersonal relationships, self-concept, cognitive functioning, physiological status, and other aspects of life. The identification of nursing problems should be as complete as possible to ensure an adequate plan of care and intervention. Nursing diagnoses related to the range of possible maladaptive responses of the patient are identified in Table 11-5.

Nursing diagnoses can be formulated for any patient experiencing anxiety. It may be a coping response to a physical illness, a psychological illness, or a perceived threat to one's physical integrity or self-system. The patient may or may not also have been medically diagnosed.

■ Related medical diagnoses

Many patients experiencing mild or moderate anxiety have no medically diagnosed health problem. However, patients experiencing more severe levels of anxiety usually have neurotic disorders that fall under the category of anxiety disorders in the DSM-III-R.[2] Recent studies show that anxiety disorders occur twice as often in women as in men, and obsessive-compulsive disorder is about equally prevalent in women and men. In addition, no outstanding differences in the prevalence of anxiety disorders have been found on the basis of race, income, education, or rural versus urban dwelling.[22] Thus, these disorders affect every aspect of the population. The eight major disorders included in this category are listed in Table 11-5. Each one is now briefly described.

■ **PANIC DISORDER.** The essential features of this disorder are recurrent panic (anxiety) attacks. Although these attacks sometimes are unpredictable, they may become associated with certain situations, such as driving a car. They are manifested by sudden intense apprehension, fear, or terror and are often associated with feelings of impending doom. The most common symptoms experienced during an attack are shortness of breath, choking, palpitations, chest pain, sweating, faintness, dizziness, nausea, depersonalization, numbness, hot flashes, trembling, fear of dying, and fear of going crazy or doing something uncontrolled. Attacks usually last minutes; more rarely, hours. The individual often develops varying degrees of nervousness and apprehension between attacks.

■ **AGORAPHOBIA WITHOUT PANIC ATTACKS.** The essential features of agoraphobia are a fear of being away from a safe place or person, especially in situations where incapacitation may occur. The individ-

TABLE 11-5

MEDICAL AND NURSING DIAGNOSES RELATED TO ANXIETY

Medical Diagnostic Class	Psychiatric Nursing Diagnostic Class
Anxiety disorders	Anxiety
Related Medical Diagnoses (DSM-III-R)*	**Related Nursing Diagnoses (NANDA)**
Panic disorder	†Adjustment, impaired
Agoraphobia without panic attacks	†Anxiety
Social phobia	Breathing pattern, ineffective
Simple phobia	Communication, impaired verbal
Obsessive-compulsive disorder	†Coping, ineffective individual
Post-traumatic stress disorder	Diarrhea
Generalized anxiety disorder	†Fear
Anxiety disorder NOS	Health maintenance, altered
	Incontinence, stress
	Injury, potential for
	Nutrition, altered
	Post-trauma response
	Powerlessness
	Self-esteem disturbance
	Sensory/perceptual alterations
	Sleep pattern disturbance
	Social interaction, impaired
	Social isolation
	Thought processes, altered
	Urinary elimination, altered patterns

*From American Psychiatric Association: Diagnostic and Statistical Manual of Mental Disorder, Third Edition-Revised, Washington D.C., 1987, The Association.
†Indicates primary nursing diagnoses for anxiety

ual experiences generalized travel restrictions, often needs a companion away from home, and has a severely altered life-style. Agoraphobia has been classically described as "fear of the marketplace." More recently it is viewed as a fear of experiencing panic or anxiety away from a safe place or person and thus a "fear of fear." Agoraphobia is one of the most complex and disabling of the anxiety disorders.

■ **SOCIAL PHOBIA.** The essential feature of social phobia is a persistent, irrational fear of situations in which the individual may be exposed to scrutiny by others. This fear is accompanied by a compelling desire to avoid such situations. The person also fears behaving embarrassingly. Anticipatory anxiety occurs if the individual is faced with the possibility of such a situation and therefore attempts to avoid it. The individual recognizes the avoidance behavior as excessive or unreasonable and thus is extremely distressed. Examples include fear of speaking or performing in public, using public lavatories, eating in public, or writing in the presence of others.

■ **SIMPLE PHOBIA.** The essential feature of simple phobia is a persistent, irrational fear of an object or situation other than a panic attack or humiliation in social situations. The fear interferes with functioning and is recognized by the individual as unreasonable. The most common simple phobias involve the fear of animals, particularly dogs, snakes, insects, and mice. Other phobias include acrophobia—fear of heights; claustrophobia—fear of closed spaces; monophobia—fear of being alone; and pyrophobia—fear of fire.

■ **OBSESSIVE-COMPULSIVE DISORDER.** These reactions may be experienced singularly or in combination. The presence of either warrants the diagnosis. The essential feature of an obsessive-compulsive disorder is an incessant preoccupation with impulses and anxieties that the individual believes are groundless, senseless, and impossible. An *obsession* is a recurring thought that cannot be voluntarily removed from consciousness. They are intrusive, repetitive, and unwanted thoughts, images, or impulses that generate resistance. The content is typically repulsive, consisting of blasphemous, obscene thoughts, doubts, or fears that invade the patient's consciousness. There are five major categories of obsessions. In descending order of frequency these include: (1) dirt, germs, and contamination; (2) aggressive behavior; (3) orderliness of inanimate objects; (4) sexual behavior; and (5) religious matters.

A *compulsion* is a recurring, irresistable impulse to perform some act. It is, in a sense, an obsession in action. The two primary forms of compulsive behavior are excessive cleaning or washing and the checking of inanimate objects. Compulsive behavior tends to relieve anxiety that would be overwhelming if the individual were restrained from performing the activity.

The two behaviors may be combined in an obsessive-compulsive reaction. For example, the person who compulsively washes his hands might also experience obsessive thoughts relating to dirt and germs. Again, the repeated thought or act prevents the person from experiencing severe anxiety. The important element with these disorders is that the person does not want to repeat the act or thought but feels compelled to do so.

■ **POST-TRAUMATIC STRESS DISORDER.** The essential feature of this disorder is the development of characteristic symptoms following a psychologically traumatic event. The events that precede these symptoms are generally outside the range of usual human experience. The characteristic symptoms involve reexperiencing the event; a numbing of responsiveness or reduced involvement with the external world; recurrent, distressing dreams of the event; and autonomic, depressed, or anxious symptoms.

■ **GENERALIZED ANXIETY DISORDER.** The essential feature is generalized, persistent anxiety lasting at least 6 months. The anxiety involves two or more life circumstances. The specific symptoms that characterize panic disorders, obsessive-compulsive disorders, or anorexia nervosa are absent. The diagnosis is not made if the disturbance is caused by another physical or mental disorder. Mild depressive symptoms are common.

■ **ANXIETY DISORDER NOS.** This is a residual category for disorders involving prominent anxiety or phobic avoidance that are not classified as a specific anxiety disorder or as an adjustment disorder with anxious mood.

❦ Planning and implementation

■ Goal setting

The overall goal of the nurse working with an anxious patient is not to free him totally from anxiety.

The patient needs to develop the capacity to tolerate mild anxiety and to use it consciously and constructively. In this way his self will become stronger and more integrated. As he learns from these experiences, he will move on in his development. The patient will be able to meet anxiety constructively if he has sound, firm, flexible values. He must also be convinced that the values to be gained in moving ahead are greater than those to be gained by escape. Anxiety can be considered a war between the threat and the values a person identifies with his existence. Maladaptive behavior means that the struggle is won by the threat. The constructive approach to anxiety means that the struggle is won by the person's values. Thus a general nursing goal is to help the patient develop sound values. This does not mean that the patient assumes the nurse's values. Rather, the nurse works with the patient to sort out his own values, which go beyond the present situation and extend toward the good of the community.

Anxiety can also be an important factor in the patient's decision to seek treatment. Since anxiety is undesirable, the individual will seek ways to reduce it. If the patient's coping mechanism or symptom does not minimize his anxiety, his motivation for treatment will be increased. Conversely, anxiety about the therapeutic process can delay or prevent the individual from seeking treatment.

The patient should actively participate in the phases of planning and implementation. If the patient is actively involved in identifying relevant stressors and planning possible solutions, the success of the implementation phase will be maximized. Patients in extreme anxiety initially will not be able to participate in the problem-solving process. However, as soon as their anxiety is reduced, the nurse should encourage their involvement to stress the importance of their participation. This will also reinforce that they are responsible for their own growth and personal development.

In formulating a plan of care for the patient, the nurse first develops nursing goals. Goals such as "decrease anxiety" and "minimize anxiety" lack specific behaviors and evaluation criteria. These goals therefore are not particularly useful in guiding nursing care and evaluating its effectiveness. The long-term goals for the patient should relate to the nursing diagnosis. They should focus on significant reduction or elimination of the problematic behavior identified in the nursing diagnosis. They should also include learning new, more constructive coping mechanisms. The short-term goals should break this down into readily attainable steps. Short-term goals are important to provide smaller but measurable progress toward the long-term goal. Both these factors allow the nurse and patient to see

PSYCHIATRIC NURSING CARE PLAN

Precautions:

_____
_____
_____

Special nursing needs:
Consistency in daily routine;
adherence to behavioral program;
supportive limit setting

Visitors: { } No restrictions
         { } Family only
         {x} Restricted to:
         Individuals specified in behavioral plan
         { } No visitors

Telephone: {x} Limited
             { } Unlimited

Privileges: { } Restricted to unit
          {x} Off unit accompanied by staff
          { } Off unit accompanied by family/visitor
          { } Off unit unaccompanied
          { } Out of hospital leave (dates) _____

Assessment data summary: First admission although has had symptoms for over 7 years; employed as bank teller but on leave of absence due to symptoms of hadwashing (over 30 times/day); prolonged showering (up to 2 hours/shower) and frequent changing of clothing; obsessional concern about contamination

Nursing diagnoses: 1. Severe level of anxiety related to fear of contamination evidenced by cleanliness rituals.
2. Altered family processes related to fear of contamination evidenced by withdrawal and repusion of contact with family.
3. Impaired skin integrity related to excessive washing evidenced by chapped, bleeding skin.
4. Altered role performance related to obsessional thinking evident by inability to work and avoidance of public places.

Treatment goal: Support and protect patient and reduce his anxiety to a moderate-mild level.

Date	Problem/need	Expected outcome (objective)	Target Date	Nursing Intervention
4/1	Excessive cleanliness behaviors	Handwashing limited to 3× day; bathing and changing clothes once/day	4/21	Gradual desentization techniques per behavioral therapy program. Supportive but consistent approach that emphasizes his strengths.
4/1	Skin healing on hands, face and skin folds	Skin will be less chapped with no evidence of bleeding or scabs	4/15	Observe skin for integrity and infection. Apply ointments as prescribed. Encourage adequate nutrition.

Room	Patient's name	Age	Doctor	Primary nurse	Admit date
104	Mr. P	35	Dr. B	Ms. S	3/30/90

Continued.

Fig. 11-6. Sample nursing care plan for a patient with obsessive-compulsive disorder. (This nursing care plan includes examples of the elements of a total plan as it might appear at a particular time in the patient's course of treatment. It should not be considered all inclusive.)

Date	Medications	Date	P.R.N. Medications	Diagnostic & psychiatric tests	Req.	Done
4/1/90	Anafronil	4/1/90	Zanax			
	25 mg ×3 days		0.5 mg tid			
	50 mg ×3 days					
	100 mg ×4 days					
	then increase					
	dose as indicated					
		Date	Treatments	Special orders and concerns		
		4/1/90	Lubriderm	Adherence to interdisciplinary		
			for chapped	behavioral program		
			hands			

Allergies:	Medical diagnosis: (axis I-III)	Diet:
None	Obsessive-compulsive disorder	Regular

Fig. 11-6, cont'd. Sample nursing care plan for a patient with obsessive-compulsive disorder.

progress even if the ultimate goal still appears distant (Fig. 11-6).

When the nursing diagnosis describes the patient's anxiety at the severe or panic levels, the highest-priority short-term goals should address lowering the anxiety level. Only after this has been achieved can additional progress be made. The reduced level of anxiety should be evident in a reduction of behaviors associated with the severe or panic levels. The reduction of these behaviors thus forms part of the content for the short-term goals. Following are examples of short-term goals for a particular patient.

After 10 days Mr. Jones will:

1. Attend and remain seated during all ward meetings.
2. Participate at least three times during each meeting.
3. Discuss one topic for a minimum of 10 minutes when meeting with his nurse.
4. Attend all occupational therapy sessions.
5. Sleep a minimum of 6 hours a night.

When these goals are met, the nurse can assume and validate that the patient's level of anxiety has been reduced. The nurse may then develop new short-term

goals directed toward insight or relaxation therapy. Throughout the nursing process, the nurse must continually reevaluate the level of the patient's anxiety. Kristic[11] studied the anxiety level of psychiatric patients throughout their total hospitalization. She found three specific crisis periods of increased anxiety: on admission, after the fifth day of the hospitalization, and on discharge. She notes that not only is intensive intervention needed at these times, but that nurses have the greatest opportunity for implementing them. Studies such as these may provide a basis for predicting periods of particular stress for patients. This knowledge would have direct implications for the planning and implementing of therapeutic nursing care.

■ **Intervening in severe and panic levels of anxiety**

■ **ESTABLISHING A TRUSTING RELATIONSHIP.** The patient experiencing severe or panic levels of anxiety may be hospitalized. To reduce this patient's level of anxiety, most nursing actions are supportive and protective. Initially the nurse needs to establish an open, trusting relationship. To accomplish this, she should actively listen to the patient and encourage him to discuss his feelings of anxiety, hostility, guilt, and frustration. She should answer his questions directly and offer unconditional acceptance of him. Both her verbal and her nonverbal communications should convey awareness of the patient's feelings and acceptance of them. The patient might express himself in rapid, disjointed speech, hostile outbursts, or crying episodes. The nurse should remain available to the patient and respect his use of personal space. Research indicates that a 6-foot distance in a small room may create the optimum condition for openness and discussion of fears.[13] The more this distance is increased or decreased, the more anxious the patient may become.

■ **SELF-AWARENESS.** The nurse's own feelings are of particular importance when working with a highly anxious patient. The nurse may find herself being unsympathetic to the patient, impatient with him, and frustrated by him. These are common feelings of reciprocal anxiety that the nurse should be aware of and accept. If the nurse is alert to the development of anxiety in herself, she can learn from it and use it therapeutically within the nurse-patient relationship. For example, it may indicate some important emotional issue that the patient is unable to identify and verbalize, or it may reflect a conflict within the nurse that is interfering with her ability to be therapeutic. She should therefore be alert to the signs of anxiety in herself, accept them, and attempt to explore their cause. What is threatening her? Is this patient a source of reflected esteem for her? Has she failed to live up to what she imagines is the patient's ideal? Is she comparing herself to a peer or another health professional? Is the patient's area of conflict one that she has not resolved for herself? Is her anxiety related to something that will or may happen in the future? Is her patient's conflict really one of her own that she is projecting onto him?

If the nurse denies her own anxiety, it can have detrimental effects on the nurse-patient relationship. Because of her own anxiety, she may be unable to differentiate between levels of anxiety in others. She may also transfer her own fears and frustrations to the patient, thus compounding his problem. Finally, her anxiety will arouse defenses in other patients and staff that will severely interfere with her therapeutic usefulness. She should strive to accept her patient's anxiety without reciprocal anxiety by continually clarifying her own feelings and role (see Clinical example 11-1).

■ **PROTECTING THE PATIENT.** Another major area of intervention is protecting the patient and reassuring him of his safety. One way of decreasing his anxiety is by allowing the patient to determine what stress he can handle at the time. The nurse should not force or probe the severely anxious patient into situations he is not able to handle. She should not attack

CLINICAL EXAMPLE 11-1

Ms. R was a 35-year-old married woman and mother of three children, ages 4, 6, and 9. She was a full-time housewife and mother. Her husband was a salesman and spent about two nights each week out of town. She came to the clinic complaining of severe headaches that "come upon me very suddenly and are so terrible that I have to go to bed. The only thing that helps is for me to lie down in a dark and absolutely quiet room." She said that these headaches were becoming a real problem for everyone in the family, and her husband told her that she "just had to get over them and get things back to normal."

Mr. W, a psychiatric nurse, offered to see Ms. R in therapy once a week. After 4 weeks, he was asked to present his evaluation, treatment plans, and progress report to the clinic staff at their regular weekly team conference. Mr. W began his presentation by stating, "This case is really a tough nut to crack. I'll start with the progress report and say that there is none, because I can't seem to get past all the complaining this patient does!" He then went on to discuss his evaluation and treatment plan in depth. It became obvious to the other members of the staff that Mr. W saw his patient as a woman who was not living up to her roles and responsibilities. He defended Ms. R's husband even though the husband had refused to come to the sessions with his wife. When the psychiatrist asked about the possibility of a medication evaluation for Ms. R, the nurse replied, "Everyone gets headaches. I don't think we should reward or reinforce this woman's complaints."

In reviewing this case, the staff noted that Mr. W appeared to have problems relating empathically to his patient because of her particular set of problems and some of his own values and perceptions. Mr. W agreed with this and said he had thought of asking someone else to work with Ms. R. Mr. W's supervisor observed that the nurse had problems with this type of patient in the past, and a more constructive approach would be to increase his supervision on this case, focusing on the dynamics between the patient and nurse that were blocking learning and growth for both of them. Mr. W and his supervisor then set a time when they could begin to meet with this purpose in mind.

his coping mechanism or attempt to strip him of it. Rather, she should attempt to protect his defenses. The coping mechanism or symptom is attempting to deal with an unconscious conflict. The patient does not understand why the symptom has developed or what he is gaining from it. He only knows that the symptom relieves some of the intolerable anxiety and tension. If he is unable to release this anxiety, his tension mounts to the panic level and he could lose control. It is also important to remember that the severely anxious patient has not worked through his area of conflict. He therefore has no alternatives or substitutes for his present coping mechanisms.

This principle also applies to severe levels of anxiety, such as obsessive-compulsive reactions and phobias. The nurse should not initially interfere with the repetitive act or force the patient to confront the phobic object. She should not ridicule the nature of his defense. Also, she should not attempt to argue with him about it or reason him out of it. He needs this coping mechanism to keep his anxiety within tolerable limits. The nurse must not reinforce the phobia, ritual, or physical complaint by focusing attention on it and talking about it a great deal. With time, however, the nurse can place some limits on the patient's behavior and attempt to help him find satisfaction with other aspects of life.

■ **MODIFYING THE ENVIRONMENT.** If the patient is hospitalized, the nurse can consult with other members of the health team to identify anxiety-producing situations for the patient and attempt to reduce them. She can set limits by assuming a quiet, calm manner and decreasing environmental stimulation. Limiting the patient's interaction with other patients will minimize the contagious aspects of anxiety. Supportive physical measures such as warm baths, massages, or whirlpool baths may also be helpful in decreasing a patient's anxiety.

■ **ENCOURAGING ACTIVITY.** The nurse should also encourage the patient's interest in activity outside himself. This limits the time he has available for his destructive coping mechanisms and increases his participation in and enjoyment of other aspects of life. Within the hospital setting he may become engaged in simple games, concrete tasks, or occupational or art therapy. The nurse can share some of these activities with him to provide him with support and reinforce socially productive behavior. She might also schedule vigorous physical activities for him, such as walking, a sport, or an active hobby. This form of physical exercise helps to relieve anxiety because it provides an emotional release or discharge and directs the patient's attention outward. In one study, participation in a jog-

ging program resulted in the reduction of anxiety for chronically distressed community clients. These gains were maintained 15 months after the completion of the study.[14]

Similar interventions can be implemented with the severely anxious patient who is not hospitalized. The nurse and patient can plan a daily schedule of activities that he can carry out in the community. Family members may be involved in the planning, since they can be very supportive in setting limits and stimulating outside activity.

Some nursing interventions can be detrimental and increase anxiety in severely anxious patients. These include pressuring the patient to change prematurely, being judgmental and verbally disapproving of the patient's behaviors, and asking the patient a direct question that places him on the defensive. Focusing in a critical way on the patient's anxious feelings with other patients present, lacking awareness of one's own be-

TABLE 11-6

ANTIANXIETY DRUGS

Chemical class generic name (Trade name)	Usual dosage range (mg/day)
Antianxiety drugs	
Benzodiazepines	
alprazolam (Xanax)	0.5–4
chlordiazepoxide (Librium)	20–100
chlorazepate (Tranxene)	7.5–60
clonazepam (Klonopin)	1.5–2.0
diazepam (Valium)	10–0
halazepam (Paxipam)	80–60
lorazepam (Ativan)	2–6
oxazepam (Serax)	15–90
prazepam (Centrax)	10–60
Antihistamines	50
diphenhydramine (Benadryl)	
hydroxyzine (Atarax)	100–300
Beta-adrenergic blocker	10–40
propranolol (Inderal)	
Anxiolytic	10–40
buspirone (Buspar)	
Tricyclic antidepressant drugs	
chlomipramine (Anafranil)	50–200

haviors and feelings, and withdrawing from the patient can also be detrimental to the anxious patient.

■ **INTERVENING WITH MEDICATION.** Nursing intervention may include the administration of antianxiety medications to the highly anxious patient (Table 11-6). Because anxiety is a pervasive problem, large portions of the population take these drugs. Americans are now spending more than $500 million each year for drugs to relieve anxiety. Among these drugs, the benzodiazepines are the medication of choice in the management of anxiety and are the most widely prescribed drugs in the world. They have almost replaced the barbiturates in the treatment of anxiety because of their effectiveness and wide margin of safety. Use of these drugs in combination with alcohol, however, may result in a serious or even fatal sedative reaction. Antipsychotic drugs are frequently prescribed for those patients experiencing a panic level of anxiety of psychotic proportions.

Although some patients may need to take antianxiety drugs for extended periods these drugs should always be used in conjunction with nonpharmacological treatments. Potential dangers of these drugs include withdrawal syndrome side effects and addiction. It should be emphasized that psychopharmacology is not a substitute for an ongoing therapeutic relationship. When used together, psychopharmacology can enhance the therapeutic relationship. Chemical control of painful symptoms allows the patient to direct his attention to the conflicts underlying his anxiety. More detailed information on antianxiety and antipsychotic medications is presented in Chapter 23.

Table 11-7 summarizes the principles, rationale, and nursing interventions in severe and panic levels of anxiety.

■ Intervening in a moderate level of anxiety

The nursing interventions previously mentioned are supportive and directed toward the general short-term goal of reducing severe or panic-level anxiety. When the patient's anxiety is reduced to a moderate level, the nurse can begin helping him with problem-solving efforts to cope with the stress. Long-term goals focus on helping the patient understand the cause of his anxiety and learn new ways of controlling it.

Education is an important aspect of promoting the patient's adaptive responses to anxiety. The nurse can identify relevant health teaching needs of each patient and then formulate an individualized teaching plan to meet those needs. The plan should be designed to increase the patient's knowledge of his own predisposing and precipitating stressors, coping resources, and adaptive and maladaptive responses. Alternative coping strategies can be identified and explored. Health teaching should also address the beneficial aspects of mild levels of anxiety in motivating learning and producing growth and creativity.

The specific nursing interventions for a moderate level of anxiety were originally described by Peplau[19] and Burd[4] and reflect the problem-solving process. Short-term goals may be written for each step of this process. Goals include recognition of anxiety, insight into the anxiety, and coping with the threat. These interventions can be implemented in any setting—psychiatric, community, or general hospital.

■ **RECOGNITION OF ANXIETY.** After analyzing the patient's behaviors and determining his level of anxiety, the nurse helps the patient to recognize he is anxious. She helps him explore his underlying feelings with such questions as "Are you feeling anxious now?" or "Are you uncomfortable?" It is also helpful for the nurse to identify the patient's behavior and link it to the feeling of anxiety (e.g., "I noticed you smoked three cigarettes since we started talking about your sister. Are you feeling anxious?"). In this way the nurse acknowledges the patient's feeling, attempts to label it, encourages the patient to describe it further, and relates it to a specific behavioral pattern. She is also validating her inferences and assumptions with the patient.

The patient's goal, however, is often to avoid or negate his anxiety. He therefore might use any of the following resistive approaches described by Meares[16]:

1. **Screen symptoms.** In this case the patient focuses his attention on minor physical ailments. The purpose of these apparently unrelated complaints is to avoid acknowledging his anxiety and conflict areas.
2. **Superior status position.** The patient attempts to control the interview by questioning the nurse's abilities or asserting the superiority of his own knowledge or experiences. It is important that the nurse not respond emotionally to this approach. She should not accept the patient's challenge and compete with him, since such a conflict would only further avoid the issue of anxiety.
3. **Emotional seduction.** The patient attempts to manipulate the nurse and to elicit feelings of pity or sympathy.
4. **Superficiality.** The patient relates on a surface level and resists the nurse's attempts to explore underlying feelings or analyze issues.

TABLE 11-7

SUMMARY OF NURSING INTERVENTIONS IN SEVERE AND PANIC LEVELS OF ANXIETY
Goal—Support and protect the patient and reduce his anxiety to a moderate or mild level

Principle	Rationale	Nursing interventions
Establish an open, trusting relationship	Reduce the threat that the nurse poses to the highly anxious patient	Listen to the patient Encourage the patient's discussion of feelings Answer questions directly Offer unconditional acceptance Be available to the patient Respect his use of personal space
Become aware of and control nurse's own feelings	Anxiety is communicated interpersonally; reciprocal anxiety in the nurse can interfere with her therapeutic ability	Become open to one's own feelings Accept both positive and negative feelings, including the development of anxiety Explore the cause of one's feelings Use this understanding of one's feelings therapeutically
Reassure the patient of his safety and protect his defenses and coping mechanisms. Do not focus on or reinforce the presenting maladaptive behaviors	Severe and panic levels of anxiety can be reduced by initially allowing the patient to determine what stress he can handle If the patient is unable to release his anxiety, his tension may mount to the panic level and he may lose control. At this time, he has no alternatives for his present coping mechanisms	Initially accept and support, rather than attack, the patient's defenses Acknowledge the reality of the pain associated with the patient's present coping mechanisms. Do not focus on the phobia, ritual, or physical complaint itself Give feedback to the patient about his behavior, stressors, appraisal of stressors, and coping resources Reinforce the idea that one's physical health is related to one's emotional health and that this is an area which will need exploration in the future In time, begin to place limits on the patient's maladaptive behavior in a supportive way
Identify and attempt to reduce anxiety-provoking situations for the patient	The patient's behavior may be modified by altering his environment and his interaction with it	Assume a calm manner with the patient Decrease environmental stimulation Limit the patient's interaction with other patients to minimize the contagious aspects of anxiety Identify and modify anxiety-provoking situations for the patient Administer supportive physical measures, such as warm baths and massages
Encourage the patient's interest in activity outside himself	By encouraging outside activities, the nurse limits the time the patient has available for his destructive coping mechanisms, while increasing his participation in and enjoyment of other aspects of life	Initially share an activity with the patient to provide support and reinforce socially productive behavior Provide for physical exercise of some type Plan a schedule or list of activities that can be carried out daily Involve family members and other support systems as much as possible
Promote the patient's physical health and well-being	The effect of a therapeutic relationship may be enhanced if the chemical control of symptoms allows the patient to direct his attention to underlying conflicts	Administer medications that help reduce the patient's discomfort Observe for medication side effects and initiate relevant health teaching

5. **Circumlocution.** The patient gives the pretense of answering questions, but he succeeds instead in talking around the topic and actually avoiding it.

6. **Amnesia.** This is a type of purposeful "forgetting" of a certain incident or event to avoid confronting and exploring it with the nurse.

7. **Denial.** The patient may use this approach only when discussing significant issues with the nurse or may generalize his denial to all others, including himself. His purpose is often to avoid humiliation.

8. **Intellectualization.** The patient who uses this technique usually has some knowledge of psychology or medicine. He is able to express appropriate insights and analysis yet lacks personal involvement in the problem he describes. He is not actually participating in the problem-solving process.

9. **Hostility.** The patient believes that offense is the best defense. He therefore relates to others in an aggressive, defiant manner. The greatest danger in this situation is that the nurse will take his behavior personally and respond with anger. This serves to reinforce the patient's avoidance of exploring his anxiety.

10. **Withdrawal.** The patient may resist the nurse by replying in vague, diffuse, indefinite, and remote ways.

All these resistive approaches may create feelings of frustration, irritation, or reciprocal anxiety in the nurse. She must recognize her own feelings and identify the patient's behavior pattern that might be causing them (see Clinical example 11-2).

In attempting to deal with these patient defenses and intervene successfully, the importance of a trusting relationship becomes evident. If the nurse establishes herself as a warm responsive listener, gives the patient adequate time to respond, and is supportive of his self-expressions, she will become less threatening to him. In helping him recognize his anxiety, the nurse should use open questions that move from nonthreatening topics to central issues of conflict. It may be helpful to vary the amount of anxiety to enhance the patient's motivation. In time, supportive confrontation may be used with the patient to address his repeated use of a particular resistive pattern. If, however, the patient's level of anxiety begins to rise rapidly, the nurse might choose to refocus the discussion to another topic.

■ **INSIGHT INTO THE ANXIETY.** Once the patient is able to recognize his anxiety, subsequent nursing interventions strive to expand the present context

CLINICAL EXAMPLE 11-2

Mr. T was a 28-year-old male who was transferred from the neurological unit to the psychiatric unit, where Ms. P was assigned to be his primary nurse. Ms. P was 24 years old and had been working on the unit for 3 years. In completing her nursing assessment of Mr. T, the nurse noted that he was experiencing a paralysis of his legs, which began gradually approximately 4 weeks previously. All neurological tests were negative, and he was transferred to the psychiatric unit for evaluation and treatment. He was an only child, unmarried, and had been living at home with his parents. He had completed college and was employed in the postal service. He had been dating one girl for 2 years and had recently proposed to her. She had told him that she was not ready to get married yet but she did want to continue seeing him. Mr. T had a small group of close friends, males and females, and they visited him often in the hospital, as did his family.

Ms. P had established a good relationship with her patient and spent much time with him. She found his friends to be kind and jovial and noted that one of Mr. T's strengths was his sense of humor and "ready smile." She observed, however, that his girlfriend never visited with him alone. Mr. T, meanwhile, had many cards, gifts, and visitors and appeared to be most appreciative of everything done for him.

A physical therapist came to work with Mr. T regularly, and this was a very difficult time of the day for him. While watching them work together one day, Ms. P remarked how impersonal and brusque the physical therapist was in relating to her patient. In discussing this observation in nursing rounds the next day, Ms. P began to realize that some of her actions were being influenced by her feelings of sympathy and pity for the patient and by the blame she had been unconsciously projecting onto his girlfriend. She wondered if his joviality, agreeable nature, and professed signs of gratitude were not indications of his manipulation of her and emotional seduction of her feelings toward him. The more she thought about this possibility, the more likely it seemed. At the end of the nursing rounds that morning, she requested that she be able to present his case in the staff treatment meeting the next day. Other staff were also feeling frustrated in their care for him and agreed that the conference would be most valuable.

of the patient. The patient may be asked to describe the situations and interactions that immediately precede the increase in anxiety. Together the nurse and patient make inferences about the precipitating causes or biopsychosocial stressors.

The nurse then helps the patient see which of his values are being threatened. It is possible to link the threat with underlying causes and to analyze how the conflict developed. To do this, the patient's present experiences are related to his past ones. The depth of this analysis depends on the nurse's educational and professional experiences. It is also important to explore how the patient reduced anxiety in the past. How did he handle anxiety, and what kinds of actions produced relief?

■ **COPING WITH THE THREAT.** If previous coping responses have been adaptive and constructive, the patient should be encouraged to use them. If not, the nurse can point out their maladaptive or destructive effects. She can point out to the patient that his present way of life appears unsatisfactory and distressing to him and that he does not attempt to improve the situation. The patient needs to assume responsibility for his own actions and realize that he has placed limitations on himself. He must not blame other people. In this phase of intervention the nurse assumes an active role as she interprets, analyzes, confronts, and correlates cause and effect relationships. She should proceed clearly so that the patient can follow while maintaining his anxiety within appropriate limits. If his anxiety becomes too severe, she may change topics temporarily.

The nurse can help the patient in his problem-solving efforts in various ways. One way of helping the patient cope is to reevaluate the nature of the threat or stressor. Is it as bad as the patient perceives it? Is his cognitive appraisal realistic? Together they might discuss his fears and feelings of inadequacy and analyze his projective identification. Does he fear others are as critical, perfectionistic, and rejecting of him as he is of others? Is his conflict based in reality, or is it the result of unvalidated, isolated, and perhaps distorted thinking? By sharing his fears with family members, peers, and staff, the patient frequently sees his own misperceptions. With their support he can validate his ideas, values, and goals.

Another approach is to help the patient modify his behavior and learn new ways of coping with stress. He may decide to restructure his goals or develop different values based on feedback from those around him, or he might consider alternatives to mastering the situation. The nurse may act as a role model in this regard or engage the patient in role playing. This can decrease his anxiety about new responses to problem situations.

One nursing function therefore is to teach the patient how aspects of mild anxiety can be constructive and growth producing. Physical activity should be encouraged as a way to discharge anxiety. Interpersonal resources such as family members or close friends should be incorporated into the nursing plan of care to provide the patient with support.

Frequently the cause for anxiety arises from an interpersonal conflict. In this case, it is much more constructive to include the persons involved when analyzing the situation with the patient. This helps to open communication between them. In this way cause and effect relationships are more open to examination. Coping patterns can be examined in light of their effect on others, as well as on the patient.

Working through this problem-solving or reeducative process with the patient will take time. He has to accept it both intellectually and emotionally. Breaking previous behavioral patterns can be difficult. Throughout the implementation phase the nurse needs to be patient and consistent in her approach and continually reappraise her own anxiety.

■ **PROMOTE THE RELAXATION RESPONSE.** In addition to problem-solving, one can also cope with stress by regulating the emotional distress associated with it. Long-term goals directed toward helping the patient regulate emotional distress are supportive or palliative. Distress can be regulated in maladaptive ways such as taking drugs, denying the facts, or withdrawing. Only the adaptive responses, however, are described in this chapter. These include the relaxation techniques of systematic desensitization, meditation, and biofeedback. All human beings have a natural and protective mechanism against "overstress," which Benson calls the "relaxation response."[3] This response produces a decreased heart rate, lower metabolism, and decreased respiratory rate. Relaxation, therefore, is the ultimate stress management technique. The relaxation response is the physiological opposite of the fight or flight, or anxiety, response.

Relaxation techniques are useful nursing interventions when the patient's level of stress interferes with his ability to function and be productive. They have long been used in helping women deal with childbirth. Relaxation techniques are being used in new ways with all kinds of people in various stress situations. These include helping patients handle pain; overcome test anxiety; sleep better; and overcome side-effects related to chemotherapy, surgery, or myocardial infarctions. Relaxation techniques are also being used to help patients handle various medical, nursing, and dental procedures; monitor the emotional triggers associated with chronic illnesses, such as asthma, muscle tension, ulcers, hypertension, tension headaches, or colitis; and deal with anger more constructively.

Relaxation can be taught individually, in small groups, or even in larger group settings. A mental health education plan for teaching the relaxation response is presented in Table 11-8. It is within the scope of nursing practice, requires no special equipment, and does not need a physician's supervision. As a group of interventions, relaxation can be implemented in various settings. A major benefit for the patient is that after several training sessions, he can practice the techniques on his own. This puts the control in the patient's hands and increases his self-reliance.

In 1929, relaxation training was originated by physiologist Edmunt Jacobson.[10] He developed a method of combating tension and anxiety by instructing patients to tense and relax various muscle groups in the body systematically. The philosophy of the method was that it was physically impossible to be "nervous" in a part of the body that was completely relaxed. The aim of the training was not to eliminate stress, but rather for people to feel comfortable with

themselves and alert to their internal and external environment. Relaxation did not become popular in psychiatric circles until the late 1950s, when Wolpe[28] developed the procedure called "systematic desensitization." He produced research evidence demonstrating its effectiveness in treating phobic patients.

The various relaxation procedures are very similar. They all involve rhythmic breathing, reduced muscle tension, and an altered state of consciousness. Clinical experience suggests there are individual differences in people's experiences of relaxation. Not everyone will demonstrate all characteristics of a relaxed psychophysiologic state. The physiological, cognitive, and behavioral manifestations of relaxation are presented in Table 11-9.

All these relaxation techniques require a thorough assessment of oneself and one's patient. The nurse must learn how to relax herself because it is impossible for a tense person to teach another tense person to relax. The nurse should also remember that relaxation is a learned skill that develops over time. Trying "too hard" is a deterrent and can actually create tension. An

TABLE 11-8

MENTAL HEALTH EDUCATION PLAN—THE RELAXATION RESPONSE

Content	Instructional activities	Evaluation
Describe the characteristics and benefits of relaxation	Discuss physiological changes associated with relaxation and contrast these with the behaviors of anxiety	Patient identifies own responses to anxiety Patient describes elements of a relaxed state
Teach deep muscle relaxation through a sequence of tension-relaxation exercises	Engage the patient in the progressive procedure of tensing and relaxing voluntary muscles until his body as a whole is relaxed	Patient is able to tense and relax all muscle groups Patient identifies those muscles that become particularly tense for him
Discuss the relaxation procedure of meditation and its components	Describe the elements of meditation and assist the patient in using this technique	Patient selects a word or scene with pleasant connotations and engages in relaxed meditation
Assist in overcoming anxiety-provoking situations through systematic desensitization	With patient, construct a hierarchy of anxiety-provoking situations or scenes Through imagination or reality, work through these scenes using relaxation techniques	Patient identifies and ranks anxiety-provoking situations Patient exposes himself to these situations while remaining in a relaxed state
Allow the rehearsing and practical use of relaxation in a safe environment	Role play stressful situations with the nurse or other patients	Patient becomes more comfortable with new behavior in a safe, supportive setting
Encourage patient to use relaxation techniques in life	Assign homework of using the relaxation response in everyday experiences Support success of patient	Patient uses relaxation response in life situations Patient is able to regulate anxiety response through use of relaxation techniques

TABLE 11-9

MANIFESTATIONS OF RELAXATION

Physiological	Cognitive	Behavioral
Decreased pulse	Altered state of consciousness, usually	Lack of attention to and concern for
Decreased blood pressure	alpha level	environmental stimuli
Decreased respirations	Heightened concentration on single	No verbal interaction
Decreased oxygen consumption	mental image	No voluntary change of position
Decreased metabolic rate	Receptivity to positive suggestion	Passive movement easy
Pupil constriction		
Peripheral vasodilation		
Increased peripheral temperature		

From DiMotto J: Am J Nurs 84:754, 1984.

open willingness to relax is most effective. A complete assessment of the patient should focus on where the patient experiences anxiety in his body. Relevant muscle groups should be identified and given emphasis in the relaxation interventions.

Systematic desensitization. The goal of systematic desensitization is to help the patient change his response to the threatening stimulus. To be successful, the person must have sufficient skills for coping with whatever he fears. For example, a person may be afraid of driving but can drive and is limited only by his fear. This is different from the person who fears heterosexual contacts and actually lacks the necessary social skills. Systematic desensitization involves combining deep muscle relaxation with imagining scenes of situations that cause anxiety. The assumption is that if the person is taught to relax while imagining such scenes, the real-life situation that the scene depicted will cause much less anxiety.

One of the important parts of systematic desensitization is deep muscle relaxation. As a therapeutic tool it is very effective and can be used alone to decrease tension and anxiety. It can also be combined with other types of interventions such as supportive or insight therapy. The basic premise is that muscle tension is related to anxiety. If tense muscles can be made to relax, anxiety will be reduced. The method used involves the tensing and relaxing of voluntary muscles in an orderly sequence until the body, as a whole, is helped.

Rimm and Masters[21] describe systematic desensitization. The patient should be seated open and unrestricted in a comfortable chair. Soft music or pleasant visual cues may be present. Before beginning the exercises, a brief explanation should be given that relates anxiety to muscle tension. The relaxation procedure should also be described. The patient should take a deep breath and exhale slowly. A sequence of tension-relaxation exercises is then initiated. The patient is instructed to tense each muscle group for about 10 seconds while the nurse describes how tense and uncomfortable this body part feels. He then is asked to relax this muscle group as the nurse comments, "Notice how all the hardness and tension is draining from your hands. Now notice how they feel warm, soft, and calm. Compare this feeling to when they were tense and see how much better they feel now." The patient should be reminded to tense only the muscle group named.

The patient then proceeds to the next muscle group in the following sequence.

1. **Hands.** First the fists are tensed and relaxed. Then the fingers are extended and relaxed.
2. **Biceps and triceps.** These are tensed and relaxed.
3. **Shoulders.** They are pulled back and relaxed and then pushed forward and relaxed.
4. **Neck.** The head is turned slowly as far to the right as possible and relaxed, then turned to the left and relaxed. It is then brought forward until the chin touches the chest and relaxed.
5. **Mouth.** The mouth is opened as wide as possible and relaxed. The lips form a pout and then relax. The tongue is extended out as far as possible and relaxed, then retracted into the throat and relaxed. It is pressed hard into the

roof of the mouth and relaxed, then pressed hard into the floor of the mouth and relaxed.

6. **Eyes.** They are opened as wide as possible and relaxed, then closed as hard as possible and relaxed.
7. **Breathing.** The patient inhales as deeply as possible and relaxes. He then exhales as much as possible and relaxes.
8. **Back.** The trunk of the body is pushed forward so the entire back is arched, then relaxed.
9. **Midsection.** The buttock muscles are tensed and relaxed.
10. **Thighs.** The legs are extended and raised about 6 inches off the floor and then relaxed. The backs of the feet are pressed into the floor and relaxed.
11. **Stomach.** It is pulled in as much as possible and relaxed, then extended and relaxed.
12. **Calves and feet.** With legs supported, the feet are bent with the toes pointing toward the head and then relaxed. Feet are then bent in the opposite direction and relaxed.
13. **Toes.** The toes are pressed into the bottom of the shoes and relaxed. They are then bent to touch the top inside of the shoes and relaxed.

The final exercise asks the patient to become *completely* relaxed, beginning with his toes and moving up through his body to his eyes and forehead. When the patient learns the procedure, he can employ the exercises only on the muscles that usually become tense. This is individual for each person and may include the shoulders, forehead, back, or neck. He may also eliminate the tensing exercises and perform only the relaxation ones.

Systematic relaxation may be followed or replaced by another approach to evoke the relaxation response *meditation.* The basic components for meditation include the following[3]:

1. A quiet environment
2. A passive attitude
3. A comfortable position
4. A word or scene to focus on

The first three components are necessary for any relaxation procedure. The fourth component refers to the process in which the patient selects a cue word or scene with pleasant connotations. He is then instructed to close his eyes, relax each of the major muscle groups, and then begin repeating the word silently to himself each time he exhales.

Another method of tension reduction is the use of *biofeedback.* During a biofeedback training session small electrodes connected to the biofeedback equipment are attached to the patient's forehead. The patient is then instructed to concentrate on relaxing. This will reduce the pitch of the biofeedback tone created by his tension. The higher the pitch, the greater is the muscle tension. Once he has developed the ability to relax, the patient is encouraged to apply the technique in stressful situations.

If systematic desensitization is employed, the patient must be able to relax his muscles. Additional steps are then undertaken. A hierarchy, or graded series, of feared situations or scenes is identified. They must be realistic, concrete situations created by the patient. They are then ranked from 1 to 10, with 1 evoking little or no anxiety and 10 evoking intense or severe anxiety. These feared situations may then be worked with either through imagination (in vitro) or in reality (in vivo). In vivo exposure is widely considered to be the treatment of choice for simple and social phobias, as well as obsessive-compulsive disorders.

For example, with in vitro exposure the patient is asked to imagine the scenes and use his ability to relax. He begins with the first anxiety-provoking scene. If he experiences no anxiety, he continues on to the next scene. If he experiences anxiety, he stops and restores himself to the state of relaxation. This procedure is repeated until the hierarchy is completed. This method appears to be successful because it indirectly encourages patients to expose themselves to objects or situations that are actually feared. It is most effective in the treatment of phobias.

Additional steps may also be taken. The patient may role play the stressful situation with the nurse or other patients. While role playing, he is asked to identify the location and level of his anxiety and practice relaxing it away. The patient can practice relaxing at home, as well as when he is approaching feared situations. These exercises teach the practical use of relaxation and allow the patient to rehearse them with some safety. Ideally, he will learn to recognize when and how his body responds to stress and will initiate relaxation exercises accordingly. The final step is to control one's response when actually coping with the stressor and to maintain these new relaxation skills. This will require nursing care feedback and follow-up and perhaps the development of personalized stress management programs for the patient.

As with any other nursing intervention, problems can arise in the teaching, learning, and practicing of these relaxation techniques. If a little is good, it should not be assumed that a lot is even better. It has been observed that when the relaxation response was elic-

TABLE 11-10

COMMON PROBLEMS AND SOLUTIONS ASSOCIATED WITH RELAXATION TRAINING

Problem	Solution	Problem	Solution
Muscle cramps	Ask the patient to generate less tension in these areas for shorter periods and to tense and relax the muscles more slowly. If cramps do occur, let the patient manipulate the cramped muscle, wait a few minutes, and then continue.	Inability to relax certain muscle groups	Work with the patient to evaluate the technique and develop an alternate tensing strategy.
Movement, such as stretching, yawning, or shifting position	Sometimes this helps the patient assume a more relaxed position and should be encouraged. If it is disruptive, review the specific relaxation technique being used and evaluate its effectiveness.	Strange or unfamiliar feelings, such as floating or lack of body perception	This is a common occurrence if relaxation techniques are new to the patient. Convey this to him and ask him to open his eyes and look around to become oriented. Encourage the patient to respond to relaxation as an enjoyable, rather than fearful, experience.
Laughter or talking	Initially this may indicate embarrassment or nervousness over a new situation. Since doing the facial exercises may create "funny-looking" expressions, it may be helpful for the nurse to do them with the patient.	Sense of "losing control"	Sometimes these exercises focus directly on issues of control that may be problematic in themselves for the patient. If so, spend more time discussing his subjective experience, introduce the exercises more gradually, and spend more time ensuring that the positive expectancies established earlier are fulfilled.
Noise	Initially a quiet room is best, which minimizes the disruptions associated with phones ringing, clocks ticking, and doors slamming. Gradually, the patient should be helped to relax with some background noise, since the everyday world is filled with sounds.	Sense of "internal arousal" or inside tension despite external relaxation	Explain to the patient that these exercises effect voluntary muscle control, whereas internal tension results from involuntary muscles as well. However, voluntary and involuntary control are interrelated; with practice, the patient should feel decreased internal tension.
Intrusive thoughts	If intrusive thoughts result in anxiety or discomfort for the patient, the nurse can either increase dialogue or help the patient select a new group of thoughts or images. If the intrusive thoughts involve sexual arousal, the nurse can note that this is not unusual and continue to focus on other images.	Failure to follow instructions	Identify and analyze the underlying cause. Has the patient forgotten or misunderstood the directions, or is he trying to control the nurse and therapy situation?
Sleep	This is *not* a desired outcome; the nurse should be careful not to use the word sleep, but rather "relaxed but very awake." The patient can also be asked to focus on the sound of her voice	Problems with practicing	Assist the patient in arranging his work and home schedules to allow for two 20-minute sessions per day. If a problem continues, the patient's lack of cooperation and resistance should be discussed
Coughing and sneezing	This is usually only a problem with heavy smokers. In this case the nurse should not encourage very deep breaths because they might cause the smoker to cough	Words and phrases to avoid	Assess the patient before and during the exercises for phrases that appear to be annoying or tension producing for him. These should be avoided in the first few sessions

Adapted with permission from Bernstein D and Borkovec T: Progressive relaxation training, Champaign, Ill, 1973, Research Press.

TABLE 11-11

SUMMARY OF NURSING INTERVENTIONS IN A MODERATE LEVEL OF ANXIETY

Goal—Help the patient in his problem-solving efforts to cope with stress

Principle	Rationale	Nursing interventions
Establish and maintain a trusting relationship	Reduce the threat the nurse poses to the patient	Be a warm and responsive listener Give the patient adequate time to respond Be supportive of the patient's self-expressions
Become aware of and control the nurse's own feelings	Resistance by the patient may produce negative feelings in the nurse that can block future progress	Recognize own feelings Identify the patient's behavior pattern or resistive approach that might be causing them Explore the patient's behavior and the nurse's response to them with the patient to learn and grow from them
Help the patient recognize his anxiety	To adopt new coping responses, the patient first needs to be aware of his feelings and to overcome his conscious or unconscious denial and resistance	Help the patient to identify and describe his underlying feelings Link the patient's behavior with his feeling Validate all inferences and assumptions with the patient Use open questions to move from non-threatening topics to issues of conflict Vary the amount of anxiety to enhance the patient's motivation In time, supportive confrontation may be used judiciously
Expand the patient's insight into the development of his anxiety	Once the patient recognizes his feelings of anxiety, he needs to be helped to understand its development, including precipitating stressors, appraisal of the stressor, and resources available to him	Help the patient describe the situations and interactions that immediately precede his anxiety Review with the patient his appraisal of the stressor, which of his values are being threatened, and the way in which the conflict developed Relate his present experiences with relevant ones from the past
Help the patient learn new adaptive coping responses	New adaptive coping responses can be learned through analyzing coping mechanisms used in the past, reappraising the stressor, using available resources, and accepting responsibility for change	Explore how the patient reduced anxiety in the past and what kinds of actions produced relief Point out the maladaptive and destructive effects of present coping responses Encourage the patient to use adaptive coping responses effective in the past Focus responsibility for change on the patient Assume an active role with the patient, correlating cause and effect relationships while maintaining his anxiety within appropriate limits Assist the patient in reappraising the value, nature, and meaning of the stressor when appropriate Help the patient identify ways he can restructure goals, modify behavior, use resources, and test new coping responses Use role playing if appropriate Educate the patient in the growth-producing aspects of mild anxiety Encourage physical activity to discharge energy Include significant others as resources and social supports in helping the patient learn new coping responses Allow the patient time to implement new adaptive coping responses
Promote the relaxation response	One can also cope with stress by regulating the emotional distress that accompanies it through the use of stress management techniques	Use relaxation techniques to reduce the patient's level of stress Teach the patient relaxation exercises to increase his control and self-reliance

ited for two daily periods of 20 to 30 minutes, no adverse side effects resulted. However, when elicited more frequently, some patients might experience a "withdrawal from life" that can complicate or compound previous psychiatric problems. Furthermore, relaxation techniques should not be used to insulate oneself from the outside world. Mild levels of anxiety are growth producing, and the fight or flight response is often appropriate and essential for survival. Other common problems specific to relaxation training are summarized in Table 11-10. Table 11-11 summarizes the nursing interventions that help the moderately anxious patient in his problem-solving efforts to cope with stress.

🔼 Evaluation

Evaluation is an ongoing process engaged in by the nurse and patient that is part of each phase of the nursing process. Even before she begins to formulate the nursing diagnosis, the nurse should ask herself: "Did I critically observe my patient's physiological and psychomotor behaviors? Did I listen to his subjective description of his experience? Did I fail to see the relationships between his expressed hostility or guilt and his underlying anxiety? Did I assess his intellectual and social functioning?" After collecting the data, the nurse should analyze it. Was she able to identify the precipitating stressor for the patient? What was his perception of the threat? How was this influenced by his physical health, past experiences, and present feelings and needs? Did she correctly identify the patient's level of anxiety and try to validate it with him? Was she able to identify the patient's coping mechanisms and determine if they were constructive or destructive? The diagnosis should be stated clearly and precisely. It should include the patient's problematical behavior pattern and his level of anxiety.

Nursing goals should be mutually determined and should describe what the nurse wishes to accomplish within a designated time. Her plan of action explains how and why. When using the criteria of adequacy, effectiveness, appropriateness, efficiency, and flexibility in judging the nursing goals and actions, the following questions can be raised:

- Were the planning and implementation a mutual process as much as possible?
- Were my goals and actions adequate in number and sufficiently specific to minimize my patient's level of anxiety?
- Did I work through all the stages of the problem-solving process with my patient?

- Were his maladaptive responses reduced?
- Did he learn new adaptive coping responses?
- Was the care plan reasonable in terms of our mutual constraints of time, energy, and expense?
- Were my many inferences, such as anxiety level, stressors, and coping patterns, appropriately validated with the patient and other staff members?
- Was I accepting of the patient and did I critically monitor my own anxiety level throughout the relationship?
- Was I able to modify my interventions on the basis of the patient's changing needs and feelings?
- Did I include the patient in the evaluation process?

Answering these questions enables the nurse to review the total care she provided. Additional patient needs may become evident at this time. The nurse will also identify personal strengths and limitations in

DIRECTIONS FOR FUTURE RESEARCH

The following are some of the nursing research problems raised in Chapter 11 that merit further study by psychiatric nurses:

1. Empirical validation of the four levels of anxiety and their effects on the individual as described by Peplau
2. Exploration of the relationships between anger and anxiety and self-esteem and anxiety
3. Early life experiences that predispose the individual to high levels of anxiety later in life
4. Personality characteristics associated with use of the various types of coping mechanisms
5. The relationship between medical and nursing diagnoses associated with anxiety
6. The ability of psychiatric nurses to distinguish among anxiety, depression, and fear
7. Levels of anxiety of patients during the course of the nurse-patient relationship
8. The effectiveness of various types of supportive physical measures in decreasing a patient's anxiety
9. Effective nursing actions for dealing with the resistance of patients in recognizing anxiety and conflict areas
10. Evaluation of the short- and long-term effectiveness of relaxation techniques with different patient groups

working with the anxious patient. Plans may then be made for overcoming the areas of limitation and further improving the nursing care. Throughout this process the nurse supports the belief that the "clarification of anxiety makes possible expanded awareness and an expansion of the self, which means the achievement of emotional health."[15:150]

■ SUGGESTED CROSS-REFERENCES ■

The nursing model of health-illness phenomena, with a detailed discussion of precipitating stressors, appraisal of the stressors, and coping resources, is discussed in Chapter 3. Interventions related to preventive mental health nursing are discussed in Chapter 8. Crisis intervention is discussed in Chapter 9. Physical illness as a response to stress is discussed in Chapter 12. Nursing interventions in psychotic panic states are discussed in Chapters 13 and 16. Psychological responses to physical illness are discussed in Chapter 21. Antianxiety drugs are discussed in Chapter 23.

■ SUMMARY ■

1. Anxiety is defined as diffuse apprehension that is vague and associated with feelings of uncertainty and helplessness. It is an emotion without an object that is subjective and communicated interpersonally. The capacity to be anxious is necessary for survival. Four levels of anxiety were identified and described: mild, moderate, severe, and panic.

2. There are two major types of precipitating factors: threats to one's physical integrity and threats to one's self-system.

3. Data collection by the nurse should include both behavioral responses and coping mechanisms. Physiological responses associated with anxiety are predominantly sympathetic in nature and serve to activate body processes in a "fight or flight" reaction. Behavioral responses reflect increased activity and restlessness. Affective responses convey apprehension, and vague fears and may also include feelings of anger, boredom, depression, worthlessness, and helplessness. As anxiety increases, cognitive functioning is characterized by a decreased perceptual field, poor concentration, and errors in judgment.

4. The individual uses various coping mechanisms to deny or allay his anxiety.

　　a. **Task-oriented reactions are conscious attempts to meet realistically the demands of the stress situation. They are action-oriented responses and include** *attack, withdrawal,* **and** *compromise.*

　　b. Ego-oriented reactions, or *defense mechanisms,* serve as one's first line of psychic defense, since they protect the person from feelings of inadequacy and anxiety.

5. The position of anxiety within the larger perspective of the model of health-illness phenomena is described. Constructive coping mechanisms lead to adaptive responses, whereas destructive coping mechanisms lead to maladaptive responses and can be expressed as either neurotic or psychotic health problems.

6. Nursing and medical diagnoses of anxiety are related. The overall goal of the nursing intervention is to help the patient develop the capacity to tolerate mild anxiety and use it consciously and constructively.

7. The highest-priority nursing goals should address lowering the patient's severe or panic levels of anxiety. Related nursing interventions should be supportive and protective. The development of a therapeutic relationship in which the nurse critically monitors her own anxiety level is necessary. The patient's needs are met through the protection of his defenses and providing for the discharge of anxiety through physical activity. Supportive medications may also be administered.

8. When the patient's anxiety is reduced to the mild or moderate level, insight-oriented or reeducative nursing interventions may be implemented. This involves the patient in a problem-solving process that includes the following steps: recognition of anxiety, insight into the anxiety, and coping with the threat. Nursing interventions that help the patient cope with stress by regulating the emotional distress associated with it include the relaxation techniques of systematic desensitization, meditation, and the use of biofeedback.

■ REFERENCES ■

1. Akiskal H: Anxiety: definition, relationship to depression, and proposal for an integrative model. In Tuma A and Maser J, editors: Anxiety and the anxiety disorders, Hillsdale, NJ, 1985, Lawrence Erlbaum Associates Publishers.
2. American Psychiatric Association: Diagnostic and Statistical Manual of Mental Disorder, Third Edition-Revised, Washington, D.C., 1987, The Association.
3. Benson H: The relaxation response, New York, 1975, William Morrow & Co, Inc.
4. Burd S: Effects of nursing intervention in anxiety of patients. In Burd SF and Marshall MA, editors: Some clinical approaches to psychiatric nursing, New York, 1963, Macmillan, Inc.
5. Dollard J and Miller N: Personality and psychotherapy, New York, 1950, McGraw-Hill Book Co.
6. Dzegede S, Pike S, and Hackworth J: The relationship between health-related stressful life events and anxiety: an analysis of a Florida metropolitan community, Community Ment Health J 17(4):294, 1981.
7. Elliott S: Denial as an effective mechanism to allay anxiety following a stressful event, J Psychiatr Nurs 18(10):11, 1980.
8. Freud S: Problem of anxiety, New York, 1936, WW Norton & Co, Inc.
9. Freud S: A general introduction to psychoanalysis, New York, 1969, Pocket Books.
10. Jacobson E: Progressive relaxation, ed 3, Chicago, 1974, University of Chicago Press.
11. Kristic J: Anxiety levels of hospitalized psychiatric pa-

tients throughout total hospitalization, J Psychiatr Nurs 17(7):33, 1979.

12. Lagina S: A computer program to diagnose anxiety level, Nurs Res 20:491, 1971.

13. Lassen C: The effect of proximity in the psychiatric interview, J Abnorm Psychol 82:226, 1973.

14. Long B: Stress-management interventions: a 15-month follow-up of aerobic conditioning and stress innoculation training, Cognitive Ther Res 9(4):471, 1985.

15. May R: The meaning of anxiety, New York, 1950, Ronald Press Co.

16. Meares A: The management of the anxious patient, Philadelphia, 1963, WB Saunders Co.

17. Menninger K, Maymann M, and Rugyser P: The vital balance, New York, 1963, The Viking Press.

18. Oden G: Individual panic: elements and patterns. In Burd S and Marshall M, editors: Some clinical approaches to psychiatric nursing, New York, 1963, Macmillan, Inc.

19. Peplau H: Interpersonal techniques: the crux of psychiatric nursing, Am J Nurs 62:53, 1962.

20. Peplau H: A working definition of anxiety. In Burd S and Marshall M, editors: Some clinical approaches to psychiatric nursing, New York, 1963, Macmillan, Inc.

21. Rimm D and Masters J: Behavior therapy, New York, 2nd ed, 1979, Academic Press, Inc.

22. Robins L et al: Lifetime prevalence of specific psychiatric disorders in three sites, Arch Gen Psych 41:949, 1984.

23. Shand J and Grau B: Perceived self and ideal self ratings in relation to high and low levels of anxiety in college women, J Psychol 87:55, 1977.

24. Sullivan HS: The interpersonal theory of psychiatry, New York, 1953, WW Norton & Co, Inc.

25. Tillich P: The courage to be, New Haven, Conn, 1952, Yale University Press.

26. Weissman M: The epidemiology of anxiety disorders: rates, risks and familial patterns. In Tuma A and Maser J, editors: Anxiety and the anxiety disorders, Hillsdale, NJ, 1985, Lawrence Erlbaum Associates Publishers.

27. Will O: Psychotherapy in reference to the schizophrenic reaction. In Stein M, editor: Contemporary psychotherapies, New York, 1961, The Free Press of Glencoe.

28. Wolpe J: The practice of behavior therapy, New York, 1973, Pergamon Press, Inc.

■ ANNOTATED SUGGESTED READINGS ■

Barlow D: The anxiety disorders: the nature and treatment of anxiety and panic, New York, 1988, Guilford Press.

Comprehensive overview of the medical diagnoses and treatment of the anxiety disorders written by an expert in the field.

*Bond M: Stress and self-awareness: a guide for nurses, Rockville, Md, 1986, Aspen Publishers.

Unique contribution is that it is written to help nurses manage their own stress and enhance their adaptive coping abilities. Good reading for all nurses.

*Burd S: Effects of nursing intervention in anxiety of patients. In Burd SF and Marshall MA, editors: Some clinical approaches to psychiatric nursing, New York, 1963, Macmillan, Inc.

Follows approach outlined by Peplau. Uses the problem-solving and learning process to develop a framework for intervening with anxious patients; reports the results of a small study conducted to examine the framework. Describes principles as well as techniques.

*Davis J: Treatment of a medical phobia including desensitization administered by a significant other, J Psychosoc Nurs Ment Health Serv 20(8):6, 1982.

Account of a young woman's fear of physicians and medical treatments and how it was helped through teaching her boyfriend systematic desensitization techniques.

*Dossey B et al: Holistic nursing: a handbook for practice, Rockville, MD, 1988, Aspen Publishers.

Describes the holistic and healing traditions within nursing with clear descriptions on the use of relaxation, imagery, and music therapy with patients. Recommended to all nurses.

*Garrison J and Scott P: A group self-care approach to stress management, J Psychiatr Nurs 17(6):9, 1979.

Describes a procedure for teaching patients relaxation as a coping skill. Clearly defines each of the three components of this group training, including progressive relaxation and clinical meditation.

*Hays D: Teaching a concept of anxiety, Nurs Res 10:108, 1961.

Summarizes a small study on teaching patients about anxiety. Relates levels of anxiety, perceptual and behavioral changes, and learning tasks of the anxious person.

Jenike M et al, editors: Obsessive compulsive disorders: theory and management, St Louis, 1989, Mosby–Year Book, Inc.

Presents recent treatments for patients with obsessive-compulsive disorders. Researchers and clinicians describe various therapies, neurobiology, management issues, and related illnesses. Highly recommended.

*Jones P and Jakob D: Nursing diagnosis: differentiating fear and anxiety, Nurs Papers 3:20, 1981.

Describes a research project to collect data related to nurses differential diagnosis of fear and anxiety. Summarizes the literature and explores the implications for nursing care of patients experiencing either human coping response. Additional such studies are needed to define further and validate accepted nursing diagnoses.

*Karl G: Survival skills for psychic trauma, J Psychosoc Nurs 27(4):15, 1989.

Explores general behavioral responses to severe and traumatic stress, including the protective processes of coping and adaptation.

*Laraia M: Biological correlates of panic disorder with agoraphobia: practice perspectives for nurses, Arch Psych Nurs. In press.

A concise, clear description of the latest biological theories

---

*Asterisk indicates nursing reference.

pertaining to anxiety disorders, with implications for nursing practice and research.

*Laraia M, Stuart G, and Best C: Behavioral treatment of panic-related disorders: a review, Arch Psych Nurs 3(3):125, 1989.

Behavioral theories and therapy techniques for panic-related disorders are reviewed. Reading for the advanced nurse. An excellent, inclusive article.

May R: The meaning of anxiety, New York, 1950, Ronald Press Co.

Brings together various theories of anxiety, synthesizes common elements of these theories, and suggests some constructive methods for dealing with anxiety. An excellent text and a classic in the field.

*Oden G: Individual panic: elements and patterns. In Burd SF and Marshall MA, editors: Some clinical approaches to psychiatric nursing, New York, 1963, Macmillan, Inc.

Explores the questions, "What is panic?" and "What happens during a panic episode?" Reviews the literature on both individual and group panic and presents the results of research related to the identification of the elements and patterns of individual panic. Describes seven case studies.

*Olson L: Intervention in a pathological cycle of anxiety, J Psychiatr Nurs 12:21, 1974.

Case presentation of a 13-year-old girl hospitalized with myasthenia gravis and experiencing high levels of anxiety. Describes the plan of care developed with the aid of a nursing consultant and includes problems, goals, and nursing approaches.

*Roncoli M: Bantering: a therapeutic strategy with obsessional patients, Perspect Psychiatr Care 12:171, 1974.

Explores the strategy of the therapist as a psychological humorist who assists the obsessional patient to gain insight through the use of bantering. Bantering is defined as ridiculing lightly and good naturedly. The purpose is to release the patient's aggression and anger and the therapist's feelings of exasperation.

Roy-Byrne P and Katon W: An update on treatment of the anxiety disorders, Hosp Community Psych 38(8):835, 1987.

Reviews developments since 1983 in the pharmacological, psychological, and behavioral treatments of the anxiety disorders as defined in the DSM-III-R. Excellent medical update.

*Sheer B: The effects of relaxation training on psychiatric inpatients, Issues Ment Health Nurs 2(4):1, 1980.

Attempts to determine if psychiatric inpatients who receive relaxation training as a part of their nursing care show a decrease between pretest and posttest scores on an anxiety scale. Although results do not support this hypothesis, worth reading for the research process described.

*Tilley S and Weighill V: How nurse therapists assess and contribute to the management of alcohol and sedative drug use among anxious patients, J Adv Nurs, 11:499, 1986.

Describes a nursing research study on patients with anxiety disorders and assessment of their substance use by nurse therapists. Implications for nursing education and practice are included.

Tillich P: The courage to be, New Haven, Conn, 1952, Yale University Press.

Addresses anxiety, its conquest, and the meaning of courage. Anxiety comes from the loss of the meaning of life, whereas the "courage to be" involves participation as well as individualization. A distinguished classic in the field.

White R and Gilliland R: Elements of psychopathology, New York, 1975, Grune & Stratton, Inc.

Collects all the basic information needed to understand the mechanisms of defense from a psychoanalytical viewpoint. Organizes each defense mechanism into general comments, definition, clinical examples, clinical syndromes that illustrate the mechanism, and examples of the use of the mechanisms in normal behavior. Valuable to the student and an excellent review for the clinician.

*Whitley G: Anxiety: defining the diagnosis, J Psychosoc Nurs 27(10):7, 1989.

Highly recommended. Reviews the body of knowledge about the nursing diagnosis of anxiety through nurse expert and clinical validation studies. Includes recommendations for future work in the area.

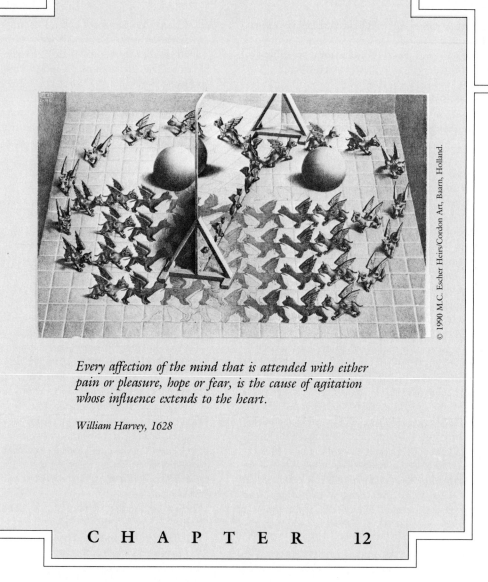

Every affection of the mind that is attended with either pain or pleasure, hope or fear, is the cause of agitation whose influence extends to the heart.

William Harvey, 1628

C H A P T E R   12

PSYCHOPHYSIOLOGICAL ILLNESS

DIAGNOSTIC PREVIEW

MEDICAL DIAGNOSES RELATED TO PSYCHOPHYSIOLOGICAL ILLNESS

- Somatization disorder
- Somatoform pain disorder
- Body dysmorphic disorder

- Conversion disorder
- Hypochondriasis
- Psychological factors affecting physical condition

LEARNING OBJECTIVES

After studying this chapter, the student should be able to:

- describe the stress response.

- discuss the relationship among intrapsychic conflict, anxiety, stress, and psychophysiological illness.

- discuss the predisposing factors that have been proposed for psychophysiological illnesses.

- analyze precipitating stressors that contribute to the development of psychophysiological illness.

- identify the physiological, psychological, and interpersonal behaviors associated with the development of psychophysiological illnesses.

- identify and describe coping mechanisms commonly used by persons with psychophysiological illnesses.

- analyze psychophysiological illness relative to the nursing model of health-illness phenomena.

- formulate individualized nursing diagnoses for patients with psychophysiological illnesses.

- assess the relationship between nursing diagnoses and the medical diagnoses of somatoform disorder and psychological factors affecting physical condition.

- develop long-term and short-term individualized nursing goals with patients experiencing psychophysiological illness.

- apply therapeutic nurse-patient relationship principles with an appropriate rationale in planning the care of a patient with a psychophysiological illness.

- describe nursing interventions appropriate to the needs of the patient experiencing a psychophysiological illness.

- develop a mental health education plan to assist a patient to develop more effective methods of coping with stress.

- assess the importance of the evaluation of the nursing process when working with patients who have a psychophysiological illness.

- identify directions for future nursing research.

- select appropriate readings for further study.

Continuum of psychophysiological responses

Throughout history, philosophers and scientists have debated the nature and extent of the relationship between the mind *(psyche)* and body *(soma)*. In ancient times, physical illness was thought to result from possession by evil spirits, possibly because of misbehavior by the victim. Shamans, witch doctors, and medicine men used potions and spells to drive out the evil. That these approaches continue to be used in some parts of the world shows that they do work in many cases. The cures resulting from these primitive methods have not been explained. However, it is possible that absolute belief in the power of the healer can cure a physical disorder, through some undefined mind-body interaction.

The Greek philosophers searched for the meaning of life, or *logos*. Plato pursued meaning through mathematics, and Aristotle focused his search on language. According to Lynch,[15] these various belief systems had a major effect on the development of medical theory. During the Renaissance, Descartes and Pascal continued the studies begun by Plato and Aristotle. Pascal believed the emotional side of the human experience to be most important. Descartes focused on the mathematical, or the rational. Descartes concluded that people differ from animals in their ability to think, which he related to the existence of the soul. However, physiological functioning of both people and animals was thought to be about the same and based on mechanical principles. The result of this widely accepted approach was to separate the thinking and feeling aspects of humans from the physical side. This attitude is still seen today, when physical disorders are treated with little or no thought given to the interaction of mind and body.

Barsky[4] cites the contribution of Freud in linking physical and mental processes. Freud's theory of psychosexual development describes developmental tasks related to specific areas of physical functioning. For instance, the meeting of oral needs for nurturance is related to the development of the capacity to trust. Freud also studied disorders that he labeled "conversions." These were physical illnesses that had no observable organic pathology. Freud demonstrated that psychoanalysis was an effective treatment for these patients. He concluded that the physical illness symbolized an intrapsychic conflict resulting from failure to successfully resolve conflicts associated with an earlier developmental stage. For example, a young woman whose legs became paralyzed the day after her engagement had not resolved issues related to the oedipal stage of development. She became paralyzed so she could not "walk down the aisle" and assume the sexual role of an adult woman.

Recently, there has been a renewed interest in studying the Aristotelian approach to human nature. Holistic health practices, based on the idea that mental processes influence physical well-being and vice versa, are becoming increasingly popular. Research is attempting to identify the links between thoughts, feelings, and body functioning. Great interest has arisen about the role of the endocrine and immune systems in the development of psychophysiological disorders. Some even believe that all illness has a psychophysiological component—that physical disorders have a psychological component and mental disorders a physical one.

Much of the current thinking about psychophysiological behavior is related to an increased understanding of the role of stress in human life. In 1929 Walter Cannon[7] published his landmark work, *Bodily Changes in Pain, Hunger, Fear and Rage*. Based on research on animal physiology, he described the "fight-or-flight" response. The physiological behaviors associated with this reaction to stress are described in Chapter 11 (see Table 11-1). In response to Cannon's research, other investigators began to study physical responses to a variety of stressors, including psychological ones. For instance, in 1951, Wolf and colleagues[22] reported their research on the connection between stress and hypertension. They found that emotional arousal did lead to elevations in blood pressure.

Stress theory was significantly advanced when Hans Selye[19] published *The Stress of Life* in 1956. Selye described the stress response in detail, creating a greater understanding of the effect of stressful experiences on physical functioning. He identified a three-stage process of response to stress that has overwhelmed localized adaptation. This generalized response is called the general adaptation syndrome (GAS). These levels of response are:

1. *The alarm reaction*. This is the immediate response to a stressor that has not been eliminated in a localized area. Adrenocortical response mechanisms occur, resulting in behaviors associated with the fight-or-flight response.
2. *Stage of resistance*. There is some resistance to the stressor. The body adapts and functions at a lower than optimal level. This requires a greater than usual expenditure of energy for survival.
3. *Stage of exhaustion*. The adaptive mechanisms become worn out and fail. The negative effect

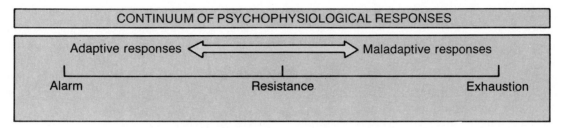

Fig. 12-1. Continuum of psychophysiological responses.

of the stressor spreads to the entire organism. If the stressor is not removed or counteracted, death will ultimately result.[19]

Selye's theory has aided investigators in psychophysiology as they attempt to identify more specific mental-physical interactions and interventions in stress responses.

Any experience believed by the individual to be stressful may cause a psychophysiological disorder. The stress does not have to be recognized consciously, and in fact, most often it is not. If the person does recognize that he is under stress, he is often unable to connect the cognitive understanding of feeling stress with the physical symptoms of the psychophysiological disorder. Fig. 12-1 illustrates the range of possible psychophysiological responses to stress, based on Selye's theory.

 Assessment

■ **Predisposing factors**

A number of biopsychosocial factors are believed to influence the individual's psychophysiological response to stress. Most of the specific relationships between physical and mental processes are still not well described. Thus it is important for the nurse to consider all possibilities when assessing factors that might predispose the patient to a particular disorder.

■ **BIOLOGICAL FACTORS.** It is thought by some that biological factors may predispose one to psychophysiological illness. Endocrine activity has been noted by Oken[17] to have an effect on the person's personality. However, although efforts have been made to link specific hormones and emotions, little success has been achieved. Genetic factors have also been considered.[4] It has been proposed that a biological tendency for particular psychophysiological responses could be inherited. Unanswered questions related to this theory include concerns about the specificity of the biological tendency. Alexander[1] believed that target organs were

related to specific stressors. He theorized that conflict was experienced as stress, and this resulted in transmission of nerve impulses to the associated organ. This theory has not been supported by research, but it does represent an early effort to establish a mind-body connection.

Recently research on the biological factors causing psychophysiological illness has been done. One focus has been on the new field of psychoneuroimmunology.[3] It has been demonstrated that the immune response can be modified by behavior modification techniques. Researchers are now investigating the possibility of modifying the immune response in the treatment of autoimmune illnesses such as rheumatoid arthritis, systemic lupus erythematosus, myasthenia gravis, and pernicious anemia. Other related research is exploring the relationship among the immune system, stress, and cancer. It has been suspected that high stress, especially if prolonged, can decrease the immune system's ability to destroy neoplastic growths. Unfortunately, this is an extremely difficult area in which to conduct research. There has not been enough time to conduct prospective studies of this hypothesis. Retrospective studies are compromised by the person's stress response to the diagnosis of cancer, which makes it impossible to measure preexisting stress levels accurately.

■ **PSYCHOLOGICAL FACTORS.** Clinical observation has led to the theory that there is a relationship between personality type and specific psychophysiological disorders. Probably the best known of these descriptions is the "type A" personality, identified by Friedman and Rosenman.[10] The type A person is more likely than others to develop stress-related cardiac symptoms. This person is described as tense, ambitious, impatient, achievement oriented, irritable, and aggressive. He tends to be successful in work but is frequently less successful interpersonally. Most type A's tend to be men. However, as women's roles change, more of them are beginning to fit this personality type. Initially, a type B was identified as the polar opposite of the type A. It has become apparent that to try to group all people into one of two personality types is impossible. Type B identification is seldom used.

Lynch[15] has described the personality characteristics often observed in people who have migraine headaches. They tend to be "meticulous, perfectionistic, conscientious, intelligent, neat, inflexible, rigid, resentful, guilt-ridden, and compulsive." In another study, migraine sufferers were described as "unguarded, anxiety-prone, depressive, lacking in interpersonal warmth, and somewhat alienated from peers."[6] Lynch also described the hypertensive person as being in conflict over the expression of hostile and aggressive feelings. The person also struggles with dependency needs, which are at odds with his need to achieve. Interpersonally, he fears exposure of these conflicts, so he represses them, leading to hypertension. As one reviews the adjectives used to describe the heart disease–prone person, the migraine sufferer, and the hypertensive person, the role of stress in the psychophysiological reaction again becomes clear. None of these people can be described as relaxed, calm, or secure.

Siegel[20] has developed a psychological profile of patients with cancer. This includes a lack of childhood closeness to parents; an extroverted personality that allows the person to seek validation from others; and loneliness and a feeling of inadequacy during adolescence. Siegel also describes the person with cancer as having an unrealistic view of himself. Whereas he may see himself as a person of many accomplishments, he fears that others will not like him if they know about his opinion of himself. Therefore he downgrades his real abilities and achievements. The patient, as a young adult, may establish relationships and appear to be well adjusted. However, if a loss occurs, his ability to cope is limited. The pain of the loss is hidden. Siegel refers to cancer as "the disease of nice people."

People with psychophysiological disorders resist admitting the role that emotions play in their illnesses. This led Sifneos[21] to coin the term *alexithymia,* which means "no words for feelings." These individuals can describe feelings and discuss them intellectually, but they do not experience them and therefore do not convey the affective experience. Interpersonally, they are perceived as being cold and aloof. It is not possible to empathize with them, because the emotional component is missing.

Some people show symptoms of physical illness but have no evidence of organic impairment. These disorders, which are termed "somatoform" by psychiatrists, are thought to be a response to an underlying psychological conflict. Psychoanalysts believe that the physical symptoms of a conversion reaction symbolize unacceptable impulses that have been repressed. For instance, a woman who becomes angry with her child experiences paralysis of her arm. This prevents her from acting on her rage, which she unconsciously believes to be murderous. The symptom protects her from feeling overwhelming anxiety. Another psychoanalytic approach focuses on a patient's dependency needs. In such a case, the person is not aware of his wish to be dependent and to recreate the mother-infant relationship. Physical illness is an acceptable expression of that need.

■ **SOCIAL FACTORS.** Lynch[15] has been investigating the effect of interpersonal interaction on various psychophysiological disorders, particularly hypertension and migraine headaches. He has discovered that most of his patients are out of touch with their bodies. They are unaware of the response of body functions to social interaction and resist admitting that they have interpersonal problems. When hypertensive persons are attached to a monitor, they are able to see their blood pressure rise when they are talking. It rises still more if they discuss stressful experiences. Observations such as this help individuals recognize the need for life-style changes to control their physical problems. Similarly, migraine patients are amazed to see the changes in skin temperature that take place as their peripheral blood vessels constrict in response to interpersonal interactions.

■ Precipitating stressors

Any experience that the individual interprets as stressful may lead to a psychophysiological response. Some of these are relatively mild and short-lived, related to the stimulation of the fight-or-flight reaction. Examples include diarrhea before an examination or a dry mouth when speaking before a large group of people. Sometimes the response is more serious and indicates a higher level of anxiety. For instance, a person might feel panicky and experience tachycardia when boarding an airplane. Because the psychophysiological disorder is an attempt to deal with anxiety, it is recommended that information on stressors related to anxiety (Chapter 11) be reviewed.

One type of stressor that has been shown to cause physical illness and even death is the loss of a significant interpersonal relationship. Siegel[20] has noted that "one of the most common precursors of cancer is a traumatic loss or a feeling of emptiness in one's life." An increased mortality rate has been found among recently widowed people. Similar observations have been made about people admitted to institutions such as nursing homes, who are separated from significant others. Children who have been separated from their mothers, especially if placed in an impersonal environment, also show a decline in physical health. The effect of a loss may cause both physical and psychological symptoms for an extended period of time. Moore, Gilliss, and Martinson[16] studied parents of children who had died from cancer. They observed an increased incidence of symptoms 2 years after the loss. Illnesses and deaths related to loss of a loved person seem to represent the exhaustion phase of the general adaptation syndrome.

Sometimes a psychophysiological problem is a response to an accumulation of rather small stressors. A patient may find it hard to identify one specific stressor that preceded his problem. Careful assessment may reveal a pattern of overwork and overcommitment or a series of seemingly minor events that all required extra effort. The use of a tool such as the Holmes and Rahe Social Readjustment Rating Scale described on page 73 may be helpful in assessing the impact of accumulated stressors. Most of the psychophysiological disorders come and go. This may be related to changes in the person's stress level. When the cumulative stress gets too high, the body "calls time out" by developing physical symptoms.

■ Behaviors

■ PSYCHOLOGICAL FACTORS AFFECTING PHYSICAL CONDITION. The primary behaviors observed with psychophysiological illnesses are the physical symptoms. These disruptions experienced by the patient lead him to seek health care. Psychological factors affecting the physical condition may involve any body part. The most common reactions involve the following:

Skin (allergic eczema, hives, and acne)
Respiratory system (asthma, sinusitis, and bronchial spasms)
Cardiovascular system (hypertension and migraine headaches)
Musculoskeletal system (backaches and muscle cramps)
Gastrointestinal system (colitis, gastritis, constipation, hyperacidity, duodenal ulcer, obesity, and anorexia)
Genitourinary system (menstrual disturbances, impotence, and vaginismus)

Some would add cancer to this list. The list changes from time to time because no specific psychological-biological connection has been scientifically established for any of them. All the above disorders are related to organic disease. It is suspected that most result from difficulties in coping with psychological stress.

The person is usually reluctant to believe that the problem is related to psychological factors. In part, this occurs because being physically ill is much more socially acceptable than being mentally ill. The problem is compounded because the patient really does have physical symptoms. Denial of the psychological component of the illness may lead to "doctor shop-

---

CLINICAL EXAMPLE 12-1

Mr. R was a successful 42-year-old executive who had risen quickly to the top of his company. He worked long hours and had difficulty delegating any of his responsibilities. He set high standards for his employees and was believed to be insensitive to human concerns. He viewed himself as "tough, but fair." However, he had little sympathy for a worker who requested extra time off for personal business.

Mr. R was married but saw little of his family. He expected his wife and children to do their part to maintain his standing in the community by associating with "the right people." He seldom interacted with his children except to reprimand them if they disturbed his concentration while he was working. His wife reported that their sexual relationship was unsatisfying to her. Mr. R used it for physical release for himself but was not concerned about meeting her needs. She suspected that he was involved in an extramarital affair but did not want to endanger the marriage by confronting him.

Mr. R was expecting to be named to the board of directors of a prestigious philanthropic foundation. He anticipated that this would add to his social prominence in the community. Shortly before the announcement was to be made, his 14-year-old son was arrested in a drug raid in a lower middle class part of town. Mr. R did not get the appointment. He was furious with his son but dealt with his anger by withdrawing still more. One day at work, he experienced an episode of dizziness, followed by a severe headache. He attributed it to tension, took some aspirin, and continued to work. However, after several similar episodes, he decided to consult his family doctor. The physician arrived at a diagnosis of essential hypertension. He tried to discuss work, family, and social behavior with Mr. R but was frustrated by superficial responses. Although concerned about Mr. R's condition and stress level, the doctor gave in to Mr. R's demand for medication to lower his blood pressure. He also advised Mr. R to exercise and to find a relaxing activity. However, he did not really expect him to comply with those suggestions.

ping." The patient searches for someone who will find an organic cause for the illness. Clinical example 12-1 illustrates this problem.

Mr. R is typical of many people with stress-related psychophysiological disorders. He is reluctant to admit to a lack of control over his mind and body. He expects a magical cure that will let him follow his usual life-style without interruption. He will probably stop taking his medication as soon as he feels better. Distance from the stressor will probably allow him to function for a while without noticeable symptoms of his hypertension. Sooner or later, however, new stressors will lead to another dizzy spell, headaches, or possibly myocardial infarction or cerebrovascular accident.

In his studies of hypertension, Lynch[15] found that people with psychophysiological problems are unable to share feelings with others. The person who is not aware of or comfortable with his own feelings has trouble communicating, because sharing of personal pain would result. Speech is used to hide rather than reveal. When that mechanism fails, the cardiovascular system goes out of control. Lynch describes this as the "loneliest loneliness."

Pines[18] has reported work done by Kobasa and Maddi to define "hardiness," a behavioral characteristic that seems to assist people to resist stress. Hardiness consists of three components. First, change is seen as a challenge rather than a threat. Second, a sense of commitment to people or a cause is present. Finally, hardy people have a sense of control over their lives. One study compared hardiness and frequency of illness in lawyers and businesspeople. Lawyers had the lower rate of illness episodes. Lawyers may be taught to expect stress and to function in a stressful environment. One can also speculate that a person who selects a law career is already someone who enjoys working under stress. On the other hand, businesspeople are influenced by mass media information that defines stress as harmful and to be avoided. This research seems to indicate that attitude toward stress influences the individual's response. A study conducted by Lambert et al.[14] indicated that hardiness and satisfaction with social supports lead to increased feelings of well-being in women with rheumatoid arthritis.

■ **SOMATOFORM DISORDERS.** Some people have physical symptoms without any organic impairment. These are termed *somatoform disorders.* They include somatization disorder, in which the person has many physical complaints; conversion disorder, in which a loss or alteration of physical functioning occurs; somatoform pain disorder, in which pain is the only symptom; hypochondriasis, the fear of or belief that one has an illness; and body dysmorphic disorder,

the concern by a person with a normal appearance that he has a physical defect. Clinical example 12-2 is a case history of a person with a medical diagnosis of somatization disorder.

Ms. O shows the dependent behavior that is often typical of people with somatization disorder. Her

---

CLINICAL EXAMPLE 12-2

Ms. O, a 28-year-old single woman, was admitted to the medical unit of a general hospital for a complete medical workup. When asked about her main problem during the nursing assessment, she replied, "I've never been very well. Even when I was a child I was sick a lot." Ms. O listed multiple complaints during the physical assessment. These included palpitations, dizzy spells, menstrual irregularity, painful menses, blurred vision, dysphagia, backache, pain in her knees and feet, and a variety of gastrointestinal symptoms including stomach pain, nausea, vomiting, diarrhea, flatulence, and intolerance to seafood, vegetables of the cabbage family, carbonated beverages, and eggs. Except for the food intolerances, none of the symptoms was constant. They occurred at random, making her fearful of going out of her home.

The psychosocial assessment revealed that Ms. O lived with her parents. She was the youngest of three children. Her siblings were living away from the parental home. She had graduated from high school but had poor grades because of her frequent absences. She had tried to work as a clerk in a retail store but was asked to leave because of absenteeism. She did not seem particularly bothered about the loss of her job. She had never tried to find other work, although she had been unemployed for 8 years. When asked how she spent her time, she said that she did some gardening and some housework when she felt well enough. However, she spent most of her time watching television.

Ms. O's parents visited her most of every day. Her mother asked whether she could spend the night in her daughter's room and was displeased when told no. The O family had many complaints about the quality of the nursing care, most about failures to anticipate the patient's needs. Extensive diagnostic studies failed to reveal any organic basis for her physical complaints. When informed that the problem was most likely psychological and advised to obtain psychotherapy, the O's protested angrily and refused a referral to a psychiatric clinic. Ms. O was discharged and returned to her parents' home.

many symptoms allowed her to be taken care of and to avoid the demands of adult responsibility. Her needs to be cared for fit with her mother's needs to nurture. Therefore she received little encouragement to give up her symptoms. A periodic hospital stay served to reinforce the seriousness of her problem. Secondary gain related to the gratification of dependency needs is a powerful deterrent to change in many patients.

Another type of somatoform disorder is the conversion disorder. Symptoms of some physical illness appear without an underlying organic cause. The organic symptom reduces the patient's anxiety and usually gives a clue to the conflict. For example, a patient who has an impulse to harm his domineering mother may develop paralysis of his arms and hands. The primary gain this patient receives is that he is unable to carry out his impulses. He also may experience secondary gain in the form of attention, manipulation of others, freedom from responsibilities, and economic benefits. Conversion symptoms might include the following:

1. Sensory symptoms, such as areas of numbness, blindness, or deafness
2. Motor symptoms, such as paralysis, tremors, or mutism
3. Visceral symptoms, such as urinary retention, headaches, or difficulty breathing

It is often difficult to diagnose this reaction. Other patient behaviors may be helpful. Often patients display little anxiety or concern about the conversion symptom and its resulting disability. The classic term to describe this lack of concern is *la belle indifference*. The patient also tends to seek attention in ways not limited to the actual symptom.

Hypochondriasis is another type of somatoform disorder. The person has an exaggerated concern with physical health that is not based on any real organic disorders. He fears presumed diseases and is not helped by reassurance. These people tend to seek out and use information about diseases to convince themselves that they are probably ill or about to become so. Unlike the conversion reaction, no actual loss or distortion of function occurs. Patients appear worried and anxious about their symptoms. This concern may be based on physical sensations overlooked by most people or on symptoms of a minor physical illness that the patient magnifies. This is frequently a chronic behavior pattern and is often accompanied by a history of visits to numerous physicians.

Hypochondriacal behavior is not related to a conscious decision. If a person decides to fake an illness, the behavior is called *malingering*. This is usually done to avoid responsibilities the person views as burdensome. Many otherwise healthy people malinger at one time or another. For instance, a person involved in an automobile accident may feign neck pain to receive insurance money. Frequently, the person exaggerates his symptoms, is evasive, and contradicts himself.

Many behaviors are associated with psychophysiological disorders. Careful assessment is needed so that actual organic problems are defined and treated. This type of illness should never be dismissed as "only psychosomatic" or "all in his head." Serious psychophysiological disorders can be fatal if not treated adequately.

■ Coping mechanisms

The psychophysiological disorders may be seen as attempts to cope with the anxiety associated with overwhelming stress. Unconsciously, the person links the anxiety to the physical illness. Secondary gain then adds to the psychological relief experienced.

Several of the defense mechanisms described in Chapter 11 may be seen in psychophysiological disorders. Repression of feelings, conflicts, and unacceptable impulses often leads to physical symptoms. The maintenance of repression over long periods of time requires a great deal of psychic energy. As the system approaches a state of exhaustion, physical symptoms occur. When a psychological basis for his illness is suggested, the patient denies it. This indicates that the person is unable to handle the anxiety that would be released if he admitted the psychic conflicts being repressed. The need for this defense should be respected.

Some individuals respond to psychophysiological illness with compensation. They attempt to prove that they are actually healthy by being more active and exerting themselves physically even if told to rest. This coping style is typical of the type A person, who needs desperately to prove that he is in control of his body, not controlled by it. The opposite of this reaction is the person who uses regression as a coping mechanism. This individual becomes dependent and embraces the sick role to avoid responsibility and dealing with conflict.

Common to each of these coping mechanisms is the need not to confront the basic conflict that is leading to stress and anxiety. This need is so strong that premature attempts to convince the person of his psychological conflicts may result in the substitution of a less adaptive coping mechanism for a more adaptive one. In extreme cases, if the person is stripped of all his efforts to cope and not provided with a substitute, death can result, either from worsening of the organic disorder or from suicide.

Nursing diagnosis

The nursing diagnosis must reflect the complex biopsychosocial interaction that is the hallmark of psychophysiological disorders. The individual's effort to cope with stress-related anxiety may result in many somatic and emotional disorders. All the possible disruptions must be considered when formulating a complete nursing diagnosis.

The model of health-illness behavior (Fig. 12-2) may help in the diagnostic process. A thorough interview will reveal many of the predisposing factors and precipitating stressors present for the individual. The nurse must use good communication skills during the interview to enable the patient to share his experience as completely as possible. Areas of resistance and gaps in information should be noted as possible indicators of a conflict. These may be explored more completely

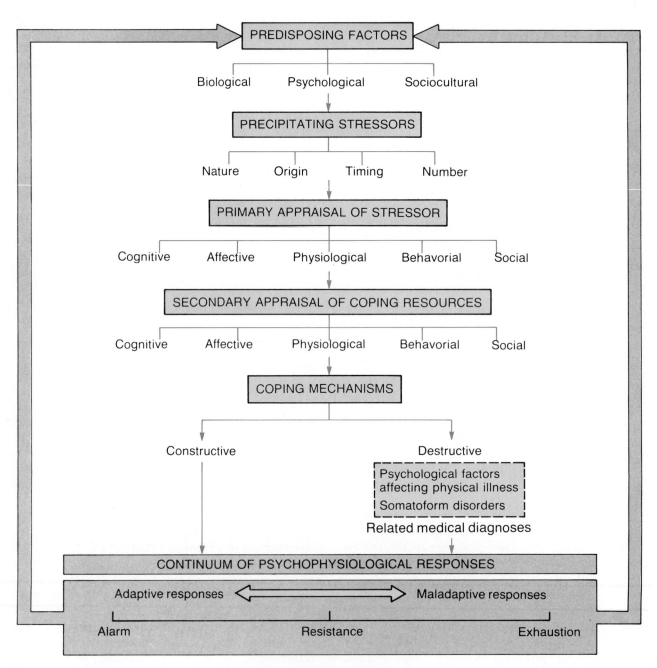

Fig. 12-2. Nursing model of health-illness phenomena with psychophysiological responses.

as trust is established in the nurse-patient relationship. Questions related to life-style and usual activities may help identify precipitating stressors and coping behaviors. It is particularly important to have the patient give his view of what is happening to him. This will provide valuable information about his awareness of the relationship between his mind and body. Nonverbal behaviors also give clues about the patient's concerns. Apparent lack of concern may reveal the use of denial that is typical of a person with a conversion disorder.

As the diagnosis is formulated, the nurse must consider the individual's coping in the context of the stress response. Is he in a stage of alarm with many coping resources at hand? Or is he in the stage of re-sistance, using coping mechanisms but depleting his energy resources? Has he reached the stage of exhaustion, needing intensive intervention to maintain life? The determination of the level of stress and coping being used will influence the interventions begun for patient care. The box on page 362 lists primary NANDA diagnoses and complete nursing diagnoses for patients with psychophysiological disorders. Medical and nursing diagnoses for these patients are described in Table 12-1.

■ Related medical diagnoses

Medical disorders related to psychophysiological illnesses are classified under the general headings of "somatoform disorders" and "psychological disorders

TABLE 12-1

MEDICAL AND NURSING DIAGNOSES RELATED TO PSYCHOPHYSIOLOGICAL ILLNESS

Medical Diagnostic Class	**Psychiatric Nursing Diagnostic Class**
Somatoform disorders	Psychophysiological illness
Psychological factors affecting physical condition	
Related Medical Diagnoses (DSM-III-R)	**Related Nursing Diagnoses (NANDA)***
Somatization disorder	Adjustment, impaired
Conversion disorder	Anxiety
Somatoform pain disorder	Constipation
Hypochondriasis	†Coping, ineffective individual
Body dysmorphic disorder	Denial, ineffective
Psychological factors affecting physical condition	Diarrhea
	Diversional activity deficit
	Family processes, altered
	Fear
	Gas exchange, impaired
	Health maintenance, altered
	Home maintenance management, impaired
	Hopelessness
	Mobility, impaired physical
	Nutrition, altered: less than body requirements
	Pain, chronic
	Powerlessness
	Self-care deficits
	Self-esteem, chronic low
	Self-esteem disturbance
	Self-esteem, situational low
	Skin integrity, impaired
	Sleep pattern disturbance
	Social isolation
	Spiritual distress
	Swallowing, impaired

*From American Psychiatric Association: DSM-III-R, American Psychiatric Association, October 1987.
†Indicates primary nursing diagnosis for psychophysiological illness

<table>
<tr><td>

Nursing Diagnoses Related to Psychophysiological Illness

Primary NANDA nursing diagnosis
Coping, ineffective individual

Examples of complete nursing diagnoses
Ineffective individual coping related to inability to express hostile and aggressive feelings evidenced by labile hypertension
Ineffective individual coping related to fear of assuming adult responsibilities evidenced by multiple somatic complaints
Ineffective individual coping related to repressed sexual impulses evidenced by urinary retention with no organic cause

</td></tr>
</table>

affecting physical condition." Specific diagnostic criteria for disorders classified as "psychological factors affecting physical condition" in DSM-III-R[2] are found in the International Classification of Diseases, edition 9 (ICD-9). These disorders and related nursing care are described in detail in medical and surgical nursing textbooks and will not be repeated here.

■ **SOMATIZATION DISORDER.**[2] The essential features include the following: There is a history of multiple somatic complaints beginning before age 30 and potentially involving several organ systems. There must be no organic cause found. Symptoms do not occur only during a panic attack. Symptoms cause an alteration in life-style or require medical attention or medication.

■ **CONVERSION DISORDER.**[2] The essential features include lost or altered physical functioning suggestive of a physical disorder that apparently expresses a psychological conflict or need. The disorder is not intentionally produced, and no organic cause is found. It is not limited to pain or alterations in sexual functioning.

■ **SOMATOFORM PAIN DISORDER.**[2] The essential features include pain persisting for more than 6 months with no organic cause or pain in excess of that usually found with the disorder.

■ **HYPOCHONDRIASIS.**[2] The essential features include preoccupation with fear of illness or the belief that one has an illness based on interpretation of physical signs or sensations. No evidence of a related illness

is found on physical examination, but the concern persists. The symptoms do not result from panic attacks. The disturbance must have lasted at least 6 months and be unrelated to any major mental illness.

■ **BODY DYSMORPHIC DISORDER.**[2] The essential feature is preoccupation with perceived physical abnormality by a person who appears normal. The belief is not delusional in nature and is not exclusively related to anorexia nervosa or transsexualism.

■ **PSYCHOLOGICAL FACTORS AFFECTING PHYSICAL CONDITION.**[2] The essential features include a temporal relationship between psychologically meaningful stimuli and the development of organic pathology (recorded on Axis III). The condition must not meet the criteria for any of the somatoform disorders.

Goal setting

The primary goal for the patient with a psychophysiological disorder is to consciously experience feelings and to be able to share them with others. This is a very long-term goal; some may never reach it. However, an increased level of self-awareness is beneficial and should be achievable to some extent by all patients. An improved ability to deal with conflict will reduce the need to use repression. This in turn will decrease stress and allow the patient to function with fewer episodes of physical illness.

The establishment of mutual goals with these patients is a problem. The patient's primary goal is to ease the physical symptoms of his illness. He expects this to be done by medical or surgical treatment. Exploration of psychological conflicts is likely to be seen as unnecessary. This resistance is related to the need to maintain defenses against the extreme anxiety that has led to the illness. The nurse must identify common treatment goals. The nurse also wants the patient to obtain relief from physical symptoms. Many patients will receive medical or surgical treatment and related nursing care. At the same time, the nurse should try to build a trusting relationship, so she can help the patient begin to feel safe in exploring interpersonal conflicts and feelings. Samples of short term goals for a patient with a psychophysiological disorder are included in Fig. 12-3.

Significant others must also be considered in developing the plan of care. It is important to explore their understanding of the patient's problem. They can be valuable allies in encouraging the patient to change his life-style, if this is necessary. At the same time, the nurse must recognize that a change in one family member requires a change in all the others. The family may be active participants in the patient's pathological

PSYCHIATRIC NURSING CARE PLAN

Precautions: _____

_____

_____

Special nursing needs: Assign consistent staff whenever possible; spend time with family _____

_____

Visitors: {x} No restrictions
　　　　 { } Family only
　　　　 { } Restricted to:
　　　　 _____
　　　　 { } No visitors

Telephone: { } Limited
　　　　　 {x} Unlimited

Privileges: { } Restricted to unit
　　　　　 { } Off unit accompanied by staff
　　　　　 {x} Off unit accompanied by family/visitor
　　　　　 { } Off unit unaccompanied
　　　　　 { } Out of hospital leave (dates) _____

Assessment data summary: Lives at home with parents; identifies herself as a person who is usually sick; many food intolerances; lacks insight into role of psychological factors in her illness; family is very protective

Nursing diagnoses: 1. Ineffective individual coping related to low self-esteem, evidenced by description of herself as always sick. 2. Ineffective family coping, disabling, related to failure to resolve dependence/independence conflict, evidenced by overinvolvement of parents.

Treatment goal: Expression of feelings verbally rather than through the development of physical symptoms.

Date	Problem/need	Expected outcome (objective)	Target Date	Nursing Intervention
5/29	Low self-esteem	To name at least one thing she values about herself	6/5	Establish a trusting relationship; give verbal feedback about attributes.
5/29	Outpatient psychotherapy	To accept an appointment at the community mental health center	6/5	Encourage to discuss feelings about referral; introduce to therapist.

Room 312	Patient's name Ms. O	Age 28	Doctor Dr. K	Primary nurse Mrs. G	Admit date 5/29/90

Fig. 12-3. Sample nursing care plan for a patient with psychophysiological illness. (This nursing care plan includes examples of the elements of a total plan as it might appear at a particular time in the patient's course of treatment. It should not be considered all inclusive.)

Date	Medications	Date	P.R.N. Medications	Diagnostic & psychiatric tests	Req.	Done
		5/29	Milk of	Upper GI series	5/30	6/2
			magnesia	Lower GI series	5/30	6/4
			30 ml qhs	ECG	5/30	6/1
			for constipation	EEG	5/30	6/1

Date	Treatments	Special orders and concerns
		Parents may visit during
		visiting hours only

Allergies: None	Medical diagnosis: (Axes I-III) Somatization disorder	Diet: Regular; no seafood, cabbage, carbonated drinks, eggs

Fig. 12-3, cont'd. Sample nursing care plan for a patient with psychophysiological illness.

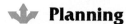

Planning

Care plans for these patients may be rather lengthy. The nurse must attend to the whole complex of the patient's biopsychosocial needs. Most patients, while having needs in all spheres, have their most urgent needs in a limited area of functioning. Patients with psychophysiological disorders are likely to have urgent needs in all three functional areas. Physical disorders are usually disabling and may be life threatening. Psychosocial problems will hinder recovery from the physical illness and so must also be given immediate attention. Fig. 12-3 presents a sample nursing care plan for Ms. O, the patient with a medical diagnosis of somatization disorder who was described in Clinical example 12-2.

Educational approaches may also be helpful in providing nursing care to patients with psychophysiological illnesses. Stress reduction techniques may help the patient to be able to reduce his anxiety and decrease his symptoms. Table 12-2 presents a mental health education plan for teaching coping strategies in a group setting.

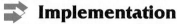

Implementation

Patients with psychophysiological illnesses are most frequently seen in general hospital and outpatient settings. They usually seek health care because of symptoms related to physiological functioning. Only after a thorough medical examination can the role of psychosocial stressors in the disorder be evaluated. In some cases, a pathophysiological disruption will require physical nursing intervention. If the physical condition is life-threatening, this intervention is given highest priority. For instance, a person with a bleeding ulcer needs intensive care to maintain his life. However, once the physical crisis is past, the nurse can assist the patient in avoiding similar problems in the future. For physical illnesses with psychosocial etiologies, this requires psychiatric nursing approaches using interpersonal relationships.

Skilled and compassionate nursing care directed to the patient's physical needs is the first step in establishing the trusting relationship. A person who is in pain,

TABLE 12-2

MENTAL HEALTH EDUCATION PLAN—TEACHING COPING STRATEGIES

Content	Instructional activities	Evaluation
Definition of stress	List feelings that indicate stress Discuss behaviors associated with elevated stress	The student will identify behaviors associated with stressful situations
Recognition of stressful situations	Ask learners to describe situations they have experienced as stressful Role play the situation (with videotape if possible) Discuss stress-related behaviors observed and feelings experienced	The student will correctly identify a stressful experience
Description of common life stressors	Ask each learner to describe one situation in his life that produces stress Conduct discussion about common elements of stressful experiences	The student will identify stressful aspects of his life
Identification of coping mechanisms	Review the role-played stressful situations Discuss alternative ways to cope with the stressors Role play at least one coping mechanism Provide feedback about the effectiveness of the selected coping mechanism	The student will identify and practice alternative coping mechanisms The student will select an appropriate coping mechanism when experiencing stress

Adapted from Hoover RM and Parnell PK: J Psychosoc Nurs 22:17, 1984.

bleeding, or covered with a rash is unable to discuss emotions or interpersonal relationships. The cardinal principle for patients with psychophysical disorders is to assess the patient's stress level and, whenever possible, act to reduce it. Stress and anxiety are at the root of the patient's problem. The nurse must care for immediate needs before addressing less obvious ones.

■ **INTERPERSONAL APPROACHES.** The psychophysiological symptom defends the person from overwhelming anxiety. It provides some patients with a way to receive help and nurturance without admitting the need for it. Others are protected from expressing frightening aggressive or sexual impulses. Recognizing the defensive nature of the symptom, the nurse should never try to convince the patient that his problem is entirely psychological. Likewise, the attitude that the patient only needs to get his life under control to get better is not therapeutic. The patient has not made a conscious choice to be hypertensive or to develop a conversion disorder. The dilemma of these disorders is that the patient consciously would like nothing more than to be cured, but unconsciously he is unable to give up the symptom. Conscious recognition of the psychological role of the symptom defeats its purpose and is therefore vigorously resisted. An example of this resistance is illustrated in Clinical example 12-3.

CLINICAL EXAMPLE 12-3

Ms. W was a 20-year-old woman who was admitted to the general hospital with a history of sudden onset of blindness. There was no evidence of any pathophysiological process affecting her eyes. Assessment revealed that she had witnessed her father's suicide by gunshot at the age of 5, although she claimed to have no memory of this. Her boyfriend had recently been expressing suicidal thoughts to her.

It seemed clear that the blindness was a conversion reaction. In order to confirm the diagnosis, the physician decided to interview Ms. W while she was sedated with amobarbital sodium. The interview was videotaped. During the interview, Ms. W was able to see. She read the day's menu and told the time by looking at a clock across the room. She also described the incident with her father. However, when the sedation wore off, Ms. W was again blind. The decision was made to show her the videotape, so she would recognize the psychogenic nature of her blindness. As she watched the tape, she did indeed regain the ability to see. However, when it reached the part in which she described her father's suicide, she became deaf.

It is not unusual for a person with a conversion disorder to substitute another symptom if the original one is taken away. This happens because the basic conflict remains. The ego still needs to be defended from experiencing repressed anxiety. The patient really needs assistance in dealing with the conflict. When this is resolved, the symptom will disappear because there is no longer a need for it.

Great skill is needed to intervene psychotherapeutically with these patients. Graduate education in psychiatric mental health nursing is required to be qualified to give insight-oriented psychotherapy. The nurse who is not prepared at this level can be supportive and available to talk with the patient and provide physical nursing care. He or she should be familiar with the therapeutic process in order to encourage the patient and understand behavioral changes that may occur. (See Table 12-3 for nursing interventions used in psychophysiological illnesses.)

Kaplan[13] described the process of insight-oriented therapy for patients with psychophysiological disorders. The patient's underlying anger must be recognized and confronted supportively. As the patient becomes aware of anger, he may have difficulty expressing it appropriately. The nurse should accept the patient's attempts to express anger as healthy and provide feedback. Sometimes patients in this phase of therapy are labeled as hostile or demanding and avoided by nursing staff. This only reinforces their conviction that angry feelings are unacceptable.

The next step in therapy is to identify and explore the patient's defenses. The therapist proceeds very carefully, helping the patient discover and test new, more adaptive coping mechanisms as the dysfunctional ones are given up. The nurse can help by supporting the patient in using new behaviors. Spending time with the patient and appreciating his positive qualities will help build his self-esteem and give him confidence. The nurse should be alert to signs of increased anxiety and report these immediately to the psychotherapist. The physical disorder may worsen if the therapy moves too rapidly. The therapist may decide to recommend changes in the patient's environment to assist him to function more comfortably. If the patient must consider a job change or another change in life-style, the nurse can offer time to talk about alternatives.

The patient may also need help in explaining changes in himself or his life-style to his significant

---

TABLE 12-3

SUMMARY OF NURSING INTERVENTIONS IN PSYCHOPHYSIOLOGICAL ILLNESSES

Goal—Assist the patient to consciously experience feelings and to be able to share them with others

Principle	Rationale	Nursing interventions
Maintain biological integrity	Highest priority is given to nursing interventions that preserve life and safety	Based on the patient's physical disorder, provide for adequate nutrition, hygiene, elimination, and safety needs
Establish a trusting relationship	Psychosocial nursing intervention is based on the therapeutic nurse-patient relationship	Meet the patient's stated needs; establish mutual goals; empathize with the patient; use therapeutic communication skills
Support the psychotherapeutic process	Conflict aroused in psychotherapy leads to increased anxiety and possible increase in psychophysiological symptoms	Schedule time to interact with the patient; encourage to continue to work in therapy; observe changes in symptoms; report increases to therapist; give patient positive feedback for new, healthier behaviors
Assist the patient to develop new ways to cope with stressful situations	Inability to deal with intrapsychic conflict leads to anxiety and stress, resulting in physiological dysfunction	Assist to identify stressful situations; explore alternative coping behaviors; teach various approaches to stress management; support patient in testing new behaviors
Assist significant others to support the patient's behavioral changes	Change in one part of a system affects all the other parts; systems tend to resist change	Explain the plan of care to significant others; involve them in the patient's care whenever possible; teach stress management techniques

others. The family is a system, and a change in one component of the system requires adjustment of all the other parts. For instance, a man who was very involved in his job and out several nights a week agreed to limit himself to 8-hour work days. This affected the rest of the family. Although his wife had protested for years that he spent too much time away from home, in reality she built her life around his schedule. She spent several evenings a week in other activities. If he were to be at home every evening, she would have to reevaluate her activities and decide whether she should go out or be with him. These are not easy decisions for family members to make. It is important that any underlying feelings of resentment be revealed and discussed to prevent indirect expression, which would create a new stressor for the patient. Family therapy may be necessary if family members have been supporting the patient's disorder. For instance, families sometimes become adjusted to having a dependent member and unwittingly sabotage efforts to foster independence. Since social support systems may help patients cope with their illnesses, the nurse may need to look for alternatives when the family is not supportive. Self-help groups often provide the needed social support. Corbin and associates[9] found that group interventions were helpful in decreasing overuse of health care services by patients with somatoform disorders.

Nurses must be aware that countertransference frequently occurs with these patients. They may be impatient and demanding. In general, it is easier to care for them when they are seriously physically ill. It is easy to become impatient with a demanding patient who is not acutely ill when there are sicker patients also needing nursing care. Reacting to this behavior by avoidance or anger only adds to the patient's anxiety and makes the situation worse. Clinical supervision by an experienced psychiatric nurse is highly recommended for nurses who work with these difficult patients. Frequent nursing care conferences are also helpful. If possible, a limited number of staff members should be assigned to the care of these patients. This fosters the development of a trusting relationship.

■ **EDUCATIONAL APPROACHES.** Health education is important in caring for the patient with a psychophysiological disorder. The patient with an organic pathologic condition usually needs instruction about medications, treatments, and life-style changes. He and his family will need information about follow-up care and crisis management. In addition, patients should be offered education about ways to cope with stress. It may be possible to increase acceptance of this idea by linking it to the general concern about stress management in American society. Group classes on stress management may be productive. They may enable pa-

tients to share experiences and make suggestions to each other about coping behaviors. Former patients who have made successful life adjustments can also be effective teachers of coping strategies. Table 12-2 presents a mental health education plan for stress management. This approach would be most effective with a small group of patients. However, it could be used with an individual if the nurse participated actively in suggesting and demonstrating coping strategies.

■ **ALTERNATIVE APPROACHES.** The approach to relaxation described by Benson[5] and presented in Chapter 11 is helpful for patients with psychophysiological disorders. The relaxation response helps reduce tension. Physiologically, it is the opposite of the fight-or-flight response. Therefore it decreases the sympathetic nervous system activity that leads to many of the physiological problems these patients have. It is also helpful to patients who dislike the idea of medication and want to be able to counteract stress when it occurs. Relaxation requires no special equipment and is not difficult to learn. The nurse will find this a useful intervention with many patients having various nursing care problems. Nurses may find it helpful to practice relaxation when they themselves are under stress.[11]

Meditation and hypnosis are closely related to relaxation therapy. Both involve the induction of deep states of relaxation by altering the state of consciousness. In meditation, the person concentrates on a word or phrase and clears his mind to convey a sense of peace to himself. Hypnosis may be induced by oneself or another. Posthypnotic suggestions are often effective in strengthening healthy coping mechanisms. Hypnosis should not be attempted by anyone who has not had extensive training and supervision in its use. Zahourek[23] describes the use of hypnosis with patients who are having pain. She found that it was most helpful in cases of acute pain. People with psychogenic pain were too fearful of giving up their pain, but it was sometimes possible to modify it. The best candidates for hypnosis were emotionally healthy, intelligent, and motivated persons.

Biofeedback may also be used successfully in conjunction with the relaxation response. This approach is used by Lynch[15] in work with hypertensive and migraine headache patients. The blood pressure and pulse of hypertensive patients are monitored during an interpersonal interaction. Fluctuations in these values are pointed out. As the patient is able to tolerate the information, the connection is made between the content of the conversation and the change in vital signs. This helps him recognize the role played by stress in his problem. He is then taught to express the feelings he has been repressing and to accept social support. Improvement is demonstrated by positive changes in the monitored physical signs. A similar approach is used with migraine headache patients, except that peripheral skin temperature is monitored.

Other approaches to stress management have been described by Charlesworth and Nathan.[8] For instance, physical activity is very relaxing for some people. Ideally, it is an activity that the person enjoys and can share with others. Patients need medical permission before participating in strenuous physical activity. Diet may also be helpful in building the person's coping ability. People under stress should not overuse dietary stimulants, such as caffeine. They may need education about the elements of a healthful diet. If the patient has been relying on alcohol or other drugs to cope with stress, he should be encouraged to find less destructive coping mechanisms. Specific information on alcohol and drug abuse is found in Chapter 19.

 Evaluation

The evaluation of the nursing care of the patient with psychophysiological illness is based on the identified patient care goals. If goal achievement is not attained, the nurse must ask the following questions:

Was the assessment complete enough to correctly identify the problem?
Did the patient agree with the goal?
Was enough time allowed for goal achievement?
Was I skilled enough to carry out the desired intervention?
Were there environmental constraints that affected goal accomplishment?
Did additional stressors change the patient's ability to cope?
Was the goal achievable for this patient?
What alternative approaches should be tried?

It is very important that neither the patient nor the nurse interpret the lack of goal achievement as a failure. The nurse should try to look at it as a challenge and convey that attitude to the patient. It is not at all helpful to add failure to achieve a goal to the patient's collection of stressors. The care of these patients is exceedingly complex. The nurse may expect to modify the treatment plan several times before finding a successful approach. The most important thing is to keep trying and to encourage the patient to persist in his efforts to find health.

■ SUGGESTED CROSS REFERENCES ■

The nursing model of health-illness behavior is discussed in Chapter 3. The therapeutic nurse-patient relationship is discussed in Chapter 4. Anxiety and

DIRECTIONS FOR FUTURE RESEARCH

The following are some of the nursing research problems raised in Chapter 12 that merit further study by psychiatric nurses:

1. The effect of feeling states on biological parameters
2. The relationship between the stress state of the nurse and her response to patient demands
3. Nursing interventions that assist Type A patients to modify their behavior
4. Validation of nursing diagnoses related to level of coping ability
5. Behaviors that patients interpret as indicating increased stress
6. The relationship between personality characteristics and acceptance of various stress management approaches
7. Impact of having family members participate in a stress management program with the patient
8. Characteristics of activities perceived as being relaxing
9. Responses of nurses to patients with psychophysiological illnesses in medical as opposed to psychiatric settings
10. Analysis of the effect of offering relaxation training to all patients on a general hospital unit

coping responses are discussed in Chapter 11. Problems with the expression of anger are discussed in Chapter 17. Psychological responses to physical illness are discussed in Chapter 21. Liaison nursing is discussed in Chapter 26.

■ SUMMARY ■

1. A historical perspective was provided on the progression of understanding of the relationship between the mind and the body. A dualistic approach was identified as being the major influence on modern medical thinking. More recently, a holistic influence has begun to be accepted.

2. The stress response was described as identified by Selye. It consists of three phases: alarm, resistance, and exhaustion.

3. Predisposing factors were discussed relative to biological, psychological, and sociocultural influences. Biological factors included the target organ theory and the possibility of genetic influences. Psychological factors included the possible influence of developmental experiences, unresolved dependency needs, and the inability to recognize, identify, or express feelings. Personality traits thought to be related to

selected psychophysiological disorders were described. Sociocultural factors included lack of social support systems and the loss of significant others.

4. Precipitating stressors were related to the experiencing of a crisis or to the gradual accumulation of a number of small stressors. Loss of defense mechanisms can also lead to the development of physical disorders.

5. Behaviors were discussed in terms of the meaning of the primary symptom to the patient. Somatoform disorders, which do not involve organic impairment, were compared to psychological factors affecting physical condition, which do. Feelings associated with psychophysiological disorders included anger, dependency, and sexual impulses that are unacceptable to the person. The presence of depression and anxiety was also discussed.

6. Coping mechanisms associated with psychophysiological illnesses were identified as repression, regression, denial, and compensation. The function of the illness itself as a coping mechanism was also discussed.

7. Nursing and medical diagnoses related to psychophysiological illnesses were presented.

8. Long- and short-term goals were suggested for patients with psychophysiological illnesses.

9. A sample nursing care plan and a mental health education plan related to psychophysiological illness were provided.

10. Nursing interventions were discussed. These included interpersonal approaches of a supportive nature, educational approaches, and alternative approaches of relaxation, meditation, hypnosis, biofeedback, activity, and nutrition.

11. Evaluation of the nursing care is based on the identified goals. Several questions were proposed that will assist the nurse in assessing lack of goal accomplishment.

■ REFERENCES ■

1. Alexander F: Psychosomatic medicine: its principles and application, New York, 1950, WW Norton.
2. American Psychiatric Association: DSM-III-R, Washington, DC, 1987, The Association.
3. Anderson A: How the mind heals, Psychol Today 16:50, 1982.
4. Barsky AJ: Somatoform disorders. In Kaplan HI and Sadock BJ, editors: Comprehensive textbook of psychiatry/V, ed 3, Baltimore, 1989, The Williams & Wilkins Co.
5. Benson H: Behavioral medicine: a perspective from within the field of medicine, Nat Forum 60:3, Winter 1980.
6. Brandt J et al: Personality and emotional disorder in a community sample of migraine headache sufferers, Am J Psychiatry 147:303, 1990.
7. Cannon WB: Bodily changes in pain, hunger, fear and rage, New York, 1929, Appleton-Century-Crofts.
8. Charlesworth EA and Nathan RG: Stress management: a comprehensive guide to wellness, New York, 1984, Atheneum.
9. Corbin LJ et al: Somatoform disorders: how to reduce overutilization of health care services, J Psychosoc Nurs Ment Health Services 26:31, 1988.
10. Friedman M and Rosenman RH: Type A behavior and your heart, Greenwich, Conn, 1974, Fawcett.
11. Hartl DE: Stress management and the nurse, Adv Nurs Sci 1:91, 1979.
12. Hoover RM and Parnell PK: An inpatient education group on stress and coping, J Psychosoc Nurs 22:17, 1984.
13. Kaplan HI: Treatment of psychosomatic disorders. In Kaplan HI, Freedman AM, and Sadock BJ, editors: Comprehensive textbook of psychiatry, ed 3, Baltimore, 1980, The Williams & Wilkins Co.
14. Lambert VA et al: Social support, hardiness and psychological well-being in women with arthritis, Image 21:128, 1989.
15. Lynch JJ: The language of the heart, New York, 1985, Basic Books, Inc.
16. Moore IM, Gilliss CL, and Martinson I: Psychosomatic symptoms in parents 2 years after the death of a child with cancer, Nurs Res 37:104, 1988.
17. Oken D: Current theoretical concepts in psychosomatic medicine. In Kaplan HI and Sadock BJ, editors: Comprehensive textbook of psychiatry/V, ed 5, Baltimore, 1989, The Williams & Wilkins Co.
18. Pines M: Psychological hardiness: the role of challenge in health, Psychol Today 14:34, Dec 1980.
19. Selye H: The stress of life, New York, 1956, McGraw-Hill Book Co.
20. Siegel BS: Love, medicine and miracles, New York, 1986, Harper & Row, Publishers, Inc.
21. Sifneos P: The prevalence of "alexithymic" characteristics in psychosomatic patients, Psychother Psychosom 22:255, 1973.
22. Wolf S et al: Life stress and essential hypertension, Baltimore, 1955, The Williams & Wilkins Co.
23. Zahourek RP: Hypnosis in nursing practice—emphasis on the "problem patient" who has pain, Part II, J Psychosoc Nurs 20:21, Apr 1982.

■ ANNOTATED SUGGESTED READINGS ■

Charlesworth EA and Nathan RG: Stress management: a comprehensive guide to wellness, New York, 1984, Atheneum.

A useful reference for the nurse looking for information on a variety of approaches to stress management. Particularly helpful for patients who are interested in learning more about stress.

Cousins N: Anatomy of an illness, New York, 1979, WW Norton Co.

Account of a personal experience showing that patients should assume a partnership role in the health care relationship. Discusses author's participation in own recovery from a progressive and potentially fatal illness through use of a stress management approach. Contains many provocative observa-

tions about the health care system.

Dager SR et al: Mitral valve prolapse and the anxiety disorders, Hosp Community Psychiatry 39:517, 1988.

Demonstrates the complexity of establishing relationships between physcial and psychiatric disorders.

*Dossey B et al: Holistic nursing: a handbook for practice, Rockville, MD, 1988, Aspen Publishers.

Describes the holistic and healing traditions within nursing with clear descriptions on the use of relaxation, imagery, and music therapy with patients. Recommended to all nurses.

*Hartl DE: Stress management and the nurse, Adv Nurs Sci 1:91, 1979.

Suggest stress management approaches that nurses might find helpful in their personal and professional lives.

*Kunzer MB: Marital adjustment of headache sufferers and their spouses, J Psychosoc Nurs Ment Health Serv 25:13, 1987.

Recommends an assessment of the marital relationship when providing nursing care to headache sufferers. In some cases, marital therapy may be a useful adjunct to biofeedback therapy.

*Lessman M: A painful chronicle, Am J Nurs 85:551, 1985.

Nursing student reflects on experience as an adolescent being treated for Crohn's disease. He reminds the reader of the need to reach out to frightened adolescents and to allow them the time to understand the alien experience of hospitalization and surgery.

*Lewis MC: Attribution and illness, J Psychosoc Nurs Ment Health Serv 26:14, 1988.

Application of concepts of attribution related to the cause of illness in a study of patients with inflammatory bowel disease. Identified three subcategories of attribution: scientifically inclined, stress, and I don't know.

---

*Asterisk indicates nursing reference.

Lynch JJ: The language of the heart, New York, 1985, Basic Books, Inc.

Contains author's observations of patients who suffer from psychophysiological disorders and his approaches to their treatment. Describes his partnership with a clinical nurse specialist who carries out much of the intervention.

Miller TW: Advances in understanding the impact of stressful life events on health, Hosp Community Psychiatry 39:615, 1988.

Discusses the relationship between body chemistry and personality related to resiliency or vulnerability to stressors. Cites relevant research and identifies topics for further study.

Neppe VM and Tucher GJ: Modern perspectives on epilepsy in relation to psychiatry: behavioral disturbances of epilepsy, Hosp Community Psychiatry 39:389, 1988.

Delineates similarities between some cases of epilepsy and schizophrenia. Describes current research exploring the relationship, if any, between the disorders.

Selye H: The stress of life, New York, 1956, McGraw-Hill Book Company.

Classic work setting forth the description of the stress response. A pioneering work with which every nurse should be familiar.

Sontag S: Illness as metaphor, New York, 1977, Vintage Books.

Small but thought-provoking book that uses the examples of tuberculosis and cancer to demonstrate the many meanings attributed to illness. Suggests that metaphorical thinking relative to illness may stand in the way of successful coping.

*Sparacino J et al: Psychological correlates of blood pressure: a closer examination of hostility, anxiety, and engagement, Nurs Research 31:143, 1982.

Describes nursing research related to blood pressure in response to hostility and anxiety. Describes a possible relationship and recommends further research in this area.

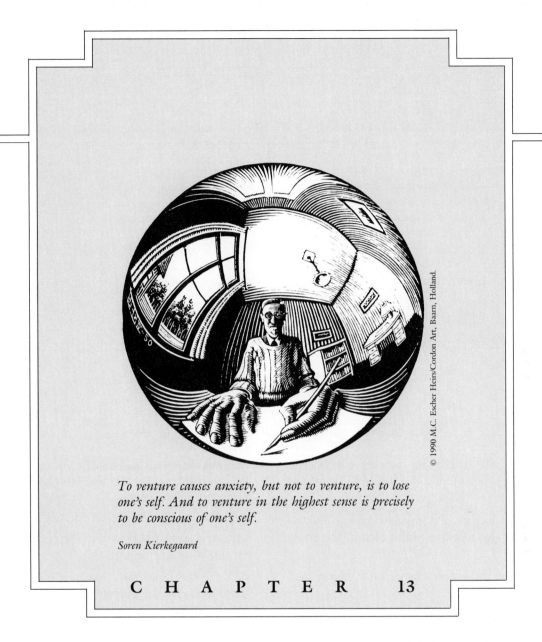

To venture causes anxiety, but not to venture, is to lose one's self. And to venture in the highest sense is precisely to be conscious of one's self.

Soren Kierkegaard

C H A P T E R   13

ALTERATIONS IN SELF-CONCEPT

DIAGNOSTIC PREVIEW

**MEDICAL DIAGNOSES RELATED
TO ALTERATIONS IN
SELF-CONCEPT**

- Multiple personality disorder

- Psychogenic amnesia

- Dissociative disorder

- Borderline personality disorder

- Bulimia nervosa

- Psychogenic fugue

- Depersonalization disorder

- Narcissistic personality disorder

- Anorexia nervosa

LEARNING OBJECTIVES

After studying this chapter, the student should be able to:

- define the following terms: self-concept, body image, self-ideal, self-esteem, role, and identity.

- discuss factors and experiences throughout the life cycle that influence each of the above concepts.

- describe the characteristics of a healthy personality.

- analyze the predisposing factors and precipitating stressors affecting self-concept.

- identify and describe behaviors and coping mechanisms associated with alterations in self-concept.

- formulate individualized nursing diagnoses for patients with alterations in self-concept.

- assess the relationship between nursing diagnoses and medical diagnoses associated with alterations in self-concept.

- develop long-term and short-term individualized nursing goals for patients with alterations in self-concept.

- apply therapeutic nurse-patient relationship principles in planning care of the patient with an alteration in self-concept.

- describe the progressive levels of nursing interventions for the patient with an alteration in self-concept.

- develop a mental health education plan to promote a patient's adaptive self-concept.

- assess the importance of the nursing process when working with alterations in a patient's self-concept.

- identify directions for future nursing research.

- select appropriate readings for further study.

Of all human attributes, the self appears to be the most complex and most intangible. One can neither see nor touch a self-concept, yet it has been a topic of concern to behavioral scientists since the late 1800s. The concept of self is not clearly defined, has various meanings, and is used in many different ways.

The self is the most real aspect of one's experience, however, and it is the frame of reference through which a person perceives, conceives, and evaluates the world around him. Self-concept can be defined as all the notions, beliefs, and convictions that constitute an individual's knowledge of himself and influence his relationships with others. It includes the perceptions of one's characteristics and abilities, one's interaction with other people and the environment, one's values associated with experiences and objects, and one's goals and ideals.

Helping professionals of all backgrounds have increasingly come to view the self-concept as a critical and central element for the understanding of people and their behavior, and it is now the subject of an enormous body of theory and research. This inquiry has given rise to a theoretical school known as "self theory," which is based on the principle that human behavior is always meaningful and that a person reacts to the world in terms of the way he perceives it. No two people have identical self-concepts. The self-concept emerges or is learned as a result of each person's experiences within himself, with other people, and with the realities of the world. Because it is the frame of reference through which the person interacts with the world, it is a powerful influence on human behavior. Self theorists believe it is impossible to understand a person fully or to predict his behavior accurately without understanding his internal frame of reference. This involves sharing his perceptual world and his views of himself. Thus understanding a patient's self-concept is a necessary component of all nursing care.

Continuum of self-concept responses

■ Developmental influences

Although theories of self-concept development vary considerably, most theorists agree that the self-concept does not exist at birth. The self develops gradually as the infant recognizes and distinguishes others and vaguely begins to differentiate himself as a separate individual. The boundaries of the self are defined as the result of exploratory activity and experience with the person's own body. At first self-differentiation is slow, but with the development of language it accelerates. Language helps to clarify the concept of the self, and the child's own name is a major linguistic aid. The use of a proper name helps the child identify himself and perceive himself as someone special, unique, and independent. In general, the ability to use language enables the child to make clear distinctions between himself and the rest of the world and to symbolize and understand his experiences. Once the infant has begun to differentiate himself from other people and the environment, the continued process of self-concept development is greatly benefited by the following:

■ Interpersonal and cultural experiences that generate positive feelings and a sense of worth

■ Perceived competence in areas valued by the individual and society
■ Self-actualization, or the implementation and realization of one's true potential

■ **SIGNIFICANT OTHERS.** The self-concept is learned in part through accumulated social contacts and experiences with other people. Sullivan[34] called this development "learning about self from the mirror of other people." What a person believes about himself is a function of his interpretation of how others see him, as inferred from their behavior toward him. His concept of self therefore rests partly on what he thinks others think of him. "Significant others" in the life of a child particularly affect the development of self-concept, and for a young child the most significant others are his parents. How they help him grow and react to his experiences has a tremendous influence on him. According to Combs and Snygg:

No experience in the development of the child's concepts of self is quite so important or far-reaching as his earliest experiences in his family. It is the family which introduces a child to life, which provides him with his earliest and most permanent self definitions. Here it is that he first discovers those basic concepts of self which will guide his behavior for the rest of his life.[12:134-135]

Combs and Snygg believe that the family provides the individual with his earliest experiences of (1) feelings of adequacy or inadequacy, (2) feelings of acceptance or rejection, (3) opportunities for identification, and (4) expectancies concerning acceptable goals, values, and behaviors. Research indicates that parental influence is strongest during early childhood and continues to have a significant impact through adolescence and young adulthood. Over time, however, the power and influence of friends and other adults increase, and they become significant others to the individual. Parents and immediate family members therefore are crucial to the initial development of the self-concept, and continuing development and change in self-perceptions are influenced by countless experiences with many other people.

Culture and socialization practices also affect self-concept and personality development. The dominant cultural patterns of the individual's environment give important clues to the sources of personality formation. General culture patterns as well as cultural subdivisions, such as social class membership, have formative influences on the individual's view of self. According to Combs and Snygg:

The culture in which we move is so completely a part of our experience as to overshadow almost all else in determining the nature of the self. Even our definitions and values are not left entirely to our own experience but are colored, interpreted and valued one way or another by the culture into which we are born, as they are interpreted to us by the acts of the people who surround us.[12:86]

■ **SELF-PERCEPTIONS.** A person's view of himself is not exclusively a collection of the views, expectations, and desires of others. Each person can observe his own behavior the same way that others do and form opinions about himself. One's perception of reality is selective, however, according to whether the experience is consistent with one's current concept of self. The way a person behaves is a result of how he perceives the situation, and it is not the event itself that elicits a specific response but rather the individual's subjective experience of the event. An individual's needs, values, and beliefs strongly influence his perceptions. One more readily perceives that which is meaningful and consistent with present needs and personal values. Similarly, people behave in a manner consistent with what they believe to be true. In this case, a fact is not what is but what one believes to be true. Once perceptions are acquired and incorporated into one's self-system, they can be difficult to change. Ways exist to change or modify one's perceptions, however, including modification of cognitive processes, exposure to drugs, sensory deprivation, and biochemical changes within the body.

As the self-concept develops, it brings a unique perspective of one's relationship with the world. What a person perceives and how he interprets what he perceives are conditioned by his concepts of self. A person with a weak or negative self-concept and who is unsure of himself is likely to have narrowed or distorted perception. Because he feels easily threatened, his anxiety level will rise quickly and he will become preoccupied with defending himself. In contrast, a person with a strong or positive self-concept can explore his world openly and honestly because he has a background of acceptance and success. Positive self-concepts result from positive experiences leading to perceived competence.

In conclusion, self-concept is a critical and central variable in human behavior. Individuals with positive self-concepts function more effectively, as evident in interpersonal competence, intellectual efficiency, and environmental mastery. In contrast, negative self-concept is correlated with personal and social maladjustment. As with the other nursing problems described in this text, it is possible to view one's self-concept responses along the health-illness continuum of coping responses described in Chapter 3. Fig. 13-1 describes the range of self-concept responses from the most adaptive state of self-actualization to the most maladaptive response of depersonalization.

Because one's self-concept pervades every aspect of life, therapeutic interventions related to self-concept are a core element in psychiatric nursing. This requires an understanding of various components of the self, including body image, self-ideal, self-esteem, role, and identity, which are now briefly discussed. This chapter then focuses on the nursing therapeutic process model for maladaptive responses related to self-concept.

■ **Body image**

The concept of one's body is central to the concept of self. The body can be thought of as a capsule in which one is permanently enclosed and through which one interacts with the world. One lives with his body 24 hours a day from birth until death. It is the most material and visible part of the self, and, although it alone never accounts for one's entire sense of self, it remains a lifelong anchor for self-awareness. An individual's attitude toward his body may mirror important aspects of his identity. A person's feelings that his body is big or small, attractive or unattractive, or weak or strong also reveal something about his self-concept. Numerous research studies have documented the close positive relationship between self-concept and body image. This association appears to exist both within American society and across other cultures.[4]

Body image can be defined as the sum of the conscious and unconscious attitudes the individual has toward his body. It includes present and past perceptions as well as feelings about size, function, appearance,

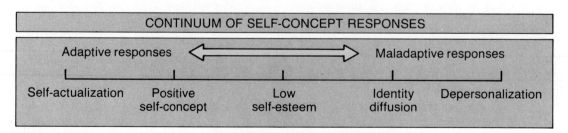

Fig. 13-1. Continuum of self-concept responses.

and potential. Body image is a dynamic entity because it is continually being modified by new perceptions and experiences. It serves as a target or screen on which the person projects significant personal feelings, anxieties, and values.

■ **DEVELOPMENTAL INFLUENCES.** One is not born with a body image. The infant receives input from his body but reacts to it in a global, undifferentiated way. As he gradually explores parts of his body, receives sensory stimulation from others, and begins to manipulate the environment, he becomes aware of the separateness of his own body. In the development of body awareness, the external body, that is, the body that can be seen and felt, is easier to learn about and is discovered earlier than the inner body. This recognition grows out of pleasurable and painful experiences. Actually, pain becomes the more dominant learning experience because pain sensory endings are distributed over the total surface of the body, whereas sensations of pleasure are concentrated in a few erotic zones. For the preschooler, the exploration of genitals and the discovery of anatomical differences between the sexes becomes especially important. The body occupies a middle position between the external world and the self as the agent of one's perceiving, thinking, and acting. The body can be viewed more externally and objectively than one's inner tensions, thoughts, and feelings. With increasing age there is a further differentiation of the self as a body and the self as a mind that can solve problems, make decisions, and experience feelings.

During adolescence the physical self is a focus of concern more than during any other period of life, except perhaps old age. Basic physical changes force the body into the adolescent's awareness. He has lost the security of a familiar body. New sensations, features, and body proportions have emerged. Height, weight, and physical strength increase, and the growth of secondary sex characteristics may be troublesome or embarrassing. The development of breasts, menarche, growth of pubic and facial hair, and voice changes must be integrated into the individual's evolving body image. Physical changes at adolescence also symbolize the end of childhood; maturity is just over the horizon. Adult proportions begin to emerge, but it is impossible to be certain of the nature, extent, or duration of changes still to come. Soon the outline of mature features will be complete. So the adolescent is anxious—will his mature physical self become reasonably close to his ideal? One's body image during adolescence is a crucial element in shaping his self-concept and in facilitating or retarding his attainment of status and adequate social relations.

Early adulthood brings some stability to body change. For the healthy adult, the body experience is a moment-to-moment, highly flexible aspect of his daily life pattern. As he has grown older, the importance of his body experience has changed. It can be said that the child "lives in his body," as compared to the adult, who "lives in his mind." To the child, eating, crawling, walking, and defecating can be all consuming, as can coughing and being febrile, congested, or constipated. They can occupy his sense of reality totally. The intensity of the child's involvement with his body, however, must diminish and develop into a broadening sense of what is real. The diminution must be selective, since the emerging adult needs to retain awareness of direct body sensation and a blending of body awareness into all aspects of his life. Many factors in his body experience must achieve the autonomy of automatic responses, such as walking and breathing. Other aspects of the body experience must emerge as flexibly adjusted pleasures, such as eating, orgasm, and exercise.

Middle age brings new challenges as different body parts age at different rates. The individual realizes his body is not functioning as well as it previously had. The later years of life accelerate the decline in physical abilities and can severely influence one's lifestyle and self-concept. As one's body image develops, extensions of the body become important, and anything that extends the effectiveness or control of one's body function can be called one's own. Clothes become identified closely with the body, and in the same way toys, tools, and possessions serve as extensions of the body and help to widen one's sense of self. Still later, position and wealth serve similar functions.

When the individual values his body and acts to preserve and protect it, the body image becomes the basis of sympathy through which the bodies and possessions of others are also valued. Body image, appearance, and positive self-concept are related. Studies indicate that the more a person accepts and likes his body, the more secure and free from anxiety he feels. It has also been shown that people who accept their bodies are more likely to manifest high self-esteem than people who dislike their bodies.[18,22] Thus the concept of body image is a central one to understanding self theory, and the relationship between the two will have implications for developing and implementing nursing care.

■ **Self-ideal**

The self-ideal is the individual's perception of how he should behave based on certain personal standards. The standard may be either a carefully constructed image of the type of person one would like to be or merely a number of aspirations, goals, or values that one would like to achieve. The self-ideal creates self-expectations based in part on society's norms and to which the person tries to conform. Formation of the self-ideal begins in childhood and is influenced by significant others who place certain demands or expectations. With time, the child internalizes these expectations, and they form the basis of his own self-ideal. New self-ideals that may persist throughout life are taken on during adolescence, formed from identification with parents, teachers, clergy, and peers. In old age additional adjustments must be made that reflect diminishing physical strength and changing roles and responsibilities.

Various factors influence one's self-ideal. First, a person tends to set goals within a range determined by his abilities. One does not ordinarily set a goal that is accomplished without any effort or that is entirely beyond one's abilities. Self-ideals are also influenced by cultural factors as the person compares his self-standards with those of his peers. Other influencing factors include one's ambitions and the desire to excel and succeed, the need to be realistic, the desire to avoid failure, and feelings of anxiety and inferiority. Based on these factors, one's self-ideal may be clear and realistic and thus facilitate personal growth and relations with others, or it may be vague, unrealistic, and demanding. The adequately functioning individual, however, demonstrates congruence between his perception of self and his self-ideal. That is, he sees himself as being very similar to the person he wants to be.

In summary, self-ideals are important in maintaining mental health and balance. They serve as internal regulators and help a person maintain an even course in the face of conflicting or confusing circumstances. For mental health the self-ideal must neither be too high and demanding nor too vague and shadowy, yet it must be high enough to give continuous support to self-respect.

■ Self-esteem

Self-esteem is the individual's personal judgment of his own worth obtained by analyzing how well his behavior conforms to his self-ideal. The frequency with which his goals are achieved will directly result in feelings of superiority (high self-esteem) or inferiority (low self-esteem) (Fig. 13-2). If a person is repeatedly successful, he tends to feel superior, but if he fails to live up to his expectations, he feels inferior. High self-esteem is a feeling rooted in unconditional acceptance of self, despite mistakes, defeats, and failures, as an innately worthy and important being. It involves accepting complete responsibility for one's own life.

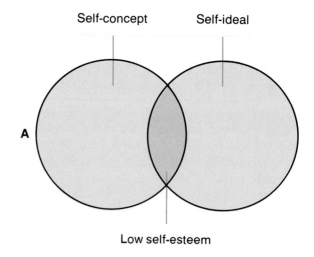

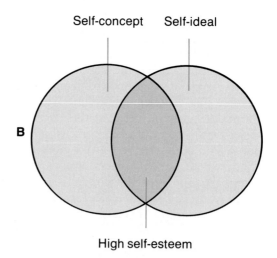

Fig. 13-2. A, Individual with a low level of self-esteem caused by a large discrepancy between self-concept and self-ideal. **B,** Person with greater conformity of self-concept and self-ideal and therefore a person with a high level of self-esteem. (From Sundeen SJ et al: Nurse-client interaction: implementing the nursing process, ed 4, St Louis, 1989, Mosby–Year Book, Inc.)

Self-esteem is derived from two primary sources: the self and others. It is first a function of being loved and of gaining the respect of others. Self-esteem is lowered when love is lost and when one fails to receive approval from others. Conversely, it is raised when love is regained and when one is applauded and praised. The origins of self-esteem can be traced to childhood and are based on acceptance, praise, and respect. Coopersmith[13] described the four best ways to promote a child's self-esteem:

1. Providing him with success
2. Instilling ideals

3. Encouraging his aspirations
4. Helping him build defenses against attacks to his self-perceptions

These should provide the child with a feeling of significance, or success in being accepted and approved of by others; a feeling of competence, or an ability to cope effectively with life; and a feeling of power, or control over one's own destiny.

Self-esteem increases with age and is most threatened during adolescence, when concepts of self are being modified and many self-decisions need to be made. The adolescent has to choose an occupation and decide if he is good enough to succeed in a given career. He has to decide whether he is able to participate or is accepted in various social activities. Heterosexually, is he attractive enough to interest and attract a desirable member of the opposite sex? Will he succeed in marriage? Does he have the courage to carry out his convictions? Is he capable of performing the roles assigned to him?

With adulthood the self-concept stabilizes, and maturity provides a clearer picture of self. The adult tends to be more self-accepting and less idealistic than the adolescent. He has learned to cope with many of his self-deficiencies and to maximize his self-strengths. Not all adults attain maturity; some continue to function as adolescents for many of their adult years.

In later life, self-esteem problems again arise because of the new challenges posed by menopause, retirement, loss of spouse, and physical disability. The impact of aging on self-esteem is also affected by the status of older people in American society. Being old in a society that values youth often leads to an assignment of low status and prejudicial attitudes toward old age and the aged themselves. The negative stereotypes of the elderly and the stigmatization that result can decrease self-esteem. Two other potential negative factors are the decreased social interaction of the elderly and the loss of control the elderly are able to exert over their environment, both of which can result in fewer opportunities for the elderly to validate and confirm their self-concepts.[35]

Research shows a clear relationship between self-reported physical health and self-esteem.[3] The report of a health problem, regardless of its type or severity, is associated with significantly lower self-esteem than is the report of no health problem. Severity of reported health problems is also related to lower levels of self-esteem. Finally, perception of ill health is negatively related to self-esteem.

High self-esteem has similarly been correlated with low anxiety, effective group functioning, and acceptance of others. According to Maslow, it is a prerequi-site to self-actualization; once self-esteem is achieved, the individual is free to concentrate on achieving his potential.[27] Low self-esteem has been correlated with poor interpersonal relations and is particularly prominent in schizophrenia and depressive disorders.

■ Role performance

Roles are sets of socially expected behavior patterns associated with an individual's function in various social groups. Identity emerges from self-concept and is evident as role behavior. Roles can provide social participation and a test of identities for consensual validation by significant others. The individual assumes various roles that he attempts to integrate into one functional pattern. Because these roles overlap and intertwine, an understanding of the person requires the nurse to see him in the context of the several roles he occupies. On the basis of his perception of role adequacy in the most "ego-involved" roles, the individual develops a level of self-esteem. High self-esteem results from roles that meet needs and are congruent with one's self-ideal. Many factors, including the following, influence an individual's adjustment to the role he occupies:

1. The clarity of the behaviors appropriate to the role and his knowledge of specific role expectations
2. The consistency of the response of significant others to his role
3. The compatibility and complementarity of his various roles
4. The congruency of cultural norms and his own expectations for role behavior
5. The segregation of situations that would create incompatible role behaviors

There are two basic types of roles. The first is ascribed; the individual has no choice over this role. Examples of ascribed roles include age and sex. The second is assumed; the person selects or achieves the role by choice. These include occupational and marital or family roles.

Sex roles affect one's performance in other roles. They are particularly significant to family roles but permeate most others as well and are frequently the cause of role conflict or disturbance. Another difficult problem faced by the individual growing up in contemporary society is that of emancipation from one's parents and establishment of an independent life. This primarily occurs during adolescence and early adulthood, when great ambiguity in role definitions occurs. The social roles of child and adolescent make it difficult to prepare oneself for adulthood. The child is not expected to be responsible; the adult is. The child is expected to be submissive; the adult dominant. The child is expected to be asexual; the adult is expected to be sexually mature and maintain intimate sexual relationships. However, few transitions or "rites of passage" exist to help the adolescent shift his role behavior. A final crisis is faced during old age when role behavior must again be changed by aging parents. They rely on their children yet strive to balance their lives with a sense of independence and a high level of self-esteem. Role behavior is intimately related to self-concept and identity, and role disturbances frequently involve conflicts between independent and dependent functioning.

■ Personal identity

The word identity is derived from the Latin root *idem,* meaning the same. It is the organizing principle of the personality system that accounts for both the unity and the continuity of the personality. Identity is the awareness of "being oneself," as derived from self-observation and judgment. It is the synthesis of all self-representations into an organized whole and is not associated with any one accomplishment, object, attribute, or role. Identity is different from self-concept in that it refers to a feeling of distinctness from others. It implies consciousness of oneself as an individual with a definite place in the general scheme of things. The person with a sense of identity feels integrated, not diffuse. When a person acts in accordance with his self-concept, his sense of identity is reinforced; when he acts in ways contrary to his self-concept, he experiences anxiety and apprehension. Behavior conforming with self-concept may thus be viewed as behavior preserving one's sense of identity.

The person with a strong sense of identity sees himself as a unique individual. Indeed, the very word individual, as a synonym for person, implies a universal need to perceive oneself as separate from others. This depends in part on a sense of self-perceived consistency, not only at a particular moment but also over time. One needs to perceive the person he is today as, if not the same person he was yesterday, at least similar to and having links with the person he was yesterday. This does not imply, however, that one attains a stable, fixed identity. Rather, as Bugenthal says, "to be human is . . . to be incomplete, needing; for life to be ever open, uncertain. Only as I allow full awareness of my needs and wants can I approach real wholeness."[11:276]

Identity combines many conscious and unconscious elements. It connotes autonomy based on understanding of and confidence in self. In this sense autonomy arises from feelings of self-respect, competency, and mastery over one's destiny. Autonomy implies self-government and self-acceptance with a tendency toward self-assertion and self-expansion. Identity also includes a person's body image, his own perceptions of his role performance, and the definitions of self contained in these roles.

■ DEVELOPMENTAL INFLUENCES.

The concept of ego identity was developed by Erikson[16] and built within his formulation of the eight stages of human development. For each stage, Erikson describes a "psychosocial crisis" that must be resolved for further growth and personality development. Chapter 8 describes these developmental stages over the life span. In adolescence the crisis of "identity versus identity diffusion" occurs. Identity formation, however, does not begin in adolescence. Rather, the groundwork is laid in infancy and evolves through the steps of introjection and identification. Introjection, or incorporation, depends on a mutually satisfying relationship between the infant and the mothering figure. The safety of this relationship allows the child to reach out for his first "love objects." The child further broadens and expands his sense of self as he identifies with parents, peers, teachers, and folk heroes. However, identity is more than the process of successive identifications. It is rather the capacity to synthesize successive identifications into a coherent, consistent, and unique whole.

Identity formation begins where the usefulness of identification ends and is the major task of adolescence. At no other phase of life are the promise of finding oneself and the threat of losing oneself so closely aligned. The adolescent's task is one of self-definition as he strives to integrate significant identifications and previous roles into a unique and reasonably consistent sense of self. Just as the process of identity formation did not begin in adolescence, neither does it end there. It is an evolving configuration, and circumstances in later periods greatly influence one's sense of identity.

Important in achieving identity is the issue of sexuality, the image of oneself as a male or a female and convictions about what that implies. "What does it feel like to be a girl?" "Do I like being a boy?" The answers to these questions are built up gradually from infancy as the result of learned conceptions about males and females. Society's ideals of masculinity and femininity provide important standards for judging oneself as good, bad, inferior, superior, desirable, or undesirable. These ideals are passed down from generation to generation and become an important part of the culture that transmits expectations to males and females. If males are defined as superior, this idea becomes part of the self-image of both males and females. If passivity and obedience are feminine ideals in a society, most little girls will be taught to be unassertive and obedient.

Men and women differ anatomically, hormonally, and genetically. Anatomical differences involving strength, ratio of muscle to fat, and reproductive organs are obvious. Hormonal and chromosomal differences are less obvious. The relationship of these differences to personality, sexual behavior, and conceptions of masculinity and femininity is controversial. How much effect do chromosomal and hormonal factors have versus environment and learning? This area merits further research, which will hopefully yield greater freedom and experimentation in the expression of sexuality in society. This is an important element of the personality because the security of one's sexual identity is a cardinal factor in achieving a stable ego identity.

In addition, much of one's identity is expressed in relationships with others. How a person relates to other people is a central personality characteristic. This presents a paradox in that everyone is a part of humanity yet each person is also separate from all others. Achieving identity is both the precursor to and the partial prerequisite for establishing an intimate interpersonal relationship. Research has shown that only after a stable sense of identity has been established can one engage in genuinely intimate, mature, and successful relationships.

Meier identified the following six attributes of ego identity, which can serve to summarize this discussion:

1. The individual recognizes himself as an intact body organism, separate from other organisms.
2. The individual acknowledges his sexuality.
3. The individual regards the various aspects of himself, such as roles, values, and actions, as compatible.
4. The individual's regard for himself is congruent with the way in which he is regarded by society.
5. The individual is aware of the relationships between past, present, and future.
6. The individual has goals of value that can be realized.[28:65]

Meier notes that not all these attributes are of equal importance and that they are not always present to the same degree. Rather, the individual's quest for identity is an evolving one in which new elements of identity are being added or changed as one attempts to answer the question "Who am I?"

■ The healthy personality

It is possible to describe the healthy personality according to developmental theory and the dynamics of the self. This description may help give perspective to the many aspects of self previously discussed. An individual with a healthy personality would experience the following:

1. **Positive and accurate body image.** Body image is the sum of the conscious and unconscious attitudes the individual has toward his body. It includes present and past perceptions, as well as his feelings about size, function, appearance, and potential. A healthy body awareness would be based on self-observation and appropriate concern for one's physical well-being.
2. **Realistic self-ideal.** Self-ideal is the individual's perception of how he should behave or the standard by which he appraises his behavior. An individual with a realistic self-ideal would have attainable life goals that are valuable and worth striving for.
3. **Positive self-concept.** Self-concept consists of all the aspects of the individual of which he is aware. It includes all his self-perceptions, which direct and influence his behavior. A positive self-concept implies that the individual expects to be successful in life. It includes the acceptance of the negative aspects of the self as part of the individual's personality. Such a person believes he can master his environment. He does not fear rejection but feels secure and accepted. He faces life openly and realistically and affirms his own existence.
4. **High self-esteem.** Self-esteem is the individual's personal judgment of his own worth, which is obtained by analyzing how well he matches up to his own standards and how well his performance compares with others. It evolves through a comparison of the individual's self-ideal and self-concept. A person with high self-esteem views himself as someone worthy of respect and dignity. He believes in his own self-worth and approaches life with aggressiveness and zest. The individual with a healthy personality is one who sees himself as very similar to the person he wants to be.
5. **Satisfying role performance.** The individual with a healthy personality can relate to others intimately and receives gratification from social and personal roles. Through open and honest communication he can trust others and enters into mutual and interdependent relationships. His capacity for sharing enables him to experience love, freedom, interdependence, and high role adequacy.

6. **Clear sense of identity.** Identity is the integration of inner and outer demands in the individual's discovery of who he is and what he can become. It is the realization of personal consistency. The person with a clear sense of identity experiences a unity of personality and perceives himself to be a unique individual. His "sense of self" gives his life direction and purpose.

An individual with these qualities is able to perceive himself and his world accurately. His insight into himself creates a feeling of harmony and inner peace.

 # Assessment

■ Predisposing factors

■ **AFFECTING SELF-ESTEEM.** Predisposing factors that originate in early childhood can contribute to problems with self-concept. Because the infant initially views himself as an extension of his parents, he is very responsive to both parents' self-hate and any feelings of hatred toward himself. Parental rejection causes the child to be uncertain of himself and other human relationships. As a result of his failure to be loved, the child fails to love himself and is unable to reach out with love to others.

As he grows older, the child may experience lack of recognition and appreciation by parents and significant others. He may learn to feel inadequate because he is not encouraged to be independent, to think for himself, and to take responsibility for his own needs and actions. Overpossessiveness, overpermissiveness, or overcontrol, exercised by one or both parents, can nurture a feeling of unimportance and lack of esteem in the child. Harsh, demanding parents can set unreasonable standards, often raising them before the child has developed the ability to meet them. Parents may also subject their children to unreasonable, harsh criticism and inconsistent punishment. These actions can cause early frustration, defeatism, and a destructive sense of inadequacy and inferiority. Another factor in creating such feelings may be the rivalry or unsuccessful emulation of an extremely bright sibling or of a prominent parent, often generating a sense of hopelessness and inferiority. In addition, repeated defeats and failures can destroy one's sense of self-worth. In this instance the failure in itself does not produce a sense of helplessness, but internalization of the failure as proof of personal incompetency does.

Unrealistic self-ideals. With age, additional factors emerge that can cause and perpetuate feelings of low self-esteem. The individual who lacks a sense of meaning and purpose in life also fails to accept responsibility for his own well-being. He becomes dependent on others, self-indulgent, and fails to develop his capabilities and potential. He denies himself the freedom to full expression, including the right to make mistakes and fail, and becomes impatient, harsh, and demanding with himself. He sets standards that cannot be met. Examinations are constructed that cannot be passed. Self-consciousness and observation then turn to self-contempt and self-defeat. This results in a further loss of self-trust.

These self-ideals or goals are often silent assumptions, and the person may not be immediately aware of them. They reflect high expectations and are unrealistic in relation to one's proved capacities. When the individual judges his performance by these unreasonable and inflexible standards, he cannot live up to his ideals and, as a result, experiences guilt and low self-esteem. Horney[20] has described these inner dictates as the "tyranny of the shoulds" and has identified some of the common ones:

1. I should have the utmost generosity, considerateness, dignity, courage, and unselfishness.
2. I should be the perfect lover, friend, parent, teacher, student, and spouse. Everyone should love me.
3. I should be able to endure any hardship with equanimity.
4. I should be able to find a quick solution to every problem.
5. I should never feel hurt; I should always be happy and serene.
6. I should know, understand, and foresee everything. I should be competent in all ways.
7. I should always be spontaneous; I should always control my feelings.
8. I should assert myself; I should never hurt anybody else.
9. I should never be tired or get sick.
10. I should always be at peak efficiency. I should not make mistakes.

The person who overemphasizes these rules or ideals often makes, for example, the following series of deductions: "Everyone should love me . . . If he doesn't love me, I have failed . . . I have lost the only thing that really matters . . . I am unlovable . . . There is no point in going on . . . I am worthless." This inner punishment results in feelings of depression and despair because the demands on self are those no human being could fulfill, and they reflect a disloyalty to what one can feel or do at present. Slavishly striving for these ideals interferes with other activities, such as living a reasonably healthy, tranquil life and having satisfying relationships with other people. These predisposing factors lay the groundwork for feelings of low self-esteem.

■ AFFECTING ROLE PERFORMANCE

Sex roles. A particularly relevant source of strain in contemporary America comes from values, beliefs, and behaviors about sex roles. Differences between male and female body structures have given rise to various theories or propositions. Freud ascribed much weight to biological factors in sexuality. Erikson supported his belief that anatomy predestined the individual to certain types of behavior. These psychoanalytical views have come under attack in recent years for their theories of femininity and masculinity and for the negative effects these theories are believed to have had on sexuality and role behavior. They largely ignore the influence of culture and learning on one's self-perceptions.

Unfortunately, research demonstrates that society continues to have clearly defined sex-role stereotypes for men and women. The work of Broverman and coworkers[10] indicates that women are perceived as relatively less competent, less independent, less objective, and less logical then men. Men are perceived as lacking interpersonal sensitivity, warmth, and expressiveness in comparison to women. Moreover, stereotyped masculine traits are more often perceived as desirable than are stereotyped feminine characteristics.

To the extent that these results reflect societal standards of sex-role behavior, both women and men are put in role conflict by the difference in the standards. If a woman adopts behaviors desirable for a man, she risks censure for her failure to be appropriately feminine; if she adopts behaviors designated as feminine, she is deficient in the values associated with masculinity. So, too, if a man adopts the behaviors specified as desirable for a woman, his masculinity and sexuality may be questioned and his contributions may be devalued or ignored; if he adopts the behaviors associated with masculinity, he risks alienating attributes of his personality associated with warmth, tenderness, and responsiveness. Thus when a woman steps out of her home, where her sex role has traditionally been defined and confined, and enters the world of work, she may expect to experience heightened role strain. Similarly, the man who arrives home from work in the evening may feel uncertain or in conflict about how he should relate to his school-age son, infant daughter, or working wife.

Most importantly, both men and women incorporate the positive and negative traits of the stereotype into their self-concepts. Since more feminine traits are negatively valued than are masculine traits, women tend to have more negative self-concepts than do men. Women also have higher rates of mental illness than men and are more likely to become depressed. Grove and Tudor[17] suggest several possible reasons for this:

1. Many women are restricted to a single, major social role as housewife, whereas most men have two roles—household and work—and therefore two sources of gratification.
2. Some women find their role expectations regarding raising children and keeping house to be limiting and frustrating. They wish to work but are unable to, whereas other women are forced to work for financial reasons at jobs that are not gratifying and would rather remain at home caring for their house and children. In either situation, one's role preferences are not being met.
3. The housewife role is unstructured, invisible, and often perceived to be of low status, particularly with the current value and status placed on "career women."
4. Even when a married woman works, she is often in a less satisfying position than a man because of discrimination and limited opportunity.
5. Expectations confronting women are unclear and diffuse and may result in an unclear female identity.

Role conflict and role ambiguity therefore arise from the biological factors and social expectations set for men and women. Role overload can also occur for the woman who has numerous, often conflicting, roles imposed on her. The existence of a women's movement in many countries can be viewed as an attempt by women to examine their own identities and determine appropriate role behavior.[7] Thus the interaction of marriage, parenting, and employment emerges as a likely source of role strain for women.

Work roles. Work does not imply, however, a singular social role. It is possible to distinguish between women who perceive their employment as careers and those who view their work as a job. Women are still in the minority of most high-status occupations and are clustered near the bottom in terms of professional status and financial reward. Holahan and Gilbert[19] conducted a study that compared conflict experienced by career and noncareer (job) women in relationship to the roles of worker, spouse, parent, and self as a self-actualizing person. Greater role conflict was reported by the job versus career group, particularly involving the parent versus self and spouse versus self roles. The career group reported receiving significantly more life satisfaction from both work and self roles than the job group.

This and other studies suggest that work viewed as desirable, valuable, and adequately compensated can bring greater life satisfaction. Hunt has listed the needs that may be met by work as those for "money, identity, achievement, status, personal pride, inner joy, and for many a woman, whether she realizes it or not, a means of achieving a lasting peace rather than a cease-fire within marriage."[31] Furthermore, a large-scale study conducted by the Department of Health, Education and Welfare found housewives had higher symptom rates than employed women, and professionally employed women had lower symptom rates than those in other occupational categories.

The problem appears to be the lack of support for women performing multiple roles. This lack is reflected in payment received, willingness by other family members to share family tasks, and encouragement for the woman pursuing her own goals. At present in American society, women are socialized to seek an ideal that includes marriage, children, higher education, and satisfying work outside the home. They are increasingly expected to perform in both "feminine" and "masculine" spheres.

This situation has both positive and negative aspects. First, it can be argued that it merely replaces the traditional woman's role with another equally confining one. By valuing the new role, the traditional roles of wife and mother become devalued. Second, although women are expected to assume more "masculine" qualities, a corresponding trend for men to assume more "feminine" behaviors is not apparent. Third, the woman who seeks such an expanded role is faced with reconciling the often conflicting goals of work, marriage, homemaking, and parenting. Little organized support by society exists to aid the woman, however, and thus her task can be formidable or overwhelming.

Despite social and economic changes, there is often little sharing of tasks when men and women are both gainfully employed. Rather, most industrial societies have witnessed a gradual change in the obligations of women, who now perform a double, or "dual," role—outside employment and continued responsibility for home and children. The expectation exists that the woman will make the adjustments needed both at home and in her career, including housekeeping and managing; arranging meals, lessons, and appointments; entertaining; caring for the sick; and communicating with the family. There is also the traditional expectation that the wife will be the primary caretaker of the child and will subsume other activities to this end. Johnson and Johnson[21] report that the wives and mothers of dual-career families with young children experience difficulties with growing demands in both home and job situations. The greatest strain was in the maternal role, where guilt and anxiety predominated.

Although it may appear that attitudes toward sex roles are changing, the division of household labor within the family is not. In the study of Berk, Berk, and Berheide,[6] wives reported that they did 86% of the kitchen cleaning, 92% of the laundry tasks, 88% of the meal preparation, 89% of the straightening tasks, 74% of the outside errands, and 76% of "other" household tasks. Even the stereotypically husbandly duties of taking out the garbage and paying the bills were generally done by wives (60% and 62%, respectively). Furthermore, married women employed outside the home were not found to do a significantly smaller proportion of household work. Also, the presence of preschool children did not affect the division of labor. The authors concluded that women with small children at home just work harder.

Given these factors, Weissman and co-workers[36] understandably found that the search for work by young educated housewives was associated with a moderate degree of stress and mild depressive symptoms. On the one hand, these women wanted to find self-expression through work outside the home; on the other, they held traditional values about marriage and children. Thus career adaptations had to be made to fit personal and family needs. One attempted solution to this role strain is for the woman to become "superwoman" and do everything well. Not only is this impossible, but the attempt is exhausting and self-defeating.

Bailyn[5] compares this situation to that of a man. He, too, is faced with different values in his work and family, and some degree of conflict along the same lines also exists for him. His situation is eased, however, by a hierarchy of values that precludes the necessity of conscious decision. Unless family needs reach crisis proportions, the demands of his work come first. Very little is written about paternal role strain, accommodation, or the career and homemaking changes made by men in a dual-career family. Comparatively, the role set of women appears far more complex, and thus the increased susceptibility of women to role strain is not surprising.

One might conclude, therefore, that sex and work roles will continue as a source of stress (1) until care of children, home, and career are viewed as equally valuable and important by both sexes and (2) until gender is regarded as irrelevant to the abilities, personalities, and activities of the individuals involved. Such a change in attitude should begin with nurses and other mental health clinicians who, by accepting the stereotyped views of society, indirectly increase role strain. The research of Broverman and co-workers[9] shows that clinicians have different concepts of health for men and women and that these differences parallel the sex-role stereotypes prevalent in our society. The cause of mental health might be better served if psychiatric clinicians encouraged both men and women to maximize individual potential rather than adjust to existing restrictive sex roles.

■ **AFFECTING PERSONAL IDENTITY.** Constant parental intervention interferes with adolescent choices. In our culture this is related to the lack of a cutoff point and fixed limit to parental intervention. Parental distrust leads a child to wonder whether his own choices are correct and to feel guilty if he goes against parental ideas. Parental distrust implies belittlement because it devalues the child's opinions and leads to indecisiveness, feelings of nothingness, exasperated impulsiveness, and acting out in an attempt to achieve some identity. When the parent does not trust the child, the child ultimately loses respect for the parent. It has been found that parents and children do not disagree on significant issues, such as war, peace, race, or religion. Instead, personal and narrow concerns—fads, dating, a party, the car, curfews, homework—create the conflict between parents and youth. Here parental intervention interferes with options and identity.

Peers also add to the problems of identity. The adolescent wants to belong, to feel needed and wanted. The peer group, with its rigid standards of behavior, gives him this feeling and provides a bridge between childhood and adulthood. The adolescent loses himself in the fads and the language of the group. However, because all peer group members are searching to define their identity and are beset by the pressures and frustrations of a complex society, the group is often a cruel testing ground that hurts as much as it helps. Taught to be competitive, the young person competes with his friends, "putting them down" to bring himself up. Membership in the peer group is bought at a high price; the adolescent must surrender much of his identity to belong. Often there is open destruction of self-esteem and ferocious insistence on conformity. In sexual relationships adolescents introduce further uncertainty into their lives, which can interfere with developing a stable self-concept.

■ **Precipitating stressors**

Specific problems with self-concept are initiated by almost any difficult situation to which the person does not have the capacity to adjust. During his lifetime, the individual is faced with numerous role transitions. These transitions may require the person to incorporate new knowledge and alter his behavior. Meleis[29] has identified three categories of role transitions: (1) developmental, (2) situational, and (3) health-illness. Developmental transitions are normative changes associated with growth. Situational transitions involve the addition or subtraction of significant others, occurring through birth or death; an example is the change from nonparental to parental status. Health-illness transitions involve moving from a well state to an illness state. Each of these role transitions can precipitate a threat to the individual's self-concept.

■ **ROLE STRAIN.** People who experience stress associated with expected roles or positions are said to experience role strain. Role strain is experienced as frustration, since the person may feel torn in opposite directions or feel inadequate and unsuited to certain roles. Over time, role strain places a considerable burden on the person, who will act to alleviate role strain and increase the gratification of high role adequacy. Role strain, as a general term, incorporates the concepts of role conflict, role ambiguity, and role overload.[7]

Role conflict occurs when a person is subjected to two or more contradictory expectations that he cannot simultaneously meet. Conflict can arise because two internal needs, drives, or motives are incompatible, or because an internal need, drive, or motive opposes an external demand. For example, role conflict can occur because there are cultural expectations that certain attributes go with certain roles. In this case the role conflict is caused by the incongruency between the individual's and society's expectations for specific role behavior. This is evident in a society's sex-role stereotyping and may be experienced by the woman who enters a traditionally male occupation, or vice versa. Another source of conflict is different perceptions of appropriate behavior. An example of this is evident in family roles. Each adult brings to marriage a set of perceived family roles greatly influenced by his or her own upbringing. Often the individuals' perceptions may be contradictory and pose problems within the marriage.

Role ambiguity appears when shared specifications set for an expected role are incomplete or insufficient to tell the individual what is desired or how to do it. This confusion regarding role expectations and appropriate behavior can be very stressful. It is particularly evident among adolescents, since society's demands have become stronger, more diversified, and more immediate, often producing confusion, frustration, alienation, and violence. Adolescents are pressured to play different roles by their parents, the mass media, and their peers. They are expected to "earn their own keep" but are unable to find jobs in times of high unemployment and economic inflation. They are confused by the discrepancy between the morality practiced by society and the morality they learned as a child. Some young people turn to violence as a way of asserting themselves, whereas others become apathetic and alienated.

A final type of strain is **role overload,** occurring when a person faces a role set that is too complex. The person lacks the physical, intellectual, emotional, or economic resources to perform the necessary role. Each of the roles may be making legitimate discrete demands, but together the expectations are overwhelming and perhaps impossible. An example is the numerous roles of the contemporary woman—wife, cook, mother, employee, chauffeur, maid, lover, and so on.

■ **DEVELOPMENTAL TRANSITIONS.** Various developmental stages can precipitate threats to one's identity. Adolescence is perhaps the most critical, since it is a time of upheaval, change, anxiety, and insecurity. Adolescents are modifying their concepts of self and are analytical about not only themselves but also the world in general. Adolescents are faced with many decisions. They must decide if they are good enough to succeed in a given career. They must determine if they have the ability to participate in various social activities. Are they attractive enough heterosexually to interest and succeed with a member of the opposite sex? Will they succeed in marriage? Do they have the courage to carry out their convictions apart from the crowd while remaining a member of it? Are they a leader, a follower, or a coward? Are they satisfied with their roles, and can they implement them comfortably?

An adult's problems of identity are simpler than those of an adolescent. Maturity stabilizes self-concept and provides a firmer picture of self. A serious threat to identity in adulthood is cultural discontinuity. This occurs when a person moves from one cultural setting to another and experiences emotional upheaval. Faced with differing cultural standards, many people have difficulty maintaining their self-system. In addition, problems within the social structure, such as political upheavals, economic depression, and high unemployment, can pose threats to identity.

Cultural stressors confront a person in challenging personal values: conforming versus individuality, cowardice versus bravery, winning versus losing, career versus marriage, equality versus superiority, cooperation versus competition, dependence versus independence, intelligence versus feeling. Although these values are not necessarily opposite or mutually exclusive, they raise fundamental questions that the individual must resolve and integrate. One's sexual identity can also be influenced by cultural pressures, which can control both how one expresses sexuality and how it fits into one's self-system. Definitions of acceptable approaches to both sexes, the values placed on virility and procreation as proof of virility, definitions of suitable sex partners, and the values concerning marital fidelity may all be culturally determined.

In late maturity and in old age, identity problems again arise. New problems and roles result from the process of aging and from the view of the elderly held by the more youthful members of society. Menopause, retirement, and increasing physical disability are problems for which the aging person must work out adaptive behavior.

■ **HEALTH-ILLNESS TRANSITIONS.** Some stressors can cause disturbances in body image and related changes in self-concept. One threat is the loss of a major body part, such as an eye, breast, or leg. Disturbances also may occur following a surgical procedure in which the relationship of body parts is disturbed. The results of the surgical intervention may be either visible, as with a colostomy or gastrotomy, or invisible, as with a hysterectomy or gallbladder removal. Changes in body size, shape, and appearance can threaten one's self-perceptions. These changes can result from rapid weight gain or loss, a skin infection, or even plastic surgery. Threats to body image can occur from a pathological process that causes changes in the structure or function of one's body, such as arthritis, multiple sclerosis, Parkinson's disease, cancer, pneumonia, and heart disease. The failure of a body part, as experienced by the paraplegic or stroke victim, is particularly difficult to integrate into one's self-perceptions. The physical changes associated with normal growth and development may pose problems, as may some potentially threatening medical or nursing procedures, such as enemas, catheterizations, suctioning, radiation therapy, dilation and curettage, and organ transplantation.

All these stressors can pose a threat to one's body image, with resultant changes in self-esteem and role perception. Any threat to body integrity is interpreted as a threat to self. How the individual perceives the threat determines the coping mechanism summoned. Factors that influence the degree of threat to one's body image have been identified by Norris[30]:

1. The meaning of the stressor for the individual. Does it threaten his ideal of youth and wholeness and decrease his self-esteem?

2. The degree to which his pattern of adaptation is interrupted. Does it jeopardize his security and self-control?
3. The coping capacities and resources available to him. What response is elicited from significant others, and what help is offered him?
4. The nature of the threat, extent of change, and rate at which it occurs. Is the change one of many small adjustments over time or a great and sudden readjustment?

Finally, physiological stressors may also disturb one's sense of reality, interfere with an accurate perception of the world, and threaten one's ego boundaries and identity. Such stressors include oxygen deprivation, hyperventilation, biochemical imbalances, severe fatigue, and sensory and emotional isolation. Alcohol, drugs, and other toxic substances may also produce self-concept distortions. Usually these stressors produce only temporary changes within the individual.

Whether the problem in self-concept is precipitated by psychological, sociological, or physiological stressors, the critical element is the patient's perception of the threat. As the nurse assesses pertinent behaviors and formulates a nursing diagnosis, she must continue to validate her observations and inferences to establish a mutual, therapeutic relationship with the patient.

■ Behaviors

Assessing the various components of a patient's self-concept will present a challenge to the nurse. Because self-concept is the cornerstone of the personality, it is intimately related to states of anxiety and depression, problems in relationships, acting out, and self-destructive behavior. All behavior is motivated by a desire to enhance, maintain, or defend the self; thus the nurse will have extensive information to evaluate. However, the nurse must delve beyond objective and observable behaviors to the patient's subjective and internal world. Only when the nurse explores this realm will the patient's actions be given meaning.

The nurse can begin the assessment by observing the patient's appearance. Posture, cleanliness, makeup, and clothing provide data. The nurse might discuss the patient's appearance with him to determine his values related to body image. Observing or inquiring about his eating, sleeping, and hygiene patterns gives clues to his biological gratifications and tendencies toward self-preservation. These initial observations should lead the nurse to ask, "What does my patient think about himself as a person?" The nurse might ask the patient to describe himself or how he feels about himself. What strengths does he think he has? What areas of weakness? What is his self-ideal? Does he conform to it? Does fulfillment of his self-ideal bring him satisfaction? Does he value his strengths? Does he view his weaknesses as important personality deficits, or are they relatively unimportant to his self-concept? What are his priorities? Is he a participant in life or an observer? Does he feel unified and self-directed or diffuse and other directed?

The nurse can then compare the patient's responses to his behavior, looking for inconsistencies or contradictions. How does he relate to other people? How does he respond to compliments and criticisms? The nurse can also examine his or her affective response to the patient. Is it one of hopelessness, despair, anger, or anxiety? The nurse's own response to the patient is often a good indication of the quality and depth of the patient's pain.

■ **ASSOCIATED WITH LOW SELF-ESTEEM.** Low self-esteem is a major problem for many people and can be expressed in moderate and severe levels of anxiety. It involves negative self-evaluations and is associated with feelings of being weak, helpless, hopeless, frightened, vulnerable, fragile, incomplete, worthless, and inadequate. Low self-esteem is a major component of depression, which acts as a form of punishment and anesthesia for the individual. Low self-esteem indicates self-rejection and self-hate, which may be a conscious or unconscious process expressed in direct or indirect ways.

Direct expressions of self-hate or low self-esteem may include any of the following:

1. **Self-derision and criticism.** The patient has a negative cognitive set and believes he is doomed to failure. Although the expressed purpose of the criticism may be self-improvement, there is no constructive value to it and the underlying goal is to demoralize oneself. This occurs when the individual places himself in a situation he cannot handle and then subjects himself to ridicule. He might describe himself as "stupid," "no good," or a "born loser." He views the normal stressors of life as impossible barriers and becomes preoccupied with self-pity.
2. **Self-diminution.** The minimizing of one's ability by avoiding, neglecting, or refusing to recognize one's real assets and strengths.
3. **Guilt and worrying.** Destructive activities by which the individual terrorizes and punishes himself. They may be expressed through nightmares, phobias, obsessions, or the reliving of painful memories and indiscretions. They indicate self-rejection.

4. **Physical manifestations.** These might include hypertension, psychosomatic illnesses, and the abuse of various substances, such as alcohol, drugs, tobacco, or food.

5. **Postponing decisions.** A high level of ambivalence or procrastination produces an increased sense of insecurity.

6. **Denying oneself pleasure.** The self-rejecting person feels the need to punish himself and expresses this through denying himself the things he finds desirable or pleasurable. This might be a career opportunity, a material object, or a desired relationship.

7. **Disturbed relationships.** The person may be cruel, demeaning, or exploitive with other people. This may be an overt or a passive-dependent pattern of relating, which indirectly exploits others. Another behavior included in this category is withdrawal or social isolation, which arises from feelings of worthlessness.

8. **Withdrawal from reality.** When anxiety resulting from self-rejection reaches severe or panic levels, the individual may dissociate and experience hallucinations, delusions, and feelings of suspicion, jealousy, or paranoia. Such withdrawal from reality may be a temporary coping mechanism or a long-term pattern indicating a profound problem of identity confusion.

9. **Self-destructiveness.** Self-hatred can be expressed through accident proneness or attempting dangerous feats. Extremely low levels of self-esteem can lead to the ultimate act of rejection, suicide.

10. **Other destructiveness.** People who have overwhelming consciences may choose to act out against society. This activity serves to paralyze their own self-hate and displaces or projects it on victims in their environment.

Indirect forms of self-hate complement and supplement the direct forms. They may be chronic patterns and difficult to change in therapy:

1. **Illusions and unrealistic goals.** Self-deception is the core element; the individual refuses to accept a limited here and now. Illusions increase the possibility of disappointment and further self-hate. The illusions or goals frequently involve money, love, power, prestige, marriage, sex, children, family, success, and parenthood. Examples of illusions are "If I were married, I would be happy" and "Money brings fulfillment." This indirect form of low self-esteem may make the person sensitive to criticism or overresponsive to flattery. It may also be evident in the defensive mechanisms of blaming others for one's failures and becoming hypercritical to create the illusion of superiority.

The individual may also attempt to compensate by expressing an exaggerated opinion of his ability. He may continually boast, brag of his prowess and exploits, or claim possession of extraordinary talents. An extreme compensatory behavior for low esteem is grandiose thinking and related delusions. Another example of unrealistic goals is evident in the perfectionist. Such individuals strain compulsively and unremittingly toward impossible goals and measure their own worth entirely in terms of productivity and accomplishment. The result of such striving, however, is often vulnerability to emotional turmoil and impaired productivity. This tendency may further serve as a predisposing factor toward the development or recurrence of depressive illnesses.

2. **Boredom.** This involves the rejection of one's possibilities and capabilities. The individual may neglect or reject aspects of himself that have great potential for future growth.

3. **Polarizing view of life.** In this case the individual has a simplistic view of life in which everything is worst or best, wrong or right. He tends to have a closed belief system that acts as a defense against a threatening world. Ultimately this view of life will lead to confusion, disappointment, and alienation from others.

The behaviors associated with low self-esteem are described in Clinical example 13-1 and are summarized in the box on page 387.

In this clinical example, Mrs. G's favorable perception of self was closely related to her ability to work. Her retirement created role changes difficult to adapt to. This example points out the close relationship between feelings of low self-esteem and role strain. The situation was further compounded by her husband's retirement. Mrs. G's feelings of low self-esteem were evident in her self-criticism, refusal to recognize her own strengths, worrying, physical complaints, reduced social contacts, and unrealistic expectations of her family. Her diagnosis of major depressive episode was based on the severity of her feelings of self-depreciation, somatic problems, saddened emotional tone, history of losses, and absence of a manic episode.

Low self-esteem is also a major dynamic element of disturbed body image. Clinical example 13-2 illus-

Behaviors Associated with Low Self-Esteem

Criticism of self and/or others	Physical complaints
Decreased productivity	Polarizing view of life
Destructiveness toward others	Rejection of personal capabilities
Disruptions in relatedness	Self-derision
Exaggerated sense of self-importance	Self-destructiveness
Feelings of inadequacy	Self-diminution
Guilt	Social withdrawal
Irritability or excessive anger	Substance abuse
Negative feelings about one's body	Withdrawal from reality
Perceived role strain	Worrying
Pessimistic view of life	

trates the effect of the loss of a body part on a person's self-concept.

■ **ASSOCIATED WITH IDENTITY DIFFUSION.** The term "identity diffusion" was first used by Erikson to denote certain individuals' failure to integrate various childhood identifications into a harmonious adult psychosocial identity.[15] Individuals with identity diffusion manifest incompatible personality attributes. For example, they can exhibit both great tenderness and extreme indifference toward others. Other contradictory character traits that coexist include naivete and suspiciousness, greed and self-denial, and arrogance and timidity.[1]

Important behaviors that relate to identity diffusion include disruptions in relationships or problems of intimacy. The initial behavior may be withdrawal or distancing. If a person is experiencing an undefined identity, he may wish to ignore or destroy those people who threaten him. The problem is one of gaining intimacy, but it is reflected in isolation, denial, and withdrawal from others. Such patients lack the condition for normal empathy.

A contrasting behavior that may be evident is personality fusing. Erikson has pointed out that true intimacy involves a sense of mutuality, which implies a firm self-delineation of the partners and not a diffused merger of two people. If a person is struggling to cope with a weak or undefined identity, however, he may try to establish his sense of self by fusing or belonging to someone else. This may occur in formal relationships, intense friendships, or brief affairs, since each can be seen as a desperate attempt to outline one's own identity. This non-autonomous fusion, however,

leads to a further loss of identity. Some of these behaviors are evident in Clinical example 13-3.

Many of the behaviors displayed by Mrs. P reflect the problem of identity diffusion. She married at an early age before defining her own sense of self as an autonomous individual. Her only experience in a close relationship was with her husband, and she attempted to establish her own identity by living through his. Within the security of the marriage, she managed to avoid any self-analysis, but the impending separation brought forth her fears and self-doubts. She displayed a low level of self-esteem and an unresolved conflict between dependence and independence.

Personality fusion and problems with identity also have serious implications for the larger family system. Dysfunctional families are frequently characterized by a fusion of ego mass that may be evident in severe symptomatology by one or more family members. This may be expressed in some form of family violence or abuse (see Chapter 32) or in the scapegoating of one family member, who becomes the "diagnosed" or "symptomatic" psychiatric patient (see Chapter 29).

Identity diffusion can also be expressed as pathological narcissism, in which the individual has an exaggerated sense of self-importance manifested as extreme self-absorption. The person has an unrealistic idealized self based in illusion. He believes he has solved his search for identity, but his idealized notion of self reflects an alienation of his own being. In narcissism, according to Kernberg, "The normal tension between actual and ideal self . . . is eliminated by the building up of an inflated self-concept in which the actual self and ideal self . . . are confused."[24:238] Thus, unlike

CLINICAL EXAMPLE 13-1

Mrs. G was a 66-year-old woman admitted to the psychiatric hospital with a major depressive episode. She told the admitting nurse that "things have been building up for some time now" and she had been seeing a private psychiatrist for the past 6 months who suggested she enter the hospital. Mrs. G slowly recounted an extensive medical history with numerous gastrointestinal problems. These did not, however, significantly interfere with her functioning. She had been employed in a community college as a librarian until 18 months previously when she was forced to retire. Mrs. G said she had been married for 39 years and had two grown children who were married and lived out of state. Her husband worked as an accountant but had retired a month previously. She said that since her retirement she had felt "useless and lost and closed in by their apartment." She seldom left the apartment, however, and had lost contact with many of her friends. She said she worried a great deal about their financial situation, especially now that her husband was also retired. He has repeatedly reassured her that they have sufficient funds, but she cannot stop worrying about it. She said her children called her weekly, but she thought they did this only out of duty and were not "really interested" in her or her husband. She thought that if they did love her and were concerned about her, they would never have moved out of state.

Mrs. G said that she liked her job very much and thought she was good at it. A younger woman took her place at the library, and Mrs. G was very bitter when talking about her. She said that, little by little, this woman took over duties Mrs. G was responsible for and one day even cleaned out Mrs. G's desk and took it as her own. Since her retirement, she said "things have been going downhill steadily." She said she is not a good housewife and dislikes cooking. These tasks had become even more difficult since her husband retired because he is "always underfoot and criticizing what I do." In the past couple of weeks, she had had great difficulty sleeping, a decreased appetite, fatigue, and little interest in her personal appearance. She said it seemed that all she had to do was "wait around to die."

CLINICAL EXAMPLE 13-2

Mrs. M was a 29-year-old married woman admitted to the general hospital for a total hysterectomy. Her history was presented in a nursing care conference because she was making many demands and the head nurse noticed that many of the staff were avoiding caring for her. Mrs. M had been married for 2 years and did not have any children. It was observed that Mr. M seldom visited his wife, although she spoke to him over the phone almost daily. Mrs. M complained that she was unable to sleep at night and often rang for the nurses with apparently minor requests. She appeared to have established a relationship with one of the evening nurses who was able to describe some of Mrs. M's concerns.

Mrs. M appeared to have a severe level of anxiety about her hysterectomy. She feared the effect of the surgery on her sexual desires, attractiveness, and ability to have intercourse and respond to her husband. Without her reproductive organs she said she felt "inadequate and no longer like a woman." She said that she and her husband always planned on having children, and she wondered if her husband might leave her in the future. She also feared that having the hysterectomy would cause her to lose her beauty and youth.

When the nursing staff became aware of Mrs. M's many fears and concerns, they were better able to understand her behavior and plan nursing care. They discussed with her the physiological implications of a hysterectomy and encouraged her to verbalize her feelings. Mr. M was not aware of his wife's concerns, and the nursing staff supported open discussions between them. As the staff were able to identify Mrs. M's concerns, they realized that some of their previous avoidance behavior resulted from their own fears and discomfort. The female nurses had identified with her as a patient, and the hysterectomy, in some ways, threatened their own concepts of self, body integrity, and sexual identity.

the person with low self-esteem who keenly perceives the discrepancy between his actual self and self-ideal, the narcissist rejects the reality of who he is by subscribing to an idealized self. His resulting state of identity confusion may be characterized by fantasies of un-

limited success, an insatiable need for attention and admiration, exploitative relationships, feelings of entitlement, and lack of empathy for others.

An additional behavior is the lack of temporal continuity in oneself. The past, present, and future are not integrated into a smooth continuum of remembered, felt, and expected existence. Time is fragmented, and all real experience is confined to the present. This may be manifested as an inability to

CLINICAL EXAMPLE 13-3

Mrs. P was seen by a psychiatric nurse in the psychiatric outpatient department of a general hospital. She was a well-dressed 24-year-old woman who had numerous somatic complaints, including decreased appetite, frequent headaches, fatigue, and difficulty falling asleep. She reported she had no energy or interest in doing anything or being with people. She said she dreaded each day and felt abandoned and all alone.

She was married at the age of 17 to the only boy she ever dated in high school. He was 19 at the time and she "looked up to him tremendously." He established a successful career in the insurance business, and she stayed at home to care for the house. She described herself as "centering my whole world around him." Three months previously he had told her that he wanted a separation and suggested she begin making a new life for herself. He said he intended to move out of the house at the end of the present month, but Mrs. P said she hoped he would not do that when he saw how much she loved and needed him.

Mrs. P also described feelings of being unloved and unlovable. She said she "felt empty inside" and "didn't really know who she was." She complained about her appearance and expressed much fear about living alone, finding a job, and getting along with people, especially men.

make goals and to project into the future. Fragmentation is also evident in these patients' lack of authenticity and susceptibility to external influence. These experiences result in a sense of inner aloneness and emptiness. These should be distinguished from the feeling of loneliness that is alive with fantasies and emotions. In contrast, emptiness in this sense is a more deeply frightening and dehumanizing experience.

Individuals with identity diffusion display weak gender identity or more apparent gender confusion. They also lack an historical-cultural basis of identity and thus display a peculiar lack of ethnicity. This is evident in their sense of history, cultural norms, group affiliations, object choices, life-style, and child-rearing practices. A related behavior is the absence of an inner moral code or of any genuine inner value. These behaviors characteristic of identity diffusion are summarized in the box below.

■ **ASSOCIATED WITH DEPERSONALIZATION.** A more maladaptive response to problems in identity involving withdrawal from reality occurs when the individual experiences panic levels of anxiety. This panic state produces a blocking off of awareness, a collapse in reality testing, and feelings of depersonalization. Depersonalization is a feeling of unreality in which one is unable to distinguish between inner and outer stimuli. It is, in essence, a true alienation from oneself. The individual has great difficulty distinguishing self from others, and his body has an unreal or strange quality. Depersonalization is the subjective experience of the partial or total disruption of one's ego and the disintegration and disorganization of one's self-concept. Because of this, it is the most frightening of human experiences. It develops as an outcome of uncertainties in human relationships. The individual has a not-loved feeling and, as a result of his failure to be loved, he fails to love himself. Depersonalization serves as a defense, but it is destructive because it masks and immobilizes anxiety without diminishing its intensity. It can occur in a variety of clinical illnesses, including depression, schizophrenia, manic states, and organic brain syndromes, and it represents the advanced state of ego breakdown associated with psychotic states.

Behaviors Associated with Identity Diffusion

Absence of moral code
Contradictory personality traits
Exploitative interpersonal relationships
Feelings of emptiness
Fluctuating feelings about self
Gender confusion
High degree of anxiety

Inability to empathize with others
Lack of authenticity
Pathological narcissism
Problems of intimacy
Temporal fragmentation and discontinuity
Unrealistic idealized self

Many behaviors are associated with depersonalization. Primarily, the patient experiences feelings of estrangement as though he were hiding something from himself. He experiences a lack of inner continuity and sameness and feels as if life is happening *to* him rather than his living by his own initiative. The patient may say that the world appears queer, dreamlike, or frightening. He may experience a loss of identity and express confusion regarding his own sexuality. He may describe related feelings of insecurity, inferiority, frustration, fear, hate, shame, and a loss of self-respect and be unable to derive a sense of accomplishment from any activity.

In depersonalization there may be a loss of impulse control and an absence of feeling and emotion that is manifested in impersonality, stiffness, formality, and rigidity in social situations. The individual may become lifeless and lack spontaneity and animation. He may plod through each day in a state of numbness and may respond to situations ordinarily eliciting emotion without characteristic love, hate, anxiety, or guilt. A heightened sense of isolation may mark his interpersonal relationships. The individual may become increasingly passive, as shown by withdrawing from social contacts, failing to assert himself, losing interest in his surroundings, and allowing others to make decisions for him.

Another sign of depersonalization is a disturbance in the individual's perception of time and space. He may become disoriented and be unable to recognize events as pertaining to yesterday or tomorrow or to plan his activities with reference to a schedule. A disturbance of memory may be characterized by aphasia, amnesia, or memory distortion. His thinking and judgment may be impaired and may reflect great confusion and distortion or focus on trivial details. Problems in information processing may be evident in visual hallucinations, and disturbed interpersonal relationships may be reflected in delusions, auditory hallucinations, and incongruent or idiosyncratic communication.

A final common behavior associated with depersonalization is a confused or disturbed body image. The person may have a feeling of unreality about parts of his body. He may feel that his limbs are detached or that the size of his body parts is changed, or he is unable to tell where his body leaves off and the rest of the world begins. Some patients describe the feeling that they had stepped outside their bodies and were observing themselves as detached and foreign objects. The many behaviors associated with depersonalization are summarized in Table 13-1. Clinical example 13-4 may further clarify depersonalization.

This example and the previous discussion show that the various feelings and perceptions associated with depersonalization represent extreme defenses against threats to self that do not serve to alleviate the anxiety and may add to it because of the frightening experience. The patient views his own behavior as foreign and sees himself as a strong, unknown, and unpredictable being whom he does not recognize. As both a participant and a spectator, he observes himself with great fear, since he is unable to control his own impulses. He cannot completely escape the pain of self-awareness. He therefore disowns his behavior, feelings, thoughts, and body and becomes alienated from his true self.

TABLE 13-1

BEHAVIORS ASSOCIATED WITH DEPERSONALIZATION

Affective	Perceptual	Cognitive	Behavioral
Experiences loss of identity	Auditory and visual hallucinations	Confusion	Blunting of affect
Feelings of alienation from self	Confusion regarding one's sexuality	Disoriented to time	Emotional passivity and nonresponsiveness
Feelings of insecurity, inferiority, fear, shame	Difficulty distinguishing self from others	Distorted thinking	Incongruent or idiosyncratic communication
Feelings of unreality	Disturbed body image	Disturbance of memory	Lack of spontaneity and animation
Heightened sense of isolation	Experiences the world as dreamlike	Impaired judgment	Loss of impulse control
Lack of sense of inner continuity			Loss of initiative and decision-making ability
Unable to derive pleasure or a sense of accomplishment			Social withdrawal

CLINICAL EXAMPLE 13-4

Mr. S was a 40-year-old man with no history of psychiatric hospitalization. Two months before his present admission, he was severely burned while on the job in a steel-making plant. He received second- and third-degree burns over his face, hands, chest, and back, and was treated in the burn center of a large university hospital. Three days before he was to be discharged from the burn unit, he experienced a psychotic episode. He reported hearing voices telling him to kill himself, and he was unable to recall any events surrounding the accident that produced his burns. He said he "felt his arms were withering away and his eyes were falling into his skull." He was unable to change the dressing on his burns even though he had done this previously. When looking at his arms or chest, his face remained impassive and he showed no emotion. He began to talk continuously about returning to work but was unable to identify how long he had been out on sick leave or the amount of time recommended by his physician for recovery.

With the onset of these symptoms, he was transferred from the burn unit to the psychiatric unit of the hospital. He remained socially isolated on the unit and refused to participate in ward meetings and group activities. At times he would wander into other patients' rooms and take pieces of their clothing. He would later be seen wearing this clothing, and the staff would intervene to return it to its owner.

■ Coping mechanisms

Erikson identified the normative crisis of **identity confusion** as a normal phase of increased conflict occurring during adolescence that is characterized by a high growth potential.[15,16] The transitory stage of acute identity confusion poses the possible failure to achieve integration and continuity of one's self-images. Adolescents may appear excessively self-conscious because of their extreme self-doubt. They may also display a diffused time perspective, which consists of a sense of great urgency and also a loss of consideration for time as a dimension of living. They may feel very young and very old simultaneously and ambivalently hope and fear that change will come with time. These contradictory feelings may be displayed in a general slowing of activities, which reflects an underlying despair. A diffused sense of industry is also often present, evident in inability to concentrate on the work they are

supposed to be doing. This may be accompanied by a distaste for competition. Although they may be intelligent and previously successful in office work, schoolwork, and sports, adolescents may lose the capacity for work, exercise, and sociability.

■ **SHORT-TERM DEFENSES.** The identity crisis of adolescence is transitory and may be resolved in various ways. One can view these resolutions as either short-term or long-term ego-oriented coping mechanisms used to ward off the anxiety and uncertainty of identity confusion. Logan[26] has described the following four categories of short-term defenses:

- Activities that provide temporary escape from the identity crisis
- Activities that provide temporary substitute identities
- Activities that serve temporarily to strengthen or heighten a diffuse sense of self
- Activities that represent short-term attempts to make an identity out of meaninglessness and identity diffusion itself—that try to assert that the meaning of life is meaningless itself

The first category of temporary escape includes any of several activities that seem to provide intense immediate experiences. These experiences so overwhelm the senses that the issue of identity literally does not exist because one's entire being is taken up with "right now" sensations. Examples of this might include drug experiences, loud rock concerts, fast car and motorcycle riding, some forms of hard physical labor, exercise or sports, and even obsessive television watching.

The category of temporary substitute identity is derived from being a "joiner;" the identity of a club, group, team, movement, or gang may function as one's basis for self-definition. The individual temporarily adopts the group definition as his own identity in a type of totalistic devotion to the larger entity. The adolescent's need to join and "belong" makes him particularly vulnerable to being manipulated by various religious groups and political sects. Being a devoted "follower" and imitator of an idolized figure, such as guru, rock star, sect leader, or life-style rebel, can also provide a temporary substitute identity for those who may not actually "join" a group. Temporary substitute identities can also be obtained by playing a certain role within a group, such as clown, bully, or chauffeur, or by purchasing objects that are marketed with ready-made identities. Thus a certain type of cologne, make of car, or article of dress implies built-in personalities the person can adopt as his own.

The third category of defenses involves "putting

oneself up against something" to feel more intensely alive. This is evident in risk taking for its own sake, which creates a feeling of heroic bravado and notoriety. Competitive activities, such as sports, academic achievement, and popularity contests, can also fit into this category. The idea is that competition and comparison with an outsider more sharply define one's own sense of self. Another example of this is bigotry and prejudice. By adopting a bigoted stance toward some outgroup or scapegoat, one can temporarily strengthen one's own sense of esteem or ego integrity. Superpatriots, youth gangs, and cliques are all examples of this temporary defense.

The final category helps to explain the fads that adolescents indulge in with such fervor and that seem so meaningless to others. The sheer force of commitment to the fads is an attempt to transform them into something meaningful.

All these categories of short-term coping mechanisms overlap, which can compound the overall effect. Logan emphasizes this point in analyzing the problem of drug abuse and the powerful hold it has on some adolescents:

One may take drugs for the intense, immediate experience and the escape from worldly concerns into heightened sensations that they provide. The very acts of procuring, smuggling, selling, and taking drugs provide challenging risks of harm, arrest, and illness that may make one feel more daringly and rebelliously alive. The taking of drugs may also be the initiation ceremony for "joining," and the badge of membership for belonging to the group and life-style from which one derives a temporary identity. A sense of identity may also be derived from the role of freak, head, or pusher that one plays within the drug culture. The drug culture may also be a vehicle for bigotry and prejudice—the contemptuous "put-down" of the "straight" world for its narrow-minded rejection of drugs helping to boost the self-esteem of drug users. One might speculate that a kind of identity might be derived from the kind of "stuff" one habitually purchases and uses. Finally, one even might argue that drugs may be taken because of the faddish meaninglessness of the act—as a kind of final affirmation and flinging in the face of society that, yes, life is meaningless, so meaningless, in fact, that the drug-taker makes a career of meaninglessness.[26:506-507]

■ **LONG-TERM DEFENSES.** Any of these short-term defenses may develop into a long-term one that will be evident in maladaptive behavior. Other resolutions or long-term defenses are also possible for the adolescent. A positive resolution or adaptive response produces an integrated ego identity and unified self, as previously described. Another type of long-term resolution has been identified as **identity foreclosure**. This occurs when a young person adopts "ready made" the type of identity desired by his elders without really coming to terms with his own desires, aspirations, or potential. This is a less desirable long-term resolution, as is adopting a deviant or negative identity.

A **negative identity** is one that is at odds with the values and expectations of society. This choice of delinquent roles may be caused by pressing demands made on the adolescent by parents or significant others to adopt a particular self-definition. The individual may think his autonomy is in jeopardy, or he may not value social norms. He then attempts to define the self in a nonprescribed or antisocial manner. The choice of a negative identity represents an attempt to retain some mastery in a situation in which a positive identity does not seem possible or desirable. The person may be saying, "I would rather be somebody bad than nobody at all." Clinical example 13-5 describes the negative identity assumed by an adolescent with a medical diagnosis of "conduct disorder—undersocialized, aggressive."

Ken displays many of the behaviors characteristic of a negative identity. His actions seem to challenge the accepted activities of youth. The nurse working with Ken explored his underlying feelings and self-perceptions. Great anger with his father began to surface, and Ken was able to verbalize it. Because he was the only son, he believed he was competing with his father and had to live up to his father's ideals. Ken feared failing in trying to adopt a positive identity and resented the identity his father was trying to impose on him. He thought he had no part in defining it and that it did not represent his real self.

This example demonstrates that although identity confusion is a normative crisis of adolescence, the adoption of a negative identity can establish a maladaptive coping response that continues throughout life. Problems of identity diffusion also may emerge at any point during one's adult years.

■ **EGO DEFENSE MECHANISMS.** In later life, patients with alterations in self-concept may use a variety of defense mechanisms to protect themselves from confronting their own inadequacies. However maladaptive, the defenses represent attempted solutions to inner problems and perceived deficiencies. Typical ego defense mechanisms include fantasy, dissociation, isolation, projection, displacement, splitting, turning anger against the self, and acting out.

Other, more damaging compensatory mechanisms can also be used to protect the self-esteem of the individual.[33] When self-esteem is threatened, the individual chooses a behavior that will protect it. These include a variety of behaviors that may be characteristic of individual maladjustment of social deviance including the following:

Psychosis	Delinquency
Neurosis	Crime
Obesity	Drug use
Anorexia nervosa	Cult membership
Promiscuity	Rape
Chronic overworking	Family violence
Suicide	Incest

These are not adaptive coping responses, but they provide the individual with an excuse for failure. They are all a function of inferiority or lack of goal accomplishment. One's choice of the specific compensatory mechanism is shaped by one's early developmental experiences, family environment, life-style, peer network, and cultural norms.

 ## Nursing diagnosis

▪ Identifying nursing problems

An individual's self-concept is a critical aspect of his overall personality adjustment. Problems with self-concept are associated with feelings of anxiety, hostility, and guilt. These often create a circular, self-propagating process that ultimately results in maladaptive coping responses (Fig. 13-3).

Most individuals who express dissatisfaction with life, display deviant behavior, or have difficulty functioning in social or work situations have problems related to self-concept. The nature of the patient's problem, the degree of disruption, and his level of anxiety will be determined by the patient and nurse together on the basis of the behavioral or objective data the nurse has collected, as well as the patient's subjective responses and description. In completing an assessment, the nurse attempts to identify relevant stressors and link these to the problem the patient is experiencing related to self-concept.

A nursing diagnosis should specify the nature of the nursing problem, the relevant stressors, and the patient's maladaptive coping response. The primary NANDA nursing diagnoses related to alterations in self-concept are body image disturbance; self-esteem disturbance; role performance altered; and personal identity disturbance.

Examples of complete nursing diagnoses related to self-concept are presented in the box on page 395. However, alterations in self-concept affect all aspects of an individual's life. One would expect, therefore, that many additional nursing problems would be identified by the nurse. Nursing diagnoses related to the range of possible maladaptive responses of the patient are identified in Table 13-2.

CLINICAL EXAMPLE 13-5

Ken was a 17-year-old boy referred to the local community mental health center by his high-school nurse. She made the referral after attending a team conference at school concerning Ken's repeated behavioral problems. He had a history of aggressive and destructive behavior in school, poor peer relationships, and low academic performance. The school had suspended him on three occasions previously, and the result of the team conference was to expel him for the remainder of the school year.

Mr. P, a psychiatric nurse at the mental health center, established a contract to work with Ken and his family. He noted that Ken was an obese young man (112.5 kg [250 pounds]) who took little interest in his appearance. His dress was sloppy, his complexion unclean, and his hair oily. He sat slumped in the chair in a disinterested and slightly defiant posture.

As Ken talked about himself, he complained of many pressures he experienced in his part-time job at a local hardware store. He thought the work was too difficult and tiring and that he was qualified for better and more prestigious work. When asked for specifics, he could not identify another job in particular. He also expressed a great deal of harassment from his family. His mother and father had been married for 31 years, and he was the only child of the marriage. His mother worked part time at a bakery, and his father was recently retired from his job as a supervisor at a local utility company, where he was highly regarded.

Ken said that his father "always had things for me to do." He described how his father signed him up for various team sports—baseball, basketball, football—without acknowledging how much Ken hated sports and how uncoordinated he was. His father also stressed good grades and "the necessity of college" for success in life. Ken described his mother as passive and polite and said he had little respect for her. He said his aggressive outbursts occurred both at home and at school—whenever he was frustrated. People reacted by staying out of his way. He said he never hurt anyone with his temper. He mostly destroyed property and objects.

Ken avoided the subject of peers but, when asked about friends, said he "hung out with" a couple of boys in the neighborhood. They were older than he was. Most had dropped out of high school and were employed in odd jobs. He denied drug use but said they drank heavily, especially on the weekends. He said he had no girlfriends and "wasn't interested in complicating my life with some broad."

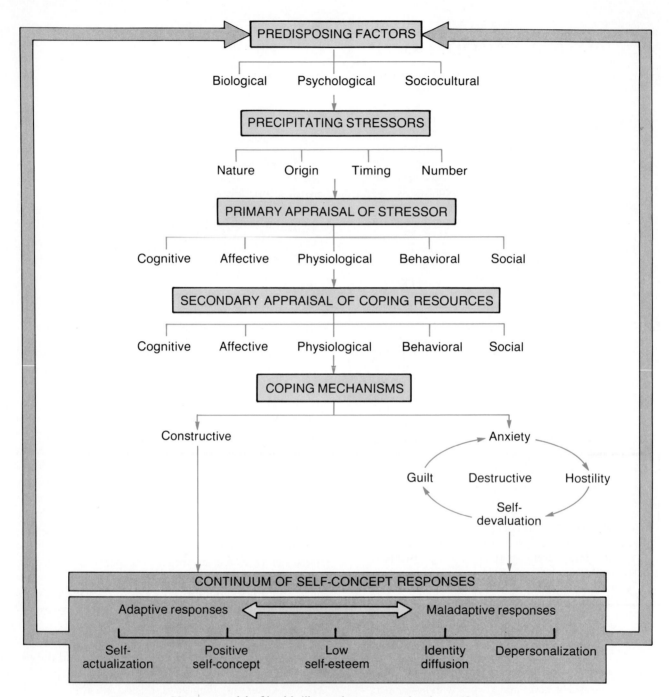

Fig. 13-3. Nursing model of health-illness phenomena related to self-concept responses.

■ Related medical diagnoses

In practice, maladaptive responses indicating alterations in self-concept can be seen in a variety of people experiencing threats to their physical integrity or self-system. This nursing diagnosis is not limited to the psychiatric setting, and it does not have a discrete category of medical diagnoses associated with it. Because it pertains to one's basic personality structure and feelings about oneself, this nursing diagnosis can emerge with many neurotic and psychotic disorders. Potentially, it could be related to all the diagnostic categories identified in the DSM-III-R[2] since the psychodynamics of all these disorders ultimately reflect on one's view of self. Several specific medical diagnoses deserve

Nursing Diagnoses Related to Self-Concept

Primary NANDA nursing diagnoses

Body image disturbance; self-esteem disturbance; role performance, altered; personal identity disturbance

Examples of complete nursing diagnoses

Body image disturbance related to fear of becoming obese, evidenced by refusal to maintain body weight at normal limits

Body image disturbance related to leukemia-chemotherapy, evidenced by negative feelings about one's body

Body image disturbance related to cerebrovascular accident, evidenced by lack of acceptance of body limitations

Self-esteem disturbance related to death of spouse, evidenced by withdrawal from others and feelings of hopelessness

Self-esteem disturbance related to overly high self-ideals, evidenced by depressed mood and withdrawal from activities

Role performance, altered, related to incompatibility of newly assumed work and family roles, evidenced by self-criticism and feelings of inadequacy

Role performance, altered, related to incongruency of cultural and self role expectations about aging, evidenced by feelings of frustration and criticism of others

Personal identity disturbance related to unrealistic parental expectations, evidenced by running away from home

Personal identity disturbance related to drug toxicity, evidenced by confusion and loss of impulse control

---

TABLE 13-2

MEDICAL AND NURSING DIAGNOSES RELATED TO SELF-CONCEPT

Medical Diagnostic Class	Psychiatric Nursing Diagnostic Class
Dissociative disorders	Alterations in self-concept
Personality disorders	

Related Medical Diagnoses (DSM-III-R)*	Related Nursing Diagnoses (NANDA)
Multiple personality disorder	Adjustment, impaired
Psychogenic fugue	Anxiety
Psychogenic amnesia	†Body image disturbance
Depersonalization disorder	Communication, impaired verbal
Dissociative disorder NOS	Coping, ineffective individual
Narcissistic personality disorder	Grieving, dysfunctional
Borderline personality disorder	Hopelessness
Anorexia nervosa	†Personal identity disturbance
Bulimia nervosa	Powerlessness
	†Role performance, altered
	Self-care deficit
	†Self-esteem disturbance
	Sensory-perceptual alteration
	Sexuality patterns, altered
	Social interaction, impaired
	Social isolation
	Spiritual distress
	Thought processes, altered
	Violence, potential for

*From American Psychiatric Association: Diagnostic and Statistical Manual of Mental Disorder, Third Edition–Revised, Washington D.C., 1987, The Association.
†Indicates primary nursing diagnoses for alterations in self-concept.

particular attention, however, since their dominant features include alterations in self-concept. They are listed in Table 13-2 and are now briefly described.[2]

■ **MULTIPLE PERSONALITY.** The essential feature is the existence within the individual of two or more distinct personalities or personality states. Each personality has a full or almost full range of mental functions, each with its own pattern of perceiving, relating to, and thinking about the environment and one's self. Each personality state at some time takes full control of the individual's behavior, and the transition from one to the other is sudden. Amnesic barriers are found between one personality and another.

■ **PSYCHOGENIC FUGUE.** The essential feature of psychogenic fugue is sudden, unexpected travel away from home or one's customary place of work, with an inability to recall one's past. A partial or complete new identity is assumed, and the patient is unaware that he has forgotten anything.

■ **PSYCHOGENIC AMNESIA.** The essential feature of psychogenic amnesia includes a temporary disturbance in the ability to recall important personal information that is too extensive to be explained by ordinary forgetfulness. It typically has a sudden onset and is the most common dissociative disorder.

■ **DEPERSONALIZATION DISORDER.** The essential feature of depersonalization disorder is an alteration in the perception or experience of the self, with loss of one's own sense of reality and associated changes in body image. All a person's mental operations and behavior may become alien to him. The person loses the capacity to express emotions, and feelings of unreality and strangeness invade his perceptions of the objects and people around him.

■ **DISSOCIATIVE DISORDER NOS.** This residual category is used for disorders in which the predominant feature is a dissociative symptom that does not meet the criteria for a specific dissociative disorder.

■ **NARCISSISTIC PERSONALITY DISORDER.** The essential feature of narcissism is excessive self-involvement, hypersensitivity to the evaluation of others, and lack of empathy. The person has a grandiose sense of self-importance, demands constant attention, and takes advantage of others to achieve his own ends.

■ **BORDERLINE PERSONALITY DISORDER.** The essential feature is instability of mood, interpersonal relationships, and self-image. The person with a borderline disorder shows an extreme, persistent lack of a consistent sense of identity, recurrent suicidal threats and self-destructive acts, and problems expressing anger and impulse control. Interpersonal relationships are exploitive and characterized by manipulation and splitting, with intense shifts between the extremes

of overidealization and devaluation. This disorder has received greater attention recently because of the challenge it presents to the psychiatric clinician.

■ **ANOREXIA NERVOSA.** The essential features are refusal to maintain body weight over a minimal normal weight for age and height; an intense fear of gaining weight or becoming fat, even though underweight; a distorted body image; and amenorrhea in females.

■ **BULIMIA NERVOSA.** The essential features are recurrent episodes of binge eating (the rapid consumption of a large amount of food in a discrete period of time); a feeling of lack of control over eating behavior during the eating binges; self-induced vomiting, use of laxatives or diuretics, strict dieting or fasting, or vigorous exercise in order to prevent weight gain; and persistent overconcern with body shape and weight. In order to qualify for the diagnosis, the person must have had, on average, a minimum of two binge eating episodes a week for at least 3 months.

❧ Planning and implementation

■ Goal setting

Research indicates that patients with negative self-concepts believe their illnesses have a greater negative effect on their lives, have less hope and optimism about the future, and are more anxious about their illnesses. These findings support the need for effective nursing intervention related to problems with self-concept.

The general goal of the nursing intervention is to facilitate the person's self-actualization by helping him grow, develop, and realize his potential while compensating for his impairments. The nurse's focus is to help the individual understand himself more fully and accurately so he can direct his own life in a more satisfying way. In a sense, nursing intervention concerns all that is involved in promoting the patient's self-realization. This means helping him strive toward a clearer, deeper experience of his feelings, wishes, and beliefs; toward a greater ability to tap his resources and use them for constructive ends; and toward a clearer perception of his direction in life, assuming responsibility for himself and his decisions. It involves replacing repression with consciousness and unreality with reality. Sustaining, protecting, and enhancing the self results in increased self-esteem and self-acceptance, the essence of personality integration. A positive therapeutic outcome results in greater self-direction, tolerance, flexibility, and risk taking. A reorganization of the self results in a change in behavior, the outcome of alterations in the concept of the self.

Self-awareness is a crucial aspect in bringing about changes in self-concept, but people usually spend little time in introspection. Certain conditions or events, however, do stimulate self-awareness. This may occur when stimuli from the body are intensified, as in states of pain, fatigue, or anger, or when stimuli from the environment are decreased, as in sensory deprivation or states of isolation. Self-awareness may be triggered when something unexpected or extraordinary takes place, when the person has succeeded well or failed miserably, or when the person is confronted with himself by looking in a mirror, listening to his voice on a tape recorder, or reading an old letter. Special occasions, such as birthdays, anniversaries, New Year's Eve, or a death may stimulate introspection. It may also be initiated when others direct their attention to the person through conversation or touch.

Once the person begins to look at and analyze himself, changes in the self become possible. Frequently they are the result of feelings of failure, unhappiness, anxiety, inadequacy, doubt or perplexity, or perceived discrepancies between one's concept of self and the demands of the environment or the expectations of others. Usually changes in the self occur only as a result of experiences and occur gradually. Occasionally, however, a change may take place suddenly. A traumatic experience may force a person to face that he is inadequate or out of step with his peers and that something drastic must be done.

The nurse should take all these factors into consideration when planning nursing care. An example of a short nursing care plan is presented in Fig. 13-4. Since the goal is to increase the patient's self-realization and acceptance, he must be an active participant in the formulation and implementation of plans. The nurse therefore must move with the patient and assess his readiness for growth within the therapeutic relationship. Together they formulate long-term goals that should reflect a positive resolution of the problem and of the stressor identified in the nursing diagnosis. Short-term goals should be as clear and explicit as possible. They should identify realistic steps that the patient can accomplish. In this way the patient's self-confidence will increase, and this will directly affect his feelings of self-esteem. These goals should emphasize his strengths instead of his pathological condition. If they are mutually identified, they will serve to motivate the patient and help him assume increased responsibility for his own behavior. Following are examples of goals related to role performance:

Long-term

Mrs. P will resolve role conflict by achieving greater congruency between work and family roles.

Short-term

After 1 week:

1. Mrs. P will describe her responsibilities in both her work and home roles.
2. She will identify aspects of these roles that provide her with satisfaction.
3. She will identify areas of role incompatibility.

After 2 weeks:

1. She will describe three alternative ways of increasing the complementarity of the roles.
2. She will discuss the advantages and disadvantages of each alternative.

After 3 weeks:

1. Mrs. P will take the necessary measures to implement one of the previous alternatives.

Following are examples of goals related to body image disturbance:

Long-term
Mr. B will accept his modified body image after treatment with chemotherapy for leukemia.
Short-term
After the first phase of chemotherapy:

1. Mr. B will identify the medications he is receiving.
2. He will describe the effect they have on his illness and related body systems.
3. He will express his feelings (e.g., anger, sadness) about his illness and therapy.
4. He will identify three positive aspects of his modified body image.

■ **Intervening in alterations in self-concept**

The mutually identified goals can be reached by a problem-solving approach that focuses primarily on the present, removes much of the responsibility from the nurse, and actively engages the patient in working on his difficulties. This approach increases the patient's self-confidence and self-esteem. It requires that the patient first develop **insight** into his problems and life situation and then take **action** to effect lasting behavioral changes. The nurse must thus incorporate both the responsive dimensions (insight oriented) and the action dimensions (action oriented) of the therapeutic relationship described in Chapter 4.

The focus of this approach is on the patient's cognitive appraisal of his life, which may contain faulty perceptions, beliefs, and convictions. His awareness of his feelings and emotions is also important, since they may be subject to misconceptions that arise from the acceptance of his cognitive analysis. Often the patient's display of affect is a clue to significant problem areas.

PSYCHIATRIC NURSING CARE PLAN

Precautions: Special nursing needs:
Evaluate for suicidal risk   Supportive limit setting
_____   Adherence to behavioral contract
_____   Monitoring of bathroom activities

Visitors: { } No restrictions   Telephone: {x} Limited
          {x} Family only   { } Unlimited
          { } Restricted to:

          { } No visitors

Privileges: { } Restricted to unit
            {x} Off unit accompanied by staff
            { } Off unit accompanied by family/visitor
            { } Off unit unaccompanied
            { } Out of hospital leave (dates) _____

Assessment data summary: First admission; 7 year history of eating disorders; one suicide attempt 2 years ago; separated from husband; attending college; conflictual relationship with parents but close to sister; history of poor compliance with treatment plan; alternately expresses anger, sadness, arrogance, and contempt for others.

Nursing diagnoses: 1. Self-esteem disturbance related to unrealistic self-expectations evidenced by feelings of guilt and negative verbalizations. 2. Body image disturbance related to fear of becoming obese evidenced by binging and self-induced vomiting. 3. Altered nutrition, less than body requirements related to fasting and vomiting evidenced by recent weight loss. 4. Impaired social interaction related to her view of others as all good or all bad evidenced in her lack of supportive relationships.

Treatment goal: Expanded self-awareness and self-evaluation that promotes self-esteem and adaptive coping responses.

Date	Problem/need	Expected outcome (objective)	Target Date	Nursing Intervention
9-11-90	Unrealistic expecta-tions of self/others	Intregration of positive and negative aspects of self	9-25-90	Elicit perceptions of self strengths and weaknesses. Identify faulty beliefs, misperceptions, and unfounded criticisms.
9-11-90	Lack of control over eating behavior	Elimination of binging and purging activities	9-30-90	Provide nutrition education. Assist in setting realistic goals. Help patient identify sources of stress. Explore alternative coping mechanisms.

| Room 305 | Patient's name Ms. T | Age 24 | Doctor Dr. R | Primary nurse Ms. P | Admit date 9-10-90 |

Fig. 13-4. Sample nursing care plan for a patient with bulimia. (This nursing care plan includes examples of the elements of a total plan as it might appear at a particular time in the patient's course of treatment. It should not be considered all inclusive.)

Date	Medications	Date	P.R.N. Medications	Diagnostic & psychiatric tests	Req.	Done
9-10-90	Fluoxetine					
	20 mg. qd in					
	AM					

		Date	Treatments	Special orders and concerns		
		9-10-90	Daily weight	Daily meal planning with dietician		
			Daily I/O	Maintain observation of patient		
				during meals / 1 hour following		

Allergies:	Medical diagnosis: (axis I-III)	Diet:
None	Bulimia nervosa (Axis I) Borderline Personality Disorder (Axis II)	(See special orders)

Fig. 13-4, cont'd. Sample nursing care plan for a patient with bulimia.

Only after examining his cognitive appraisal of the situation and related feelings can he gain insight into the problem and bring about behavioral change. Adaptive behavior is based both on insight and on carrying out the solution to the initial problem.

Therefore one can describe principles of nursing care that are applicable to the various problems with self-concept. These principles are incorporated here within a problem-solving approach and are presented as progressive levels in the sequence in which they occur. They focus primarily on the level of the individual. They may, however, be implemented in conjunction with group- or family-level interventions, and the nurse is expected to include the patient's family, significant others, and community supports whenever possible. Such a mobilization of the patient's coping resources can have both preventive and curative effects.

■ **LEVEL 1—EXPANDED SELF-AWARENESS.** A consistent picture of the self is necessary for security; to avoid anxiety, most people resist change. The ego resists change as a threat to its stability and integration. Furthermore, the closer a deviant perception of the self is to the core of the self-concept, the more difficult it is to change. In general, change in the self is easier when threat is absent. Threat forces a person to defend himself; perceptions are narrowed, and the person has difficulty forming new perceptions of himself.

To expand the patient's self-awareness and reduce the element of threat, the nurse should adopt an accepting attitude. Acceptance allows the patient the security and freedom to examine all aspects of himself as a total human being with positive and negative qualities. The basis of a therapeutic relationship will be established by listening to the patient with understanding, responding nonjudgmentally, expressing genuine interest, and conveying a sense of caring and sincerity. Creating a climate of acceptance allows previously denied experiences to be brought into consciousness and explored. This broadens the patient's concept of self and helps him to accept all aspects of his personality. It also indicates to him that he is a valued individual who is responsible for himself and is able to help himself. This is important because the nurse must work through whatever ego strength the patient possesses. To the extent that a person has certain elements of ego strength—the capacity for self-control, some adeptness at reality testing, and a degree of ego integration—there is a foundation on which to build.

Most patients seen in clinics, the general hospital, and the community setting possess considerable ego strength. Hospitalized individuals, however, might have limited ego resources with which to work. Psychotic patients experiencing depersonalization and identity confusion often present difficult challenges for the nurse. They tend to isolate themselves and withdraw from reality, so little ego strength is available for problem solving. For this type of patient, expanding self-awareness means first confirming the patient's identity. The nurse should attempt to provide supportive measures to decrease the panic level experienced by this patient. Her nursing will be more active while exerting less pressure. Additional interventions related to anxiety and psychotic states are described in Chapters 11 and 16.

The nurse can spend time with the patient in an undemanding way and approach him nonaggressively. Initially she may accept his need to remain nonverbal or attempt to clarify and understand his verbal communication even though it may be distorted or lack apparent logic. She should prevent him from isolating himself and establish a simple routine for him. If the patient displays bizarre behavior, such as inappropriate laughing or mannerisms, she can set limits on his behavior. It is important to orient him frequently to reality and reinforce appropriate behavior.

The patient should be helped to increase the activities that provide positive experiences for him. This may involve the use of occupational therapy, recreational therapy, or activity groups because success at tasks and increased involvement with objects can increase self-esteem. Movement therapy or body ego technique provides a goal-directed way to develop identity, body image, and ego structure. It is predominantly a nonverbal therapy because the emphasis is on movement and not on what the person says.

Depersonalization often leads to poor hygiene and an unkempt personal appearance. The nurse who is aware of her own value system regarding cleanliness and grooming can assist the patient unable to care for himself. She can use patience and repetition to establish health routines and can kindly but firmly encourage the patient to care for himself. By her verbal and nonverbal messages, she can encourage the patient to take pride in his appearance and reinforce any progress made. Another possible nursing intervention is photographic self-image confrontation. This involves taking photographs of the patient and discussing them with him. Spire[32] found that this intervention produced positive behavioral changes with schizophrenic patients and provided a means for establishing a nurse-patient relationship and mutually exploring some aspects of the self.

Mutuality is often difficult to establish with a pa-

tient experiencing depersonalization. Initially the nurse will determine appropriate activities and incorporate the patient into them without asking for a response. Gradually, however, the nurse can expect greater participation and can involve the patient in decision making. Table 13-3 summarizes the nursing interventions appropriate to level 1.

Sometimes the nurse's attitude or behavior can block the patient from expanding his self-awareness. This can be in the form of criticism, belittlement, condemnation, condescension, indifference, or insincerity. An impersonal attitude or ignoring the patient can decrease his self-esteem. Excessive demands or direct challenges to self-concept can result in his further withdrawal. The nurse should not allow him to remain alone or inactive, attempt to shame him into improving his habits, or assume total care for him. If she avoids these behaviors and strives for acceptance, she removes herself as a source of threat and encourages the patient to lower his defenses. He is then prepared to undertake the next step in problem solving.

■ **LEVEL 2—SELF-EXPLORATION.** At this level of intervention the nurse encourages the patient to examine his feelings, behavior, beliefs, and thoughts, particularly in relationship to the current stressful situation. The patient's feelings may be expressed verbally, nonverbally, symbolically, or directly. Acceptance continues to be important because when the nurse accepts the patient's feelings and thoughts, she is helping him to accept them as well. The nurse should facilitate the expression of strong emotions, such as anger, sadness, and guilt. In a sense, the patient's emotions or affect serve as clues to inner thoughts and current behavior.

As the patient is helped to focus his attention on the meaning that experiences have for him, he is clarifying his perceptions and concept of himself and his relationship to the people and events around him. The nurse can elicit his perception of strengths and weaknesses and have him describe his self-ideal. He can be made aware of his self-criticisms. Frequently, recognition in itself is a powerful therapeutic tool that motivates the patient to change. Jourard[23] has noted that many patients will experience a reduction in anxiety following the experience of full self-disclosure to an interested nurse. He believes patients withhold self-disclosure because of anxiety and the belief that no one is really interested in them.

It is important for the nurse to accept and deal with his or her own feelings before becoming involved in the self-exploration of others. Self-awareness will limit the potential negative effects of countertransference in the relationship. It will also allow the nurse the freedom to manifest authentic behavior that, in turn,

TABLE 13-3

SUMMARY OF NURSING INTERVENTIONS IN ALTERATIONS IN SELF-CONCEPT AT LEVEL 1

Goal—Expand the patient's self-awareness

Principle	Rationale	Nursing interventions
Establish an open, trusting relationship	Reduces the threat that the nurse poses to the patient and helps him to broaden and accept all aspects of his personality	Offer unconditional acceptance Listen to the patient Encourage discussion of his thoughts and feelings Respond nonjudgmentally Convey to the patient that he is a valued individual who is responsible for himself and able to help himself
Work with whatever ego strength the patient possesses	Some degree of ego strength, such as the capacity for reality testing, self-control, or a degree of ego intragration, is needed as a foundation for later nursing care	Identify the ego strength possessed by the patient Guidelines for the patient with limited ego resources are as follows: 1. Begin by confirming his identity 2. Provide support measures to reduce his panic level of anxiety 3. Approach him in an undemanding way 4. Accept and attempt to clarify any verbal or nonverbal communication 5. Prevent him from isolating himself 6. Establish a simple routine for him 7. Set limits on inappropriate behavior 8. Orient him to reality 9. Reinforce appropriate behavior 10. Gradually increase activities and tasks that provide positive experiences for him 11. Assist him in personal hygiene and grooming 12. Encourage the patient to care for himself
Maximize the patient's participation in the therapeutic relationship	Mutuality is necessary for the patient to assume ultimate responsibility for his own behavior and maladaptive coping responses	Gradually increase the patient's participation in decisions that affect his care Convey to the patient that he is a responsible individual

can be elicited and reinforced in the patient. Often patients will experience great difficulty in discussing or describing their feelings, possibly because society tends to discourage self-revelation or because the patient is honestly out of touch with his inner self. In this case the nurse can use himself or herself therapeutically by sharing feelings, verbalizing how he or she might feel in the situation, or mirroring his or her perception of the patient's feelings. In this way the nurse can help the patient explore his maladaptive thinking, including:

- Catastrophizing—the tendency to think the worst about what will happen in the future
- Minimizing and maximizing—the tendency to minimize the positive and magnify the negative

- Black-and-white thinking—the tendency to see things as belonging to one of two extremes without any middle ground
- Overgeneralization—the tendency to believe that since something happened once, it will always happen
- Self-reference—the tendency to believe that everyone is concerned with his thoughts and actions and is particularly aware of his mistakes
- Filtering—the process of supporting one's beliefs by selectively pulling certain details out of context and neglecting other more positive facts[15]

The nurse can facilitate the patient's thinking by using reflection to paraphrase and sharpen the meanings in the patient's discussion. Validation and empathic responses are essential to guide the patient to the next level of nursing intervention. In all these ways the nurse provides encouragement, since most patients have strong tendencies to avoid thinking and talking about disturbing problems. In addition, the nurse's reflections or clarifications of meaning help the patient to perceive more precisely what he has been discussing. Verbalized thoughts that the nurse responds to often become more concrete and tangible. Reflected responses can also provide subtle guides because they often emphasize verbal content whose significance may have escaped the patient's attention.

The nurse must be careful not to reinforce the patient's self-pity by responding with sympathy. Patients frequently disclaim any personal responsibility for their "plight," and they fail to see how their own behavior precipitates the problem about which they complain. Examples include patients who seek treatment because of things that happened *to* them, such as their wife left them, their husband beats them, or their boss fired them, and patients who seek help because of things that have *not* happened, such as not being happy or not having friends. These patients fail to see that they have a choice in life and that personal growth and satisfaction involve both risk and responsibility.

The nurse can clarify with the patient that he is not helpless or powerless. He is powerless when he sees himself as such and gives up control and responsibility for his behavior. Each person is responsible for his own behavior, including the things he decides to do or not to do. One must also accept responsibility for logical consequences. Only if a patient fully understands the implications of his actions and the scope of his choices can he set goals, explore alternatives, and effect change.

In stressing the importance of behavior, the nurse helps the patient see that he chooses to behave in certain ways. If the patient projects his problems onto the environment, the nurse can discuss with him the difficulty in changing other people and instead explore the possibilities of changing his own self. This means helping the patient realize that when he says, "I can't," he really means "I don't want to." The nurse should not give the impression that he or she has the power to change a patient's life. That power lies with him alone. The nurse can, however, help him to maximize his strengths, use available resources, and see that there is more to life than being involved with misery and pain.

Self-exploration need not take place solely within the one-to-one relationship. Family sessions and group meetings can help clarify how the individual appears to others. These meetings can supplement the individual sessions with the patient, or similar nursing interventions can be applied within regular family therapy or group therapy. Regardless of the setting, the nurse collects information on the patient's thinking about himself, logical or illogical reasoning, and reported or observed reactions. Interventions at this level should see the patient progress from denying or attributing contradictory feelings to the external situation, and to realizing his own conflict in the particular situation, to recognizing a major conflict within himself (Table 13-4).

Patients with borderline personality disorder present particular challenges to the nurse in encouraging the patient's self-exploration. These patients display unsatisfactory interpersonal relationships, mood instability, suicide threats, and splitting, which is the failure to integrate and accept positive and negative aspects of oneself and others. Such behaviors reflect a variety of nursing care problems (see Chapters 14, 15, and 16), including issues related to low self-esteem and identity diffusion. In addition, one of the therapeutic dynamics is the active resistance of the patient to self-exploration and the development of insight.

Working with these patients can be very difficult and challenging for nursing staff. Nursing interventions should be organized around maintaining consistency and minimizing the patient's experience of fragmentation and anxiety. This requires an open communication and support system among staff members. Often, designating one staff member to work with the patient is helpful. A consistent nursing treatment approach is also essential to minimize the patient's success in undermining the efforts of the other staff. A matter-of-fact, consistent, nonpunitive approach allows these patients to assume a degree of control over their behavior. A behavioral contract with the patient can also be helpful in assuring a consistent nursing approach. Setting clearly defined limits for these patients is essential, while providing a supportive environment in which the patients are able to explore aspects of themselves is also important to successful nursing care.

■ **LEVEL 3—SELF-EVALUATION.** This level involves hard work for the patient as he critically examines his own behavior, accepts the consequences for it, and judges whether it is his best possible choice. At this point, the problem should be clearly defined, and the patient should be helped to understand that his beliefs influence both his feelings and his behavior. Only by actively and systematically challenging his faulty beliefs and perceptions can he hope for change. Previously identified misperceptions and distortions should be evaluated. Irrational beliefs, such as the following, should be identified and analyzed:

■ Everyone must love me.
■ I must be competent and adequate in all ways.

TABLE 13-4

SUMMARY OF NURSING INTERVENTIONS IN ALTERATIONS IN SELF-CONCEPT AT LEVEL 2

Goal—Encourage the patient's self-exploration

Principle	Rationale	Nursing interventions
Assist the patient to accept his own feelings and thoughts	When the nurse shows interest in and accepts the patient's feelings and thoughts, she is helping him to do so as well	Attend to and encourage the patient's expression of his emotions, beliefs, behavior, and thoughts—verbally, nonverbally, symbolically, or directly Use therapeutic communication skills and empathic responses Note his use of logical and illogical thinking and his reported and observed emotional responses.
Help the patient to clarify his concept of self and his relationship to others through self-disclosure	Self-disclosure and understanding one's self-perceptions are prerequisites to bringing about future change; this may, in itself, produce a reduction in anxiety	Elicit his perception of self-strengths and weaknesses Assist him to describe his self-ideal Identify his self-criticisms Help him to describe how he believes he relates to other people and events
Be aware and have control of your own feelings	Self-awareness allows the nurse to model authentic behavior and limits the potential negative effects of countertransference in the relationship	Openness to one's own feelings Acceptance of both positive and negative feelings Therapeutic use of self by: 1. Sharing one's own feelings with the patient 2. Verbalizing how another might have felt 3. Mirroring one's perception of the patient's feelings
Respond empathically, not sympathetically, emphasizing that the power to change lies with the patient	Sympathy can reinforce the patient's self-pity; rather, the nurse should communicate that the patient's life situation is subject to his own control	Use empathic responses and monitor oneself for feelings of sympathy or pity Reaffirm to the patient that he is not helpless or powerless in the face of his problems Convey verbally and behaviorally that the patient is responsible for his own behavior, including his choice of maladaptive or adaptive coping responses Discuss with him the scope of his choices, his areas of ego strength, and coping resources that are available to him Use the support systems of family and groups to facilitate the patient's self-exploration Assist the patient in recognizing the nature of his conflict and the maladaptive ways in which he tries to cope with it

- I am unable to control my own happiness and destiny.
- I should condemn myself for making mistakes.
- I am better off if I avoid responsibilities rather than trying to face them.
- I am controlled by my past and can never break free of it.

- If I worry about potential problems, my anxiety will prevent their occurrence.
- My life is a disaster if it doesn't work out exactly as I had planned.

The patient's hopelessness should be countered by exploring areas of realistic hope. It is important to point out the mature part of the patient's personality and contrast it to the childhood part that causes problems. The behaviors that interfere with effective functioning should be put in perspective; thus the patient can see that his maladaptive behavior is only a small part of his total personality.

Sometimes the patient is unable to identify any strengths, and few may be obvious to the nurse. This requires additional thinking. All people, no matter how disturbed their behavior, have some areas of personal strength. The nurse should examine:

1. Hobbies
2. Skills
3. School
4. Work
5. Character traits
6. Interpersonal skills
7. Personal qualities, such as loyalty and honesty
8. Appearance

As the nurse is able to see positive aspects of the individual, he or she should share them with the patient to expand his own awareness.

Success and failure must be placed in perspective. Failures occur every moment of every day and are a natural consequence of human activity. As long as people strive to achieve, they will frequently not reach their goals. The only way to avoid failure is to do absolutely nothing. Failure may be caused by one's own mistakes; it may be a result of lack of motivation; or it may result from circumstances beyond one's control. Whatever the reason, failure is the unavoidable outcome of human effort. The problem arises when individuals are labeled or label themselves as failures. This is illogical and potentially destructive. As an inherent aspect of life, failure should be viewed either as a neutral concept or a positive one for the learning experience it has provided, rather than a negative one. If such misperceptions and unrealistic goals can be changed to reflect reality more accurately, maladaptive behavior and feelings of self-depreciation are likely to be reduced.

Unrealistic self-ideals, dependency patterns, and denial are all potential areas that can be analyzed. The patient can be helped to realize that all behavior and coping responses have positive and negative consequences. Contrasts can be drawn between behavior that is destructive, inhibitory, or sabotaging and behavior that is productive, enhancing, or growth producing. The patient must see that he acts in self-defeating ways because some "payoff" or personal gain is in it for him. The drawbacks or disadvantages to the patient's maladaptive coping responses will probably be

well known to him. The payoffs, or secondary gains, may be more obscure and well repressed. Following are some frequently experienced payoffs[25]:

- Procrastination
- Avoiding risks
- Retreating from the present
- Evading responsibility for one's actions
- Avoiding working or having to change

More specific payoffs should be identified by the nurse and patient together, relative to his particular problem. For example, possible secondary gains from being obese include having people feel sorry for you, having an excuse for not dating or being married, being the focus of dieting attention, or being easily recognized and noticed when with other people. Possible secondary gains for an adult remaining dependent on his parents might include not having to make one's own decisions, having someone else to blame if things go wrong, being protected from risks and venturing out in the world, not establishing lasting intimate relationships, or not having to establish one's own identity, but rather adopting the values and goals of others. Such payoffs can be identified for each nursing diagnosis.

The nurse becomes more active at this level of intervention. He or she begins confronting, interpreting, persuading, and challenging. The goal is to increase the patient's objectivity in dealing with stressors. For example, the nurse can show the borderline patient that the negative and positive characteristics of people can be integrated. Thus the same person can nurture and gratify as well as anger and frustrate, since both negative and positive qualities coexist in the same person.

Various techniques may be used at this time. In interpretation and confrontation, the nurse offers information that the patient may not have or does not recognize as relevant. Supportive confrontation may be particularly effective in calling to the patient's attention inconsistencies in words and actions. The climate of acceptance established by the nurse in level 1 and the empathic communication developed in level 2 provide a basis for confrontation in level 3. This groundwork is necessary to prevent premature confrontation, which can be destructive.

The use of reflection allows the nurse to restate the meaning or emphasize the significance of the patient's revelations. It functions to inform the patient that the nurse understands what is being said, and it encourages him to continue his self-evaluation. Reflections and confrontations are often phrased in the form of questions, which can also encourage the patient to search for additional information. In this regard the questions should be specific and not overwhelming, which occurs when one repeatedly asks, "Why?" Suggestion can introduce alternative ways of thinking or behaving.

The nurse may use various aspects of role theory during this level of intervention. He or she may assist the patient in role clarification, which is the gaining of knowledge, information, and cues needed to perform a role. It involves identification of behaviors, clarification of expectations, and specification of goals relative to the role, taking into consideration the influence of significant others and the context of the situation. Role clarification therefore reduces the potential for or existence of role strain. The nurse can also encourage the patient to participate in any activity in which he can observe his own behavior. Role playing may be particularly effective in providing the patient with feedback and increasing his insight. Through it, he may be able to gain objectivity toward the irrationality and self-destructiveness of his self-criticisms.

The nurse-patient relationship provides a rich source of information for the patient. Within this relationship he is enacting and experiencing many of his problem areas, and the nurse can use this as a "study in miniature." He or she can assist the patient in observing how he reacts in the one-to-one situation and share reactions with him to give him feedback on how he affects others and openly disclose some of his or her own feelings about the patient's behavior. The analysis and use of transference and countertransference reactions comprise the nurse's "therapeutic use of self." When a block arises within the relationship or the nurse experiences increased anxiety, he or she should explore its meaning with the patient. The nurse should confront the problem and openly discuss it with him. This can also be done in family or group therapy sessions.

Psychodrama, a special form of group therapy, provides the patient with an additional opportunity to gain self-insight. In psychodrama the therapist organizes events so that the patient has an audience to whom he plays a role structured for him by the therapist. In this modality the audience acts as a standard against which the patient can judge the social adequacy of his own reactions and behavior.

During this level of intervention the patient and nurse critically evaluate his behavior (Table 13-5). Misperceptions, unrealistic goals, and distortions of reality are explored. This provides the patient with sufficient knowledge to progress to the next level of problem solving.

■ **LEVEL 4—REALISTIC PLANNING.** The nurse and patient are now ready to formulate possible solutions or alternatives. This begins by investigating what solutions were attempted in the past and evaluating their effectiveness. When inconsistent perceptions are held by the individual, he is faced with several choices. He can change his perceptions and beliefs to bring them closer to a reality that cannot be changed. Alternately, he may seek to change his environment to bring it in line with what he believes. When his behavior is not consistent with his self-concept, he can change his behavior, change the beliefs underlying his self-concept so that they include his behavior, or change his self-ideal while leaving his self-concept intact.

At this time, all possible solutions should be openly discussed with the patient. The nurse must be careful not to use his or her influence to persuade the patient to do anything that represents his or her values rather than the patient's. The nurse should help him conceptualize his goals. If they are within his reach, his efforts can be supported. If the patient has conflicting goals, the nurse helps him identify which are more realistic or obtainable by discussing emotional and practical consequences.

The nurse can work with the patient in various ways. The patient may be encouraged to give up superhuman standards by which he judges his behavior. These standards may set him up for failure and create a pathological cyclical pattern. Together they may work at destroying illusions not part of his authentic self. The patient may need to lower his self-ideal and limit his goals to what is humanly possible. He should be encouraged to renew involvement with life and enter new experiences for their growth potential.

Role rehearsal, role modeling, and role playing may be employed. In role rehearsal the person imagines how a particular situation might take place and how his role might evolve. He mentally enacts his role and tries to anticipate the responses of significant others. Role rehearsal is important in anticipating and planning the course of future action. Role modeling occurs when the individual observes someone else playing a certain role so that he is able to understand and emulate those behaviors. The person he observes may be the nurse, a family member, a group member, or a peer. The nurse can be important in assisting the patient in his role learning. He or she can model behavior that may be posing problems for the patient, such as expression of feelings, specific socialization skills, or realistic self-expectations. Proceeding one step further, the nurse and patient may role-play certain situations to conceptualize alternative solutions.

Visualization can also be used to enhance self-esteem through goal setting.[14] Through the conscious

---

TABLE 13-5

SUMMARY OF NURSING INTERVENTIONS IN ALTERATIONS IN SELF-CONCEPT AT LEVEL 3

Goal—Assist the patient's self-evaluation

Principle	Rationale	Nursing interventions
Help the patient to define the problem clearly	Only after the problem is accurately defined can alternative choices be proposed	Identify relevant stressors with the patient and his appraisal of them Clarify that the patient's beliefs influence both his feelings and behaviors Mutually identify faulty beliefs, misperceptions, distortions, illusions, and unrealistic goals Mutually identify areas of strength Place the concepts of success and failure in proper perspective Explore the patient's use of coping resources
Explore the patient's adaptive and maladaptive coping responses to his problem	It is then necessary to examine the coping choices the patient has made and evaluate both the positive and the negative consequences of them	Describe to the patient how all coping responses are freely chosen and have both positive and negative consequences Contrast adaptive and maladaptive responses Mutually identify the disadvantages of the patient's maladaptive coping responses Mutually identify the advantages or "payoffs" of the patient's maladaptive coping responses Discuss how these payoffs have perpetuated the maladaptive response Use a variety of therapeutic skills, such as the following: 1. Facilitative communication 2. Supportive confrontation 3. Role clarification 4. The transference and countertransference reactions occurring in the one-to-one relationship 5. Psychodrama

---

programming of desired change with positive images, expectations are molded. Strong, positive expectations can then become self-fulfilling. To use visualization, the nurse should:

1. Ask the patient to select a positive, specific goal, such as: "I will call a friend and suggest we go out together."
2. Help the patient to relax using a relaxation technique (see Chapter 11).
3. Have the patient repeat the goal phrase several times slowly.
4. Instruct the patient to close his eyes and visualize the goal written on a piece of paper.
5. Have the patient, while relaxed, imagine accomplishing the goal.

The patient should then describe how he feels when the desired goal is reached and how other people are responding to him. In this way the patient can be helped to gain positive control over his life.

Nursing actions at this level of intervention are summarized in Table 13-6. Ultimately, the patient should decide on a plan that includes a clear definition of the change to be achieved. Converting a "talking decision" into an "action decision" is the final, but most important, step.

■ **LEVEL 5—COMMITMENT TO ACTION.** The nurse assists the patient to become committed to his decision and then achieve his goals. The patient's development of self-awareness, self-understanding, and insight is not the ultimate desired outcome of the nursing therapeutic process. Insight alone does not make problems disappear or transform one's world in magical ways. Although a patient may have obtained a high level of insight, he may nevertheless continue to function at a minimum level. Such a patient may be

TABLE 13-6

SUMMARY OF NURSING INTERVENTIONS IN ALTERATIONS IN SELF-CONCEPT AT LEVEL 4

Goal—Assist the patient in formulating a realistic plan of action

Principle	Rationale	Nursing interventions
Help the patient identify alternative solutions	Only when all possible alternatives have been evaluated can change be affected	Help the patient understand that he can only change himself, not others If the patient holds inconsistent perceptions, help him to see that he can change the following: 1. His beliefs or ideals to bring them closer to reality 2. His environment to make it consistent with his beliefs If his self-concept is not consistent with his behavior, he can change the following: 3. His behavior to conform to his self-concept 4. The beliefs underlying his self-concept to include his behavior 5. His self-ideal Mutually review how coping resources may be better used by the patient
Help the patient conceptualize his own realistic goals	Goal setting that includes a clear definition of the expected change is necessary	Encourage the patient to formulate his own (not the nurse's) goals Mutually discuss the emotional, practical, and reality-based consequences of each goal Help the patient clearly define the concrete change to be made Encourage the patient to enter new experiences for their growth potential Use role rehearsal, role modeling, role playing, and visualization when appropriate

able intellectually to discuss with great ease the nature of his problem and the contributing influences, but the problem continues to be unresolved. Some patients actually use their insights to resist moving forward and avoid the hard work involved in making behavioral changes. The value of having the patient gain insight and increase his self-understanding is that he can gain perspective on why he behaves the way he does and what must be done to break maladaptive patterns.

Providing opportunity for the patient to experience success becomes essential at this time. To help him commit himself to his goal, the nurse can relate to the patient how he or she sees him, correcting his own poor self-image. In this mirroring technique, he or she can openly and honestly describe to the patient the healthy parts of his personality and how, by using these parts, he can achieve his goal. The nurse should reinforce his strengths or skills and provide him with opportunities to use them whenever possible.

Sometimes the lack of vocational or social skills may be a causative factor for low self-esteem. If so, nursing intervention can be directed toward gaining vocational assistance for the patient. Group involvement may be instrumental in raising self-esteem. The experience of being accepted by others, the sense of belonging and being important to others, and the opportunity to develop interpersonal competence can all enhance self-esteem.

Similarly, the family of origin is the source of most people's self-esteem. The key relationships for improving basic self-differentiation are those with parents and siblings, even in adulthood. These relationships involve the unresolved emotional fusion that influences many interactions. Adult contact with parents and siblings can correct misconceptions underlying low self-esteem and allow more positive beliefs. Learning to interact with family members with closeness, but without counterproductive forms of fusion and

TABLE 13-7

MENTAL HEALTH EDUCATION PLAN—FAMILY RELATIONSHIPS[8]

Content	Instructional activities	Evaluation
Define the concept of self-differentiation within one's own family of origin	Discuss the differences between high and low levels of self-differentiation Ask the patient to identify level of functioning among own family members	Patient identifies his functioning level in his family of origin
Describe the characteristics of emotional fusion, emotional cutoff, and triangulation	Analyze types and patterns of family relationships Use paper and pencil to diagram family patterns	Patient describes interactional patterns within his own family Patient identifies his own roles and behavior
Discuss the role of symptom formation and symptom bearer in a family	Sensitize the patient to family dynamics and manifestations of stress Encourage communication with family of origin	Patient recognizes family contribution to the stress of individual members Patient contacts family members
Describe a family genogram and show how it is constructed	Use a blackboard to map out a family genogram Assign family genogram at homework	Patient obtains factual information about own family Patient constructs family genogram
Analyze need for objectivity and responsibility for changing one's own behavior and not that of others	Role-play interactions with various family members Encourage testing out new ways of interacting with family members	Patient demonstrates a higher level of differentiation in family of origin

TABLE 13-8

SUMMARY OF NURSING INTERVENTIONS IN ALTERATIONS IN SELF-CONCEPT AT LEVEL 5

Goal—Assist the patient to become committed to his decision and achieve his own goals

Principle	Rationale	Nursing interventions
Help the patient take the necessary action to change maladaptive coping responses and maintain adaptive ones	The ultimate objective in promoting the patient's insight is to have him replace the maladaptive coping responses with more adaptive ones	Provide opportunity for the patient to experience success Reinforce the strengths, skills, and healthy aspects of the patient's personality Assist the patient in gaining the assistance he might need (vocational, financial, social services) Use groups to enhance the patient's self-esteem Promote the patient's self-differentiation in his family of origin Allow the patient sufficient time to change Provide the appropriate amount of support and positive reinforcement for the patient to help him maintain his progress

emotionality, can enable a more mature pattern to develop. Family relationships would therefore be an appropriate focus for patient education. A mental health education plan using Bowen's theory of family systems is presented in Table 13-7.[8] Chapter 29 has a more detailed discussion of family systems theory and family therapy.

At this point the individual needs much support and positive reinforcement in effecting and maintaining change. For many patients, this will mean breaking chronic behavior patterns and exposing themselves to real risk. A person must actively maintain the processes learned to avoid slipping back to the previous behavior. Doing this is difficult and requires that the patient build on the progress he has made in the other levels. Successful change is a continuing process of modifying not only one's behavior but one's environment to help ensure that the change to new ways of behaving is permanent. Otherwise a relapse will occur.

The nurse serves as a transition between the pain of the past and the positive gratification of the future. Both nurse and patient must allow sufficient time for change. A significant period may be required for patterns that developed over months or years to be broken and new ones established. The nurse's role now becomes less active and directive and more confirming of the value, potential, and accomplishments of the patient (Table 13-8).

 Evaluation

Problems with self-concept are prominent in many psychological disorders. Changes in self-concept are accompanied by greater self-realization and self-acceptance and lead to behavioral changes and improved personality adjustment. To evaluate the success or failure of the nursing care given in this area, each phase of the nursing process should be reviewed and analyzed by the nurse and patient.

The nurse's assessment should include both the objective and the observable behaviors as well as the subjective perceptions of the patient. Did the nurse explore the patient's strengths and weaknesses and elicit his self-ideal? Was information obtained on his body image, feelings of self-esteem, role satisfaction, and sense of identity? Did the nurse compare her responses to his behavior, and were any inconsistencies or contradictions identified? Was the nurse aware of his or her own affective response to the patient, and how did this affect his or her ability to be therapeutic?

Before formulating a nursing diagnosis, the nurse should have discussed with the patient his appraisal of stressful life events and the nature of the threat they

posed to him. Did they determine his level of anxiety, and was he able to express related feelings, such as hostility, sadness, or guilt? Were the therapeutic goals realistic, explicit, adequate, and efficient? Were the patient's coping resources well assessed and utilized?

The nurse should have adopted a problem-solving approach that placed responsibility for growth on the patient. The most fundamental nursing action should have been to create a climate of acceptance that confirmed the patient's identity and conveyed a sense of value or worth. In expanding the patient's self-awareness, how effective was the nurse in promoting full and pertinent self-disclosure? Was the patient able to listen more fully to himself and others? What behaviors or attitudes did the nurse display that prevented the patient from expanding his self-awareness? Was the nurse able to manifest authentic behavior in the relationship and share thoughts and reactions? What interventions were used, and which ones proved benefi-

DIRECTIONS FOR FUTURE RESEARCH

The following are some of the nursing research problems raised in Chapter 13 that merit further study by psychiatric nurses:

1. Nursing interventions that enable patients to facilitate a child's development of a positive self-concept
2. The relationship between role strain and nurse burnout
3. Educational strategies that will prepare mental health clinicians to recognize role strain and intervene in a health-promoting manner
4. Nursing interventions that assist the individual to recognize ego strengths and to build on existing strengths
5. Effective ways to promote positive self-esteem for individuals and groups in different life situations
6. The ability of mental health clinicians to recognize patient strengths
7. Exploration of the concept of empowerment as a self-enhancing nursing intervention
8. Nurses' awareness of role modeling as an intervention and their self-awareness relative to this concept
9. The correlation between nurses' and patients' perceptions of improvements in patients' self-concept
10. The relationship between the self-concept of the nurse and the effectiveness of interventions with patients experiencing self-concept alterations

cial—validation, reflection, confrontation, suggestion, role clarification, role playing? Did the nurse progress on the basis of the patient's readiness and motivation?

What was the outcome of the patient's cognitive analysis and exploration of feelings? Was he able to transfer his new perceptions into possible solutions or alternative behavior? How did the nurse help the patient implement his plans? What success did he experience? Did they both allow sufficient time for changes to occur?

The degree of overall success achieved through nursing care can be determined by eliciting the patient's perception of his own growth and comparing his behavior to the healthy personality described in this chapter. Not everyone will achieve all these characteristics, but success has been achieved if the patient's potential has been maximized.

■ SUGGESTED CROSS-REFERENCES ■

Definitions of mental health are discussed in Chapters 2 and 3. Therapeutic relationship skills are discussed in Chapter 4. Interventions with family and group support systems and other coping resources are discussed in Chapters 8 and 10. Interventions related to anxiety are discussed in Chapter 11. The relationship of role strain and low self-esteem to depression is discussed in Chapter 14. Self-destructive behaviors, including anorexia, obesity, and suicide, are discussed in Chapter 15. Nursing intervention in psychotic panic states is discussed in Chapter 16. Family therapy is discussed in Chapter 29. The family dysfunctions of violence and abuse are discussed in Chapter 32.

■ SUMMARY ■

1. Self-concept is defined as all the notions, beliefs, and convictions that constitute an individual's knowledge of himself and influence his relationships with others. One's self-concept is learned as a result of a person's unique experiences within himself, with significant others, and with the realities of the world.

2. Body image is the sum of the conscious and unconscious attitudes the individual has toward his body. It includes present and past perceptions, as well as feelings about size, function, appearance, and potential.

3. Self-ideal is the individual's perception of how he should behave based on certain personal standards, aspirations, goals, or values. Mental health is associated with a clear, realistic self-ideal and congruence between one's perception of self and his self-ideal.

4. Self-esteem is the individual's personal judgment of his own worth obtained by analyzing how well his behavior conforms to his self-ideal. High self-esteem is a feeling rooted in unconditional acceptance of self, despite mistakes, defeats, and failures, as an innately worthy and important being.

5. Roles are sets of socially expected behavior patterns associated with an individual's function in various social groups. Ascribed roles are assigned roles over which the person has no choice. Assumed roles are those selected or chosen by the person.

6. Identity is the organizing principle of the personality that accounts for the unity, continuity, consistency, and uniqueness of the individual. In connotes autonomy and includes perceptions of one's sexuality.

7. Individuals with positive self-concepts function more effectively, which is evident in interpersonal competence, intellectual efficiency, and environmental mastery. Negative self-concept is correlated with personal and social maladjustment.

8. Predisposing factors and precipitating stressors related to alterations in self-concept were identified and briefly described.

9. Data collection by the nurse should include objective and observable behaviors as well as the subjective and internal world of the patient.

10. Nursing diagnosis should specify the nature of the nursing problem, the related stressor, and the patient's maladaptive coping response. Nursing diagnoses associated with alterations in self-concept were presented and related to selected medical diagnoses.

11. The goal of nursing intervention is to facilitate the person's self-actualization by helping him grow, develop, and realize his potential while compensating for his impairments. Changes in the self occur only as a result of experiences and occur gradually.

12. Nursing intervention helps the patient examine his cognitive appraisal of the situation and his related feelings to help him gain insight and then take action to bring about behavioral change. This problem-solving approach includes the following levels of intervention: (a) expanded self-awareness, (b) self-exploration, (c) self-evaluation, (d) realistic planning, and (e) commitment to action. It can be used with individuals, families, or groups.

13. A climate of acceptance was noted to be of particular importance in broadening the patient's concept of himself, helping him to accept all aspects of his personality, and conveying that he is a valued individual responsible for and able to help himself. Confirming the patient's identity is particularly important with problems of identity confusion and depersonalization.

14. The nurse and patient together evaluate the success of the nursing care in each step of the nursing process. The degree of overall success can be determined by eliciting the patient's perception of his own growth and comparing his behavior to the characteristics of the healthy personality described in this chapter.

■ REFERENCES ■

1. Akhtar S: The syndrome of identity diffusion, Am J Psychiatry 141(11):1381, 1984.
2. American Psychiatric Association: Diagnostic and Statistical Manual of Mental Disorder, Third Edition—Re-

vised, Washington, DC, 1987, The Association.

3. Antonucci T and Jackson J: Physical health and self-esteem, Fam Community Health 6(2):1, 1983.

4. Austin J, Champion V, and Tzeng O: Cross-cultural relationships between self-concept and body image in high school boys, Arch Psych Nurs 3(4):234, 1989.

5. Bailyn L: Notes on the role of choice in the psychology of professional women. In Lifton R, editor: The woman in America, Boston, 1967, Beacon Press.

6. Berk S, Berk R, and Berheide C: The non-division of household labor. In Fisher A, editor: Women's worlds, NIMH Supported Research on Women, Rockville, Md, 1978, National Institute of Mental Health.

7. Biddle B: Role theory: expectations, identities, and behaviors, New York, 1979, Academic Press, Inc.

8. Bowen M: Family therapy in clinical practice, New York, 1978, Jason Aronson, Inc.

9. Broverman I et al: Sex-role stereotypes and clinical judgments of mental health, J Consult Clin Psychol 24:1, 1970.

10. Broverman I et al: Sex-role stereotypes: a current appraisal, J Soc Issues 28:59, 1972.

11. Bugenthal J: The search for existential identity, San Francisco, 1976, Jossey-Bass, Inc, Publishers.

12. Combs A and Snygg D: Individual behavior: a perceptual approach, New York, 1959, Harper & Row, Publishers, Inc.

13. Coopersmith S: The antecedents of self-esteem, San Francisco, 1967, WH Freeman & Co, Publishers.

14. Crouch M and Straub V: Enhancement of self-esteem in adults, Fam Community Health 6(2):65, 1983.

15. Erikson E: The problem of ego-identity, J Am Psychoanal Assoc 4:56, 1956.

16. Erikson E: Childhood and society, New York, 1963, WW Norton & Co, Inc.

17. Grove W and Tudor J: Adult sex roles and mental illness, Am J Sociol 78:812, 1973.

18. Hamachek D: Encounters with the self, New York, 1971, Holt, Rinehart & Winston, Inc.

19. Holahan C and Gilbert L: Interrole conflict for working women: careers versus jobs, J Appl Psychol 64:86, 1979.

20. Horney K: Neurosis and human growth, New York, 1950, WW Norton & Co, Inc.

21. Johnson C and Johnson F: Attitudes toward parenting in dual-career families, Am J Psychiatry 134:391, 1977.

22. Jourard S: Personal adjustment: an approach through the study of the healthy personality, New York, 1963, Macmillan, Inc.

23. Jourard S: The transparent self, New York, 1971, Litton Educational Publishing, Inc.

24. Kernberg O: Borderline conditions and pathological narcissism, New York, 1975, Jason Aronson, Inc.

25. Kottler J: Promoting self-understanding in counseling: a compromise between the insight and action-oriented approaches, J Psychiatr Nurs 17(12):18, 1979.

26. Logan R: Identity diffusion and psychosocial defense mechanisms, Adolescence 13(51):503, 1978.

27. Maslow A: Motivation and personality, New York, ed 2, 1970, Harper & Row, Publishers, Inc.

28. Meier E: An inquiry into the concepts of ego identity and identity diffusion, Soc Casework 13:63, 1964.

29. Meleis A: Role insufficiency and role supplementation: a conceptual framework, Nurs Res 24:264, 1975.

30. Norris C: The professional nurse and body image. In Carlson C, editor: Behavioral concepts and nursing intervention, Philadelphia, 1970, JB Lippincott Co.

31. Rostow E: Conflict and accommodation. In Lifton R, editor: The woman in America, Boston, 1967, Beacon Press.

32. Spire R: Photographic self-image confrontation, Am J Nurs 73:1207, 1973.

33. Steffenhagen R and Burns J: The Social Dynamics of Self-Esteem, New York, 1987, Praeger.

34. Sullivan HS: The interpersonal theory of psychiatry, New York, 1963, WW Norton & Co, Inc.

35. Taft L: Self-esteem in later life: a nursing perspective, Adv Nurs Science, 8(1):77, 1985.

36. Weissman M et al: The educated housewife: mild depression and the search for work, Am J Orthopsychiatry 43:565, 1973.

■ ANNOTATED SUGGESTED READINGS ■

*Anderson G and Ross C: Strategies for working with a patient who has multiple personality disorder, Arch Psych Nurs 2(4):236, 1988.

Uses the nursing process to organize treatment strategies in caring for the patient with multiple personality disorder. A thorough, practical, and well-written article.

Berne E: Games people play, New York, 1964, Grove Press, Inc.

Presents the theory behind transactional analysis, contains descriptions of various interpersonal games, and explores the possibility of being game free. Has implications for problems with self-concept and is recommended reading for all nurses.

*Bonham P and Cheney A: Concept of self: a framework for nursing assessment. In Chinn P, editor: Advances in nursing theory development, Rockville, Md, 1983, Aspen Systems Corp.

Reviews the literature and proposes a model to define a nursing focus for self-concept. With a systems approach, applies the model to nursing and addresses future implications.

Dellas M and Gaier E: The self and adolescent identity in women: options and implications, Adolescence 10:399, 1975.

Explores three possible female identity patterns—traditional role and stereotype, achievement and role success, and bimodal—and problems related to each.

Erikson E: Identity: youth and crisis, New York, 1968, WW Norton & Co, Inc.

Presents extensive formulations on the adolescent crisis of identity. Reviews stages of the life cycle and explores the pathology of identity confusion through theory and case history. An

*Asterisk indicated nursing reference.

important work on a previously unexplored developmental stage.

Family and Community Health 6(2), 1983.

> *Entire volume devoted to self-esteem. Highly recommended reading for the various articles:*
> *Physical health and self-esteem*
> *Self-esteem through the life span*
> *The evaluation of self-esteem*
> *Enhancement of self-esteem in children and adolescents*
> *Enhancement of self-esteem in adults*
> *Future needs for self-esteem research and services*

*Freeman S: Inpatient management of a patient with borderline personality disorder: a case study, Arch Psych Nurs 2(6):360, 1988.

> *Examines the inpatient behavior of a patient diagnosed with borderline personality disorder. Nursing management techniques are presented along with the crucial aspect of staff reactions.*

Gara M, Rosenberg S, and Cohen B: Personal identity and the schizophrenic process: an integration, Psychiatry 50:267, 1987.

> *Explores the relation between identity theory and the schizophrenic process. Also discusses the effects of medication in establishing a patient identity and preventing psychotic relapse. Advanced reading.*

*Hauser M: Cognitive commands change, J Psychiatr Nurs 19(2):19, 1981.

> *Reviews three specific techniques for working with parent-child interpersonal and behavioral problems: (1) Ellis' restructuring beliefs, (2) Meichenbaum's coping via internal speech, and (3) Gordon's problem solving. All these cognitive techniques are aligned with social learning theory.*

*Johnson M and Silver S: Conflicts in the inpatient treatment of the borderline patient, Arch Psych Nurs 2(5):312, 1988.

> *Uses a case study to examine conflicts that arise in the inpatient treatment of the borderline patient with recommendations to decrease or avoid such problems.*

*Kadner K: Resilience: responding to adversity, J Psychosocial Nurs 27(7):20, 1989.

> *Analyzes the psychosocial resources of ego strength, social intimacy, and resourcefulness and the role they play in the resilience of individuals to stress. Suggests implications for both primary and secondary prevention nursing activities.*

Kanfer F and Goldstein A, editors: Helping people change, New York, 1975, Pergamon Press, Inc.

> *Deals with such topics as cognitive change, self-management, modeling, and role play.*

*Kerr N: Pathological narcissism, Perspect Psychiatr Care 18(1): 29, 1980.

> *Reviews the many facets of narcissism including its development, psychodynamics, and interpersonal aspects and includes a good bibliography.*

*Knowles R: A guide to self-management strategies for nurses, New York, 1984, Springer.

> *Describes self-control strategies nurses can use to increase feelings of self-esteem, lower anxiety, heighten belief in self, and promote achievement of personal and professional goals. Has application for patients as well.*

*Lego S: Multiple personality disorder: an interpersonal approach to etiology, treatment and nursing care, Arch Psych Nurs 2(4):231, 1988.

> *Describes the diagnosis, treatment, and nursing care issues related to patients with multiple personality disorder from the perspective of interpersonal theory.*

*Piccinino S: The nursing care challenge of borderline patients, J Psychosocial Nurs 28(4):22, 1990.

> *Describes behaviors of patients with borderline personality disorder, their effect on the nursing staff and recommendations for nursing care. Good overview article.*

Raimy V: Misunderstandings of the self, San Francisco, 1975, Jossey-Bass, Inc, Publishers.

> *Premise is that misunderstandings of the self may be major hindrances to personal and social adjustment. Presents an approach to psychotherapy that is an application of self-concept theory and describes faulty beliefs or misconceptions as responsible for psychological disturbances. Easy to read, and integrates sophisticated features of various psychotherapies that involve cognitive change. Provocative for the advanced reader.*

Rogers C: On becoming a person, Boston, 1961, Houghton Mifflin Co.

> *Discusses personal growth from the individual's and therapist's point of view. Compilation of important papers that address a variety of mental health disciplines. Highly recommended.*

Salkin J: Body ego technique, Springfield, Ill, 1973, Charles C Thomas, Publisher.

> *An educational and therapeutic approach to the normal development of body image and self-identity. Provides an in-depth account of procedures, materials, and technique and describes how to use the elements of movement, rhythm, space, and force to facilitate the development of ego strength. Useful reference for interventions related to dance and body movement.*

Steffenhagen R and Burns J: The social dynamics of self-esteem, New York, 1987, Praeger.

> *Discusses the characteristics of current culture that contribute to the enhancement of or act as a deterrent to self-esteem development. Stimulating reading for the advanced practitioner.*

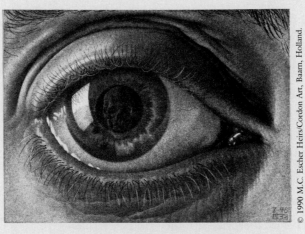

Lying awake, calculating the future,
Trying to unweave, unwind, unravel
And piece together the past and the future,
Between midnight and dawn, when the
past is all deception,
The future futureless . . .

T.S. Eliot

C H A P T E R   14

DISTURBANCES OF MOOD

DIAGNOSTIC PREVIEW

MEDICAL DIAGNOSES RELATED TO DISTURBANCES OF MOOD

- Bipolar disorder
- Major depression
- Cyclothymia
- Dysthymia

LEARNING OBJECTIVES

After studying this chapter, the student should be able to:

- define mood, its four adaptive functions, and the continuum of emotional responses.

- identify the characteristics that lead to the recognition of severe disturbances of mood.

- describe the concepts of grief, the delayed grief reaction, depression, and mania.

- discuss the predisposing factors proposed for the origin of disturbances of mood.

- analyze precipitating stressors that contribute to the development of disturbances of mood.

- state the value of a unified multicausal model of disturbances of mood.

- identify and describe behaviors and coping mechanisms associated with uncomplicated grief reactions, delayed grief reactions, depression, and mania.

- formulate individualized nursing diagnoses for patients with disturbances of mood.

- assess the relationship between nursing diagnoses and medical diagnoses associated with disturbances of mood.

- develop long-term and short-term individualized nursing goals for patients experiencing disturbances of mood.

- apply therapeutic nurse-patient relationship principles with appropriate rationale in planning the care of a patient experiencing a disturbance of mood.

- describe nursing interventions appropriate to the needs of the patient experiencing an uncomplicated grief reaction, depression, or mania.

- develop a mental health education plan to promote a patient's adaptive emotional responses.

- assess the importance of evaluating the nursing process when working with patients with disturbances of mood.

- identify directions for future nursing research.

- select appropriate readings for further study.

Variations or fluctuations in mood are a dominant feature of human existence. They indicate that a person is perceiving his world and responding to it. Extremes in mood have also been linked with extremes in human experience, such as creativity, madness, despair, ecstasy, romanticism, personal charisma, and interpersonal destructiveness. These moods have fascinated scientists, philosophers, and novelists alike, who romanticize, study, and exaggerate the possible alliance between mood, deep emotional experience, and talent.

In this text, **mood** refers to a prolonged emotional state that influences one's whole personality and life functioning. It pertains to prevailing and pervading emotion and is synonymous with the terms "affect," "feeling state," and "emotion." As with other aspects of the personality, emotions or moods serve an adaptive role for the individual.

The four adaptive functions of emotions are social communication, physiological arousal, subjective awareness, and psychodynamic defense. The components of social communication, such as crying, posture, facial expression, and touch, promote early mother-child attachment and the formation of other interpersonal bonds. Depressive mood states also initiate physiological arousal involving the central nervous system, biogenic amines, and neuroendocrine systems. The subjective components of human emotions are believed to play important functions in goal setting and in the monitoring of current behavior, particularly in judging personal reality against internalized values and goals. Finally, the fourth adaptive function of emotion is in aiding psychodynamic defense on both conscious and unconscious levels.

Continuum of emotional responses

The variety of emotions one can experience, such as fear, joy, anxiety, love, anger, sadness, and surprise, are all normal accompaniments of the human condition. The problem arises in trying to evaluate when a person's mood or emotional state is maladaptive, abnormal, or unhealthy. Grief, for example, is a healthy, adaptive, separative process that attempts to overcome the stress of a loss. Grief work, or mourning, therefore, is not a pathological process. It is an adaptive response to a real stressor. The absence of grieving in the face of a loss is suggestive of maladaptation.

Note the continuum of health and illness in Fig. 14-1. At the adaptive, or healthy, end is emotional responsiveness. This involves being affected by and an active participant in one's internal and external worlds. It implies being open to one's feelings and aware of them. If used in such a way, feelings provide us with valuable learning experiences. They are barometers that give a person feedback about himself and his relationships, and they help a person function more effectively. Also adaptive in the face of stress is an uncomplicated grief reaction. Such a reaction implies that the person is facing the reality of his loss and is immersed in the work of grieving.

A maladaptive response would be the suppression of emotions. This may be evident as a denial of one's feelings, a detachment from them, or an internalization of all aspects of one's affective world. A transient suppression of feelings may at times be necessary to cope, such as in an initial response to a death or tragedy. Prolonged suppression of emotion, however, such as in delayed grief reaction, will ultimately interfere with effective functioning.

The most maladaptive emotional responses or severe mood disturbances can be recognized by their intensity, pervasiveness, persistence, and interference with usual social and physiological functioning. These characteristics apply to the severe emotional states of depression and mania, which complete the maladaptive end of the continuum of emotional responses.

Nursing intervention in disturbances of mood requires understanding a range of emotional states. To assist in this process, grief, the delayed grief reaction, depression, and mania are briefly described.

■ Grief

Grief is the subjective state that follows loss. It is one of the most powerful emotional states experienced by an individual and affects all aspects of one's life. It forces the person to stop his normal activities and to focus on his present feelings and needs. Most often, it is the response to loss of a loved person through death or separation, but it also occurs following the loss of something tangible or intangible that is highly regarded. It may be a valued object, a cherished possession, an ideal, a job, or status. As a response to the loss of a loved one, grief is a universal reaction. As one's interdependence on others grows, the chance increases that one must face loss, separation, and death, which elicit intense feelings of grief. The capacity to form

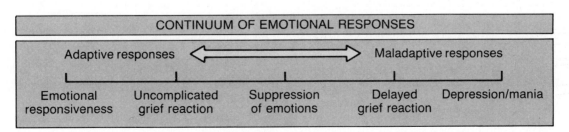

Fig. 14-1. Continuum of emotional responses.

warm, satisfying relationships with others also makes one vulnerable to sadness, despair, and grief when those relationships are terminated.

As a natural reaction to a life experience, grief is universal. It involves stress, pain, and suffering and an impairment of function that can last for days, weeks, or months. Thus the understanding of grief and its manifestations has become of great practical importance for its impact on both physical and emotional health.

The ability to experience grief is gradually formed in the course of normal development and is closely related to the capacity for developing meaningful object relationships. The process of growth and development is a series of goal attainments marked by emotional withdrawals from previous positions and reinvestment in new prospects that are thought to offer increased security. Progress is stimulated by physiological growth, which provides new abilities, strengths, and skills, as well as by encouragement and reinforcement from parents and significant others. Goals become more complex, and conflicts in life's choices create inner stress, turmoil, pressure, and unrest. Energies previously turned inward are projected to external objects. If the gratification obtained from the external object is relatively complete and fulfilling, the external object is valued as necessary to the self and is loved. If there is a change in the object, gratification ceases and readjustment is necessary. The person may withdraw within himself, feel isolated, and become preoccupied with his own person and feelings. This is a part of the grieving process. It is resolved only when the lost object is internalized, bonds of attachment are loosened, and new object relationships are established.

Grief responses may be either uncomplicated and adaptive or morbid and pathological. Uncomplicated grief runs a consistent course that is modified by the abruptness of the loss, one's preparation for the event, and the significance of the lost object. It is a self-limited process of realization; it makes real the fact of the loss.

■ Delayed grief reaction

A maladaptive, or pathological, response to loss implies that something has prevented it from running its normal course. Two types of pathological grief reactions have been identified by Lindemann—the delayed reaction and the distorted reaction.[36] Depression is one type of a distorted grief reaction.

Persistent absence of any emotion may signal an undue delay in the work of mourning, or a delayed grief reaction. The delay may occur in the beginning of the mourning process or become evident in a re-

tarding of the process once it has begun, or both. The delay and rejection of grief may occasionally involve many years. The underlying emotions associated with the loss may be triggered by a deliberate recall of circumstances surrounding the loss or by a spontaneous occurrence in the patient's life. A classic example of this is the anniversary reaction in which the person experiences incomplete or abnormal mourning at the time of the loss, only to have the grieving response recur at anniversaries of the original loss.

■ Depression

The individual who does not mourn can experience a pathological grief reaction known as depression, or melancholia. It is an abnormal extension or overelaboration of sadness and grief. Depression is the oldest and most frequently described psychiatric illness. It has been described as early as 1500 BC, and it appears to be part of the human condition familiar to all yet mysterious to many. The term "depression" is used in a variety of ways. It can refer to a sign, symptom, syndrome, emotional state, reaction, disease, or clinical entity. In this chapter it is viewed as a clinical condition that is severe, abnormal, maladaptive, and incapacitating.

The Wall Street Journal called depression the disease of the 1970s, and some mental health workers consider it to cause more total suffering and anguish in the world than any other single medical or psychiatric illness. Depression may range from mild and moderate states to severe states with psychotic features. Psychotic depression is relatively uncommon, however, accounting for less than 10% of all depressions. It is estimated that 15% to 30% of adults experience clinical depressive episodes, most often of moderate severity, at some point in their lives, with the onset of depressive illness peaking in the 40s and 50s. However, only 25% of persons with depressive symptoms seek mental health professional attention. Furthermore, 50% to 80% of all suicides are attributed to depression, and perhaps as much as 75% of all psychiatric hospitalizations.[14]

There is also an almost universal world trend toward greater prevalence of depression among women than among men in a ratio of 2:1. Other risk factors for depression are having a family history of depression or alcoholism; having childhood experiences in a disruptive, hostile, and generally negative home environment; having had recent negative life events, particularly deaths or losses; lacking an intimate, confiding relationship; and having had a baby in the past 6 months.[14,44]

Research has also revealed the high incidence of

depression among patients hospitalized for medical illnesses. These depressions are largely unrecognized and thus are untreated by health care personnel. Depression is found in all severities of medical illness, although its intensity and frequency are higher in patients more severely ill. Available studies suggest that about one-third of medical inpatients report mild or moderate symptoms of depression and up to one fourth may suffer from a depressive illness. Certain medical conditions are frequently associated with depression, especially cancer, strokes, epilepsy, multiple sclerosis, Parkinson's disease, and a variety of endocrine disorders.[49] Thus, research suggests depression is a common accompaniment of many major medical illnesses.

Despite its prevalence, most people with a depressive illness do not seek treatment because many of them do not know that they have a treatable disease. As a result of this, in 1988 the National Institute of Mental Health (NIMH) initiated a national education campaign, called Depression/Awareness, Recognition, and Treatment (D/ART), about depressive illnesses. The campaign's goal is to reduce unnecessary suffering by encouraging people with depressive illness to get appropriate treatment. The D/ART campaign is directed toward providing health care practitioners and the general public with the latest treatment information.[45]

At first glance, the grieving person and the depressed person may seem indistinguishable. Both are in despair. Both are unable to be interested in the world around them. Neither can believe the pain and sadness will ever cease. Both may feel life is finished or wish it were, and for both, time is meaningless.

However, differences exist between mourning and depression. Drake and Price[18] believe the difference is the quality of an individual's attachment to the loved object. The degree and nature of the attachment determines the type of loss phenomenon and the extent of the depressive reaction. The disruption of a "normal" attachment results in a sense of loss and grief that is resolved in simple mourning and bereavement. In contrast, disruption of an "inordinate" attachment results in grieving that leads into a cycle of depression, since the person is unable to cope with life and function effectively.

Another difference is apparent in the acknowledgment of loss. The mourner attends to all things that are connected in any way with the person he mourns. Although his pain is heightened, it is not meaningless; rather, it is an acknowledgment of the loss, and positive feelings toward the lost object predominate. The depressed individual wishes to deny the loss and sepa-

ration. Even though his affective responses express sorrow, he continues to deny his need to mourn or even that a need to mourn exists.

■ Mania

In addition to a severely depressed disturbance of mood, one may also experience manic episodes. These episodes, as with those of depression, can vary in intensity and accompanying level of anxiety from moderate manic states to severe and panic states with psychotic features. Basically, mania is characterized by a mood that is elevated, expansive, or irritable. **Hypomania** describes a clinical syndrome similar to, but not as severe as, that described by the terms mania or manic episode.

In the DSM-III-R,[3] both manic and depressive episodes fall under the category of mood (affective) disorders. Mania, however, is not given a separate category as is depression. Rather, the major affective disorders are separated into two subgroups—bipolar and depressive disorders—based on whether manic and depressive episodes are involved longitudinally (Table 14-1).[3] In this classification, major depression may involve a single episode or a recurrent depressive illness, but without manic episodes. When there has been one or more manic episodes, with or without a major depressive episode, the category of bipolar disorder is used. Bipolar disorders are subdivided according to the symptoms of the current episode as manic, depressed, or mixed.

Thus, if one experiences a depressive episode with no manic episodes, it would be classified as a "depressive disorder." If one experiences a depressive episode with manic episodes in the past or present, it would be classified as a "bipolar disorder."

Although bipolar affective disorders occur less often than depressive disorders, it is estimated that 0.6% to 0.88% of the adult population, or approximately 2 million Americans, suffer from bipolar disorder. Risk factors are being female and having a family history of bipolar disorder. The data suggest that people under age 50 are at higher risk of a first attack, whereas someone who already has the disorder faces increased risk of a recurrent manic or depressive episode as he or she grows older.[14,44]

Assessment

Severe disturbances of mood, such as in depressive and manic episodes, have been accounted for by numerous theories or models of causation. These models identify predisposing and precipitating factors that may affect the individual's coping re-

TABLE 14-1

CLASSIFICATION OF MOOD (AFFECTIVE) DISORDERS IN DSM-III-R* RELATIVE TO DEPRESSIVE AND MANIC EPISODES

	Depressive disorders		Bipolar disorders		
	Single	Recurrent	Manic	Depressed	Mixed
Depressive episode	Yes	Yes	—	Yes-present	Yes-present
Manic episode	No	No	Yes-present	Yes-past	Yes-present

*American Psychiatric Association: Diagnostic and Statistical Manual of Mental Disorder, Third edition–Revised, Washington, D.C., 1987, The Association.

sponse and adjustment. Some of the theories are in conflict with each other, some are not supported by research, and certainly all of them are not applicable to each person. Rather, they present causative factors that may operate in severe disturbances of mood.

■ Predisposing factors

■ **GENETIC FACTORS.** The first theory addresses genetic aspects of depression. There is wide agreement that both heredity and environment play an important role. Genetic factors related to severe mood disturbances have been investigated in Scandinavia, Germany, Great Britain, and the United States. Four techniques of investigation are used: (1) familial aggregation studies, comparing illness rates within and between generations of a particular family; (2) studies comparing illness rates in monozygotic and dizygotic twins; (3) general population surveys, comparing illness rates of relatives of depressed patients with those of the general population; and (4) linkage studies, using known genetic markers such as blood type or color blindness.

Studies using only familial aggregations do not necessarily demonstrate the role of genetics, since disturbances may be the result of nutritional, infectious, or psychological factors. Some studies using genetic markers such as color blindness suggest that bipolar affective disorder is transmitted by an X-linked dominant gene. Controversy surrounds the mode of genetic transmission in affective disorders, however, since the findings from other studies contradict this hypothesis and suggest a multifactorial mode of transmission. Most recent research suggests there are different forms of genetic transmission.

Other evidence includes (1) an increased frequency of the illness in relatives of the patient compared with the general population; (2) a greater concordance rate in monozygotic twins than in dizygotic twins; (3) an increased frequency of psychiatric abnormalities in relatives of the affective disorder patient than in the general population; and (4) onset of the illness at a characteristic age with no evidence of a precipitating event. Good evidence exists for the role of genetic factors in affective disturbances.[53] Studies continue in this important area.

■ **AGGRESSION-TURNED-INWARD THEORY.** The anger-turned-inward theory of Freud views depression as the inward turning of the aggressive instinct, for some reason not directed at the appropriate object and accompanied by feelings of guilt. The process is initiated by the loss of an ambivalently loved object. The person feels angry and loving at the same time. He is unable to express his anger because he thinks it is inappropriate or irrational. Also, he may have developed a pattern throughout life of containing feelings, especially those he views negatively. He then directs his angry feelings inward. Freud believed that if one went so far as to commit suicide, the act was a strike against the hated and loved object as well as against the self.

This theory does not lend itself to empirical verification. Although it is one of the most widely quoted theories of depression, little systematic evidence substantiates it. Some researchers have identified depressed patients who outwardly express anger and hostility. Furthermore, the redirection of hostility at outside objects has not been consistently correlated with clinical improvement. In some instances it may actually have negative effects on the patient's view of self and problem resolution. It should therefore be viewed as one possible theory of causation that is not applicable to all people.

■ **OBJECT LOSS THEORY.** The object loss theory of depression has been advanced by Bowlby,[8,9] Robertson and Robertson,[47] and Spitz.[54] It refers to traumatic separation of the person from significant objects of attachment. Two issues are important to this theory: loss during childhood as a predisposing factor for adult depressions and separation in adult life as a precipitating stress.

The first issue proposes that a child has ordinarily formed a tie to a mother figure by 6 months of age, and once that tie is ruptured, the child experiences separation anxiety, grief, and mourning. Furthermore, this mourning in the early years frequently affects personality development and predisposes the child to psychiatric illness. As Bowlby states:

Unfavorable personality development is often to be attributed to one or more of the less satisfactory responses to loss having been provoked during the years of infancy and childhood in such degree, over such length of time, or with such frequency, that a disposition is established to respond to all subsequent losses in a similar way.[9:22]

Evidence for this model was reported by Spitz[54] in 1942 when he described a deprivational reaction in infants separated from their mothers at age 6 to 12 months. The reaction was characterized by apprehension, crying, withdrawal, psychomotor slowing, dejection, stupor, insomnia, anorexia, and gross retardation in growth and development. This syndrome is called "anaclitic depression;" it has been questioned whether it is caused by the separation or the adverse effects of an orphanage. A similar separation reaction was described by Robertson and Robertson[47] and Bowlby[8] in older children. They identified three stages of response:

1. A "protest" stage in which the child appeared restless and tearful and searched for his mother
2. A "despair" stage of apathetic withdrawal
3. A "detachment" stage seen in some children who rejected their mothers on reunion

From a research point of view, the connection between early object loss and adult depression is complex. Robertson and Robertson[47] cast doubt on the universality of the responses described and suggest that appropriate mothering during the separation period can prevent their occurrence. Some studies indicate that depressive patients seem to experience more parental loss from death, separation, and other causes than do normal and other diagnostic groups. However, that factor alone does not seem sufficiently universal to account for all forms of depression. There is even discussion about the beneficial or immunizing effects of having successfully coped with an early loss in the development of resilience.

■ **PERSONALITY ORGANIZATION THEORY.** Another psychodynamic view of depression focuses on the major psychosocial variable of low self-esteem. The patient's self-concept is an underlying issue, whether expressed as dejection and depression or overcompensated with an air of supreme competence, as displayed in manic and hypomanic episodes. Threats to self-esteem arise from poor role performance, perceived low-level everyday functioning, and the absence of a clear self-identity.

Three forms of personality organization that could lead to depression have been identified by Arieti and Bemporad.[4] One, based on the "dominant other," occurs because the patient has relied on an esteemed other for self-esteem. Satisfaction is experienced only through an intermediary. Clinging, passivity, manipulativeness, and avoidance of anger characterize the person with this type of depression. There is a noticeable lack of personal goals and a predominant focus on problems.

Another form of personality results when a person realizes he may never accomplish a desired, but unrealistic, goal. This is the "dominant goal" type of depression. This person is usually seclusive, arrogant, and often obsessive. He has set unrealistic goals for himself and evaluates them with an all-or-nothing standard. He spends an inordinate amount of time in wishful thinking and introverted searches for meaning.

The third type of depression is manifested as a constant mode of feeling. These patients "inhibit any form of gratification because of strongly held taboos." They experience emptiness, "hypochondriasis, pettiness in interpersonal relationships, and a harsh critical attitude toward themselves and others."[4]

This view of depression looks at the patients' belief systems in relation to their experiences. Even in the absence of an apparent precipitating stressor, their depression appears to be preceded by a severe blow to their self-esteem. It emphasizes the crucial position of self-concept in adaptation or maladaptation, and the importance of the patient's appraisal of his life situation.

■ **COGNITIVE MODEL.** The cognitive model of Beck[5,6] proposes that people experience depression because their thinking is disturbed. He proposes that depression is a cognitive problem dominated by the patient's negative evaluation of himself, his world, and his future. This theory is in contrast to others that propose the depressive affect is primary and the negative cognitive set is secondary. Beck suggests that in the course of development certain experiences sensitize the individual and make him vulnerable to depression. The person also acquires a tendency to make extreme, absolute judgments; loss is viewed as irrevocable and indifference as total rejection.

The depression-prone person, according to this theory, is likely to explain an adverse event as a personal shortcoming. For example, the deserted husband believes "She left me because I'm unlovable," instead of considering the other possible alternatives, such as personality incompatibility, the wife's own problems, or her change in feelings toward him. As he focuses on his personal deficiencies, they expand to the point where they completely dominate his self-concept. He can think of himself only in a negative way and is unable to acknowledge his other abilities, achievements, and attributes. This negative set is reinforced when he interprets ambiguous or neutral experiences as additional proof of his deficiencies. Comparisons with other people further lower his self-esteem, and thus every encounter with others becomes a negative experience. His self-criticisms increase as he views himself as deserving of blame.

Depressed patients become dominated by pessimism; they expect future adversities and experience them as though they were happening in the present or had already occurred. Their predictions tend to be overgeneralized and extreme. Since they view the future as an extension of the present, they expect their failure to continue permanently. Thus pessimism dominates their activities, wishes, and future expectations.

Beck proposes that the constellation of negative thoughts that characterize depression remains relatively dormant until a person becomes depressed. Depressed individuals are capable of logical self-evaluation when not in a depressed mood or when only mildly depressed. When depression does occur, after some precipitating life stressors, the long-dormant negative cognitive set makes its appearance. As depression develops and increases, the negative idiosyncratic thinking increasingly replaces objective thinking.

Although the onset of the depression may appear sudden, Beck suggests it develops over weeks, months, or even years, as each experience is interpreted as further evidence of failure. As a result of this "tunnel vision," the individual becomes hypersensitive to experiences of loss and defeat and oblivious to experiences of success and pleasure. He has difficulty acknowledging anger, since he thinks he is responsible for, and deserving of, insults from others and problems in living. Along with low self-esteem, he experiences apathy and indifference. He is drawn to a state of inactivity and withdraws from life. He lacks all spontaneous desire and only wishes to remain passive. Because he expects failure, he lacks the ordinary energy to make an effort.

Suicidal wishes can be viewed as an extreme expression of the desire to escape. The patient sees his life as filled with suffering, with no chance of improvement. Given this negative set, suicide seems a rational solution. It promises to end his misery and relieve his family of a burden, and he begins to believe that everyone would be better off if he were dead. The more he considers the alternative of suicide, the more desirable it may seem, and as his life becomes more hopeless and painful, his desires become stronger to end his life.

Naturalistic, clinical, and experimental studies have provided substantial support for this model of depression. For example, Stuart and co-workers researched the early childhood experiences of women with depression in comparison with women who were free of psychiatric diagnosis. They found that the depressed women experienced both parents as rejecting and perceived less warmth from their fathers; described less rational discussion in the resolution of family conflict; experienced significant separation anxiety as children; and grew up in households with more deaths and chronic physical illness.[56] Nursing studies such as this one will assist the nurse in understanding the personal world of the depressed person and organizing her observations regarding the depressed person's logic and thinking in a way that best promotes recovery.

■ **LEARNED HELPLESSNESS MODEL.** The learned helplessness model evolved from Seligman's research with dogs, from which he postulated a theory of human depression. He defines helplessness as a "belief that no one will do anything to aid you" and hopelessness as a belief that neither "you nor anyone else can do anything."[52] His theory proposes that it is not trauma per se that produces depression, but the belief that one has no control over the important outcomes in one's life and therefore refrains from adaptive responses. Learned helplessness is both a behavioral state and a personality trait of a person who believes that he has lost control over the reinforcers in his environment. These negative expectations lead to hopelessness, passivity, and an inability to assert oneself.

Seligman suggests that people resistant to depression have experienced mastery in life. Their childhood experiences proved that their actions were effective in producing gratification and removing annoyances. In contrast, those susceptible to depression have had lives devoid of mastery. Their experiences proved that they were helpless to influence their sources of suffering and gratification or they controlled too many reinforcers that did not allow for the development of their coping responses against failure.

Abramson, Seligman, and Teasdale[1] proposed an attributional reformulation of the learned helplessness hypothesis. According to the attributional reformulation, the types of causal attributions people make for lack of control influence whether their helplessness will entail low self-esteem and whether their symptoms of helplessness will generalize across situations and time. According to the reformulation, three attributional dimensions are crucial for explaining human helplessness and depression: internal-external, stable-unstable, and global-specific.

In brief, the reformulated model postulates that attributing lack of control to internal factors leads to lowered self-esteem, whereas attributing lack of control to external factors does not. Attributing lack of control to stable factors should lead to an expectation of uncontrollability in the future and, consequently, helplessness deficits extended across time. Similarly, attributing lack of control to global factors should lead to an expectation of uncontrollability in other situations and, consequently, helplessness deficits extended across situations. Alternatively, attributing lack of control to unstable specific factors should lead to short-lived situation-specific helplessness deficits.

Abramson, Seligman, and Teasdale summarized the implications of the attributional reformulation for the helplessness model of depression:

1. Depression consists of four classes of deficits: motivational, cognitive, self-esteem, and affective.
2. When highly desired outcomes are believed improbable or when highly aversive outcomes are believed probable, and the individual expects that no response in his repertoire will change their likelihood (helplessness), depression results.
3. The generality of depressive deficits will depend on the globality of the attribution for helplessness. The chronicity of the depression deficits will depend on the stability of the attribution for helplessness. Whether self-esteem is lowered will depend on the internality of the attribution for helplessness.
4. The intensity of the deficits depends on the strength, or certainty, of the expectation of uncontrollability and, in the case of the affective and self-esteem deficits, on the importance of the outcome.[1:68]

In concluding a discussion of this model, three points are worth noting. First, the attributional reformulation of helplessness and depression bears a significant similarity to Beck's cognitive model of depression previously described. Second, this model is proposed as a sufficient, but not necessary, condition for depression. Other physiological and psychological factors can produce symptoms of depression in the absence of an expectation of uncontrollability. Finally, it must be emphasized that the reformulation model is still being empirically validated.

■ **BEHAVIORAL MODEL.** The behavioral model studied by Lewinsohn, Youngren, and Grosscup[35] is derived from a social learning theory framework in which the cause of depression is assumed to reside in the person-behavior-environment interaction. Social learning theory assumes that psychological functioning can best be understood in terms of continuous reciprocal interactions among personal factors. These include cognitive processes, behavioral factors, and environmental factors, all operating as interdependent determinants of one another. The relative influences exerted by these interdependent factors differ in various settings and for different behaviors.

This theory views people as capable of exercising considerable control over their own behavior. They do not merely react to external influences. They select, organize, and transform incoming stimuli. Thus people are not viewed as powerless objects controlled by their environments, but neither are they absolutely free to do whatever they choose. Rather, people and their environment are reciprocal determinants of one another.

The concept of reinforcement is crucial to this view of depression. Reinforcement is defined in terms of the quality of interactions with one's environment. Person-environment interactions with positive outcomes constitute positive reinforcement. Such interactions strengthen the person's behavior. Little or no rewarding interaction with the environment causes the person to feel sad or blue. Thus the key assumption in this model is that a low rate of positive reinforcement is the historical antecedent of depressive behaviors.

Two particular variables are important. One is that the individual may fail to provide appropriate responses to initiate positive reinforcement. The other is that the environment may fail to provide reinforcement and thus worsen the patient's condition. These variables are often apparent, since depressed patients have been shown to be deficient in the social skills needed to interact effectively. In turn, other people find the behavior of the depressed person distancing, negative, or offensive and avoid him as much as possible.

Depression is likely to occur if certain positively reinforcing events are absent; particularly those which fall into the following categories[34]:

Positive sexual experiences
Rewarding social interaction
Enjoyable outdoor activities
Solitude
Competence experiences

These may be described as "being sexually attractive," "being with friends," "being relaxed," "doing my job well," and "doing things my own way." Depression also occurs in the presence of certain punishing events, particularly those that fall into three categories:

Marital discord
Work hassles
Receiving negative reactions from others

This model of depression emphasizes an active, rather than passive, approach to the person and relies heavily on an interactional view of personality. Within this model, social interpersonal behavior, cognitive factors, and self-regulatory mechanisms play important roles. Treatment is aimed at assisting the person to increase the quantity and quality of positively reinforcing interactions and to decrease aversive interactions.

■ **BIOLOGICAL MODEL.** Another major area of research on depression involves a biological model, which explores chemical changes in the body during depressed states. Whether these chemical changes cause depression or are a result of depression is not yet understood. However, significant abnormalities can be demonstrated in many body systems during a depressive illness.[44] These include electrolyte disturbances, especially of sodium and potassium; neurophysiological alterations based on findings from electrophysiological studies using electroencephalography and evoked potential methods; dysfunction and faulty regulation of autonomic nervous system activity; adrenocortical, thyroid, and gonadal changes; and neurochemical alterations in the neurotransmitters, especially in the biogenic amines, which serve as central nervous system and peripheral neurotransmitters. The biogenic amines include three catecholamines—dopamine, norepinephrine, and epinephrine—as well as serotonin and acetylcholine.

Catecholamines. The catecholamine hypothesis states that depression is associated with a deficiency of catecholamines, particularly of norepinephrine, in the central nervous system. Mania is associated with an excess of catecholamine. This hypothesis is derived in part from the observations that certain drugs, such as the monamine oxidase (MAO) inhibitors and tricyclic antidepressants, which potentiate or increase brain catecholamines, stimulate behavior and relieve depression. In contrast, lithium carbonate, a drug effective in treating mania, acts by decreasing the release of norepinephrine and increasing its reuptake. One of the metabolites of norepinephrine, 3-methoxy-4-hydroxyphenylglycol (MHPG), is decreased in the cerebrospinal fluid and urine of depressed patients, further supporting this hypothesis. The biogenic amine model is par-

ticularly important, since it provides links between clinical observations and psychotrophic drugs that have emerged as effective treatments.

Endocrine dysfunction. The possibility of hormonal causes of depression has been considered for many years. Some symptoms of depression that suggest endocrine changes are decreased appetite, weight loss, insomnia, diminished sex drive, gastrointestinal disorders, and variations of mood. New assay techniques have recently detected alterations of hormone activity concurrent with depression. Mood changes have also been observed with a variety of endocrine disorders, including Cushing's disease, hyperthyroidism, and estrogen therapy. Further support for this theory is evident in the high incidence of depression during the postpartum period, when hormonal levels change.

Current study of neuroendocrine factors in affective disorders emphasize the disinhibition of the hypothalamic-pituitary-adrenal (HPA) axis. Two new tests based on the neuroendocrine theory and performed clinically may prove to be useful in diagnosing affective illnesses. The first is the corticotropin releasing factor stimulation test that evaluates the pituitary's ability to respond to corticotropin-releasing hormone (CRH) and secrete sufficient amounts of adrenal corticotropin hormone (ACTH) to induce normal adrenal activity. The second test is the thyroid-releasing hormone (TRH) infusion test that differs from the CRH infusion by assessing the pituitary's ability to secrete sufficient amounts of thyroid-stimulating hormones (TSH) to produce normal thryroid activity. These tests may be helpful in differentiating unipolar from bipolar depression and mania from schizophrenic psychosis.[57]

Cortisol. Many depressed patients exhibit hypersecretion of cortisol; this has been used in the dexamethasone suppression test (DST) (dexamethasone is an exogenous steroid that suppresses the blood level of cortisol). The DST is based on the observation that, in patients with biological depression, late afternoon cortisol levels are not depressed after a single dose of dexamethasone. However, many physical illnesses and some medications can interfere with the test results. Thus these results should be viewed only as a research tool at this time.

Biological rhythms. Mood disorders are also typified by periodic variations in physiological and psychological functions. Affective illnesses are usually recurrent, with episodes often occurring and remitting spontaneously. Two subtypes of mood disorders are specifically cyclical in nature: rapid cycling manic depressive illness and seasonal affective disorder. In the first, cycles may be days, weeks, months, or years. In seasonal affective disorder, cycles occur annually at the same time each year, as individuals react to changes in environmental factors such as climate, latitude, or light.[25]

People who are depressed or manic have certain characteristic changes in biological rhythms and related physiology. For instance, body temperature and certain hormones reach their peak earlier than normal; some depressed patients are more sensitive to light than nondepressed persons; and many depressed people describe circadian rhythm disturbances, such as diurnal variation and early morning awakening. All-night sleep studies of depressed patients show some basic abnormalities. There is decreased total sleep time, an increased percentage of dream time, difficulty in falling asleep, an increased number of spontaneous awakenings, and a shortened period between sleep onset and the first dreaming period (rapid eye movement, or REM, latency period). These and other findings in the area of biological rhythmicity may prove to be valuable diagnostic tools for depression.

Research on the biological model has been extensive and of high quality. It has lent support to a biological basis for mood disorders and suggested biological markers of clinical usefulness in diagnosis and treatment. These tests, such as the urinary MHPG, DST, and REM latency measure, are described in greater detail in Chapter 23 under the discussion of antidepressant drugs.

The discovery of neuropharmacological abnormalities neither is surprising nor precludes psychological causes. Furthermore, a biochemical model based on one amine is undoubtedly an oversimplification. Research in this model of depression is conflicting at times. Sufficient evidence suggests that a variety of precipitating stressors can induce changes in biogenic amines. The neuropharmacological mechanisms investigated might form final common pathways for both psychological and biological causes. Some depressions might be caused primarily by neuropharmacological dysfunctions, resulting in reduced norepinephrine levels. Others might result from events whose psychological effect would presumably have parallel neurophysiological phenomena, resulting in reduced release of norepinephrine. In other cases, both effects might apply, the life event tipping the balance more easily into depression because activity of the norepinephrine-producing system was already reduced.

■ **Precipitating factors**

Disturbances of mood are a specific response to stress. Although this statement is undoubtedly true, its simplicity tends to mask its full implications. For ex-

ample, two major types of stress exist. The first is the stress of major life events that are evident to other persons. The second type, the minor stress or irritations of daily life, may not be obvious to others. These are the small disappointments, frustrations, criticisms, and arguments that, when accumulated over time and in the absence of compensating positive events, produce a major and chronic negative impact. McLean notes:

Nondepressed persons also report high rates for these kinds of stressors, but the critical difference is that, on the average, nondepressed persons experience compensating numbers of positive events and outcomes within the same period that effectively offset the negative impact of the routine stressors. It is the ratio between negative and positive events and outcomes that is decisive for mood determination.[38:186]

It is appropriate, therefore, to examine in more detail some of the stressors that may produce disturbances of mood. Five such stressors include loss of attachment, major life events, roles, coping resources, and physiological changes.

■ **LOSS OF ATTACHMENT.** Loss in adult life can precipitate depression. The loss may be real or imagined and may include the loss of love, a person, physical functioning, status, or self-esteem. Many losses take on importance because of their symbolical meaning, which makes the reactions to them appear out of proportion to reality. In this sense, even an apparently pleasurable event, such as moving to a new home, may involve the loss of old friends, warm memories, and neighborhood associations. Loss of hope is another significant stressor often overlooked. Because of the actual and symbolical elements involved in loss, the patient's perception takes on primary importance.

The individual is constantly experiencing losses and thus struggling with integrating them. The intensity of a person's grief becomes meaningful only when one understands his earlier losses and separations. A person reacting to a recent loss is behaving as he did in previous separations. The intensity of the present reaction therefore becomes more understandable when one realizes that the reaction is to earlier losses as well. By definition loss is negative, a deprivation. The ability to sustain, integrate, and recover from loss, however, is a sign of personal maturity and growth.

Uncomplicated grief reactions are the process of normal mourning or simple bereavement. Mourning includes a complex sequence of psychological processes. It is accompanied by anxiety, anger, pain, despair, and hope. The sequence is not a smooth, unvarying course, however; it is filled with turmoil, regressions, and potential problems. Certain factors have been identified that influence the outcome of mourning[41]:

Childhood experiences, especially the loss of significant others

Losses experienced later in life

Previous history of psychiatric illness, especially depression

Life crises before the loss

Nature of the relationship with the lost person or object, including kinship, strength of attachment, security of attachment, dependency-independency bonds, and intensity of ambivalence

Process of dying (when applicable), including age of deceased, timeliness, previous warnings, preparation for bereavement, expression of feelings, and preventability of the loss

Social support systems

Secondary stresses

Emergent life opportunities

These should be assessed by the nurse for each person experiencing a loss. Two of the factors—the nature of the relationship with the lost person or object and the mourner's perception of the preventability of the loss—have been identified as prime predictors of the intensity and duration of the bereavement.[13] Concurrent crises, the circumstances of the loss, and a pathological relationship with the lost person or object are other factors that contribute to a failure to resolve grief.

Inhibiting factors. Loss of a loved one is a major stressor for grief reactions. Most individuals resolve this loss through simple bereavement and do not experience pathological grief or depression. Various external and internal factors, however, can inhibit mourning. An external factor may be the immersion of the mourner in practical, necessary tasks that accompany the loss but are not directly connected to the emotional fact of the loss. These tasks may include funeral arrangements, unfinished business of the deceased, or a search for immediate employment. All these tasks foster denial of the loss. Denial also may be encouraged by cultural norms that minimize or negate the finality of the loss. The American norm of "courage in the face of adversity" can prevent the mourner from an open display of grief.

Mourning may also be inhibited when the bereaved lacks support from his social network. Nonsupportiveness suppresses grieving when significant others inhibit the mourner's expression of sadness, anger, and guilt; block his review of the lost relationship; and attempt to orient him too quickly to the future. Finally, the widespread use of tranquilizers and antidepressant medications may suppress normal grief and encourage pathological reactions.

Internal factors that inhibit mourning are often fostered by a society that encourages the control and hiding of feelings. Crying, for example, may be seen as weakness, especially in men. Two emotions are particularly repressed in our society—grief and anger—and this may create many emotional problems. Another inhibitor is the belief that the quantity and quality of emotion is so unique it cannot be communicated. Both these factors lead to suppression of mourning and rely heavily on the intellectual concepts of behavior.

In concluding this discussion of loss as a precipitating stressor, it is necessary to place it in proper perspective based on research. Some studies have failed to demonstrate a relationship between loss and depression. Other studies support the relationship but suggest that depression may be the cause of alienation and object loss, and not vice versa. Thus the following conclusions may be proposed:

1. Loss and separation events are prominent among the possible precipitating stressors of depression.
2. Loss and separation are not universal in all depressions.
3. Not all people who experience loss and separation will develop depressions.
4. Loss and separation are not specific to depression but may serve as precipitating events for a variety of psychiatric and medical illnesses.
5. Loss and separation may result from depression.

■ **MAJOR LIFE EVENTS.** Holmes and Rahe[27] did the pioneering work in life events with the Social Readjustment Rating Scale described in Chapter 3. Subsequently, others have used this approach for measuring stress concentrations in people who have become depressed shortly thereafter.

Research conducted by Paykel and co-workers[43] on life events and depression reveals that, on the average, depressed patients reported almost three times as many important life events during the 6 months before onset of clinical depressive episode as did normal subjects. The events included loss of self-esteem, interpersonal discord, socially undesirable occurrences, and major disruptions of life patterns. The authors found that those events perceived as undesirable were most often the precipitants of depression. They further categorized the events into "exit" events, or separation and interpersonal losses, and "entrance" events, or the introduction of a new person into the social sphere of the subject. Analysis of the data showed that exit events more frequently than entrance events were followed by worsening of psychiatric symptoms, physical health changes, impairment of social role performance, and depressive illnesses in particular. The concept of exit events in their study overlaps with the psychiatric concept of loss.

Most psychiatric clinicians are convinced that a relationship does exist between stressful life events and depression. Some believe that life events play the primary role in depression; others are more conservative, limiting the role of life events to that of contributing to the onset and timing of the acute episode. Any definitive conclusions, however, should be made with caution. All people experience stressful life events, but not all people become depressed. This suggests that specific events can contribute only partially to the development of depression. For example, in an analysis of loss in relation to depression, exits from the social field occurred in 25% of depressed persons and 5% of control subjects. Exits preceded depression in only a small, although substantial, number of persons. Furthermore, less than 20% of the population experiencing exits became clinically depressed. This evidence suggests that other factors must also be significant in disturbances of mood.

Another study supporting such a conclusion was conducted by Nezu and Ronan.[40] They proposed a conceptual model in which negative life events influence depression directly as well as indirectly through their impact on the frequency of current problems and one's level of problem-solving ability. Their model was supported as a strong predictor of depressive symptoms and has implications for nurses engaged in treatment and prevention.

■ **ROLES.** The relationship between role strain and depression has gained popularity with emergence of the women's movement. Women have higher rates of depression, and theories have been proposed linking depression with various aspects of women's lives. For example, Beck[7] examined learned helplessness and prejudice as possible explanations for depression in women. Very few studies, however, have explored role strain and depression.

The most notable work in this area has been done by Ilfield.[28] He developed nine scales to measure current social stressors, defined as circumstances or conditions of daily social roles that are problematic or undesirable. These scales measure ongoing stressful experiences instead of single "events" in the past. They include stressors from neighborhood, job, financial affairs, homemaking, parenting, marriage, singlehood, unemployment, and retirement. The survey population was divided into five subgroups to compare the relative potency of social stressors and the differential ef-

fects of any one stressor across each population. He found that current social stressors are significantly related to depressive symptoms for each of the five groups.

Specifically he reported that current marriage/singlehood stressors have the highest correlation with depression for all groups except single employed women. Parenting, job, and financial stressors were intermediate in association.

Marriage. It is possible to analyze each social role stressor in detail. It becomes obvious in doing so that much of the literature focuses on women. This reflects the predominance of depression among women and the increasing interest in women's changing roles. Role strain in marriage emerges as a major stressor related to depression for both men and women. Jacob and co-workers[29] studied role expectation and role performance in distressed and nondistressed couples and found that nondistressed couples reported (1) greater satisfaction, pleasure, and fidelity in sexual relationships with spouses, (2) more shared activities and positive emotional interchanges, and (3) greater influence of the wife in various areas of family decision making. Gove[22] studied the rates of mental illness among married men and women. He found higher rates of mental illness for married women, whereas single, divorced, and widowed women have lower rates than men. From this he concluded that being married has a protective effect for males but a detrimental effect for females.

Parenting. Another explanation for differing rates of mental illness, particularly depression, between men and women may be the role strain inherent in parenting. LeMasters[32] and Dyer[19] found an "extreme crisis reaction" to the birth of the first child in many young mothers, particularly those with extensive professional training or work experience. Cohen[16] found more pregnancy-related emotional problems in multiparas than in primiparas, commenting that it seemed these mothers had realized pregnancy and parenting were sources of conflict and dissatisfaction.

Ilfield[28] notes the relatively low position of parenting as a social role stressor for employed married men and unemployed married women compared to its primary ranking along with marriage as a stressor for employed married women. This finding is interesting, especially since it includes only individuals with children over 6 years of age. It suggests an interaction and possible role strain between parenting and employment for women.

Work. Additional research also shows that married career women have, or need, supportive husbands. The nature of this support, however, is not clearly described. Much of the literature on two-career families directly documents the additive nature of the mother's role, that is, the assumption of a career in addition to her domestic role.[24] Ilfield[28] in his study did not even include homemaking as a social role for men. Division of household labor did emerge as an important aspect of Rosenfield's study.[51] She examined the relationship between depressive symptoms and traditional and non-traditional sex-role relationships in terms of division of labor. In nontraditional relationships, males had higher levels of depressive symptoms than females. She suggests this gives further support to a sex-role basis for sex differences in depression.

In a nursing research study, Woods explored employment, family roles, and mental health in young married women.[61] She found that the number of women's roles was not associated with poorer mental health and that no clear relationship existed between employment or parenting and mental health. She did find, however, that women who had traditional sex roles, little task-sharing support from a spouse, and little support from a confidant had poorer mental health than their counterparts. In addition, for women who were both spouse and parent, support from a confidant was most important. Task-sharing support was the most important for women who were employed but not parents. Nontraditional sex role norms had the most important protective effects for women who had multiple roles as spouse, employee, and mother.

Clearly, the relationship between role strain and depression merits further exploration. Research in this area, however, must take into account the complexity of causal or interactive relationships. Stuart has identified these as follows[55]:

1. *Predisposing factors.* Important variables include sex, marital status, income, age, education, type of occupation, social position, level of social integration, past experiences (particularly history of disturbances of mood), and a sense of mastery over one's own fate or locus of control.
2. *Role strain as a precipitating stress.* Measurements should provide for identification of roles; type of role strain experienced (role conflict, ambiguity, discontinuity, or overload); magnitude, intensity, and unpredictability of strain; degree of control over roles; duration of role strain (short term versus habitual pattern or personality characteristic); and interaction among roles.
3. *Affective significance of role strain.* The meaning or significance of the role strain experienced should be placed within the context of the need-value system of the individual.

4. *Coping-defensive patterns available.* Focus should be placed on the individual's social support systems that might act as buffers, including family members and a community of significant others who express shared values. The marital relationship merits particular emphasis through examining the supportiveness of the spouse, ways in which this support is expressed, power relationships within the marriage, and levels of marital satisfaction and intimacy.
5. *Illness outcome.* In addition to depressive symptoms, one might assess the length and intensity of disability, areas of impaired functioning, and long-term consequences of the depression (i.e., role strain that induces depression might serve to legitimize future role failure).
6. *Adaptive outcome.* Research in this area would assess specific coping strategies to handle role strain, including division and delegation of responsibilities, changing expectations, clarification of goals, and use of social resources. Such research would have direct implications for preventive and therapeutic interventions in the future.

■ **COPING RESOURCES.** Life stress may also take the form of inadequate coping resources. Personal resources available to individuals include their socioeconomic status (income, occupation, social position, education), families (nuclear, extended), interpersonal networks, and the secondary organizations provided by the broader social environment. The far-ranging effects of poverty, discrimination, inadequate housing, and social isolation cannot be ignored or taken lightly. The results of three studies are relevant in this regard.

In the first study, Myers, Lindenthal, and Pepper[39] reported that social integration is important in the relationship between life events and psychiatric symptoms. In particular, those who described few life events but significant symptoms were less well integrated than those who reported few symptoms but many events. Three particular deficiencies in social networks or support systems serve to increase the individual's vulnerability to stress—social isolation, social marginality, and status inconsistency.

The second study investigating coping resources and related issues was reported by Brown and Harris.[10] Using data from a community survey in London, they examined the relationship between psychosocial stress and subsequent affective disorders in women. They found that working-class married women with young children at home had the highest rates of depression. They were five times more likely to become depressed than middle-class women given equal levels of stress. Four factors were found significant: loss of a mother in childhood; three or more children under age 14 living at home; absence of an intimate and confiding relationship with a husband or boyfriend; and lack of full- or part-time employment outside the home. The first three factors were found more frequently among working-class women. Confidants other than a spouse or boyfriend did not have a protective effect. Rather, an important factor in preventing depression was the amount of emotional support the husband or boyfriend gave the woman and the general levels of satisfaction and intimacy in the relationship. Employment outside the home had a protective effect by alleviating boredom, increasing self-esteem, improving finances, and increasing social contacts. This is the type of research needed regarding life stress and illness.

The third study was conducted by Warheit[59] on losses, coping resources, and depression. The major findings were:

1. Persons with high loss scores had higher depression scores than those with low to moderate loss.
2. The presence of a spouse was significantly correlated with lower depression scores for all groups. The presence of relatives nearby was not significant. Availability of friends was significantly correlated with lower depression scores for the high-loss group.
3. Low socioeconomic status (SES) was significantly correlated with higher depression scores: 64.8% of those in the low SES group were in the high-loss group, compared with 31.1% in the high SES group. The data suggest that low SES causes double jeopardy; people have fewer coping resources and experience more losses.
4. A series of regression equations showed that losses, absence of resources, and preexisting depressive symptoms were powerful predictors of depression scores. The most powerful predictor was preexisting depression, followed by absence of resources, (including personal, familial, social, cultural, and SES). Loss scores had the lowest predictive value.

These data illustrate the complex relationship between life events, coping resources, and depressive symptoms:

The findings suggest that while life-event losses and the absence of personal and social resources are related to high depression scale scores, other factors are statistically (and probably theoretically) more important sources of explanation of depressive symptomatology. The findings also suggest that for some persons, at least, depressive symptomatology is a trait condition that may predispose them to life events which in turn exacerbate their preevent levels of psychiatric distress. The data also indicate that life-event losses are mitigated somewhat by the availability of personal, familial, interpersonal, and other resources; this finding has implications for early therapeutic intervention designed to assist those experiencing significant life-event losses.[59:507]

A final, more recent nursing research study has found additional support that depression is linked with poor adaptational or coping abilities in patients. Specifically, the four subgroups of social support, confidence, problem-solving ability, and tension reduction all showed a strong negative relationship with depression in hospitalized men and women.[23] Such research suggests the importance of nursing interventions that foster the person's ability to develop capacities for coping with life's disruptions.

■ **PHYSIOLOGICAL CHANGES.** Mood may also respond to drugs or a wide variety of physical illnesses (Table 14-2). Drug-induced depressions can follow treatment with antihypertensive drugs, particularly reserpine, and the abuse of addictive substances such as amphetamines, barbiturates, and alcohol. Depression may also occur secondary to medical illnesses, for example, viral infections, nutritional deficiencies, endocrine disorders, anemias, and central nervous system disorders such as multiple sclerosis, tumors, and cerebrovascular disease. Most chronic debilitating illnesses, whether physical or psychiatric, are accompanied by depression.

The depressions of the elderly are particularly complex because the differential diagnosis often involves organic brain damage and clinical depression. Diagnostic differentiation is complicated. Persons with early signs of senile brain changes, vascular disease, or other neurological diseases of aging may be more at risk for depression than the general population. In the United States there has been a tendency to overdiagnose arteriosclerosis and senility in persons over age 65, without recognizing that depression may manifest itself by a slowing of psychomotor activity. Lowered intellectual function and a loss of interest in sex, hobbies, and activities may be taken as signs of brain disease.

Mania can also be secondary to drugs, particularly steroids, amphetamines, and tricyclic antidepressants. It can be triggered by infections, neoplasms, and metabolic disturbances. The evidence that mania can result from pharmacological, structural, and metabolic disturbances suggests that mania, as with depression, is a clinical syndrome with multiple causes. The diversity

TABLE 14-2

PHYSICAL ILLNESSES AND DRUGS ASSOCIATED WITH DEPRESSIVE AND MANIC STATES

	Depression	Mania
Infectious	Influenza	Influenza
	Viral hepatitis	St. Louis encephalitis
	Infectious mononucleosis	Q fever
	General paresis (tertiary syphilis)	General paresis (tertiary syphilis)
	Tuberculosis	
Endocrine	Myxedema	Hyperthyroidism?
	Cushing's disease	
	Addison's disease	
Neoplastic	Occult abdominal malignancies (e.g., carcinoma of head of pancreas)	
Collagen	Systemic lupus erythematosus	Systemic lupus erythematosus
		Rheumatic chorea
Neurological	Multiple sclerosis	Multiple sclerosis
	Cerebral tumors	Diencephalic and third ventricular tumors
	Sleep apnea	
	Dementia	
	Parkinson's disease	
	Nondominant temporal lobe lesions	
Nutritional	Pellagra	
	Pernicious anemia	
Drugs	Steroidal contraceptives	Steroids
	Reserpine	Levodopa
	Alpha-methyldopa	Amphetamines
	Physostigmine	Methylphenidate
	Alcohol	Cocaine
	Sedative-hypnotics	Monoamine oxidase inhibitors
	Amphetamine withdrawal	Tricyclic antidepressants
		Thyroid hormones

From Whybrow P, Akiskal H, and McKinney W: Mood disorders: toward a new psychobiology, New York, 1984, Plenum Press.

of causes probably involves more than one pathophysiological pathway and challenges any unitary model of causation, whether the proposed factor of causation is biochemical, psychological, genetic, or structural.

■ Integrative model

Debate continues throughout psychiatry over the nature of depression, that is, whether depression is a single illness with different signs and symptoms or whether several diseases exist. This discussion of the various models or theories of causation also suggests the controversies in psychiatric research and practice. Each theory contributes to an understanding of mood disturbances. Many of them overlap and interrelate. Recent research also clearly shows that there are multiple causes for mood disturbances. These involve an interactive effect among predisposing and precipitating

factors that are biological and psychosocial in origin. Thus a unitary theory is not possible, but perhaps a unified theory is. Table 14-3 summarizes these major theories on causation.

Akiskal and McKinney and Whybrow[2,60] have presented a unified model of mood disorders that attempts to integrate current conceptual models. They view depression as the feedback interaction of three sets of variables at the chemical, experiential, and behavioral levels, with the diencephalon serving as the field of action. They propose that impairment in one of the variables affects the other two. Thus any one of the three variables can contribute to a depression and produce changes in the other two areas. For example, a chemical imbalance can result in distorted perceptions, or a major life change can cause a chemical imbalance. In this model, depressive illness is the culmi-

TABLE 14-3

SUMMARY OF MODELS OF CAUSATION OF SEVERE MOOD DISTURBANCES

Model	Mechanism
Genetic	Transmission through heredity and family history
Aggression turned inward	Turning of angry feelings inward against oneself
Object loss	Separation from loved one and disruption of attachment bond
Personality organization	Negative self-concept and low self-esteem influence one's belief system and appraisal of stressors
Cognitive	Hopelessness experienced because of negative cognitive set
Learned helplessness	Belief that one's responses are ineffectual and that reinforcers in the environment cannot be controlled
Behavioral	Loss of positive reinforcement in life
Biological	Impaired monoaminergic neurotransmission
Life stressors	Response to life stress from five possible sources: loss of attachment, major life events, roles, coping resources, and physiological changes
Integrative	Interaction of chemical, experiential, and behavioral variables acting on the diencephalon

nation of various processes that converge in those areas of the diencephalon modulating arousal, mood, motivation, and psychomotor functions. As depicted in Fig. 14-2, the form the illness takes depends on the following factors:

1. Genetic vulnerability—important, particularly in recurrent and manic-depressive illnesses
2. Developmental events—early object loss that may sensitize the individual to future stress,

create negative cognitive sets, and result in learned helplessness
3. Physiological stressors—stimuli such as viral infections and childbirth that induce biochemical changes
4. Psychosocial stressors—stressful life events that overwhelm coping mechanisms

This integrative multicausal model presents a useful frame of reference for the nurse. It is holistic and encourages the assessment of behavior in developing nursing interventions. It also presents a variety of causative factors and stresses their interrelationship in explaining present behavior. Predisposing factors are important, and the way they interact with the precipitating event is crucial.

■ Behaviors

■ **ASSOCIATED WITH UNCOMPLICATED GRIEF REACTIONS.** The successful resolution of uncomplicated grief somewhat follows a sequence by which the nurse can determine if healing is occurring. Knowledge of normal mourning allows the nurse to provide support as well as identify maladaptive responses, if they should occur. Various theorists have identified stages of grief and mourning, including Bowlby,[9] Kübler-Ross,[31] and Engel,[20] and there are many similarities.

A cross-cultural study of grief and mourning in 78 cultures indicated that mourning and accompanying grief represent a universal human response.[50] The form of emotional expression varies from culture to

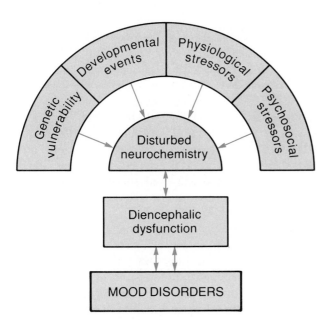

Fig. 14-2. Unified model of mood disorders.

culture, but an emotionless reaction to the loss of a loved person is rare. Bowlby's phases present a comprehensive review of the process of mourning and can be applied to losses of any type. These phases are (1) the urge to recover the lost object, (2) disorganization, and (3) reorganization. Each phase and its emotional component of mourning is briefly described.

Phase 1 is disequilibrium. The survivor experiences shock and disbelief. This reaction is followed by a numbed sensation in which the survivor does not acknowledge the reality of the death and hopes to recover his loss. Two of the major affective components of this phase are weeping and anger. Crying involves an acknowledgment of the loss and a regression to a more childlike state. Tears among the survivors are generally accepted and elicit certain types of support, although this varies greatly from culture to culture.

Anger is the other major component of this stage. It may erupt toward nurses or other health care personnel whom the survivor associates with the death. The mourner may also turn this anger on himself, particularly if he feels the death was his responsibility in any way. Guilt is a related emotion as the survivor berates himself for failing to do right by the lost one. The greater the survivor's ambivalence toward the deceased, the greater will be his sense of guilt.

Phase 2 is disorganization. When the survivor realizes the loss is permanent, despair sets in and his behavior becomes increasingly disorganized and restless. He experiences a loss of self-esteem and profound loneliness, fear, and helplessness. This phase is painful and alarming, and he might use denial to protect himself. Symptoms of somatic stress may appear. Lindemann[36] identified the most common ones: (1) sighing, (2) lack of strength and exhaustion, and (3) digestive difficulties, such as loss of appetite and a feeling of emptiness in the stomach. Previous conflicts may be reactivated, such as dependence versus independence and trust versus mistrust.

The sensorium is generally altered. There is a slight feeling of unreality, emotional distance from others, and preoccupation with the image of the deceased. Recurrent tearful longing for the deceased may be associated with thoughts, memories, or mental images. These may be triggered by any reminder of the lost one and may be especially intense and painful at night. Many survivors have illusions of seeing or feeling the presence of the dead person. In extreme cases these are intense but transient hallucinations. There may be much random activity but an inability to organize and complete tasks. Life is devoid of enthusiasm, and daily activities proceed automatically. Social interaction is greatly reduced, and feelings of helplessness

may complicate mourning in two ways: there is a sense of powerlessness over restoring the lost person and helplessness without the person's companionship.

Phase 3 is reorganization. The survivor no longer lives in the past and begins to break his attachment to the lost person. He establishes new goals and relationships. He may incorporate the values, behaviors, and goals of the deceased in an appropriate and satisfying way. He tests out new behavior and expands his own sense of identity.

Successful mourning takes 6 months to a year, with intensity of the initial reaction subsiding after a couple of weeks. As with any other process, it can take one of several courses. Those that enable the individual ultimately to relate to new objects and to find satisfaction in them are typically judged adaptive, or healthy. Those that fail in this outcome are believed to be maladaptive, or pathological.

In recent years attention has been focused on somatic illness and increased mortality caused by death of or separation from a loved object. The loss represents a precipitating factor in such diverse diseases as asthma, pulmonary tuberculosis, peptic ulcer, ulcerative colitis, diabetes, coronary occlusion, myocardial infarction, cardiac failure, thyrotoxicosis, pernicious anemia, leukemia, and multiple sclerosis.

Psychiatric illness can also be a sequel to loss. Parkes and Brown,[42] in an investigation of bereavement and mental illness, found that 2.9% of 3,245 admissions to psychiatric hospitals took place within 6 months of the death of a close relative. Frequency of admission after the death of a spouse was six times greater than would be expected by chance alone. Although the bereaved patients proved to have a variety of psychiatric illnesses, the most common diagnosis was depression. Evidence relating object loss to somatic symptom formation does not prove cause and effect. However, it strongly suggests that grief related to object loss may contribute diverse somatic reactions.

■ **ASSOCIATED WITH DELAYED GRIEF REACTIONS.** The designation of grief as pathological indicates that something has prevented it from running its normal course. Defenses used successfully in an uncomplicated grief reaction become exaggerated or maladaptive in a pathological reaction. The result may be delayed grief or a distorted reaction, such as in depression or mania. Delayed grief reactions may be manifested by excessive hostility and grief, prolonged feelings of emptiness and numbness, an inability to weep or express emotions, low self-esteem, use of present tense instead of past when speaking of the loss, persistent dreams about the loss, retention of clothing of the deceased, an inability to visit the grave of the deceased,

Mrs. G was a 38-year-old married woman with no history of depression. She came to the local community mental health center complaining of "severe throbbing headaches, difficulty falling asleep, fitful and disturbing dreams when asleep, and poor appetite." She said she felt "disgusted" with herself and "useless" to her family. At present she was living alone with her husband.

Her family history revealed she had three children—two boys and a girl. Her eldest son, age 20, was attending college out of state, and her daughter, age 19, was living with a girlfriend in the same city. Her youngest son was killed in an automobile accident 2 years ago when 15 years old. She described him as her "baby" and expressed much guilt for contributing to his death. She scolded herself for allowing him to drive to the shore for the weekend with friends, and said she now worries a great deal about her other two children. She said she was trying to protect them from the dangers of the world, but they resented her advice and concern. On questioning by the nurse, Mrs. G reported that these feelings of sadness and guilt had emerged in the last month and seemed to be triggered by the graduation of her son's high-school class.

and the projection of living memories into an object held in place of the lost one. Clinical example 14-1 illustrates some of the behaviors associated with a delayed grief reaction.

In this example Mrs. G was experiencing a delayed grief reaction precipitated by the emotionally invested event of her deceased son's would-be graduation. She had failed to progress through mourning at her son's death and was beginning "grief work" at present. The behaviors she displayed were consistent with her depression.

Because sadness, disappointment, and frustration are normal in human life, the boundary between normal and abnormal mood is often difficult to define. Behaviors associated with severe mood disturbances or affective disorders reflect an increase in the intensity or the duration of otherwise normal emotions. They may range from moderate anxiety (indicative of neurotic health problems) to panic (indicative of psychotic health problems). In severe forms, disturbances of mood are maladaptive because of their intensity, pervasiveness, persistence, and interference with daily functioning. This may be reflected in impaired body function; the inability to perform social roles, such as at work, in the family, or at school; suicidal thoughts; and interference with reality testing, such as delusions, hallucinations, or confusion.

■ **ASSOCIATED WITH DEPRESSION.** The behaviors associated with depression vary. Sadness and slowness may predominate, or agitation may occur. The key element to a behavioral assessment is change—the individual changes his usual patterns and responses. Research indicates that the individual working through normal mourning responds to his loss with psychological symptoms often indistinguishable from depression, but accepted by him and by his environment as normal. In contrast, patients with depression experience their condition as a "change" unlike their usual self, which often leads them to seek help.[15]

Many behaviors are associated with depression. These may be divided into affective, physiological, cognitive, and behavioral manifestations (Table 14-4). Obviously, some are contradictory and incompatible. The lists describe the spectrum of possible behaviors, acknowledging that not all individuals experience all of them.

The most common and central behavior is that of the depressive mood. This is not necessarily described by the patient as "depression" but as feeling sad, blue, down in the dumps, unhappy, or unable to enjoy life. Crying often occurs. On the other hand, some depressed persons do not cry and describe themselves as "beyond tears." The mood disturbance of the depressed patient resembles that of normal unhappiness multiplied in intensity and pervasiveness. Another mood that often accompanies depression is anxiety—a sense of fear and intense worry. Both depression and anxiety may show diurnal variation, that is, a pattern whereby certain times of the day, such as morning or evening, are consistently worse or better.

The literature reveals no agreement on which behaviors typically reflect depression and which are most significant for assessment, treatment, and prognosis. Also, the identified behaviors are not exclusive to depression; they may also appear in other health problems. Levitt and Lubin[33] reviewed the literature and listed the symptoms of depression cited in at least 2 of 13 sources published between 1961 and 1969. They also reviewed the symptoms appearing in at least 2 of 16 depression measurement instruments. Of the 24 self-rating measures, 5 are most frequently used: the Minnesota Multiphasic Personality Inventory (MMPI) depression scale, the Beck Depression Inventory, the Hamilton Rating Scale for Depression, the Zung Self-Rating Depression Scale, and the Depression Adjective Checklist. Beck[5] provided further data by reviewing

TABLE 14-4

BEHAVIORS ASSOCIATED WITH DEPRESSION

Affective	Physiological	Cognitive	Behavioral
Anger	Abdominal pain	Ambivalence	Aggressiveness
Anxiety	Anorexia	Confusion	Agitation
Apathy	Backache	Inability to concentrate	Alcoholism
Bitterness	Chest pain	Indecisiveness	Altered activity level
Dejection	Constipation	Loss of interest and motivation	Drug addiction
Denial of feelings	Dizziness	Self-blame	Intolerance
Despondency	Fatigue	Self-depreciation	Irritability
Guilt	Headache	Self-destructive thoughts	Lack of spontaneity
Helplessness	Impotence	Pessimism	Overdependency
Hopelessness	Indigestion	Uncertainty	Poor personal hygiene
Loneliness	Insomnia		Psychomotor retardation
Low self-esteem	Lassitude		Social isolation
Sadness	Menstrual changes		Tearfulness
Sense of personal worthlessness	Nausea		Underachievement
	Overeating		Withdrawal
	Sexual nonresponsiveness		
	Sleep disturbances		
	Vomiting		
	Weight change		

TABLE 14-5

SYMPTOMS OF DEPRESSION AND THEIR PREVALENCE

Symptom	Sources using symptom[33] (%)	Measurement instruments monitoring symptom[33] (%)	Severely depressed patients showing symptom[5] (%)
Self-devaluation	54	100	81
Dejected mood	92	87	88
Suicidal thoughts	100	81	74
Pessimism, feelings of hopelessness	77	81	87
Loss of appetite	77	75	72
Sleep disturbance	77	75	87
Loss of libido	84	44	61
Fatigability	46	81	78
Loss of interest, enjoyment	46	62	92
Guilt feelings	70	62	60
Social withdrawal	38	69	64
Crying spells	38	44	83
Indecisiveness	30	50	76
Constipation	30	44	52
Psychomotor retardation	30	81	87
Loss of motivation	46	62	86
Diurnal mood variation	40	20	37
Feelings of inadequacy, helplessness	30	20	90

the proportions of depressed patients manifesting various symptoms. Table 14-5 summarizes the findings of Levitt and Lubin and Beck. According to the findings of Beck, the cardinal symptoms of a depressive syndrome, as defined by their presence in at least 75% of patients, include feelings of inadequacy and helplessness, loss of motivation, psychomotor retardation, indecisiveness, crying spells, loss of interest and enjoyment, fatigability, sleep disturbances, pessimism, dejected mood, and self-devaluation.

Finally, the potential for suicide should always be assessed in severe mood disturbances. Suicide and other self-destructive behaviors are discussed in detail in Chapter 15. The intensity of anger, guilt, and worthlessness may precipitate suicidal thoughts, feelings, or gestures, as illustrated in Clinical example 14-2.

This example dramatically emphasizes three important points. First, medical illness frequently involves a loss of function, body part, or appearance. Therefore all patients should be assessed for depression. Second, all people experiencing depression and despair have the potential for suicide. Third, nurses can intervene to support the grieving and mourning process whether it is uncomplicated or pathological. Nursing actions can be preventive, curative, or rehabilitative, based on the nursing assessment and diagnosis.

■ **ASSOCIATED WITH MANIA.** The essential feature of mania is a distinct period of intense psychophysiological activation. Some of the associated behaviors are given in Table 14-6. The predominant mood is elevated or irritable, accompanied by one or more of

CLINICAL EXAMPLE 14-2

Mr. W was a 60-year-old man who lived alone. His son and daughter were married and lived in the same state. His wife died 2 years ago, and since that time his children had often asked him to move in with either of them. He had consistently refused to do this, believing that both he and his children needed privacy in their lives. Six months ago he was diagnosed as having advanced prostatic cancer with metastasis. After the diagnosis and because of increasing disability, he left his job and began to receive disability compensation. He visited his children and their families about twice a month and kept his regularly scheduled visits with the medical clinic. The nurses and physicians at the clinic noted he was "despondent and withdrawn," but viewed this as a normal reaction to his diagnosis and family history. No interventions were implemented based on his emotional needs. A week after attending the clinic for a routine, follow-up visit, he went to the cemetery where his wife was buried and at her gravestone shot himself in the head. A grounds keeper of the cemetery heard the shot, discovered what had happened, and called an ambulance. Mr. W was taken to the emergency room of the nearest hospital and, with prompt medical care, survived the suicide attempt.

TABLE 14-6
BEHAVIORS ASSOCIATED WITH MANIA

Affective	Physiological	Cognitive	Behavioral
Elation or euphoria	Dehydration	Ambitiousness	Aggressiveness
Expansiveness	Inadequate nutrition	Denial of realistic danger	Excessive spending of money
Humorous	Needs little sleep	Distractibility	Grandiose acts
Inflated self-esteem	Weight loss	Flight of ideas	Hyperactivity
Intolerance of criticism		Grandiosity	Increased motor activity
Lack of shame or guilt		Illusions	Irresponsibility
		Lack of judgment	Irritability or argumentativeness
		Loose associations	Poor personal grooming
			Provocativeness
			Sexual overactivity
			Social activity
			Verbosity

the following symptoms: hyperactivity, the undertaking of too many activities, lack of judgment in anticipating consequences, pressured speech, flight of ideas, distractibility, inflated self-esteem, and hypersexuality.

If the mood is elevated or euphoric, it is often infectious. Patients report feeling happy, unconcerned, carefree, and devoid of problems. Although such experiences would seem enviable, these affective moods are without any concern for reality or the feelings of others. The mood is often expansive, and some patients have extraordinary delusions about their power and importance. They characteristically involve themselves in seemingly senseless and risky enterprises.

Alternately, the mood may be irritable, especially when plans are thwarted. Patients can be contentious and provoked by seemingly harmless remarks. Self-esteem is inflated during a manic episode, and, as activity level increases, feelings about the self become increasingly disturbed. Delusional grandiose symptoms are evident, and the patient is willing to undertake any project possible.

In contrast to depressed patients, manic patients are extremely self-confident, with an ego that knows no bounds; they are "on top of the world." Accompanying this magical omnipotence and supreme self-esteem is an equally inordinate lack of guilt and shame. Often they deny realistic danger. The patient's boundless energy, cunning, planning, scheming, and inability to forecast consequences frequently lead to irresponsible enterprises and excessive spending, as well as to misdemeanors of a sexual, aggressive, or possessive nature. In contrast to depressed patients, manic patients have heightened libidinal drives, with abounding energy and heightened sexual appetite. Characteristic physical changes are inadequate nutrition, partly because manic patients have no time to eat, and serious loss of weight related to their insomnia and overactivity. Extremely manic patients may be dehydrated and require prompt attention.

In addition to mood, speech is often disturbed. As mania intensifies, formal and logical speech is displaced by loud, rapid, and confusing language. As the activated state increases, speech becomes full of plays on words and irrelevancies that can increase to loosened associations and flight of ideas. Some of these behaviors are evident in Clinical example 14-3.

Associated behaviors found in mania include lability of mood with rapid shifts to brief depression. Such behavior accounts for those patients who have loosened associations and alternately laugh and cry. In addition, hallucinations of any type, ideas of reference, and frank delusions may be present with predominant feelings of guilt and thoughts of suicide. Manic epi-

---

CLINICAL EXAMPLE 14-3

Mr. B was a 30-year-old single man who was admitted to the psychiatric unit of the local community hospital. He had been hospitalized 2 years ago for problems related to alcoholism. He was accompanied to the hospital by a friend who lived with him. His friend said that for the past 2 months Mr. B had been "running on ten cylinders instead of four." He slept and ate little and talked constantly, sometimes so fast that no one could understand what he was trying to say. He had redecorated his bedroom in the apartment twice and had gone into debt buying a new "mod" wardrobe. His friend brought him in because his behavior was becoming more erratic and his physical condition was failing.

The nurse who admitted Mr. B asked about his social relationships. He revealed that his girlfriend of 7 years had left him 6 months ago for another man. He said that initially he thought she would "see the light," but she had refused to see him since then. Mr. B said this "upset" him a little at the time, but he was sure it was "for the best and there were plenty other women out there just waiting for him."

---

sodes have a high tendency toward recurrence. Only about 25% of manic patients have just one episode, and almost all with manic episodes also have depressive episodes. However, the duration and severity of the manic episode vary, as do the intervals between relapses and recurrences.

All these clinical examples illustrate the interrelatedness of disturbances of mood with self-esteem and disrupted relationships. Multiple aspects of the individual's life are affected, including physical health. Hypertensive crises, irritable bowel syndromes, coronary occlusions, rheumatoid arthritis, migraine headaches, and various dermatological conditions can occur with severe mood disturbances.

■ Coping mechanisms

Uncomplicated grief reactions can be normal mourning or simple bereavement. Mourning includes all the psychological processes set in motion by the loss. Increased preoccupation with detailed memories of the lost object is the work of mourning. Freud described it as the painful and necessary work of readjustment to the loss. As mourning is extended over time, there is a "working through" of an affective behavior that, if released in its full strength, would overwhelm the ego.

Mourning begins with the introjection of the lost object. When a person grieves, his feelings are directed to a mental image of the loved one. Thus the mechanism of introjection serves as a buffering mechanism. Through reality testing, the individual realizes that the love object no longer exists, and he withdraws his emotional investment from it. This is accompanied by an internal struggle because he does not willingly abandon a source of personal gratification. The ultimate productive outcome is that reality wins out, but this is accomplished slowly over time. When the mourning work is completed, the ego becomes more free and uninhibited to invest in new objects.

Although specific reactions may vary, grief has to be worked out. If not, the person will continue to experience conflict. Hodge has explained it as follows:

The problem must be brought into the open and confronted, no matter how unpleasant it may be for the patient. *The grief work must be done.* There is no healthy escape from this. We might even add that the grief work *will* be done. Sooner or later, correctly or incorrectly, completely or incompletely, in a clear or a distorted manner, *it will be done.* People have a natural protective tendency to avoid the unpleasantness of the grief work, but it is necessary and the more actively it is done, the shorter will be the period of grief. If the grief work is not actively pursued, the process may be fixated or aborted or delayed, with the patient feeling that he may have escaped it. However, almost certainly a distorted form of the grief work will appear at some time in the future.[26:230]

A delayed grief reaction therefore reflects exaggerated defense mechanisms of denial and suppression in an attempt to avoid intense distress. The distorted grief reaction of depression is, in a sense, abortive grieving. Specific defenses used to block mourning are repression, suppression, denial, and dissociation. The person may even unconsciously wish to be rewarded for suffering by restoration of the lost object. Because this is impossible, the depressed person's hopelessness takes on an added dimension. Denial of the loss in depression results in profound feelings of guilt, anger, and despair that focus on one's own unworthiness. Thus the cycle of depression is reinforced and perpetuated.

Manic and hypomanic episodes occur more rarely than depressive states. Some believe that mania is a mirror image of depression and that, even though the behaviors are dissimilar, the dynamics and coping mechanisms are related. According to this view, manic behavior is a defense against depression, since the individual attempts to deny his feelings of worthlessness and helplessness. His elation and hyperactivity are an appeal for love and a protection from depression.

 # Nursing diagnosis
■ Identifying nursing problems

The diagnosis of disturbances of mood depends on an understanding of many interrelated concepts, including anxiety, self-concept, and hostility. One task of the nurse in formulating a diagnosis is to decide if the patient is experiencing primarily a state of anxiety (see Chapter 11) or depression. It is often difficult to distinguish between the two because they may coexist in one patient and are manifested by similar behaviors. Crary and Crary[17] suggest some comparative observations that may be helpful. They note that the depressed patient is often slowed down in speech and movements; the anxious patient often responds normally or actively. The depressed patient is reluctant to discuss his problems or symptoms; the anxious patient is more likely to discuss his symptoms and related topics. The depressed patient has decreased his outside interests; the anxious patient usually retains interest in some things. The depressed patient has difficulty enjoying things; the anxious patient can enjoy some activities. The depressed patient usually feels worse in the morning or after sleep; the anxious patient usually feels worse in the evening and better after sleep or rest. The depressed patient usually has decreased appetite and enjoyment of food; the anxious patient usually eats intermittently and enjoys at least some foods.

A nursing diagnosis should include the patient's maladaptive coping response and related stressor. Fig. 14-3 presents the nursing model of health-illness phenomena with the continuum of emotional responses. The maladaptive responses are a result of anxiety, hostility, self-devaluation, and guilt. This model suggests that nursing care will be centered around increasing self-esteem and encouraging expression of emotions.

Many NANDA nursing diagnoses would be appropriate for an individual experiencing a disturbance of mood. Primary NANDA nursing diagnoses and examples of complete nursing diagnoses related to mood disorders are presented in the box on page 437. A complete nursing assessment would incorporate the many human responses in diagnostic formulations. Table 14-7 presents nursing diagnoses related to possible maladaptive responses of the patient with a mood disorder.

■ Related medical diagnoses

The model also identifies some medical diagnoses appropriate to disturbances of mood or affective disor-

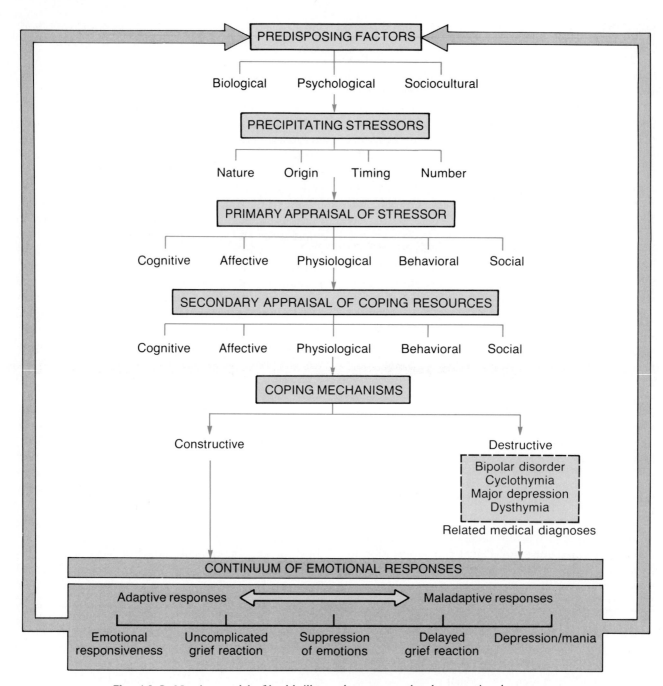

Fig. 14-3. Nursing model of health-illness phenomena related to emotional responses.

ders. The psychiatric classification of affective disorders has largely reflected the controversies surrounding the nature, cause, and treatment of these disorders. Although these traditional labels are no longer used in the DSM-III-R,[3] nurses know them because they may continue to have some research and clinical value.

One traditional distinction has been to separate patients into those with **psychotic versus neurotic affective states.** Unfortunately, these terms have acquired multiple meanings and have lost their precision in defining clinical or research practice. Another traditional distinction has been between **endogenous versus reactive, or exogenous, types of depression.** Endogenous depressions were believed to have resulted from early personality development and intrinsic biological processes, whereas exogenous, or reactive, types

Nursing Diagnoses Related to Mood Disturbances

Primary NANDA nursing diagnoses

Coping, ineffective individual
Grieving, anticipatory
Grieving, dysfunctional
Hopelessness
Powerlessness
Spiritual distress (distress of the human spirit)
Violence, potential for self-directed

Examples of complete nursing diagnoses

Ineffective individual coping related to discovery of spouse's extramarital affair, evidenced by euphoric state, hyperactivity, and lack of judgment
Anticipatory grieving related to son's impending departure from home, evidenced by sadness and loss of interest in daily events

Dysfunctional grieving related to death of sister, evidenced by self-devaluation, sleep disturbance, and dejected mood
Hopelessness related to loss of job, evidenced by feelings of despair and development of ulcerative colitis
Powerlessness related to new role as parent, evidenced by apathy, uncertainty, and overdependency
Spiritual distress related to loss of child in utero, evidenced by self-blame, somatic complaints, and pessimism about the future
Potential for self-directed violence related to rejection by boyfriend, evidenced by self-destructive acts

TABLE 14-7

MEDICAL AND NURSING DIAGNOSES RELATED TO MOOD DISTURBANCES

Medical Diagnostic Class Mood (affective) disorders	**Psychiatric Nursing Diagnostic Class** Disturbances in mood
Related Medical Diagnoses (DSM-III-R)*	**Related Nursing Diagnoses (NANDA)**
Bipolar disorder	Anxiety
Cyclothymia	Communication, impaired verbal
Major depression	†Coping, ineffective individual
Dysthymia	†Grieving, anticipatory
	†Grieving, dysfunctional
	†Hopelessness
	Injury, potential for
	Nutrition, altered
	†Powerlessness
	Self-care deficit
	Self-esteem disturbance
	Sexual dysfunction
	Sleep pattern disturbance
	Social isolation
	†Spiritual distress (distress of the human spirit)
	Thought processes, altered
	†Violence, potential for self-directed

*From American Psychiatric Association: Diagnostic and Statistical Manual of Mental Disorders, Third edition–Revised, Washington, D.C., 1987, The Association.
†Indicates primary nursing diagnoses for disturbances in mood.

were believed to have occurred in response to external environmental stress, such as recent loss or disappointment. Research, however, has failed to verify these traditional distinctions. Thus the psychotic-neurotic distinction and the endogenous-reactive dichotomy are better regarded as continuums along which patients may be placed. Most patients are intermediate on the continuum and few are at the extremes. Neither classification is used in the DSM-III-R.[3]

Robins and Guze[48] avoid the controversial endogenous-reactive and psychotic-neurotic dichotomies. They propose a distinction between **primary and secondary affective disorders** based on two criteria, chronology and the presence of associated illnesses. "Primary" affective disorders occur in patients who have been well or whose only previous episodes of psychiatric disease were mania or depression. "Secondary" affective disorders include feelings of sadness, inadequacy, and hopelessness that occur with another preexisting psychiatric disorder, such as anxiety reactions. It also includes symptoms secondary to medical illnesses.

A final distinction is the **bipolar-unipolar affective states.** It proposes the separation of depressed patients with a history of manic episodes (the bipolar group) from those who have had only recurrent episodes of depression (the unipolar group). Among newer approaches, the bipolar-unipolar distinction has achieved considerable acceptance. Two major categories of mood or affective disorders are identified in the DSM-III-R[3]: bipolar disorders and depressive (unipolar) disorders (Table 14-7). The specific disorders identified under each are now briefly described.

■ **BIPOLAR DISORDER.** The essential feature of bipolar disorder is current or past experience of a manic episode, lasting at least 1 week, when one's mood was abnormally and persistently elevated, expansive, or irritable. The episode is sufficiently severe to cause extreme impairment in social or occupational functioning. Bipolar disorders may be classified as manic (limited to only manic episodes), depressed (a history of manic episodes with a current depressive episode), or mixed (a mixed presentation of both manic and depressive episodes).

■ **CYCLOTHYMIA.** The essential feature of cyclothymia is a history of 2 years of hypomania in which the person experienced numerous periods with abnormally elevated, expansive, or irritable moods. These moods did not meet the criteria for a manic episode, and many periods of depressed mood did not meet the criteria of a major depressive episode.

■ **MAJOR DEPRESSION.** The essential feature of major depression is the presence of at least five symptoms during the same 2-week period, with one being either depressed mood or loss of interest or pleasure. Other symptoms might include weight loss, insomnia, psychomotor agitation or retardation, fatigue, feelings of worthlessness, diminished ability to think, and recurrent thoughts of death. Major depressions may be classified as single episode or recurrent.

■ **DYSTHYMIA.** The essential feature of dysthymia is at least 2 years of a usually depressed mood and at least one of the symptoms mentioned for major depression without meeting the criteria for a major depressive episode.

◆ Planning and implementation

■ Goal setting

The general goal of the nurse working with a patient experiencing an uncomplicated grief reaction is to support him in the subjective experience of his grief work or to help him mourn. This means helping the person know what has been lost, that his pain is worthy of his own respect, and that real hope lies in acknowledging rather than denying his loss. He needs to extricate himself from his bondage to the lost object and to find new patterns of rewarding interaction. In this way he copes with the loss, integrates it into his past, and grows from the experience. Mutual long-term goals will therefore refer to completing the process of grieving, mourning, or bereavement. This may take 6 months to a year or longer, since the duration of grieving varies considerably among cultural groups[3]. Short-term goals identify realistic steps the patient can take as he works through the mourning process. They should reflect progression through Bowlby's[9] phases: (1) the urge to recover the lost object, (2) disorganization, and (3) reorganization. Short-term goals may include the following:

The patient will:

1. Express feelings of sorrow caused by the loss of her husband within 10 days
2. Describe her ambivalence (love and anger) toward her husband by the end of 1 month
3. Review her relationship with her husband, including shared pleasures, regrets, and so on

When the patient is experiencing a maladaptive disturbance of mood, long-term goals may be directed toward reinitiating a delayed grief reaction or exploring areas of conflict. When nursing intervention is planned, psychotherapeutic, sociotherapeutic, and somatotherapeutic factors should be considered collectively and conjointly. An abbreviated sample care plan for a patient is presented in Fig. 14-4. The long-term

PSYCHIATRIC NURSING CARE PLAN

Precautions:
Assess for suicidal ideation

Special nursing needs:
Encourage personal hygiene

Visitors: {x} No restrictions
{ } Family only
{ } Restricted to:

{ } No visitors

Telephone: { } Limited
{x} Unlimited

Privileges: { } Restricted to unit
{ } Off unit accompanied by staff
{x} Off unit accompanied by family/visitor
{ } Off unit unaccompanied
{ } Out of hospital leave (dates) _____

Assessment data summary: Second admission; tearful; withdrawn; married with 2 adolescent children; husband is supportive but away for extended periods of time due to naval career; recently relocated to the state due to husbands career; one previous psychiatric admission in another state 4 years ago precipitated by her mother's death; works part-time in local department store; expresses being overwhelmed and despairing.

Nursing diagnoses: 1. Powerlessness related to multiple role demands evidenced by feelings of apathy and despair.
2. Self-esteem disturbance related to lack of career and problems with children evidenced by self-deprecatory verbalizations.
3. Alteration in family process related to absences and lack of involvement of husband evidenced by marital conflicts and distancing.

Treatment goal: Growth toward use of adaptive emotional responses and increased satisfaction and pleasure in daily activities.

Date	Problem/need	Expected outcome (objective)	Target Date	Nursing Intervention
7-3-90	Recognition and expression of feelings	Verbalization of positive and negative feelings	7-10-90	Assist patient to identify and describe feelings about her life situation
7-3-90	Involvement in self-enhancing behaviors	Identification of specific growth-producing activities	7-12-90	Explore positive self-attributes. Identify realistic goals. Reinforce self-enhancing behaviors and verbalizations
7-7-90	Family integration and negotiation	Increased communication and role clarification by family members	7-17-90	Facilitate clarification of family roles. Encourage discussion among family members. Support differentiation of patient from husband.

Room	Patient's name	Age	Doctor	Primary nurse	Admit date
204	Mrs. W.	45	Dr. R	Mr. M	7-2-90

Fig. 14-4. Sample nursing care plan for a depressed patient. (This nursing care plan includes examples of the elements of a total plan as might appear at a particular time in the patient's course of treatment. It should not be considered all inclusive.)   *Continued.*

Date	Medications	Date	P.R.N. Medications	Diagnostic & psychiatric tests	Req.	Done
7-3	Imipramine	7-4	Halcion	Dexamethasone	7-3	✓
	50 mg		0.5 mg H.S.	suppression test		
7-5	Imipramine			(DST)		
	100 mg					
7-7	Imipramine			ECG	7-4	✓
	150 mg					
7-9	Imipramine			Tricyclic blood	7-10	
	200 mg			level		
		Date	Treatments	Special orders and concerns		

Allergies:	Medical diagnosis: (axis I-III)	Diet:
None	Major depression	Regular

Fig. 14-4, cont'd. Sample nursing care plan for a depressed patient.

goals of nursing care for patients with severe mood disturbance have the following aims:

1. To allow for recognition and continuous expression of feelings, including denial, hopelessness, anger, guilt, blame, helplessness, regret, hope, and relief, within a supportive therapeutic atmosphere
2. To allow for gradual analysis of stressors while strengthening the patient's self-esteem
3. To increase the patient's sense of identity, control, awareness of choices, and responsibility for behavior
4. To encourage healthy interpersonal ties with others
5. To promote understanding of maladaptive emotions and to acquire coping responses to stressors

Specific short-term goals should be generated from behaviors of the patient, present areas of difficulty, and relevant stressors. Goal setting should involve a holistic view of the patient and his world. Goals probably will need to be developed regarding the patient's self-concept, physical status, behavioral performance, expression of emotions, and relation-ships. All these areas can directly relate to the disturbance of mood. The patients participation in setting these goals can be a significant first step in regaining mastery over his own life.

■ **Intervening in uncomplicated grief reactions**

The nurse's overall goal is to assist the patient who has experienced a loss work through grieving or mourning and to prevent maladaptive responses. Grieving is resolved when the lost object is internalized, bonds of attachment are loosened, and new object relationships are established. Grief most often occurs as a response to separation. Grief may also occur, however, following loss of something tangible or intangible that is highly regarded. Thus loss of a body part or function, job, opportunity, relationship, family possessions, or status and regard among one's peers can all precipitate grief reactions.

Nurses frequently care for patients who have lost body functions. Such losses include body parts (amputation, mastectomy), internal organs, sensory loss (vision, hearing), sexual function (impotence, menopause), and aging (mental functioning, physical strength). More than 40,000 limb amputations are performed annually in the United States. Breast amputation is a major approach to treating mammary cancer, which accounts for 25% of all malignancies in women. Such partial loss of the body is increasingly common and often results, at least temporarily, in a disturbance in body image (see Chapter 13). The patient's reaction to a loss of body part may be comparable to the loss of a significant person. Consequently, mourning is initiated and grief is the normal response.

In a broader sense, loss and separation are the recurrent themes of human life, and all change can be regarded as loss—the loss of the past in the movement to something new. This new area can be anticipated or feared, valued or dreaded. It can also be a normal developmental change, such as entering school or getting married. Even if society regards the event as positive, the significance of it for the individual may be quite different. Thus the nurse must assess both the nature of the change or loss and the significance of it. The principles underlying therapeutic nursing interventions in uncomplicated grief reactions are the same, however, regardless of the exact nature of the loss.

■ **SELF-AWARENESS.** Before the nurse becomes actively involved with the bereaved person, he or she must have an understanding of his or her own feelings and reactions to loss. Time should be spent recalling previous losses, examining related feelings, and resolving areas of conflict. If the nurse is uncomfortable or ambivalent about death or has delayed the grief work involved in a personal loss, he or she will be unable to work with the bereaved person. Hope is an essential quality for the nurse. Hope and commitment to the future can be transmitted to the bereaved. Hope also involves sharing and a sense of partnership. These are demonstrated in the nurse-patient relationship as the nurse shares the grief of the bereaved. Finally, nurses working with mourning persons need support systems of their own. Nursing peers, supervisors, and other professionals can provide formal or informal opportunities for ventilation and rejuvenation. This is essential because assisting the bereaved can be psychologically draining and interpersonally painful.

■ **OFFER ANTICIPATORY GUIDANCE.** Interventions can be initiated through anticipatory guidance even before the loss occurs. This involves talking about the impending loss with the individual and his family, if appropriate. Past losses may be reviewed and analyzed to clarify the meaning of the present loss. Since losses are present in all aspects of life and in all settings, any nurse may implement these interventions. For example, the industrial nurse may discuss the impending retirement of an employee; an office nurse may discuss the implications of a scheduled hysterectomy for a young woman; or a public health nurse may focus on a mother's feelings about her youngest child starting school. Many opportunities for interventions are overlooked by nurses, but their preventive potential is immeasurable.

■ **SUPPORT THE PATIENT AND FAMILY.** Engel[20] identifies several preventive actions the nurse can take in working with a dying patient and his family. He suggests that news of death or impending death should be communicated to a family group, rather than an individual alone, in a private setting. The nurse should be prepared to stay with and comfort the bereaved at least until a friend or clergyman arrives. The survivor's need to see the dying or dead patient should be met whenever possible because this helps in facing the reality of death.

When the nurse encounters an angry hostile survivor, two considerations should be kept in mind. First, the person could be justified. If not, he may be trying to deal with his own anger and guilt toward the dying person. The reaction is not directed toward the nurse but serves as an important coping mechanism in the initial stage of mourning. Second, another defense the survivor may display is disbelief and distraught behavior. The nurse should find a place for survivors to cry and express their feelings. She should also be considerate of the cultural, religious, and social customs of the mourners, regardless of how different they may be from her own. Finally, Engel stresses the need of the patient to grieve for himself. This point is emphasized by Kübler-Ross[31] in her work with the dying.

■ **IDENTIFY THOSE AT HIGH RISK.** The principal task of the nurse is to support the normal mourning. His or her effectiveness will be increased if those individuals likely to experience difficulty can be identified. The nursing assessment will be helpful. Childhood experiences and later losses provide information about early separations that predispose the individual to renewed conflicts and about unresolved feelings that may surface in the present disruption. Previous history of psychiatric illness alerts the nurse to recurrent depressive episodes or decreased coping abilities. Information about life crises before the loss reveals the stresses previously experienced and the adaptive resources available at present. The relationship with the lost person or object is a critical factor. A close relationship, a strong attachment, a high degree of dependency, and great ambivalence will all make mourning more complex and painful.

When separation occurs through death, the process of dying is also crucial. A sudden death poses greater problems, as do a denial of emotions in the early mourning phase, the death of a child or young adult, and a belief that the death was preventable. Bugen asserts that the belief the death was preventable is the "single most influential factor contributing to the prolongation of the human grief response."[13:202] The bereaved's support systems, secondary stresses, and future opportunities are relevant factors in planning interventions and promoting future growth.

■ **ASSIST IN GRIEF WORK.** The core nursing interventions are directed toward helping the patient go through the "grief work" by helping him experience the feelings and emotions connected with the loss and eventually find new patterns of rewarding interaction. He needs to accept the reality of the loss and realize that grieving is appropriate and that sharing makes it less painful. In establishing a contract, the nurse can explain that he or she would like to help the bereaved talk over any feelings and difficulties. Many people find it is easier to talk to an impartial "outsider" about painful memories, ambivalent feelings, and problems that threaten self-esteem. With the nurse the bereaved does not have to fear alienation from the family. In addition, it is important for the nurse, in establishing the contract, to convey his or her belief in the person's recovery and future coping ability.

Initially the person may be dazed or numbed. If so, he will need help in making even simple decisions. He will also need time to organize his ideas and take in what has happened. After the initial reaction has subsided, it will be possible to explore the loss, related memories, and affect of the bereaved. A useful beginning point is a discussion of the circumstances and nature of the loss. This often mobilizes the expression of significant and related feelings and reveals those that are absent or inappropriately expressed, such as sadness or anger. Many bereaved people are surprised and frightened by the intensity of their emotions. They may ask, "Is this normal?" or "Am I going mad?" Distractibility, difficulty remembering, and a sense of unreality may cause worry and concern. Reassurance that they are not going mad and that such feelings are normal is helpful, particularly if the nurse does not seem frightened or alarmed. Nurses can show by their willingness to reveal their own feelings that they are not ashamed or rendered useless by them.

Guilt, anger, and sadness are important emotions. Crying is an effective emotional release that can communicate strong feelings and drain off immobilizing energy or tension. At times, the values of the nurse or society may negate crying because it is viewed as a sign of weakness or causes discomfort in others. Nurses need to guard against these prejudices and encourage crying as an acceptable emotional release. In these in-

stances silence and companionship are often the most therapeutic responses. The universality of sadness, anger, and guilt need to be acknowledged. Asking how the person feels about a certain event, suggesting the way he may have felt ("that must have made you feel angry"), or describing how another person would feel in the situation ("that would make me feel isolated and forgotten") may help the bereaved person explore his emotions. In the beginning he may test out the nurse for clichés of reassurance used by others. The person may be exploring whether the nurse can confront the loss. If the nurse does not respond in a stereotyped and superficial way, the bereaved may begin to express "bad" memories as well as "good."

Initially, defenses need to be supported, but with time they should be analyzed and released. Denial needs to be changed to developing awareness. Reaction formation may lead to idealization of the lost one and may have to be dealt with by releasing the negative emotions involved. In projective identification the anger and guilt are acknowledged in another but not as part of oneself, and the concern is with the other. With this defense the nurse needs to promote more direct expression of feeling. The goal is to place the loss in perspective and loosen the bonds of attachment.

Various resistances may appear. Early resistance manifests as attempts to concentrate on practical or financial problems rather than on emotional ones. The bereaved may ask help in getting a job or collecting insurance. The nurse can offer assistance or referral in these areas while also encouraging the expression of grief and mourning. The nurse must not join with the bereaved in avoiding grief. Another resistance occurs when the person shuts out the nurse through such statements as "No one really knows what I'm going through" or "You're so young, how can you possibly understand what it's like?" Other resistances occur when the person focuses on the nurse's losses as a way of escaping his own or when he claims that his grief is resolved, although the nurse realizes it is a premature resolution.

■ **SUPPORT SOCIAL SYSTEMS.** It may be necessary for the nurse to work directly or indirectly to promote social network support, that is, support that will promote the expression of grief. The nurse may modify the bereaved's support system or may mobilize various significant others, such as the clergy. The nurse may hold a conjoint interview with the family to open up channels of communication and break the conspiracy of silence that frequently blocks grief.

The use of daytime sedatives and tranquilizers should be avoided. They may help the person maintain a calm appearance and avoid crying, but they artificially extend the period of denial and suppress normal mourning. With the suppression of these emotions, the balance of normal ambivalence may be tipped to its extreme, producing depression with its greater degree of maladaptation. Tranquilizers can also encourage patterns of drug dependence, sedation, and inhibition of grief.

As the grief process is resolved, the person will be seen investing himself in new situations and relationships. The loss is placed in perspective, the attachment bonds are released, and energy is directed back out into the world. New patterns of rewarding interaction should be encouraged and reinforced.

It is important that in terminating the nurse-patient relationship, sufficient time is allowed for dealing with that loss as well. The person may wish to continue the relationship as a substitute for the previous loss. Awareness of these issues will allow the nurse to confront them and encourage the independence of the bereaved.

Other therapeutic nursing interventions look to society in general. The nurse can encourage others in the community to accept the open expression of grief and the display of emotions. If these are accepted and supported, one type of stress can be avoided. In addition to changing attitudes, the nurse can facilitate the growth of organizations for the bereaved. The effectiveness of widow-to-widow groups, colostomy associations, and single-parent groups has been well established. Support groups play a significant role in preventing maladaptive responses and are an appropriate area for nursing intervention. These interventions related to uncomplicated grief reactions are summarized in Table 14-8.

■ Intervening in depression and mania

Maladaptive emotional responses may emerge at unpredicted moments, can vary in intensity from mild to severe, and can be transitory, recurrent, or more stable trait conditions. Episodes of depression and mania can occur in any setting and can arise in conjunction with existing medical problems. Also, the treatment of mood disturbances can take place in various settings—at home, at an outpatient department, or in a hospital. The choice of where the patient can be best treated depends on the severity of the illness, available support systems, and resources of the treatment center. In timing intervention, remember that help given when maladaptive patterns are developing is likely to be more acceptable and effective than help given after these patterns have been established. Thus early diagnosis and treatment are associated with more positive outcomes.

The nursing interventions that are described rela-

tive to severe mood disturbances are based on a unified, multicausal, and interactive model of affective disorders. Such a model dismisses the notion of one cause or one cure for the range of maladaptive emotional responses. Rather, it proposes that affective problems have many determinations and many dimensions that affect all aspects of a person's life. Thus a single approach to nursing care would be inadequate. Nursing interventions must instead reflect the complex nature of the model and address all maladaptive aspects of a person's life. Intervening in as many areas as possible should have the maximum effect in modifying maladaptive responses and alleviating severe mood disturbances. The ultimate aim of these nursing interventions is to teach the patient coping responses and increase the satisfaction he receives from his world.

These nursing actions can be implemented in any setting. They are described on the basis of patients' needs in the following areas:

1. Environmental
2. Nurse-patient relationship
3. Affective
4. Cognitive
5. Behavioral
6. Social
7. Physiological

The specific interventions now described are derived from the model of severe mood disturbances presented earlier in this chapter.

■ **ENVIRONMENTAL INTERVENTIONS.** Environmental interventions are useful when the patient's environment is highly dangerous, impoverished, aversive, or lacking in personal resources. In caring for the patient with a severe mood disorder, high priority should be given to the potential for suicide. Hospitalization is definitely indicated when there is suicidal risk. In the presence of rapidly progressing symptoms and in the absence or rupture of usual support systems, hospitalization is strongly indicated. Nursing care in this case means protecting and assuring the patient he will not be allowed to harm himself. Specific interventions for the suicidal patient are described in Chapter 15.

The depressed patient must always be assessed for possible suicide. He is at particular risk when he appears to be coming out of his depression, because he may then have the energy and opportunity to kill himself. Acute manic states are also life threatening. These patients show poor judgment, excessive risk taking, and an inability to evaluate realistic danger and the consequences of their actions. In an acute manic epi-

TABLE 14-8

SUMMARY OF NURSING INTERVENTIONS IN UNCOMPLICATED GRIEF REACTIONS

Goal—Assist the patient who has experienced a loss to work through the process of grieving or mourning and prevent maladaptive emotional responses

Principle	Rationale	Nursing actions
Awareness and control of nurse's own feelings	Self-awareness is a prerequisite for the "therapeutic use of self" in working with those experiencing loss	Understand one's own feelings and reactions to loss Recall previous losses and resolve areas of conflict Communicate hope in the future and commitment to the work of grieving in the nurse-patient relationship Use one's own personal and professional support systems for ventilation and rejuvenation
Grieving can be facilitated by anticipating losses and their consequences	Anticipatory guidance by the nurse can be an effective intervention in primary prevention	Discuss impending losses and their significance with the patient and family Review past losses
Support the patient and family at the time of the loss	Therapeutic interventions at the time of the loss can prevent future maladaptive responses	Be prepared to stay with and comfort the bereaved until others arrive Use the family group or significant others as a coping resource to provide initial support for those experiencing the loss Provide the bereaved a place to express their feelings Unconditionally accept the emotional responses of those grieving Incorporate the cultural, religious, and social customs of those grieving into one's nursing care
Identify those persons at high risk for maladaptive responses	Nursing interventions will be more effective if adapted to a person's unique needs	Identify individuals at high risk for maladaptive responses by assessing factors that significantly influence the outcome of mourning
Help the patient go through the "grief work"	This will help him accept the reality of the loss and realize that grieving is an appropriate and healthy response	Convey belief in the person's recovery and future coping ability Initially assist the patient in immediate decision making, if necessary Explore the circumstances and nature of the loss Facilitate the patient's expression of feelings, including guilt, anger, and sadness Offer acceptance and assurance of the appropriateness and commonality of the patient's positive and negative emotions Initially support the patient's ego defense mechanisms; with time, encourage his analysis and release of them by placing the loss in perspective and loosening bonds of attachment Work through any resistances that may occur in the nurse-patient relationship Encourage and reinforce new patterns of rewarding interactions Deal with the loss imposed by the termination of the nurse-patient relationship
Promote social network support as a coping resource	The positive role that social support plays in dealing with loss has been well established in both research and clinical practice	Mobilize a social support system for the patient that is appropriate to his needs (i.e., family, clergy, and community agency) Facilitate the formation and growth of organizations that act as support groups to others

sode, immediate measures must be instituted to prevent a fatal outcome.

Another environmental intervention involves changing the physical or social setting by assisting the patient to move to a new environment. Sometimes a change in the general pattern of living is indicated, such as a leave of absence from work, a different job, a new peer group, or leaving one's family setting. Changes such as these decrease the immediate stress and mobilize additional support.

■ **NURSE-PATIENT RELATIONSHIP.** Both depressed and manic patients present unique challenges to the nurse. Depressed patients resist involvement through withdrawal and nonresponsiveness. Because of their negative views, they tend to remain isolated, verbalize little, think they are unworthy of help, and form dependent attachments.

In working with depressed patients, the nurse's approach should be quiet, warm, and accepting. He or she should demonstrate honesty, empathy, and compassion. Admittedly, it is not always easy to give warm, personal care to a person who is unresponsive and detached. The nurse may feel angry or resentful of the patient's helplessness or fear rejection by him. Patience and a belief in the potential of each person to grow and change is needed. If this is calmly communicated, both verbally and nonverbally, in time he may begin to respond.

The nurse should avoid assuming an overaggressive or lighthearted approach with the depressed individual. Comments such as "You have so much to live for," "Cheer up—things are sure to get better," or "You shouldn't feel so depressed" convey little understanding of and respect for the patient's feelings. They will create more distance and block the formation of a potential relationship. Also, the nurse should not sympathize with the patient. Subjective overidentification by the nurse can cause him or her to experience similar feelings of hopelessness and helplessness and can seriously limit therapy.

Rapport is best established with the depressed patient through shared time, even if the patient talks little, and through supportive companionship. The very presence of the nurse indicates belief that the patient is a valuable person. The nurse should adjust to the depressed patient's pace by speaking more slowly and allowing him time to respond. The patient should be addressed by name, talked to, and listened to. By studying the patient's life and interests, the nurse might select topics that lay the foundation for more meaningful discussions.

In contrast, elated patients may be very talkative and need simple explanations and concise, truthful answers to questions. Although the manic patient may appear willing to talk, he resists involvement through manipulation, testing limits, and superficiality. His hyperactivity, short attention span, flight of ideas, poor judgment, lack of insight, and rapid mood swings all present special problems to the nursing staff.

Manic patients can be very disruptive to a unit and resist engagement in therapy. They may dominate group meetings or therapy sessions by their excessive talking and manipulate staff or patient groups. By identifying a vulnerable area in another person or a group's area of conflict, manic patients are able to exploit others. This provokes defensive and angry responses. Nurses are particularly susceptible to these feelings, since they often have the most contact with patients and the responsibility for coordinating and maintaining the psychiatric unit. When anger is generated, therapeutic care breaks down. Thus the maneuvers of manic patients serve as diversionary tactics. By alienating themselves, they can avoid exploring their own problems.

It is important for nurses to understand how manic patients are able to manipulate others and their reasons for doing so. The treatment plan for these patients should be thorough, well coordinated, and consistently implemented. Constructive limit setting on manic patients' behavior is an essential part of the plan. The entire treatment team must be consistent in their expectations of these patients, and progressive limits must be set as situations arise. Other patients may also be encouraged to carry out the agreed limits. Pressure applied by peers can sometimes be more effective than pressure applied by the staff. Frequent staff meetings are recommended to reduce faulty communication, share in understanding the manic patient's behavior, and ensure steady progress.

One goal of nursing care is ultimately to increase the patient's self-control, and this should be kept in mind when setting limits. Patients need to see that they can monitor their own behavior and that the staff is there to help them. Also, the nurse should point out that there are many positive aspects to their behavior. The ability to be outgoing, expressive, and energetic are coping strengths that can be maximized in the therapy.

■ **AFFECTIVE INTERVENTIONS.** Affective interventions are necessary because patients with mood disturbances have difficulty identifying and expressing feelings. Feelings that are particularly problematic are hopelessness, sadness, anger, guilt, and anxiety. A range of interventions is available to the nurse in meeting patient needs in this area.

Intervening in emotions requires self-understanding by the nurse. Whether the interventions will be therapeutic depends greatly on the nurse's values regarding the various emotions, his or her own emotional responsiveness, and the ability to offer genuine respect and nonjudgmental acceptance. The nurse must be able to experience feelings and express them if he or she expects to help the patient.

Initially, the nurse must express hope for depressed patients. They have a genuine need for repeated reassurance. The nurse can reinforce that depression is a self-limiting disorder and that the future will be better. This can be expressed calmly and simply. The intent is not to cheer the patient but to reassure him that, although recovery is a slow process involving weeks or months, he will feel progressively better. The nurse may acknowledge the patient's inability to take comfort from this reassurance. For him, only the depression is real; past or future happiness is an illusion. By affirming her belief, however, the nurse may make his existence more tolerable.

This initial reassurance is a way of acknowledging the patient's pain and despair while also conveying a sense of hope in his recovery. It is not the premature reassurance of "Don't worry—everything's going to be just fine." It is an openness to his feelings and acknowledgment of them. This is a very important first step. It also tells him that his present state is not permanent. For the depressed patient who lacks time perspective, it directs his thoughts beyond the present with genuine hopes for tomorrow.

Nursing actions in this area should convey that expressing feelings is normal and necessary. Blocking or repressing emotions is partly responsible for the patient's present pain. The nurse can help him to realize that his overwhelming feelings of dejection and worthlessness are defenses that prevent him from dealing with his problems. Encouraging a patient to express his unpleasant or painful emotions can reduce their intensity and make him feel more alive and masterful. Thus nursing should be directed toward first helping the patient experience his feelings and then express them. These actions are a prerequisite to interventions in the cognitive, behavioral, or social areas.

When the nurse accepts without criticism the anger, despair, or anxiety expressed by the patient, he sees that expressing feelings is not destructive or a sign of weakness. Sometimes, however, the patient's expression of anger changes his cognitive set from self-blaming to blaming others. It may allow him to see himself as more effective because it connotes power, superiority, and mastery. How this anger is expressed is important because aggressive behavior can be destructive and

serve to further isolate him. Many patients experiencing both depressive and manic emotional states have problems with expressing anger and need to learn assertive behavior. This important area of nursing intervention is explored in Chapter 17.

Relaxation techniques may also help both manic and depressed patients deal with their anxiety and tension and obtain more pleasure from life. Reducing anxiety to tolerable levels broadens the individual's perceptual field and allows the nurse to intervene in the cognitive and behavioral areas. Nursing actions to reduce anxiety are described in Chapter 11.

To successfully implement any of these nursing actions related to the patient's affective needs, the nurse must use a variety of communication skills (see Chapter 4). Particularly important are empathy skills, reflection of feeling, open-ended feeling-oriented questions, validation, self-disclosure, and confrontation. Feelings are the essence of empathy and thus make empathy an essential therapeutic quality. The various other communication skills must also focus on feelings rather than facts. The patient with a severe mood disturbance will challenge the nurse's therapeutic skills and stringently test his or her caring and commitment.

■ **COGNITIVE INTERVENTIONS.** When intervening in the cognitive area, the nurse has three major aims, which require that he or she begin with the patient's conceptualization of his problem:

1. To increase the patient's sense of control over his goals and behavior
2. To increase the patient's self-esteem
3. To assist the patient in modifying his negative expectations

Depressed patients usually see themselves as victims of their moods and environment. They do not view their behavior and their interpretation of events as possible causes of depression. They assume a passive stance and wait for someone or something to lift their mood. One task of the nurse, therefore, is to move the patient beyond his limiting preoccupation to other aspects of his world that are related to it. To do this, the nurse must progress gradually. The first step is to help him explore his feelings. This is followed by eliciting his view of the problem. In so doing, the nurse accepts the patient's perceptions but need not accept his conclusions. Together they need to define the problem to give the patient a sense of control, a feeling of hope, and a realization that change may indeed be possible.

Nursing actions may then focus on modifying the patient's thinking. Depressed patients are noticeably dominated by negative thoughts. Often, despite a successful performance, the patient will view it negatively. Cognitive changes may be brought about in various ways.[5,6,62]

Frequently, negative thinking is an automatic process of which the patient is not even aware. The nurse can therefore assist him in identifying his negative thoughts and decreasing them through thought interruption or substitution. Concurrently, the patient can be encouraged to increase his positive thinking by reviewing his personal assets, strengths, accomplishments, and opportunities. Next he can be assisted in examining the accuracy of his perceptions, logic, and conclusions. Misperceptions, distortions, and irrational beliefs become evident. The patient should be helped to move from unrealistic to realistic goals and to decrease the importance of unattainable goals. All these actions enhance the patient's self-understanding and increase his self-esteem. More detailed interventions in this area are explored in Chapter 13, which addresses alterations in self-concept, which are inherent in disturbances of mood.

Also, because the depressed patient tends to be overwhelmed by despair, it is important to limit the amount of negative evaluation in which he engages. One way is to involve the patient in productive tasks or activities; another way is to increase his level of socialization. These benefit the patient in two complementary ways: they limit the time he can spend on brooding and self-criticism, and they provide positive reinforcement.

A final consideration is that the nurse realize the meaning, nature, and value the patient places on his behavior and mood change. Most research has focused on the psychopathologic nature of affective disorders. One study that explored the positive aspects found that patients with bipolar illnesses receive pronounced short- and long-term positive effects from their manic-depressive illness.[30] The patients reported short- and long-term increases in productivity, creativity, sensitivity, social outgoingness, and sexual intensity. It is important for the nurse to understand these attributions. They suggest that disturbances of mood can produce powerful reinforcers of a maladaptive response and thus make change more difficult. For some patients, the positive consequences of an illness may outweigh their perception of negative consequences.

■ **BEHAVIORAL INTERVENTIONS.** Successful behavior is a powerful antidepressant. This idea, however, seldom occurs to depressed patients, who use their despondent mood as a rationalization for inactivity. They instead believe that once their mood lifts, they will be productive again. Such an idea is consis-

tent with a negative cognitive set and a sense of helplessness. However, inactivity prevents satisfaction and social recognition. Thus it reinforces a depressive state.

Nursing interventions therefore focus on activating the patient in a realistic, goal-directed way. Directed activities, strategies, or homework assignments mutually determined by the nurse and patient reveal alternative coping responses. Some benefits of assigning therapeutic tasks are identified by Goldberg:

1. The client continues to be involved with the therapist even when not in therapy, thus strengthening the therapeutic relationship.
2. The responsibility for change is the client's.
3. The implication is that the client can change, which instills hope.
4. If successfully completed, therapeutic tasks tend to enhance the client's self-esteem.
5. They help restructure a system.
6. They teach problem-solving skills by providing the client an opportunity for experiential learning.
7. They test the flexibility of a person or system and reveal areas of resistance to change.
8. They encourage the generalization of therapeutic gains beyond the therapy session.[21:157]

Many depressed patients benefit from nursing actions that encourage them to redirect their self-preoccupation to interests in the outside world. The timing of these interventions is crucial. The patient should not be forced into activities initially. Also, he will not benefit from coming into contact with too many people too soon. Rather, the nurse should encourage activities gradually and suggest more involvement on the basis of his energy.

For severely depressed hospitalized patients, a structured daily program of activities can be beneficial. Because these patients lack motivation and direction, they are reticent to initiate actions. The nurse should take into consideration the patient's tolerance to stress and probability of succeeding. The particular task should neither be too difficult nor too time consuming. Success tends to increase expectations of success, and failure tends to increase hopelessness.

The elated patient usually needs little encouragement to become involved with others. Because of his short attention span and restless energy, however, he cannot deal with complicated projects. He needs tasks that are simple and that can be completed quickly. He needs room to move about and furnishings that do not overstimulate him.

The ability to accomplish tasks and be productive depend on various factors. First, expectations and goals should be small enough to ensure successful performance, relevant to his needs, and focused on positive activities. Following is a positive activities list* with categories of rewarding or potentially rewarding activities.[46]

1. Planning something you will enjoy
2. Going on an outing (e.g., a walk, a shopping trip downtown, a picnic)
3. Going out for entertainment
4. Going on a trip
5. Going to meetings, lectures, classes
6. Attending a social gathering
7. Playing a sport or game
8. Spending time on a hobby or project
9. Entertaining yourself at home (e.g., reading, listening to music, watching TV)
10. Doing something just for yourself (e.g., buying something, cooking something, dressing comfortably)
11. Spending time just relaxing (e.g., thinking, sitting, napping, daydreaming)
12. Caring for yourself, making yourself attractive
13. Persisting at a difficult task
14. Completing a routine task or unpleasant task
15. Doing a job well
16. Cooperating with someone else on a common task
17. Doing something special for someone else, being generous, going out of your way
18. Seeking out people (e.g., calling, stopping by, making a date or appointment, going to a meeting)
19. Initiating conversation (e.g., at a store, party, or class)
20. Discussing an interesting or amusing topic
21. Expressing yourself openly, clearly, or frankly (e.g., opinion, criticism, anger)
22. Playing with children or animals
23. Complimenting or praising someone
24. Physically showing affection or love
25. Receiving praise, compliments, attention

Next, attention should be focused on the task at hand, not what has yet to be done or was done incorrectly in the past. Finally, positive reinforcement should be based on actual performance. If such an approach is used consistently over time, the nurse can expect the patient to demonstrate increasingly productive behavior.

Occupational and recreational tasks are usually easily identified by the nurse. These can be most valuable and are well represented in the positive activities list. Another source of accomplishment is movement and physical exercise. Brown, Ramirez, and Taub[11]

---

*From Rehm L: A self-control therapy program for treatment of depression. In Clarkin J and Glazer H, editors: Depression: behavioral and directive intervention strategies, New York, 1981, Garland Publishing, Inc.

have made the following observations about the relationship between mood and movement:

- Physical fitness is often associated with a feeling of well-being and reduced depression and anxiety.
- Fitness appears to be associated with physical and psychological benefits regardless of the subject's age.
- The biological benefits of exercise may be associated in part with changes produced among brain amines, salt metabolism, muscle neuronal activity, and striatal functions.
- A comprehensive history of the depressed patient's motor activity is useful in prescribing an exercise regimen of maximum benefit.

Jogging, walking, swimming, bicycling, and aerobics are popular forms of exercise that may be incorporated in a regular program of activity. They are beneficial because they improve the patient's physical condition and release emotions and tensions.

■ **SOCIAL INTERVENTIONS.** Social factors play a major role in the causation, maintenance, and resolution of affective disorders, particularly depression. Socialization moderates depression by providing an experience incompatible with depressive withdrawal. It also provides increased self-esteem through the social reinforcers of approval, acceptance, recognition, and support.

A major problem is that patients with maladaptive emotional responses are less accomplished in social interaction. In addition, they may be avoided by others because of their self-absorption, pessimism, or elation. One nursing action to counteract this problem is to help the patient improve his social skills. A plan for enhancing social skills is presented in Table 14-9. It involves sequential learning that includes the following:

1. Assessing the patient's social skills, supports, and interests
2. Reviewing existing and potential social resources available to the patient
3. Instructing and modeling effective social skills
4. Role playing and rehearsing troublesome social situations and interactions
5. Providing feedback and positive reinforcement of effective interpersonal skills
6. Encouraging the initiation of socialization in an expanded social arena

Number 6 often proves difficult for depressed patients, who report they are unable to meet new people and engage in an active social life. Thus increasing a patient's social activities is another area of nursing in-

---

TABLE 14-9

MENTAL HEALTH EDUCATION PLAN—ENHANCING SOCIAL SKILLS

Content	Instructional activities	Evaluation
Describe behaviors interfering with social interaction	Instruct the patient on corrective behaviors	Patient identifies problematic and more facilitative behaviors
Discuss components of social performance relevant to the patient's situation	Model effective interpersonal skills for the patient	Patient describes specific skills he could acquire
Analyze the way in which the patient could incorporate these specific skills	Use role-play and guided practice to allow patient to test out these new behaviors	Patient shows beginning skill in assumed social behaviors
Encourage patient to test out new skills in other situations	Give homework assignments for the patient to do in his natural environment	Patient discusses his ability to complete the assigned tasks
Discuss generalization of new skills to other aspects of the patient's life and functioning	Give feedback, encouragement, and praise for newly acquired social skills and their generalization	Patient is able to integrate the new social behaviors in his social interactions with others

---

tervention. Involvement with others often is a result of shared activities. The nurse can work with the patient to identify recreational, career, cultural, religious, and personal interests and how to best pursue these interests through community groups, organizations, and clubs. Women's groups, single-parent groups, jogging clubs, church groups, and neighborhood associations are all opportunities. Although this may appear to be a relatively simple nursing intervention, it is often one that taxes the nurse's creativity and knowledge of resources.

Family involvement. In addition to a one-to-one relationship, patients with maladaptive emotional responses can benefit from family and group work. For example, it has long been suggested that family relationships are critical to successful reentry of the hospitalized patient back into the community, yet conventional discharge planning and aftercare models tend to neglect the family. Buckwalter and Abraham report on a family-centered discharge nursing intervention with a cognitive behavioral orientation that helped depressed patients adjust better to their posthospital environment.[12] In their family sessions they included information on the following areas:

1. Patient's diagnosis and treatment plan, including medications
2. Relapse signs and symptoms or recurrent illness and what to do if they should appear
3. Community resources including medical, social, vocational and postdischarge follow-up

4. Positive support and knowledge to anticipate and avoid problems
5. Resocialization issues or potential problems identified by the patient

They found that inclusion of the family in predischarge planning resulted in patients making greater use of aftercare services in the community and reporting higher adjustment scores three months after discharge. They concluded that the quality of social, family and community readjustment variables were all influenced in a positive way by this nursing intervention.

In family therapy, depression can be interpreted as dependency, which is contributed to and supported by other family members. The patient's sense of powerlessness in human relationships is examined in light of family patterns, and all members are expected to take responsibility for their share of the continuing pattern.

The theory that friends and partners often reinforce and support the patient's depression has been well documented. When a person becomes depressed, he usually receives much attention and secondary gain from others, who respond by being helpful, nurturing, or annoyed. When the patient acts in a nondepressed way, however, little attention is paid to him. Therefore one goal of family therapy is to have the family reinforce adaptive, nondepressed behavior and ignore maladaptive depressive responses.

Family interventions also are needed with manic patients. In one study that followed the families of patients with bipolar manic-depressive illness, the authors noted the following:

The recurring psychopathology of manic-depressive patients has significant effects on the psychosocial adaptation of their spouse and children. Not only is the genetic predisposition handed down over generations, but the environment may have long-term detrimental effects on the children's personality.[37:1537]

The "wavering capacity for interpersonal relatedness" of the patient and other family members is a clear indication for nursing interventions at the family level.

Group treatment. Group therapy can also provide multiple benefits. Knowledge that others have ambivalence and sharing this guilt, as well as realistic sympathy and support of the group members, enable the depressed patient to lessen his guilt. He can thereby give up his maladaptive behavior patterns and develop more satisfying relationships. Van Servellen and Dull[58] developed a format for group treatment of women with major depressive illness. The overall aim is to increase self-worth and self-esteem through identification with the group and awareness of personal strengths. The depressed women in Van Servellen and Dull's group identified several general goals:

1. Learning more about their individual behavior and relationships with others based on feedback from members and group process
2. Increasing social support through group relatedness
3. Gaining a heightened sense of identity, self-understanding, and control over their own lives
4. Realizing that other people have problems similar to their own, which helps to reduce their sense of loneliness and isolation, thereby also decreasing feelings of hopelessness, helplessness, and powerlessness
5. Learning new ways to cope with stress from others in the group
6. More realistically modifying their perceptions and expectations of self and others
7. Allowing for the expression of feelings of hopelessness and frustration within the supportive context of the group

An essential part of any therapeutic intervention is the evaluation of its effectiveness. Van Servellen and Dull also present a format for evaluation that can be used to measure change in the patients in group treatment. Research comparing and evaluating therapeutic modalities used by nurses is a high priority.

■ **PHYSIOLOGICAL INTERVENTIONS.** Physiological interventions include both physical care and somatic therapies. They begin with a thorough physical examination and health history to determine present health, past and present health problems, and current treatments or medications that may be affecting the patient's mood.

In depression, physical well-being may be forgotten or the patient may not be capable of caring for himself. The more severe the depression, the more important is the physical care. For example, an anorexic patient may need to have his diet monitored. Staying with the patient when he is eating, arranging for preferred foods, and encouraging frequent small meals may be helpful. Recording his intake and output and weighing him daily will help evaluate this need.

Sleep disturbances typically occur. It is best to plan activities according to each patient's energy levels; some feel best in the morning and others in the evening. A scheduled rest period may be helpful, but patients should not be encouraged to take frequent naps or remain in bed all day. Patients with depression experience less stage III and IV sleep, and since these stages depend on the period of wakefulness, napping may worsen sleep disturbances. For many patients, eating regularly, staying active during waking hours, and cutting back on caffeine (especially late in the day) may promote more normal sleep patterns.

The patient's appearance may be neglected and all his movements slowed. The nurse may have to assist with bathing or dressing. The nurse should do this matter-of-factly, explaining that the patient is being helped because he is unable to do it for himself right now. Cleanliness and interest in appearance can be noticed and praised. The nurse must allow the patient to help himself whenever possible. Often the nurse might rush the patient or do a task herself to save time, but this does not facilitate the patient's recovery and should be avoided.

The manic patient primarily needs protection from himself. He may be too busy to eat or take care of himself. Eating problems can be handled in the same way as with the depressed patient. The patient sleeps little, so rest periods should be provided, along with baths, soft music, and whirlpools. The manic patient may also need help in selecting clothes and carrying out hygiene. Setting limits and using firm actions are effective in physical care.

Somatic and drug therapies. Over the past 25 years there has been much progress in the somatic and pharmacological treatment of patients with affective disorders. Recent developments include biological markers of clinical value in the diagnosis and treatment of disturbances in mood. One test for somatically treatable depression is the dexamethasone suppression test (DST), mentioned previously in this chapter and

TABLE 14-10

ANTIDEPRESSANT DRUGS

Chemical class generic name (Trade name)	Usual dosage range (mg/day)
Tricyclic drugs	
Tertiary (parent drug)	
amitriptyline (Elavil, Endep)	50–300
doxepin (Adapin, Sinequan)	50–300
imipramine (SK-Pramine, Tofranil)	50–300
trimipramine (Surmontil)	50–300
chlomipramine (Anafranil)	50–200
Secondary (metabolite)	
desipramine (Norpramin, Pertofrane)	50–150
protriptyline (Vivactil)	15–60
Nontricyclic drugs	
amoxapine (Asendin)	50–600
maprotiline (Ludiomil)	50–225*
trazodone (Desyrel)	50–600
Luproprion (Wellbutrin)	50–600*
fluoxetine (PROSAC)	20–80
Monoamine oxidase inhibitors	
isocarboxazid (Marplan)	30–70
phenelzine (Nardil)	45–90
tranylcypromine (Parnate)	20–60

*Antidepressants with a ceiling dose due to dose-related seizures.

TABLE 14-11

LITHIUM PREPARATIONS

Lithium salts (Trade name)	Available forms (mg)
Lithium carbonate (generic)	150,300
Lithium carbonate (Eskalith) (Lithotabs) (Lithane) (Lithonate)	300
Lithium carbonate sustained release (Eskalith C-R)	450
(Lithobid)	300
Lithium citrate concentrate (Cibalith-S)	5 ml/300

described in Chapter 23. It is an easy, relatively inexpensive test posing minimum risk to the patient. It is most useful in identifying patients who do not display all the typical behaviors of depression but who are likely to respond to somatic treatments, such as antidepressant therapy or electroconvulsive therapy (ECT). It may also be useful in monitoring recovery and in deciding when to stop antidepressant therapy.

Antidepressant medications are frequently administered to elevate the mood of the depressed patient. At this time no single drug has been found effective for all forms of depression. There are three types of antidepressant drugs commonly used—tricyclics, nontricyclics, and monoamine oxidase (MAO) inhibitors (Table 14-10). Of these, tricyclic drugs appear to be the most effective class of antidepressants. They pose a

smaller risk of side effects than the MAO inhibitors and appear to be useful against relapses. Many consider lithium carbonate the drug of choice in the treatment of mania (Table 14-11). Some believe that it not only produces a remission of symptoms, but also prevents recurrence. The overall success rate of drugs used to treat depressed patients is 60% to 80%.

Despite their success, antidepressant drugs are far from ideal. Their therapeutic effects begin only after 2 to 6 weeks, and they have numerous side effects, which deter some patients from maintenance. Patient education by the nurse is essential. Youssef reports that a directive patient-education group conducted by nurses resulted in a significant difference in medication compliance among psychiatric outpatients with affective disorders.[63] Additional programs and research by nurses in this area is needed to monitor and evaluate patient progress.

Another major problem with antidepressant medications is their toxicity. They are lethal at high doses, which makes them particularly dangerous for people most in need of them—suicidal patients. In addition, antidepressant medications do not help everyone, and it is difficult to predict who will respond to which drug. Fortunately, those who do not benefit from one type frequently do well when taking another.

ECT is also used with depressed patients, particularly those with recurrent depressions and those resistant to drug therapy. ECT is regarded by many as a specific therapy for patients with severe depressions characterized by somatic delusions and delusional

TABLE 14-12

SUMMARY OF NURSING INTERVENTIONS IN DEPRESSION AND MANIA

Goal—Teach the patient adaptive emotional responses and increase the satisfaction and pleasure he receives from his world

Principle	Rationale	Nursing action
Modify the patient's environment if it is dangerous, impoverished, aversive, or lacking in personal resources	All patients with severe mood disturbances are at high risk for suicide; environmental changes can protect the patient, decrease the immediate stress, and mobilize additional resources	Continually evaluate the patient's potential for suicide Hospitalize the patient when there is a suicidal risk Assist the patient to move to a new environment when appropriate (i.e., new job, peer group, family setting)
Establish and maintain a therapeutic nurse-patient relationship	Both depressed and manic patients resist becoming involved in a therapeutic alliance; acceptance, persistence, and limit setting are necessary	Use a warm, accepting, empathic approach Be aware of and in control of one's own feelings and reactions (i.e., anger, frustration, sympathy) With the depressed patient: 1. Establish rapport through shared time and supportive companionship 2. Allow the patient time to respond 3. Personalize his care as a way of indicating his value as a human being With the manic patient: 4. Give simple, truthful responses 5. Be alert to possible manipulation 6. Set constructive limits on negative behavior 7. Use a consistent approach by all health team members 8. Maintain open communication and sharing of perceptions among team members 9. Reinforce the patient's self-control and positive aspects of his behavior
Assist in the patient's recognition and expression of emotions	Patients with severe mood disturbances have difficulty identifying and expressing feelings	Demonstrate emotional responsiveness and acceptance Use facilitative communication skills and the responsive and action dimensions described in Chapter 4 Respond empathically with a focus on feelings rather than facts Acknowledge the patient's pain and convey a sense of hope in his recovery Help the patient experience his feelings and then express them Assist the patient in the appropriate expression of anger Reduce the patient's anxiety to mild-moderate levels
Aid the patient in modifying his negative cognitive set	This will help to increase his sense of control over his goals and behaviors, enhance his self-esteem, and modify his negative expectations	Review with the patient his conceptualization of the problem but do not necessarily accept his conclusions Identify the patient's negative thoughts and help him to decrease them through thought interruption or substitution Help him increase his positive thinking Examine the accuracy of his perceptions, logic, and conclusions

Continued.

TABLE 14-12—cont'd

SUMMARY OF NURSING INTERVENTIONS IN DEPRESSION AND MANIA

Goal—Teach the patient adaptive emotional responses and increase the satisfaction and pleasure he receives from his world

Principle	Rationale	Nursing action
Aid the patient in modifying his negative cognitive set—cont'd		Identify misperceptions, distortions, and irrational beliefs Help him move from unrealistic to realistic goals Decrease the importance of unattainable goals Limit the amount of negative personal evaluations he engages in Realize the meaning, nature, and value the patient places on his behavior and mood change
Activate the patient in a realistic goal-directed way	Successful behavioral performance counteracts feelings of helplessness and hopelessness	Assign appropriate action-oriented therapeutic tasks Encourage activities gradually, escalating them as the patient's energy is mobilized Provide a tangible structured program when appropriate Set goals that are realistic, relevant to the patient's needs and interests, and focused on positive activities Focus on present activities, not past or future activities Positively reinforce successful performance Attain mutuality whenever possible Incorporate physical exercise in the patient's plan of care
Enhance the patient's establishment of interpersonal relationships	Socialization is an experience incompatible with withdrawal and increases self-esteem through the social reinforcers of approval, acceptance, recognition, and support	Assess the patient's social skills, supports, and interests Review existing and potential social resources Instruct and model effective social skills Use role playing and rehearsal of social interactions Give feedback and positive reinforcement of effective interpersonal skills Encourage increasing socialization in an expanded social arena Intervene with families to have them reinforce the patient's adaptive emotional responses Support or engage in family and group therapy when appropriate
Promote the patient's physical health and well-being	Physiological changes occur in disturbances of mood; physical care and somatic therapies are required to overcome problems in this area	Complete a nursing assessment of the patient's physiological health status Assist the patient to meet his self-care needs, particularly in the areas of nutrition, sleep, and personal hygiene Encourage the patient's independence whenever possible Administer prescribed medications and treatments

guilt, accompanied by a lack of interest in the world, suicidal ideation, and weight loss. A more detailed discussion of antidepressant medications and ECT is presented in Chapters 22 and 23.

Sleep deprivation therapy may also be effective in treating depression. Research indicates that depriving some depressed patients of a night's sleep will improve their clinical condition. How sleep deprivation works is not known, and the duration of improvement varies. Further developments in somatic therapies will have direct implications for nursing care.

All the previously described nursing interventions in depression and mania are summarized in Table 14-12. These reflect the holistic nature of care for disturbances of mood.

 Evaluation

The effectiveness of nursing care is determined by changes in the patient's maladaptive emotional responses and the effect they have on present functioning. Problems related to self-concept and interpersonal relationships merge and overlap. Since all individuals experience life stress and related losses, the nurse can ask a fundamental question related to evaluation: "Did I assess my patient for problems in this area?"

Of particular significance are the many special aspects of transference and countertransference that may occur. The patient's heightened attachment and dependency behaviors and his lowered defensiveness can lead to intense transference reactions that should be worked through. Themes of loss and fear of loss, control of emotions and lack of control, and ambivalence predominate. Termination of the nurse-patient relationship may be difficult, since the patient experiences it as another loss that requires mourning and integration.

Countertransference can be related to the nurse's own bereavements, his or her attitudes about anger, guilt, sadness, and despair, the ability to confront these emotions openly and objectively, and most importantly, conflicts about death and loss. Difficulties with any of these issues can be evident in avoidance behavior, preoccupation with fantasies, blocking of feelings, or shortening of sessions. The nurse can expect to review and perhaps rework his or her feelings about personal bereavement. Nursing care will be more appropriate and effective if the nurse is aware of these issues and sensitive to her own feelings and conflicts regarding loss. Supervision and peer support groups can be of great help in this area.

DIRECTIONS FOR FUTURE RESEARCH

The following are some of the nursing research problems raised in Chapter 14 that merit further study by psychiatric nurses:

1. Nursing interventions that facilitate a healthy resolution of grief reactions
2. Development and validation of an assessment instrument that will identify individuals at risk for complicated grief reactions
3. Comparison of the grief process when it is mediated by psychopharmacological agents and when it is not, including behavioral outcomes
4. The relationship between various life events, the production of biogenic amines, and disturbances of mood
5. Outcomes of nursing interventions related to patients' sleep patterns
6. Identification of nursing interventions effective in primary prevention of disorders of mood
7. Description of the therapeutic characteristics of self-help groups for individuals who have experienced a loss
8. Identification of children at risk for affective disorders
9. The effect of patient education by nurses on medication compliance
10. Effectiveness of structured social interventions by nurses working with depressed and manic patients

■ SUGGESTED CROSS-REFERENCES ■

The model of health-illness phenomena, including precipitating life stressors, is described in Chapter 3. Therapeutic relationship skills and self-awareness of the nurse are discussed in Chapter 4. Strengthening coping resources through health education, environmental change, and supporting social systems is presented in Chapter 8. Interventions related to self-concept and cognitive therapy are discussed in Chapter 13. Interventions with the suicidal patient are discussed in Chapter 15. Disruptions in interpersonal relationships are discussed in Chapter 16. Problems with anger and limit setting are discussed in Chapter 17. Somatic therapy is discussed in Chapter 22. Psychopharmacology is discussed in Chapter 23. Group therapy is discussed in Chapter 28. Family therapy is discussed in Chapter 29.

SUMMARY

1. Mood refers to a prolonged emotional state that influences one's whole personality and life functioning. It pertains to one's prevailing and pervading emotion and is synonymous with the terms "affect," "feeling state," and "emotion." Severe mood disturbances can be recognized by their intensity, pervasiveness, persistence, and interference with usual social and physiological functioning.

    a. Grief is an individual's subjective response to the loss of a person, object, or concept that is highly valued. Uncomplicated grief is a healthy, adaptive, reparative response closely related to the capacity for developing meaningful object relationships. An uncomplicated grief reaction is the process of normal mourning. If grief is not worked through, delayed grief reactions and depression can occur.

    b. Depression was distinguished from grief by attachment to the loved object, degree of regression, acknowledgment of the loss, and intensity of emotions over time.

    c. Mania is characterized by a mood that is elevated, expansive, or irritable. Hypomania is similar to mania but less severe.

2. Stressors affecting the grief reaction and factors that place a person at high risk for maladaptive responses were identified. Ten models of causation of severe mood disturbances were discussed. These include genetic, object loss, aggression turned inward, personality organization, cognitive, learned helplessness, behavioral, biochemical, life stressors, and integrated models. An integrated multicausal model is the most valuable for the nurse when implementing care.

3. The phases associated with mourning, as described by Bowlby,[9] are the urge to recover the lost object, disorganization, and reorganization. They can be applied to losses of any type.

4. Maladaptive emotional responses were related to feelings of anxiety, hostility, self-devaluation, and guilt. The key element of a behavioral assessment is change in the person's usual patterns and responses. Selected nursing diagnoses were related to appropriate medical diagnoses from the DSM-III-R.[3]

5. The general goal of the nurse working with a patient who has experienced loss is to support him in the subjective experience of grief. When the patient is experiencing a maladaptive disturbance of mood, long-term goals may be directed toward reinitiating a delayed grief reaction or exploring areas of conflict underlying a depressive or manic state.

6. Interventions in uncomplicated grief reactions include anticipatory guidance, support of normal mourning, and social system intervention. Interventions in depression and mania involve the environment, nurse-patient relationship, affective, cognitive, behavioral, social, and physiological areas. Intervening in as many areas as possible should have the maximum effect in modifying maladaptive responses and alleviating severe mood disturbances.

7. When evaluating nursing care, the nurse should pay particular attention to problems with transference and countertransference. Supervision and peer support groups can be helpful in working with patients experiencing grief.

REFERENCES

1. Abramson L, Seligman M, and Teasdale J: Learned helplessness in humans: critique and reformulation, J Abnorm Psychol 87:49, 1978.
2. Akiskal H and McKinney W: Depressive disorders: toward a unified hypothesis, Science 182:20, 1973.
3. American Psychiatric Association: Diagnostic and Statistical Manual of Mental Disorder, Third Edition—Revised, Washington DC, 1987, The Association.
4. Arieti S and Bemporad J: The psychological organization of depression, Am J Psychiatry 137:1360, 1980.
5. Beck A: Depression: causes and treatment, Philadelphia, 1978, University of Pennsylvania Press.
6. Beck A et al: Cognitive therapy of depression, New York, 1979, The Guilford Press.
7. Beck C: The occurrence of depression in women and the effect of the women's movement, J Psychiatr Nurs 17(11):14, 1979.
8. Bowlby J: Grief and mourning in infancy and early childhood, Psychoanal Study Child 15:9, 1960.
9. Bowlby J: Processes of mourning, Int J Psychoanal 42:22, 1961.
10. Brown G and Harris T: Social origins of depression, London, 1978, Tavistock Publications, Ltd.
11. Brown R, Ramirez D, and Taub J: The prescription of exercise for depression, Physician Sports Med 6(12):34, 1978.
12. Buckwalter K and Abraham I: Alleviating the discharge crisis: the effects of a cognitive-behavioral nursing intervention for depressed patients and their families, Arch Psych Nurs 1(5):350, 1987.
13. Bugen L: Human grief: a model for prediction and intervention, Am J Orthopsychiatry 47:196, 1972.
14. Charney E and Weissman M: Epidemiology of depressive illness. In Mann J, editor: Phenomenology of depressive illness, New York, 1988, Human Science Press.
15. Clayton P et al: Mourning and depression: their similarities and differences, Can Psychiatr Assoc 19:309, 1974.
16. Cohen M: Personal identity and sexual identity, Psychiatry 29:1, 1966.
17. Crary W and Crary G: Depression, Am J Nurs 73:472, 1973.
18. Drake R and Price J: Depression: adaptation to disruption and loss, Perspect Psychiatr Care 13:163, 1975.
19. Dyer E: Parenthood as crisis: a restudy, Marriage Fam Living 25:196, 1963.
20. Engel G: Grief and grieving, Am J Nurs 64:93, 1964.
21. Goldberg C: Therapeutic tasks: strategies for changes, Perspect Psychiatr Care 18(4):156, 1980.
22. Gove W: The relationship between sex roles, marital status, and mental illness, Soc Forces 51:34, 1972.
23. Gulesserian B and Warren C: Coping resources of depressed patients, Arch Psych Nurs 1(6):392, 1987.

24. Hare-Mustin R: Family change and gender differences: implications for theory and practice, Family Relations 37:36, 1988.
25. Hensley M and Rogers S: Shedding light on "SAD"-ness, Arch Psych Nurs I(4):230, 1987.
26. Hodge J: They that mourn, J Relig Health 11:229, 1972.
27. Holmes T and Rahe R: The Social Readjustment Rating Scale, J Psychosom Res 2:213, 1967.
28. Ilfield F: Current social stressors and symptoms of depression, Am J Psychiatry 134:161, 1977.
29. Jacob T et al: Role expectation and role performance in distressed and normal couples, J Abnorm Psychol 87:286, 1978.
30. Jamison K et al: Clouds and silver linings: positive experiences associated with primary affective disorders, Am J Psychiatry 137(2):198, 1980.
31. Kübler-Ross E: On death and dying, New York, 1969, The Macmillan Publishing Co, Inc.
32. LeMasters E: Parenthood as crisis, Marriage Fam Living 19:352, 1957.
33. Levitt E and Lubin B: Depression: concepts, controversies, and some new facts, New York, 1975, Springer Publishing Co, Inc.
34. Lewinsohn P and Amenson C: Some relations between pleasant and unpleasant mood related activities and depression, J Abnorm Psychol 87:644, 1978.
35. Lewinsohn P, Youngren M, and Grosscup S: Reinforcement and depression. In Depue R, editor: The psychobiology of the depressive disorders, New York, 1979, Academic Press, Inc.
36. Lindemann E: Symptomatology and management of acute grief, Am J Psychiatry 101:141, 1944.
37. Mayo J, O'Connell R, and O'Brien J: Families of manic-depressive patients: effect of treatment, Am J Psychiatry 136:1535, 1979.
38. McLean P: Remediation of skills and performance deficits in depression. In Clarkin J and Glazer H, editors: Depression: behavioral and directive intervention strategies, New York, 1981, Garland Publishing, Inc.
39. Myers J, Lindenthal J, and Pepper M: Life events, social integration, and psychiatric symptomatology, J Health Soc Behav 16:421, 1975.
40. Nezu A and Ronan G: Life stress, current problems, problem solving, and depressive symptoms: an integrative model, J Consult Clin Psychol 53(5):693, 1985.
41. Parkes C: Bereavement: studies of grief in adult life, New York, 1972, International Universities Press.
42. Parkes C and Brown R: Health after bereavement: a controlled study of young Boston widows and widowers, Psychosom Med 34:449, 1972.
43. Paykel E et al: Life events and depression, Arch Gen Psychiatry 21:753, 1969.
44. Post R and Ballenger J: Neurobiology of mood disorders, Baltimore, Md, 1984, Williams & Wilkins.
45. Regier D et al: The NIHM depression awareness, recognition, and treatment program: structure, aims and scientific base, Am J Psych 145(11):1351, 1988.
46. Rehm L: A self-control therapy program for treatment of depression. In Clarkin J and Glazer H, editors: Depression: behavioral and directive intervention strategies, New York, 1981, Garland Publishing, Inc.
47. Robertson J and Robertson J: Young children in brief separation: a fresh look, Psychoanal Study Child 26:264, 1971.
48. Robins E and Guze S: Establishment of diagnostic validity in psychiatric illness, Am J Psychiatry 126:983, 1970.
49. Rodin G and Voshart K: Depression in the medically ill: an overview, Am J Psych 143(6):696, 1986.
50. Rosenblatt P, Walsh R, and Jackson D: Grief and mourning in cross-cultured perspective, New Haven, Conn, 1976, HRAF Press.
51. Rosenfield S: Sex differences in depression: do women always have higher rates? J Health Soc Behav 21:33, 1980.
52. Seligman M: Helplessness: on depression, development and death, San Francisco, 1975, WH Freeman and Co, Publishers.
53. Simmons-Alling S: Genetic implications for major affective disorders, Arch Psych Nurs IV(1):67, 1990.
54. Spitz R: Anaclitic depression, Psychoanal Study Child 2:313, 1942.
55. Stuart GW: Role strain and depression: a causal inquiry, J Psychosoc Nurs 19(12):20, 1981.
56. Stuart G et al: Early family experiences of women with bulimia and depression, Arch Psych Nurs IV(1):43, 1990.
57. Tirrell C and DeForest D: Neuroendocrine factors in affective disorders, Arch Psych Nurs I(4):225, 1987.
58. Van Servellen G and Dull L: Group psychotherapy for depressed women: a model, J Psychosoc Nurs 19(8):25, 1981.
59. Warheit G: Life events, coping stress, and depressive symptomatology, Am J Psychiatry 136(4B):502, 1979.
60. Whybrow P, Akiskal H, and McKinney W: Mood disorders: toward a new psychobiology, New York, 1984, Plenum Press.
61. Woods N: Employment, family roles, and mental health in young married women, Nurs Res 34(1):4, 1985.
62. Wright J and Beck A: Cognitive therapy of depression: theory and practice, Hosp Community Psychiatry 34(12):1119, 1983.
63. Youssef F: Compliance with therapeutic regimens: a follow-up study for patients with affective disorders, J Adv Nurs 8:513, 1983.

■ **ANNOTATED SUGGESTED READINGS** ■

Birtchnell J: Defining dependence, Br J Med Psychology 61:111, 1988.
Reviews evidence that dependence contributes to depression, and related dependence to the process of maturity, linking it

---

*Asterisk indicates nursing reference.

with such issues as competence, need for approval, use of drugs, religiousness, self-esteem and femininity.

Bowden C: Current treatment of depression, Hosp Community Psychiatry 36(11):1192, 1985.

This important article reviews current medical treatments for depression emphasizing biological therapies, including drug selection, newer antidepressants, usefulness of plasma levels, and ECT. Should be read by all nurses working with depressed patients.

*Buckwalter K and Abraham I: Alleviating the discharge crisis: the effects of a cognitive-behavioral nursing intervention for depressed patients and their families, Arch Psych Nurs 1(5):350, 1987.

Describes an experimental study focused on the reintegration of depressed patients after psychiatric hospitalization. Excellent example of clinically based nursing research.

*Burnard P: Spiritual distress and the nursing response: theoretical considerations and counseling skills, J Adv Nurs 12:377, 1987.

Examines the issues and practical skills involved in counseling people who fail to invest life with meaning. Good review of the literature on this topic.

*Field W: Physical causes of depression, J Psychosoc Nurs Ment Health Serv 23(10):7, 1985.

Summarizes the major physical causes of depression including brain diseases, drugs, electrolyte disorders, postsurgical phenomena, and other physiological relationships.

Gaylin W: Feelings: our vital signs, New York, 1979, Harper & Row, Publishers, Inc.

Attempts to analyze and describe feelings. Contends that feelings are important and serve a purpose; they provide for our survival both as individuals and as a species.

*Gifford B and Cleary B: Supporting the bereaved, Am J Nurs 1990:49, 1990.

Reviews the stages and manifestations of grief and strategies that nurses can use to help people cope.

*Goldberg C: Therapeutic tasks: strategies for change, Perspect Psychiatr Care 18(4):156, 1980.

Describes value of therapeutic, action-focused tasks through the effective use of clinical examples. Practical, pertinent, and clearly written.

*Gordon V et al: A 3-year follow-up of a cognitive-behavioral therapy intervention, Arch Psych Nurs II(4):218, 1988.

Research report on the effectiveness of a cognitive-behavioral group intervention with depressed women. Includes theoretical framework, research methodology, and outcome measure.

*Hauser M and Feinberg D: An operational approach to the delayed grief and mourning process, J Psychiatr Nurs 14:29, 1976.

Discusses Bowlby's phases of mourning and identifies psychological components related to each phase and appropriate nursing interventions. Well-written with direct clinical application.

Lindemann E: Symptomatology and management of acute grief, Am J Psychiatry 101:141, 1944.

Describes the course and management of normal and abnormal grief reactions from observations of 101 patients. Classic work in the study of grieving.

*Lum T: An integrated approach to aging and depression, Arch Psych Nurs II(4):211, 1988.

Presents a comprehensive review of depression in people over 65, including theories of causation and implications for therapy, counseling and health care for the elderly through an integrated nursing approach.

*Manderino M: Mobilizing depressed clients: cognitive nursing approaches, J Psychosoc Nurs Ment Health Serv 24(5):23, 1986.

Describes cognitive-behavioral interventions in detail. Particularly helpful to practitioners who want specific applications of the cognitive therapy approach to depression.

*McEnany G: Psychobiological indices of bipolar mood disorder: future trends in nursing care, Arch Psych Nurs IV(1):29, 1990.

Presents the biological dimensions underlying bipolar mood disorders and applies the nursing process to psychobiological aspects of patient care.

O'Connell R and Mayo J: The role of social factors in affective disorders: a review, Hosp Comm Psych 39(8):842, 1988.

Reading for the advanced student. Reviews five social factors —demographics, early childhood experiences, life events, social support, and families— in relation to affective disorders.

*Pheifer W and Houseman C: Bereavement and AIDS: a framework for intervention, J Psychosocial Nurs 26(10):21, 1988.

Applies the principles of bereavement intervention to survivors of persons with AIDS. Discusses opportunities for nursing. Timely and highly recommended reading.

*Pollack L: Improving relationships: groups for inpatients with bipolar disorder, J Psych Nurs 28(5):17, 1990.

Reviews the literature on group work for patients with bipolar disorder, and includes goals, therapeutic factors and interventions of a nurse-led group. Clearly written and very practical.

Rippere V and Williams R: Wounded healers: mental health workers' experiences of depression, New York, 1985, John Wiley & Sons.

In an interesting text, 19 contributors describe their experiences with depression, what they did about it, what they found helpful and unhelpful, and what they learned by the experience. Honest and insightful.

Rodin G and Voshart K: Depression in the medically ill: an overview, Am J Psych 143(6):696, 1986.

Reviews the epidemiology, diagnosis, clinical presentations and response to treatment of depressive symptoms in the medically ill. A thorough presentation for the advanced student.

*Rogers C and Ulsafer-Van Lanan J: Nursing interventions in depression, Orlando, Fla, 1985, Grune & Stratton, Inc.

Describes the treatment of people with affective disorders in various age groups and settings. Devoted entirely to depressed patients and recommended for its incorporation of recent research and biological aspects of affective disorders.

*Rosenbaum J: Depression: viewed from a transcultural nursing theoretical perspective, J Adv Nurs 14:7, 1989.

Depression is examined in the context of Leininger's theory of transcultural diversity. Implications for nursing care and research are included.

*Ryan L, Montgomery A, and Meyers S: Impact of circadian rhythm research on approaches to affective illness, Arch Psych Nurs I(4):236, 1987.

Describes circadian rhythm research and its implications for psychiatric treatment, nursing care, and nursing research.

Sargent M: Depressive illnesses: treatments bring new hope, Rockville, Md, 1989, US Department of Health and Human Services, National Institute of Mental Health.

This pamphlet is part of the Depression/Awareness, Recognition, and Treatment (D/ART) campaign. It is written for the public and gives a brief overview of the various depressive illnesses—their symptoms, causes and treatments.

*Simmons-Alling S: Genetic implications for major affective disorders, Arch Psych Nurs IV(1):67, 1990.

Reviews the current outcomes of twin, adoption, and family epidemiological studies that relate genetics and affective disorders, with implications for nursing practice.

*Stuart G et al: Early family experiences of women with bulimia and depression, Arch Psych Nurs IV(1):43, 1990.

Describes a research study of the early childhood experiences of women with depression focusing on parental rearing practices, family conflict resolution, sexual mistreatment, problematic childhood indicators, and childhood separation experiences.

*Thomas S, Wilt D, and Noffsinger A: Pathophysiology of depressive illness: review of the literature and case example, Issue Mental Health Nurs 9:271, 1988.

Uses a case example to explore the interaction of psychological and physiological variables in depression and the use of new laboratory tests to establish diagnosis and treatment. Implications for nurse clinicians are included.

Whybrow P, Akiskal H, and McKinney W: Mood disorders: toward a new psychobiology, New York, 1984, Plenum Press.

Reviews historical and clinical perspectives on mood disorders and present knowledge of etiologic factors. Presents a model of psychobiological integration that views affective illness as a final common path to adaptive failure. Highly recommended.

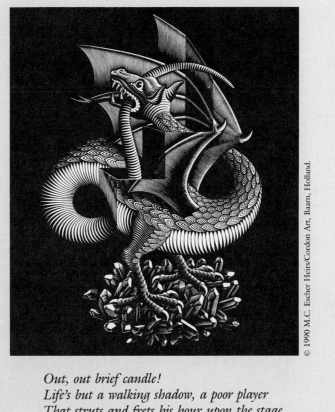

Out, out brief candle!
Life's but a walking shadow, a poor player
That struts and frets his hour upon the stage
And then is heard no more. It is a tale
Told by an idiot, full of sound and fury,
Signifying nothing.

William Shakespeare, Macbeth, Act V

C H A P T E R 15

SELF-DESTRUCTIVE BEHAVIOR

DIAGNOSTIC PREVIEW

MEDICAL DIAGNOSES
RELATED TO
SELF-DESTRUCTIVE
BEHAVIOR

- Major depression
- Anorexia nervosa
- Bulimia nervosa

- Bipolar disorder
- Noncompliance with medical treatment

LEARNING OBJECTIVES

After studying this chapter, the student should be able to:

- describe the continuum of coping responses related to self-enhancing/self-destructive behavior.

- compare and contrast indirect and direct self-destructive behavior.

- discuss the predisposing factors that place a person at risk for self-destructive behavior.

- identify individuals who represent a high suicide risk.

- analyze precipitating stressors that contribute to the development of self-destructive behavior.

- identify an individual's behaviors that are indicative of self-destructive activity.

- differentiate suicide threats and attempts as related to the concepts of ambivalence and hostility.

- analyze coping mechanisms related to indirect and attempted direct self-destructive behavior.

- formulate individualized nursing diagnoses for patients with self-destructive behavior.

- assess the relationship between nursing diagnoses and medical diagnoses associated with self-destructive behavior.

- develop long- and short-term nursing goals that take into account the need to protect the patient from self-destructive impulses and promote self-enhancing behavior.

- apply therapeutic nurse-patient relationship principles with appropriate rationale in planning the care of the patient with self-destructive behavior.

- develop a mental health education plan to assist patients and family members to understand self-destructive behavior.

- describe nursing interventions appropriate to the needs of the patient with self-destructive behaviors.

- assess the importance of the evaluation of the nursing process when working with patients with self-destructive behaviors.

- identify directions for future nursing research.

- select appropriate readings for further study.

Continuum of self-enhancing to self-destructive responses

Many daily activities involve an element of risk. For instance, riding in a car exposes a person to the risk of physical injury if the car is in an accident. Even if no accident occurs, the increased stress from exposure to hazards creates anxiety and requires the use of coping mechanisms. As another example, choice of diet may indicate a willingness to take risks. A family living on a farm and using organic methods to raise most of their food is exposed to a much lower level of potentially harmful chemicals than the family that usually eats commercially prepared foods.

Life is characterized by risk. Each individual must choose the amount of potential danger to which he is willing to expose himself. Sometimes these choices are conscious and rational. For instance, the elderly person who decides to stay in the house on an icy day has chosen not to risk falling and possibly fracturing a bone. Other risk-taking behavior is unconsciously determined. The soldier who volunteers for a suicide mission is probably unaware of his motivation. If asked, he would probably cite patriotism or concern for his comrades. Most people go through life accepting some risks as part of their daily routine while carefully avoiding others. The person who constantly takes chances while driving may refuse to fly in an airplane because he feels unsafe.

Even though life is risky, most societies have a norm that defines the degree of danger to which the person may expose himself. This norm varies according to the individual's age, sex, socioeconomic status, and occupation. For instance, there is great reluctance in contemporary American society to allow women to participate in "contact" sports with men. Although this attitude arises from many factors, the usual reason is that women are not strong enough to compete with men and would be hurt. In general, the very young, the old, and women are viewed as needing to be protected from harm.

Great ambivalence is directed at those who engage in potentially self-destructive behavior. Some risk takers are greatly admired, particularly athletes, military personnel, those with dangerous occupations, and those who place themselves in danger to help others. At the same time, feelings of admiration may be accompanied by fear and perplexity about the danger-seeking behavior. The varying attitudes toward cigarette smoking provide another example of cultural ambivalence. On one hand, smoking is viewed as mature behavior, denoting sophistication and social acceptability. On the other, it is seen as socially alienating, immature, and inconsiderate of the needs of others.

■ Types of self-destructive behavior

Self-destructive behavior may range from subtle to overt. Until recently, however, little systematic attention was given to the covert end of the continuum. Farberow[7] has differentiated indirect from direct self-destructive behavior. Direct self-destructive behavior (DSDB) includes any form of suicidal activity, such as suicide threats, attempts, gestures, and completed suicide. The intent of this behavior is death, and the individual is aware of the desired outcome. Indirect self-destructive behavior (ISDB) is any activity detrimental to the person's physical well-being that potentially may result in death. However, the person is unaware of this potential and will generally deny it if confronted. Examples of ISDB used in this chapter include eating disorders (anorexia nervosa, bulimia nervosa) and noncompliance with medical treatment. Abuse of alcohol and drugs, also self-destructive, is discussed in Chapter 19. Other ISDBs identified by Farberow include cigarette smoking, automobile accidents, self-mutilation, gambling, criminal activity and socially deviant behavior, stress-seeking behavior, and participation in high-risk sports.

Theories of self-destructive behavior overlap with those of self-concept and disturbances in mood. Careful study of Chapters 13 and 14 will help the reader understand the behaviors discussed in this chapter. To think about or attempt destruction of the self, one must have low self-regard. Low self-esteem leads to depression, which is always present in self-destructive behavior. The range of behaviors that includes self-destructive behavior is shown in Fig. 15-1.

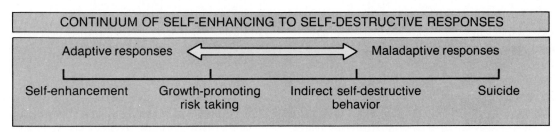

Fig. 15-1. Continuum of self-enhancing to self-destructive behaviors.

The levels of behavior in the continuum may overlap. For instance, the girl who learns and excels at gymnastics is building her self-esteem and projecting a positive self-concept. However, if she tries stunts she is not prepared for and does not take safety measures, her behavior becomes indirectly self-destructive. Similarly, at times ISDB may merge into DSDB. For instance, a diabetic who has never complied completely with his prescribed diet and medication regimen may become discouraged and intentionally take an overdose of insulin. The nurse must be aware of this tendency and be alert to subtle shifts in the mood and behavior of self-destructive patients.

 # Assessment

■ Predisposing factors

■ **AFFECTING INDIRECT SELF-DESTRUCTIVE BEHAVIOR.** ISDB may be differentiated from DSDB, or suicidal behavior, by its duration and by the person's awareness of the behavior's purpose. ISDB is usually long term and repetitive, whereas suicidal behavior, if not interrupted, leads rapidly to death. This distinction differentiates between the individual involved in numerous traffic accidents as the result of drinking and driving (ISDB) and the person who is killed while sober by driving his car into a wall at a high rate of speed (DSDB). Although the latter is usually called accidental, it may be assumed that many one-car accidental deaths are really suicidal.

The other cardinal feature of ISDB is the person's use of the mechanism of denial, frequently accompanied by rationalization. If the danger of the behavior is recognized intellectually, it is not taken seriously. For instance, a hypertensive person may avoid salting food and adding salt while cooking but eat potato chips, cured meats, and processed foods with a high sodium content. The person may respond to confrontation about this behavior by saying, "I know I shouldn't eat those foods, but I feel good. A little bit once in a while can't hurt me." Another example is the anorexic person who is a nutrition student but refuses to acknowledge her own starvation. This recognition of potential harmfulness without any change in behavior or denial of any danger is typical of the indirectly self-destructive person. Denial can help the individual to function. Everyone engages in risky activities daily. Denial controls the anxiety that would interfere with activities of daily living if one were completely aware of the dangers involved. The failure of this mechanism may lead to maladaptive neurotic behaviors, such as phobias. The nurse must assess whether the individual is using denial in a healthy adaptive manner or whether denial is interfering with adaptation so that healthier coping mechanisms should be explored.

Noncompliance. Nurses often care for patients who resist recommended self-care activities. It has been estimated that one half of patients do not comply with health care providers' recommendations. American society is characterized by an increasing elderly population. This results in an increase in the incidence of chronic diseases, such as cardiovascular disease, cancer, cerebrovascular accident, renal disease, and diabetes mellitus. The medical and nursing care of patients with these conditions requires self-care activities by the patient. Diet, activity, and medications must be controlled. Good health practices are needed to prevent complications or the development of additional illnesses. To support the patient in performing self-care, the nurse must understand the underlying emotional issues and assist the patient to deal with them.

Eating disorders. Sociocultural factors influence dietary patterns and possibly the development of eating disorders. Family eating patterns are transmitted to children even before birth. Ethnic background may affect a mother's decision to breast-feed or bottle-feed; bottle feeding has been associated with overweight. Ethnicity and economic status also influence food preferences, for example, high-carbohydrate diets versus more seafood and vegetables.

Powers[19] has applied Minuchin's description of psychosomatogenic families to eating disorders. There are four characteristics of the psychosomatogenic family configuration. The first, enmeshment, means that individuality is lost within the identity of the family group. Autonomy is not encouraged. Role confusion results from lack of clear boundaries among family members. Emotionally, there is overinvolvement and intrusion on the thoughts and feelings of other members. The second characteristic is overprotectiveness; the third is rigidity. Finally, conflict avoidance exists, and thus conflicts are not resolved. Conflict may be denied, or members may fight continuously without addressing the real problem. Family conflicts focus on the problem member, and the real issue is avoided. The true conflict may be between the parents, but it is acted out by the physiologically vulnerable child.

Pope and Hudson[17] note that most studies of the families of patients with eating disorders have not been designed scientifically. Therefore the findings must be interpreted carefully.

Anorexia nervosa has been described by Bruch as "the relentless pursuit of excessive thinness."[4] The incidence of anorexia nervosa in the United States has been increasing for the last 30 years. Before 1960, it was rarely seen. Surveys of prevalence have focused on subpopulations, such as students. This makes it difficult to generalize about the occurrence of anorexia nervosa in the total population. Pope and Hudson [17] estimate that the prevalence of anorexia nervosa is less than 1% of the adult female population. This disorder rarely occurs in males. They also note that in the past the eating disorders were thought to be more common in women from the higher socioeconomic classes. There is little evidence for that at the present time.

Researchers have developed profiles of those predisposed to developing anorexia nervosa. Doyen[5] describes them as "overly sensitive, introverted, secretive, perfectionistic, selfish, and extremely stubborn." The anorectic males studied by Andersen and Mickalide[2] were found to be perfectionistic and self-critical. Their families were of a higher socioeconomic status, and a positive history for affective or eating disorders was often found. These men were frequently involved in an occupation or sport that valued thinness. Both men and women often become anorectic when they continue with a weight reduction diet after they have achieved a normal weight.

Another eating disorder similar to anorexia nervosa is **bulimia nervosa.** The bulimic patient has episodes of binge eating, often followed by vomiting. Binge eating is compulsive intake of food that is stopped only when the person vomits, feels pain, runs out of food, or is interrupted. The age of onset is usually between 17 and 25 years, somewhat older than that of persons with anorexia nervosa. According to Pope and Hudson,[17] some anorexics become bulimic as they grow older. Unlike anorexia nervosa, severe weight loss does not generally occur and the individual is aware that her behavior is abnormal.[19] Bulimic patients usually maintain a more normal weight by alternating binging and vomiting or by eating very little between binges.

■ **AFFECTING DIRECT SELF-DESTRUCTIVE BEHAVIOR.** The ultimate self-destructive behavior is suicide. The stigma attached to suicide makes it difficult to determine the extent of the problem. The reported suicide rate in the United States in 1985 was 12.3 per 100,000 population.[25] The rate for white males of all ages was 19.9 per 100,000; black males, 11.3; for white females 5.3; and black females, 2.1. The recent increase of suicide by adolescents in the United States has been a source of great concern to mental health care providers. For females aged 15 to 25, the suicide rate per 100,000 increased from 2 in 1955 to 4.4 in 1985. For males in the same age group, the increase was from 6.3 per 100,000 in 1955 to 21.4 in 1985. It is estimated that each day 75 people in the United States commit suicide.[22]

Many deaths that appear to be accidental may really be suicidal. Inferences about the motivation for accidental death can sometimes be made based on a "psychological autopsy." This is a retrospective review of the individual's behavior for the time preceding his death. It is accomplished by tracing the person's activities and interviewing those with whom the dead person had contact just before death.

Suicidology has become an important subspecialty in psychiatry. Specialists in this field have done much work to identify groups of people at risk for suicide and have developed profiles of high-risk groups. In general, males commit suicide more frequently than females (a ratio of about 3:1), and women attempt suicide more frequently than men (also about 3:1).[23] Suicide rates also vary with age. The rate for white men increases steadily with age. Although white males over 50 years old are only 10% of the U.S. population, they represent 28% of the total deaths by suicide.[12] In contrast, the rate for white women peaks at ages 45 to 54 and then declines. In general, married people have the lowest rates, those never married are next, and divorced or widowed people have the highest rate, with the exception of older, never-married white men. Table 15-1 summarizes the risk factors associated with suicidal behavior.

In a study of adolescents who had attempted suicide, Gispert and co-workers[10] described several factors that characterized those who had made more than one attempt. These included (1) poor school performance and attendance, (2) more serious intent, (3) difficulty controlling the expression of anger, (4) more dysphoria, and (5) more total life stressors. They note that an accumulation of stressful experiences rather than acute stress seems to lead to repeated suicide attempts.

■ **Precipitating stressors**

Self-destructive behavior may result from almost any stress the individual feels as overwhelming. Stressors are somewhat individualized, as is the person's ability to tolerate stress. All self-destructive behaviors may be seen as attempts to escape from uncomfortable or intolerable life situations. Anxiety is therefore central to self-destructive behavior.

The anxiety associated with a deliberate attempt at self-destruction is overwhelming. It is difficult to imagine if it has not been experienced. Most people cringe from contemplating their own deaths, much less initiating self-destruction. Shneidman[23] believes that self-death is experienced differently from the death of another, since self-death literally cannot be experienced.

TABLE 15-1

RISK FACTORS FOR SUICIDAL BEHAVIOR*

Factor	High risk	Low risk
Age	Over 45 years or adolescent	25 to 45 years or under 12 years
Sex	Male	Female
Marital status	Divorced, separated, or widowed	Married
Socialization	Isolated	Socially active
Occupation	Professional workers (medicine, dentistry, law) or student	Blue collar workers
Employment	Unemployed	Employed
Physical illness	Chronically or terminally ill	No serious medical problems
Mental illness	Depression, delusions, or hallucinations	Personality disorder
Drug and alcohol use	Intoxicated and/or addicted	Neither intoxicated nor addicted
Previous attempts	At least one	None
Plan	Definite plan specified	Vague plan
Method	Violent means: shooting, hanging, or jumping	Nonviolent means: drugs, poison, or carbon monoxide
Availability of means	Readily available	Not yet obtained

*Risk factors are relative and intended as a guide to assessment. **Low** risk never means **no** risk.

In a sense, the person who destroys himself actually destroys everything else *but* himself.

In contrast, people engaged in gradually self-destructive behavior tend to deny their eventual deaths, usually believing that they can assume control at any time. This fantasy of being able to control, although it alleviates anxiety, also helps to perpetuate the behavior. The anxiety that leads to self-destructive behavior may evolve from a variety of sources: physiological, psychological, and sociocultural.

■ AFFECTING INDIRECT SELF-DESTRUCTIVE BEHAVIOR

Physiological stressors. No direct relationship between a biological factor and most forms of ISDB has been found. Endocrinological disorders have been explored in conjunction with anorexia nervosa. However, most studies have been done after the condition is well advanced and may be the result, rather than the cause, of starvation. Some suggest that dopamine may play a role in the development of this disorder. Dopamine is an appetite depressant, so elevated dopamine levels could contribute to anorexia nervosa.[19] Most anorectic persons experience extreme hunger, however, which would tend to negate this theory.

Psychological stressors. Psychologically, one of the antecedents of self-destructive behavior is **depres-**sion. Filstead[9] notes that despair is usually present when ISDB occurs. He describes despair as "a psychosocial state that people experience when they are trying to resolve what has become a serious personal problem . . . and realize that there does not appear to be any way to resolve it."[9] The ISDB may be serving as a defense against underlying despair. For instance, diabetics may overeat foods containing sugar to overcome anxiety related to an inadequate self-concept. However, the behavior is self-defeating and does not resolve the problem. As self-dissatisfaction increases, despair may break through into awareness. If this happens, the person is at high risk for suicidal behavior.

Adolescence is characterized by emotional upheaval. Adolescents must establish a personal identity and become independent of parental control. Bruch[4] believes that anorectic behavior may follow a new experience that is viewed as threatening. It may even be caused by a casual remark thought to be critical of the person's weight. Bruch states, "They act as if no one had ever told them that developing curves and roundness is part of normal puberty."[4] Young women who are anorectic reject their growing feminine bodies and strive for a childlike smallness. This lack of self-acceptance leads to low self-esteem and depression, which contributes to continuation of the problem. Parents of children with eating disorders may reinforce dependency through their involvement in trying to persuade the child to eat.

Another major issue in relation to ISDB is one of **control.** Whatever the risky behavior, it is under the person's control. In addition, power struggles frequently occur between the person performing the behavior and significant others who recognize the perilous nature of the behavior and try to change it. For instance, the parents of anorectic patients become very worried as their daughter becomes more emaciated. As they try to persuade or force her to eat, she becomes more determined to undo their efforts. If forced to eat, the anorectic person will vomit, take laxatives or diuretics, or exercise frantically, thus continuing to maintain control.

Control is also relevant to noncompliant behavior. The person who has a chronic illness often feels betrayed by his body, which in the past has been under his control. Compliance with a therapeutic regimen may be seen as an admission that a problem exists and that the person cannot manage it without help. Refusal to perform required self-care activities returns a sense of control. As long as overt symptoms do not occur or can be ignored, the person maintains an illusion of health. Again, significant others may become concerned about the results of noncompliant behavior and try to intervene. This increases the sense of loss of control and causes even more resistance. Powerful emotions, including anger, fear, and depression, underlie the overt behavior of self-control. If the person is not assisted to cope with these feelings, the ISDB will continue or may progress to DSDB.

Sociocultural stressors. Eating disorders are influenced by the cultural definition of ideal body image. In the contemporary United States, thinness is valued, particularly for women. Pubertal girls who begin to develop rounded body contours may interpret this as fatness and attempt to counteract the effects of normal growth and development by dieting. This behavior sometimes leads to anorexia nervosa. The idealization of slimness can also assist the anorectic girl to justify her behavior by entering modeling, the theater, or dance.

The adolescent must assimilate new behaviors and roles as a part of the developmental process. Demands from parents and peers can increase anxiety and lead to eating disorders. Doyen[5] has noted that anorexia nervosa may be caused by new social situations requiring skills that the young person has not yet mastered. Relative to young anorectic males, Andersen and Mickalide found that onset was sometimes preceded by "social disappointment, major life change, or a temporary illness that led to weight loss."[2]

Sociocultural factors also influence noncompliance with treatment. Most people develop their concept of the illness experience through childhood episodes of acute infectious diseases. Treatment is begun to cure the illness. When the symptoms disappear, the treatment is discontinued. This conceptualization does not apply to chronic illness, but it is still the expectation of many patients. Symptoms of many chronic diseases come and go, even though the disease remains. If the acute illness model is applied, the patient assumes that the periods when no symptoms are present are times of wellness. Therefore, treatment is unnecessary. Some patients also have difficulty identifying symptoms of chronic health problems, such as hypertension, except when they are severe. These behavior patterns have serious implications for the health care of the chronically ill.

Chronic illness also does not fit the pattern of sick role behavior acceptable in our society. The sick person is expected to acknowledge his illness, comply with treatment, and then recover. When recovery does not take place, the lack of conformity with cultural norms regarding sickness can lead to guilt and contribute to reluctance to comply with health care needs. Patient education programs must provide adequate information about the nature of the health problem but also recognize and attend to the patient's emotional responses to the illness experience.

■ **AFFECTING DIRECT SELF-DESTRUCTIVE BEHAVIOR.** When the sense of self-worth is extremely low, self-destructive behavior reaches its peak. At this point, suicidal behavior is likely. Suicide implies a loss of the ability to value the self at all. This in turn may be related to unresolved grief, a perceived failure in life, or anger at the self.

Psychological stressors. Unexpressed anger at others may lead a person to vent these feelings on himself. The individual may feel that his anger is not justified and become guilty, or he may not be able to direct appropriate feelings outward. Some people with this problem may exhibit masochistic behavior. Masochism is the need to inflict pain on the self. Others may derogate the self or underachieve. Still others may be so angry that they try to kill themselves.

Freudian theorists viewed self-destructive behavior as the focusing of hostile feelings on an internalized love object. Ambivalence was an important component of the theory. More recently, additional emphasis has been placed on the importance of the feelings of helplessness, hopelessness, and dependency in self-destructive behavior. These feelings are recognized as characteristics of depression. Severely depressed individuals are always suicidal risks. The extreme outcome of the self-directed anger thought to accompany depression is suicide. This is also the ultimate way of expressing hostility toward significant others. However, it is believed that some hope always exists that help will arrive, that someone will rescue the suicidal person.

Roy[21] has proposed that the fantasies of suicidal patients can reveal characteristics of the psychodynamics. Fantasies may include "wishes for revenge, power, control, punishment; wishes for atonement, sacrifice, or restitution; wishes for escape or sleep; or wishes for rescue, rebirth, reunion with the dead, or a new life."

Psyiological stressors. Another precursor to self-destructive behavior may be extreme confusion or personality disorganization. This may be related to organic mental disorder, psychosis, or use of hallucinogenic drugs. Self-destructive behavior caused by one of these problems is often unintentional. The young person under the influence of PCP (phencyclidine) may feel invincible and walk in front of a truck or jump out a window. The psychotic person may harm himself because he is hearing voices that tell him to do so. The person may be quite unaware of the implications of his behavior.

Research is taking place to identify if there are biochemical stressors related to suicidal behavior. There have been indications that low levels of serotonin are present in some people who have attempted suicide.[21] The evidence is not yet conclusive. Suicidal behavior has been associated with several mental disorders, including major depression, bipolar disorder, substance abuse disorders, and schizophrenia. As more is learned about the biochemical aspects of these disorders, more will be known about biochemical changes that may accompany suicide.

Sociocultural stressors. Patients with chronic, painful, or life-threatening illnesses may engage in self-destructive behavior. Frequently these people consciously choose to kill themselves. Quality of life becomes an issue that at times supersedes quantity of life. An ethical dilemma may arise for the nurse who becomes aware of the patient's choice to engage in this behavior. There are no easy answers to the question of how to resolve this conflict. Each nurse must do so according to her own belief system.

Self-destructive behavior may be related to many social and cultural factors. Durkheim,[6] in his pioneer study of suicidal behavior, identified three subcategories of suicide, based on the individual's motivation:

1. *Egoistic suicide* results from the individual being poorly integrated into society.
2. *Altruistic suicide* results from obedience to customs and habit.
3. *Anomic suicide* results when society is unable to regulate the individual.

Durkheim believed the structure of society has a great influence on the individual. It may either help or sustain him or lead him to destroy himself.

Social isolation may lead to loneliness and increase the person's vulnerability to suicide. People who are actively involved with others in their communities are more able to tolerate stress. Those who lose the ability to participate in social activities are more likely to turn to self-destructive behavior. Religious involvement is particularly supportive to many people during difficult times.

Interpersonal losses are especially stressful to many people. This includes losses that are real or imagined, both sudden and gradual. The suicide of someone close, either a relative or friend is particularly stressful. Family members of those who have committed suicide are at greater risk to follow suit. "Cluster suicides" have been observed in adolescents. In this case, several students from the same school or the same community, individually or in groups, will commit suicide within a short period of time, sometimes using similar methods.

Self-destructive behavior probably is determined by a variety of factors, which differ from person to person. Thus it is extremely important to assess completely the patient's medical, psychological, and social history. Identification of probable causative factors leads to individualized planning for nursing care.

■ Behaviors

■ **ASSOCIATED WITH INDIRECT SELF-DESTRUCTIVE BEHAVIOR.** The common characteristics of all varieties of ISDB are (1) it is progressively or potentially detrimental to the individual, (2) the individual is aware that his behavior is risky, and (3) he denies that he will suffer significant negative consequences from his behavior. Eating disorders, such as anorexia nervosa/bulimia nervosa, and noncompliance with prescribed health care practices, are examples of ISDB.

Eating disorders. Young women with anorexia nervosa perceive that they are fat and literally starve themselves to achieve their goal of being thin. However, because of the distortion in body image they experience, the goal is unattainable. Even when their appearance is skeletal, they maintain that they are fat and persist in their attempt to lose weight.

Bruch[4] describes the typical anorectic process as beginning with a diet. At first, the dieter feels a sense of deprivation and difficulty in maintaining the restrictions. However, she then enters a stage of pride in her accomplishment, and this perpetuates the behavior. At the same time, biological effects of starvation distort the perception of body sensations. There is a heightening of sensory experience and a feeling that has been compared to intoxication. As the condition progresses, the patient begins to feel special and different because of her superhuman effort and extraordinary accomplishment. This results in her alienation and isolation from others who fail to understand her behavior and its meaning to her. She then becomes increasingly absorbed in her own world, and her behavior assumes even greater importance to her.

Anorexia nervosa is really a misnomer. Anorexia means lack of appetite. People with anorexia nervosa do experience hunger. It is the victory over hunger that provides their reward. Anorectic persons are often fascinated with food and cooking; some become students of nutrition. They may loiter in places where food is sold or served and watch other people eat. Their life becomes centered around food and the avoidance of eating. Anorectic persons go to extremes to avoid weight gain. They will induce vomiting, take diuretics and laxatives, and exercise strenuously. If they are forced to eat, these associated behaviors are increased.

Bruch[4] also describes decreased internal awareness and a sense of ineffectiveness as characteristics of anorexia nervosa. Decreased internal awareness refers to both emotional awareness and recognition of body sensations. Bruch believes that this results from the parents' failure to respond to the patient's needs during infancy. Since feeding was not directly related to hunger when she was an infant, the adolescent is also less aware of the relationship. The sense of ineffectiveness leads to the great need of anorectic persons to control at least one aspect of their lives. Thus they focus all their attention on mastery of their weight and eating.

As the disorder continues, signs of starvation become more evident. Amenorrhea occurs early in the course of the illness. It was thought to be a symptom of anorexia nervosa; Now it is believed to result from weight loss. Early symptoms of anorexia nervosa are difficult to identify. The problem is usually not recognized until a significant weight loss has already occurred. Therefore initial assessment reveals symptoms of starvation as well as those of anorexia.

Feighner and Corvorhers have also described behaviors characteristic of anorexia nervosa. These behaviors are compared to those recommended for diagnosis of anorexia nervosa by DSM-III-R[1] in Table 15-2. The Feighner criteria are widely used in anorexia nervosa research settings. Clinical example 15-1 illustrates behaviors characteristic of anorexia nervosa.

The prognosis for anorexia nervosa is unclear at

TABLE 15-2

COMPARISON OF FEIGHNER AND DSM-III-R CRITERIA FOR THE DIAGNOSIS OF ANOREXIA NERVOSA

Feighner et al[8]	DSM-III-R[1]
Onset before 25 years old	Unrelenting fear of obesity
Loss of at least 25% of preillness weight	Disturbed body image
Distorted attitude toward food, eating, or weight	Refusal to maintain weight within norms for age and height
No known medical illness causing weight loss	In females, at least three missed menstrual periods
No known psychiatric illness causing anorexia	
At least two of the following:	
1. Amenorrhea	
2. Lanugo	
3. Bradycardia	
4. Episodic overactivity	
5. Episodic bulimia	
6. Vomiting (may be self-induced)	

present. Pope and Hudson report a mortality of about 5% to 20% according to recent studies.[24] Bruch believes that psychotherapists must identify the patient's concerns and avoid dealing only with eating patterns if any long-term change is to occur.[4] Longitudinal studies are needed to determine whether the body image distortions and disordered eating patterns are overcome when weight is gained.

The typical bulimic pattern is to eat normally for a while, then have episodes of binging and purging. For this reason, bulimic persons are able to maintain a relatively normal weight and do not experience physical symptoms of starvation. However, the binging and purging behavior leads to other physical disorders. Herzog and Copeland[13] describe these as menstrual irregularities; gastric dilation, sometimes with rupture of the stomach; and aspiration leading to pneumonia. Vomiting can also cause enlarged parotid glands, dental caries, esophagitis, and tears or rupture of the

CLINICAL EXAMPLE 15-1

Ms. L was a 17-year-old, white unmarried woman who was admitted to a general hospital medical unit with a diagnosis of malnutrition. On admission, she was 5 feet, 5 inches (162.5 cm) tall and weighed 92 pounds (40.4 kg). She told Ms. B, her primary nurse, that she was on a special diet. She ate no breakfast, a carrot for lunch, and an apple for dinner. She also said that she would be jogging in the halls twice a day. It was very important that she maintain her exercise routine of running 10 miles daily. Physical assessment revealed the presence of lanugo, especially on the arms and buttocks, amenorrhea of 8 months' duration, and dry skin and mucous membranes. At lunchtime, Ms. L offered her tray to another patient and watched her while she ate. Soon after this, she began to jog up and down the hall.

Ms. B tried to communicate to Ms. L her concern that she was starving and could die. Ms. L said, "You sound just like my parents. You want me to be fat just like they do. You're jealous that I can control my body." When her parents visited, they were observed to be a well-dressed, upper middle-class couple. They gave Ms. L a box of candy. She became furious, throwing the candy on the floor and demanding that they tell the nurses to give her the carrots and apples that she had requested. The parents told Ms. B that they were frustrated and frightened. They recognized that their daughter's irrational behavior could be fatal. They said that she began to diet after her physical education teacher told her she was getting too large to compete in gymnastics. She had always been athletic and had won several prizes for her gymnastic ability. The L's were unconcerned at first but then realized that she had nearly stopped eating. Coercion did not persuade her to eat. After many family arguments, they forced her to see the family physician, who recommended hospitalization.

A diagnosis of anorexia nervosa was made, and Ms. L was transferred to the psychiatric unit for treatment.

esophagus. Hypokalemia can result from vomiting and abuse of laxatives or diuretics. Poisoning from overdose of ipecac, an emetic agent, may lead to potentially fatal myocardial dysfunctions. Therefore, although bulimic persons may not appear to be as physically ill as anorexic individuals, they are at great risk for serious physical illness. In addition, people with eating disorders have an increased risk for suicide.

Noncompliance. People who do not comply with recommended health care activities are generally aware that they have chosen not to care for themselves. They usually have a reason for noncompliance, such as being asymptomatic, not being able to afford the treatment they need, not understanding the activity they are to perform, or not having time. These are rationalizations. They help to relieve the underlying anxiety that is really causing the noncompliance. Patients may also minimize the seriousness of their problems. Many chronic illnesses are characterized by long periods of stability, during which the person may not be aware of discomfort. This reinforces the noncompliant behavior.

Patients with chronic illnesses frequently hunt for health care providers who will prescribe other, less disruptive treatment plans than the ones they are trying to avoid. They are susceptible to questionable practices such as miracle cures and faith healing in their search for the return of complete health. Patients who are receiving chemotherapy or radiation for cancer become frustrated with the side effects of the treatment. They are easily victimized by those who promote "cures" that involve no discomfort but have no scientifically proven effectiveness. The popular literature is constantly reporting miraculous new treatments for chronic diseases. Most of these lead to more suffering for those who become hopeful and are then disappointed.

The most prominent behavior associated with noncompliance is refusal to admit the seriousness of the health problem. This denial interferes with acceptance of treatment. At the same time, however, it protects the ego from the anxiety that recognition of impaired health will create. The greater the threat imposed by the illness, the greater will be resistance to treatment. Many chronic illnesses are associated with advancing age. Anxiety is increased because admission of illness also implies recognition that one is growing older. In a society that values youth, this behavior is not surprising.

An unfortunate aspect of noncompliance is that guilt about not following health care recommendations may also interfere with obtaining regular care. The hypertensive person who has not been taking his medication will be reluctant to have his blood pressure checked because an elevated reading will undermine his defensive system. If the medical system treats these people as children and chastises them for their behavior, they feel even guiltier and are more reluctant to seek routine health care.

Noncompliant people are also struggling for control. Serious illness is often seen as an attack on the

CLINICAL EXAMPLE 15-2

Ms. C was a 61-year-old, white married woman who had been in good health most of her life. She had three grown children who had left home and established their own families. She had been a homemaker since her marriage at age 19. She and her husband were both looking forward to his retirement in 6 months. They planned to buy a recreational vehicle and travel around the United States.

Ms. C visited the gynecologist regularly. She was very concerned about having annual Pap smears. Since she was receiving no other regular health care, the nurse practitioner who worked with this physician did a complete physical examination each time Ms. C was seen. On her most recent visit, laboratory studies revealed an elevated blood glucose level. She was then referred to an internist for a more thorough examination. The new physician hospitalized her for a short time. Her diagnosis was diabetes mellitus, adult onset. Ms. C was told that her condition was not serious and could be controlled by diet. She was 20 pounds (9 kg) overweight and was advised that she needed to lose the excess weight. Before discharge, she was instructed about her diet, how to test her urine, and about possible complications of diabetes. A community health nursing referral was made.

Ms. C was frightened about her condition but did not mention this because no one else seemed very concerned. When she first arrived home, she was conscientious about following her diet and testing her urine. She felt very well and was proud when she lost 5 pounds. When the community health nurse visited, she congratulated Ms. C on how well she was doing. As time went on, Ms. C began to wonder if she was really so sick. She had never felt ill. On her husband's birthday, she fixed a special dinner and baked a cake. She decided she deserved a reward for "being good" and did not follow her diet. She anxiously tested her urine at bedtime and it was negative. Then her son and his family visited the C's for a week. She fixed all their favorite foods and ate with them. She still felt fine and decided she did not need to test her urine. When it was time for her next checkup, she postponed calling the physician. She was very busy preparing for retirement travel.

The community health nurse contacted the physician's office to find out about the results of Ms. C's visit. When she discovered that Ms. C had not been seen, she made a home visit. Ms. C talked with her but was not very receptive to her expressed concern. Ms. C said she would try to diet, but emphasized that she really felt well and was not sure if the diet was realistic in view of her travel plans. She agreed that she would see her physician immediately if she developed any signs of illness and that she would make an appointment for a physical examination at her convenience. The nurse's plan was to visit Ms. C again in a month. However, she noted that it was unlikely that Ms. C would observe her treatment plan until she experienced overt behavioral disruption related to her illness.

person and a betrayal by his body. The patient needs to reassert his control and prove that he is still the master of his fate. The diabetic who cheats on his diet is gambling that he still has control over his body and can resist his problem by will. Most chronically ill people need to test the limits of their control and the validity of the prescribed self-care regimen. Clinical example 15-2 illustrates the problem of noncompliance with a prescribed health care regimen.

■ ASSOCIATED WITH DIRECT SELF-DESTRUCTIVE BEHAVIOR (SUICIDE)

Types of suicidal behavior. Suicidal behavior is usually divided into the categories of suicide threats, suicide attempts, and successful suicide. In addition, certain suicide attempts may be referred to as **suicide gestures.** The gesture is a suicide attempt directed toward the goal of receiving attention rather than actual destruction of the self. Use of this term is questionable. It implies that it is *only* an attention-seeking behavior and should not be taken seriously. All suicidal behavior is serious, whatever the intent, and deserves the nurse's serious consideration. Therefore suicide gestures are included in the general category of suicide attempts.

The **suicide threat** may be veiled but usually occurs before overt suicidal activity takes place. The suicidal person may make a statement such as "Will you remember me when I'm gone?" or "Take care of my family for me." If taken in the context of recent stressors and the person's life situation, statements such as these may be ominous. Nonverbal communication frequently reveals the suicide threat. The person may give away prized possessions, make a will or funeral arrangements, or systematically withdraw from all friendships and social activities. Sometimes a person may make a direct verbal suicidal threat, but this occurs less often. The threat is an indication of the ambivalence that is usually present in the suicidal behavior. It represents the hope that someone will recognize the danger and rescue the person from his self-destructive impulses. It may also be an effort to discover whether anyone cares enough to prevent the individual from harming himself.

Jourard[14] has presented an interesting analysis of suicidal behavior related to the wish for rescue. He believes that suicide is sometimes the result of an "invitation to die" extended by significant others. The invitation may be communicated by failure to respond to a suicide threat or, at times, even more directly. For instance, a woman was admitted to the hospital following the ingestion of iodine. She was severely depressed and highly suicidal. After a course of electroconvulsive therapy (ECT), she recovered and went home. The social history revealed that her husband was a tombstone carver. He reportedly had prepared a tombstone for the patient with only the date of death missing and kept it in a back room of their house. A few months after discharge the patient successfully committed suicide.

Suicide attempts include any actions taken by the individual toward himself that will lead to death if not interrupted. In the assessment of suicidal behavior, much emphasis is placed on the lethality of the method threatened or used. Although all suicide threats and attempts must be taken seriously, more vigorous and vigilant attention is indicated when the person is planning or tries a highly lethal means such as gunshot, hanging, or jumping. Less lethal means include carbon monoxide and drug overdose, which allow time for discovery once the suicidal action has been begun. Assessment of the suicidal person also includes whether the person has made a specific plan and whether the means to carry out the plan are available. The most suicidal person is one who plans a violent death (e.g., gunshot to the head), has a specific plan (e.g., as soon as his wife goes shopping), and has the means readily available (e.g., a loaded gun in a desk drawer). This person is exhibiting little ambivalence about his plan. On the other hand, the person who thinks he might take a bottle of aspirin if the situation at work does not improve soon is communicating an element of hope. He is really asking for help in coping with his work situation.

Assessment instrument. Several assessment instruments, or lethality scales, have been developed by staff members at suicide prevention centers. One good example is the Assessment of Suicidal Potentiality[15]

form developed by the Los Angeles Suicide Prevention Center (see box on pages 472-473). It considers risk factors, stressors, the lethality of the method, coping mechanisms, and support systems to arrive at an overall rating of suicide potential.

Clinical example 15-3 illustrates the behavior of a suicidal person. It may be used in conjunction with the Assessment of Suicidal Potentiality if the student wishes to practice assessment skills related to the suicidal patient.

Completed suicide may take place after warning signs have been missed or ignored. Some people do not give any easily recognizable warning signs. Research done on completed suicide has of necessity been retrospective. However, it can be informative to interview survivors. This procedure is referred to as the psychological autopsy. The information obtained can be used to better understand suicidal behavior and to enhance the effectiveness of primary prevention activities.

Significant others of suicidal people, including survivors, have many feelings about this behavior. A significant element of hostility exists in suicidal behavior. Frequently the message to significant others, stated or implied, is "You should have cared more." At times, when the person survives the attempt, this message may be transmitted in a manipulative way. An example is the adolescent girl who discovers that her boyfriend is dating someone else and takes an overdose of over-the-counter sleeping pills. If she sets the scene so she will almost inevitably be discovered and makes sure that her boyfriend hears of her behavior, she is behaving in a hostile, manipulative way. A remorseful response by the boyfriend would be reinforcing and increase the likelihood that the behavior will be repeated. It is important to treat these attempts seriously and help the patient develop healthier communication patterns. Persons who do not really intend to die may do so if they are not discovered in time.

When suicide is successful, the survivors are left with many feelings that they cannot communicate to the involved object, the dead person. This may lead to an unresolved grief reaction and depression. Some suicide prevention centers have become involved in "postvention"[23] to assist people to deal with this dilemma. Survivors are assisted either individually or in groups to express their feelings and work through their grief.

■ Coping mechanisms

The most prominent coping mechanism related to ISDB is **denial.** Even though the individual may verbalize that his behavior is potentially harmful, direct

CLINICAL EXAMPLE 15-3

Mr. Y was a 52-year-old black man employed in the foundry of a large steel mill. He had worked for the company for 20 years. He lived in a rented room in a blue-collar neighborhood near the mill. Most of his neighbors were Appalachian white and southern black families who had moved to the community to work at the mill. There was an undercurrent of racial tension in the neighborhood, but Mr. Y was not involved in conflicts with his neighbors. He had separated from his wife before moving to the community and had no close friends or family. The separation resulted from his violent behavior related to drinking binges.

Mr. Y was seen by the occupational health nurse, Ms. G, when he came to the employee health clinic following a 6-week absence from work. He had been hospitalized for broken ribs and a concussion after he had been beaten and robbed by a gang of adolescents in an alley behind his home. Ms. G was familiar with this employee because he had been a participant in the company's Employee Assistance Program for alcoholics. When she saw him in the clinic, she immediately noted that he appeared depressed. His face was expressionless, his posture slumped, and he had lost weight. He appeared disheveled, which was a change from his usual neat appearance. He said he did not feel ready to return to work, but he had received a letter from the personnel office requesting that his condition be evaluated by the company's physician. His speech was slow and halting and so soft that he could barely be heard. He told Ms. G that he had a request to make of her. He knew from past conversations that she was an animal lover. He wanted her to take his pet dog because he did not feel able to care for it adequately, and the neighbors who kept it while he was in the hospital had neglected it.

Ms. G was very concerned about Mr. Y and asked him how he was spending his time. He said he kept the television on and he thought a lot. When asked, he said he felt "too shaky" to go outside unless he absolutely had to. He thought the boys who attacked him were still in the neighborhood. Ms. G asked if he had thought about harming himself. Mr. Y looked startled, then admitted that he saw no other solution to his problem. "It makes sense. I don't have anybody. If you take Rover, I can go." With further questioning, he admitted that he had a loaded revolver at home and planned to use it after he left the clinic. Ms. G realized that Mr. Y needed help immediately. She asked the clinic secretary to sit with him while she discussed his situation with the physician.

injury to the self is denied. For instance, the overweight person will remark, "I shouldn't do this—but I will," as he cuts a large slice of cake. Most obese people can recite all the risks associated with obesity but have no sense of immediate personal threat.

Other people who engage in risk-seeking behavior enjoy the feeling of challenging fate and gambling that they will overcome danger. Daredevils, soldiers, and people who participate in dangerous sports deny the importance of the risk involved. The sense of mastery they feel when they win the gamble reinforces future repetition of the behavior.

Rationalization is another coping mechanism often present with ISDB. The noncompliant patient may give many reasons for his inability to comply with his health care plan. These explanations are really ways of decreasing the anxiety and fear related to recognition of a serious illness.

Many patients also use **intellectual defenses.** Anorectic people may become students of nutrition, thus gaining a sense of mastery over their behaviors. Noncompliant patients may seek out information about their illness and then use conflicts among the experts to justify their reluctance to accept treatment.

Regression is another characteristic of these patients. Eating disorders frequently are related to the feeding patterns that the person experienced during infancy. Anorectic patients often begin dieting when confronted with the need to behave in a more adult manner. It is as if maintaining a childlike appearance will allow the continuation of childlike behavior. The occurrence of amenorrhea reinforces this perception. ISDB also invites parental interaction from significant others who try to persuade the person to behave in a self-enhancing way.

These coping mechanisms may be standing between the person and self-destruction. They are defending him from strong emotional responses to life events that are a serious threat to the ego. If they are removed, underlying depression will become overt and may lead to suicidal behavior.

Suicidal behavior indicates the imminent failure of the coping mechanisms. A suicidal threat may be a last-ditch effort to get enough help to be able to cope. Completed suicide represents the failure of the coping and adaptive mechanisms.

 ## Nursing diagnosis

When considering the nursing diagnosis of self-destructive behavior, the nurse must incorporate information about the seriousness and immediacy of the patient's harmful activity. The nurse must consider the

Assessment of Suicidal Potentiality

Name _____ Age _____ Sex _____ Date _____

Rater _____ Evaluation _____

1 2   3 4 5 6 7 8 (9)
Low Medium High

Suicide potential

Age and sex _____   Resources _____   Total _____
Symptoms _____   Prior suicidal behavior _____
Stress _____   Medical status _____   Number of categories related _____
Acute vs. chronic _____ Communication aspects _____
Suicidal plan _____   Reaction of significant other _____   Average _____

Rating for category   **Rating for category**

1. Age and sex (1-9)   ( )   **3. Stress (1-9)**   ( )

Male   Loss of loved person by   ( )
  50 plus (7-9)   ( )   death, divorce,
  35-49 (4-6)   ( )   separation (5-9)
  15-34 (1-3)   ( )   Loss of job, money,   ( )
Female   prestige, status (4-8)
  50 plus (5-7)   ( )   Sickness, serious illness,   ( )
  35-49 (3-5)   ( )   surgery, accident, loss of
  15-34 (1-3)   ( )   limb (3-7)

2. Symptoms (1-9)   ( )   Threat of prosecution,   ( )
                                                 criminal involvement,
Severe depression: sleep   ( )   exposure (4-6)
  disorder, anorexia,   Change(s) in life,   ( )
  weight loss, withdrawal,   environment, setting
  despondency, loss of   (4-6)
  interest, apathy (7-9)   Success, promotion,   ( )
Feelings of hopelessness,   ( )   increased responsibilities
  helplessness, exhaustion   (2-5)
  (7-9)   No significant stress (1-3)   ( )
Delusions, hallucination,   ( )   Other (describe):   ( )
  loss of contact,
  disorientation (6-8)   **4. Acute versus chronic**   ( )
Compulsive gambler (6-8)   ( )   **(1-9)**
Disorganization, confusion,   ( )   Sharp, noticeable, and   ( )
  chaos (5-7)   sudden onset of specific
Alcoholism, drug   ( )   symptoms (1-9)
  addiction, homosexuality   Recurrent outbreak of   ( )
  (4-7)   similar symptoms (4-9)
Agitation, tension,   ( )   Recent increase in long-   ( )
  anxiety (4-6)   standing traits (4-7)
Guilt, shame,   ( )   No specific recent change   ( )
  embarrassment (4-6)   (1-4)
Feelings of rage, anger,   ( )   Other (describe):   ( )
  hostility, revenge (4-6)
Poor impulse control, poor   ( )   **5. Suicidal plan (1-9)**   ( )
  judgment (4-6)
Frustrated dependency   ( )   Lethality of proposed   ( )
  (4-6)   method—gun, jump,
Other (describe):   ( )   hanging, drowning,
                                                 knife, poison, pills,
                                                 aspirin (1-9)

From Los Angeles Suicide Prevention Center: Assessment of Suicidal Potentiality, Los Angeles, The Center.

Assessment of Suicidal Potentiality—cont'd

	Rating for category
Availability of means in proposed method (1-9)	( )
Specific detail and clarity in organization of plan (1-9)	( )
Specificity in time planned (1-9)	( )
Bizarre plans (4-6)	( )
Rating of previous suicide attempt(s) (1-9)	( )
No plans (1-3)	( )
Other (describe):	( )

6. Resources (1-9)   ( )

No sources of support (family, friends, agencies, employment) (7-9)	( )
Family and friends available, unwilling to help (4-7)	( )
Financial problem (4-7)	( )
Available professional help, agency, or therapist (2-4)	( )
Family and/or friends willing to help (1-3)	( )
Stable life history (1-3)	( )
Physician or clergy available (1-3)	( )
Employed (1-3)	( )
Finances no problem (1-3)	( )
Other (describe):	( )

7. Prior suicidal behavior (1-7)   ( )

One or more prior attempts of high lethality (6-7)	( )
One or more prior attempts of low lethality (4-5)	( )
History of repeated threats and depression (3-5)	( )
No prior suicidal or depressed history (1-3)	( )
Other (describe):	( )

8. Medical status (1-7)   ( )

Chronic debilitating illness (5-7)	( )
Pattern of failure in previous therapy (4-6)	( )
Many repeated unsuccessful experiences with physicians (4-6)	( )

	Rating for category
Psychosomatic illness (asthma, ulcer, etc.) (2-4)	( )
Chronic minor illness complaints, hypochondria (1-3)	
No medical problems (1-2)	( )
Other (describe):	( )

9. Communication aspects (1-7)   ( )

Communication broken with rejection of efforts to reestablish by both patient and others (5-7)	( )
Communications have internalized goal (e.g., declaration of guilt, feelings of worthlessness, blame, shame) (4-7)	( )
Communications have interpersonalized goal (to cause guilt in others, to force behavior, etc.) (2-4)	( )
Communications directed toward world and people in general (3-5)	( )
Communications directed toward one or more specific persons (1-3)	( )
Other (describe):	( )

10. Reaction of significant other (1-7)   ( )

Defensive, paranoid, rejected, punishing attitude (5-7)	( )
Denial of own or patient's need for help (5-7)	( )
No feelings of concern about the patient; does not understand the patient (4-6)	( )
Indecisiveness, feelings of helplessness (3-5)	( )
Alternation between feelings of anger and rejection and feelings of responsibility and desire to help (2-4)	( )
Sympathy and concern plus admission of need for help (1-3)	( )
Other (describe):	( )

information obtained in the assessment to identify accurately the patient's need for nursing intervention. It is necessary to review the person's stressors and his coping mechanisms. Formal assessment tools may help in organizing data so that the nursing diagnosis may be formulated.

Validation of the nursing diagnosis with the patient is needed. However, denial is a prominent defense with most self-destructive disorders. The patient may not be able to agree with a statement that confronts this behavior. The primary concern is to communicate, through the diagnosis, the level of need for protection. In the case of self-destructive behavior, caution is recommended in determining the level of risk. It is better to respond to the patient more intensively than necessary than it is to allow serious injury to occur.

A complete nursing diagnosis is individualized and related to all the patient's behaviors and nursing needs. Primary NANDA nursing diagnoses and examples of complete nursing diagnoses related to self-destructive behavior are presented in the box below. Because of the nature of the disorders associated with self-destructive behavior, several other NANDA diagnoses are frequently applied in the nursing care of these patients (see Table 15-3). In addition, many of these patients will receive a psychiatric assessment and be given a DSM-III-R diagnosis. The psychiatric diagnoses most closely related to self-destructive behavior are also shown in Table 15-3.

Nursing diagnoses for these patients generally also refer to other behavioral problems, including anxiety, communication, unresolved grief, self-concept disorders, and anger. Self-destructive behavior usually evolves from other behavioral problems. Fig. 15-2 relates self-destructive behavior to the nursing model of health-illness phenomena.

■ **Related medical diagnoses**

Several medical diagnostic classifications include actual or potential self-destructive behavior among the defining criteria. Suicidal behavior is not separately identified as a diagnostic category. Therefore medical diagnoses in which this type of behavior is listed as possible are included in this section. Additional descriptions of the affective disorders are found in Chapter 14. The disorders included in this section are described in DSM-III-R[1] and are listed in Table 15-3.

■ **ANOREXIA NERVOSA.** The essential features of anorexia nervosa are fear of obesity, unrelated to actual body weight; disturbed body image; refusal to maintain weight within norms for age and height; and in females, at least three consecutive missed menstrual periods.[1]

■ **BULIMIA NERVOSA.** The essential features of bulimia nervosa include recurrent binge eating; self-induced vomiting, laxative or diuretic abuse, excessive exercise or strict dieting to counteract binging; a perceived inability to control binging; an average of at least two binges a week for at least 3 months; and persistent preoccupation with body shape and weight. Weight may vary because of binges and fasts. Bulimic persons may think that conflicts about eating dominate their lives.

Nursing Diagnoses Related to Self-Destructive Behavior

Primary NANDA nursing diagnoses

Noncompliance
Nutrition, altered: less than body requirements
Nutrition, altered: more than body requirements
Violence, potential for: self-directed

Examples of complete nursing diagnoses

Noncompliance with taking antihypertensive medication related to asymptomatic behavior evidenced by unchanged elevation in blood pressure
Noncompliance with 1,800 calorie per day diabetic diet related to denial of illness, evidenced by gain of 10 pounds since last clinic visit
Altered nutrition: less than body requirements related to conflict over sexual maturation, evidenced by loss of 30% of preillness weight
Altered nutrition: less than body requirements related to prolonged dieting, evidenced by refusal to eat any food other than green salads
Altered nutrition: more than body requirements related to maternal rejection, evidenced by hoarding and binging on food
Potential for self-directed violence related to loss of spouse, evidenced by purchase of a gun
Potential for self-directed violence related to phencyclidine (PCP) abuse, evidenced by extreme psychotic disorganization

---

TABLE 15-3

MEDICAL AND NURSING DIAGNOSES RELATED TO SELF-DESTRUCTIVE BEHAVIOR

Medical Diagnostic Class

Eating disorders
Mood (affective) disorders

Related Medical Diagnoses (DSM-III-R*)

Anorexia nervosa
Bulimia nervosa
Bipolar disorder
Major depression
Noncompliance with medical treatment

Psychiatric Nursing Diagnostic Class

Self-destructive behavior

Related Nursing Diagnoses (NANDA)

Adjustment, impaired
Anxiety
Body image disturbance
Coping, family-ineffective: compromised
Coping, ineffective individual
Denial, ineffective
Fluid volume deficit, potential
†Noncompliance
†Nutrition, altered: less than body requirements
†Nutrition, altered: more than body requirements
Self-esteem disturbance
†Violence, potential for: self-directed

*American Psychiatric Association: Draft of the DSM-III-R in Development (subject to change), as proposed by the Work Group to Revise DSM-III. American Psychiatric Association, October 1985.
†Indicates primary nursing diagnoses for self-destructive behavior.

■ **BIPOLAR DISORDER.** The essential feature of bipolar disorder is a current or past experience of a manic episode consisting of a distinct period when one's mood was abnormally and persistently elevated, expansive, or irritable. Usually major depressive episodes have also occurred. The episode of mood disturbance is sufficient to cause severe impairment in social or occupational functioning. Bipolar disorders may be classified as manic (limited to only manic episodes), depressed (a history of manic episodes with a current depressive episode), or mixed (a mixed presentation of both manic and depressive episodes).[1]

Although the outstanding characteristic of bipolar disorder in the manic phase is expansiveness, a threat of suicidal behavior is related to the extreme lability of mood, resulting in depression and thoughts of suicide. The patient's lack of control may lead to impulsive suicide attempts.

■ **MAJOR DEPRESSION.** The essential feature is the presence of at least five symptoms nearly every day during the same 2-week period, with one being either depressed mood or loss of interest or pleasure. Other symptoms might include weight loss, insomnia or hypersomnia, psychomotor agitation or retardation, fatigue, feelings of worthlessness or excessive guilt, diminished ability to think or indecisiveness, and recur-

rent thoughts of death. It is not related to an organic factor or recent bereavement. Major depressions may be classified as single episode or recurrent.[1]

■ **NONCOMPLIANCE WITH MEDICAL TREATMENT.** This category can be used when a focus of attention or treatment is noncompliance with medical treatment that is apparently not caused by a mental disorder. Examples include behavior that results from denial of illness, religious beliefs, or personal values.[1]

⚜ Planning

■ Goal setting

The overall goal for the patient with self-destructive behavior is to prevent the infliction of physical harm to the self. Careful setting of priorities is necessary with the self-destructive patient. Highest priority should be given to goals related to preservation of life. The nurse must identify goals related to immediately life-threatening behavior. For example, the actively suicidal person must first be prevented from acting on his impulses. Later, the nurse can attend to development of insight into the suicidal behavior and substitution of healthy coping mechanisms. The anorectic person must be prevented from starving to death as the highest priority goal.

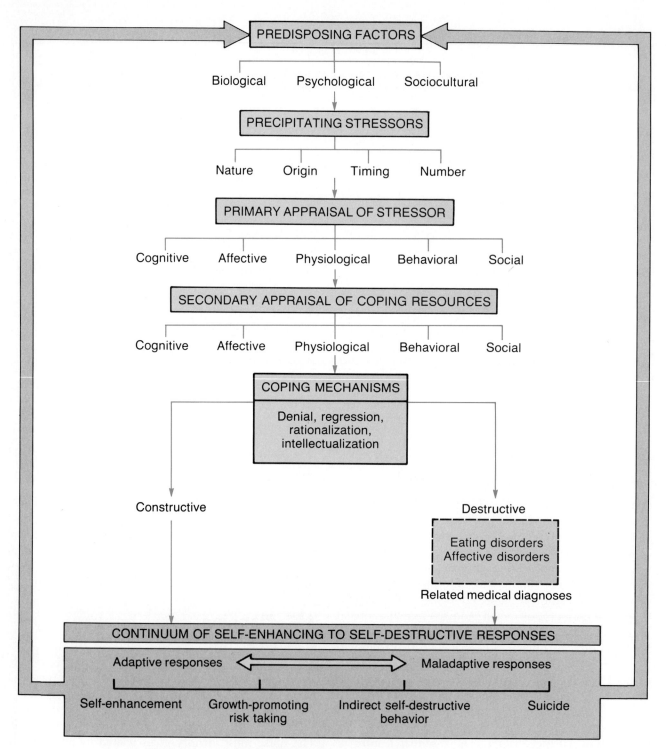

Fig. 15-2. Nursing model of health-illness phenomena related to self-destructive behavior.

Indirect self-destructive behaviors also serve as coping mechanisms. Therefore there is great resistance to changing these behaviors. Goals must include development of new ways of coping to replace the previous self-destructive ones.

In dealing with self-destructive behavior, the nurse and the patient may appear to have incompatible goals. Suicidal patients may resist attempts to protect them and may actively try to evade their observers. However, most of these patients have some ambivalence. The nurse, in setting positive, life-preserving goals, is appealing to the healthy part of the person's self that wants to survive and be better able to cope with life. The very act of seeking help is an expression of this healthy aspect of the personality. The positive attitude of the nurse in setting constructive goals conveys a sense of hope to a patient who may be feeling hopeless.

The nursing care plan for the person with self-destructive behavior must focus first on protecting the patient from harm. In addition, the plan must address the factors that contributed to the patient's dangerous behavior. Figs. 15-3 and 15-4 are examples of partial nursing care plans for the patients described in Clinical examples 15-1 and 15-3. The planning process also involves providing the patient with education about his illness. Table 15-4 is an example of a mental health education plan for a patient with noncompliance with medical treatment.

Intervening in self-destructive behavior

Common elements exist in nursing intervention with all patients who exhibit self-destructive behavior. First, the nurse must consider her own response to people who are trying to destroy themselves. It can be difficult for a person who is happy and involved in life to imagine the depth of despair that leads to suicidal impulses or the lack of caring for the self that results in physically, psychologically, and socially damaging behavior, even if not immediately lethal. On the other hand, a nurse who is depressed and dissatisfied with her own life may be threatened by interacting with patients who are more upset because she may fear similar consequences for herself. This nurse may also overidentify with the patient, which limits her ability to help the patient. One tends to assume that the pa-

---

TABLE 15-4

MENTAL HEALTH EDUCATION PLAN—COUNSELING A NONCOMPLIANT DIABETIC

Content	Instructional activities	Evaluation
Assess patient's knowledge of self-care activities	Ask patient to describe usual diet, exercise, and medication patterns. Validate whether described behaviors match self-care instruction received in the past.	Patient describes usual behavior. Patient repeats previous directions
Identify areas in which patient behavior differs from healthy self-care practices	Describe healthy self-care behavior to patient; provide written, patient education materials; encourage patient to describe reasons for not performing recommended self care.	Patient discusses problems in compliance
Discuss alternative approaches to self care	Assist patient to identify alternative self-care behaviors that would be more acceptable. Enable patient to talk about feelings related to illness and treatment regimen.	Patient decides on different approach. Shares feelings related to illness.
Agree on a reward for compliant behavior	Ask patient how he would reward himself for taking good care of himself.	Patient identifies reward.
Reinforcement	Praise patient for making a commitment to a healthier lifestyle.	Patient recognizes renewed commitment to self care.

PSYCHIATRIC NURSING CARE PLAN

Precautions: Close observation for ½ hour after meals

Special nursing needs: Provide support to parents when they visit; discourage excessive exercise

Visitors: {x} No restrictions
{ } Family only
{ } Restricted to:
_____
{ } No visitors

Telephone: { } Limited
{x} Unlimited

Privileges: {x} Restricted to unit
{ } Off unit accompanied by staff
{ } Off unit accompanied by family/visitor
{ } Off unit unaccompanied
{ } Out of hospital leave (dates) _____

Assessment data summary: Began dieting when faced with becoming too large for gymnastics; does not recognize extent of weight loss; exercises excessively; signs of starvation and dehydration; parents are concerned and supportive

Nursing diagnoses: 1. Altered nutrition: less than body requirements related to excessive dieting, evidenced by low body weight and amenorrhea. 2. Body image disturbance related to conflict about physical maturation, evidenced by verbalization that she will be fat if she does not diet.

Treatment goal: Maintenance of adequate nutrition and hydration through self acceptance

Date	Problem/need	Expected outcome (objective)	Target Date	Nursing Intervention
6/2	Inadequate food and fluid intake	To consume at least 1000 ml of fluid and 1200 calories daily	6/5	Monitor food intake; observe for vomiting; give liquid nutritional supplement.
6/2	Inability to adapt to new developmental stage	To describe her feelings about becoming a woman	6/12	Establish a trusting relationship; introduce but do not force talking about maturation.

Room	Patient's name	Age	Doctor	Primary nurse	Admit date
477	Ms. L	17	Dr. Y	Ms. B	6/2/90

Sample nursing care plan for a patient with the medical diagnosis of anorexia nervosa. (This nursing care plan includes examples of the elements of a total plan as it might appear at a particular time in the patient's course of treatment. It should not be considered all inclusive.)

Date	Medications	Date	P.R.N. Medications	Diagnostic & psychiatric tests	Req.	Done
6/2	Sustecal 250 ml	6/2	Milk of	psychological	6/2	6/7
	10 a.m., 2 p.m		magnesia	testing		
	8 p.m. observe		30 ml. qhs	Blood chemistries	6/2	6/2
	while drinking		for			6/3
	and for ½ hr		constipation			6/4
	after finished					6/5
						6/6
						6/7
		Date	**Treatments**	**Special orders and concerns**		
		6/2	Weigh qd	Restrict exercise to		
				½ hour daily		

Allergies:	Medical diagnosis: (Axes I-III)	Diet:
None	Anorexia nervosa	High fiber

Fig. 15-3, cont'd. Sample nursing care plan for a patient with the medical diagnosis of anorexia nervosa.

tient's situation and one's own are exactly alike, whereas in reality this is probably not so. A therapeutic approach is empathic and nonjudgmental, with limitation of subjective responses through awareness of one's own attitudes.

Hamel-Bissell[11] has studied the reactions of nurses to long-term work with suicidal individuals and identified four stages of reaction.

1. *Stage of naïveté*—in her first exposure to suicidal behavior, the nurse experiences feelings of "shock, lack of understanding, avoidance, and denial."[11]
2. *Stage of recognition*—in her first experience with a suicidal patient, the nurse undergoes a recapitulation of the stage I feelings, only they are stronger. The forced confrontation of these feelings leads to the next feeling cycle of "fear, anxiety, hopelessness, and confusion."[11]
3. *Stage of responsibility*—the nurse experiences conflict over the need to protect the patient combined with realization of her limitations to control the behavior of another person. The feelings associated with this stage are "responsibility, guilt, and anger."[11]

4. *Stage of individual choice*—the nurse achieves a realistic understanding of the patient's responsibility for his own life. The nurse accepts the possibility of losing a suicidal patient.

The recognition of the patient's ultimate responsibility for determining his own fate does not imply a fatalistic or unconcerned attitude by the nurse. All possible efforts are made to protect the patient and to motivate him to choose life. Blythe and Pearlmutter[3] suggest that the nurse align herself with the patient's wish to live and then assist the patient to be responsible for his own behavior. However, nurses must understand that some patients will choose death despite their best efforts to intervene. For the nurse's own emotional health, she must recognize when this has happened. Hamel-Bissell[11] found that nurses took from 2 to 10 years to reach the stage of individual choice.

■ **PROTECTION.** The highest-priority nursing activity with the self-destructive patient is to protect him from inflicting further harm on himself and, if suicidal, from killing himself. The message of protection is conveyed to the patient verbally and nonverbally.

Verbally, the patient is informed of the nurse's intention not to allow harm to come to the patient. To

PSYCHIATRIC NURSING CARE PLAN

Precautions:
Suicide precautions 1:1

Special nursing needs:
Accompany to Alcoholics Anonymous meetings

Visitors: {x} No restrictions
{ } Family only
{ } Restricted to:

{ } No visitors

Telephone: { } Limited
{x} Unlimited

Privileges: {x} Restricted to unit
{ } Off unit accompanied by staff
{ } Off unit accompanied by family/visitor
{ } Off unit unaccompanied
{ } Out of hospital leave (dates)

Assessment data summary: History of alcohol abuse; no close friends or family; concerned about pet dog; recently out of work after attack by neighborhood adolescents; recovered from injuries; recent weight loss; has made suicidal threat.

Nursing diagnoses: 1. Potential for self-directed violence related to lack of social support system, evidenced by description of suicide plan. 2. Social isolation related to neighborhood violence, evidenced by expressed reluctance to leave his house.

Treatment goal: Improvement in mood demonstrated by absence of suicidal behavior and verbalization of decrease in hopelessness.

Date	Problem/need	Expected outcome (objective)	Target Date	Nursing Intervention
2/28	High suicide risk	To refrain from suicidal behavior	ongoing	Observe 1:1; remove dangerous objects
2/28	No social support system	To accept referral to a self-help group	3/21	Accompany to AA meetings; assist to interact with other patients; invite employee health nurse to team meetings

Room	Patient's name	Age	Doctor	Primary nurse	Admit date
518	Mr. Y	52	Dr. D	Ms.J	2/28/90

Fig. 15-4. Sample nursing care plan for a suicidal patient. (This nursing care plan includes examples of the elements of a total plan as it might appear at a particular time in the patient's course of treatment. It should not be considered all inclusive.)

Date	Medications	Date	P.R.N. Medications	Diagnostic & psychiatric tests	Req.	Done
3/5	Amitriptyline		Acetaminophen	Liver function	2/28	3/1
	100 mg, po qhs		650 mg po	tests		
			q4h prn for	Blood chemistries	2/28	3/1
			pain in ribs			

		Date	Treatments	Special orders and concerns
				Observe for alcohol withdrawal symptoms

Allergies:	Medical diagnosis: (Axes I-III)	Diet:
None	Major depression Alcohol dependence	High calorie

Fig. 15-4, cont'd. Sample nursing care plan for a suicidal patient.

the anorectic patient, he or she might say, "We will not allow you to starve yourself to death. You may choose whether to eat voluntarily or to be fed by us, but you will be prevented from starving to death." To the suicidal patient the nurse might say, "I understand that you are feeling impulses to harm yourself. I will be here with you to help you control those impulses. I will do whatever is necessary to protect you. I'd like to talk with you about how you are feeling whenever you feel able to share that with me."

The nonverbal communications should reinforce and agree with the verbal. Obviously, dangerous objects such as belts, sharp implements, glass, and matches should be taken from the suicidal patient. It is impossible to make an environment perfectly safe. Even walls and floors can cause injury if the patient throws himself against them. However, the removal of dangerous objects gives a message of concern. One-to-one observation of the extremely suicidal individual also communicates caring. This observation should be carried out with sensitivity, the nurse neither hovering over nor remaining aloof from the patient. The patient's nonverbal cues can guide the one-to-one interaction. It is important to remain alert until the mental health team and the patient agree that the self-destruc-

tive crisis is over. Suicidal patients may appear to be feeling much better immediately before making an attempt. This is attributed to the feeling of relief experienced when the decision has been made and the plans finalized. Nurses have been fooled by this behavior pattern, relaxing their vigilance, only to have the patient kill himself when he is allowed to be alone for a moment.

If anorectic patients are being forced to eat, they must be observed carefully to prevent induced vomiting. Vigilance during meals is necessary because anorectic patients are usually very skilled at hiding food in napkins, giving it to other patients, burying it in plants, and otherwise disposing of it. They also require limits on activity and close observation of bowel and bladder functioning to ensure they are not secretly taking laxatives or diuretics.

■ **INCREASING SELF-ESTEEM.** Self-destructive people have low self-esteem. The nurse may intervene by treating the patient as someone deserving of attention and concern. Positive attributes of the patient should be recognized with genuine praise. An attempt to make up reasons to praise the patient is usually recognized as artificial and lowers the patient's self-esteem. The message is that the patient is so bad that one has to search for positive characteristics. Andersen and Mickalide[2] recommend that the primary therapeutic interventions with anorectic males be educational and supportive, encouraging the patient to give up his attitude of guilt and blame.

As the nurse gets to know the patient, he or she should be alert to strengths that can be built on to provide the patient with positive experiences, as illustrated in Clinical example 15-4.

■ **REINFORCING HEALTHY COPING.** Closely related to the building of self-esteem is the reinforcement of healthy coping mechanisms. Ms. P's bread making was a way for her to express her anger more productively than by pacing. If past healthy coping mechanisms can be identified, these may be reinforced. In addition, growth may take place through the learning and practice of new adaptive behaviors.

Behavior modification programs may be used to teach new coping patterns. Eating disorders are often approached in this way. For example, principles of behavior modification are recommended by some anorexia nervosa treatment programs. Privileges may be given for pounds gained. For instance, a patient may be confined to her room until she gains 2 pounds, restricted from visitors until 5 pounds have been gained, and so on. Activity limitations and constant observation by staff are unpleasant conditions that the patient can change only by altering behavior. Some programs use feeding by nasogastric intubation as a type of aversive stimulus. Tube feeding is begun if the patient does not consume the required number of calories in a specific time or if weight declines by a predetermined amount. Other programs avoid tube feeding except in emergency situations. These health care providers believe that the insertion of a feeding tube reinforces the patient's low self-esteem and may be interpreted as punishment for misbehavior rather than an effort to be helpful. Some treatment teams refuse to inform the patient of either her present or her goal weight. This avoids endless arguments about desirable weight and decreases to some extent the patient's anxiety about increasing weight. Behavior modification programs are structured to allow the patient to assume more responsibility for her behavior as she demonstrates her ability to behave responsibly. Group interaction and peer support are encouraged.

Potts[18] has suggested a behavior modification program to assist bulimic patients to gain control over their binging and purging behavior. Intake is recorded, and a regular eating pattern is maintained. Alternative activities keep the patient busy and distracted from eating. Other interventions are directed toward altering the attitude about the self and food. The patient is assisted to learn alternative coping mechanisms. The eating of small amounts of "forbidden foods" is encouraged to demonstrate that the patient can avoid binging. Self-help groups are advised to obtain peer support.

■ **EXPLORATION OF FEELINGS.** For noncompliant patients, healthy coping implies the assumption of responsibility for self-care. Interventions must be directed toward developing the patient's understanding of the illness experience.

It may be helpful to assist the patient to explore the predisposing and precipitating factors influencing his behavior. Once the acute crisis is over, understanding the underlying feelings and realizing how they developed and went out of control may help the person to change his behavior. The nurse without advanced preparation in psychiatric nursing should not probe for feelings that the patient is reluctant to discuss and should avoid making interpretations of behavior. These approaches can be very stressful and may precipitate a new crisis, which the inexperienced nurse may be unable to handle.

Group interventions have been helpful to patients with anorexia nervosa. Staples and Schwartz[24] have identified several themes that have characterized their group of anorexic patients. At first the patients simultaneously expressed a wish to change and defended their anorexic behavior. They directed anger toward the therapists. Later, the feeling tone changed to sadness. This was accompanied by self-blame and a recognition of the threat of a loss of identity if they gave up their illness. The feeling in the group then became hostility and blame, which finally yielded to an ability to develop meaningful relationships with others. Oehler and Burns [16] also advocate a group approach. They have included anorexic and bulimic patients together in their groups. The focus has been on developing adaptive social skills.

If the self-destructive behavior represents a response to other behavioral disruptions, appropriate nursing interventions should be directed toward these problems. The angry patient must be helped to deal constructively with his anger. The patient with physiological needs must be helped to meet those needs. For example, the anorectic patient who is in a state of starvation is unable to think rationally and interpret sensations correctly until she has been stabilized metabolically. Attempts to help her develop insight during the period of starvation are certain to fail. When she is physiologically stable, psychotherapy may be initiated.

■ **LIMIT SETTING AND CONTROL.** Issues of control are usually present with self-destructive behavior. A person may be so determined to demonstrate control of his life that he participates in harmful behavior because it is discouraged by others. Bruch[4] observed that this is a characteristic of anorectic patients. Schlemmer and Barnett[22] described the manipulative behavior of anorexia nervosa patients. They noted that manipulation seems to occur in response to limits. For instance, their treatment program had no limits specified for vomiting. Self-induced vomiting, which is a typical behavior of anorectic patients, occurred in only one patient. Patients who were being treated with behavior modification were more manipulative than those who were not. The behavior modification treatment plan was very structured and initially involved strict limits. The authors advised that nurses respond to manipulation with consistent enforcement of limits. They observed that as patients grew to trust the reliable response of the staff, manipulation decreased. They also made it clear that patients retained control of their weight gain or loss. The constant limit testing of a self-destructive patient can be frustrating to nursing staff. It was recommended that nursing staff meet regularly to express their feelings and provide group support.

All forms of self-destructive behavior are controlling in nature. In effect, the patient challenges others to try to stop him from harming himself. In reality, everyone knows that the patient retains the right to choose growth-promoting or harmful behavior.

■ **MOBILIZATION OF SOCIAL SUPPORT.** Frequently, self-destructive behavior reflects a lack of both internal and external resources. Mobilization of social support systems is an important aspect of nursing intervention. Significant others probably have many feelings about the patient's self-destructive behavior. They need an opportunity to express their feelings and make realistic plans for the future. Family members must be made aware of control issues and helped to encourage self-control of the behavior by the patient. Both the patient and the family may need assistance in seeing that caring can be expressed by fostering self-care, as well as by providing care. Families of suicidal patients may be frightened of future suicidal activity. They need to be aware of behavioral clues to suicide and of community resources that can assist with crises. Suicidal behavior frequently recurs. False reassurance should be avoided. A better approach is to foster improved communication patterns and an ability to cope in the family. The nurse may help people sort out their feelings and frequently may want to refer significant others for social work intervention or initiate a referral for family therapy.

If a patient commits suicide, it is important to intervene with the survivors who may be at risk for suicidal behavior. Van Dongen[26] has described approaches to work with survivors. They need someone who can listen to them and let them know that their feelings are not abnormal. They need to be able to discuss their beliefs about why the death occurred and assisted to find some meaning in the experience. Family members should be encouraged to support one another. Survivors are often stigmatized and may need assistance in dealing with this.

Community resources may also be important for the long-term care of the self-destructive person. Self-help groups may provide the recovering patient with needed peer support. Family therapy may assist in the reintegration of a family group that has been disrupted by the patient's recent experiences. Public health nurses, clergy, and other community-based helping people can provide patient and family with day-to-day support. The nurse may be active in explaining resources to the patient and in initiating referrals to other agencies.

■ **MENTAL HEALTH EDUCATION.** Patient education is another important aspect of nursing intervention. The nutrition knowledge of patients with eating disorders should be assessed. Anorexic or bulimic patients may be well informed about foods, but may have difficulty linking that information with their own self-destructive behavior. Education needs to be timed carefully. Patient readiness is essential if behavior change is to result.

Patients who are noncompliant with prescribed

health care regimens may not understand the nature of their problem. Knowledge should be assessed and appropriate teaching initiated. Many patients are willing to participate in self-care if it makes sense to them. Teaching ways to monitor health status may also be helpful. For instance, if a hypertensive patient can check his own blood pressure, he can learn to associate his health care activities with his physiological response. Powers and Wooldridge[20] studied factors influencing knowledge, attitudes, and compliance of hypertensive patients. They found that educational programs presented by nurses were effective in increasing patients' understanding of their illnesses and medications. The blood pressure of patients who participated

in the study also significantly decreased. Patients following medication regimens, such as psychotropic medication for the previously suicidal patient, should know the prescribed dosage, frequency, and side effects. Information about how to handle any future crises should be provided to the patient. If the nurse has explained the possible reason for the patient's behavior, he or she may reinforce this with him at termination of the relationship to help him integrate his experience into his self-concept. Helping a patient to work through his self-destructive behavior can be an extremely rewarding aspect of psychiatric nursing. Table 15-5 summarizes nursing interventions for patients with self-destructive behavior.

TABLE 15-5

SUMMARY OF NURSING INTERVENTIONS IN SELF-DESTRUCTIVE BEHAVIOR

Principle	Rationale	Nursing action
Goal—Prevention of infliction of physical harm to self		
The patient must be protected from harming himself	Highest priority is given to life-saving patient care activities The patient's behavior must be supervised until self-control is adequate for safety	Observe closely Remove harmful objects Provide a safe environment Provide for basic physiological needs
Increase self-esteem	Self-destructive behavior reflects underlying depression related to low self-esteem and anger directed inward	Identify patient strengths Encourage the patient to participate in activities that he likes and does well Encourage good hygiene and grooming Foster healthy interpersonal relationships
Reinforce healthy coping mechanisms	Maladaptive coping mechanisms must be replaced with healthy ones to manage stress and anxiety	Assist the patient to recognize unhealthy coping mechanisms Identify alternative means of coping Reward healthy coping behaviors
Goal—Acceptance of help from family and community support systems		
Mobilize social support systems	Social isolation leads to low self-esteem and depression, perpetuating self-destructive behavior	Assist significant others to communicate constructively with the patient Promote healthy family relationships Identify relevant community resources Initiate referrals to community resources
Patients and significant others should receive education about identified health care needs	Understanding of and participation in health care planning enhances compliance	Involve patient and significant others in care planning Explain characteristics of identified health care need, nursing care needs, medical diagnosis, and recommended treatment and medications Elicit response to nursing care plan Modify plan based on patient feedback

Evaluation

Powers and Wooldridge[20] have identified one of the difficulties in evaluating nursing intervention with noncompliant patients. The most intensive level of intervention is often the most effective in creating behavioral change. It is also the most expensive. In an era of cost containment, this is very difficult to justify. Longitudinal studies must be conducted to show the effectiveness of nursing intervention in preventing deterioration of the patient's condition and rehospitalization.

Problems have also been identified related to anorexia nervosa research. Following an extensive review of the literature, Doyen[5] identified the following factors that make it difficult to compare research studies:

1. Lack of consistent diagnostic criteria
2. Use of subjects with different levels of severity of illness
3. Different posttreatment follow-up intervals
4. Mixing a variety of treatment approaches within the same study
5. Lack of consistent criteria for recovery
6. Varied methods of collecting follow-up data; none found with the validity or reliability of the methodology established

Problems such as these must be resolved if clinical research is to be useful for evaluating patient care programs.

Hendin[12] has identified the following changes in approaches to research on suicide:

1. Exploration of the differentiation of suicidal subgroups in diagnostic categories
2. Consideration of the role of genetic factors
3. Reconsideration of the inverse relationship between overt aggression and suicide
4. Abandonment of the search for universal models of suicide
5. More attention given to cultural influences

Nurses need to contribute to research on self-destructive behavior. As more nurses with graduate preparation in clinical nursing become active researchers, they will assist all nurses to be evaluators of patient care by developing and validating criteria.

Evaluation of the nursing care of the self-destructive patient requires careful daily monitoring of the patient's behavior. Involvement of the patient in evaluation of his progress can provide reinforcement and an incentive to work toward a goal. Modifications of the care plan are frequently necessary as the patient reveals more of himself and his needs to the nurse. As soon as

possible, the patient should become a participant in the planning, evaluation, and modification process.

Unfortunately, self-destructive behavior tends to recur. Nurses sometimes become discouraged and angry with patients who return again and again with the same behavior. When this occurs, the nurse may be caught in the trap of feeling responsible for the patient's behavior. The nurse who has given the best nursing care possible has done as much as she can for the patient. It is impossible to change a patient's total life situation for him. The nurse can only help to identify alternative behaviors and provide encouragement for change. If the patient returns, the nursing process must begin again with an attitude of hope that this

DIRECTIONS FOR FUTURE RESEARCH

The following are some of the nursing research problems raised in Chapter 15 that merit further study by psychiatric nurses:

1. Longitudinal study of the eating patterns of children of women who have a diagnosis of anorexia nervosa
2. Comparison of alterations in body image, self-concept, and eating patterns to weight gain by recovering anorexia nervosa patients
3. The relationship between nurses' experiences with and attitudes toward death and their ability to intervene therapeutically with self-destructive patients
4. Health education approaches that enhance or inhibit the likelihood of compliance with a prescribed health care plan
5. The effectiveness of family therapy in decreasing the occurrence of future episodes of self-destructive behavior
6. Patient responses to one-to-one observation for the prevention of suicidal behavior
7. The relationship of various staffing patterns to the occurrence of episodes of self-destructive behavior in the hospital setting
8. Identification of behavioral responses to the physiological condition of starvation
9. Comparison of the relative effectiveness of nursing interventions with self-destructive patients when the health care process is controlled by the nurse or patient or is collaborative
10. Identification of primary prevention nursing activities that decrease the incidence of self-destructive behavior in a community

time the patient will learn and grow more and be better able to live a satisfying life.

■ SUGGESTED CROSS-REFERENCES ■

The model of health-illness phenomena is discussed in Chapter 3. Therapeutic relationship skills are discussed in Chapter 4. The phases of the nursing process are discussed in Chapter 5. Mobilization of social support systems and health education are discussed in Chapters 8, 9, and 10. Interventions related to low self-esteem are discussed in Chapter 13. Depression is discussed in Chapter 14. Substance abuse is discussed in Chapter 19. Behavior modification approaches are discussed in Chapter 27.

■ SUMMARY ■

1. Self-destructive behavior varies in degree from slow and insidious (overeating) to immediate and dangerous (suicide attempts).

2. Stereotypes of self-destructive people are usually misleading. Most people engage in some form of self-destructive behavior.

3. Descriptive information is presented about indirect self-destructive behavior. The examples of this behavior used throughout the chapter are, anorexia nervosa, bulimia nervosa, and noncompliance with a prescribed health care plan.

4. Data are presented about identification of groups at high risk for suicide.

5. The continuum of coping responses from self-enhancing behavior to suicide is presented. Anxiety and the attempt to escape from it are central to the occurrence of self-destructive behavior.

6. Other behavioral disruptions, including psychosis, may lead to self-destructive behavior.

7. Depression related to low self-esteem and unexpressed anger is intimately related to self-destructive behavior.

8. Issues of control are prominent relative to self-destructive behavior.

9. Social factors, such as loneliness, interpersonal frustration, family communication patterns, cultural changes, and patterns of a subculture may lead to self-destructive behavior.

10. Behaviors characteristic of indirect self-destructive behavior include anorexia nervosa, bulimia nervosa, and noncompliance and involve the core behavior of denial of potential personal harm.

11. Characteristics of suicidal threats, attempts, and completed suicide are discussed, including warning signs, assessment of suicidal risk, and the necessity to understand ambivalence as it relates to suicidal behavior. The function of hostility in suicidal behavior is a major theme.

12. Coping mechanisms related to indirect self-destructive behavior (ISDB) include denial, rationalization, intellectualization, and regression. Suicide represents the failure of all coping attempts.

13. Nursing diagnoses and related medical diagnoses relative to self-destructive behavior are presented.

14. Initially, it may be necessary to set goals for self-destructive patients, but they should be encouraged to participate as soon as possible. Highest priority is given to goals that preserve the person's life.

15. Examples are presented of a nursing care plan for patient's who are directly and indirectly self-destructive. A mental health education plan is presented for a patient with obesity.

16. Nursing interventions should focus on protecting the patient, increasing self-esteem, reinforcing healthy coping mechanisms, understanding the underlying problem, mobilizing environmental resources, and providing patient education.

17. The nurse must explore his or her own feelings relative to the self-destructive behavior of patients.

18. Evaluation is based on the patient's increasing ability to behave in a self-enhancing manner. An attitude of hopefulness is necessary even when patients revert to their self-destructive behaviors and require readmission.

■ REFERENCES ■

1. American Psychiatric Association: DSM-III-R. American Psychiatric Association, 1987.
2. Andersen AE and Mickalide AD: Anorexia nervosa in the male: an underdiagnosed disorder, Psychosomatics 24:1066, 1983.
3. Blythe MM and Pearlmutter DR: The suicide watch: a re-examination of maximum observation, Perspect Psychiatr Care 21:90, 1983.
4. Bruch H: The golden cage: the enigma of anorexia nervosa, Cambridge, Mass, 1978, Harvard University Press.
5. Doyen L: Primary anorexia nervosa: a review and critique of selected papers, J Psychosoc Nurs Ment Health Serv 20:12, 1982.
6. Durkheim E: Suicide, New York, 1951, The Free Press. Translated by JA Spaulding and G Simpson.
7. Farberow NL, editor: The many faces of suicide: indirect self-destructive behavior, New York, 1980, McGraw-Hill Book Co.
8. Feighner JP et al: Diagnostic criteria for use in psychiatric research, Arch Gen Psychiatry 26:57, 1972.
9. Filstead WJ: Despair and its relationship to indirect self-destructive behavior. In Farberow NL, editor: The many faces of suicide: indirect self-destructive behavior, New York, 1980, McGraw-Hill Book Co.
10. Gispert M et al: Predictive factors in repeated suicide attempts by adolescents, Hosp Community Psychiatry 38:390, 1987.
11. Hamel-Bissell BP: Suicidal casework: assessing nurses' reactions, J Psychosoc Nurs Ment Health Serv 23:20, 1985.
12. Hendin H: Suicide: a review of new directions in research, Hosp Community Psychiatry 37:148, 1986.

13. Herzog DB and Copeland PM: Eating disorders, N Engl J Med 313:295, 1985.
14. Jourard S: Suicide: an invitation to die, Am J Nurs 70:269, 1980.
15. Los Angeles Suicide Prevention Center: Assessment of Suicidal Potentiality, Los Angeles, The Center.
16. Oehler JM and Burns MJ: Anorexia, bulimia, and sexuality: case study of an adolescent inpatient group, Arch Psych Nurs 1:163, 1987.
17. Pope HG and Hudson JI: Eating disorders. In Kaplan HI and Sadock BJ, editors: Comprehensive textbook of psychiatry, vol V, Baltimore, 1989, Williams & Wilkins.
18. Potts NL: The secret pattern of binge/purge, Am J Nurs 84:32, 1984.
19. Powers PS: Obesity: the regulation of weight, Baltimore, 1980, Williams & Wilkins Co.
20. Powers MJ and Wooldridge PJ: Factors influencing knowledge, attitudes and compliance of hypertensive patients, Res Nurs Health 5:171, 1982.
21. Roy A: Suicide. In Kaplan HI and Sadock BJ, editors: Comprehensive textbook of psychiatry, vol V, Baltimore, 1989, Williams & Wilkins.
22. Schlemmer JK and Barnett PA: Management of manipulative behavior in anorexia nervosa patients, J Psychiatr Nurs 15:35, 1977.
23. Shneidman ES, editor: Suicidology: contemporary developments, New York, 1976, Grune & Stratton, Inc.
24. Staples NR and Schwartz M: Anorexia nervosa support group: providing transitional support, J Psychosoc Nurs Ment Health Serv 28:6, 1990.
25. US Department of Commerce: Statistical abstract of the US, 1988, 108th edition, Washington, 1987, Department of Commerce Bureau of the Census.
26. Van Dongen C: The legacy of suicide, J Psychosoc Nurs Ment Health Serv, 26:8, 1988.

■ ANNOTATED SUGGESTED READINGS ■

*Abercrombie RK and Thielemann P: Suicide: two views, Am J Nurs 84:597, 1984.

Compares the beliefs of two people regarding suicide as a response to chronic debilitating illness. The viewpoints are "a compassionate solution" and "a chilling encounter." The issues raised would provide material for a stimulating debate.

Alvarez A: The savage god, New York, 1971, Bantam Books.

Presents suicide against a historical and literary background. Discusses experiences with Sylvia Plath, a writer who committed suicide, and observations of her behavior.

Durkheim E: Suicide, New York, 1951, The Free Press. Translated by JA Spaulding and G Simpson.

This classic identifies demographic factors for suicidal behavior. Describes types of suicidal behavior that are still discussed in contemporary literature. One of the first attempts to apply research techniques to a sociological study.

Farberow NL, editor: The many faces of suicide: indirect self-destructive behavior, New York, 1980, McGraw-Hill Book Co.

Highly recommended as a resource on characteristics of self-destructive behaviors, including problems of noncompliance with therapeutic plans, drug abuse, alcohol abuse, hyperobesity, cigarette smoking, self-mutilation, automobile accidents, gambling, criminal and deviant activity, stress-seeking behaviors, and high-risk sports.

Frances A and Clarkin JF: Considering family versus other therapies after a teenager's suicide attempt, Hosp Community Psychiatry 36:1041, 1985.

Illustrates the possible relationship between a child's suicide attempt and family stress. Discusses the use of both family and individual therapy.

Hawton K: Assessment of suicide risk, Brit J Psychiatry, 150:145, 1987.

Good summary of the risk factors that should be considered when assessing a suicidal patient. Analyzes suicide risk related to various mental disorders.

Hendin H: Suicide: a review of new directions in research, Hosp Community Psychiatry 37:148, 1986.

Presents a thorough review of current research compared with past assumptions regarding etiology, demographics, and psychodynamics of suicidal behavior and suggests directions to pursue in the future.

Herzog DB and Copeland PM: Eating disorders, N Engl J Med 313:295, Aug 1985.

Thorough review of current research related to eating disorders. Particularly strong in analyzing the physical disruptions related to anorexia nervosa and bulimia.[1]

*Jourard S: Suicide: an invitation to die, Am J Nurs 70:269, 1970.

Connects family process to suicidal behavior. Leads the reader to consider the broader social system, which usually affects the identified patient's behavior.

*Kiecolt-Glaser J and Dixon K: Postadolescent onset male anorexia, J Psychosoc Nurs Ment Health Serv 22:11, 1984.

Uses literature review and case material to support contention that males who become anorectic following adolescence have different personality characteristics than females and younger males—an important observation for treatment planning. Further study would be beneficial.

Menninger K: Man against himself, New York, 1938, Harcourt, Brace & World, Inc.

This classic investigated self-destructive behavior long before it was fashionable to do so. Took a psychoanalytical approach to suicidal behavior and identifies several levels of attempts at self-destruction.

Morgan HG: Death wishes? The understanding and management of deliberate self-harm, New York, 1979, John Wiley & Sons, Inc.

Provides an excellent comparison of the characteristics of suicide and nonfatal deliberate self-harm. Addresses such issues as epidemiological factors, treatment, and implications for prevention and clarifies the need for further study. Particularly recommended for readers interested in research.

---

*Asterisk indicates nursing reference.

*Neville D and Barnes S: The suicidal phone call, J Psychosoc Nurs Ment Health Serv 23:14, 1985.

Discusses issues related to interacting with a suicidal person on the telephone, recommending information that should be collected and helpful and unhelpful responses. Emphasizes the need for peer support of the telephone counselor.

Niswander GD, Casey TM, and Humphrey JA: A panorama of suicide, Springfield, Ill, 1973, Charles C Thomas, Publisher.

Presents a fascinating collection of psychological autopsies. Adds depth to one's understanding of the many facets of suicidal behavior.

*Potts NL: The secret pattern of binge/purge, Am J Nurs 84:32, 1982.

Presents an overview of issues related to bulimia, including assessment, possible etiology, and treatment approaches. Includes useful information differentiating bulimia from anorexia nervosa.

Pretzel PW: Understanding and counseling the suicidal person, New York, 1972, Abingdon Press.

Takes a philosophical approach to suicide with a deeply humanistic view. Although intended for clergy, approaches to counseling are equally applicable to nursing.

Robinson R: Survivors of suicide, Santa Monica, California, 1989, IBS Press.

Excellent book directed toward the lay audience. Addresses facts about suicide, the experiences of survivors, and ways to help a suicidal person.

*Sanger E and Cassino T: Avoiding the power struggle, Am J Nurs 84:31, 1984.

Describes a treatment program that has been successful in helping anorectic patients and is structured to use a behavior modification approach with defined outcomes. Behaviors associated with anorexia are not addressed directly by nursing staff.

*Santora D and Starkey P: Research studies in American Indian suicides, J Psychosoc Nurs Ment Health Serv 20:25, 1982.

Demonstrates the value of exploring sociocultural influences on behavior. Reviews studies of suicide in several American Indian tribes, enabling the reader to identify similarities and differences.

*Stanitis MA and Ryan J: Noncompliance: an unacceptable diagnosis? Am J Nurs 82:941, 1982.

Challenges the acceptability of the nursing diagnosis of noncompliance, pointing out that this is a value-laden term that may result in the development of negative attitudes toward the patient. Also questions whether compliance with a medical regimen is always a positive behavior. Could be assigned as a stimulus for group discussion.

*White JH: Bulimia: utilizing individual and family therapy, J Psychosoc Nurs Ment Health Serv 22:22, 1984.

Demonstrates the application of individual and family therapy to a nurse psychotherapist's treatment of bulimia. Describes the use of the interpersonal individual and structural/functional family therapy models. Theory is well integrated with the clinical material.

White-Bowden S: Everything to live for, New York, 1985, Pocket Books.

A mother's account and analysis of her teenage son's suicide. Recommended for nurses and parents. Contains excellent advice related to prevention.

Wolman BB, editor: Between survival and suicide, New York, 1976, Gardner Press, Inc.

Includes chapters by several of the more controversial psychiatric theorists. Stimulating and thought provoking because of the many unique approaches.

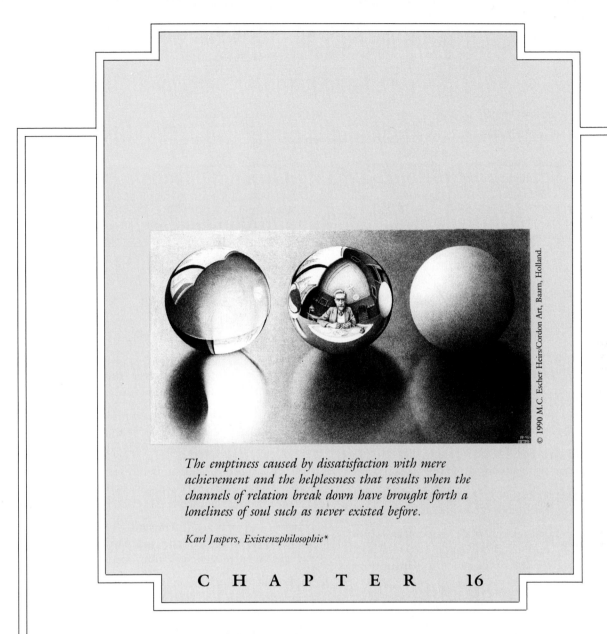

© 1990 M.C. Escher Heirs/Cordon Art, Baarn, Holland.

The emptiness caused by dissatisfaction with mere achievement and the helplessness that results when the channels of relation break down have brought forth a loneliness of soul such as never existed before.

Karl Jaspers, *Existenzphilosophie**

C H A P T E R   16

DISRUPTIONS IN RELATEDNESS

L E A R N I N G   O B J E C T I V E S

After studying this chapter, the student should be able to:

- describe the characteristics of a healthy interpersonal relationship.

- discuss the development of relatedness throughout the life cycle.

- identify five possible disruptions that can occur in the process of relatedness.

- describe predisposing factors that may lead to problems with interpersonal relationships.

- analyze the developmental, sociocultural, biochemical, and psychodynamic stressors that contribute to the development of disruptions in relatedness.

- identify and describe behaviors associated with disruptions in relatedness, including impaired communication, withdrawal, suspicion, dependency, and manipulation.

- discuss the manifestation of impaired relationship behaviors in patients with medical diagnoses of paranoid schizophrenia, catatonic schizophrenia, dependent personality disorder, borderline personality disorder, and antisocial personality disorder.

- formulate individualized nursing diagnoses for patients with disrupted relationship patterns.

- assess the relationship between the nursing and medical diagnoses of individual patients.

- identify the individual's attempts to cope with the anxiety created by the inability to establish healthy interpersonal relationships.

- develop long-term and short-term individualized nursing goals with patients experiencing disruptions in relatedness.

- develop a mental health education plan to assist patients to understand and participate in the treatment of their relationship problems.

- apply therapeutic nurse-patient relationship principles with an appropriate rationale to the care of the patient who is unable to establish healthy relationships.

- analyze nursing interventions for the patient who is suspicious, dependent, withdrawn, manipulative, or unable to communicate effectively.

- assess the importance of evaluating the nursing process for patients with disrupted interpersonal relationships.

- identify directions for future nursing research.

- select appropriate readings for further study.

Continuum of social responses

■ Positive interpersonal relationships

To find satisfaction in life, people must be able to establish positive interpersonal relationships. People involved in such relationships experience closeness to each other while keeping their separate identities. Sullivan[36] refers to this type of closeness as intimacy, characterized by being sensitive to the other person's needs. Also, there is mutual validation of personal worth. There may or may not be a sexual component of an intimate relationship. Rogers[31] has described other characteristics of healthy relatedness, including open communication of feelings, acceptance of the other person as valued and separate, and deep empathic understanding. To become this deeply involved with another person, one must be willing to risk revealing private thoughts and feelings. This can be frightening, especially if a person has found it difficult to share feelings with other people in the past. Fear of exposing private feelings often makes people reluctant to become involved in intimate relationships.

Issues of control are also involved when people relate to each other. Sometimes one must place the needs of the other person or the relationship before one's own needs. At other times, assertiveness is required. The mature person must prioritize needs and share the rationale with others.

Within a relationship, the participants usually develop a continuum of dependent and independent behavior. Ideally, these behaviors are balanced, which is described as interdependence. The interdependent person can decide when to rely on others and experience the caring that may be felt with dependency. However, at times it is appropriate and satisfying to be independent. The interdependent person can let someone else be dependent or independent without needing to control that person's behavior. In this case each person is responsible for controlling his own behavior while receiving support and help from significant others when it is needed.

Every person has the potential to be involved in relationships at many levels, from the intimacy just described to superficial passing contacts. Intimate and interdependent relationships provide a secure base that gives the person self-confidence to cope with the demands of day-to-day life. A lack of intimacy with family members and friends leaves only superficial encounters, taking away many of life's most meaningful experiences. The support of significant others frees energy for involvement with social groups, work groups, and the community. The mature adult can be involved at all these levels and feel satisfied with the quality of his relationships with others

■ Life cycle development of relatedness

■ **INFANCY.** Learning to relate to others maturely is a growth process that occurs throughout the developmental cycle. The infant depends on others for meeting all its biological and psychosocial needs. Infants must develop trust in a mothering person with whom they have a stable relationship. People who fail to establish basic trust are handicapped in relating to others as they continue to grow and develop.

■ **CHILDHOOD.** As a child grows older and develops motor skills, independence becomes a possibility. He strives to establish himself as an individual, separate from the mothering person who has been meeting all his needs. Conflict occurs as adults set limits on behavior, often frustrating the child's efforts toward independence. Loving, consistent limit setting, however, communicates caring and assists the child to develop interdependence. As the child grows older, the parents' guidelines for behavior are adopted as his own, and a value system begins to emerge. Now the child enters school and begins to learn cooperation, competition, and compromise. Peer relationships become important, as does the approval of adults from outside the family group, such as teachers, scout leaders, and parents of friends.

■ **PREADOLESCENCE AND ADOLESCENCE.** By preadolescence, the individual becomes involved in an intimate relationship with a friend of the same sex, a "best friend." This relationship involves sharing. It offers another chance to clarify values and recognize differences in people. This is usually a very dependent relationship. There are often active efforts to exclude others. However, as adolescence develops, the dependence on a close friend of the same sex usually yields to a dependent heterosexual relationship. While the young person is involved in these dependent relationships with peers, he is asserting independence from his parents. Friends support each other in this struggle, which often includes rebellious behavior. Parents can help the adolescent to grow by consistent limit setting and a caring tolerance of rebellious outbursts. Another step toward mature interdependence is taken as the individual learns to balance parental demands and peer group pressures.

■ **YOUNG ADULTHOOD.** The adolescent period ends when the person is able to be self-sufficient and maintain interdependent relationships with parents and peers. Decisions are now made independently, with the advice and opinions of others taken into account. The individual may marry and begin a new family unit. Occupational plans are made and begun. The mature person demonstrates self-awareness by balancing dependent and independent behavior. He allows others to be dependent or independent as appropriate. Sensitivity to and acceptance of the feelings and needs of oneself and of others is critical to this level of mature functioning. Interpersonal relationships are characterized by mutuality.

- **MIDDLE ADULTHOOD.** Parenting and adult friendships will test the person's ability to foster independence in others. This involves a need to give up some dependence on the other person so he may grow. Children gradually separate from parents as they grow, and friends may move away or drift apart. The mature person must then be self-reliant and find new supports. Pleasure can be found in the development of an interdependent relationship with children as they grow. Decreased dependent demands by children creates freedom that can be used for new activities that promote self-growth.

- **LATE ADULTHOOD.** Change continues during late adulthood. Losses occcur, such as the physical changes of aging, the death of parents, loss of occupation through retirement, and later the deaths of friends and one's spouse. The need for relatedness must still be satisfied. The mature person grieves over these losses and recognizes that others can help resolve the grief. However, new possibilities arise, even with a loss. Old friends and relatives cannot be replaced, but new relationships can develop. Grandchildren may become important to the grandparent, who may delight in spending time with them that was never available for children. The aging person may also find a sense of relatedness to the culture as a whole. Life has deeper meaning in relation to the individual's perception of his accomplishments and contributions to the welfare of society. The mature older person can accept whatever increase in dependence is necessary but also retain as much independence as possible. Even loss of physical health need not necessarily force the person to give up all independence. The ability to maintain mature relatedness throughout life enhances self-esteem.

- ### Disruptions in achieving relatedness

Disruptions can occur in the development of mature interdependent interpersonal relationships. Some people have trouble establishing or maintaining close relationships. They may **withdraw** from other people, sometimes to the point where they are unable to remain in the community. A similar situation can occur when a person is isolated by others. Sometimes, individuals may have a problem with too much **dependency** on other people. This can lead to rejection by friends and relatives because it becomes exhausting to try to meet a dependent person's demands. A third disruption in relatedness is **manipulation** of other people. In this case, closeness is not established. Other people are treated as objects to be maneuvered to meet the manipulator's needs. People having problems in relatedness may find it difficult to trust others. Therefore **suspicion** is usually present with any of the behaviors described. Another behavior that may accompany disruptions in relatedness is **impaired communication.** Verbal and nonverbal communication patterns may be distorted or incongruent. This keeps others at a safe distance and prevents the development of intimacy.

In addition, loneliness is likely to be part of these people's lives. Copel[9] has defined loneliness as "an emotional state in which an individual is aware of the feeling of being apart from another or others, along with the experience of a vague need for individuals." The characteristics of loneliness include a feeling of being separate from others, a perception or experience of unsatisfactory relationships, and recognition of a difference between the desired relationship and the existing one. Loneliness from a lack of intimacy with others is pervasive and painful. This is difficult to imagine if it has not been experienced. The pain of loneliness can be shared empathically to some extent. It often causes anxiety in the person with whom it is shared. Biographical accounts of experiences of a psychiatric patient, such as *I Never Promised You a Rose Garden* by Joanne Greenberg or *The Bell Jar* by Sylvia Plath, also communicate some of this pain. Fromm-Reichmann[13] identified extreme loneliness as she worked with many withdrawn patients. She believed that it should be differentiated from anxiety and that it may even be a more frightening experience than anxiety. She describes loneliness as a state in which past relationships are forgotten and there is little hope of any future relationship. It is a difficult feeling to study because the lonely person cannot talk about it or may not want to remember it. Persons studying loneliness become anxious when they try to understand it. Loneliness of this type must be differentiated from aloneness and solitude.

Welt[39] has related healthy aloneness to the internalization of a consistent, caring parent. This provides the person with a sense of security because he feels protected. Welt has also described premature aloneness. In this case the child is left to meet his own needs before the caring parent has been internalized. This leads to loneliness. Some people try to avoid recognition of loneliness through defensive aloneness. They stay away from others so they do not have to confront

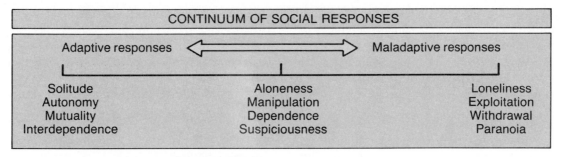

Fig. 16-1. Continuum of social responses.

their inability to participate in a close relationship. These conditions may be sought out by individuals from time to time and may foster thought, creativity, and the growth of self-awareness.

■ Continuum of social responses

Interpersonal relationship behaviors may be represented on a continuum that ranges from healthy interdependent interactions to those involving no real contact with other people. This continuum of coping responses is illustrated in Fig. 16-1.

Progression from the adaptive to the maladaptive end of the continuum reflects an increase in the seriousness of the relationship disorder. The medical diagnoses used in this chapter to demonstrate these behaviors include schizophrenia, paranoid type; schizophrenia, catatonic type; schizophrenia, disorganized type; schizophrenia, undifferentiated type; schizophrenia, residual type; schizoid personality disorder; schizotypal personality disorder; paranoid personality disorder; borderline personality disorder; antisocial personality disorder; and dependent personality disorder. These illnesses also present the patient with problems of varying intensity. The goal of nursing intervention is to help the patient shift his interpersonal behavior toward the adaptive end of the continuum.

Assessment

■ Predisposing factors

A variety of factors—within the individual, between the individual and significant others, and environmental—may lead to disrupted interpersonal relationships. Although much research has been done on disorders that affect interpersonal relationships, there are no specific conclusions about their causes. A combination of factors probably is involved. The nurse must recognize this and explore all relevant areas during the nursing assessment.

■ **DEVELOPMENTAL FACTORS.** The capacity for relatedness results from a developmental process. Anything that interferes with that process decreases the person's ability to develop healthy interpersonal relationships. The first experiences with closeness to others occurs within the family. Lack of maternal stimulation or attention deprives the infant of a sense of security; the infant then fails to establish basic trust. This can lead to a suspicious attitude toward others that may continue throughout life. The quality of mothering attention is also important. A child may be adequately fed and receive perfect physical care but without any communication of maternal caring. A child who is treated as an object may become an adult who treats others as objects. Rather than respond to personal expressions of caring, the person may rely on material possessions to feel secure. Early experiences of maternal deprivation also frequently lead to severe depression in the child, as demonstrated in the studies of Spitz.[35] Without corrective experiences, and if he survives, the child will probably develop into a withdrawn and chronically depressed adult. Early experiences such as these can lead to the most serious of psychiatric disorders and frequently to chronic institutionalization.

Between the ages of 3 and 18 months, the infant is in the symbiotic stage of development.[26] During this time, it is very important for the mothering person to perform ego functions for the child, including orienting him to reality. This forms the basis for future interpersonal relationships in terms of being able to empathize and understand the position of others.

More potential problems arise as the child begins to strive for independence. Masterson[26] calls this the separation-individuation stage, occurring between 18 months and 3 years of age. The goal of this phase is to develop autonomy. If the toddler's efforts to become autonomous are not supported, excessive dependency may lead to the development of a fearful, clinging adult. Inconsistent limits or lack of limits can interfere with the person's ability to perceive the needs and rights of others. This inhibits the ability to achieve intimacy in relationships. The mothering person and child must learn to tolerate separation from each other for periods of time. The child must develop confidence that the nurturer will return after an absence. At the same time, the mothering person must adjust to the child's increased independence that comes with walking and increased mobility. The child must also learn to perceive significant others as whole objects, with both good and bad characteristics. Interference with the process at this stage may result in severe interpersonal limitations. These limitations are typical of the person with the medical diagnosis of borderline personality disorder. By the end of this phase of development, the child differentiates himself from others. The ego functions that have developed include reality testing, impulse control, frustration tolerance, and the beginning of object constancy.[26]

The parents' value system is communicated to the preschool and school-age child. As school begins, the child's world expands to include more of the community. He is exposed to new ideas, which contributes to the development of his value system. The developmental process is easier if parental and community values are consistent. If the person is unclear about his values, he may become a confused adult. He is more likely to follow the lead of others than to make healthy decisions for himself. Also, value confusion may result in antisocial behavior. In this case the person has a flexible value system, and behavior is based on self-interest.

■ **FAMILY COMMUNICATION FACTORS.** Family communication patterns may lead to disruptions in relationships. It is important to emphasize that communication problems in a family *may* contribute to the development of disturbed behavior. It is unlikely that this is the only cause. However, the nurse needs to assess the nature of family communications as part of complete data collection.

Patients with a medical diagnosis of schizophrenia may be members of families with identifiably disturbed communication patterns. In a survey of family research relative to schizophrenia, Wynne, Toohey, and Doane[47] identify the following three types of family communication patterns being investigated by schizophrenia researchers: (1) communication deviance studies, initiated by Wynne and his associates;[46,47] (2) the expressed emotion studies of Vaughn and Leff;[38,47] and (3) the family relationship test investigated by Scott and colleagues.[47] The communication deviance studies use projective tests, such as the Rorschach and the Thematic Apperception Test (TAT), to study the communication patterns of identified schizophrenic patients and their immediate family members. These studies show that deviant patterns of communication exist in families in which a child becomes schizophrenic.

The expressed emotion studies[38] analyze interviews with family members of schizophrenic patients in terms of the frequency of critical comments about the patient. They also assign a global rating for the amount of hostility, warmth, or overinvolvement expressed by the relative. These characteristics are related to the future course of the illness. Studies show that high expressed emotion by relatives is associated with more relapses. Kanter, Lamb, and Loeper[21] have questioned the use of hostility, warmth, and overinvolvement as a single measure of family emotional climate, since these are really unrelated characteristics. They also point out that patient and family interactions are constantly changing and related to other life events. Categorizing or labeling has led to conflict between families and professionals in the past. Recent application of expressed emotion research has been leading to new stigmatization and stereotyping of families.

More research is needed to identify helpful family responses to specific behaviors of the schizophrenic member. The Family Relationship Test[47] measures family members' perceptions of interpersonal relationships using an adjective checklist. Patients who view their parents as "well" have a better prognosis than those who perceive their parents as "ill."

In the past the development of impaired interpersonal relationships was frequently attributed to family communication problems. For instance, Bateson and associates[3] developed the **double-bind theory,** speculating that mixed messages were given to children by their parents. For instance, a parent might verbally complain that the child never expressed affection by touching the parent. Then, when the child tried to hug the parent, he would be pushed away. This placed the child in a no-win situation. The double-bind theorists believed that repeated messages such as this would cause lack of trust in others and avoidance of close interpersonal relationships. Schizophrenic symptoms were viewed as a way of keeping others at a distance.

Unfortunately, many mental health care providers used theories such as this to blame families, especially mothers, for the child's schizophrenia. This alienated families and providers, causing serious interference in the treatment process. It also caused unnecessary pain for families who were trying to cope with the knowledge that their child had an illness that was poorly understood and probably chronic. More recently the focus has shifted to a search for biological causes for schizophrenia. Mental health care professionals have come to believe that the illness has a reciprocal relationship with interpersonal relationships, including those in the family. However, it is difficult to identify how much family stress contributes to the intensification of the illness as opposed to how much the characteristics of the illness create family conflict. It is known that families who understand as much as possible about the illness and work as a part of the health care team are better able to cope. Also, patients who live in families with adaptive coping skills apparently function better. The National Alliance for the Mentally Ill and other advocacy groups have been very active in working with professionals to develop educational and mutual support programs for families.

Social relationships outside the family may also be disrupted and have a lasting effect on behavior. Families of persons who develop a borderline personality disorder often discourage relationships with others. Failure to develop intimacy with peers, first of the same sex and later of the opposite sex, leads to social isolation in adulthood. Such an individual may appear cool and aloof. This person is likely to become involved in superficial relationships. The person is apt to have a romanticized idea of heterosexual relationships and be disappointed when this does not happen. An isolated person may also become depressed as an adult because of a vague sense of what an intimate relationship could be compared to his own reality. Involvements with others may be brief and characterized by approach-avoidance behavior as the person tries to pursue closeness. A person who has trouble with closeness may also be very dependent. This is a clinging person who refuses to give up a relationship but is afraid to risk self-disclosure. Thus truly mature involvement does not occur.

■ **SOCIOCULTURAL FACTORS.** Sociocultural factors can also influence the person's ability to establish and maintain relatedness. Many forces in our culture make the individual feel isolated and lonely. Cultural mores discourage making casual acquaintances. Friendships are often short term because of the mobility involved in many occupations. Packard[28] studied transient populations and found higher rates of mental hospital admissions, more aggressive behavior, and more marital problems in this group. Family relationships are more distant as children move from place to place, seeing parents only occasionally. Friends are often closer than siblings, in contrast to the "good old days" of the close-knit extended family.

Certain groups within the culture are particularly vulnerable to isolation. The elderly are frequently ignored in our work-oriented culture. Older people are takers of goods, and the young are the givers. We have little tolerance as a society for those who are not actively involved in the economic system. Paradoxically, even if older people have the ability to be active, they are forgotten to make room for the young. This may change as the average age of Americans increases with the aging of the "baby boom" generation.

Involuntary social isolation also affects the handicapped and chronically ill of any age. People with terminal illnesses or disfiguring disorders are frequently avoided by others. This is also true for people with long-term psychiatric problems. Although an effort has been made to decrease chronic institutionalization, many strongly resist integrating disabled persons into the community. This involuntary isolation may result in withdrawal, depression, dependency, suspicion, impaired communication, manipulative behavior, or any combination of these as the individual tries to cope with loneliness.

Other sociocultural factors are related to society's cultural norms. For instance, the media reinforce the idea that people will always be involved in idealized "meaningful relationships." Romanticized heterosexual relationships seen on television and in the movies may contribute to high rates of adolescent pregnancy as well as early marriages that end in divorce. This cultural attitude leads to the experience of loneliness as described by Gordon: "the sense of deprivation that comes when certain *expected* human relationships are absent."[14:26] The term "aloneness" is used here to differentiate this degree of loneliness from the existential kind of loneliness described earlier. The dynamics of aloneness as experienced by many Americans include the following[15]:

1. Feelings of hopelessness
2. Escape into unsatisfying relationships
3. Fear of experiencing lonely feelings
4. Denial of loneliness
5. Feelings of worthlessness and failure

Increased repetitive behavior often results. Feelings of helplessness, hopelessness, and worthlessness accumulate until the person, in desperation, may resort to self-destructive behavior.

Some groups in society prey on the alone and the lonely. In recent years a flood of various planned group experiences has been advertised as therapeutic. Most of them promise a degree of intimate human experience. Encounter groups, when under the direction of a skilled therapist, can be helpful to the isolated person. However, the danger exists that the group leader may be untrained and unsophisticated in dealing with emotional problems. Religious cults attract those who are lonely, particularly the young. These cults offer the attraction of a close-knit community and a sense of common belief and effort. This sense of belonging is so important that cult members may sever all ties with family and friends. They behave according to the group's demands, even if these conflict with a previous value system.

Closeness is a positive ideal in U.S. culture. At the same time, people are given the message that one needs to be careful in deciding whom to trust. This can cause confusion and a feeling of insecurity. In a relatively short time, people have gone from leaving houses unlocked all the time to installing several locks on each door, burglar alarms, and guard dogs. Rising crime rates cause fear and more reluctance to risk closeness or contact with strangers. Some urban residents, particularly the elderly, become prisoners in their homes. They experience loneliness and all the associated behaviors.

■ **BIOLOGICAL FACTORS.** Biological factors include genetic tendencies that may predispose the person to experience interpersonal problems. Genetic factors have been explored to try to identify populations at risk for developing schizophrenia. Cloninger[8] reports that studies have demonstrated a higher incidence of schizophrenia in family members of schizophrenic patients. Inheritance of schizophrenia is most likely when both parents are schizophrenic. It has been found that even when monozygotic (identical) twins are adopted at birth by different parents, in 58% of cases, if one develops schizophrenia, both will. This same proportion occurs with identical twins who are raised together and develop schizophrenia. However, this is not true with dizygotic (fraternal) twins. Eighty percent of schizophrenics have no parent or sibling who has the illness. Based on this information, it seems that genetic factors play a part in the development of schizophrenia, but their role is unknown.

In recent years, significant research has been done concerning the brain's structure and function as related to the development of mental disorders. Much research has focused on schizophrenia. Brain structure can be observed directly during post-mortem examinations. Berman and Weinberger[4] have described some of the findings of such studies. It is important to note that no consistent defects have been found. This supports the theory that schizophrenia is not one, but several, disorders sharing some symptoms. In some cases, there is brain atrophy with enlargement of the ventricles, a decrease in the brain's gross weight, and decreased volume of the deeper midline and limbic structures. Some studies have also noted distorted size and shape (dysmorphism) of cells in the cortical and limbic areas.

Brain imaging is used to study the brains of living subjects. More information about the various brain imaging techniques is included in Chapter 6. Computed tomography (CT) scan has provided the most information about brain structure. Studies reveal enlarged lateral and third ventricles and widened cortical sulci. Berman and Weinberger[4] note that assessment of observable behaviors in addition to CT studies is necessary to make a diagnosis of schizophrenia. Some relationship has been noticed between enlarged lateral ventricles and negative (decreased or absent behaviors, e.g., lethargy, lack of motivation) symptoms, poor social adjustment before the illness, poor treatment outcome, and disordered cognitive functioning. Magnetic resonance imaging (MRI) techniques and applications are being developed. It is expected that these will provide even more information about structural changes.

Physiological brain function in people with schizophrenia is also being investigated. New techniques are being developed. Berman and Weinberger[4] note that it is difficult to design adequately controlled studies because of the many intervening variables. These variables include the patient's activity level, medications being taken, environmental influences, and concurrent medical disorders. One technique being explored is the study of regional cerebral blood flow (rCBF) using xenon-133. There have been some reports that prefrontal cortical blood flow is reduced in schizophrenia. Positron emission tomography (PET) has also been used, with results similar to those with rCBF. Replication of these studies is needed before any definite conclusions can be drawn.

■ **Precipitating stressors**

Disruptions in relatedness are the result of experiences that influence the individual's growth. In most instances a series of life events predisposes a person to difficulty with interpersonal relationships. Many people cope with their interpersonal problems and say they are reasonably satisfied with this aspect of life. However, additional stress can cause a somewhat satisfying interpersonal life to become grossly disrupted. Response to various stressors is highly individual. However, the factors discussed next may cause some interpersonal disruption for most people. One must also remember that the individual experiences an increase in stress as anxiety. This is at the root of the behavioral disruptions.

The mature person who can participate in healthy interpersonal relationships is still vulnerable to the effects of psychological stress. Either a series of losses or a single significant loss may lead to problems establishing future intimate relationships. The pain of a loss can be so great that the individual will avoid future involvements rather than risk more pain. This response is more likely if the person had difficulty during any developmental tasks pertinent to relatedness. Losses of significant others may cause difficulty with future relationships, but other types of losses may do the same. The loss of a job decreases a person's self-esteem. This can also result in future withdrawal and problems with relatedness unless the person has a well-established interpersonal support system.

■ **SOCIOCULTURAL STRESSORS.** Stressors leading to interpersonal relationship difficulties may be sociocultural. For instance, signs indicate that the family unit is becoming less stable. The divorce rate has been rising. Mobility has broken up the extended family, depriving people of all ages of an important support system. Less contact occurs between the generations. Tradition, which provides a powerful link with the past and a sense of identity, is less observable when the family is fragmented. Interest in ethnicity and "roots" may reflect the efforts of isolated people to associate themselves with a specific identity. The many stresses on the family have made it more difficult for family members to accomplish the developmental tasks related to intimacy.

Nurses who work in general hospitals frequently encounter patients with behaviors related to disrupted interpersonal relationships. Even a reasonably well-adjusted person may have difficulty maintaining a satisfactory level of intimacy while hospitalized. The patient's feeling of isolation is enhanced by the impersonal hospital environment. Sometimes patients need to be isolated because of infection or, in the psychiatric setting, to control behavior. They are susceptible to the effects of sensory deprivation. Creative nursing care is needed to lessen this problem. On the other hand, sensory overload may be a problem for patients in critical care units. This can also lead to loneliness and separation from others.

■ **BIOCHEMICAL STRESSORS.** A strong probability exists that biochemical stressors are associated with difficulty in establishing and maintaining effective interpersonal relationships. For instance, people with a medical diagnosis of some type of schizophrenia are generally withdrawn and dependent and exhibit unusual communication patterns. They may be suspicious of other people. Current research is attempting to uncover a biochemical disorder or disorders associated with some schizophrenic disorders. This research tends to be confusing because studies contradict each other. Also, even if a particular biochemical disruption is discovered, it will not explain the origin of schizophrenia; it will indicate a more basic problem that may still be unidentified. For example, knowing that a person who exhibits the behaviors associated with diabetes mellitus has hypoglycemia does not define the real cause of the problem, which is a deficit in insulin production by the pancreas related to heredity, diet, or some other basic stressor.

Dopamine theory. Currently, a rapidly growing amount of evidence seems to indicate that some cases of schizophrenia are related to an excess of dopamine in key areas of the brain, probably the mesocortical and mesolimbic nerve tracts. The excessive dopamine may result from increased production, increased release, or turnover of dopamine. It could also come from an increased number or activity of receptors.[5] Identification of the cause of dopamine excess would assist greatly in discovering the cause of schizophrenia. The dopamine hypothesis[45] has been supported by (1) noting that the administration of dopaminergic agents (amphetamines, L-dopa, or apomorphine) leads to initiation or exacerbation of psychotic behavior and (2) discovering that neuroleptic drugs act at the synapse by binding dopamine receptor sites. This theory is the most promising one and is being studied intensively by biochemical researchers.

Norepinephrine theory. Norepinephrine is another neurotransmitter that may be involved in the pathophysiology of schizophrenia. It is most highly concentrated in the hypothalamus, thalamus, limbic system, and cerebellum. According to Wyatt, Kirch, and DeLisi,[45] some studies imply that norepinephrine levels may increase in some schizophrenic patients. However, this could be a result of neuroleptic medication rather than illness. At this time, no conclusive evidence supports this theory.

Indolamine hypothesis. This theory suggests that a defect in the metabolism of the indolamine serotonin causes schizophrenia.[45] This was based on similarities between byproducts of the metabolic process and hallucinogenic substances. It is currently believed that a relationship exists between serotonin and some cases of schizophrenia. The exact nature of the relationship is unknown.

Gamma-aminobutyric acid (GABA). Some research has noted a relationship between GABA and dopamine.[45] In some cases, decreased GABA has been associated with increased dopamine levels; in others the reverse has been true. This could be evidence that there is more than one type of schizophrenia. Other biogenic amines and amino acids that have been studied to determine if they are related to schizophrenia include methionine, serine, phenylalanine/tyrosine, asparagine, and histamine.

Endogenous hallucinogens. This hypothesis suggests that abnormal methylation of catecholamines could create a hallucinogenic substance.[45] Thus far, no research solidly supports this hypothesis.

Central nervous system peptides. Wyatt, Kirch, and DeLisi[45] note that more than 25 small peptides have been found in neurons. These are sometimes called neuroregulators. Some are similar to neuroleptic medications and may influence their action. They include cholecystokinin, vasoactive intestinal peptide, somatostatin, opioids (endorphins) and their precursors, neurotensin, and bombesin. Because of their influence on neuronal functioning, they are being investigated regarding their relationship to schizophrenia.

■ **ENDOCRINE FACTORS**

Pituitary function. Low levels of follicle-stimulating hormone (FSH) and luteinizing hormone (LH) have been noted in patients with schizophrenia.[45] Dopamine inhibits prolactin function. Some studies have revealed low prolactin levels. This tends to support the dopamine hypothesis.

Other endocrine factors. Hypothyroidism and both increased and decreased levels of adrenocortical hormones have been associated with psychotic behavior.

■ **VIRAL HYPOTHESIS.** Some have proposed that a viral infection could be a stressor related to schizophrenia.[45] It is known that some viruses cause psychotic symptoms. The human immunodeficiency virus (HIV) is an example of this. Some structural changes have been seen in the brain cells of schizophrenics that are similar to those caused by viral infections. This hypothesis is being explored further. No conclusion about the role of viruses in schizophrenia has been reached at this time.

Although the cause of schizophrenia is a puzzle, it is becoming clear that the answer depends on increased understanding of neurobiology and neurochemistry. Research in these areas will eventually lead to better treatment of schizophrenic patients. In addition, identification of measurable biochemical imbalances could result in simple tests to identify people at risk for developing psychotic behavior. This would increase prevention by allowing early intervention to decrease known stressors.

■ **BIOLOGICAL-SOCIOENVIRONMENTAL MODELS.** Researchers emphasize that schizophrenia is most likely to occur as a result of the interaction between the individual and the environment. This is supported by the results of socioenvironmental and biological research. For instance, the identical twin of a schizophrenic person does not always become schizophrenic. This implies that some interaction occurs between the environment and the person's inherited bio-

logical makeup. Liberman and colleagues[23] describe the *stress-diathesis* model of schizophrenia. This states that symptoms develop based on the relationship between the stress that a person experiences and an internal stress tolerance threshold.

The *vulnerability-stress* model described by McGlashan[25] is similar. The person's degree of vulnerability to schizophrenia is seen as relatively stable. It may be based on such factors as genetics and perinatal experiences. McGlashan has identified several areas of vulnerability to schizophrenia:

1. Cognitive, including deficits in information processing, attention span, differentiating relevant and irrelevant stimuli, and abstraction
2. Psychophysiological, including deficits in sensory inhibition; and autonomic responsiveness, especially to aversive stimuli
3. Social, including deficits in eye contact, assertiveness, carrying on a conversation, and understanding interpersonal messages
4. General coping deficits, including overassessment of threat, underassessment of personal coping resources, and overuse of denial

Fig. 16-2 demonstrates the relationship between stress, vulnerability, personal strengths, and environmental supports and the occurrence of schizophrenia.

■ **PSYCHOLOGICAL STRESSORS.** Many psychological theories have been proposed as causes of disturbed ability to establish and maintain satisfying relationships. It is known that high anxiety levels result in an impaired ability to relate to others. As described in Chapter 11, the level of anxiety experienced determines the degree of difficulty that may occur. A combination of prolonged and/or intense anxiety with limited coping ability is believed to cause severe relationship problems of a psychotic type. This theory now is explored further from the psychoanalytical and interpersonal points of view.

Psychoanalytical theory states that schizophrenic behavior results when the ego can no longer withstand the pressures from the id and from external reality. The ego of the psychotic person has limited ability to cope with stress because of serious problems in the symbiotic mother-child relationship that inhibited psychological development. The initial response to high levels of stress and anxiety is to use ego defense mechanisms pathologically to control unacceptable impulses and thoughts. An example of this is the development of paranoid delusions, a symptom related to the mechanism of projection. So much libido (psychic energy) is used to maintain repression that little is left for activities of daily living. Therefore the person withdraws

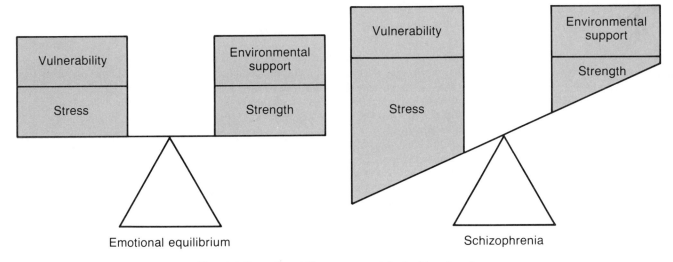

Fig. 16-2. Vulnerability-stress model of schizophrenia.

from usual activities and has difficulty meeting basic physiological needs such as nutrition and hygiene. If stress continues and the anxiety level stays high, ego functioning may deteriorate more. The person then has difficulty maintaining repression and may be flooded with frightening and primitive thoughts and impulses. There is also difficulty separating self from environment as ego identity disintegrates. Communication at this point is confused, garbled, and highly symbolic. It reflects primary process thought, which is usually kept unconscious. Little capacity exists for relatedness with others.

Will states the interpersonal view of schizophrenia as "the expression of complicated patterns of behavior adopted by the organism in an effort to deal with a gross inadequacy in relating to other humans."[42] Will further states that the behavior is a response to stress, demonstrates a disordered personality structure, involves communication, and provides some degree of security and comfort.

The mother-infant relationship sets the stage for later behavioral problems. If the mother is extremely anxious, this is communicated empathically to her child. The child receives confusing and sometimes conflicting messages from significant others before developing the ability to clarify meanings. Behavior that seems to be unacceptable is incorporated into the "not-me" component of the self-system. The person cannot remember information that is "not-me." Therefore he has a distorted view of reality. Anxious family members teach the child a distorted perception of other people. Fear of people develops, which inhibits learning and restricts the use of consensual validation. Ado-

lescence brings many anxiety-provoking experiences related to the need to develop a firm sense of identity. Normal developmental experiences lead this person to extreme anxiety and loneliness. The person is then trapped in a conflict between longing for intimacy and fearing the loss of the limited human contact he has.[42]

Masterson[26] has described the development of the borderline personality disorder as rooted in the mother-child relationship. The mother, who frequently is borderline herself, resists signs of independence and autonomy in the child. If the child tries to express individuality, the mother withdraws from him emotionally. This creates a conflict for the child, who wants to grow in autonomy but fears losing his mother's love. In most cases the child suppresses his individuality and clings to his mother. In later life the borderline person relates to others in a hostile, dependent, or manipulative way. The dilemma of dependence versus independence continues to be reflected in his interpersonal relationships.

Stressors that may lead to impairments in interpersonal relationships have been discussed. The interplay among these factors leads to the behavior that the nurse observes while relating to an individual, family, or group. It is essential to consider each of these areas when performing a thorough nursing assessment.

■ **Behaviors**

The behaviors observed in response to disruptions in relatedness represent the individual's attempt to cope with anxiety arising from the feeling of loneliness, fear, anger, shame, guilt, and insecurity. Frequently occurring behaviors include impaired commu-

CLINICAL EXAMPLE 16-1

Mr. D is a 24-year-old single man who was admitted for the third time to the psychiatric unit of an acute general hospital. His diagnosis was chronic schizophrenia, paranoid type. His other admissions had been at ages 19 and 22 and had each lasted a month. His outpatient treatment since the last admission had consisted of individual supportive therapy provided by the clinical nurse specialist, chemotherapy, and family therapy provided by the social worker. He had also been referred to the vocational rehabilitation counselor and was about to start a job training program.

Mr. D was brought to the hospital by his parents. They expressed great disappointment in his readmission because they had hoped that he was "finally going to lick this thing." They thought that the recurrence of his psychotic behavior was probably related to his impending involvement in the job training program. They could identify no other recent stressors that might have upset him.

Mr. D's nurse therapist, Ms. T, evaluated his condition soon after his admission to the hospital. He appeared frightened and was curled up in a chair when she approached him. He did not look at her when she greeted him and seemed preoccupied with his own thoughts. Ms. T was not sure that he was aware she was there. She sat down a few feet away from him and again stated his name. He looked at her blankly for a brief moment, said, "Hello," and then went back to staring into space. When asked what brought him to the hospital, he replied, "My father's car." Ms. T observed that Mr. D seemed rather upset and asked if something was bothering him. He told her nothing could bother him because God had told him that he was invincible. He knew many people were jealous of his powers and were trying to destroy him, but he had special protection. He then showed her a rabbit's foot that was sent to him by God to protect him from "evil forces." As Ms. T reached out to touch the rabbit's foot, Mr. D pulled it away and shouted angrily, "Don't touch that! It's mine! They want you to take it away to destroy my powers, but I won't let you!" Ms. T assured Mr. D that she would not take away his rabbit's foot, since it had great importance to him. He gradually relaxed. She asked if he could say more about the contact he thought he had had with God. He replied that God had spoken to him and told him about the evil forces. He knew these forces existed because they put bad thoughts in his head. He also heard people talking about him and commenting on his behavior. There were several voices, and he thought he recognized the voices of his father and Dr. M, who saw him

once a month to evaluate his medications. He denied any visual hallucinations. His speech was disjointed and at times difficult to follow because of loose associations. For instance, he said, "Mother brought me here . . . birth . . . rebirth . . . deliverance . . . didn't like that movie." As Ms. T attempted to explore his feelings about his parents' returning him to the hospital, he turned away and angrily told her to leave him alone because she was "one of them, those g ___ d ___ f ___ liars." Ms. T responded that she would continue to work with him to help him regain control of his life while he was in the hospital. However, she added that she could see he was tired and upset so she would leave and see him again later.

For his first 3 days in the hospital, Mr. D continued to be hostile, refusing to eat or drink and not sleeping except when under the influence of medication, which he took reluctantly when presented with the clear alternative of state hospital commitment. The content of his speech revolved around the messages he received from God and the evil forces who were trying to destroy him. He would tolerate only brief interactions with his therapist and other staff members. He did not interact at all with other patients, whom he believed to be staff members and "undercover agents" who were supposed to report on his behavior. He refused to see his parents, consistently referring to his mother as "That b ___."

With the assistance of consistent interpersonal support and medication, Mr. D gradually began to gain control over his thoughts. There was a steady decline in the amount of delusional speech, and although the auditory hallucinations continued, he was able to ignore them or block them out by talking with someone. He revealed to Ms. T that he became upset after his parents had a violent argument and threatened to divorce each other. They pulled him into their conflict by demanding to know with whom he would choose to live. He was unable to respond to that demand except by becoming psychotic. He was disappointed that he had missed the beginning of his job training program and was hopeful that he would still be able to start vocational rehabilitation soon. Ms. T gently helped Mr. D to look at his feelings toward his parents and also informed the family therapist of the events preceding his admission. His discharge plan was for referral to a day treatment program for a short stay until the vocational rehabilitation referral was again available. Individual therapy, pharmacotherapy, and family therapy were all to continue.

nication, withdrawal, suspicion, dependency, and manipulation.

BEHAVIORS ASSOCIATED WITH SCHIZOPHRENIA

Schizophrenia, paranoid type. Disruptions in communication accompanied by withdrawal and suspicion are evident in the thought process and interaction patterns of patients who have the medical diagnosis of schizophrenia, paranoid type.[1] Clinical example 16-1 illustrates this disruption.

The description of Mr. D's hospital experience demonstrates how disrupted communication can interfere with the ability to function. When Mr. D was forced to choose between his parents, he was placed in an impossible communication situation. The timing of this family crisis might be related to Mr. D's recent improvement and his behaving independently by entering the vocational rehabilitation program. If the family equilibrium was based on Mr. D's illness, his parents would pressure him to stay dependent. This hypothesis is supported by their explanation of Mr. D's behavior. They blamed the vocational rehabilitation program, which pulled him away from the family, rather than their argument, which pulled him into it.

Mr. D, in his distress, most likely had ambivalent feelings toward his parents. He was very dependent on them so feared angering them and risking rejection. At the same time he became very angry because of the demands they made on him but was blocked in expressing his anger by his need for them. He was able to resolve this problem only by withdrawing. At an unconscious level, he relied on repression, regression, and projection to handle the conflict.

HALLUCINATIONS.
Hallucinations, such as Mr. D's experiences of hearing God and hearing people talk about him, frequently occur in schizophrenic patients. A hallucination is a sensory perception that takes place without external stimuli. The biochemical theorists suspect that hallucinations result from a metabolic response to stress causing the release of hallucinogenic neurochemicals. Psychoanalytical theorists view hallucinations as an attempt by the ego to defend against repressed impulses threatening to enter awareness. The mechanism of projection allows the ego to deal with the impulses as threats from the outside, thus alleviating some of the anxiety. In the framework of interpersonal psychiatry, the hallucination is the autonomous expression of a specific zone of interaction, usually auditory, which symbolically represents the dissociated processes of the person's personality.[27] These dissociated experiences are included in the "not-me" component of the personality, which includes those experiences arousing such great anxiety that they were not integrated into awareness. When the self-system is flooded with anxiety, as it is during an acute schizophrenic episode, the usual security operations are not adequate. The person then deals with the dissociated thoughts that come into awareness by means of projecting them as the words of others.[27]

DELUSIONS.
Both psychodynamic theories relate hallucinations to efforts to alleviate panic levels of anxiety. Both identify projection as the mechanism used to accomplish this goal. Delusions may be similarly explained. A delusion is a fixed false belief. Some delusions are suspicious in nature, or **paranoid,** such as Mr. D's belief that evil forces wanted to destroy him. In this instance, unacceptable (ego-alien) aggressive impulses are projected outside the individual and perceived as being directed toward him. Paranoid delusions may also include a sexual component if the ego defense is directed toward sexual impulses. For instance, a woman who believes that the man next door wants to break into her house and rape her may be projecting her own unconscious sexual feelings for him. Paranoid delusions with homosexual content also occur with schizophrenic patients. This indicates a defense against an onslaught of homosexual impulses that are very frightening to the patient. If the patient is confronted with unavoidable close contact with a member of the same sex, homosexual panic can occur. When this happens, the patient enters a panic state with lack of impulse control and frequently very aggressive behavior.

Other delusions are **grandiose** in nature. Mr. D's belief that God had singled him out and given him special powers was a grandiose delusion. Grandiosity occurs in schizophrenic patients but is particularly severe in patients with a diagnosis of manic episode; bipolar disorder, mixed; or bipolar disorder, manic. Delusions of grandeur may endow the person with a special power or talent or may identify him with a famous or powerful person, such as God, a political leader, or a sports hero. This is an example of the pathological use of the mechanism of identification. It usually reflects a low self-esteem and a poorly formed ego identity. In this person, increased anxiety creates a sense of powerlessness. Identification with a powerful entity such as God allows the ego to acquire some of the power lacking within the personality structure. It is also a means of dealing with extreme fear. People with grandiose delusions may feel invincible and involve themselves in dangerous situations. It is important to keep in mind that the identification process takes place at an unconscious level and that the patient really believes he is God or the president of the United States.

Somatic delusions focus on the body and usually

include the belief that the person is the victim of a frightening disease. The person may believe that he is becoming incapacitated or that parts of his body are dead or rotting away. A variation of the somatic delusion is the belief that all or part of the body is distorted or malformed. An attractive young male patient with this type of delusion refused to turn on the light when he used the bathroom because he feared what he might see in the mirror. Bizarre somatic delusions are associated with schizophrenia. Delusions of fatal or debilitating illness are frequently associated with depression, as are **delusions of poverty.** The person is convinced that he is penniless and is responsible for the downfall of his family. This is a reflection of a strong sense of guilt and low self-esteem. These patients may make remarks such as, "Everything I touch turns to ashes."

The nature of delusional thinking is hard to understand. Its function is a protective one in helping the person cope with anxiety that would otherwise be overwhelming.

Schizophrenia, catatonic type. Clinical example 16-2 deals with Ms. W, who is psychotically withdrawn and has a medical diagnosis of schizophrenia, catatonic type.[1]

Ms. W was a rigid, inhibited young woman who had built her personal security around her relationship to her parents, assuming the role of a perfect daughter. Any threat to that relationship threatened the foundation of her security as well, causing extreme anxiety. This dependency on her parents interfered with Ms. W's ability to develop an adult level of relatedness. She was unable to establish intimacy with anyone outside her own family circle. Intellectually, she was aware of this problem. She had rationalized that she owed a great deal to her aging parents and should repay them by continuing to share her life with them. She therefore placed plans for marriage and a family far into the future. The conflict between her wish for closeness and her wish not to displease her parents by leaving them created anger. This was not compatible with her self-concept of the dutiful and obedient daughter. She defended against the anxiety this aroused by using repression and reaction formation. However, when an attractive young man began to act interested in her, her usual defenses crumbled and she was overwhelmed by anxiety and primitive anger. She then resorted to extreme withdrawal to control her frightening feelings. Unconsciously she feared that any voluntary movement would lead to uncontrolled eruption of all her feelings, which she viewed as exceedingly destructive. Her behavior therefore was self-protective.

Ms. W's behavior is characteristic of a conflict that

CLINICAL EXAMPLE 16-2

Ms. W is a 26-year-old single childless woman who lives with her parents. She was brought by ambulance to the emergency room of a large university hospital and referred to the psychiatric service for evaluation. The evaluator, a psychiatric nurse, observed Ms. W immobile, lying propped up in a hospital bed. She was totally mute and kept her eyes fixed straight ahead. She did not move voluntarily, and when moved by the examiner, offered some resistance. However, when she had been moved, she would maintain the new position. For instance, the nurse raised Ms. W's right arm 6 inches above the bed. When she let go of the arm, the patient did not move it for 5 minutes, at which time the nurse moved it back to a resting position on the bed.

Ms. W had been accompanied to the hospital by her parents, who gave the following history. Mr. and Mrs. W had been married for 20 years before their daughter was born and they had despaired of ever having a child. They had given her anything she wanted. They also set high standards for her behavior. She had always been a well-behaved child, rarely needing punishment by her parents. In fact, she was very sensitive to criticism and would burst into tears at a harsh word. She had had few friends, sharing the family belief that most other people did not have their high standards for behavior. She was particularly uncomfortable around young men, although she spoke of wanting to marry someday. She had attended an exclusive women's college, majoring in biology. At the time of her hospitalization, she was working as a research assistant in a cancer research laboratory. She was responsible for the care of laboratory rats being used for a study of suspected carcinogenic agents. She was a steady worker and apparently had performed adequately on the job, since she had recently received a merit raise.

About a month before admission Ms. W had mentioned that a new laboratory assistant had been hired. This was a young man who began asking her to have lunch with him. She had told her parents that she mistrusted his motives, and she started to find reasons not to eat lunch. The quality of her work began to deteriorate. She attempted to avoid this man at work, but he persisted in his attentions. The day before her admission he asked her out to dinner and a movie the following weekend. She refused. That evening she seemed preoccupied and spent the evening reading. Her parents noticed that she rarely turned a page. The next morning she did not get up when called for work. When her parents entered her room, they found her much as she was on admission, immobile and mute. They tried all day to arouse her but finally called their family physician, who advised them to take her to the emergency room.

Burnham, Gladstone, and Gibson have called the **need-fear dilemma.**[6] She is strongly drawn toward wanting intimacy and dependency on others (the need) but is ambivalent because she also fears being engulfed and losing her own identity. This is an example of the approach-avoidance type of conflict described in Chapter 11. This dilemma is one of the most common characteristics of most types of schizophrenia.

Many theorists have tried to identify patterns of behavior that would be diagnostic of schizophrenia. However, these efforts have been hindered by the identification of a variety of types of schizophrenia. In the DSM-III-R,[1] the American Psychiatric Association has divided schizophrenia into the following types: paranoid, catatonic, disorganized, undifferentiated, and residual. Further description of the characteristics of each of these categories, as well as of schizophrenia in general, is included in the nursing diagnosis section of this chapter.

The behaviors described as criteria for the medical diagnosis of schizophrenia have evolved over the course of many years and will continue to evolve. Because of this evolutionary process, nurses will hear discussions of other classifications of behavior. Some with historical or current significance include Bleuler's primary (the four A's) and secondary symptoms of schizophrenia, Schneider's first- and second-rank symptoms, and the diagnostic criteria developed by the International Pilot Study of Schizophrenia.

■ **BLEULER'S FOUR A'S.** The first effort to identify a group of behaviors typical of schizophrenia was that of Eugen Bleuler. He also renamed schizophrenia, once known as "dementia praecox." Bleuler identified primary and secondary symptoms of schizophrenia. Primary symptoms, frequently called the four A,s, include an *a*ffective disturbance, disordered *a*ssociation of thought, *a*utism, and *a*mbivalence.[15]

Affect. The term affect refers to feelings. One type of disturbance in the expression of feelings is a "blunting" or shallowness of expression. The characteristics of this include minimal changes in facial expression and the use of a monotonous tone of voice. Hostility may be expressed if the patient feels threatened. This may be expressed directly or symbolically. It may seem out of proportion to the situation. Some patients use cursing or obscene language to express hostile feelings. Another affective disturbance is the expression of affect inappropriate to the subject being discussed. For instance, a patient describing her impulse to murder her children begins to giggle.

Associations. Associations between thoughts are often disrupted in schizophrenic patients. Sometimes

blocking of thoughts occurs. In this case the patient begins to speak but then stops and loses track of the statement's meaning. **Looseness of association** is revealed when the patient makes a statement that sounds jumbled, such as in the following example:

NURSE: **How can we improve your nursing care, Mr. J?**
MR. J: **Improve? Can't improve. Can't prove a thing. Got me in this jail, but can't prove anything.**

Mr. J seems to drift away from the topic, but reveals that he views the hospital as a jail and suspects he is there because he has been accused of something. The nurse must explore the meaning of his statement. This loosely connected speech is frequently symbolical, but the speech of others is interpreted very literally. An example follows:

NURSE: **How are you feeling, Mr. J?**
MR. J: **(Touches various parts of his body) I guess I feel OK.**

This is often referred to as **concrete** thought and speech. Speech may also be lacking in goal direction, as in **tangential speech,** when the person begins to respond to a question but follows with a series of related topics. The patient never really gets to the point of the original statement. **Circumstantial speech** is when the person does get to the point but only after adding many unnecessary details to the response. **Perseveration** is a pattern of speech in which the person repeats the same word or phrase over and over again. The word or phrase chosen may have symbolical significance to the patient. In other speech patterns it is more difficult to grasp the patient's meaning. Sometimes patients respond by rhyming, which is called **clang association.** A patient might say, "Play ball, call, fall, tall," and so on. Another disrupted attempt at communication is **echolalia,** in which the patient repeats whatever he hears. The following is an example of echolalia:

NURSE: **How are you today, Mr. J?**
MR. J: **How are you today, Mr. J?**

A related behavior is **echopraxia,** in which the patient mimics the body position of another person. In **word salad** the patient expresses a random jumble of words, apparently meaningless.

Autism. Autism refers to a preoccupation with the self and with inner experience. The person may withdraw from any voluntary contact with others and seem to go inside a shell. Speech is highly personalized and may include **neologisms,** which are made-up words understood only by the patient. Some patients create imaginary worlds. An example of this is Yr, created by Debbie in *I Never Promised You a Rose Garden*

As Debbie became more involved in the real world, she found that she had to give up Yr and its people. Nonverbal behaviors associated with autism include rocking, head banging, stroking or fondling the self, and sometimes curling up in a fetal position.

Ambivalence. Ambivalence results in difficulty with decision making. Schizophrenics may debate endlessly about the alternatives in a situation that requires making a choice. They may also have strong simultaneous positive and negative feelings about a situation, which can be confusing and frightening. This may be reflected particularly in their response to significant others, who may be loved and hated with equal intensity at the same time.

■ **FUNCTIONS OF SYMPTOMS.** All these behaviors reflect the amount of ego function disruption that the patient is experiencing. Problems of affect demonstrate that the ego has decreased ability to inhibit impulses. Sometimes inappropriate feelings are allowed to be expressed. At other times, absolute control is enforced, resulting in no expression of feeling at all. Problems with thought association are related to the intrusion of primary process thoughts from the id into consciousness. This results in use of symbolism and in problems maintaining a logical sequence of thoughts. Autism reveals a disturbance of ego boundaries. This leads to decreased ability to distinguish between reality and fantasy. There is also a need to identify the self in concrete ways, such as touching and feeling. Autism also represents an effort to decrease stimuli by withdrawing. Ambivalence represents an inability to use secondary process thought for logical decision-making purposes. It also indicates confusion and fear about strong conflicting feelings, which may give rise to frightening impulses.

By keeping other people away, these behaviors may protect the patient from the risks involved in interpersonal relationships. It is easier to control impulsive behavior if other people keep their distance. Some schizophrenic patients have trouble deciding where they end and the other person begins, called **loss of ego boundaries.** Because of difficulty trusting people, the patient may fear being harmed by others. Communication patterns that are difficult to understand and sometimes threatening tend to drive people away. The problem here for the ambivalent schizophrenic is that he feels less threatened with people at a distance but abandoned if they get too far away.

Bleuler also listed secondary symptoms of schizophrenia. He considered them less specific to the condition and less essential for making the diagnosis. They include such behaviors as delusions, hallucinations, stupor, and negativism.[15]

■ **SCHNEIDER'S FIRST- AND SECOND-RANK SYMPTOMS.** Another description of behaviors typical of schizophrenia has been developed by Kurt Schneider. He has divided them into first- and second-rank symptoms. Schneider's first-rank symptoms include hearing one's thoughts spoken aloud, auditory hallucinations commenting on one's behavior, somatic hallucinations, the belief that one's thoughts are controlled, the belief that one's thoughts can be spread to others, delusions, and outside control or influence of one's actions.[15]

Second-rank symptoms include other hallucinations, depression, euphoria, perplexity, and emotional blunting.[15] Schneider has emphasized that none of these behaviors is absolutely indicative of schizophrenia. However, the presence of several in the absence of any other identifiable pathological condition makes the diagnosis of schizophrenia probable. The clinical and family history must also be considered. It seems unlikely that specific behavioral criteria for schizophrenia will be developed until more is understood about the stressors that cause it.

■ **INTERNATIONAL PILOT STUDY OF SCHIZOPHRENIA.** The International Pilot Study of Schizophrenia (IPSS) was initiated by the World Health Organization.[43,44] It was an effort to obtain new knowledge about the epidemiology of schizophrenia. The countries involved included Denmark, India, Colombia, Nigeria, England, the Soviet Union, Taiwan, the United States, and Czechoslovakia. A major problem in cross-cultural epidemiological studies has been doubt as to whether similar diagnostic criteria have been used. For instance, schizophrenia is diagnosed much more frequently in the United States than in Great Britain. Therefore one of the major objectives of the IPSS was to develop and standardize diagnostic criteria to be used in all nine countries with the highest possible degree of reliability and validity. Bartko[2] reports a 12-point diagnostic system derived from the work of the IPSS. The 12 signs and symptoms are restricted affect, poor insight, hearing one's thoughts spoken aloud, absence of early waking, poor rapport, lack of depressed facial expression, lack of elation, widespread delusions, incoherent speech, unreliable information given, bizarre delusions, and nihilistic delusions. Carpenter[7] has pointed out that the need to know the patient as a person is not replaced by the use of a detailed set of diagnostic criteria. Knowledge of both strengths and symptoms is necessary to provide help. Table 16-1 summarizes the criteria cited by Bartko, Bleuler, and Schneider.

The IPSS[43,44] was a major advance in the epidemiological study of mental illnesses. There was a 2-

TABLE 16-1

BEHAVIORS CHARACTERISTIC OF SCHIZOPHRENIA ACCORDING TO BLEULER, SCHNEIDER, AND THE IPSS

Bleuler[15]	Schneider[15]	IPSS[2]
Primary behaviors	**First-rank behaviors**	Bizarre delusions
Affective disturbance	Auditory hallucinations commenting on behavior	Hearing thoughts spoken aloud
Ambivalence	Belief that actions are controlled or influenced from outside	Incoherent speech
Autism	Belief that one's thoughts are controlled	Nihilistic delusions
Disordered thought association	Belief that one's thoughts can spread to others	No depressed facies
Secondary behaviors	Delusions	No early waking
Delusions	Hearing thoughts spoken aloud	No elation
Hallucinations	**Second-rank behaviors**	Poor insight
Negativism	Depression	Poor rapport
Stupor	Emotional blunting	Restricted affect
	Euphoria	Unreliable information given
	Other hallucinations	Widespread delusions
	Perplexity	

year follow-up of the patients included in the initial study. A high percentage of patients were interviewed a second time. This provided valuable information about the course of the illness in the nine cultures. One interesting conclusion was that subjects who live in developing nations seemed to do better than those from more highly developed societies. This study has laid the foundation for future epidemiological studies.

Investigators are looking for other ways to differentiate possible subtypes of schizophrenia. Pfohl and Andreasen[29] have noted a trend toward basing differentiation on positive and negative symptoms. Positive symptoms are related to abnormal or excessive mental functioning, such as hallucinations, delusions, or agitation. Negative symptoms reflect decreased or absent function, such as lack of energy, poverty of speech, lack of affect, and decreased socialization. Pfohl and Andreasen describe positive-symptom schizophrenics as having "a relatively acute onset, a course marked by exacerbations and remissions, good premorbid functioning and reasonably intact social functioning."[29] They also have a normal brain structure, normal cognition, and respond well to neuroleptic medications. This type of schizophrenia may be related to an increased dopamine level. In contrast, negative-symptom schizophrenics have "an insidious onset, a history of poor premorbid functioning, and a chronic or deteriorating course."[29] There is evidence of cognitive impairment, more frequently enlarged brain ventricles, and

less response to neuroleptics. It is suspected that this group of behaviors could be related to decreased dopamine levels. Clearly, research linking brain structure, neurochemical functioning, and behavior will play an important role in identifying and classifying the various types and manifestations of schizophrenia.

■ **BEHAVIORS ASSOCIATED WITH SUSPICION.** Schizophrenia is a severe mental disorder. Many people experience disruptions in interpersonal relationships that are less severe. Sometimes these disruptions are characterized by suspiciousness. A suspicious person has a problem with the ability to trust. This may come from early life experiences related to the basic sense of trust described by Erikson. It could also be the result of disruptive experiences later in life, as demonstrated in Clinical example 16-3.

Sociocultural and environmental stressors were the main causes of Mr. J's suspiciousness. He believes that he lives in a hostile environment because of his experience with being mugged. This is reinforced by what he sees on the television news. Much of his suspiciousness is probably also based on reality. The nurse can complete an accurate assessment by validating as much of Mr. J's information as possible. His feelings of vulnerability are probably also related to the frailty associated with aging. This was reinforced by his recent illness and hospitalization. In some ways, his suspiciousness serves a useful function. It protects him from the dangers in his environment and reduces the anxiety that

CLINICAL EXAMPLE 16-3

Mr. J is an 80-year-old man who lives alone in the ghetto of a large city. He was referred to a community health nurse following a 2-week hospital stay. He was admitted to the hospital after being arrested for "intoxication" when he was found unconscious on the street. Fortunately, it was discovered that he was comatose because of diabetic acidosis. An attempt was made to refer Mr. J to a nursing home, but he insisted on returning to his own home. The purpose of the community health nursing referral was to evaluate his ability to cope at home and to assess his ability to manage his American Dietetic Association diet and oral hypoglycemic medication.

Ms. B, the community health nurse, made her first visit the day following Mr. J's discharge from the hospital. When she knocked at his door, there was a long pause. Then a feeble voice asked who was there. When she identified herself, the door opened a crack and Mr. J peeked out at her. He said he recognized her blue uniform and would let her in his apartment. Ms. B then heard several locks being undone. At last Ms. B was face-to-face with a withered old man. His apartment was sparsely furnished but neat. The one comfortable chair faced a battered black-and-white television set. The shades at the window were drawn, leaving most of the room in shadows. Kitchen cupboards were sparsely stocked. There was no evidence of insects or rats. A scrawny cat rubbed against the nurse's leg. Mr. J introduced him as "Tiger."

Ms. B sat down to talk with Mr. J and learn more about his perception of his condition. He knew about his diabetes and seemed to understand his diet but doubted that he could comply with it. He said that he usually ate sweet rolls and coffee for breakfast, soup for lunch, and cereal with milk for dinner. He shopped at a small corner grocery store and bought only what he could carry home.

Meats were expensive and he had little money left for food after he paid his rent and utility bills. He was also hesitant to go out very often because he had been knocked down and robbed earlier in the year.

Mr. J said he had lived in the neighborhood many years and stayed there because of his memories of happier times. However, he thought the area had gone downhill. Most of his friends had died or moved away. His children lived in the suburbs, and were "too busy" to see him often, although they had asked at times for him to live with them. He doubted their motives, saying that he thought they probably wanted control of his Social Security checks, his only income.

Ms. B asked if he knew about the senior citizens center two blocks away where they served a hot meal daily and had many activities. He said he had heard about it but had no desire to socialize with the people who went there, since the others in the neighborhood were "not his kind." He also suspected that they would not serve foods that he liked. He again expressed his feelings about the lack of safety in the neighborhood and said that was the reason for his many locks. He watched the news on television every day and there were always stories about thefts and muggings of elderly people. He then confided that he also kept a gun near his bed so if "they" came in at night he would be able to defend himself.

Ms. B spent a little more time on diabetic teaching, trying to help Mr. J find ways to manage his diet within his real social and economic limitations. She planned eventually to introduce the idea of "Meals on Wheels" but realized that she needed to gain his trust first. As she left, she promised to return in 2 days to see how he was doing. Mr. J's response was, "That's up to you. I don't know why you should bother. Nothing will change much."

---

comes from his feeling of vulnerability. His suspiciousness related to his children is not helpful. They could be more supportive to him if they knew he was in need. If they could convince him of their caring and concern, he possibly could be persuaded to live with one of them. Owning a gun is also potentially harmful to him. A young intruder could probably overpower Mr. J and would be more likely to harm him if he were armed.

Many people in this society, both young and old, are isolated from others. This can lead to fear and mis-understanding, resulting in an attitude of suspicion. This can develop into a vicious circle, thus leading to a major social problem.

Suspiciousness may be thought of as a continuum from completely trusting to completely distrusting. Of course, most people fall somewhere between the extremes. Behavior at either extreme can be a problem. Others can take advantage of a completely trusting person. Such people are usually described as gullible. They are not effective in influencing others. On the other hand, extreme suspiciousness results in psy-

CLINICAL EXAMPLE 16-4

Ms. R, the psychiatric liaison nurse, was called to see Ms. J, a patient on the medical service of a general hospital. Ms. J had been admitted to the hospital complaining of attacks of dizziness, shakiness, dyspnea, and diaphoresis. She feared that she was "losing her mind." Even after she was told that the medical examinations results were all negative, the patient continued to complain of the same symptoms. The nurses on the medical unit then decided to call Ms. R. They were frustrated because Ms. J was constantly asking to have her bed adjusted, her water refreshed, her bedroom slippers found, and similar requests. In addition, she would have attacks of panic with hyperventilation. At these times she needed close nursing observation and help rebreathing into a paper bag to prevent loss of consciousness. The nurses observed that the panic attacks occurred most frequently during visits from family members. They also happened when her demands of the hospital staff were not complied with readily. The nurses were also aware that they were frustrated by her constant demands and lack of response to their interventions. This interfered with their ability to give good nursing care.

When Ms. R interviewed Ms. J, she observed that the patient lay curled on the bed and spoke in a soft, barely audible tone. She had tears in her eyes during the conversation. She spoke of her past when questioned but quickly refocused the discussion to her present complaints. Ms. J revealed that she was 45 years old, married, and the mother of a daughter, age 23. She said that she felt very close to her daughter, who had married and moved away from home 3 months ago. The attacks began soon after she left. Her daughter now lived about a mile from Ms. J and was described as devoted to her mother. Mr. J was employed as a pharmacist and was required to work some evenings. Ms. J said she had not minded this until her daughter had left home. Then she began to feel lonely on the evenings that her husband worked. She did not want to bother her daughter with visits or phone calls. She said that her family was her whole life. Ms. R asked Ms. J if she had other interests. She said that her main hobby was watching television, although she also read a few magazines and did a little sewing. She enjoyed cooking for others but not herself. She usually did not eat when her husband was working. She was on speaking terms with her neighbors but not really friendly with them. Because of her husband's objections, she had never worked outside of the home.

As she spoke with the nurse, Ms. J began to appear more and more anxious. She became shaky and started to breathe rapidly. Ms. R helped her to rebreathe and comforted her by talking soothingly and patting her on the shoulder. After Ms. J seemed calmer, Ms. R asked if she thought her behavior was related to their conversation. Ms. J said that she could see no connection. She stated that her symptoms were real to her, not just in her head, as people kept telling her. Ms. R assured her that she could see that she was indeed uncomfortable but that very nervous people sometimes showed their nervousness in physical ways. Soon after this Ms. R had to leave. As she left the room, Ms. J asked her if she would be back.

chotic, paranoid behavior. The paranoid person projects his own unacceptable impulses to other real or imaginary people and thinks he is being persecuted.

■ **BEHAVIORS ASSOCIATED WITH DEPENDENCY.** Behaviors of withdrawal and suspiciousness reduce anxiety by decreasing interpersonal contacts. Sometimes people who have disrupted intimate relationships deal with their anxiety by behaving in an excessively dependent way. This type of behavior is demonstrated by Clinical example 16-4 of a patient with a medical diagnosis of dependent personality disorder and panic disorder.[1]

Ms. R later discussed Ms. J with the nursing staff. She explained that the patient was a very dependent woman. For many years she had depended on her family, especially her daughter. When her daughter married, Ms. J felt abandoned but could not express her feelings directly. Her dependent style of relating kept her from participating in other activities. Her frustration and loneliness caused anxiety. Her coping response took the form of a physiological conversion (see Chapter 11). This behavior was reinforced when she received much attention focused on her illness. Her hospitalization was providing her with the primary psychological gain of knowing that her symptoms were being explored and treated. There was also the secondary gain of the renewed attention and consideration from her family. Her symptoms were not conscious behaviors but were her response to her anxiety. Therefore she could not understand why people kept suggesting that there was really no physical basis for her illness. Any increase in her anxiety level, therefore, increased her symptoms and her dependent behavior. Ms. J needed help with this problem. Although people were initially sympathetic to her need for de-

pendency gratification, they would soon become frustrated with her, as did the nursing staff.

■ **BEHAVIORS ASSOCIATED WITH MANIPULATION.** The disruptions in relatedness discussed so far have involved either too much distance from other

---

CLINICAL EXAMPLE 16-5

Mr. Y is a 20-year-old single man who was committed to an inpatient psychiatric unit by a judge for a psychiatric evaluation. He had been charged with sale of illicit drugs, statutory rape of his 15-year-old pregnant girlfriend, and contributing to the delinquency of a minor. He had been arrested on the grounds of a junior high school, where he was selling PCP and barbiturates to a group of young teenagers.

In jail, Mr. Y had been observed to be "crazy" by the guards. He paced his cell, chanted, and threw his food on the floor. Because of this behavior, the judge agreed to order a psychiatric evaluation. On arrival at the psychiatric unit, Mr. Y continued to behave in the same manner. However, his behavior did not seem typical of psychosis. There was no evidence of hallucinations or disorders of thought or affect. When unaware that he was observed, Mr. Y seemed relaxed and was noted at one time to be talking with another patient. By the day after admission he seemed to be free of his symptoms. At this point the staff began to describe him as a "nice guy." He complimented female staff members and behaved toward them in a pleasantly seductive manner. He was respectful to the physicians and agreed to abide by all the rules. He was helpful with other patients. In group meetings he admitted that he had behaved badly in the past and described how he had been led astray by his friends. He said he became involved in drugs because he wanted to be "one of the gang" and he "needed the bread" so he "had to" start selling drugs. By the end of his first week in the hospital he had received the sympathy of all the other patients and the staff. However, an interview with his parents revealed that he had had a stormy adolescence. This included arrests for vandalism and expulsion from school at age 14 for drug use and fighting. They said he had become involved with friends who were a bad influence. His family was glad he was getting help, because they had always known he was "sick."

Nine days after admission, following visiting hours, it was noted that Mr. Y and two other patients looked lethargic. Their speech was slurred,

and their gaits were ataxic. The nursing staff immediately collected urine and blood specimens for toxicological analysis. The unit was searched for hidden drugs, but none was found. The results of the toxicology screening tests, however, were positive for barbiturates. Suspicion was immediately focused on Mr. Y, since the other patients involved were young adolescents with no history of drug abuse. When confronted, he seemed amazed that he could be suspected and pointed out his past behavior as a model patient. He acknowledged that he had behaved strangely and said he had wondered if someone had "slipped" him some drugs. He was convincing but was warned that if he was involved in any way with drugs, he would be sent directly back to jail.

As part of the evaluation, the social worker had been working with Mr. Y's pregnant girlfriend. As the girl began to trust the social worker, she confided that she was not sure that Mr. Y had fathered her child, since she had had to turn to prostitution to help support them. Mr. Y, who had been unemployed for a year, had been angry when told of her pregnancy because it meant a reduction in his income. He had pressured her to have an abortion. She had refused because she hoped it was his baby and that he would decide to marry her once he saw the child. When she told him that her decision to have the baby was final, he assaulted her and then told her he did not want to see her again.

Mr. Y began to pressure the physicians for their decision on his ability to be held responsible for his actions. He seemed to be actively engaged in therapy and promised to continue with outpatient treatment if recommended for probation. He also convinced his family of his good intentions, and they agreed to allow him to move into their house. On the basis of these indications of positive behavioral change, Mr. Y did receive a recommendation for probation, which was carried out by the judge.

Three months after discharge from the hospital, Mr. Y and a friend were arrested for operating a PCP-manufacturing laboratory in the friend's garage.

people or the need for too much closeness to others. Another disruption in relatedness focuses on people superficially involved with others. These people use manipulative behaviors, treating others as objects. The patient who demonstrates this in Clinical example 16-5 has a history of multiple drug abuse and a medical diagnosis of antisocial personality.[1]

The manipulative person presents a particularly difficult nursing problem. There is frequently little motivation for change because manipulative behavior has rewards to the individual with antisocial personality disorder. It helps him accomplish a desired goal. The manipulator is goal oriented or self oriented, not other oriented. However, this person is skilled at giving the impression of involvement with others. Mr. Y was able to gain the confidence of the staff. He knew that he needed to do so to have the support he needed in court. The antisocial personality is unaware of the lack of relatedness to others. He assumes that all interpersonal relationships are formed to take advantage of other people. This person cannot imagine an intimate, sharing relationship. He believes that he must be in control at all times to avoid being controlled. Shostrom[34] sees this issue of controlling or being controlled as central to manipulative behavior. He notes that manipulative behavior can also be positive, if it is used for useful purposes.

Individuals with the medical diagnosis of border-

CLINICAL EXAMPLE 16-6

Ms. S is a 23-year-old woman who was admitted to an acute psychiatric unit in a general hospital following superficially lacerating her wrists three times within the week before admission. Each time she cut herself, she had telephoned her therapist, a psychiatric clinical nurse specialist. Because her therapist was about to leave for a month's vacation, she decided to arrange to have Ms. S hospitalized.

On admission, Ms. S appeared mildly depressed. She gave the impression of a guilty child who had been punished. She denied any current self-destructive thoughts. During the physical examination, it was noted that there were many scars on her body. When asked about these, she claimed to have been abused as a child. The records of the referring therapist described the scars as the result of many instances of self-mutilation, beginning at the age of 16. This had been the main reason for her seeking therapy. There was also a history of sexual promiscuity. She had been arrested 2 years earlier for possession of cocaine. She described herself as a failure, stating that she had "the best parents in the world, but they did not get the daughter they deserve." She said she was a drifter, who had never been able to settle on a career, a lifestyle, or any consistent friends. She didn't know who or what she was. When asked how she felt, she responded, "Most of the time, I don't feel anything, just empty." She had no signs of psychosis.

Ms. S was placed on constant observation, to prevent further cutting. All sharp objects were removed from her room. Initially, she was very cooperative and superficially friendly to the other patients. Because of her smooth adjustment, the constant observation was discontinued after 3 days. She was also given a schedule of activities and in-

formed that she was responsible for following it. The next day, an Exacto knife was missing from the activities therapy room. When a search was initiated, Ms. S was found in the bathroom, bleeding from several small cuts on her ankles. This sequence was repeated several times. Each time the constant observation was discontinued, she would find a sharp object and cut herself.

She was also observed to be very labile emotionally. In particular, she had unpredictable outbursts of anger, which were similar to temper tantrums. However, these outbursts passed as quickly as they came, never lasting more than several minutes. In addition, she began to categorize the staff as "good guys and bad guys." When she was around staff members she liked, she was generally pleasant, complimenting them on their kind and understanding attitudes toward her. With the staff she disliked, she was sullen and uncooperative, comparing them unfavorably to the other staff members. Eventually, the staff began to bicker about her care, some believing she was spoiled and others that she was neglected. When her parents visited, they also complained about the staff that Ms. S disliked, bringing small gifts to those she liked.

Ms. S remained in the hospital for the whole month of her therapist's absence. When she returned, the patient initially refused to see her. The frequency of angry outbursts increased dramatically. However, following regular and frequent visits from her therapist, Ms. S began to request discharge. Behavioral criteria for discharge were set, including at least a week of no self-mutilation and no temper tantrums. She met the criteria and was discharged back to outpatient treatment.

line personality disorder[1] are also frequently perceived as manipulative. This type of disruption in interpersonal relatedness is illustrated by Clinical example 16-6.

Borderline patients become manipulative because of an arrest in psychosocial development. This leads to an inability to participate in mature interpersonal relationships. Ms. S demonstrates this problem when she describes herself as a drifter and when she divides the staff into good and bad. Gunderson[17] describes the behaviors characteristic of the borderline personality as follows:

1. Interpersonal relationships are intense and unstable at the same time. Interpersonal behavior is characterized by devaluation, manipulation, dependency, and masochism.
2. Manipulative suicide attempts are designed to ensure rescue by significant others.
3. An unstable sense of self leads to failure to develop a sense of object constancy and fear of abandonment. These contribute to fear of aloneness.
4. Negative affects, including anger, sustained dysphoria, and depression, reflect a basic sense of "badness."
5. Occasional psychotic experiences are characterized by paranoia, regression, and dissociation.
6. Impulsiveness occurs, with episodic substance abuse and promiscuity.
7. A history of low achievement is present.[17]

Masterson[26] also notes the failure of the borderline person to achieve object constancy during the separation-individuation stage of psychosocial development. Because of this, the person relates to others as parts rather than wholes. When the other person fails to meet the borderline's needs, the relationship is likely to end. In addition, the borderline person cannot recall the image of a significant other who is absent. He is not able to mourn the loss of another person. Individuals who fail to complete separation from the mother and develop autonomy often repeat this developmental crisis at adolescence. Behaviors characteristic of this phase include clinging; depression accompanied by rage and defended by acting out or neurotic behavior; and detachment and withdrawal.

Many of these behaviors can be seen in the description of Ms. S's hospitalization. Because of their tendency to be manipulative and their inability to become involved in reciprocal interpersonal relationships, these patients are frustrating for nursing staff. It must be remembered that their behavior is not con-

sciously planned but is an attempt to defend against a fear of loneliness.

The major behaviors representative of disruptions in relatedness have been presented. Individual patients frequently experience combinations of these behaviors. The nurse must be able to identify the complex behavior that any person may exhibit when confronted with high levels of stress and anxiety. In some cases a usual mode of behavior, such as manipulation, may be exaggerated or combined with a change in behavior. For instance, a manipulative person may withdraw when confronted by his manipulations and may be rejected by those he has been trying to manipulate. In other instances the behavior resulting from stress may be different from the individual's usual style of relatedness. A person who is usually outgoing may withdraw when under great stress. It is helpful to include a description of the patient's usual interpersonal relationships in the nursing assessment. This provides a baseline of normal behavior for that person against which the nurse measures the patient's progress.

■ Coping mechanisms

Behaviors associated with disruptions in relatedness are attempts to cope with the anxiety associated with threatened or actual loneliness. However, the case studies in this chapter demonstrate some of the ways that these attempts to cope lead to relationship problems. Sometimes they even drive people farther away. Thus the person is always caught in the approach-avoidance conflict of the need-fear dilemma. He seeks some degree of human contact on the one hand and pushes people away on the other.

The dependent person copes by clutching others and refusing to let go. This invites rejection when others feel smothered by clinging behavior. This person has no faith in his ability to rely on himself. Reaction formation may be a coping mechanism used to avoid facing the anger that results from feeling unable to participate in growth-promoting activities. The withdrawn person craves interpersonal contact but fears rejection even more. Retreat into a shell is protective but is also lonely and therefore not rewarding. Extremely withdrawn people are using the mechanism of regression.

Suspicious people keep others at arm's length by refusing to believe that they can be trusted. This is frequently a defense against confronting the lack of more basic trust in one's self. Such a confrontation would result in intolerable anxiety and ego disintegration. Projection is the coping mechanism underlying suspicious behavior.

Manipulative people view other people as objects. Their defenses protect them from potential psychological pain related to the loss of a significant other. Reid[30] has described the defenses used by the individual with antisocial personality disorder as projection and splitting. Projection allows the person to deny responsibility for negative consequences of his antisocial behavior. For instance, a patient may excuse his use of drugs by saying, "Everybody I know uses heroin. Why shouldn't I?" Splitting is characteristic of individuals with borderline personality disorder as well. Gunderson[17] defines this as the inability to synthesize the good and bad aspects of oneself and of objects. An object is anything outside of the self, animate or inanimate, to which the person has an attachment. An object could be a parent, a friend, or a teddy bear. Gunderson describes Kernberg's description of the characteristics of splitting:

1. Alternately expressing opposite sides of a conflict while appearing unconcerned about the contradiction
2. Inconsistent lack of impulse control with periodic expression of primitive impulses that do not cause anxiety at the time
3. Dividing external objects into those that are "all good" and those that are "all bad"
4. Fluctuation between "all good" and "all bad" perceptions of others[17]

Masterson adds several other defense mechanisms characteristic of individuals with borderline personality disorder. These include "acting out, reaction formation, obsessive-compulsive mechanisms, projection, isolation, detachment and withdrawal of affect."[26] Danziger[10] has identified another set of coping mechanisms related to the borderline personality. In addition to splitting, she includes the following:

1. Denial of responsibility for acting out behavior and denial of painful or threatening feelings
2. Devaluation of another, which makes the borderline person appear good by contrast
3. Projective identification, in which the individual criticizes his own shortcomings in another
4. Idealization of positive traits of others, which when combined with identification, results in good feelings[10]

Several approaches exist to defining the defensive structure of the borderline patient. All reflect the person's severe difficulty separating himself from others and participating in close relationships.

People with schizophrenia rely on coping mechanisms that tend to be primitive and sometimes only somewhat effective in controlling their interpersonal anxiety. Searles[33] has described several coping mechanisms present in schizophrenic communication.

The first mechanism is displacement. This results in directing communication toward a person or thing that is not the real stimulus for the response. There may also be a time difference between the conscious and unconscious objects. For example, a patient who is angry at the nurse may talk about a past quarrel with a close friend. Searles[33] relates this to the person's poor differentiation of "perceptual-conceptual" experience, which leads him to perceive similar objects as identical.

Projection is a mechanism discussed earlier as it relates to the development of paranoid delusions and auditory hallucinations. Schizophrenic patients also frequently project meaning to the nonverbal communication of others. This reflects the meaning attached to the person's own nonverbal behavior. Projection can reveal much about a person's world view and about what things are difficult for him to handle.

Another coping mechanism used by schizophrenic patients is introjection. Searles believes that this mechanism is the cause of the patient's feeling he is controlled or influenced by others. The behavior and even sometimes the unconscious impulses of the other person are experienced by the patient as his own and reflected in his behavior. For instance, the patient may act out a significant other's unconscious wish that is transmitted nonverbally.

Condensation involves the concentration of several thoughts and feelings into a relatively simple verbal or nonverbal message. This may be expressed as a repeated statement or gesture, with a variety of meanings. It is as if the person has very limited resources of communication. For example, a statement that seems to be clear and straightforward may also be highly complex and symbolic.[33] The patient may be unaware of the hidden meanings. The nurse may need supervisory help to interpret the communication.

Patients may unconsciously protect themselves from experiencing overwhelming emotion by means of isolation. Much of this may be related to ambivalent feelings. It helps the individual cope with the anxiety aroused by these conflicting feelings.[33]

As can be seen from this discussion, many coping mechanisms may appear in impaired communication patterns. Behavior related to a high level of anxiety may also reflect the person's attempt to cope with the anxiety. The nurse must understand this complex interrelationship between anxiety, coping, and observable behavior to plan appropriate nursing interventions.

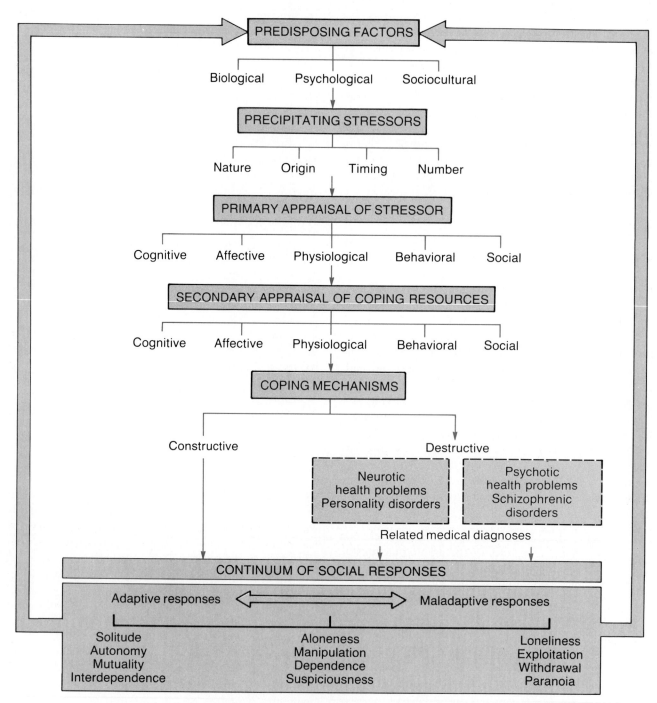

Fig. 16-3. Nursing model of health-illness phenomena related to interpersonal relationships.

Nursing diagnosis

When diagnosing a disruption in an individual's relatedness, the nurse should consider the patient's degree of disruption, the behaviors that demonstrate the disruption, and the predisposing factors and the precipitating stressors leading to the disruption. Generally, many patient problems must be considered when planning nursing care. The diagnosis should be thorough and reflect depth in understanding the patient's life situation. The nurse may formulate a nursing diagnosis by using the model of health-illness phenomena (Fig. 16-3) as a guide. When usual coping mechanisms fail, the patient will exhibit behaviors related to a personality disorder or to a psychosis. The category of behavior is not directly related to its severity. A person with a first episode of a psychosis who receives adequate treatment may be less disabled than someone who has a severe personality disorder. Accurate observation of behavior and data analysis ensure that appropriate nursing intervention may be initiated promptly.

A complete nursing diagnosis includes the statement of the nursing problem, the identified stressor related to that problem, and the observed behavioral response. The essential features of the diagnosis should be validated with the patient, whenever possible. The patient may be too suspicious or withdrawn to participate actively. Significant others may be involved, unless it is decided that this is not in the patient's best interest, as with a borderline person who refuses to participate in treatment planning. It is known that borderline people become confused about the boundaries between themselves and others. Including family members in treatment planning would add to the boundary confusion. Primary NANDA nursing diagnoses and examples of complete nursing diagnoses related to disruptions in relatedness are presented in the box that follows. Persons with serious mental disorders frequently have other health problems. Only those nursing diagnoses often related to interpersonal problems are presented here. However, the nurse is responsible for identifying and documenting all relevant nursing diagnoses for each patient. Table 16-2 identifies nursing and medical diagnoses related to disorders leading to disruptions in relatedness.

■ Related medical diagnoses

The major categories of medical diagnosis that relate to disruptions in relatedness are schizophrenia and several of the personality disorders. General criteria exist for the diagnosis of schizophrenia (see the box on page 515). Subtypes of schizophrenia are further de-

Nursing Diagnoses Related to Disruptions in Relatedness

Primary NANDA nursing diagnoses

Coping, ineffective individual
Social isolation
Thought processes, altered

Examples of complete nursing diagnoses

Ineffective individual coping related to lack of trust in others, evidenced by refusal to take medicine

Ineffective individual coping related to lack of confidence in decision-making ability, evidenced by referring all questions to husband

Social isolation related to inadequate interpersonal skills, evidenced by inappropriate sexual advances

Social isolation related to inability to accept shortcomings in others, evidenced by excessive criticism of friends

Altered thought processes related to projection of aggressive impulses, evidenced by delusion that the communists are looking for him

Altered thought processes related to physiologic changes, evidenced by neologisms and dissociated speech

fined in terms of the essential features that differentiate one from the other.

■ **SCHIZOPHRENIA, PARANOID TYPE.** The essential features include preoccupation with a system of delusions or auditory hallucinations with a single theme. There is no evidence of incoherence, loose associations, affective disturbances, catatonia, or gross disorganization.[1]

■ **SCHIZOPHRENIA, CATATONIC TYPE.** The clinical picture is dominated by any of the following:

1. Catatonic stupor or mutism
2. Catatonic negativism (resistance to all instructions or attempts to be moved)
3. Catatonic rigidity
4. Catatonic excitement
5. Cataonic posturing (voluntary assumption of inappropriate or bizarre posture)[1]

■ **SCHIZOPHRENIA, DISORGANIZED TYPE.** The essential features include incoherence, loose asso-

---

TABLE 16-2

MEDICAL AND NURSING DIAGNOSES RELATED TO DISRUPTIONS IN RELATEDNESS

Medical Diagnostic Class	**Psychiatric Nursing Diagnostic Class**
Schizophrenia	Disruptions in relatedness
Personality disorders	**Related Nursing Diagnoses (NANDA)**
Related Medical Diagnoses (DSM-III-R)*	Adjustment, impaired
Schizophrenia	Anxiety
Paranoid type	Communication, impaired verbal
Catatonic type	Coping, ineffective family
Disorganized type	†Coping, ineffective individual
Undifferentiated type	Family processes altered
Residual type	Personal identity disturbance
Personality disorders	Role performance, altered
Paranoid	Social interaction, impaired
Schizoid	Self-care deficit, specify
Schizotypal	Self-esteem disturbance
Antisocial	Sensory/perceptual alterations
Borderline	†Social isolation
Dependent	†Thought processes, altered

*American Psychiatric Association: Diagnostic and statistical manual of mental disorders, ed 3, rervised (DSM-III-R) Washington, DC, 1987, American Psychiatric Association.
†Indicates primary nursing diagnoses for disruptions in relatedness.

---

ciations, gross disorganization of behavior, and flat or inappropriate affect.[1]

■ **SCHIZOPHRENIA, UNDIFFERENTIATED TYPE.** The essential features include delusions, hallucinations, incoherence, or grossly disorganized behavior.[1]

■ **SCHIZOPHRENIA, RESIDUAL TYPE.** The essential features include the presence of residual symptoms as described in the box on page 515, without evidence of delusions, hallucinations, incoherence, or gross disorganization.[1]

■ **GENERAL CHARACTERISTICS OF PERSONALITY DISORDERS.** Personality disorders are defined by Hirschfeld[19] as "mental disorders in which personality traits are inflexible and maladaptive and cause either significant impairment in social or occupational functioning, or cause subjective distress." Personality is composed of temperament, which includes the inherited aspects, and character, which is learned. In general, the distinguishing characteristics of the personality disorders are that they are (1) chronic and long-standing, (2) not based on a sound personality structure, difficult to change, and not distressing to the person. The schizoid, schizotypal, paranoid, borderline, antisocial, and dependent types are described here by the DSM-III-R in diagnostic criteria.

■ **SCHIZOID PERSONALITY DISORDER.** The essential features include social detachment and restricted expression of emotions. Specific symptoms may include lack of close relationships, aloofness, indifference, interest in solitary activities, little interest in sexual experiences, no evidence of experiencing strong feelings, and lack of interest in others' responses or feelings.[1]

■ **SCHIZOTYPAL PERSONALITY DISORDER.** The essential features include relationship deficits combined with peculiar ideation, affect, and behavior.[1]

■ **PARANOID PERSONALITY DISORDER** The essential features include an unwarranted tendency to interpret the actions of people and events as deliberately demeaning or threatening. Typical behaviors may include suspicion of the actions or motivations of others, holding grudges, and sensitivity to perceived slights.[1]

■ **BORDERLINE PERSONALITY DISORDER.** The essential features include instability of mood, interpersonal relationships, and self-image. Characteristic behaviors may include unstable relationships, exploitation of others, impulsive behavior, labile affect, problems expressing anger appropriately, self-destructive behavior, and identity disturbances.[1]

■ **ANTISOCIAL PERSONALITY DISORDER.** The essential features include current age at least 18 years and evidence of conduct disorder before that age.

Diagnostic Criteria for Schizophrenia

A. Presence of characteristic psychotic symptoms in the active phase: either (1), (2), or (3) for at least one week (unless the symptoms are successfully treated):
  (1) two of the following:
    (a) delusions
    (b) prominent hallucinations (throughout the day for several days or several times a week for several weeks, each hallucinatory experience not being limited to a few brief moments)
    (c) incoherence or marked loosening of associations
    (d) catatonic behavior
    (e) flat or grossly inappropriate affect
  (2) bizarre delusions (i.e., involving a phenomenon that the person's culture would regard as totally implausible, e.g., thought broadcasting, being controlled by a dead person)
  (3) prominent hallucinations [as defined in (1)(b) above] of a voice with content having no apparent relation to depression or elation, or a voice keeping up a running commentary on the person's behavior or thoughts, or two or more voices conversing with each other
B. During the course of the disturbance, functioning in such areas as work, social relations, and self-care is markedly below the highest level achieved before onset of the disturbance (or, when the onset is in childhood or adolescence, failure to achieve expected level of social development).
C. Schizoaffective Disorder and Mood Disorder with Psychotic Features have been ruled out, i.e., if a Major Depressive or Manic Syndrome has ever been present during an active phase of the disturbance, the total duration of all episodes of a mood syndrome has been brief relative to the total duration of the active and residual phases of the disturbance.
D. Continuous signs of the disturbance for at least six months. The six-month period must include an active phase (of at least one week, or less if symptoms have been successfully treated) during which there were psychotic symptoms characteristic of Schizophrenia (symptoms in A), with or without a prodromal or residual phase, as defined below.
  Prodromal phase: A clear deterioration in functioning before the active phase of the disturbance that is not due to a disturbance in mood or to a Psychoactive Substance Use Disorder and that involves at least two of the symptoms listed below.
  Residual phase: Following the active phase of the disturbance, persistence of at least two of the symptoms noted below, these not being due to a disturbance in mood or to a Psychoactive Substance Use Disorder.
  Prodromal or Residual Symptoms:
  (1) marked social isolation or withdrawal
  (2) marked impairment in role functioning as wage-earner, student, or homemaker
  (3) markedly peculiar behavior (e.g., collecting garbage, talking to self in public, hoarding food)
  (4) marked impairment in personal hygiene and grooming
  (5) blunted or inappropriate affect
  (6) digressive, vague, overelaborate, or circumstantial speech, or poverty of speech, or poverty of content of speech
  (7) odd beliefs or magical thinking, influencing behavior and inconsistent with cultural norms, e.g., superstitiousness, belief in clairvoyance, telepathy, "sixth sense," "others can feel my feelings," overvalued ideas, ideas of reference
  (8) unusual perceptual experiences, e.g., recurrent illusions, sensing the presence of a force or person not actually present
  (9) marked lack of initiative, interests, or energy
  Examples: Six months of prodromal symptoms with one week of symptoms from A; no prodromal symptoms with six months of symptoms from A; no prodromal symptoms with one week of symptoms from A and six months of residual symptoms.
E. It cannot be established that an organic factor initiated and maintained the disturbance.
F. If there is a history of Autistic Disorder, the additional diagnosis of Schizophrenia is made only if prominent delusions or hallucinations are also present.

From American Psychiatric Association: DSM-III-R, Washington, DC, 1987, American Psychiatric Association. Used with permission.

Conduct disorders are characterized by truancy, school behavior problems, arrests, running away, lying, substance abuse, and general disregard for rules. After age 18, characteristic behaviors include a poor work record, disregard for social norms, aggressiveness, financial irresponsibility, impulsiveness, lying, recklessness, and inability to maintain close relationships or to meet responsibilities for significant others.[1]

■ **DEPENDENT PERSONALITY DISORDER.** The essential features include dependent and submissive behavior.

❧ Planning
Goal setting
■ Mutuality

It can be difficult to set mutual goals with a patient in the area of relatedness. This is partly because mutuality must be based on a strong nurse-patient relationship. It is, of course, difficult to develop a strong relationship with a patient who has problems establishing intimacy. In addition, setting a goal implies a commitment to change. Many patients who have disruptions in human relationships are reluctant to commit themselves to change. Since most of these behavioral disruptions also serve as coping mechanisms, there is additional resistance to change.

For these reasons, even though it is desirable to have the patient's full participation in goal setting, it may be necessary for the nurse to set initial goals. Consideration must be given to all the data collected in the nursing assessment and should be based on the nursing diagnosis. Environmental constraints also need to be considered. To overcome a problem with relatedness, the person must be involved with others. At first, the other person may be the nurse, but eventually others will take her place.

■ **LONG- AND SHORT-TERM GOALS.** The long-term nursing goal for nursing care of the patient with disruptions in relatedness is to promote growth toward achieving maximum interpersonal satisfaction. This is achieved by establishing and maintaining self-enhancing relationships with others. Short-term goals are more specific to the individual's problems. They may develop from simpler to more complex changes in behavior. See the sample nursing care plans for patients with disruptions in relatedness presented in Figs. 16-4 and 16-5.

■ **REALISTIC EXPECTATIONS.** Goals developed with patients who have impaired relationships may take a long time to accomplish. These patients frequently use bizarre communication patterns to avoid intimate relationships. They are usually reluctant to risk communicating more directly. However, it is still possible to develop goals to change disrupted communication patterns.

Goals with these patients may focus on modifying specific communication patterns. For example, "The patient will use nonverbal communication congruent with the verbal content of his speech." Another example of a goal for a patient with impaired communication is, "The patient will verbally identify angry feelings when they occur during a one-to-one interaction." These goals need to be developed with the patient's active participation. Learning to relate more directly and openly causes anxiety. Therefore the patient's ability to tolerate anxiety must be considered when determining goals. Increasing the anxiety level before the patient has increased coping ability and environmental supports may reinforce his use of dysfunctional coping behaviors.

The data collected during the assessment, the nursing diagnosis, and the goals for nursing care are combined into the nursing care plan. The nurse adds nursing interventions that are related to the goals of nursing care. The nursing care plan provides a guide for intervention. It also adds to consistency among the various nursing staff members who provide care to the patient. Fig. 16-4 provides an example of a nursing care plan for Mr. D, the patient with a medical diagnosis of schizophrenia, paranoid type, presented in Clinical example 16-1. Fig. 16-5 is a sample nursing care plan for Ms. S, the patient with a medical diagnosis of borderline personality disorder described in Clinical example 16-6. It should be noted that these are not detailed nursing care plans. They are intended to provide examples of the various components of a plan.

Planning also includes attending to the patient's educational needs. A sample mental health education plan is presented in Table 16-3. This particular plan is for a dependent patient. However, it is a nursing responsibility to assist patients and their families to understand the nature and treatment of any of the disorders that cause disturbed interpersonal relationships.

⇒ Implementation
■ Intervening in withdrawal

The interpersonal relationship between the nurse and the patient is central to the practice of psychiatric nursing. It is very challenging to establish and maintain a therapeutic relationship with a patient who has problems with relatedness. The nurse must use sensitivity and self-awareness to overcome the patient's concerns about closeness and create trust. Kahn[20] has de-

PSYCHIATRIC NURSING CARE PLAN

Precautions:
Assaultive behavior

Special nursing needs:
Fequent brief contacts
Monitor family visits
Do not touch rabbit foot

Visitors: {x} No restrictions
{ } Family only
{ } Restricted to:
_____
{ } No visitors

Telephone: { } Limited
{x} Unlimited

Privileges: {x} Restricted to unit
{ } Off unit accompanied by staff
{ } Off unit accompanied by family/visitor
{ } Off unit unaccompanied
{ } Out of hospital leave (dates) _____

Assessment data summary: Third admission; planning to start a job training program soon; parents do not seem to support this plan. Withdrawn; auditory hallucinations; believes God has spoken to him; feels invincible; loose associations; thinks concretely. Has a trusting relationship with Ms. T, C.N.S.

Nursing diagnoses: 1. Social isolation related to lack of trust in others, evidenced by belief that people are trying to destroy him. 2. Altered thought processes related to increased stress, evidenced by loose associations and and concrete thought. 3. Ineffective individual coping related to family conflict, evidenced by parent's threat of divorce.

Treatment goal: Growth toward achieving maximum interpersonal satisfaction by establishing and maintaining self-enhancing relationships with others.

Date	Problem/need	Expected outcome (objective)	Target Date	Nursing Intervention
1/10	Improved social relationships	To interact with others without talking about delusions	1/17	Inform him that his thoughts are real to him but are not shared. Emphasize that the hospital is safe. Change the subject.
1/10	Refusal to eat or drink	To maintain admission weight. To achieve normal blood chemistries.	1/13	Allow family to bring food. Offer favorite food and fluids

Room	Patient's name	Age	Doctor	Primary nurse	Admit date
211	Mr. D	24	Dr. J	Ms. T	1/10/90

Fig. 16-4. Sample nursing care plan for the patient with schizophrenia, paranoid type. (This nursing care plan includes examples of the elements of a total plan as it might appear at a particular time in the patient's course of treatment. It should not be considered all inclusive.)

Date	Medications	Date	P.R.N. Medications	Diagnostic & psychiatric tests	Req.	Done
1/10	Haloperidol					
	20 mg qid					
		Date	Treatments	Special orders and concerns		
				Vocational rehab consultation		

Allergies:	Medical diagnosis: (Axes I-III)	Diet:
None	Schizophrenia, paranoid type	Regular

Fig. 16-4, cont'd. Sample nursing care plan for the patient with schizophrenia, paranoid type.

scribed the therapeutic approach to the schizophrenic patient as characterized by "non-intrusive availability, compassionate limit setting, establishment of realistic expectations, and self-care."

One of the most frustrating, but also one of the most potentially rewarding, experiences for the psychiatric nurse is that of intervening therapeutically with a withdrawn patient, particularly one who is psychotic. Withdrawn patients do not often respond quickly to nursing intervention. They usually need consistent, repeated approaches by the nurse to convince them of sincere concern.

■ **MEETING BIOLOGICAL NEEDS.** The extremely withdrawn patient may be mute and immobile. Nursing care must meet all biological, psychological, and social needs. In her classic article on the nursing care of the withdrawn patient, Will[41] cites three general focuses for nursing intervention: (1) fulfilling the patient's needs, (2) facilitating communication, and (3) facilitating social participation.

Frequently the highest priority must first be given to fulfilling biological needs. Food and fluid intake must be carefully monitored to maintain adequate nutrition and hydration. If the patient is relatively immobile, intravenous or tube feeding may be necessary.

The nurse should explain to the patient that this is being done to maintain his health. Many patients believe that they are being punished when invasive treatments are given. It is equally important to record urinary output and frequency of defecation. Urinary retention with bladder distention and fecal impaction are complications that can be avoided by good nursing care. If the patient refuses to move voluntarily, positioning and skin care are other nursing concerns. Even if the patient responds to direction from the nurse, reminders to attend to personal hygiene will probably be required.

The nurse must remember that the indifference to others seen in withdrawn patients is probably a defense. Even people who seem completely out of contact with their surroundings are likely to be aware of everything that happens. Frequently a patient who has recovered from a state of catatonic stupor is able to describe in detail conversations and events that occurred during the stupor. Empathy can help the nurse to understand what the patient may think about being fed, bathed, and dressed. These activities are best carried out matter-of-factly. The nurse should communicate sensitivity. Patients who do not perform self-care should still be given a chance to do so by being in-

PSYCHIATRIC NURSING CARE PLAN

Precautions:
Self mutilation
Suicide

Special nursing needs:
Assign consistent staff whenever
possible

Visitors: { } No restrictions
{x} Family only
{ } Restricted to:

{ } No visitors

Telephone: { } Limited
{x} Unlimited

Privileges: {x} Restricted to unit
{ } Off unit accompanied by staff
{ } Off unit accompanied by family/visitor
{ } Off unit unaccompanied
{ } Out of hospital leave (dates) _____

Assessment data summary: Upset about vacation of outpatient therapist; three episodes of self-mutilation in last week; history of sexual promiscuity; history of arrest for cocaine possession; lack of goals; no friends.

Nursing diagnoses: 1. Potential for self-directed violence related to low self-esteem, evidenced by description of herself as a failure. 2. Social isolation related to inadequate self-concept, evidenced by statement that she does not know who or what she is.

Treatment goal: Growth toward achieving maximum interpersonal satisfaction by establishing and maintaining self-enhancing relationships with others.

Date	Problem/need	Expected outcome (objective)	Target Date	Nursing Intervention
4/23	Improved social relationships	To interact with others without splitting.	5/14	Clearly explain nursing care plan; be sure that staff are consistent in following plan.
4/23	Cutting self	To express feelings verbally instead of acting out.	4/30	Observe closely. Prohibit access to sharp objects. Offer chance to talk when upset.

Room	Patient's name	Age	Doctor	Primary nurse	Admit date
128	Ms. S	23	Dr. W	Ms. S	4/23/90

Fig. 16-5. Sample nursing care plan for the patient with borderline personality disorder. (This nursing care plan includes examples of the elements of a total plan as it might appear at a particular time in the patient's course of treatment. It should not be considered all inclusive.)

Date	Medications	Date	P.R.N. Medications	Diagnostic & psychiatric tests	Req.	Done
		4/30	Acetaminophen			
			650 mg q4h for			
			pain in lacerated			
			areas			
		Date	Treatments	Special orders and concerns		
		4/30	Dry sterile			
			dressing for			
			right wrist bid			

Allergies:	Medical diagnosis: (Axes I-III)	Diet:
None	Borderline pesonality disorder	Regular

Fig. 16-5, cont'd. Sample nursing care plan for the patient with borderline personality disorder.

structed to perform simple tasks. For example, the patient who is being bathed can be given a soaped washcloth and asked to wash himself. In this way the nurse may assess the patient's progress. As the patient can perform one task, another task should be introduced. Each new task is more complex than the one that has been mastered previously. This continues until the patient has met the goal of maximum independence in meeting his biological needs. The amount of independence that is reached will depend on the patient's strengths and disabilities. However, the nurse should continuously challenge the patient to develop new skills.

■ **VERBAL COMMUNICATION.** Communicating with the withdrawn patient demands great patience. It can be uncomfortable to sit in silence with a mute person if one is used to the action-oriented role of the nurse. It may be tempting to chatter aimlessly or to fidget. As always, the nurse needs to analyze her own response to the situation and be sure that her nursing interventions are goal directed. For instance, if the nurse has assessed the patient's interests and knows that he is a football fan, telling him about a big game can stimulate his interest in his environment. However, relating details of her date the night before is

probably an attempt to make herself less anxious by filling up the silence. Constant chatter also gives the patient the message that he is not expected to talk. It is much more therapeutic to make open-ended statements followed by pauses so the patient may respond if he wishes. The patient may be frightened by direct questions. These should be used carefully. Questions giving a choice should be used only if a choice is to be made. Asking a patient if he wants his medication when he should definitely take it is not a clear message and should be avoided. Statements should be brief, clear, and concise, without treating the patient as a child. Information from the nursing assessment can guide the nurse in selecting language appropriate to the patient's sociocultural background.

■ **NONVERBAL COMMUNICATION.** It is especially important to be aware of nonverbal communication when interacting with a withdrawn patient. Even a totally silent patient may communicate much through body language and gestures. Feelings may be communicated nonverbally, sometimes more accurately than by words. For instance, a tense person who holds his body rigidly and glares at the nurse may be angry but may not think he can tell her this. Depressed people often communicate the depth of their despair

TABLE 16-3

MENTAL HEALTH EDUCATION PLAN FOR A DEPENDENT PATIENT

Content	Instructional activities	Evaluation
Identify common concerns related to open and honest expression of real feelings and ideas.	Identify a recent situation in which the patient had difficulty stating real feelings or ideas. List alternative ways to express thoughts and feelings. Role-play each alternative. Select the one that was most effective.	The patient will identify feelings and ideas and express them directly to others.
Explain the decision-making process.	Describe the steps of decision making: Identify the problem. List alternatives. Evaluate alternatives. Test selected alternative.	The patient will apply the decision-making process when offered a choice.
Practice the decision-making process.	Offer the patient a choice. Guide the patient through the steps of the process.	
Explore the meaning of experiencing pleasure.	Discuss the difference between pleasurable and unpleasurable experiences. Identify one activity that has the potential for enjoyment. Participate in the activity together. Share feelings of pleasure at the time that they occur. Repeat on a regular basis. Assist the patient to identify and practice a solitary pleasant experience.	The patient will describe one activity that has been enjoyable. The patient will identify feelings of pleasure related to specific activities.
Describe behaviors that characterize anxiety.	List behaviors that indicate the various levels of anxiety.	The patient will identify behaviors and the related level of anxiety.
Explore situations that create anxiety.	Role-play situations that require independence and monitor anxiety level.	The patient will identify anxiety related to specific situations.
Explain stress reduction techniques.	Describe the stress response. Demonstrate relaxation exercises (see Chapter 11). Assist the patient to return the demonstration. Role-play anxiety-provoking situation. Assist patient to use relaxation when early signs of anxiety appear.	The patient will perform relaxation exercises when signs of anxiety appear.

by a body position that looks tired, droopy, and bent. Anxiety is communicated nonverbally and may contribute to the nurse's discomfort when interacting with a withdrawn patient.

The withdrawn person may also show increased openness to others nonverbally. When a person who has avoided eye contact looks directly at the nurse, it is a sign that he is ready to become involved in the relationship. Reaching out or the acceptance of a touch may have the same meaning. Relaxation of a usually tense body posture can be the first sign of increased comfort with the nurse. Other nonverbal signs of decreasing withdrawal include attention to personal ap-

pearance and participation in groups that focus on physical activity.

The nurse's own nonverbal activity is also an important part of the relationship. Many times, gestures and facial expressions are automatic, but they send a message. The withdrawn patient is usually very sensitive to events in the environment. The nurse must become aware of habitual body language. Feedback from colleagues and supervisors can be helpful and should be encouraged by the nurse. Videotape, if available, can provide immediate input about nonverbal and verbal communication; this can be a helpful tool in supervision. If videotaping is done with a patient, it should be carefully planned and done only with the patient's informed consent. Role-play with other professionals can often be equally useful. This eliminates concern about disturbing the therapeutic relationship.

Nonverbal communication can be therapeutic in the nursing care of the withdrawn patient. Looking directly at a patient when greeting him may express concern. A gentle touch can establish contact with a withdrawn depressed person. Leaning toward a patient but keeping a comfortable distance screens out other people and transmits the message that the nurse is focusing all of her attention on the patient. Caring for physiological needs is a powerful way to express caring. An attitude of concerned, but not intrusive, interest lets the patient control the development of closeness. The process of relating to a withdrawn patient requires much sensitivity.

■ **INVOLVING OTHERS WITH THE PATIENT.** At first, a one-to-one nurse-patient relationship is usually most helpful to a patient who is socially isolated or withdrawn. However, the goal is to help the patient establish healthy interpersonal relationships with a variety of other people. As the nurse and patient begin to relate more comfortably, others should gradually be included in the patient's social network. The nurse can help the patient try to relate to others. Another person can be invited to join a card game or to share in a discussion. The hospital nurse can use her knowledge of all the patients to introduce people who seem to have something in common. The community nurse can use her knowledge of community resources to make a referral to a social group that seems appropriate to the patient's interests. Sometimes patients interpret encouragement to meet other people as rejection. The nurse can use this as an opportunity to talk about change and loss in life. It is also important to remind the patient of the nurse's role in helping the patient to move ahead with his life. She can then review the elements of their interpersonal relationship and assess progress toward the patient's goals.

■ **FAMILY INTERVENTION.** For many patients the family is the focus of many interpersonal problems. Frequently family therapy is indicated. It should be undertaken only by a therapist who has special training. However, the nurse who is working with the patient can help the family understand the patient's needs. If the patient does not want to visit with the family, the nurse may help them to maintain the relationship by expressing concern for the family members. She may suggest things they can do for the patient, such as bringing favorite foods or taking care of errands. Sometimes a family needs help in seeing small signs of progress. Often family members have ques-

tions about the patient's care. The nurse can educate the family about the treatment process. The patient should be included in this teaching. He should always be informed about contacts between the nurse and the family.

Nursing intervention with the withdrawn patient should be directed toward the accomplishment of reasonable goals. A shy person should not be expected to become outgoing. Knowledge of the person's usual personality is helpful in setting expectations. However, the patient is the best source of information about goal accomplishment. The individual's comfort or discomfort with his life-style and interpersonal relationships should always be the primary criterion for therapeutic progress.

■ **TERMINATING THE RELATIONSHIP.** Terminating a relationship with a withdrawn patient may be difficult for the nurse. The patient is likely to resist separating from a person to whom he has become close after a time of loneliness and isolation. He may fear not being able to maintain the ability to form healthier relationships. New problems are often brought up at termination. This usually indicates an attempt to prolong an important relationship. The nurse, too, will have many feelings about terminating with a patient after working so hard to build a relationship. Even the satisfaction of contributing to the growth of another person cannot erase the pain of ending the relationship. However, the experience of a well-handled termination can be therapeutic by helping the patient learn to deal with a loss in a healthy, mature way.

■ Intervening in suspiciousness

■ **FOSTERING TRUST.** Nursing interventions with a suspicious patient are in many ways similar to those with the withdrawn patient. The primary long-term goal with the suspicious patient is that the patient will demonstrate trust in the nurse. It is hoped the patient will then become able to trust others who deserve to be trusted. People demonstrate trust by being open to others, both physically and emotionally. Thus the trusting patient will not avoid contact with the nurse. He will also share thoughts and feelings with her. This process develops gradually in any relationship. It may be particularly slow when the patient has difficulty trusting other people.

Reliability is one factor that helps to foster trust. The nurse must follow through on promises made to the patient. The nurse should keep the paranoid or suspicious patient informed of her scheduled appointments. Reliability is demonstrated by keeping appointments on time or informing the patient if a change is necessary. Very suspicious people are constantly on guard. They fear that others will attack them. Long interpersonal contacts make them anxious. The nurse can help by planning several brief meetings spaced throughout the day. This offers several chances to demonstrate reliability.

■ **MEETING BIOLOGICAL NEEDS.** Sometimes suspicious patients may have difficulty in maintaining their physiological well-being. Fear may interfere with sleep. A light in the room at night can help. Sleeping medication may be offered. If the paranoid patient refuses to take it, insistence by the nurse will only increase the insomnia by upsetting the patient. It is probably better to try to persuade the patient to take prescribed antipsychotic medications. Many of these have the side effect of drowsiness. In addition, the medication will reduce anxiety enabling the patient to sleep. The suspicious patient may refuse to eat and/or drink. Attempts to force oral intake usually fail and are frustrating to both nurse and patient. Sometimes a suspicious patient will eat food brought by his family, food he prepares himself, or packaged food. Whenever possible, these preferences should be respected. As the patient learns to trust the nurse and the hospital, he will begin to eat and drink. If the patient is in danger from dehydration or malnutrition, the physician may prescribe tube feeding or intravenous therapy. If this does occur, careful explanations should be given as the treatment takes place. The patient will view treatment as an assault on his physical being. Much supportive nursing care will be required.

■ **PACING THE RELATIONSHIP.** Since suspicious people do fear intrusion from others and question their motives, care must be taken to respect the patient's right to privacy. The patient may appreciate time alone that can be worked into the daily schedule. A warning should be given when approaching a suspicious person. This avoids startling him. The patient should be allowed to control the amount of self-revelation that takes place in the interaction with the nurse. A probing approach will only alienate the patient. This will retard the development of trust. As trust grows, anxiety will decrease and the patient will have less need of his suspicious defenses. The growth of the patient's ability to confide in the nurse is one way to measure the success of nursing intervention with the suspicious patient.

Most people interact with a variety of therapeutic team members, especially in the hospital setting. When the patient has difficulty establishing trust, it is best if one or two people are assigned to work consistently and closely with him. However, other staff members should be aware of the treatment plan. Their approach to the patient should be consistent with that of the primary caregivers. Significant others should also be made aware of the care plan and should be encouraged to participate in it. Consistency among those who have close contact with the patient also promotes the development of trust.

■ **TRUSTWORTHINESS OF THE NURSE.** The nurse's openness and honesty show the patient that she can be trusted. For instance, if the nurse plans to meet with the patient's family, she should inform the patient of this plan. Then she should discuss confidentiality of information with both patient and family. Families of suspicious patients often have many family secrets. The nurse should not become involved in this communication pattern. The best way to avoid this problem is to include the patient in family meetings. The patient may refuse to attend or the family may attempt to exclude the patient by telephoning or intercepting the nurse during a visit. In this instance, it is best to have a plan of action prepared. Generally the nurse should inform the patient and the family that information shared between the nurse and family members will also be shared with the patient. Open communication is a characteristic of a trusting relationship. Families often try to keep information from the patient to protect him. The patient usually learns the hidden information. Then he feels justified in his lack of trust.

■ **ADMINISTERING MEDICATIONS.** The nurse should also be honest with the patient who asks questions about the plan of care. The patient has a right to participate in the care planning. He should know the rationale for any treatment. For example, suspicious persons may believe that others are trying to control them or hurt them. For either of these reasons, they may be reluctant to take medication. Taking medication is important because it should decrease the patient's anxiety. When anxiety is lower, the person is more able to trust others.

Even though the nurse knows that a patient has been refusing medication, she should approach the patient with confidence and expect him to take it. A hesitant approach may arouse the patient's suspicion. Spoken directions should be clear; for example, "Here is your medication, Mr. Jones." If the patient hesitates, this can be followed by "Put it in your mouth and swallow it." Nonverbal communication should reinforce the verbal. Also, to prevent confusion, the patient should be offered the same form of medication each time. For instance, if the order is for chlorpromazine, 150 mg, the nursing staff should agree to always give one 100 mg and one 50 mg tablet or three 50 mg tablets. If the liquid concentrate form of medication is used, it should be used consistently. If it is mixed with fruit juice, it should be mixed with the same flavor each time. Attention to these details can save much time and discussion when medications are given. The patient may become confused when the medication dosage is changed. The physician should inform the patient when a dosage change is made.

The nurse who is giving medicine to psychiatric patients should observe the patient's behavior carefully while the medicine is being taken. A suspicious patient may hide tablets or capsules in the cheek or under the tongue and spit them out as soon as the nurse looks away. If the nurse suspects this behavior, a mouth check should be done. The nurse asks the patient to open his mouth and uses a tongue depressor to look thoroughly for hidden medication. If possible, a better solution to this problem is to give the medication in liquid form. Occasionally a patient will swallow medication when it is given and then go into the bathroom and make himself vomit. Failure to respond to a medication as expected is a clue that the patient is not taking it. When this happens, the nurse should watch the patient closely after medication is given. It may be necessary to stay with the patient until enough time has passed for the medicine to be absorbed.

Sometimes patients absolutely refuse to take any medication by mouth. The nurse should never try to trick the patient to take medicine by putting it in food or fluids. If the patient discovers this, it will destroy his trust in the staff. It will give his suspicions a basis in reality. It could also cause the patient to stop eating and drinking, leading to problems with nutrition and hydration.

Sometimes a patient who refuses oral medication needs to be given an injection. This requires a physician's order. The nurse should also be aware of laws concerning the patient's right to refuse treatment. Generally, only life-saving treatments may be given without the patient's permission. The patient will sometimes take medication by mouth if given the choice of "by mouth or by needle." However, the nurse should not become involved in a long debate to persuade the patient to take oral medicine. If the patient must have the medicine and refuses it by mouth, the injection should be given quickly. There should be only as much physical restraint as needed for the patient's safety. The procedure should also be carried out with regard for the patient's right to dignity. Injections should be discontinued as soon as the patient accepts oral medication. When they are feeling better, patients rarely object to having been medicated when they were very disturbed.

As with a withdrawn patient, the nurse must help the suspicious person to trust her and others as well. The nurse helps the patient identify characteristic behaviors of trustworthy people. The goal is for the patient to be able to recognize trustworthy and untrustworthy people. It is not for him to trust everyone. Thomas[37] has described the trusting person as one who (1) expands his self-awareness and shares this awareness with others, (2) accepts others without needing to change them, (3) is open to new experiences, (4) is consistent in words and actions over time, and (5) can delay gratification. By sharing these characteristics with the patient, the nurse can teach a rational basis for deciding whom to trust. Discussion of these criteria with the patient also helps him identify his progress toward becoming a trusting person.

■ Intervening in impaired communication

Good communication skills, empathy, and creativity are necessary for providing good nursing care to patients with impaired communication. The relationship principles discussed in Chapter 4 also apply. Impaired communication can keep participants in interpersonal relationships at a distance. Transmitting unclear messages or not revealing feelings allows the receiver to perceive only part of the information available to the sender. At other times, inadequate or inaccurate perception and evaluation may interfere with clear communication.

■ **RESPONDING TO SYMBOLISM.** To understand the unclear messages of a schizophrenic patient, the nurse must listen carefully and observe the patient. She must also be aware of the communication context. Much of the patient's speech may be symbolical. For example, a patient who was feeling pressured by a nurse to accept a visit from his wife remarked, "It sure looks hot outside." This was interpreted to mean that the patient was feeling "hot" (angry) because of the nurse's pressure. The nurse chose not to share the interpretation with the patient, who had difficulty handling anger. Instead, she responded to his message by easing the pressure she was placing on him. Interpreting the meaning of symbolical communication must be done cautiously. The patient is speaking indirectly for a reason. The symbolism may screen thoughts and feelings that would be difficult to control if stated directly. The patient is usually not consciously aware of his symbolical meaning. At best, the patient may respond to a poorly timed interpretation with denial. At worst, the interpretation may arouse the patient's anxiety and cause him to lose control and enter a panic state. The responsible nurse should not create behavior that she and the patient cannot handle.

■ **EXPRESSING FEELINGS.** A supportive approach often works well with patients who have impaired communication. Many of these patients distrust the meaning of words. They have had past experiences with incongruent communications. They are very sensitive to nonverbal behavior and its meanings. They immediately perceive whether the nonverbal behavior supports the verbal message. The nurse must be self-aware and use both verbal and nonverbal communication purposefully in the nursing intervention. Openness can be supportive to the patient. Real people become angry, sad, happy, contented, and fearful. The nurse can show the patient how to acknowledge feelings and how to express them appropriately. Feelings are part of human relationships. Consider Clinical example 16-7.

Contrast these two possible approaches that Ms. S could choose to take with Ms. A:

EXAMPLE 1

MS. S: **Ms. A, you seemed to be ignoring me.**
MS. A: **I was just interested in my story.**
MS. S: **Well, that's all right. I know your story's important to you—and we just have 2 weeks left.**
MS. A: **Uh-hum. I won't be here much longer myself.**

EXAMPLE 2

MS. S: **It seemed hard for us to get together today.**
MS. A: **I was just interested in my story.**
MS. S: **I know. I was feeling impatient with you because you seemed to be avoiding me. Then I realized that I'll be leaving in 2 weeks. That's really very frustrating to me.**
MS. A: **Every time I get so I can talk to somebody, they leave.**
MS. S: **Sounds like you're frustrated, too.**

```
╔═══════════════════════════════════╗
║    CLINICAL EXAMPLE 16-7           ║
```

Ms. S was a nursing student who had been relating to Ms. A, a patient in a psychiatric unit, for 6 weeks. The relationship would terminate in 2 more weeks, when Ms. S's clinical experience in psychiatric nursing was to end. Ms. S arrived on time for her appointment with Ms. A and went to their usual meeting place. Ms. A was across the room watching television. Ms. S waited 10 minutes and then approached Ms. A, who agreed to talk with her. Ms. S was aware that she was annoyed because she had been looking forward to talking with Ms. A. She was also aware of the possible effect of the termination process on Ms. A's behavior.

In the first example, Ms. S maintains a "you-me" focus throughout the interaction sample. She hints at her annoyance but does not state it to Ms. A, who then indirectly expresses her annoyance. Ms. S also gives a double message when she says, "That's all right," then clearly indicates why it is not all right: "We just have 2 weeks left." This is likely to confuse Ms. A. In the second example, Ms. S puts the interaction into an "us" context. She shares her thoughts about the reason for her behavior and the patient's behavior. She expresses her frustration in a nonthreatening way, letting Ms. A know she could understand that Ms. A might have similar feelings. Ms. S has set the stage for a productive discussion of termination.

Some patients, particularly schizophrenics, take time to reach a level of trust where they can tolerate the nurse's feelings toward them. The nurse can show the patient how to express feelings by interacting with other staff members in his presence. She can then discuss the situation with the patient. People who are frightened of feelings need to see that they can be expressed without causing the expected destruction. When patients take a risk and share a feeling with another person, they need feedback about how the other person was affected. Expressing caring can be even more difficult than anger because caring leaves one vulnerable to rejection. Patients often need to experience socially acceptable ways of giving and receiving both positive and negative feelings.

■ **MANAGING RESISTANCE TO CLOSENESS.** Many behaviors indicate the patient's resistance to closeness. Wildman[40] describes some of these behaviors seen in schizophrenic patients: physical and psychological withdrawal, verbal threats or rejections, physical attack, and symbolic derogations or gestures. She states that the nurse must be sensitive to the meaning of these communications and direct nursing intervention to reduce the interpersonal anxiety. This will reduce the patient's resistance to involvement. The nurse may decide to overlook behavior that would be socially unacceptable to other situations. For instance, a patient may use grossly obscene language to drive the nurse away. Inexperienced nurses may take the patient's remarks personally and respond with a lecture. A therapeutic response is to assure the patient that his need for distance is understood and that the nurse will respect this. It is also important that the nurse continue to act interested in the patient. If the nurse is driven away, the patient's negative self-concept and antisocial behavior will be reinforced. When the patient gains some trust in the nurse, she can give feedback about the effect of his behavior on other people. As the patient continues to improve, the nurse can remind him that he is responsible for his behavior and its consequences.

■ **USING TOUCH.** Because the schizophrenic patient fears closeness, touch should be used carefully. Touch is a powerful communicative tool. Patients who are afraid of closeness may experience a casual touch as an invasion or as a sexual advance. A schizophrenic patient may think that a touch from a person of the same sex is a homosexual advance. This may precipitate a panic reaction. If a procedure requires physical contact, careful explanations should be given both before and during the procedure. A businesslike approach to physical nursing care may be least threatening to an anxious patient.

Touch may also have meaning for patients with poorly defined ego boundaries. Sometimes these patients touch other people to convince themselves that they are separate. Patients with diffuse ego boundaries cannot separate themselves from others. When they are touched, they think they are a part of the other person. Very regressed patients may cuddle and rock as if they are trying to find the symbiosis of infancy. Ego boundaries may be reinforced by clearly separating self from other in communication. Statements such as "It's time for us to take our bath" are confusing to a patient who does not know where his self ends and the nurse's self begins. The use of "I" and "you" helps the patient understand.

■ **INTERVENING IN DELUSIONS.** Confusion about ego boundaries is one problem that schizophrenic patients often have with reality orientation. Delusional thinking is another behavior related to this problem. When the ego is overwhelmed with anxiety, the person's ability to test reality is limited. The delusional patient is convinced that his beliefs are real even when logic and feedback from others contradict them. Nursing intervention with a delusional patient requires great sensitivity. Communication channels must be kept open while the nurse avoids supporting and reinforcing the delusion. Stripping the patient of his delusion removes his desperate attempt to defend himself from overwhelming anxiety. This could cause an outburst of uncontrolled assaultive behavior. A direct attack on the delusion usually makes the patient feel angry and misunderstood. It is better to use tact and express doubt in the reality of the delusion. A patient who fears that gangsters are planning to kill him may be able to accept the response, "You are safe here in the hospital, and I would like to help you learn more about what makes you so afraid." This shifts the focus from the imaginary gangsters to the patient's fear, which is real. Involvement in a consistently accepting nurse-patient relationship will slowly ease the patient's anxiety and allow him to give up his delusions. The nurse helps the patient explain the delusion and the purpose it served. For example, she may say, "When you first came here, you were very frightened and did not know what was happening to you. Your idea about the gangsters was a way of explaining your feelings. Now you are beginning to learn more about yourself, and you are finding other explanations." Some patients' delusions are so strongly established that they cannot give them up. These patients may function well if they talk about their delusions only in therapeutic sessions or with significant others who can tolerate such a discussion.

■ **INTERVENING IN HALLUCINATIONS.** Auditory hallucinations are another problem in reality testing. As with delusions, they originate in the unconscious and represent high interpersonal anxiety. They are caused by projection of repressed thoughts and feelings to objects outside the self. Field and Ruelke[12] identify seven phases of hallucinatory behavior. Understanding these can help guide nursing intervention.

The first phase is recollecting interactions with a person who has been helpful to the patient in the past. This results in decreased anxiety. The second phase, establishing a pattern, is a repetition of the first phase. During the third phase, the person begins to worry that the anxiety-relieving experience will not continue. This leads to more frequent repetition of the experience and decreased ability to distinguish fantasy from reality. This requires withdrawal from interaction with real people. Phase 4 occurs when other people notice and comment on the person's behavior. This causes increased anxiety and more need for the hallucinated reassurance. At phase 5 the experience becomes less pleasant. When the voice (or voices) becomes accusing and threatening, the anxiety level rises again. The person may tend to agree with the voice or may try to convince himself that it is wrong. At Phase 6, others usually intervene because there is serious interference with the patient's ability to function. He becomes extremely withdrawn and preoccupied with the hallucinations. At this point the patient also rejects responsibility for his behavior and feels controlled by outside forces. Compromise takes place at phase 7. The patient tries to bargain for a return to the earlier anxiety-relieving experience. According to this explanation, the patient's goal is relief of anxiety. This principle must be kept in mind when nursing intervention is planned. As with the delusional patient, attempting to discredit the hallucination could increase the patient's anxiety, creating an even greater need for the hallucination.

Schwartzman[32] has identified several principles for intervening with the hallucinating patient. Before intervening, the nurse should assess the need that is being met by the hallucination. According to the process just described, the need is related to the cause of the underlying anxiety. It is important to recognize and acknowledge the feelings associated with the hallucination. Being alert to nonverbal communication can help the nurse recognize these feelings. Nonverbal cues can also help the nurse identify when the patient is hallucinating and when to intervene. The nurse should recognize that the experience is real to the patient. She tries to cast doubt on it by telling the patient that she does not share the experience. For example, the nurse might say, "I know that the voices are frightening to you. I want you to know that I do not hear them." In this way, she becomes the patient's link with reality. Encouraging the patient to talk about reality-based issues is also helpful. Many patients report that their auditory hallucinations are most bothersome when they are alone and there are no competing stimuli.

Field[11] conducted research regarding the incidence of hallucinatory experiences of hospitalized patients. He found that most of the patients did have auditory hallucinations, although they did not readily admit to this. He also found that verbally dismissing the voices by saying "Go away" or "Be quiet" was effective for most patients. The patient must understand that this should take place in private or in the presence of a person who knows what he is doing. It may take some time before the patient can gain enough ego strength to test reality independently. Some patients continue to hallucinate indefinitely but learn to live and function with the voices in the background.

■ **PROVIDING STRUCTURE.** In addition to reality testing, patients who have trouble sorting out messages need help with organization. Schizophrenic patients are often disorganized. Sometimes behavior is so fragmented that nursing help is needed to accomplish even familiar tasks, such as eating and dressing. Step-by-step instructions should be given in clear simple language, such as "Put your right arm in the right sleeve; put your left arm in the left sleeve," until the person is fully dressed. Performing the task for the patient can save time. However, helping the patient to perform whatever activities he can helps to maintain his self-esteem. Another way to help the patient structure his day is to give him a schedule of planned activities. He then knows what to expect and can prepare for events before they occur. Nursing contacts should be included in the schedule. Regular brief contacts are less threatening to the patient who fears closeness than a single long interaction with the nurse. The length of nurse-patient interactions can be increased as the patient is able to tolerate this.

■ **DECISION MAKING.** Decision making is another problem for patients who have difficulty processing complex messages resulting in ambivalence. Psychotic patients have trouble focusing their attention because they have lost the ability to screen stimuli. They feel overwhelmed by the inputs they receive from inside themselves and from the environment. Even a simple task like filling out a menu form becomes impossible because of these distractions. The nurse can help by limiting the need to make choices. Family members can provide information about the patient's likes and dislikes and his usual routine so that nursing care can be individualized. As the patient's anxiety decreases, choices can be offered, beginning with two alternatives, such as "Do you want a ham sandwich or a roast beef sandwich?" As decision-making ability grows, the nurse can help the patient to identify and evaluate alternatives. Patients may try to persuade the nurse to make major life decisions for them. It should be kept in mind that decision making also includes responsibility for the outcome of the decision. A more appropriate role for the nurse is to assist the patient to study all aspects of a decision and then to support the strength that he demonstrates by making his own choice.

Nursing intervention with a patient experiencing impaired communication is challenging. The nurse must find ways to overcome the communication barriers erected by the patient. This requires alertness, keen observation, and openness to the subtle messages the patient transmits. The nurse's communication skills become her most important tools in engaging the patient in a helping relationship.

■ **Family intervention**

Families are often the primary care providers for people with schizophrenia. They must know how to respond to the patient's disturbed behavior and unusual communication patterns. An organized psychoeducation program can be very helpful to families as they prepare to take the patient home. Greenberg and coworkers[16] have described a successful interdisciplinary education program for schizophrenic patients and their families. Although their program was developed in an acute care setting, it can also be applied in other settings.

The program elements included an overview of current information related to schizophrenia, education about symptoms and medications, and stress management. The program focused on building positive relationships among staff, patients, and families, as well as encouraging families to network with each other. It also focused on identifying patient strengths and teaching coping strategies combined with practice of adaptive skills. The presentation of current research on schizophrenia provided realistic hope. Finally, referral was made to community providers who were known to be supportive of family involvement.

This program identified the roles of various staff members. The psychiatrist was the program coordinator and reviewed the diagnosis with the patient and family. Nursing staff provided education about schizophrenia, its treatment, and stress management. Day-to-day experiences were used as examples to reinforce the teaching. The occupational therapist taught life skills, using both formal teaching and learner experiences. The social worker conducted family discussion sessions. This program provided a good example of multidisciplinary team functioning to provide a well-rounded educational program.

■ **Intervening in dependency**

At first the dependent patient may appear to be too trusting. However, this person is not sure that others are willing to be available to him and to meet his needs. In addition, he is not sure that he can be self-sufficient. Therefore he clings to others, fearing that if they are allowed any distance, they will not return.

■ **THERAPEUTIC GOALS.** Hill[18] has identified four therapeutic goals in her work with dependent women: (1) to express real feelings and ideas, (2) to make decisions comfortably, (3) to accept pleasurable experiences, and (4) to be able to control panic. She also states that unless the patient has threatened or attempted suicide, it is best to help him remain out of the hospital, since being cared for impedes progress toward these goals. Hill's goals have been incorporated into the mental health education plan presented in Table 16-3.

It is difficult for dependent people to identify feelings accurately. They are used to reacting to other people's feelings rather than their own. The nurse must help the patient identify, express, and accept his feelings. Nonverbal communication may provide clues about the patient's feelings. It can be helpful to draw the patient's attention to gestures, body posture, and facial expression. The nurse should listen for recurring themes in the patient's conversation and attempt to articulate these. Another approach is to consistently ask the patient, "What do you think about . . .?" or "How do you feel about . . .?" This communicates the expectation that the patient does have opinions and feelings to share. Role modeling can also help. The nurse can share her own feelings with the patient if they have had an experience that aroused an emotional response. For instance, the nurse might say, "I was annoyed when the head nurse called me away just as we were getting into a good discussion."

■ **ROLE CLARIFICATION.** Dependent people try to place the nurse in the parental role, which is also a comfortable role for most nurses to assume. Therefore the nurse must take care to relate to the patient as an adult. This communicates that he is a mature person who can manage his own life. The patient will probably resist this and try to prove his helplessness to the nurse. She must resist the urge to act as a parent. This part of the dependent patient's nursing care can be frustrating, since the patient becomes demanding and seeks attention. Reasonable requests should be consistently met. Limits of acceptable behavior should be discussed with the patient. Involving the patient in developing the plan of care improves the chances for successful goal accomplishment.

■ **MEDICATIONS.** Contemporary culture is drug oriented. Pills are promoted as the cure for all problems. It is not surprising that many patients expect to find relief from their problems in a "magic pill." It is hard to convince them that pills may ease pain but rarely take it all away. Hard work is necessary to resolve psychosocial problems. A pill will not mend a broken marriage or a broken heart, however much one longs for that to happen.

Dependent people are prone to be seekers of the perfect pill. Sometimes this search can lead to overdependency on medication, even to the point of addiction. The nursing problem presented by these patients is twofold. They persistently demand medication and, at the same time, refuse to examine their behavior. The following interaction demonstrates this dilemma.

Mr. M is a 45-year-old man who is mildly depressed, is anxious, and has multiple somatic complaints. A thorough medical workup has ruled out any physiological basis for his symptoms. He is receiving diazepam (Valium), 5 mg, PO, q4h, prn for anxiety. He approaches a staff nurse, Ms. J.

MS. J: **May I help you, Mr. M?**
MR. M: **I need my Valium.**
MS. J: **Tell me how you're feeling.**
MR. M: **I feel bad. Just get me my Valium.**
MS. J: **You feel bad?**
MR. M: **Look, I need my pill now!**
MS. J: **Your Valium is ordered to help you when you're anxious. I want to try to understand how you're feeling when you ask for the pill.**
MR. M: **Well, I'm anxious and I'm getting more anxious standing here talking to you about whether I'm anxious. Now, how about my pill?**
MS. J: **Well, it has been just 4 hours since your last one. Do you think you could try to hold out for a few**

minutes longer? Perhaps we could talk or play ping-pong to take your mind off your anxiety.

MR. M: **Look, the doc says I can have Valium every 4 hours. For the last hour, I've been counting the minutes. My head aches, my stomach is in knots, and look how my hands are shaking. Please get me my pill.**

MS. J: **OK. If you can't wait, I'll get it for you. I'd like to talk to you later, though, to see if we can come up with some ideas of other ways you can handle your anxiety. Pills don't get to the root of the problem, you know.**

MR. M: **Sure, sure. I'll talk to you sometime when I'm calm. I'll wait right here while you get my pill.**

In this interaction the nurse and the patient were pursuing different goals. This resulted in frustration for both. The nurse's concern about Mr. M's dependence on his medication was well founded. Her timing in approaching the idea of alternative coping mechanisms was not ideal. However, she was acting responsibly in asking Mr. M to describe his feelings before giving him medication. It can be tempting with dependent patients such as Mr. M to give medicine automatically every 4 hours without question and avoid conflict. Medication that is ordered "whenever necessary" can be withheld by the nurse if the patient does not seem to need it. If the nurse is dealing with an annoying patient, she must also evaluate whether her feelings are influencing her decision not to give medicine.

Close communication within the health team is helpful when working with patients such as Mr. M. Frequency of medication should be reviewed regularly. All team members should be supportive and encourage the patient to confront his problems and to explore other coping mechanisms.

Placebos are sometimes given to dependent patients. This is done only with a physician's order. This plan of care should be thoroughly discussed and evaluated by the health care team before it is initiated. It involves deception and could cause the patient to lose trust in caregivers. This course of action should never be taken as a retaliation against a frustrating patient. As a professional, the nurse should explore her own feelings about the use of a placebo and make her own decision about participating in this treatment.

Patients who are dependent on medication have great potential for addiction. Nursing care of the addicted patient is addressed in Chapter 19. Nurses have a role in combating addiction by discouraging unnecessary use of medication and by helping patients explore healthier ways of meeting their needs.

■ **BEHAVIOR MODIFICATION.** Behavior modification can be therapeutic when caring for a dependent patient. Appropriate behavior, such as making decisions, helping others, or caring for personal needs, is rewarded by attention and warm praise. Inappropriate requests and behaviors are ignored. Mature behavior should increase as the patient realizes that dependent behavior results in little gratification.

Sometimes nurses try to avoid dependent patients because they expect them to be clinging and demanding. This reinforces the patient's expectation that others will not be available to help him. His anxiety level then rises, and he becomes even more demanding of attention. This reinforces the nurse's frustration with him. This cycle must be broken by the nurse. If the patient receives attention without having to make demands, the anxiety decreases. Gradually the patient will make fewer demands. The nurse can then begin to help the patient learn better ways to cope with his high anxiety. As the patient behaves more maturely, the nurse must help significant others learn to interact with him as an adult. This is another instance in which family therapy is often an important part of the treatment plan.

■ **Intervening in manipulation**

■ **FAMILY INVOLVEMENT.** Significant others must be involved in the plan of care for the manipulative patient. Their involvement is needed because manipulative people often shift attention away from themselves by creating conflict between the family and the staff. For instance, the patient may complain to his family about his treatment, leading them to complain to the staff about poor nursing care. At the same time the patient may be telling the staff about mistreatment by his family. The staff interprets the family's complaint as their guilt related to past mistreatment of the patient. Staff and family are then in conflict. Attention is distracted from the patient, who avoids the discomfort of looking at his own behavior. When the staff finally realizes what is happening, the result is usually anger at the patient. Nurses should be aware of this tendency and avoid a punitive response. Often, when manipulative patients are hospitalized, this scenario is played out many times. The patient is sent home, still successfully relating to others as objects.

■ **INPATIENT TREATMENT.** Because it is difficult and takes a long time to change manipulative behavior, most patients are treated in the community. However, sometimes hospitalization is needed. For instance, the person with a borderline personality disorder may be self-destructive, or the antisocial person may require a structured environment with limit setting. Kernberg and Haran[22] recommend the following nursing roles in caring for the hospitalized borderline patient:

1. Provide a structured environment.
2. Serve as an emotional sounding board.
3. Clarify and diagnose conflicts.

The authors emphasize the need for clinical supervision.

Countertransference is usually an issue when caring for these patients. Positive countertransference by some staff members, and negative by others, leads to staff conflict. Whenever these behavioral patterns emerge while there is a manipulative patient on the psychiatric unit, the staff must examine their level of involvement with the patient.

Reid[30] addresses countertransference issues as they relate to the antisocial patient. Countertransference feelings may include "impulses to rescue, support, hurt, admire, identify with, or accept compliments from, the patient."[30] The principles of inpatient treatment for antisocial patients include the following:

1. Establish control with no option to escape involvement.
2. Provide an experienced, consistent staff.
3. Implement a strict hierarchical structure, with rules that are firm, not necessarily fair, and rigidly interpreted.
4. Provide support while the patient learns to experience painful feelings.[30]

■ **LIMIT SETTING AND STRUCTURE.** Manipulative patients must be held responsible for their own behavior. They are skilled at placing responsibility on others. Staff members must communicate with each other so that consistent messages are given. These patients recognize any inconsistency and use it to focus attention on others. They usually resist rules. Staff and family members must consistently enforce clear limits.

Masterson[26] describes guidelines for treating borderline patients that incorporate several of these principles. He emphasizes the need for availability of staff attention combined with structured discipline. There must be an expectation that the patient will meet standards of healthy behavior. Failure to meet the standard is identified, and acting out is confronted. Loss of control may be dealt with by room restriction, with the patient instructed to think about the episode so that it may be discussed in therapy. The length of the restriction should be based on the seriousness of the behavior. These approaches usually lead to depression. The depressed feelings should be directed into formal psychotherapy sessions, but the staff can act as role models for appropriate behavior. A school program, occupational therapy, and the milieu may be used to teach age-appropriate social and achievement skills. Reality orientation may also be necessary.

■ **PROTECTION FROM SELF-HARM.** The deliberate self-destructive or self-mutilating behavior of the borderline patient is very difficult to treat. Often the nursing staff must observe the patient constantly to prevent serious physical harm. At the same time these patients have intense dependency needs related to an unresolved separation-individuation developmental phase. This makes it extremely difficult to wean them from constant staff attention, and contact must be decreased very gradually. Observation may need to be increased again if the patient seems out of control. Patient involvement in planning for decreased observation may be helpful. The patient must be reassured that less contact does not equal no contact. Consistent, scheduled time with a staff member is recommended. Primary nursing is particularly effective with a patient who needs to work through these separation issues.

■ **FOCUSING ON STRENGTHS.** Manipulative patients often are effective leaders within the patient group. A useful nursing approach is encouraging them to identify and use their strengths. They may be given responsibilities within the patient care unit and can help other patients with hygiene, eating, and other activities. They are often intelligent and can participate actively in planning their own care. However, they are extremely resistant to recognizing or dealing with feelings and need consistent encouragement to attempt this. Nurses become frustrated with manipulative patients because they seem to be so aware of what is happening and so in control of most situations, yet so unaware of others needs. It must be remembered that they have little tolerance for intimacy. Their maneuvering of others is a way to keep them at a safe distance. Manipulative people are often charming, and it is easy to become involved with them. However, as soon as the other person makes demands or shows signs of emotional closeness, the patient will dilute the relationship by withdrawing, by frustrating the other, or by distracting attention from himself.

■ **BEHAVIOR MODIFICATION.** Behavior modification techniques can help decrease antisocial behavior. The patient is usually impatient with delays in gratification. He prefers material, rather than emotional, rewards. Reinforcers used in a behavior modification program should be concrete and readily available. For example, points may be accumulated to qualify for privileges, such as a weekend at home or a trip to the canteen. Other reinforcers might be a visit or a favorite food. In the past, cigarettes have been used as reinforcers. This is no longer recommended because it adds to the attraction of an unhealthy habit. Ignoring undesirable behavior is the least reinforcing but is not always possible. If behavior is disruptive and there must be a response, it should be matter of fact and one not desired by the patient. For instance, removal from contact with others for a predetermined period may discourage undesirable behavior, whereas a lecture that entails great attention may be a reinforcer.

Behavioral contracting has been tried with borderline patients. McEnany and Tescher[24] describe the goals of behavioral contracting as (1) involving the patient in care planning, (2) decreasing regression, and (3) assisting the patient to maintain control. When a contract is negotiated, control is shared between the nurse and the patient. The nurse-patient contract is negotiated based on patient-identified strengths, learning needs, and goals. However, the patient must agree to basic expectations. These usually include agreement to refrain from harmful behavior, as well as defining the length of time that the contract will be in effect.

No matter what type of disruption in relatedness the patient is experiencing, nursing care is based on accessibility. The nurse must be physically accessible to the patient on a regular basis so that an opportunity exists for interaction. There must also be psychological accessibility. This means that the nurse exhibits interest in the patient. She tries to understand him and clarify communication. She also demonstrates an empathic attitude. If the nurse-patient relationship is a healthy one, the patient can learn how to find satisfaction in other human relationships.

Table 16-4 summarizes some nursing interventions for the patient experiencing disruptions in relatedness.

 ## Evaluation

Evaluating the success or failure of a nursing intervention is difficult when the intervention focuses on the therapeutic relationship. Since the relationship is central to effective delivery of nursing care, it is threatening for many nurses to examine their ability to relate to others. This type of evaluation must take place at two levels. One level focuses on the nurse and her participation in the relationship. Introspection may be useful in accomplishing this, particularly if a nurse stops to review an interaction immediately after it takes place. Blind spots about one's own feelings that may be present while one is involved with the patient may become clearer in retrospect. However, self-evaluation is colored by one's self-perceptions. Supervision from an experienced nurse therapist can be very helpful in identifying aspects of the relationship that may be less obvious to the nurse herself. Constructive su-

pervision can help the nurse to identify the dynamics of the relationship. It can also help her deal with the patient's resistance to change. No matter how experienced a nurse becomes, her own perception of her participation in a relationship is affected by her self-concept. The need for supervision is never lost.

The second level of evaluation focuses on the patient's behavior and the behavioral changes that the nurse works to facilitate. Input about these changes is collected from several sources, with the patient as the primary source. He should be encouraged to discuss experiences with relationships, past and present. Changes in behavior should be validated with the patient to see if he is also aware of change. When the nurse and patient discuss their views of their relationship, the patient is again participating in evaluating its usefulness. Sharing feelings and intimate thoughts denotes increased trust and a willingness to risk self-revelation. Nonverbally the patient also reveals responses to the therapeutic relationship. Accessibility to the nurse for scheduled meetings indicates trust and involvement in the relationship. Eye contact usually occurs more often when one person is comfortable with another. Touching may communicate closeness. Initiation of activities with others indicates more openness to relatedness. Increased decision making and assumption of leadership roles imply improved self-esteem and increasing self-confidence. Such behaviors can be observed, documented, and validated with other staff members. Therefore these are useful evaluation criteria.

Significant others may also contribute to the evaluation. They have known the patient before the occurrence of any behavioral problem and can provide information about the patient's behavioral norms. They are particularly helpful in providing information about changes that continue when the patient is in the community. Some patients have difficulty transferring new behavior to their usual life settings. Involving families in this type of assessment helps to teach the family the behaviors learned by the patient. It gives them an idea of what is reasonable to expect from the patient.

Evaluation takes place continually throughout the course of the relationship. The nurse must review the assessment and add more information as gaps become apparent. Knowledge of past relationship experiences can explain much about present behavior. This should be explored as the relationship grows. Observation of the patient's interaction with significant others may reveal areas that require further exploration. As new behaviors are observed, the nursing diagnosis will be refined. Evaluation of the nursing diagnosis should lead the nurse to revision of the goals. Also, as the nurse

TABLE 16-4

SUMMARY OF NURSING INTERVENTIONS WITH DISRUPTIONS IN RELATEDNESS

*Goal—Growth toward achieving maximum interpersonal satisfaction by establishing
and maintaining self-enhancing relationships with others*

Principle	Rationale	Nursing interventions
Establish a trusting relationship	An atmosphere of trust facilitates open expression of thoughts and feelings; risk taking is necessary when sharing thoughts and feelings; basic trust offers the patient the support needed to take interpersonal risks; support is also important when attempting new behaviors	Initiate a nurse-patient relationship contract mutually agreed on by nurse and patient Develop mutual, behaviorally stated goals for nursing intervention Maintain consistent behavior by all nursing staff members Demonstrate honest communication of responses to the patient's behavior Provide honest, immediate feedback to the patient concerning behavioral change Provide for privacy and comfort during interactions Maintain confidentiality Demonstrate accessibility
Identify and support the patient's strengths	Success in self-care, interpersonal relationships, and activities promotes enhanced self-esteem; recognition of strengths by trusted people helps the patient recognize his positive attributes; attention given to positive behavior is a reward and reinforces the behavioral pattern	Assess the patient's constructive coping behaviors Encourage the patient to perform self-care and make decisions to the extent of his ability Maintain the patient's dignity while providing needed assistance with activities of daily living Offer genuine praise for the patient's accomplishments Initiate activities that allow the patient to experience success Educate the patient and significant others about health care needs and treatment
Promote clear, consistent, and open communication	Healthy interpersonal relationships require open communication; patients with disordered thinking need assistance in identifying and understanding reality; close relationships are often frightening at first and must be encouraged by a supportive environment; clear and consistent limits on behavior reduce the successful use of manipulative behavior	Individualize communication based on the patient's educational level, cultural background, and mental state Use congruent verbal and nonverbal communications Validate the meaning of communications with the patient Recognize the symbolic content of communication Act as a role model by sharing here-and-now feelings, perceptions, and reactions with the patient Give empathic encouragement of self-exploration by the patient Set limits as required in a clear, consistent manner

TABLE 16-4—Cont'd

SUMMARY OF NURSING INTERVENTIONS WITH DISRUPTIONS IN RELATEDNESS

*Goal—Growth toward achieving maximum interpersonal satisfaction by establishing
and maintaining self-enhancing relationships with others*

Principle	Rationale	Nursing interventions
Alleviate high levels of interpersonal anxiety	Severe and panic levels of anxiety result in thought fragmentation, self-absorption, difficulty interpreting internal and external stimuli, impaired judgment, and a shortened attention span; these behaviors interfere with interpersonal relationships; a structured, predictable environment and minimum interpersonal pressure alleviate anxiety	Whenever possible, respond to the patient's stated needs Maintain a calm, supportive approach Minimize environmental stimuli Explain procedures and other events Recognize defensive behaviors used by the patient (e.g., delusions, hallucinations, ego defense mechanisms) Assist the patient to use healthier coping responses, but avoid premature challenge of less healthy ways of coping Teach anxiety-relieving techniques (e.g., relaxation techniques, physical activities) Provide external controls when necessary Provide prescribed medications Promote structure by providing a schedule of activities, giving specific step-by-step instructions, minimizing the need to make choices, and having frequent brief contact with the patient Encourage self-control, but protect the patient from impulsive destructive behavior Respect the patient's need for control of his personal space
Maintain biological integrity	Use of the mechanisms of regression or projection may result in lack of attention to basic biological needs; lack of adequate rest and nutrients can endanger the patient; deficiencies in personal hygiene interfere with the development of interpersonal relationships; psychotropic medications may cause alterations in blood pressure and pulse, sometimes resulting in syncope; these medications also are associated with several distressing side effects, which are usually reversible if appropriate intervention occurs	Assess the patient's eating, sleeping, elimination, and hygiene habits Identify food and fluid preferences If necessary, offer food and fluids at regular intervals Assist patient with eating and drinking if necessary Identify usual elimination patterns Assist to bathroom if necessary Record intake and output if a problem is suspected or identified Record bowel movements and offer prescribed laxatives if needed Monitor vital signs Encourage bathing when needed; assist if necessary Ensure the availability of clean clothing, preferably the patient's own street clothing Ensure the availability of toiletries and cosmetics Encourage appropriate care of hair and teeth Facilitate shaving as desired Provide a restful environment for sleep Initiate sleep-promoting nursing measures Offer prescribed sedation if required Observe for medication side effects and initiate relevant health teaching

and patient become more involved in a mutual relationship, the patient will become more active in identifying nursing needs and setting goals. Nursing actions need constant revision based on feedback from the patient, the patient's family, peers, the clinical supervisor, and self. The nursing approach must be modified as the nurse-patient relationship grows and as the patient moves toward autonomy and the ability to establish and maintain mature interpersonal relationships.

■ **SUGGESTED CROSS-REFERENCES** ■

Therapeutic relationship skills are discussed in Chapter 4. The model of health-illness phenomena is presented in Chapter 3. The phases of the nursing process are discussed in Chapter 5. Nursing interventions related to severe and panic levels of anxiety are described in Chapter 11. Building social skills is described in Chapter 13. Working with dysfunctional families is discussed in Chapter 29.

■ **SUMMARY** ■

1. In a healthy interpersonal relationship, the individuals involved experience intimacy with each other while maintaining separate identities. There should also be a balance between dependent and independent behavior, described as interdependence.
2. The capacity for relatedness develops throughout the life cycle. The normal process of the development of relatedness is described.
3. Possible disruptions that can occur in the process of relatedness include impaired communication, withdrawal, suspicion, dependency, and manipulation.
4. The concept of loneliness is presented as an existential experience involving profound emotional pain and a feeling of total alienation from human relationships. This is differentiated from aloneness and solitude, which may be sought out by those who also are able to relate to others.
5. Predisposing factors and precipitating stressors that lead to disruptions in relatedness include any disruption in the normal interpersonal developmental process; sociocultural factors, including value conflicts, isolation of certain societal groups, and fragmentation of family systems; biochemical formulations, particularly the dopamine hypothesis of schizophrenia; genetic theories; and psychodynamic processes, including the psychoanalytical, interpersonal, and family process models.
6. The behaviors associated with disruptions in relatedness are presented. Behavioral responses include impaired communication, withdrawal, suspicion, dependency, and manipulation. These are examined through presentation of case studies related to the medical diagnoses of paranoid schizophrenia, catatonic schizophrenia, dependent personality disorder, panic disorder, antisocial personality disorder, and borderline personality disorder. An additional case example is provided of an isolated elderly man.
7. Examples of nursing diagnoses and descriptions of medical diagnostic criteria are presented.
8. Coping mechanisms are discussed as they apply to disruptions in the ability to maintain relatedness. The behaviors of impaired communication, withdrawal, suspicion, dependency, and manipulation function as coping mechanisms.
9. Long- and short-term nurse-patient goals pertaining to relatedness emphasize the importance of patient involvement as soon as the nurse-patient relationship has matured to the level that the patient can trust the nurse with his goals.
10. The planning of nursing care is demonstrated by

the presentation of two sample nursing care plans and a mental health education plan.

11. The therapeutic nurse-patient relationship for a patient who has problems with relatedness is important. Withdrawn persons require a consistent, patient approach, with attention given to biological, psychological, and social needs.

12. Trust is the central issue in working with a suspicious patient. Reliability and consistency are essential for the growth of trust, as is respect for the patient's need for privacy. The nursing role in terms of the patient's biological integrity must also be considered.

13. Nursing intervention with the dependent patient focuses on helping the patient to express feelings and ideas, make decisions, accept pleasure, and control panic. A behavior modification approach may be helpful with a dependent person.

14. Consistency and limit setting are primary nursing interventions with manipulative patients. Possible nursing approaches include the patient's involvement in care planning, protection from destructive behavior, and behavior modification.

15. Nursing interventions are suggested for patients who are unable to communicate clearly. The nurse must attend to both verbal and nonverbal levels of communication and understand the symbolic nature of psychotic communication.

16. Accessibility of the nurse to the patient is of primary importance when the problem is one of relatedness.

17. Evaluation of nursing care must involve the patient, the nurse, other staff, and significant others. The need for validation of observations is essential, as is the ongoing need for clinical supervision of nursing care by an experienced nurse therapist.

REFERENCES

1. American Psychiatric Association: Diagnostic and statistical manual of mental disorders, ed 3, revised (DSM-III-R), Washington, DC, 1987, American Psychiatric Association.
2. Bartko JJ: Statistical basis for exploring schizophrenia, Am J Psychiatry 138:941, 1981.
3. Bateson G et al: Toward a theory of schizophrenia. In Howells JG, editor: Theory and practice of family psychiatry, New York, 1971, Brunner/Mazel, Inc.
4. Berman KF and Weinberger DR: Schizophrenia: brain structure and function. In Kaplan HI and Sadock BJ, editors: Comprehensive textbook of psychiatry, ed 5, Baltimore, 1989, Williams & Wilkins.
5. Brown RP and Mann JJ: A clinical perspective on the role of neurotransmitters in mental disorders, Hosp Community Psychiatry 36:141, 1985.
6. Burnham D, Gladstone A, and Gibson R: Schizophrenia and the need-fear dilemma, New York, 1969, International Universities Press.
7. Carpenter WT, Jr: The phenomenology of schizophrenia, Am J Psychiatry 138:948, 1981.
8. Cloninger CR: Schizophrenia: genetic etiological factors. In Kaplan HI and Sadock BJ, editors: Comprehensive textbook of psychiatry, ed 5, Baltimore, 1989, Williams & Wilkins.
9. Copel LC: Loneliness: a conceptual model, J Psychosoc Ment Health Serv 26:14, Jan 1988.
10. Danziger S: Major treatment issues and techniques in family therapy with the borderline adolescent, J Psychosoc Nurs Ment Health Serv 20:27, Jan 1982.
11. Field WE: Hearing voices, J Psychosoc Nurs Ment Health Serv 23:9, Jan 1985.
12. Field WE and Ruelke W: Hallucinations and how to deal with them, Am J Nurs 73:638, 1973.
13. Fromm-Reichmann F: On loneliness. In Bullard DM, editor: Psychoanalysis and psychotherapy, Chicago, 1960, University of Chicago Press.
14. Gordon S: Lonely in America, New York, 1976, Simon & Schuster, Inc.
15. Grebb JA and Cancro R: Schizophrenia: clinical features. In Kaplan HI and Sadock BJ, editors: Comprehensive textbook of psychiatry, ed 5, Baltimore, 1989, Williams & Wilkins.
16. Greenberg L et al: An interdisciplinary psychoeducation program for schizophrenic patients and their families in an acute care setting, Hosp Community Psychiatry 39:277, 1988.
17. Gunderson JG: Borderline personality disorder, Washington, DC, 1984, American Psychiatric Press, Inc.
18. Hill D: Outpatient management of passive-dependent women, Hosp Community Psychiatry 21:402, 1970.
19. Hirschfeld RMA: Personality disorders: foreword. In Frances AJ and Hales RE, editors: Psychiatry update, vol 5, Washington, DC, 1986, American Psychiatric Press, Inc.
20. Kahn EM: Psychotherapy with chronic schizophrenics: alliance, transference and countertransference, J Psychosoc Nurs Ment Health Serv 22:20, July, 1984.
21. Kanter J, Lamb HR, and Loeper C: Expressed emotion in families: a critical review, Hosp Community Psychiatry 38:374, 1987.
22. Kernberg O and Haran C: Milieu treatment with borderline patients, J Psychosoc Nurs Ment Health Serv 22:29, Apr 1984.
23. Liberman RP et al: The nature and problem of schizophrenia. In Bellack AS, editor: Schizophrenia: treatment, management and rehabilitation, New York, 1984, Grune & Stratton, Inc.
24. McEnany GW and Tescher BE: Contracting for care: one nursing approach to the hospitalized borderline patient, J Psychosoc Nurs Ment Health Serv 23:11, Apr 1985.
25. McGlashan TH: Schizophrenia: psychodynamic theories. In Kaplan HI and Sadock BJ, editors: Comprehensive textbook of psychiatry, ed 5, Baltimore, 1989, Williams & Wilkins.
26. Masterson JF: Treatment of the borderline adolescent, New York, 1985, Brunner/Mazel, Inc.

27. Mullahy P: Psychoanalysis and interpersonal psychiatry: the contributions of Harry Stack Sullivan, New York, 1970, Science House, Inc.

28. Packard V: A nation of strangers, New York, 1972, The David McKay Co.

29. Pfohl B and Andreasen NC: Schizophrenia: diagnosis and classification. In Frances AJ and Hales RE, editors: Psychiatry update, vol 5, Washington, DC, 1986, American Psychiatric Press, Inc.

30. Reid WH: The antisocial personality: a review, Hosp Community Psychiatry 36:831, 1985.

31. Rogers C: On becoming a person, Boston, 1961, Houghton Mifflin Co.

32. Schwartzman ST: The hallucinating patient and nursing intervention, J Psychiatr Nurs 13:23, Nov-Dec 1975.

33. Searles HF: Collected papers on schizophrenia and related subjects, New York, 1965, International Universities Press, Inc.

34. Shostrom E: Man, the manipulator, Nashville, Tenn, 1967, Abingdon Press.

35. Spitz RA: The first year of life: a psychoanalytic study of normal and deviant development of object relations, New York, 1965, International Universities Press.

36. Sullivan H: The interpersonal theory of psychiatry, New York, 1953, WW Norton & Co, Inc.

37. Thomas M: Trust in the nurse-patient relationship. In Carlson C, editor: Behavioral concepts and nursing intervention, Philadelphia, 1970, JB Lippincott Co.

38. Vaughn C and Leff J: The measurement of expressed emotion in the families of psychiatric patients. Part 2, Br J Soc Clin Psychol 15:157, 1976.

39. Welt SR: The developmental roots of loneliness, Arch Psych Nurs 1:25, 1987.

40. Wildman LL: Reducing the schizophrenic patient's resistance to involvement, Perspect Psychiatr Care 3:26, 1965.

41. Will GT: A sociopsychiatric nursing approach to intervention in a problem of mutual withdrawal on a mental hospital ward, Psychiatry 15(2):193, 1952.

42. Will OA: Human relatedness and the schizophrenic reaction. In Stein MI, editor: Contemporary psychotherapies, New York, 1961, The Free Press.

43. World Health Organization: Report of the International Pilot Study of Schizophrenia. Vol 1: results of the initial evaluation phase, Geneva, 1973, The Organization.

44. World Health Organization: Schizophrenia: an international follow-up study, New York, 1979, John Wiley & Sons, Inc.

45. Wyatt RJ, Kirch DG, and DeLisi LE: Schizophrenia: biochemical, endocrine, and immunological studies. In Kaplan HI and Sadock BJ, editors: Comprehensive textbook of psychiatry, ed 5, Baltimore, 1989, Williams & Wilkins.

46. Wynne LC: Current concepts about schizophrenics and family relationships, J Nerv Ment Dis 169:82, 1981.

47. Wynne LC, Toohey ML, and Doane J: Family studies. In Bellak L, editor: Disorders of the schizophrenic syndrome, New York, 1979, Basic Books, Inc, Publishers.

■ ANNOTATED SUGGESTED READINGS ■

Bellack AS, editor: Schizophrenia: treatment, management and rehabilitation, New York, 1984, Grune & Stratton, Inc.

Collection of papers on many aspects of schizophrenia by experienced investigators, who present the most recent findings of their research. Written at a level that requires understanding of more basic concepts; particularly recommended for advanced practitioners, faculty, and graduate students.

Brown RP and Mann JJ: A clinical perspective on the role of neurotransmitters in mental disorders, Hosp Community Psychiatry 36:141, 1985.

Provides a complete overview of biological theories of etiology of schizophrenia and affective disorders. The charts linking pharmacological actions with neurotransmitter activity are particularly useful.

Bullard DM: Psychoanalysis and psychotherapy: selected papers of Frieda Fromm-Reichmann, Chicago, 1959, The University of Chicago Press.

Provides insight into the philosophy of an outstanding psychotherapist. Includes a section on schizophrenia that provides application of psychoanalytical theory to therapy with schizophrenic patients.[1]

*Chesla CA: Parents' illness models of schizophrenia, Arch Psych Nurs 3:218, 1989.

Identifies four models of schizophrenia described by parents who are primary care providers: strong biological, rational control, normalizing, and survival through symptoms. Nurses can be more helpful to families if they understand these models and their influence on the parent's response to the child.

Cleckley H: The mask of sanity, ed 5, St Louis, 1976, Mosby–Year Book, Inc.

Classic presentation of the characteristics of the antisocial personality. Detailed case histories are a rich source of graphic descriptive data on these patient's behavior. Does not focus greatly on treatment.

*Danziger S: Major treatment issues and techniques in family therapy with the borderline adolescent, J Psychosoc Nurs Ment Health Serv 20:27, 1982.

Presents a clear description of the complex behaviors and defenses of the borderline patient. Demonstrates, through the use of case-study vignettes, the interactive process between the adolescent and the family. Suggests techniques for therapeutic intervention. The interventions are beyond the level of the generalist, but the explanation of the defenses would be very helpful to all psychiatric nurses.

*Field WE and Ruelke W: Hallucinations and how to deal with them, Am J Nurs 73:638, 1973.

Describes developmental phases related to auditory hallucinations and postulates nursing intervention based on this developmental process.

Fromm-Reichmann F: On loneliness. In Bullard DM, editor: Psychoanalysis and psychotherapy, Chicago, 1960, University of Chicago Press.

Classic presentation of loneliness as experienced by the psychotic person. Written compassionately and includes thoughts about therapy with these patients.

---

*Asterisk indicates nursing reference

*Gallop R: The patient is splitting: everyone knows and nothing changes, J Psychosoc Nurs Ment Health Serv 23:6, Apr 1985.

Describes the consultation/supervision process as it relates to nursing staff working with borderline patients. Uses a case study to illustrate the staff splitting that these patients often cause, and discusses approaches to dealing with countertransference.

Goldman CR and Quinn FL: Effects of a patient education program in the treatment of schizophrenia, Hosp Community Psychiatry 39:282, 1988.

Reports on a study of a structured education program's effects on the positive and negative symptoms of schizophrenia as well as on knowledge of resources and of the illness. The experimental group had increased knowledge and decreased negative symptoms. No significant effect on positive symptoms occurred.

Gorton G and Akhtar S: The literature on personality disorders, 1985-88: trends and controversies, Hosp Community Psychiatry 41:39, 1990.

Discusses problems differentiating disorders, research needs, and treatment issues. Recommended for advanced practitioners.

Gunderson JG: Borderline personality disorder, Washington, DC, 1984, American Psychiatric Press, Inc.

Written by a psychotherapist with extensive experience in providing therapy to borderline personality disorder patients. Invaluable description of the problem's etiology and suggestions regarding interventions. Highly recommended for any nurses who provide care to these difficult patients.

Kanas N: Therapy groups for schizophrenic patients on acute care units, Hosp Community Psychiatry 39:546, 1988.

Describes use of open, homogeneous therapy groups as a part of the treatment program for schizophrenic patients in a short-term acute care setting. Presents practical information on structure and process.

*Kroah J: Strategies for interviewing in language and thought disorders, J Psychiatr Nurs 12:3, Mar-Apr 1974.

Identifies several disordered communication patterns and therapeutic nursing approaches. Particularly helpful for the neophyte.

Leete E: The treatment of schizophrenia: a patient's perspective, Hosp Community Psychiatry 38:486, 1987.

Recommended for all students and practitioners of psychiatric nursing. Describes experiences of a psychiatric patient and suggests ways to be helpful to a person with schizophrenia.

Lovejoy M: Recovery from schizophrenia: a personal odyssey, Hosp Community Psychiatry 35:809, 1985.

Not only describes the author's feelings, but also presents some techniques that she devised to deal with her symptoms. Calls on mental health professionals to be flexible and open to individualizing approaches according to patient needs.

*McEnany GW and Tescher BE: Contracting for care: one nursing approach to the hospitalized borderline patient, J Psychosoc Nurs Ment Health Serv 23:11, 1985.

Contracting with borderline patients provides structure and accountability in the treatment process. Case example demonstrates the use of contracting. Also describes a case in which this approach did not work.

Masterson JF: Treatment of the borderline adolescent, New York, 1985, Brunner/Mazel, Inc.

Explains the disruption in the developmental process that leads to borderline personality disorder. Also provides a thorough discussion of treatment in hospital and outpatient settings, including the identified patient and his parents.

*O'Brien P, Caldwell C, and Transeau G: Destroyers: written treatment contracts can help cure self destructive behaviors of the borderline patient, J Psychosoc Nurs Ment Health Serv 23:19, Apr 1985.

Describes the application of treatment contracting to nursing intervention with borderline patients. A case study illustrates the use of a contract with a patient who had been self-destructive.

Ruesch J: Disturbed communication, New York, 1972, WW Norton & Co, Inc.

Applies classic work in communication theory to communication patterns associated with various psychiatric disorders. Helpful for conceptualizing communication problems and planning appropriate interventions.

*Runyon N, Allen CL, and Ilnicki SH: The borderline patient on the med-surg unit, Am J Nurs 88:1644, 1988.

Provides a practical approach to the potentially disruptive behavior of the borderline patient in a medical-surgical setting. Includes sample interactions and a care plan.

Satir V: Peoplemaking, Palo Alto, Calif, 1972, Science & Behavior Books, Inc.

Focuses on family development and role structure as it describes roles that facilitate or block healthy communication. Shows how the use of blocking roles contributes to manipulative behavior.

Searles HF: Collected papers on schizophrenia and related subjects, New York, 1965, International Universities Press, Inc.

Presents views on psychotherapy with schizophrenic patients. Impressive because of the empathy with patients that is shown.

Shostrom EL: Man, the manipulator, Nashville, Tenn, 1967, Abingdon Press.

Comprehensive analysis of manipulative behavior in terms of the development, manifestations, and implications of manipulation. Specifically relates theory to various interpersonal situations and describes the therapeutic approach.

Torrey EF: Surviving schizophrenia: a family manual, New York, 1983, Harper & Row, Publishers, Inc.

Written for a lay audience but also worthwhile reading for professionals. Physician advocate for high-quality treatment for the seriously mentally disabled views schizophrenia as a brain disease and presents supporting evidence.

*Vogel CH et al: Exploring the concept of manipulation in psychiatric settings, Arch Psych Nurs 1:429, 1987.

Describes two studies undertaken to determine how nurses define the concept of manipulation. Cites need for additional research, including the development of a reliable definition and related nursing definitions.

Walsh M: Schizophrenia: straight talk for families and friends, New York, 1985, William Morrow and Co, Inc.

Excellent presentation of schizophrenia's impact on the family. Describes the author's experiences with the mental health care system and those of other families. Nurses should recom-

mend this book to families of patients. Contains much information and advice, including a list of rehabilitation resources.

*Will GT: A sociopsychiatric nursing approach to interven-
tion in a problem of mutual withdrawal on a mental hospital ward, Psychiatry 15(2):193, 1952.

Should be read and reread by every student of psychiatric
nursing. Demonstrates the use of the nursing process to problem-solve and provide therapeutic nursing care for withdrawn
patients.

Will OA: Human relatedness and the schizophrenic reaction.
In Stein MI, editor: Contemporary psychotherapies, New
York, 1961, The Free Press.

Absorbing account of psychotherapy with schizophrenic patients is based on the interpersonal theory of psychiatry. Includes
excellent descriptions of Sullivan's theory applied to the etiology
and course of schizophrenia.

World Health Organization: Report of the International Pilot Study of Schizophrenia. Vol 1: results of the initial
evaluation phase, Geneva, 1973, The Organization.

World Health Organization: Schizophrenia: an international
follow-up study, New York, 1979, John Wiley & Sons,
Inc.

Present's the results of a longitudinal epidemiological study
of schizophrenia in nine countries. Detail's the study's construction, as well as data collected and conclusions. Highly recommended for nurses interested in research, education, or advanced clinical practice.

Zimmerman M and Coryell W: DSM-III personality disorder diagnoses in a nonpatient sample, Arch Gen Psychiatry
46:682, 1989.

Examines relatives of patients for Axis I and Axis II disorders. Analyzes personality disorders related to comorbidity and
demographics. Raises questions related to the distinguishing
features of the various personality disorders and the relationships among the personality disorders as well as Axis I disorders.

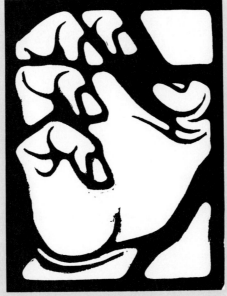

© 1990 M.C. Escher Heirs/Cordon Art, Baarn, Holland.

Healthy children raised in decent conditions among loving people in a gentle and just society where freedom and equality are valued will rarely commit violent acts toward others.

Ramsay Clark, A Few Modest Proposals to Reduce Individual Violence in America*

C H A P T E R   17

PROBLEMS WITH THE EXPRESSION OF ANGER

DIAGNOSTIC PREVIEW

MEDICAL DIAGNOSES RELATED TO PROBLEMS WITH THE EXPRESSION OF ANGER

- Disruptive behavior disorders
  Conduct disorder
  Oppositional defiant disorder

- Delusional (paranoid) disorder

- Organic personality syndrome, explosive type

- Paranoid personality disorder

LEARNING OBJECTIVES

After studying this chapter, the student should be able to:

- define anger in relationship to anxiety resulting from a threat.

- describe the continuum of behavior related to the feeling of anger.

- compare and contrast the biological/instinctual, frustration-aggression, and social learning theories concerning the predisposing factors related to anger.

- identify precipitating stressors related to the expression of anger.

- analyze biological responses to anger relative to high levels of anxiety and the fight-or-flight response.

- differentiate among passive, aggressive, and assertive behaviors.

- identify coping mechanisms relative to the experience of angry or aggressive feelings.

- formulate individualized nursing diagnoses for patients with problems with the expression of anger.

- assess the relationship between nursing diagnoses and medical diagnoses associated with anger.

- develop long- and short-term individualized nursing goals with patients who are having problems with the expression of anger.

- develop a mental health education plan to help the patient express anger assertively.

- examine one's own responses to anger.

- describe the process involved in developing assertive behavior.

- apply therapeutic nurse-patient relationship principles with appropriate rationale in planning the care of the angry patient.

- set appropriate limits on acting-out behavior.

- describe safe procedures for intervention in potential or actual violent behavior.

- assess the importance of the evaluation of the nursing process when working with patients with problems with the expression of anger.

- identify directions for future nursing research.

- select appropriate readings for further study.

Anger is a feeling of resentment that occurs as a response to anxiety when the individual perceives a threat. It is characterized by a feeling of tension. It is possible to suppress the overt expression of anger, but sooner or later, perhaps in a very different form, the tension will be released. The chronically angry person may develop a duodenal ulcer, become depressed, or react inappropriately at a minor mishap. These are all signs that anger has not been expressed productively. Other persons may deal with anger by joining the armed forces, kneading bread, or writing a symphony. These expressions are examples of sublimation and may be constructive for the individual. However, the basic issue is still avoided.

Immediate expression of anger at its cause is healthy and satisfying. This is also the most difficult response. Culturally, direct expression of anger is discouraged. Children are taught to "play nice." Little boys who fight are chastised; little girls should never even think of fighting. Because of these attitudes, many people grow up fearing anger and viewing it as abnormal. Angry feelings are then often expressed indirectly.

Fear of expressing anger is related to fear of rejection. Parental disapproval is a powerful influence on the child's behavior. The expectation of similar disapproval from significant others influences adults. Yet it is hard not to become angry at those on whom we depend. We expect that our needs will be anticipated and met. Sometimes we even believe that our needs will be recognized without direct expression. When needs are not met, disappointment and, frequently, anger result. An inner conflict exists, because direct expression of anger to the other person may result in rejection, thus further reducing the possibility of gratification. On the other hand, failure to express the feeling leads to resentment and interferes with the relationship. Rothenberg[29] states, "When anger is accompanied by a clear communication, it is a sign of basic respect for a loved person."

People also become angry at life situations. If the car breaks down or the bank is closed or the taxes go up, an individual becomes angry. However, this anger seems to be much easier to express. In fact, the person may repeat the story several times, apparently becoming more emotionally aroused each time. This kind of experience can help the person express stored up anger and is a displacement of angry feelings from a threatening to a less threatening situation.

For some people, life situations become so overwhelming that anger is expressed as violent behavior.

Poverty, unemployment, and family instability are known to contribute to a higher incidence of family violence and violent crime.

Continuum of responses to anger

Anger may be described on a continuum. Mild anger, felt as annoyance, is a part of everyday life. Small annoyances may be forgotten almost immediately. For instance, most people have had the experience of undressing, discovering a small bruise, and not remembering how it happened. Earlier in the day they probably bumped themselves, cried out, and then forgot the incident.

At the next level is interference with accomplishment of a goal, resulting in frustration. For example, a sudden thunderstorm may cause cancellation of a family picnic. Temporary confusion results as those affected share their feelings of angry disappointment. However, when feelings have been expressed, alternatives are considered and modified goals are set. The feelings associated with the experience will be remembered but are quickly resolved.

Further along the continuum, anger is more intense when frustration occurs and acceptable alternatives cannot be found. The person who has lost a job or has been told he has a terminal illness may feel anger related to impotence. This level of anger is more difficult to express and to resolve. This anger may preoccupy much of the person's attention and interfere with his ability to function productively. Concerned support from significant others, and sometimes professional counseling, may be necessary.

The extreme experience of anger is rage or fury. Rothenberg[29] differentiates anger from violence, hostility, and revenge, which involve destructiveness. At this level the person is totally consumed by angry feelings and unable to control their expression. At this point violence may occur, and there is a danger to the angry person and to others who are nearby. Rage may result from a long series of frustrating experiences that have depleted the person's coping abilities. It is also seen in psychotic states when the person is completely unable to cope with frustration. Rage is a primitive response. It is, in fact, seen in babies and small children who have not yet developed adaptive mechanisms. The fury of a 2-year-old having a temper tantrum would be difficult to control in an adult. This extreme degree of anger is frightening. Fear of losing control and becoming violent inhibits many people from overtly expressing anger.

Anger is not necessarily negative. As a feeling it

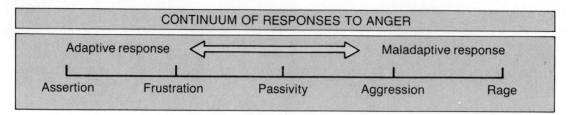

Fig. 17-1. Continuum of coping responses related to feelings of anger.

has a neutral value. Anger may be used in positive ways. For instance, a person who is frustrated by inability to accomplish a goal can use anger as a motivator to seek alternatives. A citizen who is angry about conditions in his community can use that anger to involve others in seeking change. Open expression of anger can strengthen a relationship by communicating mutual respect and confidence in the other person.

Awareness of the positive aspects of anger is important to a therapeutic nurse-patient relationship. Rather than discouraging the expression of anger, the nurse may help the patient use its positive functions constructively. Fig. 17-1 illustrates the continuum of responses to anger.

Nurses encounter anger frequently in the course of providing patient care. A disruption in health is a frustration, and frustration results in anger. In addition, the health care system is complex and may add to the patient's frustrations, leading to still more anger. Therefore nurses must understand anger, become aware of their own responses to angry feelings, and help patients express anger in a healthy and productive way.

Unfortunately, nurses may also encounter instances in which the anger of a staff member is expressed inappropriately toward a patient. Patient abuse is a persistent problem in health care settings, particularly if staff are working under stressful conditions. Abuse may be physical, ranging from handling a patient roughly to actual physical assault. It may also be psychological, including speaking rudely, cursing, using sarcasm, or ignoring a patient's needs. Whenever a nurse encounters this upsetting situation, she has a legal and ethical obligation to intervene directly if the patient is in immediate danger. If no immediate danger is present, the nurse may choose to report the incident to the appropriate supervisory nurse. The principles discussed in Chapter 32 on the abusive family may also be applied to abuse that occurs in a health care setting.

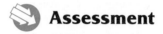 **Assessment**

There are several theories on the nature of the process of anger. In general, they may be categorized as biological, psychological, and social. No definite evidence gives one theory more validity than any other. There is a strong probability that anger really results from a combination of all these factors and the person's unique personality structure.

■ **Predisposing factors**
■ **BIOLOGICAL FACTORS**
Instinctual drive theory. Two major theorists, Sigmund Freud and Konrad Lorenz, have hypothesized that human aggression evolves from instinctual drives. Late in the development of his psychoanalytical theory, Freud came to believe that the person was under the influence of two basic drives. The first was the life drive, Eros, expressed through sexuality. The second was the death drive, Thanatos, expressed through aggression. Freud believed that life was a struggle to maintain a balance between the two drives. He hypothesized that destructive behavior such as suicide occurred when the death drive gained supremacy. Because of the strength of the drive, humans were always pressured to behave destructively, with the aim being either toward the self or toward others. This was described by Fromm as the "tragic alternative."[11:15]

Konrad Lorenz is a physician and naturalist. His theory of aggression is based on observations of animals, from fish and birds through the evolutionary ladder to humans. He believes an instinctual aggressive drive is common to all animals. Lorenz[16] acknowledges that this theory may be difficult to accept because of the comparison between human beings and other species. However, he maintains that human aggression derives from the same type of instinctual force as that of other species. He also states that modern man "suffers from insufficient discharge of his aggressive drive."[16:243] This inability to release aggression may result in various self-destructive behaviors, including neuroses and accidents.

An interesting and controversial aspect of the instinctive theories is the fact that they do not allow for the exercise of individual control. Essentially, they state that aggression will occur no matter what the person does. For some this idea is repugnant, since it implies that humans are simply the slaves of their drives. To others it is appealing because of the implication that the individual need not assume responsibility for his behavior. However, the hypothesis that aggression originates instinctively does not preclude the choice of its expression. The related behavior may be constructive or destructive according to individual choice.

Neurobiological theories. Montague[21] describes the biological mechanisms that are believed to be associated with anger. She describes stimulus complexes that activate neural circuits, causing a tendency for the individual to behave aggressively. The involved neurons are located in various areas of the brain and may be facilitated or inhibited by inputs from other neural systems. The limbic system plays a central role in both stimulating and inhibiting the aggressive responses. Research in this area is being pursued. This research is difficult because the affective areas tend to be buried deep in the primitive areas of the brain; therefore much of the research so far has been performed on animals. Fromm[11] links this neural response to the "fight-or-flight" mechanism and views it as an innate method of self-preservation. Eichelman has identified four theories involving neurotransmitters and other mechanisms that are being investigated:

1. In animals, stimulation of the gamma aminobutyric acid (GABA) seems to decrease aggressive behavior. Administration of benzodiazepines enhances the GABA system and has been noted to decrease aggression in people.
2. Animal studies suggest that norepinephrine increases aggression. There is some evidence that this is also true in people. Lithium carbonate decreases the functional availability of norepinephrine and has been shown to decrease aggressive behavior. Propranolol, a beta adrenergic receptor blocker, has had the same effect.
3. Serotonin appears to inhibit aggression. Lithium carbonate also affects the uptake of tryptophan, a serotonin precursor. It is possible that the lithium effect on aggression could be related to this factor. Some studies have reported a decrease in aggression related to administration of tryptophan and related compounds.
4. Epilepsy has been reported to be associated with some instances of impulsive aggression. The anticonvulsant drugs phenytoin and primidone have been effective at times in decreasing aggressive behavior. Recently, several studies have demonstrated a good response to carbamazepine.

Ochitill[24] has identified additional factors that predispose the individual to violent behavior. Substance abusers are prone to violent outbursts, especially if deprived of their supply of drugs. The experience of pain results in irritability, sometimes progressing to violence. Also, some types of organic brain disorder may lead to violent behavior, particularly if a lesion is present in the part of the brain responsible for mediating anger.

■ **PSYCHOLOGICAL FACTORS**

Frustration-aggression theory. One psychological approach to the evolution of aggressive behavior is the frustration-aggression theory developed by Dollard and co-workers.[6] According to this theory, all aggression results from frustration. Frustration occurs when the person is thwarted in an attempt to achieve a desired goal. The sense of frustration, and thereby the degree of aggression, is increased if the goal is highly valued or if the person has made repeated attempts to achieve it. According to Fromm,[11] this theory has been criticized recently because no allowance is made for stressors other than frustration that might lead to aggression.

Frustration may be experienced as a threat, and the anxiety that results from a threat may be experienced as anger. In addition to frustration, other threats lead to anger. One is the threatened loss of self-esteem. In this case the stressor may be real, as in the threatened loss of a job, or imagined, as when a mother interprets her child's leaving home for college as a rejection of herself. Conflict may also be viewed as threatening and lead to an aggressive response. An important element of a threatening situation is the person's perceived lack of control. Aggression can be an attempt to overcome the threat by taking control of the situation.

Behavioral theory. Behaviorists view aggression as a learned response that has been reinforced by goal achievement. For instance, 4-year-old Johnny wants a cookie just before dinner. When his mother refuses, Johnny has a temper tantrum. If his mother then gives him a cookie, Johnny has learned that an aggressive outburst will be rewarded. If similar situations continue to occur, Johnny will use an aggressive approach to need satisfaction. It is important to note that others learn that nonaggression is rewarded. Thus the behaviorists explain the range of aggressive behaviors that exist.

Existential theory. Erich Fromm[11] presents a different psychological theory. He believes that behavior is based on several existential needs, which must be met. These include the needs for an object of devotion, relatedness, unity and rootedness, effectiveness, and stimulation and excitation. For each need there are both positive and negative approaches to satisfaction. The need for effectiveness may be met by loving, productive behavior or by sadistic, destructive behavior. When the person is not able to meet his needs through positive constructive behavior, he will resort to negative destructive behavior. Fromm describes the latter person as an "existential failure, a man who has failed to become what he could be according to the possibilities of his existence." The failure is a result of social conditions, combined with the individual's reason and will.

■ **SOCIOCULTURAL FACTORS.** Social and cultural factors may also influence angry behavior. Cultural norms help to define acceptable and unacceptable means of expressing aggressive feelings. Sanctions are applied to violators of the norms through the legal system. By this means society controls violent behavior and attempts to maintain a safe existence for its members. Unfortunately, this prohibition against violent behavior is often extended to include any form of expression of anger. This inhibits people from healthy expression of angry feelings and leads to suppression.

Social environment theory. The social environment in which the person lives influences his attitude toward expressing anger and the means he chooses to do so. A cultural norm that supports verbally assertive expressions of anger will help persons deal with anger in a healthy manner. A norm that reinforces violent behavior will result in physical expression of anger in destructive ways. Madden[18] notes that persons who have a history of being victimized are more likely to become violent. They have internalized a norm legitimizing aggressive acting out of anger. He also links a history of deprivation, inadequate social adjustment, and a lack of interpersonal relationship skills with increased incidence of violent behavior.

Urban life tends to foster increased aggressive behavior. In part, this may be related to the theory of personal space. Crowding is prevalent in cities. When people have little privacy or when they feel that their area of personal space has been invaded, their response

is frequently aggressive. In ghetto areas, where overcrowding is common, this anger becomes a smoldering resentment that can erupt into violence.

Fast[9] reports on a study by Kinzel in which personal space needs of men who were imprisoned for violent behavior were compared with those of prisoners with no history of violent behavior. It was found that the violent group required twice the personal space of the nonviolent group. What would seem to most people to be a comfortable interpersonal distance would for these men be a provocation to a violent outburst. When combined with alcohol use, this tendency is particularly explosive, since usual social inhibitions are decreased as a result of drinking.

Issues related to personal space are also pertinent in a hospital setting. Nursing and medical care that involves touching is a direct invasion of intimate space. Patients may attempt to identify areas that belong to them, usually including the area immediately surrounding the bed, but sometimes extending to other areas, such as a particular chair in the day area or dining room. Intentional or accidental use of this space by another can lead to an angry outburst.

When aggressive behavior occurs in a hospital setting, it is important to analyze the characteristics of the milieu, as well as those of the patient. Intervention in staff behaviors sometimes results in positive behavioral change for patients.

Social learning theory. According to Roberts, the social learning theory was originated by Miller and Dollard and later extended first by Rotter and then by Bandura and Walters.[27] According to these theorists, aggressive behavior is learned as a part of the socialization process. This is essentially a behaviorist model of personality development. Children who grow up in violent settings learn to use aggression as an acceptable means of meeting their needs. Aggressive behavior may be learned by imitation or by direct experience.[27] Imitation may be related to the family, subculture, or symbolical models. It has been noted that parents who were victims of child abuse are more likely to abuse their own children. This is an example of imitation of a familial pattern. Subcultural patterns that lead to imitation of aggressive behavior involve the acceptance of violence as a means of achieving status. These include such diverse activities as violent crime, aggressive sports, and war. The probable influence of television on violent behavior is an example of symbolical modeling. There have been court cases in which the defense for a violent crime was the fact that the assailant had watched a similar act on television. It has also been observed that following a well-publicized act of violence, such as an assassination or mass murder, frequently a spate of similar assaults or threats of assaults occurs. A cultural paradox in the United States is the contrast between the generally stated value that peace is good and the fascinated attention that is given to violence.

According to the social learning theory, another way of learning aggressive behavior is by direct experience.[28] This aspect of the theory draws heavily on behavioral theory: behavior that is rewarded will recur. This approach has been discussed as a psychological predisposing factor related to aggression. Social learning theorists also accept the premise that biological components of aggressive behavior interact with the psychosocial aspects. Overt acts of aggression occur most likely as a result of the interaction of the person's biological, psychological, and sociocultural characteristics, and each of these factors must be considered as components of the nursing assessment.

■ Precipitating stressors

Specific reasons for angry behavior vary from person to person. The nurse needs to communicate with the patient to understand the events that he perceives as anger provoking. In general, anger occurs in response to a perceived threat. This may be a threat of physical injury, or more common, a threat to the self-concept. When the self is threatened, the person may not be entirely aware of the source of his anger. In this case, the nurse and patient need to work together to identify the nature of the threat.

A threat may be external or internal. Examples of external stressors are physical attack, loss of a significant relationship, and criticism from others. Internal stressors might include a sense of failure at work, perceived loss of love, and fear of physical illness. Anger is only one of the possible emotional responses to these stressors. Some individuals might respond with depression or withdrawal. However, those reactions are usually accompanied by anger, which may be difficult for the person to express directly. Depression is sometimes viewed as anger directed toward the self, and withdrawal may also be a passive expression of anger.

Frequently anger seems out of proportion to the event that seemed to cause it. A relatively insignificant stressor may be "the last straw" and result in the release of a flood of feelings that have been stored up over time. Nurses need to be aware of this and to refrain from personalizing anger expressed by a patient. The nurse may seem to be a safer target than significant others with whom the patient may also be angry. If an angry experience is to be understood, stressors must be evaluated in terms of number, intensity, and meaning to the patient.

Violence or the threat of violent behavior may be the result of fear of loss of control and a search for external limits. Nigrosh[23] relates this to two factors. The first is a need to accomplish the developmental task of self-control. Lack of control is thus associated with infantile behavior. The second factor is the internalization of values opposing violence. Violation of this norm results in guilt. Patients who communicate imminent loss of control need prompt provision of external controls.

The risk of loss of control may also be assessed based on the patient's history of threatening violent behavior. McNiel and Binder[17] found that 58% of patients who made threats prior to hospitalization required seclusion and 32% assaulted someone. In particular, schizophrenic patients who had made threats tended to have violent episodes. If the patient is unable or unwilling to provide information about threats the nurse should try to obtain it from significant others.

Other events may precipitate violent behavior in hospitalized patients. Conn and Lion[4] have documented that assaults on staff were most likely to occur during seclusion of a patient, in the course of a verbal argument, or following denial of a privilege by a staff member. Depp[5] found that assaults in a public mental hospital were more common when there was a high level of demand for patients to increase their activity. This tended to happen between 6 and 8 A.M., on Mondays, and when a larger than usual number of staff was working. Another finding was that the communication to the patient of low staff expectations for positive change and improvement appeared to lead to violent behavior. In planning care and in preventing aggressive behavior, nurses need to consider these possible precipitants of the violent expression of anger.

■ Behaviors

■ **PHYSIOLOGICAL.** The cardiovascular response includes increased blood pressure and heart rate. It has been demonstrated that the tachycardia does not result from vagal stimulation. It is therefore believed to result from epinephrine secretion. Blood composition is also altered, with fewer lymphocytes and increased free fatty acids. Gastrointestinal behaviors reveal a combination of sympathetic and parasympathetic innervation. Behaviors include an increase in salivation, nausea, either increased or decreased secretion of hydrochloric acid, and decreased gastric peristalsis.

Fight-or-flight response. When the individual perceives a threat, two alternative reactions are available. One is to confront the threat—to stand and fight. Many animals choose this response only when cornered. Because of social learning, humans may place a value on fighting and may choose this response even if it is not essential. The alternative is flight—to escape from the threat. Flight may involve leaving the scene of the threat or may be accomplished by emotional withdrawal. In the flight situation the individual's emotional response would probably be fear rather than anger.

The physiological response in fear and in anger is similar. Essentially, the person is prepared for the activity that is about to take place. Hyperalertness helps him to analyze the situation, including assessing the extent of the threat and scanning the environment for any additional threatening circumstances. Since the anxiety level is increased, mental activity is stimulated—at first productively—but the person's responses may become fragmented and confused if anxiety reaches panic levels (Chapter 11). Blood flow is diverted from the viscera to the skeletal muscle groups and the brain, since more activity will be required of these areas. In addition, the rate of blood flow is greater to speed nutrients to the cells. The respiratory rate increases in proportion to the body's increased need for oxygen. Gastrointestinal behaviors result from a combination of sympathetic and parasympathetic innervation. They include increased salivation, nausea, decreased peristalsis and constipation or diarrhea. Frequency of urination and pressure to urinate may occur. The pupils may be dilated. Subjectively, the person generally feels tense and flooded by feelings of resentment and hostility. When overwhelmed by intense anger, the person may act spontaneously without conscious planning. Clinical example 17-1 illustrates the operation of the fight or flight response in a patient who feels that he has lost control of the situation.

This patient demonstrates the following attributes of violence identified by Nigrosh[23]:

1. *A subjective threat to the self.* This person had felt threatened as a result of his delusional ideas about his neighbors. He was then threatened further by the demand that he remove his clothing.
2. *Loss of control.* The patient became overwhelmingly anxious and resorted to a fight-or-flight response, first fleeing and then, when cornered, fighting.
3. *Levels of self-control.* The range of violent actions extends from attacks on inanimate objects to homicide. This person's behavior escalated from letting air out of tires to attempting to assault staff members.
4. *Diminished capacity to think and speak.* This pa-

CLINICAL EXAMPLE 17-1

Mr. B was a 32-year-old man with a medical diagnosis of paranoid personality disorder. He was admitted to the locked ward of a psychiatric hospital because he had been arrested after his neighbors complained that he was letting the air out of their tires. He said that he did this because the neighbors laughed at him and talked about him when he was out walking his dog. He was angry about being arrested and wanted to leave the hospital, but was held under commitment because he also threatened to burn down the house of the neighbor who had called the police.

Mr. B resisted the admission procedure. He belligerently demanded to be released, threatening to call the governor and "sue everybody in the place." When he was asked to undress for a physical examination, he ran down the hall and barricaded himself in the dining room. As staff forcibly entered the room, he began to lash out. Several staff members removed him to a seclusion room, where he was given intramuscular medication and isolated until he regained control of his behavior. He paced the floor and pounded on the door for 30 minutes before he began to appear calmer.

Several days later, when Mr. B was used to the staff and felt more comfortable in the hospital, he related to a nurse, "I hope I didn't hurt you the other night, but I didn't know what you wanted to do to me. A man has to protect himself, you know."

tient was impaired in his ability to reason. This interfered with his capacity for reasoning out his anger and his alternatives for response to it. The use of cognitive processes can mediate violent behavior by allowing anticipation of consequences, prediction of the possible response of others, and devaluation of the importance of the antagonist.

Had the staff applied this approach to understanding violent behavior, the patient could have been given time to adjust to his new situation and to establish a degree of control before being confronted with a new threat.

■ **ASSERTIVENESS.** Wolpe is one of the major behavioral theorists. He has provided the impetus for the development of the theory of assertiveness as a positive behavioral expression of one's rights. The basic assumption of assertiveness theory is that every individual has a right to behave in a way that meets his needs, as long as he does not impinge on the rights of another person. The primary obligation is to oneself. However, assertiveness theorists believe that this approach to need gratification also enhances the esteem of the other. The assertive person assumes that the other person also has the right and the ability to act in his own best interest.

Passive behavior. Assertiveness is at the midpoint of a continuum that runs from passive to aggressive behavior. The passive person consistently subordinates his own rights to his perception of the rights of others. When the passive person becomes angry, he tries to camouflage it, thereby creating increased tension in himself. In addition, if the other person becomes aware of the anger by observing nonverbal cues, he is unable to confront the issue. This can also increase his tension. This pattern of interaction can seriously impair interpersonal growth. Clinical example 17-2 illustrates passive behavior.

Although Ms. J had thought that she was acting in a healthy way, she was actually negating her own

CLINICAL EXAMPLE 17-2

Ms. J was a staff nurse on a busy surgical unit. She enjoyed her work and liked the patients. She also placed a high value on getting along with her co-workers. Other staff members always spoke positively of her. Ms. C, the head nurse, valued Ms. J as an employee, stating particularly, "She's not like the rest of them. She never complains."

Ms. J made it a practice never to refuse a request made by a patient or another staff member. If a patient who was assigned to another nurse asked her to explain his diet or straighten his bed, she would do so, even if she was then behind in her own work. She never asked for help from others, since she felt that her assignment was her responsibility. If a co-worker asked to change days off with her, Ms. J always agreed, even if she had plans, rationalizing that the other person probably had more important plans.

Ms. C began to sense a tenseness when she was around Ms. J. Since she could not think of any problem at work, she assumed that Ms. J must have been having a problem at home. She was concerned and asked Ms. J if she could help. To her amazement, Ms. J recited a long list of angry feelings related to the work situation. Ms. C then felt guilty when she realized that she and the other staff members had been taking advantage of Ms. J.

needs and diminishing her self-respect. Her co-workers, who superficially liked her, in reality felt uncomfortable with her because they were never allowed to reciprocate when she had been helpful. Ms. C's guilty response quickly changed to anger when she realized that she had been a victim of Ms. J's passivity. If Ms. J had informed Ms. C of her feelings, she would have treated her more equitably.

Chenevert[3] has listed 10 basic rights for women in the health professions. They are the rights to

1. Be treated with respect
2. Have a reasonable workload
3. Be paid an equitable wage
4. Determine one's own priorities
5. Ask for what is wanted
6. Refuse without making excuses or feeling guilty
7. Make mistakes and assume responsibility for them
8. Give and receive information as a professional
9. Act in the best interest of the patient
10. Be human

Nurses like Ms. J tend to ignore these basic rights, which leads to passive, rather than direct, expression of anger.

A passive response to anger usually results in an indirect expression of the angry feelings. This was the source of the tension that Ms. C felt. Frequently passive-aggressive people are superficially concerned, interested, and sympathetic. However, an underlying tone of hostility contradicts the superficial message. For example, a therapist may tell a patient in a condescending tone of voice, "You're doing very well—much better than I expected." Although the verbal message is overtly supportive and complimentary, the tone of voice conveys the hostile message, "You're such a loser, I'm amazed that you get along as well as you do." The patient is at a real disadvantage in this situation. If he passively accepts the statement, he keeps peace with the therapist but decreases his own self-esteem. If he challenges the hostile undertone, he runs the risk of bringing the therapist's anger to the surface and of being labeled "paranoid." This is an example of a double-bind situation (Chapter 16), which involves a passive-aggressive message.

Passivity is also expressed nonverbally. The person may speak softly, frequently in a childlike manner. There is little eye contact. Body language communicates diffidence and self-denial. The person may be slouched in posture and generally holds his arms close to his body. Fidgeting also communicates passivity. Gestures are seldom used, although the head may be nodded in agreement (even when the person really disagrees).

Sarcasm is another indirect expression of anger. This usually provokes anger in the person who is the target. It is differentiated from assertive behavior because it usually infringes on the rights of the other. A sarcastic remark generally conveys the message "You are not worthy of my respect." Sarcasm may be disguised as humor. Confrontation may then be responded to with a disclaimer such as "Can't you take a joke?" Humor that derogates another person is hostile and is indulged in for the purpose of self-enhancement. It tends to backfire because the joker is revealed as insecure.

Aggressive behavior. At the opposite end of the continuum from passivity is aggression. The aggressive person ignores the rights of others. He assumes that every person must fight for his own interests, and he expects the same behavior from others. Life is a battle. An aggressive approach to life may lead to physical or verbal violence. The aggressive behavior frequently covers a basic lack of self-confidence. The person enhances his self-esteem by overpowering others and thereby proving his superiority. Clinical example 17-3 describes aggressive behavior.

Aggressive adults are not unlike Suzy. They try to cover up their insecurities and vulnerabilities by acting aggressive. The behavior is self-defeating because it drives people away, thus reinforcing the low self-esteem and vulnerability to rejection.

Maier and colleagues[19] have described the physical and verbal aggression cycles. These describe the interaction between patient aggression and staff response. In the physical aggression cycle, when aggression occurs the staff first work to prevent further activity ("talking down"). If this fails, physical control is applied ("taking down"). Following the episode staff members typically ask each other about physical injury but do not discuss feelings. Future interactions with the patient then take place in the context of unexpressed feelings. This tends to interfere with communication and may result in social isolation of the patient. This increases the potential for a repetition of the aggressive behavior.

The verbal aggression cycle is similar. In this case the aggressive action takes the form of a threat. The staff response is to assess the probability of the threat being carried out and talking with colleagues. Eventually the staff member may discuss the incident with the patient. Sometimes the feelings associated with the threat are unresolved. In this case, the staff member avoids the patient, resulting in the patient's resentment or sometimes enjoyment of being able to control the staff.

Aggressive behavior is also communicated nonver-

CLINICAL EXAMPLE 17-3

Suzy was a 9-year-old girl brought to the child psychiatric clinic by her mother on referral from the school nurse. She was described as a "tomboy" who loved active play and hated school. She was the first girl to make the neighborhood Little League baseball team and had proved her right to be there by beating up several male team members. Suzy was sent to the clinic after the teacher caught her forcing younger children to give her their lunch money.

When Suzy came to the clinic, she presented a facade of toughness. She did not deny her behavior and explained it by saying that the "little kids don't need much to eat anyway. I let them keep some of the money." Suzy was saving money for a new baseball glove. When she was asked about school, she said angrily, "I'm not dumb. I could learn that junk, but who needs it. I just want to play ball."

Psychological testing revealed that Suzy's IQ was slightly below average. She attended school with a group of upper middle class college-bound children. Even in the fourth grade she was feeling insecure and unable to compete. She masked her insecurity with her bullying behavior, striving for acceptance in sports, where she did have ability. The medical diagnosis was conduct disorder, undersocialized, aggressive. When Suzy's problem was explained to her parents and the school, some of the pressure for academic achievement was alleviated. Her parents spent extra time helping her with her homework. Also, she was given genuine recognition for her athletic ability, demonstrated by the gift of a new baseball glove. Suzy gradually responded to the positive input from others by developing a sense of positive regard for herself. As she did so, she no longer needed to bully other children and began to grow into some real friendships.

---

bally. The aggressive person may invade personal space. He speaks loudly and with great emphasis. He usually maintains eye contact over a prolonged period of time so that the other person experiences it as intrusive. Gestures may be emphatic and often seem threatening (e.g., the person may shake his fist, stamp his foot, or make slashing motions with his hands). Posture is erect and often the aggressive person leans forward slightly toward the other person. The overall impression is one of power and dominance.

Assertive behavior. Assertive behavior conveys a sense of self-assurance but also communicates respect for the other person. The assertive individual speaks clearly and distinctly. He observes the norms of personal space appropriate to the situation. Eye contact is direct but not intrusive. Gestures emphasize speech but are not distracting or threatening. Posture is erect and relaxed. The body language may be symmetrical with that of the other party. The overall impression is one of strength, but not threatening.

The assertive person feels free to refuse an unreasonable request. He will, however, share his rationale with the other person. He will also base the judgment about the reasonableness of the request on his own priorities. On the other hand, the assertive person does not hesitate to make a request of others, assuming that they will inform him if his request is unreasonable. If the other person is unable to refuse, the assertive individual will not feel guilty about making the request.

Assertiveness also implies communicating one's feelings directly to others. As a result, anger is not allowed to build up and the expression of feeling is more likely to be in proportion to the situation. If dissatisfaction is verbalized, the reason for the feeling is included. Assertive people also remember to express love to those to whom they are close. Compliments are given when deserved. Assertion also involves acceptance of positive input from others. Think about the real message in this brief interaction:

MARY: **That's a pretty dress, Jane. Is it new?**
JANE: **This old thing? I've had it for years. I couldn't find anything else to wear today.**

What did Jane really say to Mary? The implication is that Mary has poor taste to admire a dress that Jane thinks so little of. If Jane were assertive, she would thank Mary for the compliment and perhaps even agree with her that it really is a pretty dress.

Palmer and Deck[25] have described several assertive communication techniques. Negotiation involves expressing a feeling related to a situation; making a specific request; identifying the benefit that is to be gained; and requesting help in solving the problem. The broken record technique refers to stating the same message repeatedly in various ways until the other person indicates that it has been heard. "I" messages communicate that the person is responsible for his own thoughts, feelings, and needs.

Within each person lies the capacity for passive, assertive, and aggressive behavior. In a threatening situation the choices are to be passive, fearful, and to flee; to be aggressive, angry, and to fight; or to be assertive, self-confident, and to confront the situation directly. None is inherently good or bad. Rather, the situation and the characteristics of the individuals involved define the appropriate response. When confronted by a mugger on a deserted street, one may assertively explain why the mugger should change his mind. However, if flight is available, it might be a better choice, or passive submission might be safer. Similarly, if the children are being persistently annoying and getting on mother's nerves, aggressively telling them to stop may be most effective. The problem related to assertiveness is not that people are sometimes passive or aggressive but that they do not have the option of being assertive because they have not learned how. Table 17-1 summarizes the major characteristics of passive, assertive, and aggressive behaviors.

TABLE 17-1

COMPARISON OF PASSIVE, ASSERTIVE, AND AGGRESSIVE BEHAVIORS

	Passive	Assertive	Aggressive
Content of speech	Negative Self-derogatory "Can I?" "Will you?"	Positive Self-enhancing "I can" "I will"	Exaggerated Other derogatory "You always" "You never"
Tone of voice	Quiet, weak, whining	Modulated	Loud, demanding
Posture	Drooping, bowed head	Erect, relaxed	Tense, leaning forward
Personal space	Allows invasion of space by others	Maintains a comfortable distance; claims right to own space	Invades space of others
Gestures	Minimal, weak gesturing, fidgeting	Demonstrative gestures	Threatening, expansive gestures
Eye contact	Little or none	Intermittent, appropriate to relationship	Constant stare

CLINICAL EXAMPLE 17-4

Peter was a 16-year-old boy who was referred to a halfway house for adolescents because he could not get along in a foster home setting. He refused to obey rules, used drugs, and constantly argued with the foster parents. He was consistently truant from school, where he had completed the eighth grade. He had been arrested once for stealing hubcaps, but the charges were dropped. Peter's family of origin had fallen apart when his parents divorced when he was 5 years old. His father left town and had no further contact with Peter. His mother was alcoholic and lost custody of her children to the city Department of Social Services when neighbors reported her for neglect. Although she never tried to regain custody of Peter, even after she remarried, she also never agreed to his adoption. Peter had spent 11 years moving from foster home to foster home—eight in all. At first, he had tried to get along, but he soon discovered that his behavior had little effect on how he was treated. He then began to use whatever means he could to meet his own needs.

When Peter entered the halfway house, he was initially agreeable, followed the rules, and seemed to be making a good adjustment. He was particularly close to a young male counselor and spent hours talking with him about his thoughts, feelings, and past experiences. However, after about 3 weeks, several small, mysterious fires were discovered in the house. They had obviously been set. After the group of residents were confronted with the situation, another boy approached a counselor and said he had seen Peter setting a fire. When presented with the evidence, Peter acknowledged that he had been the culprit and asked when he would have to leave. He seemed disbelieving when he was told that he could remain if he assumed responsibility for his behavior. He questioned why he was being trusted. Later, when talking with his counselor, he related that he had felt a need to get away from the house because he was beginning to like it. He feared that he would be hurt if he stayed and was later rejected. At a deeper level, his counselor believed that Peter was testing to see if the counselor really cared about him as he seemed to or if he would abandon him as his parents had when he was a small child. Unconsciously, Peter had always thought that he was responsible for his parents' divorce, since he had been told regularly that he was a bad person. Peter's medical diagnosis was conduct disorder, socialized, aggressive.

■ **ACTING-OUT BEHAVIOR.** A variation on the indirect expression of angry feelings is acting-out behavior. Acting out may also convey such feelings as love, fear, or guilt, but frequently it involves anger. Acting out refers to behavior that attracts the attention of others. It represents the feelings or conflicts the person is experiencing. Adolescents often use this behavior as they deal with the crises of that developmental stage, but acting out is by no means limited to teenagers. Loomis[15] points out that acting out is not a controllable behavior until the person understands the reason or learns alternative behaviors. In therapy it is frequently related to transference feelings. Clinical example 17-4 illustrates this concept.

Peter's acting-out behavior was complex and in part unconsciously motivated. He was particularly frightened by feelings of caring, which made him vulnerable to hurt when the relationship ended. His response to this imagined threat of loss was to take the initiative and assume control of the situation by causing his dismissal from the home. If the sequence had gone as he expected, Peter would have also reinforced his beliefs about his own worthlessness and the vindictiveness of other people. When trust and concern were conveyed to Peter, he was able to reassess some of his beliefs about himself and other people. Because the staff in this facility was used to working with acting-out behavior, Peter's experience became the beginning of a time of growth in self-awareness.

Misdirected anger also contributes to other emotional problems. In particular, anger that is redirected toward the self and experienced as guilt is a prominent feature of depression, as described in Chapter 14. At other times internalized anger may be expressed physiologically as a psychosomatic illness. This mechanism has been considered in depth in Chapter 12.

■ **Coping mechanisms**

Many everyday activities meet the demands of the aggressive drive. The competition that is so valued in Western cultures is fueled by aggression. Accomplishment of work often requires a degree of aggressiveness. People cope with aggressive feelings by using the energy they provide for productive accomplishments.

When aggression is uncontrolled, problems result. The anger that is then felt requires psychological coping mechanisms. Since the anger is an expression of anxiety aroused by a threat, the ego defense mechanisms described in Chapter 11 are helpful. Angry feelings are frequently displaced. For instance, the man who was treated unfairly by his boss complains to his wife about the dinner she prepared. Sublimation also helps one to cope with angry feelings. Some great works of art reflect the anger that was felt by the composer or artist at the time the work was created. Music, in particular, can also help listeners to dispel some of their anger.

A less healthy means of coping with anger is projection. In this case the angry feelings are attributed to someone or something else. As an example, the person who is flooded with unconscious hostile impulses may believe that others are plotting to kill him. The person essentially trades his anger for fear. Repression may also apply to anger. However, repressed anger builds up in the unconscious and later reappears as hostility, explosiveness, bigotry, manipulation, and many other distorted expressions.

Madden[18] has identified denial as a prominent defense mechanism related to violent behavior. Denial is in operation when a person with a history of violent behavior asserts that he has no problem with violence. It is also apparent when an individual expresses lack of concern about the consequences of his behavior. This show of bravado is really protecting a very low self-esteem.

Reaction formation is the mechanism that underlies passive-aggressive behavior. Although the person seems ingratiating, this is a defense against anger that the person is unable to express directly. Other defense mechanisms may also be used as an unconscious response to anger. Because the response is unconscious, its usefulness is limited. The person is not able to examine his behavior and modify it.

Direct, conscious responses also may help one to cope with anger. One is physical activity. Sometimes angry people need a time to work off the excess physical energy associated with the biological response. Hitting a punching bag or taking a brisk walk is preferable to punching a friend and is also healthier than trying to set the feeling aside. An activity break also allows the person to review the situation and gain perspective before assertively confronting it.

Nurses also use coping mechanisms when they are confronted with angry behavior. This is revealed in a countertransference response to the patient. Because it may not seem acceptable to express anger at a patient, the nurse may deny anger, which is then reflected indirectly in her relationships with the patient and others. A related mechanism is projection.[10] In this case the nurse may provoke the patient to act out her own anger, resulting in scapegoating. Both denial and projection may lead to increased angry behavior by the patient, who senses the nurse's inability to deal with this feeling. Therefore the nurse must be aware of her own response to anger.

Dubin[7] has suggested that it is the responsibility of the unit administrative staff to help staff members identify and deal with their feelings about aggression by providing good role models. Staff cohesion is very important. Staff meetings can be used to provide an opportunity for expressing feelings. Educational programs should be provided frequently.

Each person develops an individual style for coping with anger. This results from past experiences, parental modeling, and cultural expectations. The key point to consider in assessing the person's coping ability is whether this personal style facilitates the expression of the angry feelings. If they are allowed to accumulate and fester or if they are expressed explosively, the person needs help in developing new, more satisfying coping mechanisms.

Nursing diagnosis

When formulating a nursing diagnosis relative to a patient's angry behavior, the nurse should consider the nature of the threat or physiological disruption involved. This would include the predisposing factors and circumstances discussed as stressors. In addition, the observable response to the threat should be stated as the nursing care problem. The model in Fig. 17-2 summarizes the relationship between anger, anxiety, low self-esteem, and guilt. It indicates the two possible modes of expression of the anger—externally in either constructive or aggressive behavior, or internally in either nonassertive or self-destructive behavior. This model may be helpful to the nurse in formulating a nursing diagnosis.

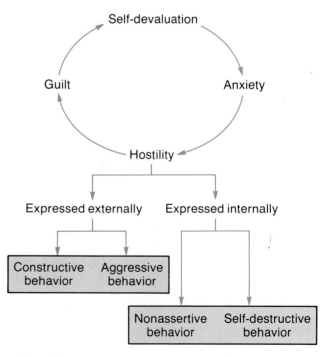

Fig. 17-2. Model representing the expression of anger.

Nursing Diagnoses Related to Problems with the Expression of Anger

Primary NANDA nursing diagnoses

Violence, potential for: directed at others
Coping, ineffective individual

Examples of complete nursing diagnoses

Potential for violence directed at others related to the delusional perception that his life is in danger evidenced by verbal statements that the staff wants to kill him

Potential for violence directed at others related to need to control others evidenced by refusal to follow hospital rules

Potential for violence directed at others related to brain tumor evidenced by confusion and hypersensitivity to interpersonal stimuli

Ineffective coping related to inability to confront others directly with angry feelings evidenced by excessive use of sarcasm

Ineffective coping related to denial of angry feelings evidenced by statement, "I never get angry."

The nursing diagnostic statement includes the identification of the nursing problem, the stressor that is responsible for the problem, and a statement of the behavior that provides evidence that the problem exists. Whenever possible, the patient should participate in the process of formulating the nursing diagnosis. However, a person who has a problem with the expression of anger may feel too threatened to describe the problem clearly. Some patients who are using the coping mechanisms of denial and projection may actively resist identifying that their problem is related to anger.

Primary NANDA nursing diagnoses and examples of complete nursing diagnoses related to problems with the expression of anger are presented in the accompanying box. Since these patients are likely to experience associated disruptions in behavior, other nursing diagnoses that are frequently applicable and

TABLE 17-2

MEDICAL AND NURSING DIAGNOSES RELATED TO PROBLEMS WITH THE EXPRESSION OF ANGER

Medical Diagnostic Class

Disruptive behavior disorders
Delusional disorder

Related Medical Diagnoses (DSM-III-R*)

Oppositional defiant disorder
Conduct disorder
Delusional (paranoid) disorders
Organic personality syndrome (explosive type)
Paranoid personality disorder

Psychiatric Nursing Diagnostic Class

Problems with the expression of anger

Related Nursing Diagnoses (NANDA)

Anxiety
Communication, impaired verbal
Coping, defensive
†Coping, ineffective individual
Fear
Grieving, dysfunctional
Injury, potential for
Post-trauma response
Powerlessness
Self-esteem disturbance
Social interaction, impaired
Social isolation
†Violence, potential for, directed at others

*American Psychiatric Association: DSM-III-R. American Psychiatric Association, October 1987.
†Indicates primary nursing diagnoses for problems with the expression of anger.

relevant medical diagnoses from DSM-III-R[2] are presented in Table 17-2. These should not be interpreted as exhaustive but should serve as a guide in assessment and diagnosis. The comprehensive plan of care will reflect the total range of the patient's biopsychosocial needs for nursing care.

There are multiple possible individualized nursing diagnoses related to anger. They will vary according to the source of anger, degree of anger, frequency of angry feelings, direction of anger, chosen mode of expression, and the person's physical condition. Because people often mask their anger and redirect it, it may be difficult to recognize the behavior and to identify the stressors involved. Good communication among health team members helps to accomplish this part of the assessment. Fig. 17-3 illustrates the nursing model of health-illness phenomena related to the expression of anger.

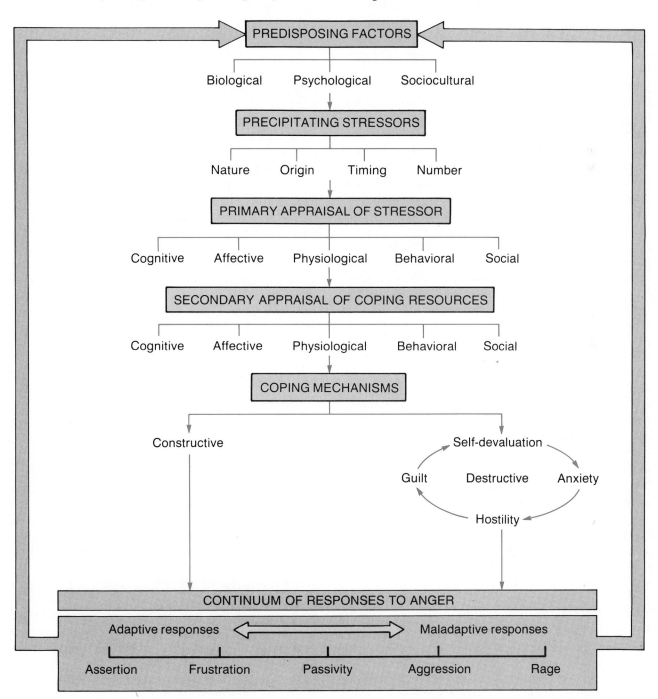

Fig. 17-3. Nursing model of health-illness phenomena related to the expression of anger.

Related medical disorders

Several medical diagnostic categories include behaviors that may indicate problems with the expression of anger. These include the affective disorders, organic mental disorders, schizophrenic disorders, anxiety disorders, and personality disorders. These are discussed in other chapters of this book. The classifications of medical disorders that are primarily characterized by problems expressing anger are briefly described.

OPPOSITIONAL DEFIANT DISORDER. The essential features are at least five of the following: argumentativeness, defiance, resentfulness, irritability, vindictiveness, bullying, use of obscene language, blaming others and frequent loss of temper for at least 6 months.[2]

CONDUCT DISORDER. Conduct disorders are associated with childhood and adolescence. The essential feature is a repetitive and persistent pattern of conduct characterized by at least three antisocial behaviors such as truancy, unauthorized use of belongings of others, running away, fighting, physical cruelty to animals or people, destruction of property, breaking into someone's property, arson, sexual activity not within the cultural norm, lying, and theft.[2]

DELUSIONAL (PARANOID) DISORDER. The essential feature is a nonbizarre delusion that focuses on everyday life experiences, such as a feeling of persecution, jealousy, a physical disorder (somatic), grandiosity, or that a higher status person is in love with one (erotomanic).[2]

ORGANIC PERSONALITY SYNDROME (EXPLOSIVE TYPE). The essential feature includes unstable affect, recurrent outbursts of aggression without adequate provocation, impaired social judgment, apathy, or suspiciousness and with evidence of abnormal brain function or structure.[2]

PARANOID PERSONALITY DISORDER. The essential feature is a persistent tendency to view others as purposely demeaning and threatening, characterized by at least three behaviors such as expecting with no apparent reason to be exploited by others, doubting the loyalty of others, finding hidden meanings in the normal activities of others, holding grudges, unwilling to confide in others, angers quickly in response to perceived slights, and questions fidelity of significant others without justification.[2]

Planning

Goal setting

Mutually set long- and short-term nurse-patient goals are essential to guide the intervention process. Long-term goals will be directed toward the recognition of feelings of anger and, when appropriate, asser-

tively communicating these feelings to other people. Short-term goals serve as guideposts along the way, helping the nurse and the patient to identify the progress of the therapeutic experience.

Progression of behavioral goals gives the patient the sense of mastery and control that is sometimes the objective of aggressive behavior. It also makes a task that may at first appear overwhelming seem manageable. This is particularly important in working with a patient who becomes frustrated easily. It also meets the need for patient education, since the patient is a full participant in the therapeutic plan.

The nursing care plan for the person who has problems expressing anger must place highest priority on the safety of the patients and others in the environment. In addition, it is important to explore with the patient options for expressing anger assertively. Fig. 17-4 is a partial nursing care plan for Mr. B, the patient who was presented in Clinical Example 17-1.

Mental health education related to problems with the expression of anger should focus learning appropriate means of communicating this feeling. Table 17-3 presents a mental health education plan that is based on a model developed by Maynard and Chitty.[20] These authors advocate encouraging the patient to evaluate the experience and the feedback by the nurse. The model focuses on the readiness of the patient for each step of the process. The role of the nurse is to guide the patient and to provide emotional support and honest feedback.

➡ Implementation

Intervening in problems with the expression of anger

SELF-AWARENESS. Angry patients are frequently labeled as problem patients because of the responses of the nurses who are assigned to care for them. The attempt to provide nursing care may deteriorate into a power struggle as the nurse and the patient each strive to be the person in control. To avoid this outcome, the nurse should use the data collected about the patient to help identify the nature of his behavior and the reason for it.

If the person is angry for primarily physiological reasons (e.g., an endocrine imbalance, a brain lesion), the nurse may find it easier to accept angry behavior. She can explain the reason for the patient's anger and may conclude that he "can't help it," circumventing the power struggle aspect. This is particularly true if medical intervention is expected to soon bring the patient's behavior under control.

TABLE 17-3

MENTAL HEALTH EDUCATION PLAN FOR THE PATIENT WHO HAS PROBLEMS WITH THE EXPRESSION OF ANGER

Content	Instructional activities	Evaluation
Help the patient identify anger	Focus on nonverbal behavior Role play nonverbal expression of anger Label the feeling using the patient's preferred words	The patient can demonstrate an angry body posture and facial expression
Give permission for angry feelings	Describe situations in which it is normal to feel angry	The patient describes a situation in which anger would be an appropriate response
Practice the expression of anger	Role play fantasized situations in which anger is an appropriate response	The patient participates in role play and identifies behaviors associated with expression of anger
Apply the expression of anger to a real situation	Help the patient identify a real situation that makes him angry Role play a confrontation with the object of the anger Provide positive feedback for successful expression of anger	The patient identifies a real situation that has made him angry He is able to role play expression of anger
Identify alternative ways to express anger	List several ways to express anger, with and without direct confrontation Role play alternative behaviors Discuss situations in which alternatives would be appropriate	The patient participates in identifying alternatives and plans when each might be useful
Confrontation with a person who is a source of anger	Provide support during confrontation if needed Discuss experience after confrontation takes place	The patient identifies the feeling of anger and appropriately confronts the object of the anger

Adapted from the model of intervention developed by Maynard CK and Chitty KK: Dealing with anger: guidelines for nursing intervention, J Psychiatr Nurs 17:36, 1979.

More often, the reason for the patient's behavior is hidden or not really related to the nurse. It is then harder to deal with the anger and more difficult not to take it personally, especially if it is expressed as an attack on the nurse's competency. Because it is threatening to be the recipient of anger, the nurse needs to develop an awareness of her own usual response to anxiety, threatening situations, and anger. Several responses are not therapeutic or productive.

Nontherapeutic responses. One nontherapeutic response to patient anger is **defensiveness.** The defensive nurse interprets the patient's anger as a personal attack and immediately tries to explain her actions to prove that the perceived attack is unjustified. For example, Ms. B, a nurse, awakened Ms. R, a patient who was hospitalized for control of her diabetes mellitus. When Ms. B told the patient that she had to give her an injection of insulin, Ms. R said, "You people here don't know anything. All you do is wake me up. I'm here for a rest, you know. Some rest!" Ms. B responded with a detailed explanation of why it was important for Ms. R to have her insulin at the correct time and also offered explanations for the possible reasons for the behavior of other staff members. The more she talked, the angrier Ms. R became. Following the interaction, the nurse described the interaction to her head nurse, who pointed out that Ms. R was probably responding to multiple feelings about hospitalization. That, combined with the interruption of her plan to withdraw for awhile by sleeping, led to an attack that was not really directed toward Ms. B. The nurse's response was a result of her own insecurity and discomfort with anger.

Retaliation is a response by the nurse that is det-

PSYCHIATRIC NURSING CARE PLAN

Precautions:
Assault precautions
Elopement precautions

Special nursing needs:
Assign consistent staff
Primary nurse to make all nursing care decisions

Visitors: {x} No restrictions
{ } Family only
{ } Restricted to:

{ } No visitors

Telephone: { } Limited
{x} Unlimited

Privileges: {x} Restricted to unit
{ } Off unit accompanied by staff
{ } Off unit accompanied by family/visitor
{ } Off unit unaccompanied
{ } Out of hospital leave (dates) _____

Assessment data summary: Arrested for disorderly conduct; made threat to burn down neighbor's house; brother and sister are concerned about him; works as a computer programmer; no history of drug or alcohol abuse; no suicidal ideation; mental status exam normal except for poor impulse control and paranoid thoughts.

Nursing diagnoses: 1. Potential for violence directed at others related to lack of basic trust, evidenced by actions and threats against neighbors. 2. Ineffective individual coping related to lack of trust, evidenced by stated need to protect himself.

Treatment goal: Recognition and appropriate expression of angry feelings by learning reality testing and trust in others.

Date	Problem/need	Expected outcome (objective)	Target Date	Nursing Intervention
9/7	Assaultive behavior	To verbalize ability to control aggression	9/7	Provide seclusion; check q15 min; assess for release q2h
9/7	Difficulty trusting others	To establish a trusting relationship	9/14	Meet with him at scheduled times; maintain a comfortable distance; teach assertiveness skills to check out meaning of communications

Room	Patient's name	Age	Doctor	Primary nurse	Admit date
215	Mr. B	32	Dr. J	Ms. S	9/7/90

Fig. 17-4. Sample nursing care plan for a patient with problems expressing anger. (This nursing care plan includes examples of the elements of a total plan as it might appear at a particular time in the patient's course of treatment. It should not be considered all inclusive.)

Date	Medications	Date	P.R.N. Medications	Diagnostic & psychiatric tests	Req.	Done
		9/7	Haloperidol	Psychological	9/7	9/11
			5 mg IM	test battery		
			q4h prn for	Routine blood	9/7	9/8
			assaultive	chemistries		
			behavior			
		Date	**Treatments**	**Special orders and concerns**		
		9/7	Seclusion			
		1 pm	Order expires			
			at 8 pm			

Allergies:	Medical diagnosis: (Axes I-III)	Diet:
Penicillin	Paranoid personality disorder	Regular

Fig. 17-4, cont'd. Sample nursing care plan for a patient with problems expressing anger.

rimental to the patient. The nurse "pulls rank" or asserts herself as the one with the authority. For instance, Ms. T, an elderly patient, requested a bedpan. She had already called the nurse to her bedside several times with small requests that were not really urgent. The nurse labeled her behavior as indirectly aggressive. After she gave the patient the bedpan, she went to check on another patient at the other end of the hall. Fifteen minutes later she returned to Ms. T, who had finished with the bedpan long before her return. When Ms. T mentioned this fact, the nurse responded by saying, "I do have other patients. I can't spend all my time here with you." In reality, she could have removed the bedpan before looking in on the other patient. She, too, was responding to the superficial meaning of the patient's behavior. The nurse believed that the patient was irritable and deliberately seeking attention to annoy her. Actually the patient was frightened, lonely, and angry because she knew she would be going to a nursing home instead of her own house. The nurse's retaliatory behavior only reinforced the patient's feelings.

Somewhat related to retaliation is an attitude of **condescension.** The nurse assumes an attitude of superiority and discounts the patient's concerns. Mr. J

was in the coronary care unit after a myocardial infarction. He was a hard-driving executive who was very frustrated because his physician had forbidden any contact at all with his business. When the nurse brought his lunch, he angrily refused to eat it and referred to the food as "garbage." The nurse replied, "Now really, Mr. J, you're acting like a child. Surely Dr. A has told you that it's important for you to eat. Let's have no more of this silliness." Mr. J then sat straight up in bed and shouted at the nurse, "Get out of my room! Right now!" After the nurse left, she told a co-worker, "He certainly is obnoxious. He'll kill himself unless he controls that bad temper." This nurse's approach only increased the patient's anxiety and ultimately his anger. He was already feeling impotent and did not need to hear himself compared to a child. Furthermore, he was given the message that his anger was unjustified and should not be expressed. On the other hand, the nurse later acknowledged that Mr. J's anger could be destructive but did not recognize that suppression of his feelings could be equally as harmful. Had she realized this, she would have spent some time helping him to explore his feelings and acquire some sense of mastery in the situation.

Another commonly noted nontherapeutic response to patient anger is **avoidance.** In avoidance, the nurse simply refuses to recognize or to deal with the patient's feelings. For instance, Mr. M said to his nurse as she changed his dressing, "You know, I think my doctor is botching my case. That infection is no better. I think he's a real quack." The nurse continued with the procedure and after a moment said, "Did your wife visit yesterday, Mr. M? She seems like such a nice person—so concerned about you." Mr. M sighed and closed his eyes as the nurse completed the procedure. Later she said to a friend, "That Mr. M is a strange one. He hardly responds at all when you talk to him." This nurse was prevented by her own defensive system from even acknowledging Mr. M's angry statement. He felt more frustrated and resorted to withdrawal when she did not acknowledge his statement. He also extended his assessment of the physician's ability to include the nurse.

■ **ASSERTIVENESS TRAINING.** The effective nurse needs to be aware of her own response to anger in others. Otherwise her feelings may actually interfere with her ability to provide effective patient care. The nurse who responds to anger either passively or aggressively needs to take steps to modify her approach. Assertiveness training for the nurse can help to fulfill this need. Not only will she grow in self-awareness and be better able to respond therapeutically to her patients, but she will also be more likely to experience job satisfaction.

Alberti and Emmons[1] recommend to the nurse the following process for the development of assertiveness:

1. Observe your behavior.
2. Keep a record of assertive and nonassertive behavior.
3. Select one situation for examination.
4. Review your behavior in the selected situation.
5. Observe an effective person in action in a similar situation.
6. Identify alternative responses.
7. Put yourself in the place of the effective person; imagine how you would act.
8. Practice the new approach by role playing.
9. Provide yourself with feedback; repeat step 4. Get feedback from others if available.
10. "Behavior shaping"—practice the new response until you begin to feel comfortable.
11. Practice the new approach in a real situation.
12. Repeat training if necessary or apply to other problem areas where you wish to change.
13. Take note of social reinforcement—the positive response of others to your new assertive behavior.

A nurse who develops assertive behavior is also learning a process that can be helpful to patients who have difficulty in expressing anger. A healthy approach to the expression of anger is essentially a problem-solving approach. The steps to assertiveness just described are really components of a problem-solving process. The model of patient education presented in Table 17-4 describes an approach to handling angry feelings that is very similar to assertiveness training.

■ **LIMIT SETTING.** When a patient is expressing his anger in ways that infringe on the rights of others, it is necessary to set limits on the patient's behavior. Limit setting is not punitive, although the patient may feel it is. It is a nonmanipulative confrontation in which the patient is told what behavior is acceptable, what is not acceptable, and the consequences attached to behaving unacceptably. The nurse does not assume responsibility for the patient's behavior, positive or negative. It is recognized that the patient has the right to choose his preferred mode of behavior as long as the consequences are clear as well. Limits should be clarified before the negative consequences are applied. Otherwise the consequence is punitive and the patient may feel tricked.

Once a limit has been defined, the consequences must take place if the behavior occurs. Every staff member must be aware of the plan and carry it out. If this consistency is absent, the patient is likely to manipulate staff by acting out and then pointing out areas of inconsistency in limit setting. Firm, but not hostile, enforcement of limits is preferable. If the nurse responds angrily, she is less likely to see the situation clearly. This is also an indication that a power struggle is taking place. Power struggles are usually detrimental to the treatment plan.

Loomis[15] has identified three steps in the limit-setting process:

1. State expectations to the patient in a positive way.
2. Help the patient explore the reason for and meaning of his behavior.
3. Consider with the patient alternative ways to express his feelings.

This approach avoids rejection of the patient. It also conveys the attitude that the patient has the right to feel anger and the ability to express that anger appropriately. Clinical example 17-5 shows acting-out behavior and constructive limit setting.

The nurse in this example applied the problem-solving process. She planned her nursing intervention and then approached Mary in a reasonable, adult-to-adult way. Ms. T was selected by the nursing staff to work with Mary because she did not have a punitive

TABLE 17-4

SUMMARY OF NURSING INTERVENTIONS WITH A PATIENT WHO HAS PROBLEMS WITH THE EXPRESSION OF ANGER

Goal: To recognize feelings of anger and, when appropriate, assertively communicate these feelings to other people

Principle	Rationale	Nursing intervention
Assertive expression of feelings	Passive behavior reinforces low self-esteem; anger builds up internally and may lead to depression; aggressive behavior also indicates insecurity and low self-esteem; the person may become isolated from others, leading to more hostility; violent behavior can result from pent-up anger; assertive behavior reinforces high self-esteem by protecting the individual's rights without violating the rights of others	Establish a trusting relationship Help the patient recognize and label anger Communicate that angry feelings are normal Identify usual means of coping with anger Support effective coping mechanisms Explore alternative behaviors Help the patient practice assertive expression Provide feedback
Promote respect for the rights of others	Adherence to reasonable limits on acting-out behavior promotes socialization; expression of feelings is a reciprocal process and involves awareness of and respect for the rights of others; anger related to limit setting can be used to teach the person more effective coping behaviors	Inform the patient of acceptable limits for behavior, including rationale Clarify the patient's responsibility for his behavior Define the consequences for failure to observe rules Achieve staff agreement on definition of reasonable limits Enforce limits by implementing consequences if violations occur Explore reasons for acting out and identify alternative behaviors Give positive feedback for adherence to limits
Protection from harm to self or others	Violent behavior entails a high risk of physical injury to the patient and to others with whom he comes into contact; psychological damage may also occur as a result of guilt related to the patient's concern that he injured someone while out of control; outbreaks of violence decrease the sense of security that is important for people to feel while they are confronting their own disturbing behaviors, thoughts, and feelings	Maintain a calm, controlled, and consistent milieu Be alert to signs of tension If possible, remove an agitated patient from a stimulating situation Give antianxiety or antipsychotic medication for agitation Avoid challenges to the patient's self-esteem If restraining the patient is necessary: 1. Maintain the patient's dignity 2. Explain the procedure to the patient 3. Gather adequate trained staff to handle the situation 4. Avoid unnecessary force 5. Protect the patient and staff from injury 6. Review the situation with the patient and staff after calm has returned Discuss episodes of violent behavior with other patients who were present

CLINICAL EXAMPLE 17-5

Mary was a 17-year-old girl who was admitted to the hospital for suspected hyperthyroidism. She quickly became bored with the hospital routine and phoned several of her friends to visit her. When the nursing staff was making rounds at the shift change, they found several teenagers in Mary's room. There was also a strong aroma of marijuana. Since there was a hospital limit of two visitors at a time, some were asked to leave. The group was also informed that marijuana smoking was not allowed in the hospital.

After visiting hours Ms. T, a young staff nurse, sat down to talk with Mary. She initiated a discussion of Mary's restlessness and irritability, which had led to the suspicion that she had a hyperthyroid condition. Mary readily shared her frustration with being in the hospital and her anxiety about her condition. Then she said, "I suppose you guys are mad at me for the pot, but that's a dumb rule. It's healthier than cigarettes, you know." Ms. T replied that she and the other nurses were not mad, but that they did expect Mary to obey the rule, now that she knew it. She also told Mary that she was responsible for telling her friends the rule. The consequence, if the behavior occurred again, would be restriction of visitors to her parents only. The nurse then initiated a discussion of what Mary might do to help out on the unit and thereby use some of her excess energy. Mary began to look excited and shared her love for plants. She proposed that she might visit other patients and help them care for their plants and flowers.

response toward marijuana use. This facilitated her being able to help Mary look at the reasons for her behavior and to select a constructive alternative. The interaction also served as the foundation for a therapeutic nurse-patient relationship between Mary and Ms. T.

■ **CONTROL OF VIOLENCE.** Unfortunately, some patients have more difficulty controlling their feelings and using angry energy constructively. A patient who loses control of his anger becomes violent. Violence refers to behavior that is physically assaultive and risks injury to the self, others, and the environment. The nurse in the psychiatric setting must develop the ability to deal with violent behavior in a way that minimizes the danger.

Prevention of violence is preferable if it is possible. The intense anxiety associated with violent feelings is communicated interpersonally. By empathizing and carefully observing patients' behavior, the nurse may be able to anticipate a violent outburst. Sometimes when a patient is on the verge of losing control, the atmosphere of the nursing unit is filled with tension. When the nurse becomes aware that tension is mounting, intervention may avoid an outburst. The nurse may isolate the disturbed patient from the rest of the patient group, may talk with the patient if he is receptive to this approach, and may give prescribed medication. Some patients respond to vigorous physical activity to express their anger, but this approach should be used with care, since it may also precipitate loss of control.

A patient who is on the verge of violent behavior is usually experiencing a panic level of anxiety. Nursing interventions related to patients who are in panic are described in Chapter 11. Kronberg[12] has recommended several interventions with the patient who is threatening to lose control. She suggests speaking softly, slowly, and with assurance. Directions should be clear and concise. It may be useful to help the patient verbalize his feelings. The nurse should take care to protect the patient's self-esteem and dignity.

Felthous[10] suggests creating a social norm against violence. The norm should be clearly stated to the patient group and repeated periodically. Patients need to be involved in the establishment of the norm. This may be accomplished by asking them to help write an orientation manual for new patients and by discussion of the norm in community meetings. Communication should focus on the creation of a comfortable, safe environment for everyone. Any episodes of violence should be discussed in a group meeting, and alternatives should be discussed with the patient group.

Self-protection is a concern when the nurse is working with a potentially violent patient. The nurse should never fail to take adequate precautions for her own safety. Whitman[30] recommends the following precautions:

1. Never see a potentially violent person alone.
2. Call police or security staff if their help is needed.
3. Keep a comfortable distance away from the patient. Avoid intruding on his personal space.
4. Maintain a clear exit route for both the staff and patient.
5. Be prepared to move. Violent patients can strike out suddenly.
6. Be sure the patient has no weapons in his possession before approaching him.
7. If it is necessary to restrain a patient, have an adequate number of nursing staff on hand.

8. Give prescribed antianxiety or antipsychotic medication when it is needed.

9. Be supportive to the patient and intervene to increase his self-esteem.

If the patient does become violent, immediate response is essential. Morton[22] advises an initial evaluation of the situation, followed by a developing plan for intervention. Enough people should be available to ensure the safety of the patient and staff. Staff members should be taught good body mechanics and methods of holding a struggling patient without causing injury. One person should direct the group action. Also, someone should talk with the patient, explaining what is happening and the reason for the intervention. Morton recommends "disarming" the patient psychologically by acknowledging his feelings and stating one's intent to be helpful. Most violent patients are reassured if they see that they can be controlled and prevented from inflicting injury. If the person is very disturbed, one staff person should be assigned to restrain each limb and a fifth person to direct the activity and communicate with the patient. Roles should be assigned before intervention, with the person who has the best relationship with the patient acting as communicator. The nurse should also be sure that staff are available to stay with and support the other patients. They should be removed from the area if possible. Sometimes a "show of force" by the presence of several staff members will be enough to enable the patient to regain control and be able to talk about his feelings. A sense of confidence on the part of the staff is important. They should be well-informed before taking action. All staff members in a psychiatric setting should receive training in the prevention and management of violent behavior, including an opportunity to discuss feelings and attitudes about this aspect of nursing care. It can be reassuring to a violent patient to see that his uncontrollable behavior can be controlled and that he can be prevented from causing harm. The patient who has become violent may need medication or seclusion to help him gain control. These therapeutic techniques are discussed further in Chapters 22 and 23.

The last step in nursing intervention with a violent patient is to review the incident with the patient after he has achieved control. This helps the patient alleviate any guilt he might be feeling or fear that he might have harmed someone. The nurse can, in retrospect, review what happened and talk about alternatives should the patient become anxious and angry in the future.

Unfortunately, nurses are sometimes assaulted by patients. It is impossible to succeed in predicting and preventing all episodes of violent behavior in a psychiatric setting. If a staff member is assaulted, she or he needs the support and assistance of colleagues. Lanza[13,14] has studied the reactions of nursing staff to physical assault by a patient. The response is similar to that experienced during the post-traumatic stress syndrome. Surprisingly, she found that many staff members were reluctant to identify any response to the assault. The investigator thought that this might be related to a sense of guilt for not having prevented the episode and concern that others would not understand.

Ryan and Poster[28] studied the responses of 61 nurses who had experienced patient assault. Their responses included "anger, anxiety, helplessness, irritability, soreness, hyperalertness, sadness, depression, shock, disbelief that the assault occurred, feeling sorry for the patient who committed the assault, and a feeling that they should have done something to prevent the assault." Eighty-two percent of the nurses had resolved their crisis state by the sixth week post-assault. One intervention that has been helpful to nursing staff members who have been assaulted is the peer support group. This legitimizes their responses and allows expression of feelings in a supportive setting.

Recently, there has been debate about whether staff should be encouraged to file legal charges against a patient who has intentionally assaulted them. Phelan and associates[26] presented several points in support of filing charges. They included the creation of a public record of assaultive behavior, allowing a judge and jury to fulfill their duty of determining responsibility, possible deterrence of future attacks, and the potential for harsher penalties for repeat offenders. Phelan and associates attributed much of the difficulty that staff have in pursuing this course of action to the ethical dilemma of deciding whether the patient was actually responsible for his behavior. In addition, if care providers feel guilty for allowing the incident to occur, they are unlikely to take legal action against the patient. This is an issue that must be resolved by the nurse based on the situation. It would also be very helpful to seek the advice of a trusted professional mentor.

Dealing with anger is a challenge for both the nurse and the patient. Nursing interventions with patients who have problems with the expression of anger are summarized in Table 17-4. Anger is not inherently good or bad. Expression of anger is not always positive or negative. Effectively dealing with anger implies that the person can accept his right to be angry and the reciprocal right of others to be angry. It is not therapeutic to encourage a patient to express angry feelings indiscriminately. It is important that the patient feel free to choose whether to express anger and that, when he chooses to do so, he avoid abridging the rights of others.

 Evaluation

The evaluation of the nursing care provided to the patient who has problems with the healthy expression of anger should be based on observed behavioral change. The subjective response of the patient is also a helpful input. Maynard and Chitty[20] recommend that the following questions be asked of a patient:

- How do you feel about the experience?
- How did the other person behave in response to your anger?
- Was the confrontation well timed?
- Did the interaction take place in private?
- What would you change in the future?
- How would you change these aspects?

Evaluation should focus on the mode of expression of anger, the appropriateness of the object, the congruence between the degree of feeling expressed and the precipitating incident, and the patient's awareness of the process. If the patient does not change in the planned direction, the data base, goals, and nursing interventions should be reviewed and appropriate modifications made.

The staff should review any episode of violent behavior. The focus of such a discussion is to dissipate any residual staff anxiety related to the incident and to objectively evaluate their performance. The situation should be analyzed to identify the precipitating stressors and the sequence of attempts to cope with the stress. Future prevention can be directed to alleviating stressors that seem to precipitate violent outbursts and to helping the patient develop more positive ways to deal with anger when it occurs. Feedback should be given to colleagues about the process of restraining the patient. Procedural modifications may be made as a result of this review.

If the patient is involved in learning techniques of assertiveness, the evaluation process is an integral part of the training program. Thus the patient should be involved in eliciting feedback about his behavior in selected situations. He should be encouraged to practice assertive behavior until he feels comfortable and consistently is perceived as behaving assertively. Patients in an assertiveness group may also evaluate each other.

Successful problem solving in assertively expressing anger becomes a self-reinforcing process. As the patient successfully asserts himself, he has good feelings about himself and discovers that his needs are met

more frequently. The assertive nurse has similar feelings and becomes increasingly effective professionally.

■ SUGGESTED CROSS-REFERENCES ■

Therapeutic relationship skills and self-awareness are discussed in Chapter 4. The model of health-illness phenomena is discussed in Chapter 5. Nursing interventions to enhance self-esteem can be found in Chapter 13. Facilitating expression of feelings and strengthening social skills are discussed in Chapter 14, and intervening in problems with interpersonal relationships is discussed in Chapters 14 and 16. Somatic therapies are discussed in Chapter 22. Intervening in family violence is discussed in Chapter 32.

■ SUMMARY ■

1. Anger is a feeling of resentment that occurs as a response to anxiety when a person perceives a threat. Various overt and covert expressions of anger were described.

DIRECTIONS FOR FUTURE RESEARCH

The following are some of the nursing research problems raised in Chapter 17 that merit further study by psychiatric nurses:
1. The conditions that predispose to patient abuse
2. The occurrence of angry responses related to the amount of personal space allotted to the individual
3. The relationship between intrastaff dissension and episodes of angry behavior by patients
4. Nurse behaviors that promote or inhibit the expression of anger by patients
5. The effectiveness of limit-setting interventions by nurses in response to selected acting-out behavior
6. The relationship between a nurse's comfort with assertive behavior and her effectiveness in setting limits with patients
7. Primary prevention nursing interventions related to episodes of violent behavior by patients
8. Interventions with violent patients that minimize the risk of injury to the patient and to the involved staff members
9. Early identification of patients at risk for expressing anger through violent behavior
10. Interventions that help staff members who have been assaulted by patients recover from the experience

2. Anger is experienced on a continuum from mild annoyance to intense rage. Rage is destructive, but positive functions of anger also exist.

3. Biological predisposing factors include the instinctual drives postulated by Freud and Lorenz, as well as physiological disruptions such as endocrine imbalance, seizure disorders, and neoplasms.

4. Psychological predisposing factors were described, including the frustration-aggression theory of Dollard and co-workers, the behavioral theory, and the existential theory.

5. Sociocultural predisposing factors include the imposition of social sanctions on behavior, crowding and intrusion on personal space, and role modeling by significant others and through the media. The social learning theory of anger was discussed.

6. Precipitating stressors that may result in anger were identified as a physical or psychological threat.

7. Physiological behaviors associated with anger result primarily from secretion of epinephrine and stimulation of the sympathetic nervous system. The behaviors resulting from this constitute preparation for fight or flight.

8. Assertive behavior was differentiated from passive and aggressive behavior as a constructive use of anger. Assertiveness theorists state that the individual has the right to pursue the gratification of his own needs so long as he does not infringe on the rights of others.

9. One may choose to be assertive or not. Assertiveness training enables the person to choose freely because he has the ability to act assertively if he wishes to accept the consequences of this behavior.

10. Acting-out behavior is often an indirect expression of anger. It attracts the attention of others and is a representation of the feelings the person is having.

11. The coping mechanisms of goal-directed behavior and use of ego defense mechanisms were discussed.

12. Examples of nursing diagnoses relative to angry behavior were given and compared to selected medical diagnoses.

13. Long- and short-term goals for the development of healthy coping behaviors can guide the nurse and patient in their work together and provide a sense of accomplishment as progress is made.

14. Planning enables the nurse and the patient to develop approaches for goal accomplishment. Samples of a nursing care plan and a mental health education plan were provided.

15. The importance of self-awareness for the nurse was discussed. Nontherapeutic responses to a patient's expression of anger were identified as defensiveness, retaliation, condescension, and avoidance.

16. Assertiveness training is a problem-solving approach to dealing with anger that can help the nurse achieve self-awareness and improve her ability to cope with the angry patient. Steps to assertiveness were described.

17. Approaches to nursing intervention with the angry patient were introduced.

18. Limit setting is a nursing intervention that may be employed with angry, acting-out patients. The patient is assumed to be responsible for his behavior and is informed of the consequences if the limited behavior occurs.

19. Intervention with the violent patient should focus on immediate control and safety, followed by discussion to alleviate guilt and identify alternative behaviors to help prevent future episodes of violence.

20. The legal and ethical dilemma of staff response to assault by a patient was presented.

21. Evaluation of the improved ability to express anger is based on objective and subjective feedback about the increased incidence of assertive behavior. The patient's increased self-esteem related to his improved communication skills tends to perpetuate assertive behavior.

■ REFERENCES ■

1. Alberti RE and Emmons ML: Your perfect right, ed 5, San Luis Obispo, Calif, 1986, Impact Publishers.
2. American Psychiatric Association: DSM-III-R. American Psychiatric Association, October 1987.
3. Chenevert M: STAT: Special techniques in assertiveness training for women in the health professions, ed 2, St Louis, 1983, Mosby–Year Book, Inc.
4. Conn LM and Lion JR: Assaults in a university hospital. In Lion JR and Reid WH, editors: Assaults within psychiatric facilities, New York, 1983, Grune & Stratton, Inc.
5. Depp FC: Assaults in a public mental hospital. In Lion JR and Reid WH, editors: Assaults within psychiatric facilities, New York, 1983, Grune & Stratton, Inc.
6. Dollard J et al: Frustration and aggression, New Haven, Conn, 1939, Yale University Press.
7. Dubin, WR: The role of fantasies, countertransference, and psychological defenses in patient violence, Hosp Community Psychiatry, 40:1280, 1989.
8. Eichelman B: Toward a rational pharmacotherapy for aggressive and violent behavior, Hosp Community Psychiatry, 39:31, 1988.
9. Fast J: Body language, New York, 1970, Pocket Books.
10. Felthous AR: Preventing assaults on a psychiatric inpatient ward, Hosp Community Psychiatry 35:1223, Dec 1984.
11. Fromm E: The anatomy of human destructiveness, New York, 1973, Holt, Rinehart & Winston, Inc.
12. Kronberg ME: Nursing interventions in the management of the assaultive patient. In Lion JR and Reid WH, editors: Assaults within psychiatric facilities, New York, 1983, Grune & Stratton, Inc.
13. Lanza ML: The reactions of nursing staff to physical assault by a patient, Hosp Community Psychiatry 34:44, 1983.
14. Lanza ML: A follow-up study of nurses' reactions to physical assault, Hosp Community Psychiatry 35:492, 1984.
15. Loomis ME: Nursing management of acting-out behavior, Perspect Psychiatr Care 8:169, 1970.
16. Lorenz K: On aggression, New York, 1966, Harcourt, Brace & World, Inc. (Translated by MK Wilson).

17. McNiel DE and Binder RL: Relationship between preadmission threats and later violent behavior by acute psychiatric inpatients, Hosp Community Psychiatry 40:605, 1989.

18. Madden DJ: Recognition and prevention of violence. In Lion JR and Reid WH, editors: Assaults within psychiatric facilities, New York, 1983, Grune & Stratton, Inc.

19. Maier GJ, et al.: A model for understanding and managing cycles of aggression among psychiatric inpatients, Hosp Community Psychiatry 38:520, 1987.

20. Maynard CK and Chitty KK: Dealing with anger: guidelines for nursing intervention, J Psychiatr Nurs 17:36, 1979.

21. Montague MC: Physiology of aggressive behavior, J Neurosurg Nurs 11:10, 1979.

22. Morton PG: Managing assault, Am J Nurs 86:1114, 1986.

23. Nigrosh BJ: Physical contact skills in specialized training for the prevention and management of violence. In Lion JR and Reid WH, editors: Assaults within psychiatric facilities, New York, 1983, Grune & Stratton, Inc.

24. Ochitill HN: Violence in a general hospital. In Lion JR and Reid WH, editors: Assaults within psychiatric facilities, New York, 1983, Grune & Stratton, Inc.

25. Palmer ME and Deck ES: Teaching your patients to assert their rights, Am J Nurs 87:650, 1987.

26. Phelan LA, Mills MJ, and Ryan JA: Prosecuting psychiatric patients for assault, Hosp Community Psychiatry 36:581, 1985.

27. Roberts TK, Mock LAT, and Johnstone EE: Psychological aspects of the etiology of violence. In Hays JR, Roberts TK, and Solway KS, editors: Violence and the violent individual, Jamaica, NY, 1981, Spectrum Books.

28. Ryan JA and Poster EC: The assaulted nurse: short-term and long-term responses, Arch Psych Nurs 3:323, 1989.

29. Rothenberg A: On anger, Am J Psychiatry 128:454, 1971.

30. Whitman J: When a patient attacks: strategies for self-protection when violence looms, RN 42:30, 1979.

■ ANNOTATED SUGGESTED READINGS ■

Alberti RD and Emmons ML: Your perfect right, ed 5, San Luis Obispo, Calif, 1986, Impact Publishers.

Practical, straightforward presentation of assertiveness that gives clear descriptions of assertive and nonassertive behavior and suggests ways to become more assertive. Part Two is directed toward the use of assertiveness training with patients; recommended for readers who have advanced preparation in psychiatric nursing.

*Bowman C and Spadoni AJ: Assertion therapy: the nurse and the psychiatric patient in an acute, short-term psychiatric setting, J Psychosoc Nurs 19:7, 1981.

An excellent presentation of assertiveness theory as applied in a short-term hospital setting. A detailed lesson plan outlines

a six-session assertiveness therapy program. Also contains a discussion of this therapeutic approach relative to the behavioral therapy from which it was derived. Particularly recommended for nurses who have been trained to conduct assertiveness therapy and are planning to initiate a program.

*Chenevert M: Special techniques in assertiveness training for women in the health professions, St Louis, 1978, Mosby–Year Book, Inc.

Applies the principles of assertiveness theory to the experience of women, especially nurses, in health care settings. Urges nurses to develop assertive skills for the sake of their patients and themselves. Identifies many difficult situations and gives practical suggestions for constructive behavior.

Davis DL and Bostic L: Multifaceted therapeutic interventions with the violent psychiatric inpatient, Hosp Community Psychiatry 39:867, 1988.

Case study approach illustrates the integrated use of several therapeutic models to decrease violent behavior.

Engel F and Marsh S: Helping the employee victim of violence in hospitals, Hosp Community Psychiatry 37:159, 1986.

Recommends that counseling be provided for staff victims of violence counseling. Points out the need to legitimize the staff member's need for assistance following an assault by a patient and presents a model for the provision of such a service.

*Freeberg S: Anger in adolescence, J Psychosoc Nurs 20:29, 1982.

Discusses anger in the context of normal adolescent development. Also gives attention to the many manifestations of anger when direct expression is blocked. Presents nursing interventions.

Fromm E: The anatomy of human destructiveness, New York, 1973, Holt, Rinehart & Winston, Inc.

Develops an existential theory of the meaning and expression of anger and compares and contrasts the existential viewpoint with other basic theoretical frameworks.

*Gluck M: Learning a therapeutic verbal response to anger, J Psychosoc Nurs Ment Health Serv 19:9, 1981.

Description of a program developed by the author to teach nursing assistants to respond more therapeutically to angry patients. Approach emphasizes an understanding that focuses on the patient's stress and the means to relieve emotional tension.

Hays JR, Roberts TK, and Solway KS, editors: Violence and the violent individual, Jamaica, NY, 1981, Spectrum Books.

A collection of papers that comprehensively views the problem of violence in the United States. Presents various theories and examines current research. Recommended as a resource for someone who is interested in serious investigation of this subject.

*Lenefsky B, de Palma T, and Locicero D: Management of violent behavior, Perspect Psychiatr Care 16:212, 1978.

Focuses on the procedure used for restraint of a person who is threatening violent behavior. Photographs illustrate recommended techniques. Safety and the importance of a team approach by the staff are emphasized.

Lion JR and Reid WH, editors: Assaults within psychiatric facilities, New York, 1983, Grune & Stratton, Inc.

An excellent resource regarding violence in psychiatric set-

---

*Asterisk indicates nursing reference

tings. *Includes data from current research and provides direction for further study. Of particular interest to the nurse is the attention given to legal perspectives on violent behavior and issues related to prevention and management of violence in the institutional setting.*

Lorenz K: On aggression, New York, 1966, Harcourt, Brace & World, Inc. Translated by MK Wilson.

A fascinating and readable presentation of the instinctual theory of aggressive behavior presented by a physician who is also a naturalist. Bound to stimulate reflection on the behavior of humankind as seen from the vantage point of the world of nature.

* Meddaugh DI: Reactance: understanding aggressive behavior in long-term care, J Psychosocial Nursing and Ment Health Services, 28:29, 1990.

Relates the occurrence of aggressive behavior in long-term care settings to limitations on freedom of choice. Illustrates with case examples.

* Morrison EF: The tradition of toughness: a study of non-professional nursing care in psychiatric settings, Image: J of Nurs Scholarship, 22:32, 1990.

Looks at the relationship between the hospital culture and the occurrence of violence. Provides suggestions for nurse administrators and clinicians to make positive changes.

Rothenberg A: On anger, Am J Psychiatry 128:454, 1971.

Differentiates anger and its growth-producing functions from the destructive emotions of hostility and vengefulness. Helps clarify some of the hazy issues about defining aggression, anger, and other related terms.

Tavris C: Anger defused, Psychol Today 16:25, 1982.

Challenges some of the traditional ways of viewing anger, claiming that ventilation may not always be the best way to handle this feeling. Points out that anger occurs in a social context and has meaning related to the transaction. Also addresses the sex role differences in acceptable expression of anger. Would be useful in stimulating discussion.

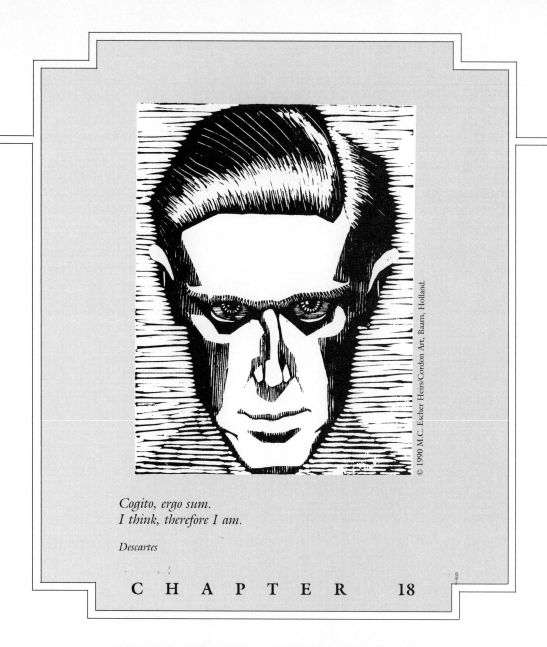

Cogito, ergo sum.
I think, therefore I am.

Descartes

C H A P T E R 18

IMPAIRED COGNITION

DIAGNOSTIC PREVIEW

MEDICAL DIAGNOSES RELATED TO IMPAIRED COGNITION

- Primary degenerative dementia of the Alzheimer type, senile onset

- Multi-infarct dementia

- Dementia

- Organic delusional disorder

- Organic mood disorder

- Organic personality disorder

- Primary degenerative dementia of the Alzheimer type, presenile onset

- Delirium

- Amnestic disorder

- Organic hallucinosis

- Organic anxiety disorder

LEARNING OBJECTIVES

After studying this chapter, the student should be able to:

- define cognition in terms of its component processes.

- identify three models of cognitive functioning.

- describe Jean Piaget's three stages of cognitive development.

- discuss predisposing factors related to cognitive impairment.

- analyze precipitating stressors that contribute to cognitive impairment.

- identify the major categories of data that should be collected regarding an individual's level of cognitive functioning.

- compare and contrast the medical diagnoses of organic mental disease versus organic brain syndrome and delirium versus dementia.

- discriminate between the characteristic behaviors of an individual who is delirious and one with dementia.

- describe the purposes of psychological testing and several frequently administered tests.

- identify coping mechanisms used by individuals with cognitive impairment.

- formulate individualized nursing diagnoses for patients with cognitive impairments.

- assess the relationship between the nursing and medical diagnoses of individual patients with cognitive impairments.

- develop long-term and short-term individualized nursing goals for patients with cognitive impairments.

- apply therapeutic nurse-patient relationship principles with appropriate rationale in planning the care of a patient with cognitive impairment characteristic of delirium or dementia.

- develop a mental health education plan for the families of cognitively impaired persons.

- assess the importance of evaluation of the nursing process when working with cognitively impaired people.

- identify directions for future nursing research.

- select appropriate readings for further study.

Continuum of cognitive responses

The ability to think and to reason is a distinguishing feature of the human being. This ability created civilization and allowed progress from the Stone Age to the Space Age. Knowledge is growing at such a rapid rate that Toffler[23] defined "future shock" as an almost overwhelming impact on the person of the need to assimilate new information. We have moved from the time when power was equated with physical strength, to the use of money to acquire power, to an era in which little power exists without information. Although strength and money play a part in the use of power, the best informed persons are the most successful. It is now thought that individual computers will be required to assist the person in effectively processing information.

Because of the importance of the ability to think rationally, intellectual functioning is highly valued by the person. Most people are threatened at the prospect of losing their cognitive abilities, which are reasoning, memory, judgment, orientation, perception, and attention. These processes allow the individual to make sense of experience and to interact productively with the environment. Impaired cognitive functioning leaves the affected person in a state of confusion, unable to understand experience, and unable to relate current to past events. Memory is a key cognitive process because to exercise judgment, make decisions, or even orient oneself to time and place, one must remember past experiences and points of reference. Therefore memory loss is a particularly frightening experience.

Cognitive impairment is so threatening that most persons, even professionals, find it difficult to relate to those who have it. Those who suffered from this problem in the past were often labeled as crazy or senile. They were often institutionalized to meet their basic needs. Custodial care was provided by caretakers who had little knowledge of their patients' needs. Only recently has significant medical and nursing research into the needs of these patients begun to emerge.

■ Associationist model of cognition

Psychology is the discipline that has historically been most involved in research on cognition. Experimental psychologists have been interested in defining the process of learning and developing models that will explain learned behavior. Learning is a persistent change in the person's behavior related to a particular situation. It results from experience rather than instinct, reflex, or maturation. The associationist model of learning relates the behavioral change to reinforcement. This is also called a behavioral model. When the

---

CLINICAL EXAMPLE 18-1

Johnny M, age 3, asked his mother for a cookie. Ms. M told Johnny that he could have a cookie after he picked up his toys. Johnny began to kick and scream. Ms. M cuddled Johnny, gave him a cookie, and picked up the toys. When she discussed this experience with her neighbor, Ms. P, the mother of four children, Johnny's mother learned that he had a temper tantrum and that the behavior was likely to continue if she gave in to Johnny's demands. The next time Johnny demanded a cookie, Ms. M again requested that he pick up his toys first. Johnny began his temper tantrum. His mother placed him in another room and informed him again that when he picked up his toys, he could have a cookie. After a few minutes, Johnny quieted, then came out and put away his toys. His mother responded with cuddling and a cookie. Over time the temper tantrums disappeared.

---

individual experiences a **stimulus,** several behavioral **responses** are available to him. He is most likely to select the response that has been **reinforced** in the past. In other words, he has learned a particular response to a given stimulus or set of stimuli. If the response is not reinforced, an alternative behavior may be substituted. If the new behavior is reinforced, the person is more likely to continue to behave in that way. Clinical example 18-1 illustrates this process.

By reinforcing Johnny's tantrums with cookies and cuddling, Ms. M had, in effect, taught him that his behavior was effective. When she stopped reinforcing Johnny's negative behavior, he learned that another behavior was more effective in meeting his needs. Gradually, with continued reinforcement, the potential for effective behavior increased. Learning theorists believe that this sequence is responsible for the development of many human behaviors. They also believe that behavior can be changed, or learning can take place, by altering the reinforcement.

This process is depicted in Fig. 18-1. Since response number 1 is not reinforced, it tends not to recur. Instead, the person tries response number 2. It is reinforced and thus will tend to recur the next time the stimulus is produced. Reinforcement need not be a reward, although rewards are certainly powerful reinforcers. Punishment can also be a reinforcer of behavior if the alternative is lack of any response. Therefore,

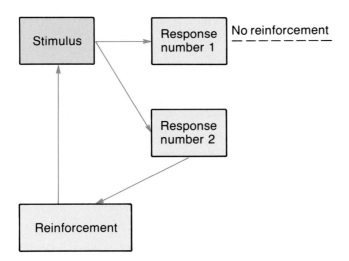

Fig. 18-1. The associationist, or behavioral, model of learning.

in the preceding example, spanking Johnny would probably have been less effective than leaving him alone, since he would still be receiving his mother's attention. Also, a reinforcer need not be a material object. The cuddling may have been as effective in reinforcing Johnny's behavior as the cookie. The associationist (behavioral) model of learning theory was developed by such theorists as Pavlov, Watson, Skinner, and Wolpe. Further information on the behavioral model and on behavior modification is found in Chapters 2 and 27.

■ Social-cognitive model of cognition

Another major group of learning theorists, including Tolman and Bandura, ascribe to a social-cognitive model.[1,24] While recognizing that reinforcement of behavior is important, they believe that behavior is based on additional information about the environment. In this case, the stimulus is perceived as a **sign** that a desired resource may be available from the environment (e.g., a cookie). This perception creates a **demand** that, when combined with knowledge about the environment, leads the person to seek gratification. The person's perception of the environment is referred to as a **cognitive map.** Cognitive learning theorists would say that the change in Johnny's cookie-seeking behavior resulted from a change in his perception of his mother's behavior as a part of his environment. Her changed behavior blocked the pathway that had previously led him to a cookie, so he had to find a new route.

Observational learning is another example of the social-cognitive model.[1] It has been shown that people learn from watching others in similar situations. If Johnny had an older brother who stole cookies when his mother was not looking, he might have tried this as an alternative path to his reward. Role modeling is a form of observational learning that is often used by nurses to teach health-related behavior.

■ Piaget developmental model of cognition

Human cognitive development has been described by Piaget[20] and is summarized in Table 18-1. His research revealed three stages in the development of thought processes. The first developmental stage is "the period of sensorimotor intelligence." This phase lasts from birth until the development of language, usually about 2 years of age. This stage is action oriented, with the actions first directed toward the self and then gradually incorporating more space and the ability to situate the self in space. Also, memory begins for objects that are out of sight. This is a necessary precursor for the development of language using words to describe objects that are not present. The baby who plays "peekaboo" is practicing this ability.

The second stage is the "period of preparation and organization of concrete operations: of categories, relations, and numbers." This period lasts from 2 to 12 years of age and is divided into two substages, which some theorists describe as separate. Early in this stage, during the preoperational substage, symbolism appears in language and in play. Greenspan and Curry[11] described five behavior patterns that are characteristic of this stage. They are: (1) imitation that starts after the model has left; (2) symbolic play or pretending; (3) drawing; (4) creation of mental images; and (5) talking about events that have already occurred. This is also the period of magical thinking, in which thoughts and words are perceived as the equivalent of action. Preoperational behavior lasts from about 2 to 5 years of age. The child then enters the substage of concrete operations. At this point, he is "capable of relatability, i.e., combinations, associations, negations and reversibility."[7] They learn to solve problems of conservation. For instance, if an object changes in shape, its weight remains the same.[11] During this period, children develop the capacity for syllogistic reasoning, which enables them to make and follow rules. They also develop the ability to quantify experience.

The third stage is "the period of formal operations."[20] This develops between ages 12 and 14 years, resulting in the ability to conceptualize at an adult level. Only at this point is the person "capable of abstract logic and has the ability to do manipulations in propositions, probabilities and permutations."[7] The

TABLE 18-1

PIAGET'S LEVELS OF COGNITIVE DEVELOPMENT

Stage	Age (years)	Characteristics
Sensorimotor	Birth to 2	Action oriented No language Develops awareness of body in space Develops memory for missing objects
Preparation and organization of concrete operations		
Preoperational phase	2 to 5	Symbolism appears Objects defined by function Magical thinking Imaginative play
Concrete operations	5 to 12	Capable of relatability Syllogistic reasoning Makes and follows rules Quantifies experience Understands conservation
Formal operations	12 to 14 and older	Abstraction Development of ideals Criticism of others Self-criticism

period of formal operations enables people to explore idealistic concepts and to measure reality against possibilities. This pertains to observations of significant others, such as parents, and of cultural institutions, such as government and religions. The same process is applied to the self in the form of self-criticism. This developmental process provides the foundation for continued cognitive growth as life experiences enrich and modify the person's perception of the world.

In some people, cognitive processes may not develop fully or, once developed, may deteriorate. When cognitive deficiencies occur during childhood, they are generally referred to as mental retardation. The reader is referred to a textbook of pediatric nursing for a discussion of cognitive deficiencies. This chapter considers cognitive disruptions in the adult. In most cases the person has developed to the level of formal operations. Although it may occur at any age, cognitive impairment is most common in the elderly. It is highly recommended that this chapter be read in conjunction with Chapter 34, because the content of the two chapters is complementary.

■ Continuum of cognitive responses

Cognitive impairments include impaired memory and judgment, disorientation, misperceptions, de-creased attention span, and difficulties with logical reasoning. They may occur episodically or be present continuously. Depending on the stressor, the condition may be reversible or characterized by progressive deterioration in functioning. Fig. 18-2 illustrates cognitive functioning as it occurs on the continuum of health-illness coping responses.

Assessment

■ Predisposing factors

Cognitive dysfunctions are usually caused by a biological disruption in the functioning of the central nervous system (CNS). The CNS requires a continuous supply of nutrients to function. Any interference with the provision of supplies to the brain will cause functional disruptions. For instance, the difficulties in cognition experienced by some elderly people result from arteriosclerotic changes in cerebral blood vessels. These changes deprive the brain of needed oxygen, glucose, and other essential basic chemicals. Other vascular abnormalities, such as transient ischemic attacks (small strokes), cerebral hemorrhage, and multiple small infarcts in brain tissue caused by chronic hypertension, can also result in cognitive impairments.

Aging itself predisposes the individual to cognitive

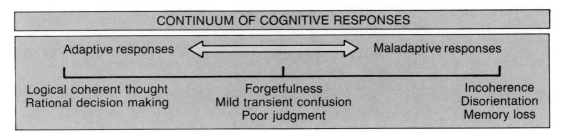

Fig. 18-2. Continuum of cognitive responses.

dysfunction. A cumulative degeneration of brain tissue is associated with aging, but it is not extensive enough to be particularly noticeable in most people. If other stressors are added, however, the person may experience difficulty. Some toxins collect in brain tissue, and a lifetime of exposure to a toxic chemical or a heavy metal may result in cognitive impairment.

Some metabolic disorders, such as chronic liver disease, chronic renal disease, and vitamin deficiencies, can result in disrupted information processing. Vitamin B−complex deficiency, particularly thiamine, is believed to cause the Wernicke-Korsakoff syndrome found in some chronic alcoholics. A prominent feature of this syndrome is a severe deficit in cognitive functioning. Malnutrition increases the person's risk of organic brain disease. This is often a problem in the elderly, who may lack the physical or financial resources needed for an adequate diet. However, young people with anorexia nervosa or bulimia nervosa are sometimes also at risk for cognitive impairment.

Genetic abnormalities may also be a cause. An example of a hereditary degenerative brain disease is Huntington's chorea, which is inherited as an autosomal dominant trait. Although a specific genetic defect has not been identified, there is evidence that Alzheimer's disease occurs more often in first-degree relatives of some victims. However, in other families there is not a consistent pattern of occurrence.[4] It does occur more frequently in people with Down's syndrome, another hereditary brain disorder.

A degree of cognitive impairment may be found along with other disruptions in mental functioning. For instance, a delusional person may seem disoriented because he misidentifies his location. People who have affective disorders may have short attention spans. Depression may also result in memory disorders, although it is often difficult to determine whether the problem is related to memory loss or lack of motivation. The predisposing factors related to these cognitive disorders are also related to the primary problem.

■ **Precipitating stressors**

Any major assault on the brain is likely to disrupt cognitive functioning. Wolanin[26] cites three major systemic problems that contribute to cognitive impairment: (1) hypoxia, (2) alterations in blood glucose content, and (3) toxicity. She further subdivides hypoxia into four types: (1) anemic; (2) histotoxic, or conditions that prevent cells from metabolizing oxygen; (3) hypoxemic, or problems with ventilation; and (4) ischemic.

■ **HYPOXIAS.** Anemic hypoxia may be insidious in onset. Possible stressors include aspirin ingestion, resulting in occult bleeding; other occult blood loss; or deficiencies of iron, folic acid, or vitamin B_{12}. Histotoxic hypoxia may be related to such stressors as dehydration, hyperthermia, or hypothermia. A possible stressor related to hypoxemic hypoxia is chronic obstructive lung disease. Others might include asthma or an acute respiratory tract infection. Ischemic hypoxia can result from congestive heart failure, atherosclerosis, hypotension, hypertension, or increased intracranial pressure resulting from a tumor, subdural hematoma, or normal pressure hydrocephalus.[26]

■ **METABOLIC DISORDERS.** Metabolic disorders often affect mental functioning, especially when severe or of long duration. Endocrine malfunctioning, whether it involves underproduction or overproduction of hormones, can adversely affect cognition. For example, the thyroid hormone greatly influences mental alertness. People with hypothyroidism are sluggish and retarded in their thinking. Those with severe hypothyroidism (myxedema) may develop psychotic behavior characterized by delusional thinking. People with hyperthyroidism, on the other hand, are frequently hyperalert and agitated. Other endocrine disorders that may cause cognitive disruptions include hypoglycemia, hypopituitarism, and adrenal disease.

■ **TOXIC AND INFECTIOUS AGENTS.** Toxic and infectious agents may also result in behavior typical of disturbed cerebral functioning. Toxins may originate within the individual or in the external environment.

An example of an internally generated toxin is the elevated blood level of urea found in a patient with renal failure. Environmental toxins include various poisonous substances, e.g., toxic wastes and animal venoms. Increased levels of aluminum have been found in the brains of people with Alzheimer's disease. However, this is now believed to be an effect of the disease rather than a cause. Acute viral and bacterial infections occur in the CNS, resulting in inflammation and impaired functioning. Infections in other body systems may also impair the CNS if temperature is extremely elevated. Chronic infections also affect the brain. One such condition is the neural manifestation of tertiary syphilis, general paresis. This is seldom seen because of the early treatment of syphilis. Some have suspected that Alzheimer's disease is caused by a viral infection. However, it is not typical of patterns related to known transmissible infections. Researchers continue to search for evidence of an atypical infectious agent.[4] It has also been determined that people who are infected with human immunodeficiency virus type 1 (HIV-1) often develop an organic brain syndrome called AIDS dementia complex.[19] This is apparently caused by invasion of non-neuronal brain cells by the virus. There are two major theories regarding the way that neurons are affected by HIV-1.[3] According to the first of these theories, the virus produces a protein that is toxic to neurons. The second theory suggests that neurotoxic substances are released by HIV-infected cells, including macrophages, microglial cells, and astrocytes. According to Barnes,[3] "the most glaring unanswered question about brain disease in AIDS is how HIV-1 infection of non-neuronal cells in the brain induces the abnormal function of brain neurons." The HIV-1 virus also causes acquired immunodeficiency syndrome (AIDS).

Wolanin[26] emphasizes the possible significance of prescription and over-the-counter drugs as toxic stressors. Thorough assessment of drug use is critical with elderly patients because of their increased sensitivity to drugs and because confusion could lead to difficulty in following directions for taking drugs. Interactions between drugs or between drugs and other substances, particularly alcohol, may also lead to disruptions in cognitive functioning.

■ **STRUCTURAL CHANGES.** Conditions that alter the structure of brain tissue are also reflected in impaired cognitive functioning. Tumors may cause proliferation or displacement of tissue, thus altering its function. Trauma, whether accidental or surgical, may result in a change in ability to process information. The specific effect depends on the location of the lesion.

■ **SENSORY STIMULATION.** Sensory underload or overload can result in cognitive dysfunction. Persons who are placed in environments with minimal stimuli seem to develop internally produced stimuli in the form of hallucinations. In contrast, the constant light and activity in intensive care units (ICUs) have led to confusion, delusions, and hallucinations, sometimes referred to as "ICU psychosis." However, it is difficult to determine how much of the cognitive impairment results from the sensory experience as opposed to other concurrent stressors, such as the introduction of multiple drugs into the system and the result of massive assaults on physical integrity.

■ **NONSPECIFIC STRESSORS.** Unfortunately, many times the specific stressor related to cognitive impairment cannot be identified. Understanding of the biochemical processes of the brain and the response of brain and nervous tissue to stressors is still limited. As knowledge grows, specific biological components may be identified in the etiology of all psychiatric disorders. The fields of psychiatry and neurology may merge at some time as knowledge grows more sophisticated. For example, deficiencies in neurotransmitters, including acetylcholine, somatostatin, substance P, and norepinephrine, have been observed in patients with Alzheimer's disease.[18] It is not known whether this is a cause or effect of the illness. Also, it is known that some chemical substances can create hallucinatory experiences and are popular in the drug culture for that reason. As more is learned about how hallucinogens such as lysergic acid diethylamide (LSD) and phencyclidine (PCP) work, more will also be understood about processes that may occur in the brains of psychotic people.

In general when assessing cognitive impairment, physiological causes are ruled out first, then psychosocial stressors are considered. Even when physiological factors are present, psychosocial stress may further compromise the person's thought process. Each patient must receive a complete assessment so that nursing care can be planned in a holistic manner.

■ **Behaviors**

Disruptions in cognitive functioning are most apparent in people who have a medical diagnosis of organic mental syndrome or disorder (DSM-III-R).[2] The use of the term "organic" is being reviewed since it is now recognized that most, if not all, of the mental disorders have a physiological component.[25] A distinction is made between **organic mental syndromes,** which are not differentiated in terms of etiology and **organic mental disorders,** in which a cause may be determined. In other words, the organic mental disorder is a defined organic mental syndrome. For example, multi-infarct dementia is an organic mental disorder. The organic mental disorders include primary degenerative dementia of the Alzheimer's type subdivided into senile (after age 65) and presenile onset, and multi-infarct dementia. Following are the categories of organic mental syndromes[2]:

1. Delirium
2. Dementia
3. Amnestic syndrome
4. Organic delusional syndrome
5. Organic hallucinosis
6. Organic mood syndrome
7. Organic personality syndrome
8. Organic anxiety syndrome
9. Intoxication
10. Withdrawal

Discussions in this chapter focus primarily on category 1, delirium and dementia, because these are the medical diagnostic categories that nurses encounter most frequently. Unless otherwise noted, discussions regarding dementia will not differentiate among the organic mental syndrome of dementia, primary degenerative dementia of the Alzheimer's type and multi-infarct dementia. The nursing approaches are the same for each of these medical diagnoses.

■ **ASSOCIATED WITH DELIRIUM.** In the past, delirium was also referred to as acute, or reversible, brain syndrome and dementia as chronic, or irreversible, brain syndrome. Acute versus chronic referred to the rapidity of the onset of the disorder and to its duration. These terms are no longer recommended because they do not discriminate between delirium and dementia. Delirium is characterized by a clouding of awareness, manifested by a limited attention span, sensory misperception, and disordered thought.[2] There are also disturbances of activity patterns and of the sleep-wake cycle. Generally, a rapid onset and a brief course of illness occurs. The disordered thought process includes disturbed attention, memory, thinking, orientation, and perception. The degree of impairment tends to fluctuate throughout the day, with periods of lucidity occurring intermittently. The disturbance is generally worse at night. Delirium usually occurs in response to a specific stressor, such as infection, trauma, a metabolic disorder, a toxin, or drug or alcohol intoxication. However, the stressor may not be immediately apparent. Clinical example 18-2 illustrates typical behaviors of a patient with delirium.

Ms. S demonstrates many behaviors often seen in patients with delirium. The behaviors are related to alterations in neurochemical and electrical responses in

the brain as a result of the stressor that causes the disruption. **Disorientation** is generally present, sometimes in all three spheres of time, place, and person. Thought processes are usually disorganized. Judgment is poor, and little decision-making ability exists. Stimuli may be misinterpreted, resulting in **illusions** or distortions of reality. An example of an illusion is the perception that a polka-dot drape is actually covered with cockroaches. Delirious patients may hallucinate. These **hallucinations** are usually visual and often take the form of animals, reptiles, or insects. They are real to the person and very frightening. Assaultive or destructive behavior may be the patient's attempt to strike back at a hallucinated image. At times, patients with delirium also exhibit a **labile affect,** changing abruptly from laughter to tearfulness, and vice versa, for no apparent reason. There may also be **loss of usual social behavior,** resulting in such acts as undressing, playing with food, and grabbing at others. Delirious patients tend to act on impulse.

Other behaviors may be specifically related to the cause of the behavioral syndrome. For example, the fever and dehydration experienced by Ms. S were a result of her systemic streptococcal infection, as was her brain syndrome. It is very important to differentiate behavioral manifestations, which help to identify the stressor. Treatment is usually conservative until a specific stressor has been isolated. Although most patients recover, it is possible for the person to die as a result of the stressor's severity. If adequate intervention does not take place, delirium may become dementia.

■ **ASSOCIATED WITH DEMENTIA.** Dementia is a cognitive disruption that features a loss of intellectual abilities and interferes with usual social or occupational activities.[2] The loss of intellectual ability includes impairment of memory, judgment, and abstract thought. The patient with dementia does not exhibit the clouding of awareness that is seen with delirium.[14] Changes in personality frequently occur. The personality change may appear as either alteration or accentuation of the person's usual character traits. The onset of dementia is usually gradual. It may result in the patient's gradual deterioration or may be stable. The process of dementia can be reversed, and the person's intellectual functioning can improve if the underlying stressors are identified and treated.

Dementia may occur at any age but most often affects the elderly. According to Horvath, et al.,[14] of the American population over 65 years old, 10% suffer from mild to moderate dementia, and slightly less than 5% have severe dementia. It is estimated that 2 million people in the United States suffer from dementia. About 55% of those with dementia have Alzheimer's

CLINICAL EXAMPLE 18-2

Ms. S was brought to the emergency room of a general hospital by her parents. She was a 22-year-old single woman who was described as having been in good health until 2 days prior to admission, when she complained of malaise and a sore throat and stayed home from work. She was employed as a typist in a small office and had a stable employment record. According to her parents, she had an active social life and there were no significant conflicts at home.

On admission, Ms. S was extremely restless and had a frightened facial expression. Her speech was garbled and incoherent. When she was approached by an unfamiliar person, she would become agitated, trying to climb out of bed and striking out aimlessly. Occasionally she would slip into a restless sleep. Her temperature on admission was 104° F (40 ° C) rectally, pulse was 108 per minute, and respirations were 28 per minute. Her skin was hot, dry, and flushed. Her mother said she had had only a few sips of water in the last 24 hours and had not urinated at all, although she had had several episodes of profuse diaphoresis.

Her ability to cooperate with a mental status examination was limited. She would respond to her own name by turning her head. When her mother asked her where she was, she said "home," but could not say where her home was. She would give only the month when asked for the date and said it was January, when the actual date was February 19. She also refused to give the day of the week. A neurological examination was negative for signs of increased intracranial pressure or for localizing signs of CNS disease.

The tentative medical diagnosis was that of delirium secondary to fever of unknown origin. Symptomatic treatment of the fever, including intravenous fluids, an aspirin suppository, and cool water mattress, was begun immediately while further diagnostic studies were carried out. Nurses caring for the patient noticed continued restlessness and disorientation. Her speech was still incoherent. In addition, they noticed that she was picking at the bedclothing. Suddenly she became extremely agitated, trying to get out of bed and crying out, "Bugs, get away, get bugs away." She was brushing and slapping at herself and the bed. As her mother and the nurse talked with her and held her, she gradually became calmer but periodically would continue to slap at "the bugs" and need reassurance and reorientation.

Later in the day additional laboratory results became available. A lumbar puncture was normal, as were skull x-ray films. Results of toxicological screening of blood were also negative. The electroencephalogram revealed diffuse slowing. There was an elevated white blood count and electrolyte imbalance consistent with severe dehydration. Cultures of her throat and blood were both positive for beta-hemolytic streptococci, so intravenous antibiotic therapy was begun at once while other supportive measures were continued.

As the infection gradually came under control and the fever decreased, Ms. S's mental state improved. A week later, when she was discharged from the hospital, her cognitive functioning was completely normal, with the exception of amnesia for the time during which she was delirious.

disease. After 75 years of age, Alzheimer's is the fourth leading cause of death. Dementia may result from accidental or surgical trauma, a chronic infection such as tertiary syphilis, cerebrovascular disruptions such as arteriosclerosis or chronic hypertension, or it may have an indeterminate cause. "Senility" is a nonspecific term and usually applies to those who have degenerative brain disease of unknown cause. Because of the negative connotation, use of the terms "senility" or "senile" is discouraged. Clinical example 18-3 demonstrates behaviors associated with dementia.

The behaviors associated with dementia reflect the brain tissue alterations that are taking place. The cognitive changes are related to the actions of stressors that interfere with the functioning of the cerebral cortex. Other areas of the brain may be affected as well, which is one reason for ensuring that the patient has a complete medical and neurological examination. Another reason is that although the condition may be irreversible, progression may be stopped by identifying the stressor and treating the underlying dysfunction. For instance, treatment of hypertension may prevent further occurrence of small hemorrhages, which are a possible cause of irreversible brain syndrome. Recent research has shown that many cases of dementia may be reversible. It has also been found that depression in the elderly is often misinterpreted as dementia and therefore not treated appropriately. This happens so

CLINICAL EXAMPLE 18-3

Mr. B is a 73-year-old widower who has resided in a nursing home for 3 years. He chose to move to the nursing home after the death of his wife, although his son encouraged him to live with him and his family. Mr. B stated that he did not want to burden his family and would be happier with others of the same age. He did well for the first 18 months. He was an active participant in social groups both in the home and in his church, where he continued to attend regularly. He also visited his son once a week and enjoyed seeing his grandchildren and puttering around his son's house.

About 18 months previously Mr. B began to seem forgetful. He would ask the same question several times and on occasion would prepare for church on a Friday or Saturday. He also became irritable and accused his son of not caring about him and abandoning him in "that place." Mr. B spent many hours taking papers from his desk and studying them. When asked what he was doing, he would say, "Attending to my business." He began to withdraw from activities, making flimsy excuses to avoid playing his favorite card game, gin rummy. When he was persuaded to play, he usually quit in frustration because he could not remember which cards had been played. At times Mr. B was quite anxious. He would periodically seem well oriented and expressed great concern about the changes he was experiencing, wondering if he was "going crazy."

Because of the concern of the nursing staff at the nursing home, Mr. B was scheduled for a complete physical examination by his family physician and for a psychiatric evaluation by the geriatric psychiatric nurse consultant who came to the nursing home weekly. The physical examination revealed generally good health for a man of Mr. B's age. He suffered from a mild hearing loss and slight prostatic hypertrophy. Hypertension had been diagnosed 10 years before this examination but was well controlled by diuretics. Neurological examination revealed normal reflexes, normal muscle strength, a slight intention tremor, normal response to sensation, normal cranial nerves, and no disturbance of gait. An electroencephalogram was normal, as were a skull x-ray film and the results of laboratory studies of blood and urine. Computed tomography studies of the brain revealed some atrophy of the cerebral cortex.

The psychiatric examination confirmed the deficits in cognitive functioning that had been observed by the nursing home staff and by Mr. B's son. He was oriented to person and place but stated that the date was April 6, 1958. The real date was March 11, 1988. He also thought the day of the week was Friday, whereas it was actually Tuesday. He correctly identified the season of the year as spring. Mr. B was able to give correctly his birth date, the date of his son's birth, and the year he began to work at his first job. He spoke at length and with great detail about his exploits as a young man. However, he could not repeat the names of three objects after 5 minutes and could not remember what he had eaten for lunch or the last name of the man who shared his room. He became distressed when he was trying to answer these questions. His vocabulary was excellent, as was his fund of general information. However, he was unable to remember the names of the two most recent presidents. He could, however, recite the names of the eight presidents preceding them.

Mr. B's judgment was somewhat impaired. When asked what he would do if he found a stamped, addressed, sealed envelope, he said he would "read it, then mail it." His ability for abstract thinking was slightly concretized. His attention span and ability to concentrate were normal. His eye-hand coordination was disrupted, as demonstrated by his difficulty in copying simple figures. His tremor was evident both when he was drawing and when he signed his name.

His affect was appropriate in quality and quantity to the content of the discussion. He appeared depressed when talking about his memory loss but cheerful and proud when describing his grandchildren. No abrupt mood swings were noted. The flow of speech was of a normal rate and volume. Content of speech was logical and coherent, except when Mr. B was trying to remember and describe recent events, when it became somewhat disjointed.

As a result of the data gathered in the physical and psychiatric examinations, he was diagnosed as having dementia of unknown cause.

Over the next several months, Mr. B's condition continued to deteriorate gradually. He became increasingly forgetful and began to confabulate (fabricate stories). He was less conforming to social norms and needed reminding about hygiene and appropriate dress. He also became seductive with female residents and staff, making suggestive remarks and occasionally fondling someone. Visits to his son's home became impossible as his behavior deteriorated. His memory of the identity of family members sometimes was confused. He would misidentify his daughter-in-law as his wife and his grandson as his son. More and more, his conversation consisted of rambling reminiscences of his life in his youth. Because he is surrounded with caring people, Mr. B continues to live with dignity and respect despite his progressively limited ability to communicate.

often that the condition has been labeled **pseudodementia.**

Depression differs from dementia in several ways.[1] A depressed person usually expresses concern about his perceived lack of cognitive ability, whereas a demented person tries to compensate for it and hide it. If motivated, a depressed person is able to perform cognitive tests, and, if not, the deficits are less consistent than those found in dementia. In addition, the date of onset of depression can usually be more specifically identified than that of dementia. However, the conditions can coexist, since a person who is somewhat aware of impaired cognitive ability may experience depression.

Alzheimer's disease is one of the most prevalent causes of impaired cognitive functioning. It is now accepted that loss of mental abilities is not automatically associated with aging, and intensive research has focused on identifying the causes, characteristics, and treatment for Alzheimer's disease. Investigators have found that characteristic alterations occur in brain tissue. Pajk[18] has summarized these as follows:

1. The presence of neurofibrillary tangles, which are "pairs of filaments wrapped around each other in the cytoplasm of the neurons"[18]
2. Neuritic plaques, which are "filamentous and granular deposits representing degeneration in the neuronal processes"[18]
3. Granulovascular degeneration, in which "fluid pockets and granular material develop in the neurons"[18]

These phenomena are found throughout the cortex but are concentrated in the hippocampus, the center for short-term memory. This is consistent with the short-term memory loss characteristic of Alzheimer's disease. In addition, there is atrophy of the associational areas of the cortex. Alterations have also been noted in the neurotransmitter systems. In particular, there is a serious deficiency of acetylcholine.[14] Other behaviors associated with this disease are found in most types of dementia.

Multi-infarct dementia is much less common than primary degenerative dementia of the Alzheimer's type. It results from disruptions in the cerebral blood supply.[14] Patients with hypertensive vascular disease may experience this type of dementia as the result of the sudden closure of the lumen of arterioles related to pressure changes. Atherosclerosis may lead to the formation of thrombi or emboli. In either case, the outcome is infarction of the brain tissue in the area supplied by the affected blood vessels. The resulting cognitive problems are related to the area of the brain that is involved.

Another organic brain disorder that results in dementia is associated with HIV-1, which also causes AIDS. Navia and Price[17] have described the course of the dementia. Early symptoms include memory impairment, decreased concentration, slowed mental responses, apathy, decreased socialization, and occasionally psychotic symptoms. Late symptoms include global cognitive impairment and psychomotor slowing. The person is alert but not spontaneous in response to others. Sometimes agitation occurs. At the end stage the person is mute, immobile, and incontinent. A computed tomographic (CT) scan reveals cortical atrophy and enlarged brain ventricles. Perry and Jacobsen[19] have identified two other behavioral patterns associated with HIV-1. The first is a mild, chronic depression, with behaviors similar to those described for a major depressive episode. The second is an acute psychotic reaction, including behaviors of "grandiosity, suspiciousness, delusional thinking, hallucinations, psychomotor agitation, rambling and repetitive speech, confusion and blunted affect."[19] The authors warn that it may be difficult to differentiate the organic and psychological aspects of these behavioral patterns.

A common behavior related to dementia is **disorientation.** Usually, time orientation is affected first, then place, and finally person. This behavior can be distressing to the patient, who may be aware of this difficulty and embarrassed or frightened by it. This is particularly true if the person's mental acuity is fluctuating. In these instances the person is aware, during periods of lucidity, of the confusion and disorientation experienced at other times.

Memory loss is another prominent characteristic of dementia. Immediate recall and recent memory are most seriously affected. Remote memory may be intact, although it will deteriorate as the condition progresses. In Clinical example 18-3, Mr. B had trouble remembering what he had eaten for lunch but gave accurate dates for significant events earlier in his life. Most aging people dwell on the past, but people with recent memory loss have difficulty shifting to the present and at advanced stages may seem to live in the past. This was exemplified by Mr. B's misidentification of his grandson and his daughter-in-law. Another behavior related to memory loss is **confabulation.** This is a confused person's tendency to make up a response to a question when he cannot remember the answer. For instance, when Mr. B was asked if he knew one of the female residents of the home, he replied, "Of course I know her. I used to play gin with her husband." Actually, the woman's husband had been dead for many years and Mr. B had never met him. This behavior should not be viewed as lying or an attempt to deceive. Rather, it is the person's way of trying to save face in an embarrassing situation. He is aware that he should know the answer to the question and gives an answer that seems reasonable, not entirely disbelieving it himself. It is not unlike the situation in which a person meets an acquaintance and cannot recall the other's name or where they met. The person acts as if these facts are remembered, hoping that the other will offer clues about his identity.

Vocabulary and general information may be less affected by dementia, at least until its very late stages. This depends on when the information was learned. Facts learned early in life may be recalled well, whereas those learned recently may be quickly forgotten, as demonstrated by Mr. B's performance in listing the last 10 presidents.

These patients may have **labile affective behavior,** particularly if the limbic system has been affected by the disease process. There may also be some **deterioration in social skills.** Impulsive sexual advances may occur. These reflect **decreased inhibition** and **impaired judgment.** Frequently this behavior is also an attempt to establish interpersonal contact and is a way of asking for caring from others. It is also a way of reinforcing an important part of the person's identity, which is becoming less secure as mental functioning declines.

Restlessness and **agitation** are other behaviors that occur with dementia. Extreme agitation may occur at night; this is sometimes referred to as the **sun-down syndrome.** It probably results from tiredness at the end of the day combined with fewer orienting stimuli, such as planned activities, meals, and contact with people.

Disorientation results in fear and agitation. Agitated behavior may also occur if the person is coerced to do something he does not understand or simply does not want to do. This may reflect an effort to keep control over the person's own life, thereby maintaining self-esteem. Change is not well accepted by these patients. Efforts to change behavior patterns will probably result in increased rigidity and, if efforts persist, agitated behavior. Routine is important, particularly a routine that fits the person's previous life-style. Table 18-2 summarizes the characteristics of delirium and dementia.

The term **confusion** is frequently used when referring to the person with cognitive impairment. Although widely accepted as nursing and medical jargon, this term has not been specifically defined. Wolanin and Phillips[27] have focused their nursing research on this topic. They define confusion as "a condition characterized by the client's disorientation to time and place, incongruous conceptual boundaries, paranormal awareness, and seemingly inappropriate verbal statements that indicate memory defects."[27:8] The term should be used with caution, however, since Wolanin and Phillips discovered a wide array of meanings when they surveyed groups of physicians and nurses.

■ **PSYCHOLOGICAL TESTING.** Often patients who have cognitive impairment are referred to a clini-

---

TABLE 18-2

CHARACTERISTICS OF DELIRIUM AND DEMENTIA

	Delirium	Dementia
Onset	Usually sudden	Usually gradual
Course	Usually brief (under 1 month), with return to usual level of functioning	Usually long term and progressive; occasionally may be arrested or reversed
Age group	Any	Most common over age 65
Stressors	Toxins, infection, hyperthermia, space-occupying lesion, trauma, and sensory deprivation/overload	Hypertension, hypotension, anemia, normal pressure hydrocephalus, vitamin deficiencies, toxins, slow viruses, hypoglycemia, tumors, hyperthermia/hypothermia, and brain tissue atrophy
Behaviors	Fluctuating levels of awareness, disorientation, restlessness, agitation, illusions, hallucinations, disorganized thought, impaired judgment and decision making, affective lability, loss of inhibitions, and diffuse electroencephalogram (EEG) slowing	Memory loss, impaired judgment, decreased attention span, disorientation, inappropriate social behavior, labile affect, restlessness, agitation, and resistance to change

cal psychologist for testing. This referral should be made for a specific purpose, since the testing is time consuming, expensive, and tiring for the patient. Some reasons for psychological testing include identification of the stressor(s) causing the disruption, understanding of the dynamics of the problem, developing guidelines for therapeutic intervention, and obtaining a prognosis for recovery. DeCato and Wicks[6] present an excellent summary of indications for psychological referral and a description of the most common psychological tests given to psychiatric patients. They divide the tests into three categories: intelligence, perceptual-motor, and projective.

Intelligence tests are used to assess the patient's general level of intellectual functioning. Those used most often are the **Wechsler Intelligence Scale for Children (WISC)** and the **Wechsler Adult Intelligence Scale (WAIS).** These tests must be evaluated by a skilled clinician, with consideration given to educational and sociocultural background of the patient. The result of the test is the person's intelligence quotient (IQ), which can serve as a guideline for understanding the person's intellectual ability. Information about psychodynamics may also be obtained by analyzing the nature of the person's behavior in the testing situation.

Perceptual-motor testing is useful in determining whether an organic mental disorder is causing disturbed behavior. The **Bender-Gestalt test** requires that the patient copy a series of geometrical figures. The accuracy and facility with which the copying is done helps to determine the presence of a biological stressor. Other factors, such as size and arrangement of the copied figures or the patient's behavior in the testing situation, provide insight into the person's psychodynamic functioning. For example, a person who uses obsessive-compulsive behavior to cope with anxiety may try hard to make an exact copy of the figure.

Projective tests are used to gain information about psychodynamics. The most widely known projective test is the **Rorschach test,** which consists of a standard series of inkblots. The patient is asked to respond to the inkblot, first generally and then in more detail. The response is then analyzed. Use and analysis of the Rorschach test is complex and must be done only by a qualified clinical psychologist. Another frequently used projective test is the **Thematic Apperception Test (TAT).** The patient is presented with drawings of people engaged in nonspecific activities and asked to describe what might be happening. In both these situations the person's response is determined by past experience, as well as current mental state. Valuable information may be gained about the person's anxiety level and the mechanisms used to cope with anxiety, which can have implications for therapy and prognosis.

Many other psychological tests are available, some used for very specialized purposes. Clinical psychologists are good resource people both for explaining specific tests and for elaborating on the results of psychological testing. Often the psychologist is asked to determine whether the person is experiencing a disruption that is organic. More information about psychological testing may be found in Chapter 6.

■ Coping mechanisms

How an individual copes emotionally with a disruption in cognitive ability is greatly influenced by past experience. A person who has developed a reservoir of effective coping mechanisms is better able to handle the onset of a cognitive problem than one who has not.

The person's response to the onset of organic brain disease often mirrors that person's basic personality. For instance, a person who has usually reacted to stress with anger directed toward other people and the environment will probably react similarly when he notices limitations in his intellectual abilities. A person who is more apt to direct anger inward and become depressed will be more likely to respond with depressive behaviors. A person who has relied on a mechanism such as intellectualization will be more threatened by loss of intellectual ability than a person who has used a mechanism such as reaction formation.

Regression is often used to cope with an advanced mental disorder. It may be caused in part by deterioration in mental function. It probably also results from the problem's behavioral manifestations, which cause the patient to become more dependent on others for the fulfillment of basic needs such as nutrition and hygiene. Encouraging patients to perform self-care also supports their use of healthier coping mechanisms.

Because the basic behavioral disruption in delirium is altered awareness, which reflects the severe biological disturbance in the brain, psychological coping mechanisms are not generally used. Therefore the nurse must protect the patient from harm and provide a substitute for his coping mechanisms by constantly reorienting him and reinforcing reality.

A characteristic of early dementia is the mechanism of denial. The person attempts to pursue his usual daily routine and makes light of memory lapses. He may be able to use some environmental resources to help him cope. For instance, a businessman who is experiencing difficulty with recent memory might ask his secretary to remind him of all his appointments and provide him with the names of the people with whom he is meeting and the meeting's purpose. As the impairment progresses, the person may become very resistant to any limits on his independence. For instance, the family of a patient with Alzheimer's disease might become very concerned about his ability to continue to drive a car safely. The patient probably would be very reluctant to give up his driver's license and would deny that he was having any problem.

As cognitive ability decreases, efforts to cope become more obvious. For instance, a family member may complain that a relative has "always been irritable, but is now belligerent when he doesn't get his way." In other cases the patient's behavior may be perceived as a personality change. Some behaviors that are probably attempts to cope with loss of cognitive ability include suspiciousness, hostility, joking, depression, seductiveness, and withdrawal. Because it is threatening to admit that a close relative has dementia, family members may focus on the coping mechanism as the real problem, thus participating in the denial of the underlying cognitive impairment.

 Nursing diagnosis

The nursing diagnosis of the person with cognitive impairment must consider both the possible underlying stressors and patient behaviors. Fig. 18-3 summarizes the nursing model of health-illness phenomena as related to cognitive functioning.

Most cognitive impairment disorders are physiological in origin. Therefore the nurse must consider the patient's physical needs, as well as the psychosocial behavioral disruptions. For instance, the delirious patient may be reacting to an infection or a drug overdose. This problem and all its effects must be reflected in a complete nursing diagnosis. Many people who are demented are also elderly. They experience many effects of the aging process in addition to impaired cognitive functioning. A thorough nursing diagnosis reflects all these influences on the patient's behavior. In addition, the nature of a cognitive impairment may inhibit the patient's ability to participate in the care planning process. The nurse must rely on observational skills and on the input of significant others to arrive at an accurate, relevant diagnosis. If the nursing diagnosis cannot be validated with the patient, a family member familiar with the person's behavioral patterns should be involved. Primary NANDA nursing diagnoses and examples of complete nursing diagnoses related to impaired cognition are presented in the box above. The range of frequently encountered NANDA nursing diagnoses and the DSM-III-R[2] medical diagnoses are included in Table 18-3.

Nursing Diagnoses Related to Impaired Cognition

Primary NANDA nursing diagnosis
Altered thought processes

Examples of complete nursing diagnoses
Altered thought processes related to severe dehydration, evidenced by hypervigilance; distractibility; disorientation to time, place, and person; and visual hallucinations

Altered thought processes related to barbiturate ingestion, evidenced by altered sleep patterns, delusions, disorientation to time and place, and decreased ability to grasp ideas

Altered thought processes related to Alzheimer's disease, evidenced by inaccurate interpretation of environment, deficit in recent memory, impaired ability to reason, and confabulation

Altered thought processes related to HIV-I infection evidenced by impaired ability to make decisions, to problem solve, to reason, to calculate, and to display appropriate social behavior

---

■ **Related medical diagnoses**

Several medical diagnostic categories are related to impaired cognitive functioning. These differ according to the cause of the disorder and the clinical manifestations. In all cases, however, the cause is organic. Each one is described briefly.

■ **PRIMARY DEGENERATIVE DEMENTIA OF THE ALZHEIMER TYPE.** This diagnosis is subdivided into presenile and senile depending on whether the onset is before or after the age of 65. The essential feature is generally progressive, deteriorating dementia that has a gradual onset. All other specific causes must be excluded. It includes loss of cognitive abilities, including memory, judgment, and abstract thought, accompanied by personality changes.[2]

■ **MULTI-INFARCT DEMENTIA.** The essential element is dementia related to cerebrovascular disease. The cognitive disorder is "patchy," with loss of some functions while others are not affected. Focal neurologic signs are present. The onset is usually abrupt.[2]

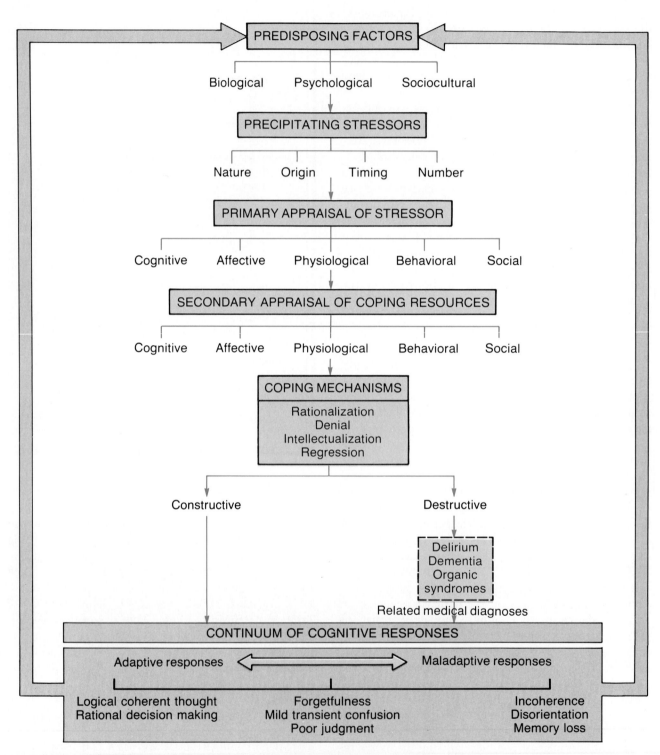

Fig. 18-3. Nursing model of health-illness phenomena related to cognitive functioning.

TABLE 18-3

MEDICAL AND NURSING DIAGNOSES RELATED TO IMPAIRED COGNITION

Medical Diagnostic Class Organic mental disorders	**Psychiatric Nursing Diagnostic Class** Impaired cognition

Related Medical Diagnoses (DSM-III-R*)
Primary degenerative dementia of the Alzheimer type, senile onset
Primary degenerative dementia of the Alzheimer type, presenile onset
Multi-infarct dementia
Delirium
Dementia
Amnestic disorder
Organic delusional disorder
Organic hallucinosis
Organic mood disorder
Organic anxiety disorder
Organic personality disorder
	Related Medical Diagnoses (NANDA)
	Anxiety
	Bowel incontinence
	Communication, impaired verbal
	Coping, ineffective family: compromised
	Coping, ineffective individual
	Diversional activity deficit
	Fear
	Fluid volume deficit, potential
	Health maintenance, altered
	Home maintenance management, impaired
	Injury, potential for
	Mobility, impaired physical
	Role performance, altered
	Self care deficit
	    Bathing/hygiene, feeding, dressing/grooming, toileting
	Sensory/perceptual alterations (specify)
	    Visual, auditory, kinesthetic, gustatory, tactile, olfactory
	Skin integrity, potential impaired
	Sleep pattern disturbance
	Social interaction, impaired
	Social isolation
	†Thought processes, altered
	Trauma, potential for

*American Psychiatric Association: DSM-III-R. American Psychiatric Association, 1987.
†Indicates primary nursing diagnosis for impaired cognition.

■ **DELIRIUM.** The essential feature of delirium is clouded consciousness with impaired ability to perceive or respond to environmental stimuli. Other behaviors include hallucinations or illusions, incoherence, agitation or somnolence, disorientation, and confusion. The onset is usually rapid; the course usually fluctuates; and duration of the episode is typically brief.[2]

■ **DEMENTIA.** The essential feature of dementia is a loss of intellectual abilities that interferes with functional ability. Memory is impaired. Other behaviors may include problems with abstraction, judgment, and higher cortical functioning and personality change. No clouding of consciousness occurs.[2]

■ **AMNESTIC SYNDROME.** The essential feature of amnestic syndrome is impairment in short- and long-term memory in the absence of clouding of consciousness or deterioration of intellectual ability. The disorder is attributed to a specific organic factor.[2]

■ **ORGANIC DELUSIONAL SYNDROME.** The essential feature is the presence of delusions that occur in the absence of clouding of consciousness, and may be attributed to a specific organic factor.[2]

■ **ORGANIC HALLUCINOSIS.** The essential feature is the presence of persistent or recurrent hallucinations that occur in the absence of clouding of consciousness and may be attributed to a specific organic factor.[2]

■ **ORGANIC MOOD SYNDROME.** The essential feature is a disturbance in mood, resembling either a manic episode or a major depressive episode, in the absence of clouding of consciousness and attributable to a specific organic factor.[2]

■ **ORGANIC PERSONALITY SYNDROME.** The essential feature is a behavioral pattern related to a specific organic factor involving labile affect, aggressive outbursts, poor judgment in social situations, apathy, OR suspiciousness.[2]

■ **ORGANIC ANXIETY SYNDROME.** The essential feature is recurrent generalized anxiety or panic in the absence of clouding of consciousness and attributable to a specific organic factor.[2]

❦ Planning

■ Goal setting

The primary goal related to the patient with cognitive impairment is to promote optimum cognitive functioning. Goals may be directed toward an improved ability to process information, if this is realistic, or toward optimum use of the abilities the patient retains if the impairment is irreversible. For example, a goal for a patient who is disoriented because of drug withdrawal might be, "The patient will verbalize the complete date within 3 days." In contrast, a goal for a patient who is disoriented because of chronic alcoholism and who is not in withdrawal might be, "Within 1 month the patient will find his own bed every night without assistance." This patient may never be able to remember the exact date but may not need that information if he is to function in a protected setting. The first patient, however, will need that information. In addition, the nurse can use the assessment of the patient's orientation to time to assess the current status of his mental functioning. Goals should be realistic to avoid discouragement. If the second patient had been required to learn the date, frequent confrontation with his deteriorated cognitive skills might result, leading to frustration, higher anxiety, and possibly less effective coping.

If an identified stressor is causing the patient's behavioral disruption, goals that focus on the stressor should also be developed. For instance, if a person is delirious because of a fever, a goal might state, "The patient's temperature will be maintained below 100° F (37.8° C)." When the cause of the elevated temperature is identified, appropriate goals will be written to address that problem. For example, dehydration may be a stressor contributing to an elevated temperature. A related nursing goal would then be, "The patient's fluid intake will be at least 3,000 ml in each 24-hour period." As the various elements of the person's behavior are explored and documented, nursing goals must be updated and modified; new goals must be added and accomplished goals deleted.

The nursing care plan for a patient with a cognitive disorder must address all of the person's biopsychosocial needs. In most cases, the person either has or is at risk for physiological problems in addition to the psychosocial disruption. Life-threatening problems al-

ways receive the highest priority for nursing intervention. Protection of the person's safety is almost always a concern with these patients. Fig. 18-4 is an example of a partial nursing care plan for Mr. B, the patient presented in Clinical example 18-3. This is a plan that might have been developed at the time Mr. B's mental status began to deteriorate.

Mental health education related to patients with impaired cognition is often directed toward the family. They are frequently the caregivers for these patients. The nurse can help them cope with this difficult and demanding responsiblity by providing them with information. Harvis and Rabins[12] found that educational approaches were helpful for caregivers or patients with dementia. One useful topic was information about problematic behaviors and problem-solving for the caregiver. Another was providing information on stress reduction, including individual ways to decrease stress, the use of respite care, and participation in a peer support group. Table 18-4 is a sample of a mental health education plan for families of cognitively impaired persons.

⇨ Implementation

■ Intervening in delirium

■ **PHYSIOLOGICAL NEEDS.** Highest priority is given to nursing interventions that will maintain life. If the individual is too disoriented or agitated to attend to basic physiological needs, nursing care must be planned to meet these needs. Nutrition and fluid balance may be maintained by intravenous therapy. If the patient is very agitated or restless, restraint may be necessary to keep the intravenous line open. However, restraints can increase agitation and anxiety and thus should be applied only when absolutely necessary. A disoriented patient should never be restrained and left alone.

Sleep deprivation may be another problem. Intervention is important because lack of sleep can add to already existing cognitive dysfunction. Since sedative medication may complicate attempts to identify the original stressor, the physician may be reluctant to prescribe sedation. Nursing measures such as a back rub, a glass of warm milk, and soothing conversation may help a less agitated patient relax and fall asleep. The presence of a family member is also reassuring to the patient. Disoriented patients need to be in a lighted room. Shadows may be misinterpreted and add to the patient's fear. Also, environmental objects help the patient orient to place and person.

■ **HALLUCINATIONS.** The disoriented patient may need to be protected from hurting himself or oth-

PSYCHIATRIC NURSING CARE PLAN

Precautions:
    Elopement precautions

Special nursing needs:
    Speak loudly — patient has mild hearing loss

Visitors: {x} No restrictions
          { } Family only
          { } Restricted to:

          { } No visitors

Telephone: { } Limited
            {x} Unlimited

Privileges: { } Restricted to unit
           {x} Off unit accompanied by staff
           {x} Off unit accompanied by family/visitor
           { } Off unit unaccompanied
           {x} Out of hospital leave (dates) every Sunday

Assessment data summary: Recent memory loss; aware of cognitive problems at times; mild intention tremor; judgment slightly impaired; disoriented to time; hypertensive; mild hearing loss; likes to reminisce; religion has been important to him; family is concerned; spends Sundays and holidays at son's house

Nursing diagnoses: 1. Altered thought processes related to dementia, evidenced by memory loss, disorientation, and impaired judgment. 2. Impaired social interaction related to decreased cognitive functioning, evidenced by refusal to participate in gin rummy games.

Treatment goal: Promotion of optimum cognitive functioning

Date	Problem/need	Expected outcome (objective)	Target Date	Nursing Intervention
3/11	Recent memory loss	To engage in activities that do not use recent memory	4/7	Involve in mild physical exercise; look at old photographs; listen to music
3/11	Disorientation to time	To be informed of date and time	3/13	Remind him of location of calendar and clock; cross out each day in his personal datebook; check orientation

Room	Patient's name	Age	Doctor	Primary nurse	Admit date
12	Mr. B	73	Dr. M	Ms. L	3/11/90

Fig. 18-4. Sample nursing care plan for a patient with dementia. (This nursing care plan includes examples of the elements of a total plan as it might appear at a particular time in the patient's course of treatment. It should not be considered all inclusive.) *Continued.*

Date	Medications	Date	P.R.N. Medications	Diagnostic & psychiatric tests	Req.	Done
3/11	Chlorothiazide	3/11	Milk of magnesia	Psychological test	3/11	
	500 mg po qd		30 ml qhs	battery		
	in am		prn for constipation	Blood chemistries	3/11	
				EEG	3/11	
				CT scan	3/11	
				Skull x-ray	3/11	
		Date	Treatments	Special orders and concerns		
		3/11	BP sitting and	Arrange for hearing evaluation		
			standing qd			
			before medication			

Allergies:	Medical diagnosis: (Axes I-III)	Diet:
None	Dementia	2 gram sodium

Fig. 18-4, cont'd. Sample nursing care plan for a patient with dementia.

ers, particularly if he is hallucinating. Visual hallucinations of delirium are often very frightening. The patient may try to run away or even jump out of a window. The patient's room must be safe, with security screens and a minimum of extra furniture or other objects placed where he might hurt himself. Frequently these patients require one-to-one nursing observation and repetitive verbal reorientation.

It is tempting to help a frightened patient eliminate the hallucinated object. For instance, the patient might request help in brushing the bugs off the sheets. Agreeing to do this is not usually therapeutic. By participating in this activity, the nurse is nonverbally communicating to the patient that the hallucinated objects are real. This can make the patient even more frightened. In reality the hallucinations will continue until the underlying stressor is eliminated. A more appropriate response is to orient the patient continually to the reality of being sick and hospitalized. In addition, the patient can be assured that the nursing staff and physician are helping him and will keep him safe. Family members should also be helped to respond in a supportive way.

■ **COMMUNICATION.** Patients with impaired cognition need clear messages and instructions.

Choices should be kept to a minimum. Independent decision making can be introduced into the plan of nursing care as the patient improves. Decisions related to orientation may be especially difficult for the patient. To respond appropriately to the question "What time would you like to take your bath?" requires knowledge of the present time and some idea of the usual routine.

Simple direct statements are reassuring and most likely to result in an appropriate response. Orienting phrases such as "here at the hospital" or "now that it's June" can be woven into a conversation. A patient who is having difficulty dressing or feeding himself needs matter-of-fact, specific direction. A very confused patient needs to be fed or dressed in a manner that allows him to maintain his dignity. Families can often assist with this. Helping the patient can lessen the family's anxiety, and the patient may be reassured by the family's physical closeness and concern.

■ **PATIENT EDUCATION.** As the patient recovers, he may be concerned about what happened to him. The health team needs to discuss this issue and arrive at a conclusion about the disruption in functioning that occurred. This should then be explained to the patient and family. The nurse should assess the patient's

TABLE 18-4

MENTAL HEALTH EDUCATION PLAN FOR THE FAMILIES OF COGNITIVELY IMPAIRED PERSONS

Content	Instructional activities	Evaluation
Explain possible causes of cognitive impairment	Describe predisposing factors and precipitating stressors that may lead to impaired cognition; provide printed reference materials	The learner identifies possible causes of the patient's disorder
Define and describe orientation to time, place, and person	Define the three spheres of orientation; role play interpersonal responses to disorientation	The learner identifies disorientation and provides reorientation
Relationship of level of cognitive functioning to ability to communicate	Describe the impact of cognitive impairment on communication; demonstrate effective communication techniques; videotape and discuss return demonstration	The learner adjusts communication approaches to the patient's ability to interact
Effect of cognitive impairment on self-care behaviors	Describe the usual progression of gain or loss of self-care ability related to nature of disorder; encourage learner to assist in providing care to patient; provide written instructional materials	The learner assists with activities of daily living as required by the patient's level of biopsychosocial functioning
Referral to community resources	Provide a list of community resources; arrange to meet with staff members of selected community programs; visit meetings of selected programs and self help groups.	The learner describes various programs that provide services relevant to the patient and family's needs; contacts appropriate programs or self help groups when needed

understanding of the nature of his problem, the stressors that were involved, any ongoing therapy that will be required, and preventive measures that will decrease the probability of a recurrence. Teaching may have to be repeated several times before the patient copes with his feelings and then understands the information. Written materials can be helpful to patients who are having residual problems processing information. The teaching should include at least one responsible family member so that the information will be reinforced when the patient goes home.

If the patient is discharged from the hospital with a residual deficit in cognitive functioning, a community health nursing referral may be helpful. The community health nurse can then continue to implement the nursing care plan and can validate the patient's compliance with the treatment plan.

■ **SUMMARY OF INTERVENTIONS WITH THE DELIRIOUS PATIENT.** Davidhizar, Gunden, and Wehlage[5] have recommended the following nursing interventions for the delirious patient:

1. Regulate lights and provide a window to show diurnal variation.
2. Verbalize orienting information, which includes name and purpose of persons entering the room.
3. Provide proper functioning of eyeglasses and hearing aids.
4. Avoid rough excessive handling of patient during procedures or turning.
5. Minimize forced feeding.
6. Elevate the head of the patient or allow him to partially sit up, since *visual hallucinations are increased when the patient is confined to his back.*
7. Provide for presence of familiar personal objects in the room.
8. Encourage visits from family members and friends as indicated by condition.
9. Assign the same personnel to give care.
10. Convey warmth and reassurance. Physical presence can have a calming effect.
11. Maintain firmness when dealing with the agitated, hostile patient.
12. Encourage verbal and nonverbal expression.
13. Provide for diversional activities and meaningful use of time.
14. Protect from situations where judgment and intellectual capacity would be overtaxed.
15. Schedule medications, treatments, or other procedures at times that will not interrupt nighttime sleep.
16. Limit treatments and procedures and schedule them in a predictable way to avoid an overwhelming situation for the patient.

17. Provide clocks and calendars.
18. Inform patient of his condition and his progress during periods of lucidity.
19. Allow patient control over aspects of his environment as he is able.
20. Recognize cultural variables that affect patient's response to stimuli.

■ Intervening in dementia

Nursing care of the patient with dementia is similar in some respects to that of the patient with delirium. Usually the stressors involved do not present an immediate threat to life; thus highest priority is given to nursing care that will help the patient maintain an optimum level of functioning. This will differ for each individual. Frequently an attitude of hopelessness evolves in those who work with chronically ill people. This can lead to stereotyping and decreased ability to see and appreciate the uniqueness of each person. It is challenging to search for this uniqueness and rewarding to find it. Individualized nursing care is probably most important for those who will be institutionalized for a long time.

Recently, gerontological nursing has been receiving more recognition as a separate specialty area. Nursing research is beginning to focus on nursing intervention with the chronically ill and the aging. One finding has been that individualized attention may stimulate enhanced functioning in people who appear to have severely limited cognitive abilities.

Nursing approaches need to address the patient's need for social interaction. Some interventions that have been helpful include discussion groups with structured agendas; exercise groups to promote physical activity; reality orientation groups; sensory stimulation; and parties appropriate to the time of the year or to recognize important events such as birthdays. Arranging for visits from community volunteer groups provides stimulation as well as an opportunity to socialize. Referral to other members of the treatment team, especially the occupational, recreational, art, music, and dance therapists may be indicated.

Gershowitz[10] recommends that therapeutic approaches with the elderly emphasize previous life experiences rather than learning new skills. She describes the essence of remotivation therapy as helping the patient to "recapture the past and apply it to the present." She stresses that remotivation must be a continuous process, not confined to episodic group or individual interactions. This approach attends to the person as a complete individual. It is a hopeful way of providing nursing care because it communicates to the patient that there is potential for activity and growth.

■ **PHARMACOLOGICAL APPROACHES.** Pharmacological approaches to the treatment of dementia are related to theories about the cause of the disorder. Much of the research seeks a treatment for Alzheimer's disease. Pajk[18] described several approaches. Substances that might promote the production of acetylcholine have not been effective. Arecoline has been tried as a substitute for acetylcholine but is too toxic. Physostigmine is being studied for its ability to decrease the breakdown of acetylcholine. Several agents that might stimulate neurotransmitter action are being investigated. Vasodilators are sometimes used to increase cerebral circulation and maximize the patient's functional level. Drugs with anticholinergic effects and benzodiazepines (which interfere with learning) should be avoided.[14]

■ **ORIENTATION.** Disorientation is a common problem of people with cognitive impairment. Nursing interventions should help the patient function in the environment. In an institution it is helpful to mark patient rooms with large, clearly printed signs indicating the occupant's name. This also reminds forgetful people of others' names. Personal possessions can also be orienting devices. A favorite rocking chair, a handmade afghan, or a family picture gives the person a sense of identity and helps to identify a personal area of the institution. Everyone needs a personal space. A light in the room at night helps the person remain oriented and decreases nighttime agitation. Some authorities recommend the use of small amounts of antipsychotic medications, such as phenothiazines and butyrophenones, to help patients rest, since barbiturate sedatives may cause paradoxical agitation in people with organic brain syndromes.

Clocks with large faces aid in orientation to time. A digital clock is not recommended, since the confused person may not identify it as a clock. Calendars with a separate page for each day and large writing also help with time orientation. Newspapers provide other orienting stimuli and also help to stimulate interest in current events. An institutional newspaper provides a creative outlet that focuses on patient strengths and also helps patients maintain awareness of the environment.

Reality orientation is a nursing approach that is generally helpful to patients with cognitive impairments. Orientation includes the dimensions of time, place, and person. Systematic reality orientation includes attention to each of these dimensions. This approach often takes place in a group. It is most effectve if the group meets daily, if possible, and at a standard time. A pattern of group activity should be established. For instance, the group might begin with each person introducing himself, followed by informing the group of the date and time. A review of the schedule for the day is frequently helpful. A brief time is allowed for questions. In general, this type of group should only last for 15-20 minutes. If the members become fatigued, their cognitive ability will deteriorate.

Mulcahy and Rosa[16] used a reality orientation approach with a group of cognitively impaired patients in a general hospital. In addition to consistent orientation to person, place, and time, their nurse-patient goals included the following: awareness of the need to be hospitalized; cooperation with treatment; maintenance of self-esteem and development of self-confidence; relatedness to the environment through the use of sight, touch, and hearing; bowel and bladder continence; interpersonal interaction; accurate identification of others; and involvement in discharge planning. The authors developed a standardized nursing care plan and taught other nurses to use it.

■ **COMMUNICATION.** Recent memory loss is another frequently encountered behavior. Patients may be frustrated when constantly confronted with evidence of failing memory. Conversational focus can be directed toward topics that the patient initiates. Most patients feel more comfortable talking about remote memories and may derive pleasure from discussing past experiences. Misperceptions of the present can be dealt with gently and diplomatically. For example, if an elderly woman who has been widowed for 10 years says that she expects her husband to come home soon, the nurse might reply, "You must have loved your husband very much. Sometimes it seems to you that he's still here." Explicitly or implicitly agreeing that her husband will "come home" is fostering false hope, perhaps leading to a disappointment. Abrupt confrontation with the reality of her husband's death is cruel and will increase her anxiety.

Farran and Keane-Hagerty[8] have recommended communication techniques for nurses who provide care for patients with dementia. The nurse introduces himself or herself at each interaction with the patient. There should be an attitude of unconditional positive regard. Empathy, warmth, and caring are important. Verbal communication should be clear, concise, and unhurried. The voice should be modulated in relationship to the patient's ability to hear. Shouting may be interpreted as anger by a person who hears well. The use of pronouns should be avoided. Questions that require a "yes" and "no" answer are best. Behavior should be requested one step at a time and if repetition is required, it should be stated in exactly the same way as originally. Nonverbal communication skills are also important. A pleasant, calm, supportive tone of voice should be used. Verbal and nonverbal communication must be congruent. Sometimes nonverbal techniques, especially touch, may be reassuring to the patient. The nurse should try to understand who the patient was in the past. This can be accomplished by encouraging reminiscence and talking with family members. Pictures or music may assist the patient to remember past experiences.

Farran and Keane-Hagerty[8] further suggest providing an environment of "sheltered freedom." This includes a predictable, unhurried schedule, and the assignment of a primary nurse. Distraction or diversion along with decreased stimulation should be used if a patient appears to becoming agitated. Appropriate use of humor and flexibility on the part of the nurse assist the patient to function in the environment. Reality orientation is important, but the nurse should avoid insisting on this if the patient is unable to recognize reality.

■ **REINFORCEMENT OF COPING MECHANISMS.** Previously helpful coping mechanisms are often used by the patient with a cognitive deficit. Sometimes these attempts to cope may be hard to understand unless placed in the appropriate context. An older man who pats and pinches the nurses and makes lewd remarks may have had past success dealing with his anxiety by behaving seductively. An elderly woman who hoards food in her room may equate food with security. An aging person who has been suspicious of others in the past may become more suspicious over time. Because of the protective nature of these behaviors, they should not be actively confronted. Rather, the nurse should try to discover the source of the person's anxiety and attempt to alleviate it, thus allowing the person to behave less defensively.

■ **WANDERING.** Wandering is a behavior that causes great concern to caregivers. In fact, it often leads to institutionalization or to the use of restraints. Fopma-Loy[9] recommends that nurses observe patients carefully to identify the situations that contribute to wandering behavior. She suggests that mapping of the behavior may be useful. In some cases, medications may cause agitation and restlessness. Some patients are extremely sensitive to stress and tension in the environment. Their wandering may be an attempt to get away. Similarly, if the patient is aware that an activity that he dislikes is about to occur, such as bathing or medication administration, he may try to avoid it. If wandering meets needs for attention, efforts to control the behavior may actually reinforce it.

Fopma-Loy suggests decreasing stress in the environment, especially at night when many people have decreased stress tolerance. Eliminating distracting background noise or shadows may help. Safe areas should be provided where patients can move about freely. If possible, this should include an outside area with adequate staff supervision to ensure safety. Environmental design can be used to camouflage doorways or to incorporate distractions. Any method of increasing orientation can also decrease the need to wander. However, it is important to base nursing intervention on observation and analysis of the motivation for the patient's behavior.

■ **DECREASING AGITATION.** Patients may also become agitated when pushed to do something unfamiliar or unclear. Expectations should be explained simply and completely. If the patient can make choices, they should be offered. An individual daily schedule of activities can help the person prepare for and plan his day. If a patient refuses to participate in an activity, continued insistence usually leads to increased agitation and sometimes loss of behavioral control. This has been called a "catastrophic response." The best approach may be to wait a few minutes and then return to see if the patient will agree to the request. In the interim the nurse can examine the approach to the patient to see if he or she might have contributed to the problem. Perhaps the patient thought the nurse was too controlling and a power struggle developed, or perhaps the nurse initiated the request abruptly, not allowing the patient a time for transition.

Richardson[21] has described several approaches to demented patients that help them deal with stress. Sin-

cerity is important. The nurse should treat the patient like an adult, offer real choices and try to maintain environmental stability. Skills should be taught in the setting in which they will be used. Encourage self-care by using the patient's strengths and abilities. If the patient becomes agitated and cannot be calmed, a change of subject and a "sign of friendship," such as a smile or a handshake, will often be effective.

■ **FAMILY AND COMMUNITY INTERVENTIONS.** Many individuals with dementia live in community settings with their families. It is important to support these care providers because the patient usually derives great benefit from being with them. Mental health education is helpful to families of people with dementia.

Teusink and Mahler[22] have identified a family reaction process in relatives of patients with Alzheimer's disease. The same sequence of responses is probably characteristic of families of individuals with other dementing illnesses. This five-stage process closely parallels the grieving process identified in the significant others of dying persons. The stages are illustrated in Table 18-5.

Families may need assistance in providing 24-hour care for the patient. Home care agencies may provide nursing and homemaking services to enable the person to remain in his own home. If family members are not available during the day, adult day-care centers are available in some communities. Mace[15] reports that these programs were first initiated in 1974. By 1984,

TABLE 18-5

PATTERN OF FAMILY MEMBERS' RESPONSES TO ALZHEIMER'S DISEASE

Stage	Family behavior	Intervention
Denial	May ignore severe memory loss; may use relatively intact remote memory as evidence of no problem; may interfere with treatment planning	Education Confrontation
Overinvolvement	Sacrifice of usual family activities; reluctance to seek help, often related to ethnicity	Determine cultural norms; help to see problems related to overinvolvement
Anger	Reaction to burden of care and feeling of abandonment by patient; often projected or displaced onto care provider	Assist to recognize and express feelings; be aware of countertransference
Guilt	Reaction to recognition of anger and wish that patient would die; may also be caused by past interpersonal experiences with the patient	Educate about the illness and what the family can and cannot control; assist to make decisions about care, even if patient objects
Acceptance	Resolution of other stages; realistic understanding of what to expect and what can be done	Provide support and knowledge as required

Adapted from Teusink JP and Mahler S: Hosp Community Psychiatry 35:152, 1984.

800 to 1,000 were operating in the United States. The services include help with activities of daily living, recreation, health supervision, rehabilitation, exercise, and nutrition. Families also receive support and assistance, particularly during the first few weeks of attendance, when the patient may be resistant because of difficulty adapting to a new experience.

■ **PRINCIPLES OF CONSERVATION.** Hirschfeld[13] recommends structuring the nursing care of the cognitively impaired older adult around Myra Levine's

---

TABLE 18-6

SUMMARY OF NURSING INTERVENTIONS IN IMPAIRED COGNITION

Goal—Promotion of optimum cognitive functioning

Principle	Rationale	Nursing action
Conservation of energy	Physiological disruptions deplete energy; energy is used to ensure survival before supporting other functions; cognitive functioning is enhanced when adequate energy is available; patient survival and safety are always the highest-priority nursing care activities	Maintain adequate nutrition Monitor fluid intake and output Monitor vital signs Provide opportunities for rest and stimulation Assist with ambulation if necessary Assist with hygiene activities if necessary Provide appropriate nursing care for identified physiological disruption Identify stressful situations to help patient avoid them Assess mood and intervene in identified disruptions (see Chapter 14)
Conservation of structural integrity	Cognitive impairment usually involves sensory and perceptual disorders that can endanger the patient's safety	Assess sensory and perceptual functioning Provide access to eyeglasses, hearing aids, canes, walkers, etc., if needed Observe and remove safety hazards (e.g., obstacles, slippery floors, open flames, inadequate lighting) Supervise medications if necessary Protect from injury during periods of agitation with one-to-one nursing care; restraints only if absolutely necessary
Conservation of personal integrity	Cognitive impairment is a threat to self-esteem; a positive nurse-patient relationship can assist the patient to express his fears and feel secure in his environment; recognition of accomplishments also raises self-esteem	Provide reality orientation Establish trusting relationship Encourage patient to be as independent as possible Identify patient's interests and skills; provide opportunities to use them Give honest praise for accomplishments Use therapeutic communication techniques to help patient communicate his thoughts and feelings
Conservation of social integrity	Caring relationships with others promote a positive self-concept; communication by significant others can often be understood more easily than that of strangers; family and friends can provide help in knowing patient's habits and preferences; involvement of significant others in caregiving often helps them cope with the stress of patient's health problem	Initiate contact with significant others Encourage patient to interact with others; involve him in group activities Teach family and patient about the nature of the problem and the recommended health care plan Allow significant others to assist in patient care if they wish Meet with significant others regularly and provide them with an opportunity to talk Involve patient and family in discharge planning

four principles of conservation:

1. Conservation of energy
2. Conservation of structural integrity
3. Conservation of personal integrity
4. Conservation of social integrity

Conservation of energy is related to the need to understand physiological disruptions that might deplete the person's energy supplies. Anxiety and depression are noted as other behaviors that use energy. Nursing intervention in these areas can free energy for other purposes, such as improving cognitive abilities. Conservation of structural integrity implies nursing attention to sensory and perceptual deficits. Patients may need to be protected from injury, and medication use may need to be supervised. Conservation of personal integrity can be accomplished through sensitivity to the person's need to maintain self-esteem. This requires awareness of one's own feelings about organic mental disorders. Encouraging self-care and establishing trust are essential. Reality orientation and listening are important nursing interventions, as are privacy and respect for personal space. Conservation of social integrity focuses on maintaining relationships with significant others. The nurse can help to interpret behavior and encourage frequent visits. Families should maintain healthy relationships with the cognitively impaired member, neither withdrawing nor fostering unnecessary dependency. These principles may be used as an organizing framework for planning the nursing care of the cognitively impaired patient (Table 18-6).

 Evaluation

Expectations of the patient who has cognitive difficulty must be realistic but not pessimistic. A brain-damaged person may never remember the correct date but may be able to find his own bedroom. However, if he is never asked to find his room, he has no opportunity to demonstrate his ability. One evaluation criterion, therefore, is the appropriateness of the nursing goal to the individual. The nurse should assess whether the expectation is too high or too low. Levels of expectation can be increased until the patient is clearly unable to function and then lowered to the realistic level.

Improved performance on tests of orientation to time, place, and person are concrete measures of the person's level of orientation. The frequency of social interaction is another criterion that may be used to evaluate patient progress. The ability to assist with or perform self-care may also be measured and compared over time. For the person with a progressive disorder,

these evaluation measures not only provide a way of assessing the effectiveness of nursing care, but also show the rate of progression over time, thus allowing the nurse to adjust interventions appropriately. Nurses in long-term care settings may wish to develop flow sheets identifying critical behaviors to facilitate this comparison.

If the disruption in behavior is reversible, knowledge of the patient's usual life-style and level of functioning is helpful. A college professor is likely to have more highly developed cognitive skills than is a laborer. A patient who is visited by numerous friends and relatives probably has different communication patterns than the person who is visited only by immediate family members. Knowledge of usual behavior serves as a gauge against which to measure progress. Friends and family are good judges of when the pa-

---

DIRECTIONS FOR FUTURE RESEARCH

The following are some of the nursing research problems raised in Chapter 18 that merit further study by psychiatric nurses:

1. Validation of nursing interventions that result in improved cognitive functioning when impairment results from hypoxia
2. Assessment of the ability of nurses who work with elderly patients to identify changes in cognitive functioning
3. The ability of nurses who work with elderly patients to assess the presence of physiological stressors related to identified cognitive impairments
4. Primary prevention measures that are effective in decreasing the incidence of dementia
5. The effects on cognitive functioning of frequently used prescription and over-the-counter medications
6. Specific stressors that lead to the occurrence of "intensive care unit psychosis"
7. Interpersonal approaches that are effective in alleviating the anxiety of delirious patients
8. The process of confabulation, including its development and the need it fulfills for the individual
9. The relationship between the existence of a consistently identified area of personal space and the level of orientation of a patient with dementia
10. Environmental characteristics of institutions that interfere with effective cognitive functioning

tient is "back to normal." However, this should also be validated with the patient. He may have different self-expectations and may use his therapeutic experience to progress beyond his pretherapy level of functioning.

Colleagues are also helpful in evaluating the nursing care plan. They may suggest alternate interventions or provide feedback about transference-countertransference issues. For instance, a nurse who is working with an aging patient with dementia may respond to concerns about her own aging or that of her parents and have difficulty seeing the patient as a unique person. Hallucinating patients frequently arouse anxiety in the nurse, who may then respond with her own defense mechanisms. Regular supervision can help the nurse to develop enhanced self-awareness and to determine when a particularly anxiety-provoking situation has bothered her and why.

■ SUGGESTED CROSS-REFERENCES ■

The health-illness model was discussed in Chapter 3. Therapeutic relationship skills were discussed in Chapter 4. The nursing process was discussed in Chapter 5. Psychological testing was discussed in Chapter 6. Depression was discussed in Chapter 14 and substance abuse in Chapter 19. The use of restraints was discussed in Chapter 22. Behavior modification was discussed in Chapter 27. Cognitive development of the child was discussed in Chapter 30. Gerontological psychiatric nursing was discussed in Chapter 34.

■ SUMMARY ■

1. Cognition is the ability to think and reason, including the processes of memory, judgment, orientation, perception, and attention.

2. Learning theorists have developed models of cognitive functioning, including the associationist model (Pavlov, Skinner, Wolpe), the social-cognitive model (Tolman), and the computer model.

3. The developmental process of cognition was described by Piaget. It has three stages: the sensorimotor stage; the stage of preparation and organization of concrete operations, subdivided into the preoperational phase and the concrete operations phase; and the stage of formal operations.

4. Predisposing factors related to impaired cognition include interference with supply of nutrients to the brain, aging, metabolic disorders, genetic abnormalities, and co-existing mental disorders.

5. Biological stressors, such as impaired delivery of nutrients to brain cells, metabolic disorders, exposure to toxic and infectious agents, tumors, and trauma, can cause cognitive impairment. In many instances the stressor cannot be identified.

6. Impairments in cognition are experienced by patients with the medical diagnoses of organic brain syndromes, including delirium and dementia.

7. Behaviors associated with delirium may include fluctuating levels of awareness, disorientation, disorganized thought processes, impaired judgment and decision making, illusions, visual hallucinations, affective lability, loss of inhibition, restlessness, agitation, diffuse EEG slowing, and behaviors directly attributable to the stressor.

8. Behaviors associated with dementia may include disorientation, memory loss, decreased attention span, labile affect, deteriorated social skills, impaired judgment and decision making, restlessness and agitation, and resistance to change.

9. Psychological testing is an assessment tool provided on consultation by a clinical psychologist. Examples of common psychological tests are presented.

10. Coping mechanisms used by patients with impaired cognition may be exaggerations of past methods of coping with anxiety.

11. Examples of nursing diagnoses of altered thought processes are presented and compared to the medical diagnostic criteria for delirium, dementia, and other organic mental disorders.

12. A sample nursing care plan for a patient with dementia and a mental health education plan focused on caregivers were presented.

13. Nursing intervention with patients who have delirium includes life support, emotional support, and protection from impulsive behavior. Family members can provide valuable assistance.

14. Nursing intervention with patients who have dementia includes reality orientation, stimulation, encouragement of independent functioning, socialization, protection from accidental injury, maintenance of optimum biopsychosocial functioning, and encouragement of relatedness with significant others.

15. Evaluation of nursing care focuses on the appropriateness of the long- and short-term goals and the adequacy and effectiveness of the nursing interventions. Feedback can be obtained from the nurse's supervisor and colleagues, the nurse's self-assessment, the patient's significant others, and the patient. A flow sheet may be useful to record behavioral change over time.

■ REFERENCES ■

1. Agras WS: Learning theory. In Kaplan HI and Sadock BJ, editors: Comprehensive textbook of psychiatry, ed 5, Baltimore, 1989, Williams & Wilkins.
2. American Psychiatric Association: DSM-III-R, third edition revised, Washington DC, 1987, The Association.
3. Barnes DM: AIDS dementia: in search of a mechanism, J NIH Research 2:23, 1990.
4. Cohen GE: Alzheimer's disease: clinical update, Hosp Community Psychiatry 41:496, 1990.
5. Davidhizar R, Gunden E, and Wehlage D: Recognizing and caring for the delirious patient, J Psychiatr Nurs 16:38, 1978.
6. DeCato CM and Wicks RJ: Psychological testing refer-

rals: a guide for psychiatrists, psychiatric nurses, physicians in general practice and allied health personnel, J Psychiatr Nurs 14:24, 1976.

7. Engelhardt K: Piaget: a prescriptive theory for parents, Maternal-Child Nurs J 3:1, 1974.

8. Farran CJ and Keane-Hagerty E: Communicating effectively with dementia patients, J Psychosoc Nursing Ment Health Services 27:13, 1989.

9. Fopma-Loy J: Wandering: causes, consequences, and care, J Psychosoc Nurs Ment Health Services 26:8, 1988.

10. Gershowitz SZ: Adding life to years: remotivating elderly people in institutions, Nurs Health Care 3:141, 1982.

11. Greenspan SI and Curry JF: Piaget's approach to intellectual functioning. In Kaplan HI and Sadock BJ, editors: Comprehensive textbook of psychiatry, ed 5, Baltimore, 1989, Williams & Wilkins.

12. Harvis KA and Rabins PV: Dementia: helping family caregivers cope, J Psychosoc Nursing Ment Health Services 27:7, 1989.

13. Hirschfeld MJ: The cognitively impaired older adult, Am J Nurs 76:1981, 1976.

14. Horvath TB et al: Organic mental syndromes and disorders. In Kaplan HI and Sadock BJ, editors: Comprehensive textbook of psychiatry, ed 5, Baltimore, 1989, Williams & Wilkins.

15. Mace N: Day care for demented clients, Hosp Community Psychiatry 35:979, 1984.

16. Mulcahy N and Rosa N: Reality orientation in a general hospital, Geriatr Nurs 2:264, 1981.

17. Navia BA and Price RW: Dementia complicating AIDS, Psychiatr Ann 16:158, 1986.

18. Pajk M: Alzheimer's disease inpatient care, Am J Nurs 84:216, 1984.

19. Perry S and Jacobsen P: Neuropsychiatric manifestations of AIDS-spectrum disorders, Hosp Community Psychiatry 37:135, 1986.

20. Piaget J: The child and reality: problems of genetic psychology, New York, 1973, Grossman Publishers.

21. Richardson K: Hope and flexibility: your keys to helping OBS patients, Nursing 12:64, 1982.

22. Teusink JP and Mahler S: Helping families cope with Alzheimer's disease, Hosp Community Psychiatry 35:152, 1984.

23. Toffler A: Future shock, New York, 1970, Random House, Inc.

24. Tolman EC: Purposive behavior in animals and man, New York, 1932, Century.

25. Tucker G et al: Reorganizing the "organic" disorders, Hosp Community Psychiatry, 41:722, 1990.

26. Wolanin MO: Physiologic aspects of confusion, J Gerontol Nurs 7:236, 1981.

27. Wolanin MO and Phillips LRF: Confusion: prevention and care, St Louis, 1981, Mosby–Year Book, Inc.

■ ANNOTATED SUGGESTED READINGS ■

Baker FM: Screening tests for cognitive impairment, Hosp Community Psychiatry 40:339, 1989.

Comparison of the usefulness of five different screening tests for cognitive impairment based on sensitivity and specificity, with attention given to sociocultural and educational factors.

*Batt LJ: Managing delirium: implications for geropsychiatric nurses, J Psychosoc Nursing Ment Health Services 27:23, 1989.

Describes nursing interventions that are helpful in providing care to a patient with delirium.

Doernberg M: Stolen mind: the slow disappearance of Ray Doernberg, Chapel Hill, NC, 1989, Algonquin Books of Chapel Hill.

The wife of a man with progressive dementia describes her experiences and his reactions to his increasing dependence. Provides insight into the impact of this illness on the family.

Frances A et al: A multidisciplinary approach to primary degenerative dementia, Hosp Community Psychiatry 39:1145, 1988.

Uses a case study approach to demonstrate the effectiveness of a multidisciplinary team in the care of a patient with dementia and in working with his wife. Describes the role of each team member.

*Jarnagan G: Taking care of mama, Johns Hopkins Magazine 33:37, 1982.

Describes nurse's experience caring for her demented mother. Conveys an understanding of the decision-making process required and the necessary psychological and life-style adjustments.

*King KS: Reminiscing: psychotherapy with aging people, J Psychosoc Nurs Ment Health Serv 20:21, 1982.

Discusses the value of reminiscence for elderly people. Includes a thorough review of relevant literature and examples of approaches in group therapy.

Klawans HL: Toscanini's fumble and other tales of clinical neurology, Chicago, 1988, Contemporary Books, Inc.

A neurologist describes some of his unusual patients. Includes discussion of the physiological disorders that lead to the behavioral impairment.

*Langston NF: Reality orientation and effective reinforcement, J Gerontol Nurs 7:224, 1981.

Identifies two aspects of reality orientation: a formal class providing specific information and 24-hour reality orientation using objects from the environment. Helpful feature is the comparison drawn between reality orientation and behavior modification.

Larson EB et al: Evaluating elderly outpatients with symptoms of dementia, Hosp Community Psychiatry 35:425, 1984.

Reports on a study of 107 elderly patients with dementia. Of 15 found to have a reversible problem with identifiable causes, only three returned to normal with treatment. Recommends a thorough physical workup for all cognitively impaired

---

*Asterisk indicates nursing reference.

patients, since even truly demented patients may improve their functioning if coexisting problems are corrected.

*Mulcahy N and Rosa N: Reality orientation in a general hospital, Geriatr Nurs 2:264, 1981.

Describes a reality orientation program for confused patients introduced in a general hospital setting. Includes an excellent example of a nursing care plan for use with a confused patient.

*Pajk M: Alzheimer's disease inpatient care, Am J Nurs 84:216, 1984.

Contains a comprehensive review of neurophysiological research regarding Alzheimer's disease. Includes sample of a nursing care plan, focusing on the functional disabilities associated with this illness, and presents a case study.

Rabins PV and Mace NL: The 36-hour day, Baltimore, 1981, The Johns Hopkins University Press.

Indispensable guide for families and other care providers for individuals with dementia. Provides practical information and explains behavioral changes in understandable terms. Excellent adjunct to health education.

*Scherer P: How AIDS attacks the brain, Am J Nurs 90:44, 1990.

Describes several possible effects of HIV-1 infection on brain functioning. Includes a table that summarizes each disorder by symptoms, treatments, and potential side effects of treatment.

*Sullivan N and Fogel BS: Could this be delirium? Am J Nurs 86:1359, 1986.

Provides an overview of delirium. Offers practical suggestions regarding assessment and nursing intervention.

*Taft LB: Conceptual analysis of agitation in the confused elderly, Arch Psych Nurs 3:102, 1989.

Identifies critical attributes of agitation. Uses case studies to illustrate the concept.

*Wolanin MO: Physiologic aspects of confusion, J Gerontol Nurs 7:236, 1981.

Well-known authority in geriatric nursing emphasizes nursing assessment as a critical factor in determining physiological causes of confusion. Also describes nursing interventions. Highly recommended for beginning students and nurses, including those in community settings who work with elderly individuals.

*Wolanin MO and Phillips LRF: Confusion: prevention and care, St Louis, 1981, Mosby–Year Book, Inc.

Attempts to clarify the concept of confusion. Understanding this concept is central to providing effective nursing care to individuals with cognitive impairment. Emphasizes nursing interventions as applied to various aspects of confusion.

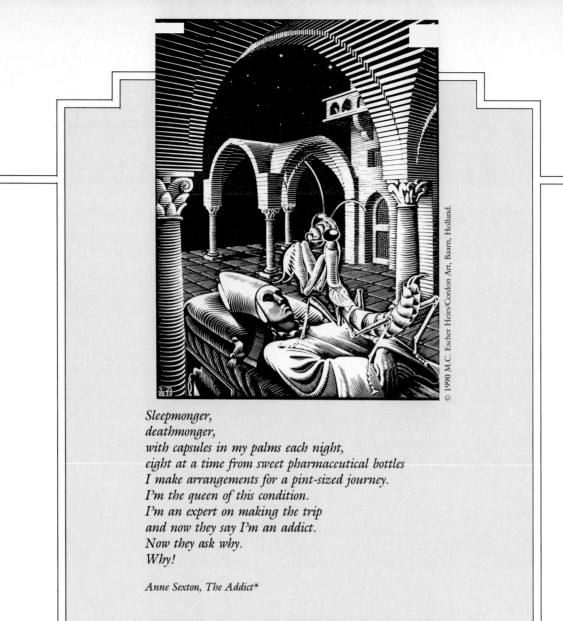

Sleepmonger,
deathmonger,
with capsules in my palms each night,
eight at a time from sweet pharmaceutical bottles
I make arrangements for a pint-sized journey.
I'm the queen of this condition.
I'm an expert on making the trip
and now they say I'm an addict.
Now they ask why.
Why!

Anne Sexton, The Addict*

CHAPTER 19

SUBSTANCE ABUSE

DIAGNOSTIC PREVIEW

MEDICAL DIAGNOSES RELATED TO SUBSTANCE ABUSE

- Psychoactive substance-induced organic mental disorders
  - Alcohol intoxication
  - Uncomplicated alcohol withdrawal
  - Alcohol withdrawal delirium
  - Alcohol hallucinosis
  - Amphetamine or similarly acting sympathomimetic intoxication
  - Amphetamine or similarly acting sympathomimetic withdrawal
  - Cocaine intoxication
  - Cocaine withdrawal
  - Hallucinogen hallucinosis
  - Opioid intoxication
  - Opioid withdrawal
  - Phencyclidine (PCP) or similarly acting arylcyclohexylamine intoxication
  - Sedative, hypnotic, or anxiolytic intoxication
  - Uncomplicated sedative, hypnotic, or anxiolytic withdrawal

- Psychoactive substance use disorders
  - Alcohol dependence
  - Alcohol abuse
  - Amphetamine or similarly acting sympathomimetic dependence
  - Amphetamine or similarly acting sympathomimetic abuse
  - Cocaine dependence
  - Cocaine abuse
  - Hallucinogen dependence
  - Hallucinogen abuse
  - Opioid dependence
  - Opioid abuse
  - Phencyclidine (PC) or similarly acting arylcyclohexylamine dependence
  - Phencyclidine (PCP) or similarly acting arylcyclohexylamine abuse
  - Sedative, hypnotic, or anxiolytic dependence
  - Sedative, hypnotic, or anxiolytic abuse
  - Polysubstance dependence

LEARNING OBJECTIVES

After studying this chapter, the student should be able to:

- define substance abuse.

- discuss the role of cultural attitudes in determining the definition of substance abuse.

- describe statistically the seriousness of the substance abuse problem.

- compare and contrast the major categories of abused substances.

- discuss the occurrence of substance abuse among members of the nursing and medical professions.

- analyze the problem of substance abuse as it relates to the stress response and the health-illness continuum.

- describe various hypotheses concerning the predisposing factors that have been proposed as influencing the occurrence of substance abuse.

- analyze precipitating stressors that may lead to episodes of substance abuse.

- compare and contrast the major categories of abused substances in terms of usual route of administration, expected behavioral responses, behaviors related to overdose, and withdrawal syndromes.

- analyze substance abuse relative to the nursing model of health-illness behavior.

- formulate individualized nursing diagnoses that incorporate the substance abused, the relevant stressors, and the behaviors observed.

- assess the relationship between nursing diagnoses and medical diagnoses associated with substance abuse.

- develop long- and short-term individualized nursing goals with substance abuse patients.

- apply therapeutic nurse-patient relationship principles with appropriate rationale in planning the care of substance abuse patients.

- analyze the biological components of intervention with the substance abuser.

- compare and contrast interactive approaches to nursing intervention with substance abuse patients.

- describe common themes in the therapy of substance abuse patients and appropriate nursing interventions.

- discuss social support systems that may be engaged to assist the substance abuse patient.

- identify five components of substance abuse prevention programs.

- develop a mental health education plan for the substance abuse patient.

- assess the importance of evaluating the nursing process when working with substance abuse patients.

- identify directions for future nursing research.

- select appropriate readings for further study.

Continuum of chemically mediated coping responses

The use of mind-altering substances is widespread in the world today. A statement such as this usually brings to mind the use of narcotics, stimulants, hallucinogens, and perhaps alcohol. However, one should also consider prescription drugs and substances containing nicotine or caffeine. To add to the complexity of the issue, some people believe that any substance use should be defined as abuse. Others maintain that abuse only exists within the norms of the culture and has no objective basis. For the purposes of this discussion, substance abuse is defined as the use of any mind-altering agent to such an extent that it interferes with the individual's biological, psychological, or sociocultural integrity.

Examples of interference with biological integrity might include the heavy smoker who develops emphysema, the anxious politician who becomes physically dependent on diazepam, or the alcoholic who is in delirium tremens. Psychological consequences of substance abuse could include the acute psychosis of a teenager who has been taking PCP (phencyclidine) or the office worker who feels unable to function without a morning cup of coffee. Sociocultural effects are experienced by the high-school student who is expelled from school following arrest for the possession of marijuana or by the young woman who prostitutes herself to make money to buy narcotics.

■ Attitudes toward substance abuse

Volumes have been written about the various types of substance abuse and much research has been conducted. Still, definitive answers to questions about the origin and nature of these problems are yet to be found. Theories cover the gamut of conceptual models of psychology, psychiatry, sociology, and the other behavioral sciences. Some drugs, such as tobacco, alcohol, caffeine, and over-the-counter remedies, are legal. Other drugs are illicit, including heroin, marijuana, cocaine, and hallucinogens. Others are legal only if obtained with a physician's prescription. The reason for these classifications is frequently unclear. Compounding the lack of clarity about the nature of substance abuse is great ambivalence in society regarding acceptance or rejection of this behavior. This is perhaps best demonstrated by considering the issues that have arisen around the use of marijuana in the United States. Many believe very strongly that marijuana use is harmful to the individual and/or society and should be strictly prohibited by law. Others believe that marijuana is harmless and should be as freely available as tobacco and alcohol. Still others advocate little or no penalty for personal use of the drug but stiff penalties for its sale. Meanwhile, marijuana is widely used and in some settings, such as rock concerts, is used openly. However, it has been extremely difficult to obtain governmental approval for the medicinal use of marijuana, even though it has demonstrated effectiveness for problems such as the alleviation of the discomfort of cancer patients receiving chemotherapy. These various attitudes reflect the confused values that exist concerning the use of mind-altering substances.

In addition, abuse of substances is viewed differently, depending on the substance being abused, the person who is abusing it, and the setting in which abuse occurs. For instance, the upper middle class businessperson who has several martinis at a dinner meeting and is therefore argumentative with the other participants is not necessarily thought of as a substance abuser. However, if a secretary keeps a bottle of wine in the desk drawer and sips it during work, that person would probably be counseled to seek help for an alcoholism problem. Is there a real difference in the behavior of these two individuals? Tobacco abuse is so widely accepted in the United States that there is serious debate about whether or not smokers have the right to inflict their habit on others, even if it may cause them physical damage. Yet, a person who smokes opium would certainly be considered deviant even if the behavior took place in private.

It is important for nurses to be aware of these cultural attitudes and to recognize their impact on the individual who abuses substances and on that person's significant others. Alcohol abuse may not be noticed because use of alcohol is generally acceptable. The great stigma attached to alcohol abuse makes the individual and the family reluctant to admit that there is a problem and seek help. Nurses must also take care that their own attitudes do not perpetuate the stigma and prevent them from providing help to the substance abuser. Self-awareness is especially critical when caring for these individuals. Substance abusers are very sensitive to the attitudes of others. They may feel guilty because of their own basic acceptance of the culture's value system that has labeled their behavior as unacceptable. The nurse must be able to help them learn to accept themselves. This is difficult if the nurse is caught up in her own value judgments.

Incidence

■ **ALCOHOL.** Substance abuse is one of the United States' major public health problems. It has been estimated that 10% of adult men who drink and as many as 3% of adult women drinkers are abusers of alcohol. About 7% of the U.S. adult population (over age 18), or approximately 9.3 to 10 million persons, are alcoholics.[8] Recently, an annual survey of drug use by high school seniors has shown an encouraging trend related to alcohol use. The percent who had used alcohol within 30 days of the survey decreased from about 72% in 1978 to about 65% in 1986. However, there

was a small increase of about 1% in 1987.[16] Alcohol abuse also affects people other than the drinker. Families of alcoholics experience increased stress and stress-related health problems as an indirect result of alcoholism. It has also been documented that alcohol is a factor in over 50% of traffic accidents. In addition, alcohol is a factor in about one third of deaths related to crashes of private planes and one third to one half of all drownings.[10] Citizen pressure in several states to legislate stiffer penalties for driving under the influence of alcohol has been increasing recently.

■ **OPIATES.** Opiate use is much less widespread than alcohol use but is still a serious problem. In 1984 less than 0.5% of 12- to 17-year-olds and 1.0% of 18- to 25-year-olds had ever used heroin.[20] Opiate use is more prevalent in urban areas, among males and minority groups, although there has been a slight increase recently in use by white middle-class adolescents and young adults. A 1985 national household survey of drug use conducted by the National Institute on Drug Abuse (NIDA) revealed that about 1% of the population admitted having ever used heroin. Projected to the total U.S. population, this would be about 1.9 million people.[16] Because of the stigma of heroin abuse, it is particularly difficult to obtain accurate data about incidence or prevalence. Further complicating the problem, many heroin abusers are homeless. Therefore, the estimate cited above is probably low.

Opiate abuse is of great concern because it leads to severely deteriorated individual functioning and frequently to criminal activity to raise money for purchasing drugs.

■ **PRESCRIPTION MEDICATIONS.** Another type of substance abuse of great concern is the habitual use of prescription medications, including sedatives and hypnotics, stimulants, and antianxiety agents. The 1985 NIDA household survey of nonmedical drug use revealed that about 9% of the population had used stimulants and that 1% were using them currently; the percentages for sedatives were 6% and 1%; for tranquilizers, 8% and 1%; and for analgesics, 7% and 1%.[16]

This problem frequently has an insidious pattern of onset. An individual may receive a prescription, like the feeling that the drug gives, and gradually take more pills at a time or take them more frequently. Next to alcohol, diazepam (Valium) is probably the most frequently abused drug. Yet it is generally viewed as a relatively harmless substance and is freely prescribed for people who are anxious as a result of day-to-day stressors.

Categories of prescription drugs that are frequently abused include narcotics, barbiturates, amphetamines, benzodiazepines, meprobamate, and occasionally tricyclic antidepressants, particularly amitriptyline. Control of these drugs is difficult because of the many legitimate medical uses for them. There have been efforts to ban production of amphetamines based on the belief that other less dangerous medications can be equally effective. They remain on the market despite these efforts. Recently, street use of methamphetamine ("ice") has been increasing. Since this drug is relatively easy for amateur chemists to synthesize, substance abuse authorities are concerned that it will be the next drug fad. Most of these substances have been placed under some degree of control by the Food and Drug Administration (FDA) of the federal government, but the black market thrives. In addition, abuse is difficult to control because patients quickly learn that they can obtain prescriptions from several physicians and have them filled at different pharmacies, thus acquiring a large supply of drugs. Multiple addiction to prescription drugs in combination with each other and/or alcohol is becoming more prevalent.

Impaired professionals. Among the groups with the highest incidence of abuse of alcohol and prescription drugs are physicians and nurses. The narcotic addiction rate for health care professionals, including nurses, pharmacists, and physicians, is estimated to be about 1%.[16] This is contrasted to the national rate for the total population of 0.7%.[16] It has been estimated that 40,000 to 75,000 of the nation's 1.7 million nurses are alcoholics.[21] 41% of all licensure discipline cases in 1985 were related to substance abuse.[4]

Known rates of substance abuse by nurses and physicians are probably artificially low. This is partially because the problem is hidden by the abuser. However, colleagues often work as enablers and fail to confront the nurse who has the problem. Whether this results from the individual's ambivalence about substance abuse or from a misguided attempt to protect the addicted nurse, it is unfortunate. It jeopardizes the well-being of the nurse and the safety of the patients under his or her care. It is the absolute responsibility of any nurse to take whatever steps are necessary to intervene when a co-worker is practicing under the influence of alcohol or drugs.

A survey conducted by Cannon and Brown[4] identified the attitudes of 376 Oregon nurses toward their impaired colleagues. The results revealed that the nurses attitudes regarding alcoholism and drug abuse differed. Relative to alcoholism, 77% said they would confront them about their behavior, 67% thought they should be allowed to return to practice, and 85% were willing to work with them. In contrast, 76%

would confront drug abusers, 54% agreed that they should return to practice, and 73% would work with them. The latter two responses indicate less tolerance among nurses for drug abuse than for alcoholism. The characteristics of the most tolerant nurses included (1) those with fewer years in nursing, (2) those with baccalaureate or higher degrees, (3) those who indicated less approval for treatment interventions, and (4) those who were more optimistic about the outcomes of treatment.

In a national survey, Sullivan[27] identified characteristics of nurses who had problems with substance abuse and who had agreed to complete a questionnaire. Of these, 65% were 26 to 40 years of age; 73% had achieved academic grades of "B" or above; 76% had been employed in nursing more than 5 years; 71% were currently employed; 61% had an alcoholic family member; 54% came from a family with a history of depression; 48% were married; 59% had been divorced at some time; 48% had children; 54% had experienced sexual trauma; 12% stated a homosexual preference; 65% had been hospitalized in the last 5 years; and 64% had a history of depression.

Of particular interest is the confirmation of the overrepresentation of males (12% versus 2% to 3% in the profession) that had also been observed in other studies of impaired nurses. Sullivan speculates that this may be related to the higher incidence of male alcoholics in the general population. The majority of the sample had received professional treatment, had been abstinent for at least 1 year, and had not relapsed. They also attended Alcoholics Anonymous (AA) or Narcotics Anonymous (NA) meetings and peer support groups. Variables that were associated with relapses included threatened or actual loss of a job, narcotics abuse, disciplinary licensure action, more than one chemical dependency treatment, and infrequent AA or NA attendance.

In recognition of the severity of substance abuse by nurses, several state nurses' associations have established peer-assistance groups to work with addicted nurses. These groups comprise volunteer nurses, many of whom are recovered addicts. They offer support and referral services to addicted nurses. This helps them to avoid loss of licensure and ultimately assists them to return to work as effective and safe practitioners. At a national level, the Council on Psychiatric and Mental Health Nursing Practice of the American Nurses' Association has expressed concern about this serious problem.

■ **PSYCHOTOMIMETICS.** Since the early 1960s, another group of substances has been abused, particularly by adolescents and young adults. These substances induce a state similar to psychosis. They include hallucinogens, the most common of which has been LSD (lysergic acid diethylamide). Another substance that is unrelated to LSD but also leads to an altered state of awareness is PCP. Other drugs included in this psychotomimetic group are tetrahydrocannabinol (THC), which is the active ingredient of marijuana; mescaline; psilocybin; and peyote. Discussion in this chapter is limited to LSD and PCP, since they are most likely to be encountered by the nurse.

In 1985, 3% of 12- to 17-year-olds and 12% of 18- to 25-year-olds had used hallucinogens.[16] In 1984, 2% of 12- to 17-year-olds and 11% of 18- to 25-year-olds had used PCP at some time.[20] Use of these drugs is of concern to society because of the erratic and unpredictable behavior they produce. They are not generally addictive but are inexpensive to produce and widely available. They may also be substituted by the seller for other more expensive drugs, thus making it difficult to determine exactly what the individual has taken.

■ **COCAINE.** The drug that is currently most popular and the use of which has the highest status in the United States is cocaine. In 1985, 5% of 12- to 17-year-olds; 25% of 18- to 25-year-olds; and 9% of those 26 and older had used cocaine at least once.[16] It is estimated that about 30 million Americans (or 1 in 10) have used cocaine.[15] Although classified as a narcotic, cocaine is really a stimulant, more similar in effect to the amphetamines than to the opiates. Habitual use can lead to deteriorated functioning, although users claim that they perform better under the influence of cocaine. A solid form of cocaine, called "crack" and which is smoked, has gained great popularity. It tends to be readily available in most cities, and its use continues to rise.

■ **MARIJUANA.** Marijuana use in the United States is pervasive. Although it is still illegal, marijuana is widely available and in some settings its use is acceptable and even expected. According to a study sponsored by the National Institute on Drug Abuse (NIDA), in 1985, 24% of 12- to 17-year-olds, 60% of 18- to 25-year-olds, and 27% of those 26 and older had used marijuana or hashish.[16] Marijuana use within the last 30 days by high school seniors has declined from about 36% in 1978 to about 21% in 1987.[16] When marijuana use began to proliferate in the 1960s, most users were young. However, years later, many of these people still use marijuana and are now struggling with the issue of how to advise their own children on the use of drugs. One serious concern about marijuana use is that it does seem to serve as a transition to the use of more harmful drugs. Most users of marijuana

do not become heroin addicts. However, a person who has never used marijuana rarely uses opiates, hallucinogens, or cocaine.

■ **MULTIPLE SUBSTANCE USE.** A serious and increasing problem related to substance abuse is the simultaneous or sequential use of more than one substance. For instance, barbiturates and amphetamines may be used alternately to achieve relaxation and then stimulation. Cocaine use is sometimes followed by heroin to moderate the stimulant effect or to ease the depression ("crash") that follows the high. Such experimentation can be dangerous, particularly if synergistic drugs, such as barbiturates and alcohol, are used. It also complicates assessment of and intervention in substance abuse, since the individual may be experiencing withdrawal from several drugs at the same time.

■ Natural opiates

Some relate the high prevalence of substance use and abuse to the need to blunt or escape from the anxiety created by the stresses of life. It is interesting to note that there have been efforts to find means of achieving a "natural high" as an alternative to the use of chemicals to achieve euphoria or relaxation. Advocates of meditation, yoga, and self-hypnosis claim that they are able to find peace from within themselves. There has been an upsurge of interest in Eastern religions, which frequently teach followers to achieve states of altered awareness. Others have found that they can relieve tension through physical activity. Joggers report the occurrence of a "runner's high." Neurochemical research has begun to reveal possible biological explanations for these experiences. Snyder[25] has reported on the discovery of enkephalins and endorphins. These naturally occurring peptides bind with opiate receptors in the brain and pituitary gland. They have been described as natural opiates. It is hypothesized that experiences resulting in a feeling of euphoria stimulate the release of these neurochemicals. Research in this area has great promise for increasing understanding of and the potential for treatment of addiction.

An individual may achieve a state of relaxation, euphoria, stimulation, or altered awareness by several means. The range of these activities is illustrated in Fig. 19-1.

Assessment

■ Predisposing factors

Much research has been conducted concerning the factors that predispose a person to become a substance abuser. This knowledge is essential to enable health

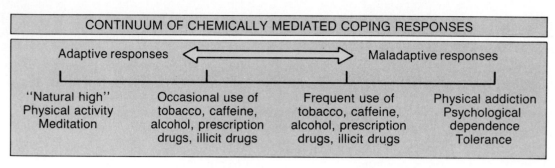

Fig. 19-1. Continuum of chemically mediated coping responses.

care providers to focus on prevention. Although some information has been provided, much work remains to be done.

■ **BIOLOGICAL FACTORS.** Factors related to substance abuse may be biological, psychological, or sociocultural but are most frequently a combination. Biological factors may include a familial tendency for substance abuse. This has been observed in the case of alcoholism. This problem also tends to occur in families that have a concurrent high incidence of bipolar disorder. About half the children of alcoholics become alcoholics even though many are repelled by their parents' behavior. This also suggests an inherited tendency for alcoholism. Another theory proposes that alcoholism is caused by an allergic response to alcohol. This is an attempt to explain that some people can control drinking behavior and others cannot. However, the only truly allergic response to alcohol that has been documented is an aversive one. A high percentage of Oriental people in particular experience a physiological response to alcohol that includes flushing, tachycardia, and an intense feeling of discomfort.[12] This response may explain the low rate of alcoholism among people of Oriental descent.

■ **PSYCHOLOGICAL FACTORS.** Various psychological theories have been proposed to explain substance abuse. For instance, it has been hypothesized that the person who becomes addicted to drugs (including alcohol and tobacco)* is dependent and unable to rely on his own resources for gratification. Freudian psychoanalytical theory describes the oral-dependent personality type. This person is fixated at the oral stage of development and seeks need satisfaction through oral behaviors, including smoking or the in-

gestion of various substances. A related theory emphasizes the low self-esteem of the substance abuser. Gold[11] has described a cycle of behavior that is illustrated in Fig. 19-2. Substance use is reinforced because it gives the individual a sense of control over the area of conflict, thus reducing anxiety. Unfortunately, the substance use itself may create a new source of conflict. Guilt or fear of discovery associated with the behavior may contribute to the individual's low self-esteem. Eventually, the substance abuse itself perpetuates the need to continue taking the drug.

Family traits that predispose the individual to drug abuse have been identified. Jaffe[16] has described a family in which the opposite sex parent may be overinvolved with the addict while the other parent is inaccessible or punitive. The family tends to focus on the addict's behavior. Stanton[26] reports a higher-than-average number of deaths in the families of drug abusers. The usual family interaction picture is that of overinvolvement of the opposite-sex parent, whereas the same-sex parent is "punitive, distant and/or absent."[26] The following characteristics are described as distinguishing the families of drug abusers from those with other types of disrupted behavior[26]:

1. A history of multigenerational addictive behaviors, including nonsubstance-related activities, such as gambling and television watching
2. More primitive and direct expression of conflict
3. Absence of schizophrenic behavior in parents
4. An illusion of the drug abuser's independence through peer group membership
5. Higher level of maternal symbiosis
6. The presence of death themes and untimely deaths
7. Immigrant parents, possibly resulting in cultural disparity between parents and children

■ **SOCIOCULTURAL FACTORS.** Advertising bombards the average person with information on the

---

*The term "drug" is used here to refer to all abused substances, including alcohol, nicotine, and caffeine. Specific agents are referred to by name or category when appropriate.

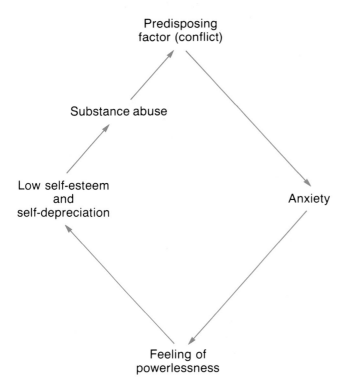

Fig. 19-2. The cycle of substance abuse. (Modified from Gold SR: The CAP control theory of drug abuse. In Lettieri DJ, Sayers M, and Pearson HW, editors: Theories on drug abuse: selected contemporary perspectives, NIDA Research Monograph 30, Rockville, Md, 1980, National Institute on Drug Abuse.)

relaxing properties of a variety of drugs. Even many illicit drugs are easily obtainable by those who are familiar with the drug culture. Marijuana and cocaine are frequently available at the social gatherings of all socioeconomic classes. A related predisposing factor is acceptance of drug use by the relevant sociocultural group.

Failure to assimilate a value system that opposes drug use is also a factor. The ambivalence of society in general about the use or abuse of various substances is perceived by the young and may be interpreted as permissiveness. Children of parents who use drugs, including alcohol and tobacco, grow up with attitudes of acceptance toward this behavior. It has been observed that members of religious groups with strong sanctions against the use of alcohol have much lower rates of alcohol use and alcoholism than members of religions that accept or encourage the use of alcohol. Cultural factors also play a role in alcohol use patterns. It has been found that Northern Europeans have higher alcoholism rates than Southern Europeans. Of the major religious groups in the United States, Roman

Catholics have the highest rate of alcoholism and Jews the lowest.

There are also sexual differences in the incidence of substance abuse. More men than women are abusers of alcohol and opiates. More women than men abuse prescription drugs such as diazepam. It must be noted, however, that the incidence of alcohol abuse by women may be higher than has been believed. Cultural attitudes toward drinking behavior differ for men and women. There is much less acceptance of female alcoholism. Therefore it is often hidden, and women tend to deny that they have a problem even longer than men do. Whereas the ability to drink large amounts is considered *macho* behavior for men, use of antianxiety drugs is viewed as weak and unmasculine. The latter behavior is acceptable for and even sometimes expected of women.

■ Precipitating stressors

The use or abuse of substances is often viewed as a way to shield the individual from the stressful events of life. Unfortunately, this attitude can lead rapidly to a spiral in which stress occurs, the substance is used, the effects wear off, more stress occurs, more substance is used, and so on. Eventually, the use of the substance becomes an additional stressor because of interference with the person's biopsychosocial functioning.

Substance abuse frequently arises during adolescence. Insecurity related to a poorly developed sense of identity may cause the young person to take drugs. In addition, adolescents are engaged in a conflict between the need to remain dependent on their parents and the need to assert their own independence. This conflict can erupt into rebellious behavior. The use or abuse of various drugs may be an expression of adolescent rebellion that is often reinforced by peer group approval.

The pleasure principle has been proposed as another explanation for substance-abusing behavior. This theory suggests that organisms are motivated to seek pleasure and to avoid pain. The use of drugs induces a pleasurable state and reduces the experience of physical or psychological pain. Since the pain returns when the effect of the drug wears off, the individual is powerfully attracted to repeated drug use. This aspect of drug use is reflected in the use of the term "high" to describe the drug experience. A related factor is the described oversensitivity of substance abusers, suggesting that they might be particularly susceptible to the euphoria-inducing effects of drugs. Some also explain the use of drugs by saying it leads to a mystical experience. They claim there is a drive to experience altered states of consciousness that is expressed through the use of drugs. This is an existential approach to drug abuse and theorizes that drug use can lead to a spiritual experience that most people achieve without the use of drugs.

Sociocultural stressors are also generally present when substance abuse occurs. The complexity and tension of modern life often cause individuals to seek avenues of escape. Drugs are readily available and provide a tempting respite from pressure. The legal drugs—alcohol, caffeine, nicotine, and over-the-counter drugs—are easily obtained and are socially approved tension-reduction agents. Illicit drugs are not usually sought by beginning users but are offered to them by others. Ease of access has also been presented as a stressor for health care professionals who abuse drugs.

Group influence and peer pressure frequently induce people to experiment with drugs. This is a particularly important factor for adolescents who are in a developmental stage where peer group acceptance is extremely important. Peer influence is also reflected in the fact that fashions in drug use change, as do fads in other areas. For instance, hallucinogen use had declined for several years but recently has begun to increase again. Cocaine particularly in its "crack" form is popular with older drug users as well as with the young, and its prevalence is increasing rapidly. In some areas of the United States, methamphetamine ("ice") is the latest fashion in drugs.

■ Behaviors associated with alcoholism

For the purpose of this discussion, the alcoholic is defined as any person whose drinking behavior interferes with his ability to carry out his usual daily activities and/or adversely affects his interpersonal relationships. This encompasses the person who indulges in episodic excessive drinking as well as the one who is addicted to alcohol. Excessive alcohol use can result in both physical and psychological dependency. **Physical dependence** occurs when there is a biological need in the body for the abused substance. If the substance is not supplied, physical withdrawal symptoms result. **Psychological dependence** is the craving for the subjective effect of the substance. The onset of alcoholism is often insidious. Many heavy drinkers fantasize that they are able to control their behavior when in reality they are addicted.

■ **IMPENDING ALCOHOLISM.** Several behaviors have been identified as warning signs of impending alcoholism. These include sneaking drinks, morning drinking, blackouts, binge drinking, arguments about drinking, missing time at work, and an alcohol-related police record. Increased tolerance, when more and more alcohol can be consumed without causing intox-

TABLE 19-1

COMPARISON OF BLOOD ALCOHOL CONCENTRATIONS TO BEHAVIORAL MANIFESTATIONS OF INTOXICATION

Blood alcohol level	Behaviors
Up to 0.1% (100 mg/ 100 ml)	Loud speech, decreased inhibitions, silliness
0.1% to 0.2%	Slurred speech, moodiness, unsteady gait, decreased coordination, shortened attention span, impaired memory
0.2% to 0.3%	Ataxia, tremor, irritability, stupor
0.3%	Unconsciousness

Modified from Butz RH: Intoxication and withdrawal. In Estes NJ and Heinemann ME: Alcoholism: development, consequences, and interventions, ed 2, St Louis, 1982, Mosby–Year Book, Inc.

ication, is also a sign that alcoholism has developed. Intoxication has been defined as a blood alcohol level of 0.1% or more. Table 19-1 compares blood alcohol levels and behaviors.

■ **PROGRESSIVE ALCOHOLISM.** Seixas[24] has identified several other behaviors that are indicative of progressive alcoholism. One is an increased incidence of suicide in alcoholics. This may also be related to the losses that alcoholics usually experience. In other cases, people who are already depressed may begin to drink as an attempt at coping and may then become alcoholics. Since drinking usually reinforces depressed feelings, suicide may result. A second behavior is increased incidence of accidental injury to alcoholics. Some of the automobile accidents involving alcoholics may also represent suicide attempts, since suicidal behavior is also greatly increased in alcoholics.[10]

Many physical behaviors are frequently related to alcoholism. Since the liver detoxifies alcohol, excessive drinking eventually results in impaired liver functioning. Fatty liver, hepatitis, and cirrhosis of the liver are frequently complications of alcohol abuse. Other problems include esophagitis, gastritis, pancreatitis, cardiomyopathy, pulmonary function changes, myopathy, osteoporosis, various anemias, disruptions of the immune system, peripheral neuropathy, and brain damage.[24] Almost no organ escapes adverse effects in the alcoholic.

Psychologically, the alcoholic may be depressed, hostile, and suspicious or exhibit many other painful emotions. Specific behaviors related to these types of disruptions may be observed. It is often debatable how much of the emotional response precedes and how much follows the development of alcoholism. Alcoholics are usually reluctant to confront or even admit to their problems. They may behave very dependently toward significant others and health care personnel. They may expect to be shielded from stress and use any conflict to justify drinking. An alcoholic patient once explained her drinking episode by saying, "It was Christmas Eve and I knew everybody in the world was drinking, so why shouldn't I?" Another person said, "If I stub my toe, it's a good enough reason to drink." This combination of dependency and rationalization can be difficult for significant others and often contributes to the breakdown of interpersonal relationships.

Socially, alcoholics may be inhibited people. Alcohol reduces the inhibitions enough to enable them to relate more comfortably to others. However, these relationships tend to be transient and superficial. The intoxicated person may also exhibit poor judgment in his selection of companions, making himself vulnerable to mugging and other forms of victimization.

Clinical example 19-1 illustrates many of the behaviors described. This person has the medical diagnoses of alcohol dependence and alcohol withdrawal delirium.

WITHDRAWAL BEHAVIORS. Alcohol withdrawal begins shortly after drinking has ended and lasts 5 to 7 days. It is characterized by various behaviors, some of which are dangerous. According to Butz, the earliest and most common behaviors are "anxiety, anorexia, insomnia, and tremor."[3] In addition, there is hyperalertness and a feeling "often described as internal shaking." There may be a mild disorientation, which usually lasts a short time. If it persists, it may be a sign of impending delirium. Tachycardia (120 to 140 beats per minute) continues throughout withdrawal and may be used to monitor the patient's condition. Alcoholic hallucinosis is another withdrawal syndrome and is characterized by auditory hallucinations in a patient who exhibits no other psychotic behavior. This condition generally lasts for only a few hours or days, although in rare instances it becomes chronic.[1] These hallucinations may be distinguished from those of alcohol withdrawal delirium because they are auditory, whereas the latter are usually visual.

Delirium tremens, now called alcohol withdrawal delirium, is a very serious withdrawal syndrome also described by Butz. Behaviors associated with this syndrome include "marked tremor, anxiety, insomnia, an-

CLINICAL EXAMPLE 19-1

Mr. H was admitted to the detoxification center of a large metropolitan hospital and was in acute alcohol withdrawal. He was delirious and having visual hallucinations of bugs crawling on his body. He was extremely frightened, thrashing around in bed and mumbling incoherently. Since he had a long and well-documented history of alcohol abuse, family members were contacted and confirmed that he had recently stopped drinking after a 2-week binge.

The patient had been a successful lawyer with a large practice. He specialized in corporate law and conducted much business over lunch or dinner. He also kept a well-stocked bar in his office to offer clients a drink. Without his really being aware of it, Mr. H's drinking gradually increased. After a few years he was drinking almost nonstop from lunchtime to bedtime. He then began to have a Bloody Mary with breakfast "just to get myself going."

His wife reported that he had become irritable, particularly if she questioned his drinking. On two occasions he had hit her during their arguments. She was seriously considering divorce. He had also become alienated from his children, who appeared frightened of him. Infrequently he would feel guilty about his neglect of his family and plan a special outing. Most of the time he was too drunk to carry out his plans. The family had also become less involved in activities with friends. Mrs. H and the children felt embarrassed about his behavior and so did not invite anyone to their home. On two occasions, Mr. H had tried to stop drinking. The first time he went to a private hospital, where he was detoxified. He remained abstinent for about a month after discharge.

He then lost an important case and decided to have "just one drink" to carry him through the crisis. Soon his drinking was again out of control. His second hospitalization was at a general hospital with an active alcoholism rehabilitation program. He was introduced to Alcoholics Anonymous and started taking disulfiram (Antabuse). This program worked until he decided that he could manage without medication. A couple of weeks later his coworkers persuaded him to "help celebrate" at an office party. This was the start of a binge that ended when he had an automobile accident on the way home from a bar. A passenger in the other car was killed, and Mr. H was charged with vehicular homicide and driving under the influence of alcohol. He stopped drinking abruptly, which resulted in his current hospital admission 3 days later.

orexia, paranoia, and disorientation."[3] Frequently these patients have episodes of uncontrolled behavior. Delusions and visual hallucinations often occur. Other symptoms may include elevated temperature, tachycardia, tachypnea, hyperpnea, vomiting, diarrhea, and diaphoresis. Occasionally, delirium tremens may lead to death. Alcohol withdrawal delirium usually occurs on the second or third day after the last drink has been taken. The episode is usually over within 48 to 72 hours after onset.[1,13]

Another serious behavioral manifestation of alcohol withdrawal is grand mal convulsions, sometimes called "rum fits." Other causes of seizure activity should be explored, including trauma and the use of other drugs. There is generally no long-term problem related to these seizures.[3] Further information on alcohol withdrawal syndromes may be found in the suggested readings at the end of this chapter.

■ **PHYSICAL DISORDERS ASSOCIATED WITH CHRONIC ALCOHOLISM.** Alcoholics frequently are malnourished and have vitamin deficiencies. Shortage of the B vitamins contributes to the occurrence of peripheral neuropathies. Thiamine deficiency may result in the development of **alcohol amnestic disorder,**[1] also referred to as Korsakoff's syndrome. Individuals with this problem exhibit severe memory problems. It frequently occurs following an episode of **Wernicke's encephalopathy,** which is manifested by neurological disturbances, such as confusion, ataxia, and abnormal eye movements. Wernicke's encephalopathy may be treated successfully with large doses of thiamine, but if it progresses to alcoholic amnestic syndrome, the prognosis for reversal of the memory loss is poor.[1]

■ **Behaviors associated with drug abuse**

Drug abuse refers to the use of any mind-altering substance (except alcohol, which has been considered separately) besides those prescribed by a physician. Categories of drugs that are commonly abused include narcotics, stimulants, depressants, antianxiety agents, and hallucinogens. All the drugs mentioned except the hallucinogens can be addictive. Drug addiction may involve physical dependency, psychological dependency, or both. The combination of these two factors is a powerful incentive to continue using drugs. It should also be remembered that many drug abusers are simultaneously addicted to more than one substance.

■ **OPIATE ABUSE.** The opiates include opium, heroin, meperidine, morphine, codeine, and methadone. The first two drugs were used for medical and, in the case of opium, religious and recreational purposes in the past, but are generally no longer used for these purposes. Meperidine, morphine, and codeine are frequently used analgesics that are found in any hospital medicine room. Methadone is a narcotic substance that is used as a treatment for addiction to other opiates. It can be used either to facilitate withdrawal or to provide a maintenance program at a stable dose. It is useful because it does not interfere with the ability to function productively as other narcotics do. Individuals receiving a methadone maintenance regimen may work and carry on a normal life, although still addicted to narcotics. Opiates may be introduced into the body by ingestion, inhalation, smoking, or intravenous, intramuscular, or subcutaneous injection.

Narcotic addiction is a great social problem. People who are addicted to opiates generally deteriorate mentally and physically to the point that they are unable to function productively. Illegal behavior that may result from addiction includes stealing or engaging in prostitution to acquire money for drugs. The obtaining and use of drugs becomes an all-consuming passion.

Users of intravenous drugs are also at a very high risk for infection by the human immunodeficiency virus, type 1 (HIV-1). This is the virus that causes the acquired immunodeficiency syndrome (AIDS). It is common for addicts to share needles when they are using drugs in a group. Since the needles are not cleaned between users, blood is transferred from one person to the other. This is an ideal situation for the transmission of HIV-1. Several approaches have been proposed to solve this public health problem. Some have tried needle exchanges, in which an addict may receive a clean needle in exchange for a used one. This has presented an ethical dilemma related to providing people with the means to engage in an illegal activity. Other programs focus on education and the provision of bleach for the purpose of cleaning needles between users. This is less objectionable to some, but drug addicts are notably unreliable in performing any activity that interferes with immediate gratification. Efforts to halt the spread of HIV-1 in this population will continue. Needle sharing and sexual relations with infected intravenous drug users are the primary routes of transmission of the virus to women. Pregnant women infected with the virus often deliver infected babies. If the mother is addicted to drugs, the baby is born with the double problem of HIV-1 infection and drug addiction. Many of these babies have been abandoned in hospital nurseries. They comprise a major, growing health care problem.

Behaviors associated with addiction to narcotics include the development of **tolerance.** Tolerance refers to the increasing need for more and more of the drug to create the same effect. This also increases the expense of the habit. Physiological effects of narcotics include decreased response to pain, respiratory depression, nausea, constriction of pupils, drowsiness, decreased response of the hypothalamus to external input, depressed pituitary functioning, decreased secretion of digestive juices, slower peristalsis, and constipation caused by increased intestinal absorption of water.[22]

The most important psychological response to opiate use is a sense of euphoria, referred to as feeling "high." It is this powerful pleasurable response that causes the individual to use the drug repeatedly, ultimately leading to addiction. Other psychological effects of narcotics include apathy, detachment from reality, and impaired judgment. The phrase "nodding out" is used to describe this complex of behaviors in combination with drowsiness. Clinical example 19-2 demonstrates the behaviors associated with opiate abuse.

Withdrawal from narcotics is extremely uncomfortable, but not usually life threatening. It may be accomplished with the aid of methadone, which can be substituted for heroin or other opiates and then gradually decreased if total withdrawal is desired. When withdrawal is not mediated by the use of drugs, behaviors may initially include anxiety, yawning, diaphoresis, abdominal cramps, lacrimation, and rhinorrhea. These are followed by mydriasis, piloerection, achiness, muscular twitching, and anorexia. Later symptoms include insomnia, hypertension, elevated temperature, increased rate and depth of respirations, restlessness, nausea, vomiting, diarrhea, spontaneous ejaculation or orgasm, and blood chemistry alterations, including hemoconcentration, leukocytosis, eosinopenia, and hyperglycemia. Overdosage of narcotics can lead rapidly to coma, respiratory depression, and death. Accidental overdoses among narcotic addicts sometimes occur, particularly when the user is uncertain of the drug's strength. Drugs are usually cut with inert substances before they are sold, thus resulting in the availability of varied strengths on the streets.

■ **BARBITURATE ABUSE.** The use of barbiturates results in a psychological experience that is very similar to that induced by alcohol. Barbiturate drugs include barbital, amobarbital (Amytal), phenobarbital, pentobarbital (Nembutal), secobarbital (Seconal), and butabarbital. These drugs are widely prescribed for their sedative and hypnotic properties. As with alcohol, they are basically depressants but induce an initial response of euphoria. For this reason, barbiturates are popular street drugs. They do lead to both physical and psychological dependence. Behaviors that result from intake of barbiturates include euphoria followed by de-

CLINICAL EXAMPLE 19-2

Mr. C was a 35-year-old black man who had been jailed for auto theft. He was believed to be a member of a large ring of automobile thieves in a major metropolitan area. His previous arrest record included several episodes of armed robbery and breaking and entering. A few hours after he had been jailed, Mr. C complained of abdominal cramps and appeared very anxious. His nose and eyes were running, there were beads of perspiration on his brow, and he was rocking back and forth on his bunk. The guard called Ms. V, the correctional health nurse.

Ms. V observed Mr. C and performed a brief physical assessment. She noted that his pupils were dilated, his blood pressure was elevated, and he had "gooseflesh." In addition, there were multiple needle "tracks" on his arms. She asked him directly about drug use, and he admitted that he had been addicted to heroin. He stated that his addiction began in 1967 while he was stationed with the army in Vietnam. When he returned to the United States, he remained in the army for 18 months and was able to stop using drugs altogether. He planned to get a job and attend school after leaving the service. He related that he was disturbed by the attitude of people toward Vietnam veterans. While he was still in the service, he was able to use peer support to cope with his feelings. However, after his discharge, he was reluctant to talk about his military experience. Others seemed disinterested, embarrassed, or hostile when he talked about it.

Mr. C had difficulty finding a civilian job. He was an artillery specialist in the army and found that it was difficult to apply this experience. He began to have nightmares and "flashbacks" of his combat experiences. Because of the anxiety associated with this, he finally returned to drugs. Without a job, he used illegal means to finance his habit and therefore repeatedly went to jail.

Ms. V discussed Mr. C's problem with the physician in the prison health department. They decided to assess Mr. C's eligibility for a methadone drug treatment program and to request consultation from a counselor at the local Vietnam veterans counseling center. He was given the medical diagnoses of opioid dependence, opioid withdrawal, and posttraumatic stress disorder.

CLINICAL EXAMPLE 19-3

Ms. W was a 34-year-old woman who was moderately overweight. She had tried various diets on her own with little success. A friend told her about a "diet doctor" who had a reputation for helping his patients lose weight with minimum deprivation from eating their usual diet. Ms. W decided to see the physician and was accepted for treatment. She was given a diuretic and appetite depressant medication. The latter contained amphetamines. She began to lose weight as soon as she started the prescribed regimen and was delighted. She also liked the additional burst of energy she felt every time she took her medication. She completed projects that she had been planning to work on for months. However, her family began to complain because she was irritable and very restless. In addition, she developed insomnia and roamed about the house at night.

On the urging of her husband, she went to her family physician. She felt guilty about seeing another physician for her weight problem, so neglected to tell her regular physician about this. With the history of insomnia, irritability, and recent weight loss, her physician thought she might be depressed. He ordered an antidepressant medication and a barbiturate sedative. Ms. W soon found that she was able to sleep well with her sedative. However, she felt slightly hung over in the morning and still wanted to lose more weight, so she continued with her diet pills as well. For a while she was able to function well. Gradually, however, she found that she needed two sedatives and then she also began to use extra stimulants. Her husband questioned her drug use. Ms. W had read about drug abuse and with her husband's help identified that she had a problem. She decided to see her family physician again and this time told him the whole story. He then advised a brief hospitalization so she could be withdrawn from both drugs under medical supervision. Ms. W was very embarrassed by her addiction. While in the hospital, she needed a great deal of nursing support to integrate this experience. The medical diagnoses that were applied to Ms. W included amphetamine dependence, amphetamine withdrawal, barbiturate dependence, and barbiturate withdrawal.[1]

pression and sometimes hostility. Inhibitions are decreased and judgment may be impaired. There is a lack of coordination and slurring of speech. The person may become quite drowsy, depending on the amount taken and the individual's level of tolerance. Barbiturates are generally swallowed or injected. Tolerance develops, resulting in the use of increasing amounts to achieve the desired effect. Because of the similarities in their actions, the use of barbiturates with alcohol is dangerous and may lead to accidental overdose.

Withdrawal from barbiturates can be dangerous and therefore is frequently conducted in the hospital. Withdrawal symptoms include postural hypotension accompanied by tachycardia, elevated temperature, insomnia, tremors, and agitation. If barbiturates are withdrawn abruptly, behaviors include apprehension, weakness, tremors, postural hypotension, twitching, anorexia, grand mal seizures, and psychosis.

■ **STIMULANT ABUSE: AMPHETAMINES AND COCAINE.** Stimulant use has been increasing rapidly in recent years because of the alertness and feeling of extra energy that they provide. Caffeine is the most pervasive stimulant in current use. It is found in coffee, tea, chocolate, and many soft drinks. The wide acceptance of caffeine use may make the use of other stimulants seem more acceptable. Amphetamines are now rarely prescribed medically for the treatment of obesity and narcolepsy. They are sometimes given to hyperactive children because of a paradoxical calming effect. As other treatments for these conditions have been found, serious questions have been raised about whether there is any legitimate medical use for amphetamines. Serious consideration has been given to placing a ban on their production. Illicit users of these drugs include truck drivers on long trips; students who are cramming for examinations; and people, such as nurses, who work night shifts.

Addiction to barbiturates and stimulants, particularly the amphetamines, frequently occurs simultaneously. Sometimes a patient who has been using "downers" finds he needs "uppers" to give him enough energy to function. Clinical example 19-3 illustrates this pattern.

Ms. W's pattern is not uncommon. Aside from street use, many people slip into drug abuse without being aware of the consequences of their behavior.

The amphetamine drugs include amphetamine, methamphetamine, dextroamphetamine, and benzphetamine. The effects of amphetamine use include euphoria, hyperactivity, irritability, hyperalertness, insomnia, anorexia, weight loss, tachycardia, and hypertension. It is not generally believed that these drugs cause physical dependence, but they do cause psychological dependence and tolerance develops. Prolonged or excessive use may result in psychotic behavior. Withdrawal of the drugs usually results in a "crash," manifested by depression and lack of energy. This discomfort provides motivation to take more drugs.

Cocaine is a stimulant drug that has become a symbol of sophistication for some. It is fashionable to inhale (snort) cocaine through rolled-up $100 bills. It may be inhaled, injected subcutaneously or intravenously, smoked, or applied topically to the genitals.[19] Those who want a more intense experience may smoke the drug after it has been processed chemically. This process is called "freebasing," and the result of the processing is called "crack." Use of cocaine has been glamorized by the publicity given to its use by movie stars, sports figures, and other well-known people. This makes it particularly inviting to adolescents who regard famous people as role models. Historically, cocaine use was advocated for a time by Sigmund Freud. He later became disenchanted with it. The drug was also a part of the life-style of Sherlock Holmes, as created by Sir Arthur Conan Doyle.

According to House,[15] cocaine is relatively short acting. Its effects last 60 to 90 minutes when it has been inhaled, 30 to 60 minutes when injected, and 5 minutes when smoked in crack form. The experience is very similar to that induced by the amphetamines. A person who is "high" on cocaine feels euphoric, energetic, self-confident, and sociable. Biochemically, cocaine blocks the reuptake of norepinephrine and dopamine. Since more neurotransmitter is present at the synapse, the receptors are continuously activated. This accounts for the euphoria that is experienced. At the same time, presynaptic supplies of dopamine and norepinephrine are depleted. This causes the "crash" that happens when the effect of the drug wears off. Other behaviors that result include tachycardia, increased systolic blood pressure, fever, increased cardiac output, and transient vasospasm.[15] Severe episodes of these behaviors can lead to serious physical illness. Sudden death has also been associated with cocaine abuse. Table 19-2 compares the behaviors that House[15] has described associated with early and prolonged use of cocaine. She also identifies the "red flags of cocaine abuse: a previously healthy young adult complains of headaches, seizures, chest pain, nasal ulcerations, chronically inflamed sore throat, chronic cough, weight loss, insomnia, depression, and/or paranoia. Problems with family, job, and/or money typically complete the picture."[15:45] Cocaine use has been known to result in sudden death. Cocaine use does not seem to result in physical dependence, but the psychological dependence is powerful.

TABLE 19-2		
CLINICAL MANIFESTATIONS OF COCAINE USE		
	Early use	Prolonged use
Neurological	Excitation Euphoria Restlessness	Depression Withdrawal Tremors Dysarthria Seizure activity
Cardiovascular	Tachycardia Hypertension Angina	Ventricular dysrhythmias Hypotension Congestive heart failure Myocardial infarction
Pulmonary	Rising respiratory rate	Chronic cough Lung congestion Productive brown/black sputum Acute respiratory distress Respiratory arrest

From House MA: Cocaine, Am J Nurs 90:41, April 1990.

■ **ABUSE OF HALLUCINOGENS AND PCP.** One behavior that became representative of the "drop-out" generation of the 1960s was the use of drugs that create experiences very similar to those typical of a psychotic state. These substances have been called hallucinogens, psychedelics, and psychotomimetics. LSD is representative of the hallucinogenic drugs. PCP use results in behaviors that are similar in many respects to those produced by hallucinogens. Because of the entirely different chemical structures, it is important to be able to compare and contrast these drugs.

LSD is generally swallowed. It is colorless and tasteless and is therefore often added to a drink or food, such as a sugar cube. It may also be given to a person without his knowledge. Pleasurable effects of hallucinogen use include intensification of sensory experiences. Colors are described as more brilliant, and sounds, smells, and tastes are heightened. Sometimes users of these drugs report **synesthesia,** or a crossover of sensory experiences during which music may be seen or colors may be heard. Space and time become distorted.

The hallucinogens have not demonstrated addictive properties. They do, however, lead to self-destructive behavior because of the impairment of judgment that results from their use. LSD, peyote, mescaline, and psilocybin are commonly used hallucinogens. Vulnerable individuals who take these drugs may experience "bad trips," which may deteriorate into psychotic episodes. The patient may experience paranoid, grandiose, or somatic delusions, usually accompanied by vivid hallucinations. The hallucinatory experience may be pleasant or frightening. The patient who is psychotic is not in contact with reality and frequently misinterprets environmental events. He may be unable to attend to any of his biological needs. He may also inadvertently hurt himself either in response to hallucinations or as an attempt to escape from the frightening experience. Since there is no physical dependence, withdrawal symptoms do not occur. Usually there is a gradual dissipation of psychotic behavior, although the patient may experience "flashbacks" for several months. These brief recurrences of the hallucinogenic experience can be frightening. Patients often express the fear that they are crazy and will never be free of the aftereffects of the drug.

PCP use has become more widespread than that of LSD and related drugs. It may be ingested and is frequently smoked in a mixture with another substance, such as marijuana or parsley flakes. PCP use may precipitate an intensely psychotic experience characterized by extreme agitation. The patient may become violent or exhibit other antisocial behaviors, such as insistence on removing his clothing or the use of profanity. Physical manifestations of PCP intoxication include hypertension, ataxia, dysarthria, increased deep tendon reflexes, and decreased pain response. Nystagmus frequently occurs and may be lateral, vertical, or sometimes rotary. At high doses, serious physiological consequences can occur, including seizures, coma, and death.[1,16] PCP use may evoke the occurrence or exacerbation of an existing and previously controlled psychosis. The unpredictability of the reaction to PCP makes it an extremely dangerous drug.

■ **MARIJUANA USE.** Marijuana is discussed briefly because it is an illicit drug. Nurses will rarely see anyone admitted to the health care system with a primary diagnosis of marijuana use. Use of marijuana generally produces an altered state of awareness accompanied by a feeling of relaxation and mild euphoria. Inhibitions are reduced and reflexes are slowed. Prolonged use may lead to a sense of apathy and loss of motivation, sometimes referred to as the **amotivational syndrome.** Psychosis may occur in individuals who are already at risk. The physiological effects of marijuana use are still being investigated but include drying of the oral and pharyngeal mucous membranes and reddening of the eyes. Pulmonary changes similar to those associated with tobacco use have also been found. Marijuana also interferes with normal functioning of reproductive hormones in both sexes. It is suspected that the altered hormonal activity increases the possibility of pregnancy and causes developmental problems in the fetus.[16] Other long-term effects are yet to be identified.

■ **ABUSE OF ANTIANXIETY DRUGS.** Antianxiety agents, particularly the benzodiazepines, constitute a large part of legal drug abuse in the United States. Chlordiazepoxide (Librium) and diazepam (Valium) were welcomed by the medical profession and the public as the answer to the stresses of life. Because they were initially described as relatively safe drugs, the benzodiazepines were prescribed and used freely. However, it has now become apparent that these agents can be physically and psychologically addictive and that tolerance to their use does occur, resulting in the ingestion of gradually increasing amounts. Long-term abuse of benzodiazepines can be debilitating with psychological and social consequences very similar to those associated with alcohol abuse. The person who takes an antianxiety drug experiences a sense of relaxation and a feeling of confidence. As with most drugs, it is this pleasurable experience that leads to repeated use of the drug. This progression is illustrated in Clinical example 19-4.

The case of Ms. T demonstrates the seductive quality of antianxiety drugs. Avoidance of anxiety is a powerful motivator of behavior. As with other drugs, as use escalates, guilt about drug taking develops. This guilt leads to anxiety that combines with the anxiety related to giving up the drug and results in increased intake. Antianxiety drugs have physiological as well as psychological effects. These may include drowsiness, hypotension, ataxia, and slurred speech. The withdrawal syndrome associated with abrupt cessation of benzodiazepines for patients who have taken the drugs for an extended time is similar to barbiturate withdrawal. Benzodiazepines have anticonvulsant properties, and withdrawal can lead to seizures, particularly in patients with a history of prior episodes of convulsive behavior.

Multiple drug abuse is becoming more common. The foregoing discussion reveals that many of the abused substances have similar effects. Abusers may use them interchangeably or simultaneously. Simultaneous use can lead to inadvertent overdose, since some of the substances are synergistic. It is extremely important that the exact nature of drug-abusing behaviors be identified so that unanticipated occurrence of withdrawal symptoms can be avoided.

CLINICAL EXAMPLE 19-4

Ms. T was a 28-year-old law student. She had always done well in school and had no difficulty with the theory portion of her law studies. However, she had always felt self-conscious and inadequate when she was required to speak before a group of people. She would become tremulous, her pulse and respiratory rate would increase, and her mouth would become dry. On occasion, she would lose track of her thoughts and be unable to continue speaking. This problem became a real handicap in her law classes. One of her professors gave her a failing grade for inadequate participation in class discussions. She went to her family physician and described her problem. He reassured her that he could give her medication that would help her overcome her "stress response." She was given diazepam, 5 mg, one tablet to be taken every 4 hours as needed for anxiety.

Ms. T was reluctant to take drugs because she recognized the danger inherent in the use of medication. However, she knew that she would never be able to stay in law school if she did not overcome her anxiety. Before her next class, she took a pill. She quickly felt relaxed and self-confident. She described the feeling as "like I had had a martini, only nicer." When the professor asked her a question, she was able to respond and was complimented for her answer. She felt a little drowsy after class but decided that she was probably tired because she had not been sleeping well.

Initially, Ms. T only took diazepam when she anticipated that she would need to speak in class. However, she was introduced to an attractive man by a friend and he asked her out for dinner. She felt anxious before the date and decided that it would do no harm to take a pill to help her relax. She was confident and charming on the date. Gradually, she began to use the drug more frequently. She rationalized that she needed the help to get through school and would stop during summer break. One day, she discovered that she had run out of pills just before she was scheduled to participate in a classroom debate. She went to the school health service, described her anxiety about the class and received another prescription for diazepam. She began to take more than one pill at a time and took them more frequently.

As her drug intake increased, Ms. T's performance in school deteriorated. She turned in papers late and missed classes. Her speech was slurred and she was uncoordinated. Her grades slipped. A year after she began to take pills to enable her to stay in school, she flunked out.

■ Dual diagnosis

As substance abuse has become more common in society, people with mental illnesses have also become victims of this problem. Caton and colleagues[6] cite studies that have identified the prevalence of alcohol abuse in psychiatric inpatients from 7.1% to 48%; of drug abuse in psychiatric patients from 14% to 66%; and of abuse of drugs, alcohol, or both by inpatients from 18% to 50%. Seriously mentally ill people are at risk to become substance abusers. Many have difficulty saying "no" to others, in part because they are lonely and fear alienation. Young mentally ill people are particularly vulnerable to substance abuse. At times, substance abuse may precipitate the first episode of a mental illness. Another contributing factor is the effect of the drug, which may alleviate the anxiety associated with the mental illness. Patients may feel energized by cocaine or amphetamines or calmed by sedatives or alcohol. If they are troubled by uncomfortable side effects from their psychotropic medication, they may prefer street drugs.

Table 19-3 summarizes the behaviors associated with substance abuse.

■ Co-dependency

In the past, substance abuse was considered an illness of the abuser. Recently it has been recognized that addiction is a family illness, particularly as it relates to alcoholism. This does not mean that all family members become addicted, although more than one may be. It means that all members of the family are affected by the addicted member's behavior. This leads family members to change their behavior in response to the addicted member. The complex of behaviors often seen in families where substance abuse is present is called **co-dependency.** Hetherington[14] identifies the cardinal rules of the alcoholic family: "Do not talk, do not trust, and do not feel."[14] She estimates that at least 28.6 million Americans or one in eight is a member of an alcoholic family. Elkin[7] points out that families of alcoholics have three choices for coping with that person. They may ignore the problem, banish the person from the family, or adapt. Most try to adapt. Elkin lists the behaviors that are typical of wives of alcoholics. These are:

1. High-level organizational ability.
2. Competence at a wide variety of tasks and the ability to learn additional ones quickly.
3. Stability and resistance to panic.
4. Skill at diplomacy and emotional manipulation.
5. Resilience with a high tolerance to pain.
6. High energy, with good resistance to fatigue.

TABLE 19-3

SUMMARY OF BEHAVIORS ASSOCIATED WITH SUBSTANCE ABUSE

Substance	Route (most common listed first)	Physical dependence	Psychological dependence	Expected behaviors
Alcohol	Ingestion	Yes	Yes	Euphoria, followed by depression and sometimes hostility; decreased inhibitions; impaired judgment; incoordination; slurred speech
Opiates				
Heroin	Injection Ingestion Inhalation	Yes	Yes	Euphoria, relaxation, relief from pain, lack of concern, detachment from reality, drowsiness, constricted pupils, nausea, constipation, slurred speech, impaired judgment
Morphine	Injection	Yes	Yes	
Meperidine	Injection		Yes	
	Ingestion	Yes		
Codeine	Ingestion		Yes	
	Injection	Yes		
Opium	Smoking Ingestion			
Methadone	Ingestion	Yes	Yes	Relieves craving for drugs without causing impaired functioning
Barbiturates	Ingestion Injection	Yes	Yes	Euphoria, followed by depression and sometimes hostility; decreased inhibitions; impaired judgment; slurred speech; incoordination; drowsiness
Amphetamines	Ingestion Injection	No	Yes	Euphoria, hyperactivity, irritability, hyperalertness, insomnia, anorexia, weight loss, tachycardia, hypertension
Cocaine	Inhalation Smoking Injection Topical	No	Yes	Euphoria, elation, agitation, hyperactivity, irritability, grandiosity, pressured speech, tachycardia, hypertension, diaphoresis, anorexia, weight loss, insomnia
Hallucinogens (psychedelics)	Ingestion Smoking	No	No	Distorted perception, heightened sense of awareness, grandiosity, hallucinations, illusions, distortions of time and space, depersonalization, mystical experiences, dilated pupils, increased blood pressure, increased salivation

TABLE 19-3

SUMMARY OF BEHAVIORS ASSOCIATE WITH SUBSTANCE ABUSE—cont'd

Behaviors related to overdose	Withdrawal syndrome	Special considerations
Unconsciousness, coma, respiratory depression, death	Tremors, halhucinosis, seizure disorder, delirium tremens (alcohol withdrawal delirium)	Chronic use leads to serious disruptions in most organ systems; malnutrition and dehydration are common; vitamin deficiency may lead to Wernicke's encephalopathy and alcoholic amnestic syndrome; alcohol-dependent people are susceptible to other dependencies as well
Unconsciousness, coma, respiratory depression, circulatory depression, respiratory arrest, cardiac arrest, death	Watery eyes, dilated pupils, anxiety, abdominal cramps, piloerection, yawning, diaphoresis, rhinorrhea, achiness, anorexia, insomnia, fever, nausea, vomiting, diarrhea	Chronic use leads to lack of concern about physical well-being, resulting in malnutrition and dehydration; criminal behavior may occur to acquire money for drugs; injection sites may become infected; multiple drug use is common
Same	Same	
Respiratory depression, coma, death	Postural hypotension, tachycardia, fever, insomnia, tremors, agitation, anxiety; rapid withdrawal causes apprehension, weakness, tremors, postural hypotension, anorexia, grand mal seizures	Frequently used alternately with stimulants; combination with alcohol enhances effects and may lead to overdosage; paradoxical responses of hyperactivity may occur in children and the elderly
Restlessness, tremor, rapid respiration, confusion, assaultiveness, hallucinations, panic	Depression, fatigue	Prolonged use can result in psychotic behavior; a paradoxical depressant reaction occurs in children; frequently used alternately with depressant substances
Seizures, respiratory depression, cardiac arrhythmias, coronary artery spasms and myocardial infarction, delirium, paranoia	Depression, fatigue, anxiety	Psychotic behavior may occur following large doses; prolonged use by inhalation may result in destruction of the mucous membranes in the nose and deterioration of the nasal septum; use in combination with other substances is dangerous
Panic, psychosis	None	A "bad trip" may result in panic, unpredictable behavior, and psychotic behaviors; "flashbacks" may occur for several months after use; self-destructive behavior may occur while under the effect of the drug

Continued.

TABLE 19-3—cont'd

SUMMARY OF BEHAVIORS ASSOCIATED WITH SUBSTANCE ABUSE

Substance	Route (most common listed first)	Physical dependence	Psychological dependence	Expected behaviors
Phencyclidine (PCP)	Smoking Ingestion	No	No	Euphoria, perceptual distortion, agitation, violence, delusions, antisocial behavior, elevated blood pressure, increased salivation, diaphoresis, ataxia, increased deep tendon reflexes, nystagmus, decreased pain response
Marijuana	Smoking Ingestion	No	Yes	Relaxation, mild euphoria, loss of inhibition, decreased motivation, red eyes, dry mouth
Antianxiety drugs (benzodiazepines)	Ingestion Injection	Yes	Yes	Relaxation, increased self-confidence, relief of anxiety, drowsiness, ataxia, slurred speech, hypotension

7. Good administrative skills.
8. The ability to defer gratification indefinitely.
9. Crisis intervention skills.
10. Strong sense of morality.
11. Loyalty and a willingness to put the needs of an important group before her own. It therefore helps if she is out of touch with her own needs and feelings.
12. Capacity to never ask "What's in this for *me?*"
13. The ability to do enormous amounts of work for a minimal payoff.
14. High level of nursing and caretaking skills.
15. Tendency toward overachievement leading to the ability to work consistently at 120% of capacity.
16. Gives low priority to her sexual needs and feelings.
17. Is symptomatic. Because drunkenness is such a powerful symptom, surviving while in constant contact with an alcoholic depends on having a "counter symptom." The necessary effect of the counter symptom is to defend the wife's boundaries without initiating dangerous conflict. Symptoms such as migraine headaches, obesity, depression, and obsessive-compulsive behaviors are common among wives of alcoholics.
18. Has low self-esteem with a very dependent personality framework.[7]

In terms of other family members, Elkin[7] describes the oldest daughter as the mother's apprentice. This child is responsible for assisting her mother to preserve the family. She learns the character traits described above. Many adult women who were raised in alcoholic families find that they need counseling and peer support group involvement to develop more functional behaviors. Twelve-step programs, based on the Alcoholics Anonymous model, have been developed for people with co-dependent problems. Many co-alcoholic women also become nurses. The behaviors that were adaptive in their families are also compatible with traditional nursing roles. Younger daughters tend to be withdrawn and may become pregnant at a young age. Incest is also a very real possibility in these families.

In contrast, the oldest son in the family is often rebellious, resulting in legal trouble that begins when he enters adolescence. According to Elkin, he almost always becomes involved in substance abuse. Younger sons, tend to get into trouble earlier in their childhood. They may also be likely to get in trouble with the law and may abuse drugs.

Nurses need to be aware of the pervasiveness of co-dependency and take this into account when performing a nursing assessment.

TABLE 19-3—cont'd

SUMMARY OF BEHAVIORS ASSOCIATED WITH SUBSTANCE ABUSE

Behaviors related to overdose	Withdrawal syndrome	Special considerations
Drowsiness, stupor, coma, grand mal seizures, death	None	Use may lead to psychotic behavior, irrationality, panic
Psychosis	None	Physiological consequences of use are under investigation
Drowsiness, confusion, hypotension, coma, death	Tremors, agitation, anxiety, grand mal seizures, abdominal cramps, vomiting, diaphoresis	Dependence may develop insidiously; users may underreport the actual amount taken because of guilt about multiple prescriptions and abuse

■ Coping mechanisms

The presence of substance abuse indicates that the person is experiencing serious difficulty coping. Healthier defense mechanisms and other adaptive behaviors are either inadequate or have not been developed. Therefore the person must resort to methods of coping that may provide temporary relief of anxiety. These methods eventually involve even more anxiety as the person becomes aware that he is harming himself. Drug and alcohol addicts tend to resist this awareness by employing ego defense mechanisms and other behaviors to delude the self. Seixas[24] describes three such defensive maneuvers characteristically used by alcoholics: denial that there is a problem, projection that the drinking behavior is the result of outside experiences beyond the individual's control, and dissociation of the drinking behavior from its effects. Drug abusers also use denial. However, in contrast to alcoholics and users of prescription drugs, who tend to isolate themselves from others, users of illicit drugs tend to band together into a drug culture. Although there may be little, if any, meaningful interaction while group members are high, there is the reinforcing effect of the group identity. This may be viewed as a justification for the behavior. A part of the group support is often an attitude of scorn and hostility toward "straight" people, which includes anyone who is not involved in drug abuse.

Nursing diagnosis

The nursing diagnosis of an individual who abuses substances must reflect the behavioral alteration, the substance used or abused, the degree to which it is used or abused, and the possible stressors involved. Jellinek[17] has proposed the following four phases of alcoholism that may assist the nurse in determining the degree to which alcohol is being used:

PHASE 1

Prealcoholic phase. This phase is characterized by social drinking, control over drinking behavior, and occasional alcohol use for stress reduction. At later stages of this phase there may be frequent drinking related to tension reduction.

PHASE 2

Early alcoholic phase. This phase begins with the first blackout. There is a slow increase in alcohol tolerance and progressive preoccupation with alcohol. The person may begin to drink alone, and his behavior may be embarrassing to others. Guilt feelings lead to excuses for drinking. There may be periods of total abstinence, which are used as evidence of the person's control over his drinking behavior.

PHASE 3

True alcoholic phase. Everything revolves around alcohol. The person is avoided by significant others and resents this. It is impossible for the individual to stop after one drink.

Nursing Diagnoses Related to Substance Abuse

Primary NANDA nursing diagnoses

Sensory/perceptual alterations (visual, auditory, tactile, kinesthetic, gustatory, olfactory)
Thought processes, altered

Examples of complete nursing diagnoses

Altered thought processes characteristic of true alcoholism related to pressures of a busy law practice and family demands, evidenced by confusion and blackouts
Altered thought processes characteristic of severe drug addiction to amphetamines related to desire to lose weight, evidenced by delusion that husband is having an affair with her mother
Sensory/perceptual alteration (visual) characteristic of complete alcohol dependence related to loss of job and rejection by family, evidenced by asking staff to "get rid of these bugs" while brushing at his clothing
Sensory/perceptual alteration (auditory) characteristic of experimentation with hallucinogens related to peer pressure, evidenced by covering ears and shouting, "Don't say those words to me," when alone in a room

PHASE 4

Complete alcohol dependence. Drinking begins in the morning and continues all day. Physical dependence is present. Severe liver damage may occur. There is usually some brain damage. If drinking continues, death will occur. The person cannot stop drinking without help.

Similar phases may be identified for abuse of drugs other than alcohol. They are as follows:

PHASE 1

Experimentation. The person takes a drug to see what it is like or to conform with peers. No further use develops from the initial experience.

PHASE 2

Early drug abuse. A specific drug or various drugs are used with some degree of regularity for the pleasurable effects or to reduce anxiety. Drugs may be used socially.

PHASE 3

True drug addiction. Drugs are used regularly, several times a day. Physical dependence begins if it is a characteristic of the drug. Psychological dependence is present. The life-style is drug focused. Social functioning deteriorates.

PHASE 4

Severe drug addiction. The person does whatever is necessary to obtain drugs. Criminal behavior occurs. There is total alienation from the non–drug-using culture. The physical condition deteriorates. Continued drug use will lead to death.

The nurse should be aware that individuals who have substance abuse problems also tend to develop multiple physical problems, particularly if the substance abuse problem is severe. The involvement with the abused agent becomes all consuming, leading to self-neglect. The complete plan of nursing care would include diagnosis of all the patient's nursing care needs. For the purposes of this discussion, the presentation of nursing diagnoses is limited to those more specifically related to substance abuse. The accompanying box presents primary NANDA nursing diagnoses and examples of complete nursing diagnoses. In Table 19-4, nursing and medical diagnoses related to substance abuse are listed.

■ Related medical diagnoses

Medical diagnoses relative to substance abuse disorders reflect the organic brain syndrome that is produced by the abused substance. Those with unique characteristics are listed and described separately. Syndromes with common characteristics are described in general, with the agents associated with the behavior listed. Table 19-3 also provides a reference to behaviors associated with these chemicals.

■ **ALCOHOL INTOXICATION.**[1] Essential features include recent ingestion of alcohol combined with maladaptive behaviors, such as interference with usual functioning. Physiological signs include slurred speech, incoordination, unsteady gait, nystagmus, and flushed face. Psychological signs include mood change, irritability, loquacity, and impaired attention. At least one physiological sign must be present.

■ **ALCOHOL WITHDRAWAL.** Essential features include recent cessation of prolonged heavy drinking

TABLE 19-4

MEDICAL AND NURSING DIAGNOSES RELATED TO SUBSTANCE ABUSE

Medical Diagnostic Class

Psychoactive substance-induced organic mental disorders

Related Medical Diagnoses (DSM-III-R*)

Alcohol intoxication
Uncomplicated alcohol withdrawal
Alcohol withdrawal delirium
Alcohol hallucinosis
Sedative, hypnotic, or anxiolytic intoxication
Sedative, hypnotic, or anxiolytic withdrawal
Opioid intoxication
Opioid withdrawal
Cocaine intoxication
Cocaine withdrawal
Amphetamine or similarly acting sympathomimetic intoxication
Amphetamine or similarly acting sympathomimetic withdrawal
Phencyclidine (PCP) or similarly acting arylcyclohexylamine intoxication
Hallucinogen hallucinosis

Medical Diagnostic Class

Psychoactive substance use disorders

Related Medical Diagnoses (DSM-III-R*)

Alcohol dependence
Alcohol abuse
Amphetamine or similarly acting sympathomimetic dependence
Amphetamine or similarly acting sympathomimetic abuse
Cocaine dependence
Cocaine abuse
Hallucinogen dependence
Opioid dependence
Opioid abuse
Phencyclidine (PCP) or similarly acting arylcyclohexylamine dependence
Phencyclidine (PCP) or similarly acting arylcyclohexylamine abuse
Sedative, hypnotic, or anxiolytic dependence
Sedative, hypnotic, or anxiolytic abuse
Polysubstance dependence

Nursing Diagnostic Class

Substance abuse

Related Nursing Diagnoses (NANDA)

Adjustment, impaired
Anxiety
Coping, ineffective individual
Injury, potential for
Self-esteem disturbance
Sleep pattern disturbance
Social interaction, impaired
†Sensory/perceptual alterations
†Thought processes, altered
Violence, potential for: self-directed or directed at others

*American Psychiatric Association: Diagnostic and statistical manual of mental disorders, third edition revised, Washington DC, 1987, The Association.
†Indicates primary nursing diagnoses for substance abuse.

---

followed by coarse tremor and at least one of the following: nausea and vomiting, malaise or weakness, autonomic hyperactivity, anxiety, depressed mood or irritability, transient hallucinations or illusions, headache, and insomnia.

■ **ALCOHOL WITHDRAWAL DELIRIUM.**[1] Essential features include delirium occurring within 1 week of ending or reducing heavy drinking, combined with autonomic hyperactivity.

■ **ALCOHOL HALLUCINOSIS.**[1] Essential features include vivid auditory or visual hallucinations following ending or reducing heavy drinking (usually within 48 hours) in an individual with apparent alcohol de-

pendence. There is no clouding of consciousness, as in delirium.

■ **SEDATIVE HYPNOTIC OR ANXIOLYTIC INTOXICATION.**[1] Essential features include recent use of a drug from this category with psychological signs that include mood lability, disinhibition of sexual and aggressive impulses, impaired judgment and impaired functioning. Neurological signs include (at least one) slurred speech, incoordination, unsteady gait, and impairment in attention or memory.

■ **SEDATIVE HYPNOTIC OR ANXIOLYTIC WITHDRAWAL.**[1] Essential features include cessation or reduction of prolonged moderate or heavy use of one of the drugs from this category. At least three of the following must occur: nausea and vomiting; malaise or weakness; autonomic hyperactivity; anxiety or irritability; orthostatic hypotension; and coarse tremor of hands, tongue, and eyelids.

■ **OPIOID INTOXICATION.**[1] Essential features include recent use of an opioid with pupillary constriction and at least one of the following neurological signs: drowsiness, slurred speech, and impairment in attention and memory. Psychological signs include: euphoria, dysphoria, apathy, and psychomotor retardation. There are also maladaptive behavioral effects.

■ **OPIOID WITHDRAWAL.**[1] Essential features include cessation or reduction of prolonged moderate or heavy use of an opioid drug. If a narcotic antagonist has been given, withdrawal may occur after briefer use. At least three of the following symptoms are present: craving for an opioid, muscle aches, lacrimation, rhinorrhea, pupillary dilation, piloerection, sweating, nausea, vomiting, diarrhea, yawning, fever, and insomnia.

■ **COCAINE INTOXICATION.**[1] Essential features include recent use of cocaine with the following psychological signs: psychomotor agitation, elation, grandiosity, fighting, impaired judgment and hypervigilance. Also, at least two from the following group of symptoms occur within 1 hour: tachycardia, pupillary dilation, elevated blood pressure, perspiration or chills, nausea and vomiting, and visual or tactile hallucinations. Maladaptive behaviors also occur.

■ **COCAINE WITHDRAWAL.**[1] Essential features include prolonged heavy use of cocaine followed by cessation or reduction. Signs include a depressed mood and at least one of the following persisting more than 24 hours after cessation: fatigue, disturbed sleep, and psychomotor agitation.

■ **AMPHETAMINE OR SIMILARLY ACTING SYMPATHOMIMETIC INTOXICATION.**[1] Essential features include recent use of a drug of this class and the following psychological symptoms: psychomotor agitation, fighting, grandiosity, impaired judgment, and hypervigilance. In addition, at least two of the following physical symptoms must occur within 1 hour: tachycardia, pupillary dilation, elevated blood pressure, perspiration or chills, and nausea or vomiting. Maladaptive behaviors also occur.

■ **AMPHETAMINE OR SIMILARLY ACTING SYMPATHOMIMETIC WITHDRAWAL.**[1] Essential features include cessation or reduction following prolonged heavy use of a drug of this class with depressed mood and at least one of the following persisting more than 24 hours after cessation: fatigue, disturbed sleep, and psychomotor agitation.

■ **PHENCYCLIDINE (PCP) OR SIMILARLY ACTING ARYLCYCLOHEXYLAMINE INTOXICATION.**[1] Essential features include recent use of a drug of this class followed within 1 hour by at least two of these physical symptoms: vertical or horizontal nystagmus, increased blood pressure and heart rate, numbness or diminished responsiveness to pain, ataxia, dysarthria, muscle rigidity, and seizures. In addition, the following psychological symptoms may occur: belligerence, assaultiveness, psychomotor agitation, impulsiveness, unpredictability, and impaired judgment. Maladaptive behaviors also occur.

■ **HALLUCINOGEN HALLUCINOSIS.**[1] Essential features include recent use of a drug of this class with perceptual changes occurring in a state of wakefulness and alertness. Psychological symptoms include marked anxiety or depression, ideas of reference, fear of losing one's mind, paranoid ideation, and impaired judgment. In addition, at least two of the following physical symptoms occur: pupillary dilation, tachycardia, sweating, palpitations, blurring of vision, tremors, and incoordination. Maladaptive behavioral effects also occur.

■ **PSYCHOACTIVE SUBSTANCE DEPENDENCE.** The essential features include at least three of the following: preoccupation with taking the substance; larger amounts of the substance taken over a longer period than intended; a great deal of time spent in activities to get the substance; tolerance to the substance; characteristic withdrawal symptoms; substance used to relieve withdrawal symptoms; desire or effort to control use of the substance; impaired social or occupational obligations; important social, occupational, or recreational activities abandoned; and continued use of the substance despite a significant social, occupational, or legal problem or a physical disorder exacerbated by use of the substance.

In summary, the model of health-illness phenomena may be applied to substance abuse, as illustrated in Fig. 19-3.

◆ Planning

■ Goal setting

The establishment of goals with a substance-abusing patient must recognize the realities of the person's life-style and habits. The ideal long-term goal is usually permanent total abstinence. However, the patient may be unable to face that level of commitment and is frequently very anxious at the thought of never again using the substance to which he is addicted. Recognition of this fact is reflected in the Alcoholics Anonymous (AA) approach to abstinence. AA members are advised

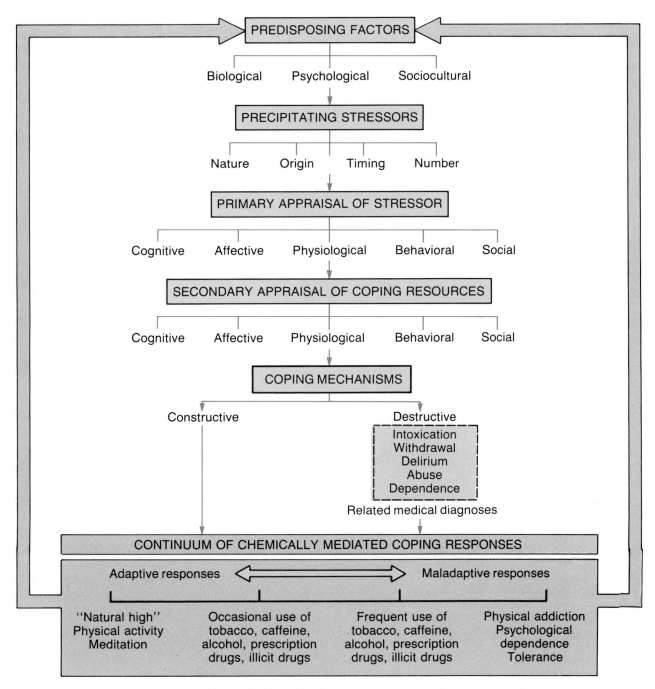

Fig. 19-3. Nursing model of health-illness phenomena related to substance abuse.

to take 1 day, or sometimes 1 hour or 1 minute, at a time. The alcoholic is then able to take satisfaction in achieving short-term goals for sobriety. The thought of never drinking again is sometimes enough to send an alcoholic out to find a drink.

The nurse must also be aware that it is rare for an addicted person suddenly to stop substance use for-

ever. Most addicts have to try at least once and usually several times to use the substance in a controlled way. Although research indicates that this may be possible for some alcoholics, it is generally not a realistic goal. It should also be noted that people who tend to become addicted to one substance, such as antianxiety drugs, also have a tendency for other types of addic-

618 UNIT II
Nursing Interventions

PSYCHIATRIC NURSING CARE PLAN FOR AN ALCOHOLIC PATIENT

Precautions:
    1:1 observation
    seizure precautions

Special nursing needs:
    Family may remain with
    patient 24 hours

Visitors: { } No restrictions
       {x} Family only
       { } Restricted to:

       { } No visitors

Telephone: { } Limited
           { } Unlimited

Privileges: {x} Restricted to unit
        { } Off unit accompanied by staff
        { } Off unit accompanied by family/visitor
        { } Off unit unaccompanied
        { } Out of hospital leave (dates) _____

Assessment data summary: Hospitalized twice in past for alcohol withdrawal; has been drinking heavily for 2 months; last drink 3 days PTA; has taken disulfiram in past; dropped out of AA; has hit wife who has considered divorce; involved in fatal auto accident; successful in business

Nursing diagnoses: 1. Sensory/perceptual alteration (visual) evidenced by stating, "Bugs are crawling on me" related to alcohol withdrawal. 2. Altered thought process evidenced by incoherence and disorientation related to alcohol withdrawal

Treatment goal: To maintain safety and an optimum level of physical comfort

Date	Problem/need	Expected outcome (objective)	Target Date	Nursing Intervention
5/5	Visual hallucinations	To describe reality based visual perceptions	5/6	Provide safe environment; provide reality orientation; encourage family to help with care
5/5	Physical safety	To remain free from injury	5/6	Restrain arms and legs as ordered; follow restraint protocol

Room	Patient's name	Age	Doctor	Primary nurse	Admit date
6	Mr. H	46	Dr. K	Ms. B	5/5/90

Fig. 19-4. Psychiatric nursing care plan for an alcoholic patient. (This nursing care plan includes examples of the elements of a total plan as it might appear at a particular time in the patient's course of treatment. It should not be considered all inclusive.)

Date	Medications	Date	P.R.N. Medications	Diagnostic & psychiatric tests	Req.	Done
5/5	Chlordiazepoxide	5/5	Chlordiazepoxide	Routine CBC	5/5	5/5
	25 mg po qid		100 mg IM q4h			
			prn for agitation			
5/5	Thiamine 100 mg					
	IM bid					

		Date	Treatments	Special orders and concerns		
		5/5	Wrist and ankle	Force fluids to 2000 ml qd		
		2 pm	• restraints for	Vital signs q2h		
			agitation			
			Renew in 8 hours			

Allergies:	Medical diagnosis: (axis I-III)	Diet:
None	Alcohol withdrawal syndrome	Regular

Fig. 19-4, cont'd. Psychiatric nursing care plan for an alcoholic patient.

tions. Substituting a new addiction for the old one will only add new problems.

In general, the long-term goals for an individual who abuses substances are to substitute healthy coping responses for substance-abusing behavior, to maintain safety and an optimum level of physical comfort, and to engage social support systems in the patient's behalf.

It is very important that goals for a substance-abusing patient be phrased so that it is clear that the patient is responsible for his behavior. Displacement of responsibility onto others is a frequent behavior of dependent people. Writing the goals into a contract to be signed by the patient and the nurse and providing the patient with a copy of the contract will also help reinforce the patient's responsibility for complying with the stated goals.

■ **Nursing care plan**

The nursing care plan for patients who are experiencing drug withdrawal must attend to any life-threatening behaviors that are present. The highest priority will be given to stabilization of the patient's physiolog-

ical status until the crisis of withdrawal is over. Emotional support will then be necessary as the person comes to terms with his behavior and begins to look to the future. The setting and constant modification of goals during this process convey to the patient the nurse's belief that there is hope for a more productive life in the future. Fig. 19-4 is a sample partial nursing care plan for Mr. H., the patient who was described in Clinical example 19-1.

Another important aspect of planning when working with patients who have substance abuse problems and their families is mental health education. The patients need to be taught about the physical and psychological consequences of their behavior. However, the most productive area for education related to this problem is prevention. A mental health education plan for prevention of substance abuse is presented in Table 19-5.

■ **Intervening in substance abuse**

Many theories have been described concerning the origin of substance abuse. There are also multiple theories about the effective treatment of this problem.

TABLE 19-5

MENTAL HEALTH EDUCATION PLAN FOR PREVENTION OF SUBSTANCE ABUSE

Content	Instructional activities	Evaluation
Elicit perceptions of substance use	Lead group discussion regarding knowledge about chemical use and experience with it; correct misperceptions	Learner will describe accurate information about substance use
Demonstrate negative effects of substance abuse	Show films of physical and psychological effects of substance abuse; provide written materials	Learner will identify and describe physical and psychological effects of substance abuse
Interaction with peer who has abused chemicals	Small group discussion with peer group member who has abused substances and quit because of negative experiences	Learner will compare and contrast advantages and disadvantages of using mind-altering substances
Obtain agreement to abstain from use of mind altering substances	Discuss future plans for refusing abused chemicals if offered	Learner will verbally agree to abstain from using mind-altering substances

The nurse will need to select the approach to intervention that seems most appropriate for each individual patient.

■ **BIOLOGICAL ASPECTS OF INTERVENTION.** Substance abusers frequently come into contact with the health care system because of a crisis in their physiological state. The crisis may be related to overdose, withdrawal, allergy, or toxicity. It may involve physical deterioration due to the deleterious effects of drugs, including such conditions as malnutrition, dehydration, and various infections, including HIV-1. When an acute physical condition is present, it takes priority over the other health needs of the patient. It is particularly important with substance abuse patients to attend to the condition that they have identified as the problem. The nurse is then perceived as potentially helpful and will have added credibility when other aspects of the addictive problem are addressed.

Withdrawal. If the person is physically dependent on a drug, withdrawal must be accomplished with medical supervision. This process is referred to as **detoxification.** Gradual weaning from the substance may be instituted, especially if the person is addicted to prescription drugs, such as barbiturates, amphetamines, or benzodiazepines. Another approach is the use of alternative drugs to block the occurrence of withdrawal symptoms. For instance, chlordiazepoxide may be given to assist with alcohol withdrawal. The dose of the substituted drug is then tapered down and eventually discontinued. The danger in this approach is that the alcoholic can become dependent on the substitute drug or may even have been taking it in addition to alcohol.

A variation on this approach is used when methadone is substituted for heroin. However, the treatment program may be aimed toward gradual withdrawal from methadone or toward indefinite maintenance at a stable dose. The decision between these two alternatives is based on assessment of the likelihood of recidivism (habitual relapsing) if the person becomes drug free. This treatment approach has been controversial because methadone is a narcotic. However, addiction to methadone does not cause impairment in functioning; thus the person can be productive while addicted. Proponents of methadone maintenance point out the benefits of avoiding the debilitating effects of heroin addiction.

Withdrawal symptoms may occur despite efforts to prevent them. Substance abusers do not always give accurate drug-use histories, although it is extremely important for the nurse to obtain as specific an assessment as possible. If the amount of substance used has been understated or if multiple abuse is undetected, withdrawal symptoms may emerge. The possibility of seizures should always be anticipated, and emergency equipment should be at hand. Drug abuse should always be considered as a possible condition when unexpected seizure activity occurs. If drug abuse is suspected, it is prudent to ensure the physician is apprised of the situation so that blood and urine specimens can be collected for laboratory analysis.

Overdose. Drug overdose is treated supportively,

depending on the characteristics of the drug taken. It is, of course, important to identify the drug. In cases of narcotic overdose, narcotic antagonists such as nalorphine may be given. After the person recovers from the acute illness, it is necessary to assess the circumstances of the overdose. It is particularly important to determine whether it was intentional or accidental. If the motivation is in doubt, it is best to assume that suicide was attempted until the nurse can obtain more information about the patient's mental state.

Toxic psychosis. Users of LSD and PCP often have an acute toxic psychosis. The behavior may be very similar to that of the schizophrenic patient. However, there may be no history of prior abnormal behavior. Careful assessment of an acute psychotic reaction, particularly in an adolescent or young adult, should include exploration of drug use. It may be necessary to interview friends of the patient to obtain this information. An attempt should be made to identify the specific drug used, although LSD and PCP may be taken without the knowledge of the person involved.

There is an important difference in the nursing approach to users of PCP as opposed to those who have an adverse reaction to LSD. Victims of PCP-induced psychosis do not respond well to attempts at interaction. They require a safe environment that has minimum stimuli. Agitated PCP users may strike out in response to their fear and panic and are potentially harmful to themselves and others.[28] LSD users experiencing a "bad trip" do respond to reassurance and may be "talked down." It seems to be most helpful if support is given by a friend or by someone who has experienced LSD. However, calm empathic reassurance and reorientation by the nurse will also help decrease the patient's panic.

Provision must also be made for the safety of these individuals because they may act impulsively out of fear and harm themselves. Adequate staff should be present to control impulsive behavior of both PCP and LSD users. Vital signs should be monitored and other physiological needs met. Excretion of PCP is aided by acidifying the urine by giving the patient cranberry juice or ascorbic acid. Gastric lavage may be necessary for persistent symptoms or if an overdose has been taken.[28]

Antabuse therapy. Another long-term biological approach to substance abuse is the prescription of disulfiram (Antabuse) for alcoholics. This drug sensitizes the person to alcohol so that an aversive physiological response occurs if the person uses alcohol in any form. The response consists of a severe headache, nausea and vomiting, flushing, hypotension, tachycardia, dyspnea, diaphoresis, chest pain, palpitations, dizziness, and

confusion. It can also lead to respiratory and cardiac collapse, unconsciousness, convulsions, and death. It is therefore important that the patient agree to take disulfiram only after careful instruction about the potential consequences of drinking while on the drug. This educational process should include a written list of alcohol-containing preparations to be avoided, including cough medicines, rubbing compounds, vinegars, aftershave lotions, and some mouthwashes. Drinking must be avoided for 14 days after disulfiram has been taken. This medication cannot prevent drinking by someone who is determined to drink. That person can simply wait until the disulfiram has been excreted. However, it helps to prevent impulsive drinking because the person does have to wait for a period of time to be able to drink safely. This treatment is used in conjunction with other supportive therapies.

Drugs in pregnancy. Since most of the drugs that are abused cross the placental barrier, women should be counseled about the possible effects of substance use during pregnancy. There have been incidents of congenital abnormalities in infants of mothers who have taken drugs. A fetal alcohol syndrome has been identified. In addition, use during pregnancy of drugs that cause physical dependency will result in the birth of an addicted baby who must then be withdrawn from the drug. The safest pregnancy is one in which the mother is totally drug free.

■ **INTERACTIVE INTERVENTIONS IN SUBSTANCE ABUSE.** Before initiating nursing intervention with a substance-abusing patient, the nurse must develop an awareness of his or her own feelings and attitudes toward the problem. It is recommended that a values clarification approach be used, as described in Chapter 4. Most people have had personal contact with substance abuse by family, friends, or colleagues. This problem evokes many negative feelings. It is important that the nurse be able to differentiate feelings associated with past situations from those aroused by professional contacts with patients and their families. A supervisor, teacher, or senior clinical nurse can be of assistance when a nurse is having difficulty sorting out feelings.

Group support. The multiplicity of stressors relative to substance abuse have been discussed. It is very important that nursing intervention be directed toward alleviating the stressors that apply to each individual patient and were identified in the nursing diagnosis. If the motivation for drug use has been peer pressure, the patient will need help in planning how to deal with the same type of pressures in the future. This may be a particularly difficult problem for adolescents who rely very much on peer group approval to maintain their self-esteem. A group support approach to treatment is helpful to these patients. They also have a tendency to deny the potential for future problems. Peers in a group setting can confront the individual with the realities of social pressure. Alcoholics also need to learn how to refuse a drink, even when urged to indulge. Role playing can be a helpful approach, especially in a group setting. Two patients can act out a social situation involving drinking and then receive feedback from the group about their behavior.

Patient education. Another nursing intervention that can be implemented effectively in a group setting is patient education. Substance abusers should be well informed about the drug they have used, its biological and psychosocial effects on the person, and community resources for future assistance. Films and other audiovisual materials reinforce important concepts. Handouts should be used for future reference.

Individual counseling. Individual counseling is frequently used with patients who are substance abusers. Liporati and Chychula[18] have described five guidelines for counseling the hospitalized drug abuser:

1. Define acceptable in-hospital behavior.
2. Make it clear that rules are set by the hospital, not the nurse.
3. Be honest about sharing information.
4. Document nursing interventions carefully.
5. Accept one's inability to cure the problem.

Niven[20] has also developed recommendations for intervention with adolescents who are substance abusers. He agrees that honesty is essential. The treatment team should be nonjudgmental and convey their concern for the patient's well-being. The diagnosis should be clearly stated and will probably need to be repeated periodically to confront the denial of the patient and the family. Treatment recommendations will also need repetition with supportive evidence of the substance-abusing behavior. Commonly encountered problems include denial, dependency, low self-esteem, manipulation, and anger. Concepts related to these behaviors are discussed elsewhere in this book. However, it is necessary to address the special application of these concepts to substance abuse.

Intervening in denial. Denial must be dealt with because it is a potential obstacle to recovery from chemical dependency. Most patients deny that they are unable to control their substance-abusing behavior even when drug-related problems have become serious. For instance, an intoxicated person who has caused an automobile accident may assert that he "just had a few beers." A barbiturate addict may claim that he can stop whenever he wants to do so. The denial is partially related to the stigma attached to drug abuse. It is difficult to apply the term "alcoholic" or "addict" to oneself. Denial also protects the person from admitting that he is unable to control his behavior. Self-control is a prized attribute that is central to the self-concept of most people. Admission of a problem is also the first step toward behavioral change. This commitment to change is very frightening to a substance-dependent person. It involves a decision to stop using a substance that has become the major focus of the person's life. Anyone who has tried to stop smoking cigarettes or diet can understand to some extent the anxiety aroused by this decision.

It is essential that denial be overcome and that the patient make the commitment to behavioral change. Repeated confrontation with evidence of substance dependence may be necessary to evoke this response. However, this must be done carefully so the patient is not antagonized. Repeated contacts with the health care system may be necessary before the patient admits to the nature of the problem.

Behavioral contracts. Many therapists use behavioral contracts when working with substance abusers. The nurse and the patient discuss and agree on realistic behavioral objectives for the patient. These are written down, and the document is signed by both the nurse and the patient. Most therapists who work with substance abuse patients insist on a provision in the contract that the patient be drug and alcohol free when attending a therapy session. This communicates the therapist's belief that the patient is able to control his behavior and take positive action in his own behalf.

Intervening in dependency. Dependency is generally a personality characteristic of people who become involved in substance-abusing behavior. This dependency may also be evident in the individual's interpersonal relationships. If the person is too dependent on others, it may drive them away, thus increasing the need to depend on alcohol or drugs. Clinical example 19-5 illustrates this problem.

Mr. B used alcohol to avoid responsibility for his actions and his life. He used his wife in a similar way. When she confronted him with her expectations, he responded in a childlike way and tried to place the nurse in the parental role. This avoidance of responsibility is one of the behaviors that is very difficult for the substance abuser to change. The nurse must be careful not to fall into the trap of co-dependent behavior by making decisions for the patient. In Clinical example 19-5, the nurse suggested that Mr. B communicate directly with his wife about how he planned to change his behavior.

Ms. B represents the co-dependency that occurs in

CLINICAL EXAMPLE 19-5

Mr. B was a 45-year-old man who was admitted to the medical unit of a general hospital with a diagnosis of gastritis. He complained of abdominal pain, nausea, and vomiting. He had a slightly elevated temperature of 37.5° C (100° F). When the admitting nurse who was completing the nursing assessment asked Mr. B about alcohol use, he said he had "a couple of beers" after work every day. He also reported that his wife had left him the day before admission. He said he was not sure why she left, but he was sure she would be back. Ms. B did come to the hospital to visit her husband. His primary nurse met with them together and asked Ms. B why she left. She said she was tired of putting Mr. B to bed every night after he passed out from drinking and did not want to continue to call his employer saying he was sick when he was really hung over. She had threatened to leave before, but Mr. B had always begged her to stay and she had relented. She had married him because she felt sorry for him. He had been living alone and was not taking good care of himself. She revealed that her first husband was also an alcoholic and her father had been one as well. She would agree to try again to make the marriage a success if he would agree to stop drinking and seek counseling. Mr. B said to the nurse, "I'll be good and do what she says. You tell her I'll be good."

CLINICAL EXAMPLE 19-6

Bobby was a 17-year-old who was admitted to the hospital acutely psychotic with a history of recent use of PCP. The emergency room nurse noted scarring of the veins in Bobby's arm and surmised that he was also a user of heroin. Blood and urine testing confirmed this suspicion. Bobby recovered from his psychotic episode in 24 hours but was then extremely uncomfortable due to opiate withdrawal. The decision was made to use titrated doses of methadone to assist with the withdrawal. Mr. L, a young nurse, established a close relationship with Bobby during this time. Bobby requested the nurse's help in planning for his future, but doubted that he had the strength to stay away from drugs. He was advised to take a day at a time. Mr. L took Bobby on a visit to a drug treatment program, and he agreed to try membership in one of the groups at this center. Bobby did well in the group and was very helpful to new members, describing his experiences and encouraging them to "take 1 day at a time." Bobby expressed an interest in finishing school and said he would like to become a drug counselor. The staff of the drug treatment program agreed that Bobby seemed to have an aptitude for that role and encouraged him to pursue his goal.

spouses of substance-abusing patients. She is a woman who appears to be drawn to dependent men. She is probably a very maternal person who likes to take care of others. This increases the possibility that she will assume the role of **enabler.** The enabler perpetuates the substance abuse problem by not confronting the substance abuser and by helping to cover up the problem. When Ms. B called Mr. B's employer to say he was sick, she was being an enabler. When significant others play an enabling role, family counseling is necessary to help the family accept and support the changing behavior of the patient. Ms. B had left her husband, but he was her second alcoholic spouse. Since she is apparently attracted to dependent men, any increase in assertiveness by Mr. B would have further disrupted their relationship.

Increasing self-esteem. Assertiveness training can be very helpful in assisting both the dependent substance abuser and significant others to accomplish a behavioral change. This therapeutic technique is de-

scribed in detail in Chapter 17. An increase in assertiveness may also have the added advantage of a positive effect on the person's self-esteem. Although some substance abusers present a facade of self-confidence, most basically have little regard for themselves. The relaxation, euphoria, or release of inhibitions imparted by the drug helps the person overcome this sense of inferiority. Another goal of nursing care must be to find ways of bolstering the person's self-esteem. This can be very difficult because many of these people have destroyed the relationships and activities that normally build self-esteem. They may have lost jobs, friends, and family. The nurse needs to help the person identify his remaining strengths and to build on them. Strengths may be related to overcoming the substance abuse problem itself. This is true in the case of Bobby in Clinical example 19-6.

Mr. L used his relationship with Bobby to convey his belief that the patient could succeed in giving up drugs. This message had a core of positive regard for

Bobby's potential strength. The staff of the drug treatment program added to this seed of self-esteem by encouraging Bobby to help others in the program and then to aim higher at becoming a counselor himself. This process taught Bobby that there were rewards in life other than those attached to drug use. Gradually, he learned to value the interpersonal rewards more than the drug rewards while making positive use of his past difficulties. Employment in drug programs has been a positive step for many ex-addicts who frequently become excellent counselors.

Intervening in manipulation. Manipulative behavior is another frequent characteristic of the substance abuser. This is often focused on obtaining access to drugs or alcohol. The hospitalized person may promise to give up the abused substance to be discharged, only to start using it again as soon as he returns home. Drug abusers sometimes manipulate the health care system by obtaining prescriptions from more than one physician or by forging prescriptions. This behavior must be confronted when it is discovered, and the patient should be helped to understand the self-defeating nature of this behavior. Although the behavior would appear to be directed toward others, the real victim is always the patient, who perpetuates his self-destructive behavior.

Intervening in anger. When substance abusers are confronted with their behavior and are pressed to assume responsibility for it, they may become angry. The root of the anger is related to the pain that is felt when the person realizes he must give up a behavior that has been central to his existence. In addition, the patient is raging over the emerging understanding of the problems he has caused for himself. Carruth and Pugh[5] have compared the loss of alcohol to the process of grieving. This comparison seems particularly applicable to the anger experienced by the addict who is mourning the loss of the abused substance and the loss of life experience during the period of addiction.

The nurse must realize that the anger felt by the patient may be directed toward him or her but generally is not related to his or her behavior. The patient should be assisted to express this anger in nondestructive ways. Exercise may be helpful. Expression through art or music may also provide an outlet for rage. A danger associated with this anger is that the patient may use it as an excuse to return to using drugs or alcohol. The substance abuser needs to learn that human support can also be of help in confronting painful feelings. It is important that the person be helped to label the feelings he is experiencing. Drug users become so accustomed to avoiding feelings chemically that they have difficulty even recognizing what it is that they are

feeling. Group counseling may also be helpful because individuals can see and identify feelings in others as well as themselves. Group support can help to decrease the sense of isolation that these patients often have.

Recidivism. Work with substance-abusing patients can be frustrating. Behavioral change is very difficult for them, so there is a high rate of recidivism. It may be very difficult for a nurse who has struggled to help someone overcome withdrawal symptoms and rebuild his life to see that person return to the health care agency readdicted. Rejection of the patient at this point is not helpful. These patients are very sensitive to rejection or criticism. They use such reactions to justify further substance abuse. They may make statements such as, "You're absolutely right. I'm not worth caring about. Nobody cares for me, so why should I care for myself?" The nurse may communicate to the patient disappointment that he did not continue to progress. However, the focus should be on beginning again, using the patient's prior success to foster an optimistic attitude toward the future.

While the nurse is establishing a helping relationship with the patient, he or she should be alert to signs of other psychosocial disruptions. Some people become substance abusers because of their efforts to deal with underlying emotional problems. Alcohol and other drugs may be used in this way. Unfortunately, most of the substances abused also have characteristics that tend to make problems worse, although there may be temporary relief. For instance, alcohol or barbiturates may be used to combat depression. There is an immediate sense of euphoria from these drugs. However, they are basically depressant substances and lead to later feelings of gloom. Amphetamines and cocaine bring about a "high," but there is also an inevitable "crash." People who use drugs to release inhibitions and relate more easily with others will find that they may develop more superficial relationships but drive away the few people to whom they have been able to feel close. The nurse needs to explore these motivations for substance abuse and help the patient find other ways to alleviate his psychological pain.

■ **SOCIAL SUPPORT SYSTEMS**

Family counseling. Reliable support from caring people is crucial to the recovery of substance abusers. Families are often frustrated with the patient's behavior. Family counseling by a qualified health care provider is likely to be necessary to assist the family in adjusting to the patient's changing behavior. Family members may need sources of support so they can be supportive to the dependent member.

Self-help groups. Formal family counseling is one approach to providing support to the social system.

Self-help groups are another way of helping the substance abuser and his significant others. AA is the prototype for self-help groups. AA is an organization that is composed entirely of recovering alcoholics. They believe that mutual support can give the alcoholic strength to abstain. AA aims for total abstinence. The member must admit to alcoholism openly and publicly by introducing himself at meetings, saying, "My name is John and I am an alcoholic." The other members promptly respond, "Hi John!" At each meeting, one or more members share their life histories with the group. This demonstrates that individual members are more alike than different, removing a resistance to involvement that is often cited by alcoholics. AA members also commit themselves to helping each other. As a member recovers, he is eventually assigned to be a sponsor for a new member. The sponsor role entails availability and accessibility to the other member whenever he feels the need to drink. This reciprocal relationship gives the new member caring support and the sponsor improved self-esteem. AA also involves a strong religious orientation that is experienced as supportive by some alcoholics.

Most cities have many AA groups. These groups often differ from each other in the characteristics of the members. There may be groups that are mostly blue collar workers, homemakers, or physicians. A nurse who is referring an alcoholic patient to a group should become familiar enough with the characteristics of that specific group to know whether the patient is likely to feel comfortable with the other members. AA meetings are frequently open. It is highly recommended that every nurse arrange to attend an AA meeting to help to understand the problem and to gain an appreciation for the work that is done by this organization.

Other support groups have developed as extensions of AA. Alanon is a self-help group that was established to meet the needs of spouses and significant others of alcoholics. The alcoholic need not be involved in AA for the significant other to join Alanon. In fact, this organization is often very helpful to spouses of alcoholics who are actively drinking. The members support each other and offer advice about moving forward with their own lives without becoming totally absorbed in the alcoholic's problem. Alateen performs a similar function for adolescents who are involved with alcoholic family members. The newest group is Co-dependents Anonymous, which exists to provide peer support to adult children of alcoholics and others who have co-dependent behavior. The message of these organizations is that the family member is not responsible for and cannot control the alcoholic's drinking. They can, however, still live meaningful lives. Bingham and Barger[2] have described the importance of a peer support group for latency-age children of alcoholics.

Transitional living programs. Many communities have transitional living programs, such as halfway houses, for alcoholics and drug abusers. These facilities serve as a transition between detoxification and complete return to the community. They usually have structured programs that include individual and group counseling, education about the addictive problem, AA meetings, and vocational rehabilitation. It is believed that this intensive program helps the patient readjust slowly to the community. These facilities are especially helpful for people who are alienated from their families.

Community treatment programs. A variety of community programs may be available for drug abusers. Drug treatment programs generally offer individual and group counseling, family counseling, vocational counseling, and drug and health education. Some also include methadone withdrawal or maintenance for opiate addicts. Methadone programs must have special licensure to operate and have specific federal guidelines to follow. Peer group relationships are an important aspect of most drug treatment programs. The clientele of these programs may differ, but many are directed toward "street people."

The nurse should know about the treatment programs that are available in the community in terms of the services offered and the characteristics of the population that is generally served. Referral of a registered nurse who has been stealing narcotics to an inner-city drug treatment program will not be effective. It is difficult to persuade a substance abuser to seek help at all. It is worthwhile to put forth the effort to find a treatment program that will meet the patient's needs as closely as possible.

Employee assistance programs. Another potential resource for the substance-abusing patient is the employee assistance program that may be part of an employee health service. Many businesses and industries have found that it is profitable for them to help substance-abusing employees. These programs generally offer counseling and health education. The employee is usually required to participate in the program to retain his job. Nurses are often key staff members in employee assistance programs. The health care system has been rather slow in developing these programs for health care providers. Since there is such a high prevalence of substance abuse among nurses and physicians, there is a great need for programs that can focus on their problems. Nurses can be advocates for the establishment of employee assistance programs in the agencies where they work.

Intervening with impaired colleagues Nurses usually find it difficult to respond to a colleague who is showing signs of a substance abuse problem. This is true of supervisors as well as peers. For the safety of the nurse and the patients under his or her care it is necessary to identify the problem and take action.

Confrontation is the recommended way to assist the impaired nurse to seek help. The nurse is presented

---

TABLE 19-6

SUMMARY OF NURSING INTERVENTIONS WITH THE SUBSTANCE-ABUSING PATIENT

Principle	Rationale	Nursing actions
Goal—To substitute healthy coping responses for substance-abusing behavior		
The nurse and patient should mutually define the problem and plan the nursing interventions	Motivation for change is related to recognition of a problem that is upsetting to the individual The patient must assume responsibility for his behavior Identification of predisposing and precipitating stressors must precede planning for more adaptive behavioral responses	Confront the patient with his substance-abusing behavior and its consequences Assist the patient to identify his substance abuse problem Encourage the patient to agree to participate in a treatment program Involve the patient in describing situations that lead to substance-abusing behavior Develop with the patient a written contract for behavioral change that is signed by the patient and nurse Assist the patient to identify and adopt healthier coping responses Consistently offer support and the expectation that the patient does have the strength to overcome his problem
Goal—To maintain safety and an optimum level of physical comfort		
Physical dependence must be managed in a safe environment with minimum withdrawal symptoms	Detoxification of the physically dependent person can be dangerous and is always uncomfortable The patient's physical safety must receive high priority for nursing intervention Withdrawal symptoms provide powerful motivation for continued substance abuse	Supportive physical care: vital signs, nutrition, hydration, seizure precautions Administer medication according to detoxification schedule Observe the patient carefully for withdrawal symptoms and report suspected withdrawal immediately
Goal—To engage social support systems in the patient's behalf		
Human support is to be substituted for dependence on chemicals Peer confrontation and support is often more acceptable than that of professionals	Substance abusers are often dependent and socially isolated people who use drugs to gain confidence in social situations Substance-abusing behavior alienates significant others, thus increasing the person's isolation It is difficult to manipulate people who have participated in the same behaviors Social support systems must be readily available over time and acceptable to the patient	Identify and assess social support systems that are available to the patient Provide support to significant others Educate the patient and significant others about the substance abuse problem and available resources Refer the patient to appropriate resources and provide support until the patient is involved in the program

with an objective description of his or her behavior by one or several colleagues. This is done in a caring way and options for help are offered. Sometimes it is effective to describe the impact of the behavior on patient care or team functioning. The nurse is likely to become defensive and angry. It is important for the confronters to maintain a calm attitude and continue to communicate their caring and concern. Families with substance abusing members are sometimes assisted to carry out a confrontation. In fact, this was the approach used by the Ford family when Betty Ford was convinced to enter addiction treatment. Although confrontation is difficult, the addicted person is usually grateful for the concern after he has been in treatment. It is essential for the friends, colleagues, or family members to continue to offer support as treatment continues. Nursing interventions with patients who abuse substances are summarized in Table 19-6.

■ **PREVENTION.** Prevention of substance abuse is an important public health problem. Nurses must be aware of the need for primary prevention and incorporate this into their professional practice. Resnick[23] suggests several components for drug abuse prevention programs. The first is to work toward improvement of the social conditions that affect families. Strengthening the family unit decreases the probability that a member will become involved in deviant behavior. The second component is to have an impact on the environment in which drug abuse takes place. There must be a focus on the schools, including their role in drug education. Legislative action may be needed. Another part of the prevention program is to strengthen the interpersonal and social skills of individuals. This leads to increased self-esteem and a positive self-concept, allowing the individual to resist peer pressure to use drugs. The fourth component is to create a strong network of interagency linkages. When different agencies work closely together, they can share resources and have a greater impact on the system. The final component is the sharing of resources between the federal and state governments.[23] This also helps to maximize the return on the investment of limited resources. Nurses can play an important part in developing and initiating policies that support the development of good substance abuse prevention programs.

 Evaluation

The evaluation of success in work with a substance abuse patient must be based on realistic expectations. Setting unreasonably high goals is discouraging to the nurse and the patient. For instance, it would be unrealistic to set a goal of total abstinence forever with a substance abuser. A more realistic goal is to lengthen periods of abstinence with the hope that the patient would eventually achieve control over his behavior.

Estes, Smith-DiJulio, and Heinemann[9] have identified evaluation criteria for the treatment of alcoholics. These criteria apply to abusers of other drugs as well:

1. Has the patient been able to progress significantly toward achieving the stated goals?
2. Can the patient usually communicate without being defensive?
3. Is the patient able to react appropriately, man-

DIRECTIONS FOR FUTURE RESEARCH

The following are some of the nursing research problems raised in Chapter 19 that merit further study by psychiatric nurses:

1. Effective strategies for sensitizing nurse administrators to the problems presented by and needs of addicted nurse employees
2. The characteristics of drug and alcohol abuse treatment programs that are effective in the treatment of addicted professionals
3. The application of knowledge about naturally induced euphoric states to the nursing care of people with addictions
4. The ability of nurses to identify the behaviors associated with withdrawal from commonly abused drugs
5. The long-term biopsychosocial effects of the therapeutic use of methadone
6. Identification and validation of nursing interventions that are effective during the acute and recovery phases of toxic psychosis resulting from hallucinogen or PCP use
7. Longitudinal study of physical and psychological development of children whose mothers used various types of drugs during pregnancy
8. Parenting behaviors of individuals who have been identified as drug abusers
9. The drug use habits of the children of individuals who have received medical treatment or been arrested as a result of drug abuse (including alcohol)
10. Nursing interventions that are effective in overcoming the denial that is generally observed as a resistance to therapy by substance abusers
11. Identification and validation of substance abuse primary prevention strategies targeted toward specific groups of potential abusers, that is, high-school students, homemakers, business people, and nurses

aging the demands of daily life without use of a drug?

4. Is the patient actively involved in a variety of activities, using external social and activity resources?

5. Does the patient use internal resources to be consistently productive at work and involved in meaningful interpersonal relationships?

The evaluation process should take place at regular intervals during the nurse-patient relationship.

■ **SUGGESTED CROSS-REFERENCES** ■

The model of health-illness phenomena is discussed in Chapter 3. The phases of the nursing process are discussed in Chapter 5. Therapeutic relationship skills are discussed in Chapter 4. Interventions in social support systems are discussed in Chapter 8. Alterations in self-concept are discussed in Chapter 13. Assertiveness training is discussed in Chapter 17. Group therapy is discussed in Chapter 28. Working with adolescents is discussed in Chapter 31.

■ **SUMMARY** ■

1. Substance abuse is defined as the use of any mind-altering agent to such an extent that it interferes with the individual's biological, psychological, or sociocultural integrity.

2. Cultural attitudes are important in determining the response to substance use or abuse.

3. Statistics are presented to demonstrate the prevalence and seriousness of the problem of substance abuse.

4. Categories of drugs that are frequently abused are described.

5. Substance abuse is a very serious problem among nurses and physicians.

6. Substance abuse is illustrated in terms of the health-illness continuum.

7. Biological, psychological, and sociocultural predisposing factors and precipitating stressors relative to substance abuse are described. There is no agreement on the existence of a specific stressor or set of stressors that is always present when substance abuse occurs.

8. The various categories of abused substances are compared, including the usual route of administration, expected behavioral manifestations, behaviors related to overdose, and withdrawal syndromes.

9. Nursing diagnosis of the substance-abusing patient is discussed relative to the stage of drug-using behavior, specific substance used, and relevant stressors. Relevant medical diagnoses are presented.

10. Goal setting must be realistic, taking into account the need for multiple short-term goals to enable the patient to experience success.

11. The biological aspects of nursing intervention include attending to physiological needs, detoxification, drug overdose, management of acute toxic psychosis, methadone treatment for opiate abusers, and disulfiram treatment for alcoholics.

12. Interactive interventions include peer group discussions, role play, patient education, and individual counseling.

13. Common themes in therapy with substance abuse patients include denial, dependency, low self-esteem, manipulation, and anger.

14. A mental health education plan for prevention of substance abuse is presented.

15. Social support systems for substance abusers include families, self-help groups, transitional living programs, drug treatment programs, and employee assistance programs.

16. Five components of drug abuse prevention programs are presented.

17. Evaluation of nursing care is described in terms of five questions to be asked about the patient's behaviors.

■ **REFERENCES** ■

1. American Psychiatric Association: Diagnostic and statistical manual of mental disorders, third edition revised, Washington DC, 1987, The Association.
2. Bingham A and Barger J: Children of alcoholic families: a group treatment approach for latency age children, J Psychosoc Nurs Ment Health Serv 23:13, 1985.
3. Butz RH: Intoxication and withdrawal. In Estes NJ and Heinemann ME, editors: Alcoholism: development, consequences, and interventions, ed 2, St Louis, 1982, Mosby–Year Book, Inc.
4. Cannon BL and Brown JS: Nurses' attitudes toward impaired colleagues, Image: J Nurs Scholarship 20:96, 1988.
5. Carruth GR and Pugh JB: Grieving the loss of alcohol: a crisis in recovery, J Psychosoc Nurs Ment Health Serv 20:18, 1982.
6. Caton CLM, et al: Young chronic patients and substance abuse, Hosp Comm Psychiatry 40:1037, 1989.
7. Elkin M: Families under the influence: changing alcoholic patterns, New York, 1984, WW Norton & Company.
8. Estes NJ and Heinemann ME, editors: Alcoholism, development, consequences, and interventions, ed 2, St Louis, 1982, Mosby–Year Book, Inc.
9. Estes NJ, Smith-DiJulio K, and Heinemann ME: Nursing diagnosis of the alcoholic person, St Louis, 1980, Mosby–Year Book, Inc.
10. Gallant DM: Alcoholism: a guide to diagnosis, intervention and treatment, New York, 1987, WW Norton & Company.
11. Gold SR: The CAP control theory of drug abuse. In Lettieri DJ, Sayers M, and Pearson HW, editors: Theories on drug abuse: selected contemporary perspectives, NIDA Research Monograph 30, Rockville, Md, 1980, National Institute on Drug Abuse.
12. Goodwin DW: The bad-habit theory of drug abuse. In

Lettieri DJ, Sayers M, and Pearson HW, editors: Theories on drug abuse: selected contemporary perspectives, NIDA Research Monograph 30, Rockville, Md, 1980, National Institute on Drug Abuse.

13. Goodwin DW: Alcoholism. In: Kaplan HI and Sadock BJ, editors: Comprehensive textbook of psychiatry, ed 5, Baltimore, 1989, Williams & Wilkins.

14. Hetherington SE: Children of alcoholics: an emerging mental health issue, Arch Psych Nurs 2:251, 1988.

15. House MA: Cocaine, Am J Nurs 90:41, 1990.

16. Jaffe JH: Drug dependence: opioids, nonnarcotics, nicotine (tobacco), and caffeine. In Kaplan HI and Sadock BJ, editors: Comprehensive textbook of psychiatry, ed 5, Baltimore, 1989, Williams & Wilkins.

17. Jellinek EM: Phases of alcohol addiction, QJ Stud Alcohol 13:672, 1952.

18. Liporati NC and Chychula LH: How you can really help the drug-abusing patient, Nursing '82 12:46, 1982.

19. Mittleman HS, Mittleman RE, and Elser B: Cocaine, Am J Nurs 84:1092, 1984.

20. Niven RG: Adolescent drug abuse, Hosp Community Psychiatry 37:596, 1986.

21. O'Connor P and Robinson RS: Managing impaired nurses, Nurs Admin Quarterly 9:1, 1985.

22. Ray OS and Ksir C: Drugs, society, and human behavior, ed 5, St Louis, 1990, Mosby–Year Book, Inc.

23. Resnick HS: It starts with people: experience in drug abuse prevention, Rockville, Md, 1978, Department of Health, Education and Welfare.

24. Seixas FA: The course of alcoholism. In Estes NJ and Heinemann ME, editors: Alcoholism: development, consequences, and interventions, ed 2, St Louis, 1982, Mosby–Year Book, Inc.

25. Snyder SH: Opiate receptors and internal opiates, Sci Am 236(3):44, 1977.

26. Stanton MD: A family theory of drug abuse. In Lettieri DJ, Sayers M, and Pearson HW, editors: Theories on drug abuse: selected contemporary perspectives, NIDA Research Monograph 30, Rockville, Md, 1980, National Institute on Drug Abuse.

27. Sullivan EJ: A descriptive study of nurses recovering from chemical dependency, Arch Psych Nurs 1:194, 1987.

28. Vourakis C and Bennett G: Angel dust: not heaven sent, Am J Nurs 79:649, 1979.

■ ANNOTATED SUGGESTED READINGS ■

*Anonymous: Interview: life with an alcoholic husband, J Psychosoc Nurs Ment Health Serv 23:30, Mar 1985.

Two women describe their experiences living with and leaving alcoholic husbands. Includes observations about their experiences in psychotherapy. Helpful to nurses working with families of alcoholics.

*Acee AM and Smith D: Crack, Am J Nurs 87:614, 1987.

Provides a good overview of facts about crack cocaine. Includes psychological and physical effects and related nursing care.

*Arneson SW, Schultz M, and Triplett JL: Nurses' knowledge of the impact of parental alcoholism on children, Arch Psych Nurs 1:251, 1987.

Report of a study which revealed that nurses learn little about the effects of parental alcoholism on children, especially the long-term effects.

*Betemps E: Management of the withdrawal syndrome of barbiturates and other central nervous system depressants, J Psychiatr Nurs 17:31 Sept 1981.

Provides information on recognition and nursing management of withdrawal from CNS depressant drugs, including a system for judging the seriousness of impending withdrawal. Discusses detoxification process in detail.

Co-dependency. Deerfield Beach, Fl, 1988, Health Communications, Inc.

Short readings that present various viewpoints on co-dependency. Provides a good overview of the many aspects of this emerging problem.

*DiCicco-Bloom B, Space S, and Zahourek RP: The homebound alcoholic, Am J Nurs 86:167, 1986.

Description of approaches to the nursing care of elderly alcoholics who are served by a home care program. The emphasis is on a positive attitude and the avoidance of enabling behavior.

*Estes NJ and Heinemann ME, editors: Alcoholism: development, consequences, and interventions, ed 2, St Louis, 1982, Mosby–Year Book, Inc.

Provides a comprehensive survey of current literature on alcoholism with broad spectrum of topics. Interesting, useful resource.

*Haack MR: Alcohol use and burnout among student nurses, Nurs Health Care 8:239, 1987.

Reports an investigation of the occurrence of burnout and the amount of alcohol use by nursing students. Identification of these signs of problems in coping with stress is important so students can receive assistance.

Hayes EN, editor: Adult children of alcoholics remember, New York, 1989, Harmony Books.

Collection of personal accounts of growing up in an alcoholic family provides an opportunity to understand the impact of parental alcoholism on the child. Nurses may also want to recommend this book to adult children of alcoholics so they can learn that others have had similar experiences and recovered.

*Jaffe S: First-hand views of recovery, Am J Nurs 82:578, 1982.

Describes experience in treating a group of alcoholic nurses. Addresses issues that concern substance-abusing nurses in particular. Recommended as a means of sensitizing nurses to the needs of their addicted colleagues.

*Jefferson LV and Ensor BE: Confronting a chemically impaired colleague, Am J Nurs 82:574, 1982.

Applies concepts related to substance abuse to the addicted nurse. Case studies illustrate the characteristics of drug- and alcohol-abusing nurses. Describes clues that should lead one to

---

*Asterisk indicates nursing reference.

suspect substance abuse. *Intervention section includes advice on confronting a nurse colleague who may be alcoholic or abusing drugs. Highly recommended for all nurses.*

*Liporati NC and Chychula LH: How you can really help the drug-abusing patient, Nursing '82 12:46, June 1982.

Presents practical suggestions for interacting with substance-abusing patients. Directed toward nurses who work in general hospitals, but pertinent to all settings. Provides examples on how to approach a patient suspected of drug abuse.

*McCoy S, Rice MJ, and McFadden K: PCP intoxication: psychiatric issues of nursing care, J Psychosoc Nurs Ment Health Serv 19:17, July 1981.

Presents patient behaviors and related nursing interventions clearly and in depth. Worthwhile reference in any setting providing health care services to adolescents and young adults.

*Morgan AJ and Moreno JW: Attitudes toward addiction, Am J Nurs 73:497, 1973.

Particularly helpful to the inexperienced nurse who needs help in analyzing his or her own feelings about working with addicted patients. Presents many realities of drug addiction that may be difficult to handle emotionally.

Niven RG: Adolescent drug abuse, Hosp Community Psychiatry 37:596, 1986.

Provides a comprehensive analysis of the assessment and care of drug-abusing adolescents. Practical suggestions, with a realistic but hopeful approach. Appendix includes information about self-help groups and sources of educational materials.

*Pisarcik G: Management of phencyclidine toxicity, J Emerg Nurs 4:35, Sept-Oct 1978.

Recommended for nurses who are likely to have contact with patients experiencing toxic reactions to PCP. Includes clear description of characteristic behaviors. Includes practical discussion of nursing intervention.

Ray OS and Ksir C: Drugs, society, and human behavior, ed 5, St Louis, 1990, Mosby–Year Book, Inc.

Highly recommended as a basic resource on all aspects of chemical dependency. Discusses both relevant psychosocial factors and pharmacological aspects.

Szasz T: Ceremonial chemistry, New York, 1974, Doubleday & Co, Inc.

Explores drug use from a cultural point of view, presenting theory that drug "abuse" is culturally defined and serves the purpose of providing society with a group of scapegoats. Views drug use as a type of religious observance in terms of its significance to the user. Thought-provoking work that forces one to reassess attitudes about drug use and abuse.

*Vourakis C and Bennett G: Angel dust: not heaven sent, Am J Nurs 79:649, 1979.

Presents a thorough overview of the manifestations of PCP use and related nursing care. Organizes the presentation of theory around primary, secondary, and tertiary prevention models. Also discusses the drug's pharmacological characteristics.

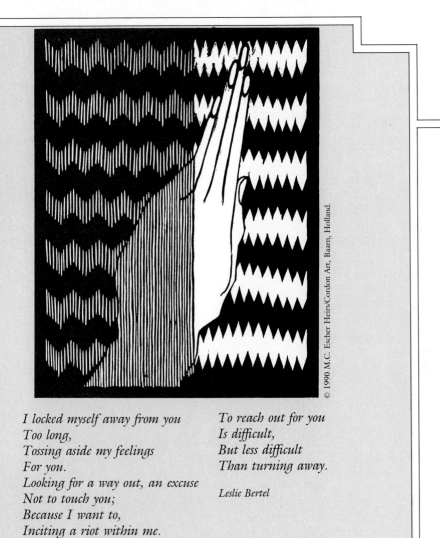

I locked myself away from you
Too long,
Tossing aside my feelings
For you.
Looking for a way out, an excuse
Not to touch you;
Because I want to,
Inciting a riot within me.

To reach out for you
Is difficult,
But less difficult
Than turning away.

Leslie Bertel

C H A P T E R   20

VARIATIONS IN SEXUAL RESPONSE

SUSAN G. POORMAN

DIAGNOSTIC PREVIEW

MEDICAL DIAGNOSIS RELATED TO
VARIATIONS IN SEXUAL RESPONSE

- Gender identity disorder of childhood, adolescences, or adulthood

- Transsexualism

- Exhibitionism

- Fetishism

- Frotteurism

- Pedophilia

- Sexual masochism

- Sexual sadism

- Transvestic fetishism

- Voyeurism

- Hypoactive sexual desire disorder

- Sexual aversion disorder

- Female/male sexual arousal disorder

- Inhibited female/male orgasm

- Premature ejaculation

- Dyspareunia

- Vaginismus

LEARNING OBJECTIVES

After studying this chapter, the student should be able to:

- discuss why nurses need knowledge of human sexuality, the type of knowledge needed, and problems encountered in obtaining it.

- describe the dimensions of sexual behavior and the continuum of adaptive and maladaptive sexual responses.

- identify two major responsibilities of the nurse in assessing variations in sexual response.

- analyze the four phases of the nurse's growth in developing self-awareness of human sexuality.

- analyze the predisposing factors and precipitating stressors associated with variations in sexual response.

- identify and describe patient behaviors and coping mechanisms associated with variations in sexual response.

- formulate nursing diagnoses for patients with variations in sexual response.

- assess the relationship between nursing diag-

noses and medical diagnoses associated with variations in sexual response.

- develop long- and short-term nursing goals with patients experiencing variations in sexual response.

- apply nurse-patient relationship principles in planning the care of a patient with a variation in sexual response.

- describe nursing interventions for the patient with a variation in sexual response.

- critique some commonly held myths regarding human sexuality.

- develop a mental health education plan to promote a patient's adaptive sexual responses.

- assess the importance of evaluating the nursing process when working with patients who have variations in sexual response.

- identify directions for future nursing research.

- select appropriate readings for further study.

As nursing moves toward a holistic approach to patient care, nurses are often called on to intervene in situations regarding patients' sexuality. As a profession, nursing has historically fallen short of its responsibility to counsel individuals in this area. Nurses have a variety of reactions to patients' concerns about sexuality. For example, some nurses claim that "nurses are not sex therapists and therefore do not understand sexual issues." Other nurses ignore or deny sexual issues that patients raise and "pass the buck" to physicians, social workers, or other health professionals. Nurses tell patients to ask their physician about sexuality questions, but physicians may not necessarily be more open or prepared. Nurses may feel embarrassed when a man talks about his fear of impotence during chemotherapy. They may be repelled or shocked by patients who "come out" and disclose their gay identity. Some nurses may hesitate to talk with a woman after her mastectomy who worries that her husband will no longer find her appealing.

Sexuality cannot be separated from being human; therefore it is imperative that nurses develop skill and confidence in addressing sexual issues if holistic care is to be provided. Education regarding sexuality provides professional nurses with theoretical knowledge.

Most nursing textbooks address sexuality as a medical model. The content primarily includes anatomy and physiology of reproductive organs and graphs of hormonal levels. Anatomical and physiological information is vital in understanding human sexuality; however, such information is available and best described in anatomy and physiology texts. This chapter departs from tradition by integrating concepts of sexual counseling in a nursing process model.

Continuum of sexual responses

Not all nurses will become experts in sexuality; however, if they are aware of basic principles, they will better understand sexual needs and problems. Nurses come in contact with sexual issues daily, regardless of their field of practice. If nurses are comfortable with sexual issues, they convey this to the patient, who can then discuss such issues. The nurse-patient relationship is intimate in many ways. Patients are often experiencing pain and change. Thus it is appropriate that the nurse-patient relationship allow for honest discussion of sexuality. In answering the question "What do nurses need to know about sexuality?" several factors must be considered.

First, nurses need to know themselves, to be aware of their own feelings and values regarding sexuality. If nurses are not aware of their feelings, they cannot help patients meet their needs. For example, nurses may become distressed when they find patients masturbating. Many people think something is innately wrong with masturbating, although they know intellectually it is a normal expression of sexual behavior. Thus a nurse who is distressed by masturbation may have difficulty talking with the patient about sexual needs.

Second, nurses need to understand that everyone's feelings and values regarding sexuality are not going to match their own. Anytime sex or an issue that hints at sex comes up, nurses frequently feel threatened and tend to lose objectivity. This may occur because of differing values between the nurse, patient, or norms of society. For example, the nurse who is staunchly opposed to abortion may have difficulty caring for a patient who has just aborted a pregnancy. Nurses may ignore patients with different beliefs and values or may become passively or even actively hostile. Nurses have been known to dehumanize patients or detach themselves from their care, then feel guilty for doing so. A vicious cycle results in which the nurse and patient both lose.

When nurses have different beliefs and values from their patients, a common response is to misunderstand, feel scared and confused, and judge others as wrong. Although textbooks tell nurses to be nonjudgmental, the ideal attitude is much easier to instruct than implement. To provide sensitive care, nurses must confront their feelings and beliefs about sexuality.

Although all nurses will not become sex therapists, all can become educated about sexual health and use sound counseling methods with patients. Specifically, nurses can:

1. Learn interviewing skills for sexual assessment and history taking.
2. Develop confidence in their ability to approach or allow patients to approach sexual issues.
3. Counsel or refer patients for counseling.

■ Dimensions of sexual behavior

Sexuality in a broad sense refers to all aspects of being sexual and is a dimension of the personality. Far more encompassing than the act of intercourse, sexuality is an integral part of every human being. It is evident in the way one looks, believes, behaves, and relates to others. Accepting a broad concept of sexuality allows the nurse to explore ways in which people are sexual beings and understand more fully his or her own feelings, beliefs, and actions.

It is difficult, if not impossible, to define "normal" sexual behavior without making value judgments. Masters, Johnson, and Kolodny caution us in defining sexuality as "normal" and "abnormal." "Normal is frequently defined as what we ourselves do and feel comfortable about, while abnormal is what others do that

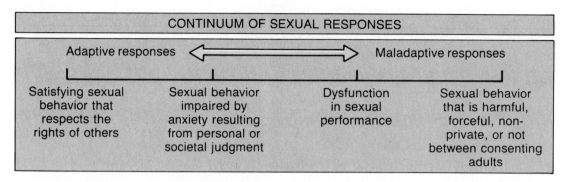

Fig. 20-1. Continuum of sexual responses.

seem different or odd to us."[18:9] One's parents, relatives, friends, and society are all likely to have different views on normal sexuality. Goldstein[8] defines normal sexual behavior as any sexual act between adults that is consensual, lacks force, and is performed in private, away from unwilling observers. If one accepts Goldstein's definition, then homosexuality, obtaining sexual pleasure from a member of the same sex, would be considered normal. Conversely, pedophilia, obtaining sexual pleasure by molesting a child, would not meet Goldstein's requirements.

Experts in sexuality do not agree on what is normal. For years many people believed that any deviation from sexual relations between married partners for procreation was problematic or abnormal. Today people view sexual behavior with a wider range of attitudes. Sexuality, on a continuum, ranges from adaptive to maladaptive (Fig. 20-1). The most adaptive responses meet the following criteria: between two consenting adults, mutually satisfying to both, not psychologically or physically harmful to either party, lacking in force or coercion, and conducted in private.

In some instances, however, sexual behavior can meet the criteria for adaptive responses but include variables that interfere with the relationship. Sexual responses that may otherwise be adaptive might be altered by what society dictates as acceptable and unacceptable. Unfortunately, society often makes these decisions based on fear, prejudices, and lack of information, rather than on data and facts. For example, the homosexual person may have the potential for healthy responses but be impaired by anxiety about societal disapproval.

Maladaptive sexual responses include behaviors that do not meet one or more of the criteria for adaptive responses. The degree to which these behaviors are maladaptive will vary. Some sexual behaviors may not meet any of the criteria mentioned. For example, incest may include force and is often psychologically harmful if a child is involved. However, other sexual responses may meet four out of five of the criteria for adaptive responses but still have a maladaptive ele-

ment. For example, a couple experiencing a sexual dysfunction (e.g., premature ejaculation) may meet Goldstein's criteria for normal behavior, but their sexual behavior may be unsatisfactory or even psychologically harmful to one or both members.

Caution must be used when attempting to label sexual behaviors as adaptive or maladaptive. There will never be total agreement and there will always be exceptions to the rule. The continuum shown in Fig. 20-1 is intended to be free of moral judgment and was developed to aid the nurse in understanding the range of sexual responses.

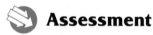 Assessment

Some people who experience stress in their sexuality may be reluctant to accept their need for help. Others seek help indirectly in that a diffuse symptom often masks an underlying sexual problem. The nurse is often the health professional who first comes in contact with these patients. The nursing process will help him other work with patients as they develop a collaborative relationship and assess problems, assign priorities, and mutually arrive at a plan of intervention.

Assessment, the first phase of the nursing process, includes two clearly defined responsibilities: (1) the development of self-awareness in relation to sexuality and (2) the assessment of the patient. The most critical element in counseling patients about sexuality is for the nurse to be aware of his or her own feelings and values. The nurse's level of self-awareness has a direct impact on the ability to intervene with patients. In developing self-awareness, nurses may progress through four phases of predictable growth experience: cognitive dissonance, anxiety, anger, and action. In assessing a patient, the nurse looks at the individual's situation and presenting problem.

■ Self-awareness of the nurse

The first step in developing self-awareness is for the nurse to clarify values about his or her own sexuality. Foley and Davies[6] identified growth experiences developed around the nursing care of rape victims. Their model is applicable in sexual counseling as well and has been adapted accordingly.

■ **COGNITIVE DISSONANCE.** The first phase of growth in developing sexual self-awareness is cognitive dissonance. Cognitive dissonance arises when two opposing beliefs exist simultaneously. For example, nurses grow up learning what society, family, and friends believe about sexual issues. If a nurse is raised in an environment that teaches her nice girls do not talk about sex, she will carry that belief into nursing practice. When a patient wants to discuss a sexual concern with her, she may experience two opposing reactions simultaneously:

1. As a professional, I should be able to discuss any problem, including sexual problems, with my patient.
2. Nice girls do not discuss sex.

Experiencing both these thoughts at the same time makes the nurse uncomfortable. This discomfort eventually forces her to examine her feelings about discussing patients' sexual problems. The nurse will resolve the cognitive dissonance by (1) denying professional responsibilities and clinging to personal beliefs or (2) examining the fact that sexuality is an integral part of the human condition.

If the nurse continues to believe that nice girls do not talk about sex, she may make excuses for unprofessional behavior by projecting blame onto the patient or rationalizing that she is "just a nurse, and can't know everything." Rationalization encourages avoidance or denial of a patient's sexual concerns. Rationalization and blaming the patient also allow the nurse to ignore her discomfort in viewing herself as a sexual human being. However, ignoring or denying one's discomfort does not allow one to understand feelings and values about sexuality.

Nurses need to examine what they believe about sexual issues and why. Environment and family background influence beliefs. In regard to sexual issues, the nurse must ask, "Do I believe this because I am knowledgeable and have researched the facts, or do I believe this because my parents or peers believe it?" Only when the nurse can say that she examined the available information and made an informed choice on values will she have truly clarified her values.

■ **ANXIETY.** If one's cognitive dissonance leads to an examination of values, a second phase of growth occurs. In the second phase, anxiety, fear and shock are experienced. Anxiety is a state of "apprehension cued off by a threat to some value which the individual holds essential to his existence as a personality."[19] It can be characterized by feelings of surprise, terror, horror or disgust.

In the second phase the nurse realizes that uncertainty, insecurity, questions, and problems regarding sexuality are experienced by everyone. Often she experiences anxiety because she realizes everyone is capable of a variety of sexual feelings and behaviors. Anyone can experience a sexual dysfunction or question one's sexual identity. The nurse experiencing anxiety may exhibit behaviors that are ineffective in discussing sexual issues, such as talking too much (not allowing patients to verbalize their feelings), failing to listen (failing to pick up on patient cues or messages), and diagnosing and analyzing (becoming preoccupied with facts rather than feelings).

■ **ANGER.** Because anxiety is uncomfortable, the nurse strives to eliminate it. Learning about sexuality and facing the ignorance of society or one's colleagues brings the nurse to a third phase of growth. Anger characterizes phase three and generally arises after anxiety and shock subside. Anger is directed at oneself, one's patients, and society. The nurse begins to recognize that issues associated with sex or sexuality are highly volatile and emotional. Rape, abortion, birth control, the equal rights amendment, child abuse, pornography, and religious issues all have an obvious or subtle connection with sexuality and give rise to vehement debates. Similarly, attempts to formulate legislation on sexual matters is often ineffective because these issues are emotion laden. The realization of society's emotionality and irrationality in relation to sex often breeds anger and contempt in the nurse. For example, the nurse may become angry at the ignorance, bigotry, or unprofessional attitude of a colleague or friend who judges homosexuals as deviants.

During this phase of anger, nurses may lecture others about the need for sex education. A nurse may develop a hostile attitude toward a patient or coworker not educated about sexuality. For instance, he or she may critically judge a patient who becomes pregnant because of ignorance about simple birth control. Furthermore, nurses are often angry with society for perpetuating ignorance about sexuality. They may not understand when others do not share their enthusiasm for changing society's beliefs.

■ **ACTION.** The final step in the growth experience is the action phase, in which the nurse experiences a decrease in anger. She begins to understand that blaming herself or society for ignorance and prejudice does not help patients with sexual concerns. During the action phase nurses often wonder, "Why didn't anyone ever teach me what I really needed to know about sexuality?" "Why aren't people educated properly?" "Where should sex education start?" and "How can I gain more knowledge for myself and others?"

Several behaviors characterize the final phase of the growth experience: data inquiry, choosing values,

CLINICAL EXAMPLE 20-1

Ms. G worked as a staff nurse at an outpatient psychiatric clinic. One day at an interdisciplinary team meeting, Ms. G presented a new case to the treatment team for review. Her case was a 29-year-old female patient who came to the clinic because she thought she was transsexual. Ms. G began to explain the patient's history to the treatment team when one of the team members interrupted, stating "If this isn't the sickest thing I've ever heard of. . . . I hope you don't expect us to treat this woman, or should I say man!" The other members of the treatment team began to snicker and continued to make jokes about the transsexual patient.

After the team meeting, Ms. G felt very confused. She usually respected her co-workers' clinical judgment and considered them to be good clinicians. However, her new patient was obviously experiencing problems with her sexuality and was serious about wanting treatment for sexual reassignment. Ms. G was also anxious because of her lack of facts and knowledge about transsexuality. She decided to do some research that evening at the library.

The next day at the office, one of the other nurse clinicians teased Ms. G about the new "half and half" patient. Another co-worker cautioned Ms. G not to see this patient in the back treatment room alone because "you never know about those perverts, they might grab you." Ms. G became irritable with her co-workers and called them ignorant bigots. Despite the problems with her co-workers, she continued to research the nature of transsexualism to help her patient. Finally, she found a psychologist in the city who worked with transsexual patients and made an appointment to talk about transsexuality.

Ms. G explained her co-workers reaction to the psychologist and her own difficulties in understanding transsexuality and in finding an appropriate referral for the patient. "This isn't the first time this has happened at our clinic," Ms. G told the psychologist. "Anytime we get a patient with sexual problems, everybody makes jokes and nothing is ever really done for them."

After the consultation appointment, the psychologist offered to do an in-service program on sexuality for the staff. Ms. G returned to the clinic, fearful that the staff would refuse the in-service program and laugh at her for suggesting the program.

The next day Ms. G told the staff at the team meeting of the psychologist's offer to talk with them about providing care to patients expressing sexual preferences that differ from their own. One of the team members responded by laughing, "We don't need anyone to teach us about sex—I think we know everything we need to know." Everyone laughed and agreed. Ms. G, although anxious, spoke up stating, "If we all know so much, why all this nervous laughter? Look, I know it's hard to talk about sex and sexual issues, but we have to admit that we don't do a very good job addressing some of the sexual issues or problems that patients present us with here. And many patients do. We just can't go on laughing and making judgments about people. Let's face it, that doesn't help anyone."

After Ms. G spoke up there was a long silence in the room until another nurse spoke up. "You know, I think Ms. G is right. There are lots of times I just don't know what to say or do for people who come in here with sexual concerns. What could it hurt to have an in-service?" After some discussion, the staff agreed to let Ms. G call the psychologist and set up the in-service program.

and prizing values. Data inquiry is demonstrated when the nurse obtains information about sexual issues. After choosing a value position, the final behavior is one of prizing the valued position. Prizing consists of an awareness and cherishing of one's feelings and values and being willing to share them publicly. Although prizing values is considered the final step in a positive growth experience, prizing does not mean that what one values now will not change. Values are never static; they evolve and shift as a person changes, grows, and acquires new experiences. Thus a person who once ascribed to pro-life values may later become understanding and empathetic toward women who

seek an abortion. Clinical example 20-1 illustrates a nurse who prizes values enough to share them publicly.

Clinical example 20-1 illustrates the phases of growth health professionals experience while increasing their awareness about sexuality. These phases are represented in Fig. 20-2. Ms. G experienced cognitive dissonance when the staff called the transsexual patient sick, and she was faced with conflicting feelings. She agreed with the staff because she respected them as expert clinicians, but she also believed the patient was not sick, weird, or perverted and had a very real problem. Ms. G experienced anxiety when she realized that she did not know anything about transsexuality. Her anxiety also stemmed from facing the reality that people express their sexuality in different ways, some totally outside her experience. Ms. G was angry at herself and the staff for ignorance and judgmental attitudes and lashed out by calling them bigots. Her anger finally motivated her into action. She decided to explore her feelings and educate herself through reading and talking with a knowledgeable professional. Finally she spoke up in a conflictive staff meeting to facilitate a staff in-service program on sexuality.

■ Assessment of the patient

Any basic health history needs to include questions regarding sexual history. Nurses are often involved in history gathering and assessments of pa-

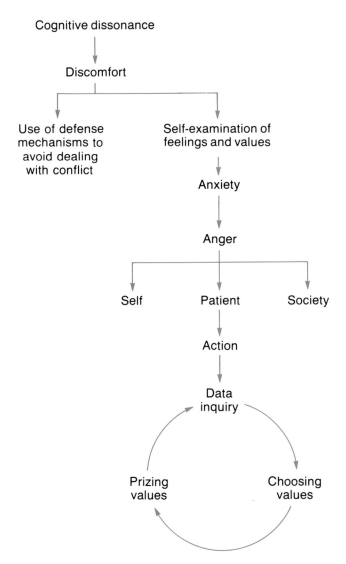

Fig. 20-2. Phases of the nurse's growth in developing self-awareness of human sexuality.

tients. Because of the possible anxiety and embarrassment associated with sexual issues, nurses react in various ways. One common reaction is to ignore the sexual questions or look at the floor and stutter while asking interview questions. Another typical reaction is to blurt out rapidly, "You don't have any sex problems, do you?" or "How's your sex life?" Patients usually respond to these statements with embarrassment and think these questions are intrusive. Each of these interview questions, when asked by the nurse, gives the patient a clear message that it is not appropriate to talk about sex. When the nurse is uncomfortable, the patient will be uncomfortable, often to the point that no sexual concerns will be discussed.

A nurse who is comfortable in discussing sexuality conveys the message that it is normal to talk about sexual health in a health assessment interview. If nurses are able to remove the attitude that "sex is dirty and should not be discussed" by presenting a calm and professional manner, questions about patients' sexual health can be asked naturally. The patient can discuss sexual matters without embarrassment.

The second requirement for a nurse to assess a patient's sexuality successfully is effective interviewing skills. Many nurses who demonstrate excellent interviewing skills become uncomfortable asking questions about sex. However, concepts of effective interviewing are the same for sexual issues as for any problem. For example, open-ended questions are often most helpful to initiate a discussion on sexuality. The question must be at the patient's level of understanding because each person is unique. The time and depth needed to complete an interview will vary. Often one or two questions may be sufficient to assess a person's sexual health. Other times, when patients have specific sexual problems, a detailed assessment needs to be done. A sexual health assessment form appears in the box on page 638.

The nurse should inform the patient that the interview is strictly confidential and that the medical chart cannot be given out without the patient's written permission. Assurance of confidentiality is important in the care of all people. Many sexual minority patients are especially sensitive about confidentiality, since they often fear family rejection or losing their jobs.

■ Predisposing factors

No one theory can adequately explain sexual development or the factors predisposing a person to maladaptive sexual responses. Several theories have been postulated, however, and some of these perspectives are now briefly described.

■ **BIOLOGICAL FACTORS.** Biological factors are initially responsible for the development of gender,

Sexual Health Assessment Form

1. When you were a child, how were your questions about sex answered? Where did your sexual information come from? (Appropriate for adolescents.) When you were a teenager, how were your questions about sex answered? (Appropriate for adults.)
2. How did you first find out about sexual intercourse (how babies are made)? (Appropriate for adolescents and young adults.)
3. How would you describe your current sexual activity?
4. What, if anything, would you change about your current sexual activity?
5. At this time in your life, how important is a sexual relationship to you?
6. Do you have any concerns about birth control?
7. Do you have any health problems that, in your opinion, affect your sexual health or happiness?
8. Are you taking any medicines that, in your opinion, affect your sexual health or happiness?
9. Is there anything about these questions that you would like clarified or explained?

From Sexuality: a nursing perspective by FH Mims and M Swenson. Copyright © 1980, McGraw-Hill Book Company. Used with the permission of McGraw-Hill Book Company.

that is, whether one is genetically male or female. One's somatotype therefore includes chromosomes, hormones, internal and external genitalia, and gonads. Sex differentiation is set off by the Y chromosome. Research in humans confirms the general rule that maleness and masculinity depend on fetal and paranatal androgens.

A biological female typically has XX chromosomes, with estrogen as the predominant hormone, appropriate internal and external genitalia, and ovaries. A biological male typically has XY chromosomes, with androgen as the predominant hormone, appropriate internal and external genitalia, and testicles. However, each of these typical configurations may vary. A person may have triple chromosomes, such as XXX, XXY, or XYY, or a single chromosome, XO. There is no YO chromosomal pattern. The triple pattern XXX and the single pattern XO (Turner's syndrome) will develop into a female body, whereas the triple patterns XXY (Kleinfelter's syndrome) and XYY will develop into male bodies. Assuming no variation occurs, the biological factors result in a single, fully developed gender, either male or female.

■ **PSYCHOANALYTICAL VIEW.** Sigmund Freud's influence on society is ever present. His psychoanalytical theory has served as the basis for contemporary psychiatry all over the world. Freud saw sexuality as one of the key forces of human life. In *Three Essays of the Theory of Sexuality,*[7] he theorized extensively about the nature of sexuality and sexual development. He was the first theorist to believe that sexuality was developed before the onset of puberty. He also believed that a person's choice of sexual expression depended on an interplay of heredity, biology, and social factors. He wrote extensively about childhood sexuality and believed infantile sexuality was central to personality development. He further believed that the development of sexuality in individuals was related to the development of object relations during the psychosexual stage.

Freud termed the sex drive *libido* and viewed it as one of the two major drives necessary for life (the other being aggression). He believed the libido was focused in various regions of the body that were extremely sensitive to stimulation (erogenous zones). The child, according to Freud, passes through a series of developmental stages in which a different erogenous zone is dominant. The first is the oral stage (birth to 12 or 18 months), in which the infant's chief sense of pleasure is derived from stimulation of the lips and mouth, that is, sucking. In the second, the anal stage (ages 1 to 3 years), the child's attention is focused on elimination functions and control over body sphincters. The third is the phallic stage (ages 3 to 5 years), in which the erotic focus is on the genitals. An important occurrence in this stage is the development of the Oedipus complex for boys and the Electra complex for girls.

In the Oedipus/Electra complex, the child experiences sexual feelings for the parent of the opposite sex and resents the parent of the same sex. According to Freud, the boy fears retaliation from his father for desiring his mother and fantasizes that the father will cut off his penis (castration anxiety). This fear is the impetus for the young boy's eventually giving up the resentment of the father and identifying with him and the male gender role. The girl, on the other hand, has no penis to fear losing. She believes that at one time she had a penis but it was cut off, and she blames her mother for this. Since she has no penis to fear losing, her motivation for resolving the Electra complex is not as strong, and her resolution remains incomplete. Thus, according to Freud, the female remains somewhat less mature than her male counterpart.[11]

After the resolution of the Oedipus or Electra complex, the child enters a prolonged stage where sexual impulses are repressed—latency. This stage lasts until adolescence, when the child enters the genital stage and sexual urges reawaken. This genital phase is triggered by the biologic focus that activates puberty. The reemergence of oedipal/electra feelings and the need to assert themselves with parents also occur during this phase of development. The adolescent then makes the final transition into mature genital sexuality. If fixation occurred at any of the earlier stages, object cathexis is incomplete and the individual may have a narcissistic object choice as a result.

In recent years there has been criticism of Freud's theory of psychosexual development. Feminists argue that psychoanalytical theory is male centered and views women as anatomically inferior to men (because they have no penis). Freud also made judgments about the quality of vaginal versus clitoral orgasms. He believed that young girls explored their clitoris in play because it was more accessible but would give up interest in it as they matured and would move their interest to the vagina. He believed the mature woman was vaginally responsive and that sexual orgasm from clitoral stimulation was immature. However, research has found no evidence to support this viewpoint.[26]

Lack of scientific evidence is one of the major problems with Freud's theory. Most of Freud's concepts cannot be studied and thus verified by any of the usual scientific methods. Other criticisms include that Freud was a victim of the Victorian era, a time of sexual repression, and that his thoughts and writings were bound by the period in which he lived. Finally, Freud's data were collected from observations of his patients, who were probably not representative of the total population and were to some degree emotionally disturbed.

■ **BEHAVIORAL VIEW.** From a behaviorist's perspective, the most legitimate data for understanding sexual reactions are observable responses to overt, quantifiable stimuli. Behaviorists are not concerned with the complex intrapsychic processes that represent early childhood and adolescent experiences. Rather, they view sexual behavior as a measurable response, with both physiological and psychological components, to a learned stimulus or reinforcement event. For example, behaviorists would consider the sexual behavior of adults caring for children to be important in the children's later sexual development.

Similarly, treatment of sexual problems involves changing behavior through direct intervention, without the need to identify underlying etiology and psychodynamics. Aversive therapy has also been used to treat socially stigmatized behavior.

■ **Precipitating stressors**

Feelings about oneself as a sexual being change throughout the life cycle. Sexual identity cannot be separated from one's self-concept or body image. Therefore, when changes occur in one's body or emotions, sexual responses change as well.

■ **ILLNESS AND INJURY.** Physical and emotional illness may alter sexuality. The patient may find that hospitalization alone changes sexual feelings and behavior. Nurses usually care for patients experiencing alterations in sexuality; they need to discuss and therapeutically intervene in a patient's response to these changes. A person with rheumatoid arthritis may experience body disfiguration and a change in body image due to swollen areas around joints. The same patient may experience decreased sexual interest because of joint and muscle pain during intercourse. Patients who suffer from depressive episodes often experience a decrease in libido. People who have had a myocardial infarction may have decreased sexual interest because they fear a heart attack from becoming sexually aroused. Psychotic patients may have hallucinations and delusions in which they become sexually preoccupied.

Some medications contribute to sexual dysfunction, failure to reach orgasm in women, and impotence or failure to ejaculate in men. Nurses should be knowledgeable about the medications they administer. They should educate patients regarding possible side effects, informing them to notify a health professional when these effects occur. For example, a patient may not be aware that his medication can cause impotence, yet he may be extremely embarrassed and hesitant to talk with the physician or nurse about the problem. Abuse of alcohol or nontherapeutic drugs may also have a debilitating effect on sexuality. Although many people believe alcohol is a sexual stimulant, prolonged use can cause erectile difficulty and other sexual dysfunctions.

Fear of contracting a sexually transmitted disease (STD) may be a stressor that creates changes in sexual behavior. The most frightening STD, acquired immune deficiency syndrome (AIDS), has reportedly changed the sexual behavior of some individuals. Among gay men who currently account for the largest proportion of AIDS cases, available evidence demonstrates a significant shift in the direction of safer sexual behavior.[27] Widely used strategies to promote safe sex include: (1) the use of condoms, (2) reducing the number of sexual partners, and (3) promoting sexual behaviors that decrease the exchange of body fluids.

Patients who become disfigured because of injury or surgery may also experience alterations in sexuality. Sudden injury leaves little or no time to prepare for the loss. People with spinal cord injuries may lose sexual functioning because of full or partial paralysis. Some sexual problems that arise from injury or surgery are organic; others are psychological. The most common surgical procedures that may cause difficulty with sexual responses include the following[21]:

1. Loss of an external body part, such as mastectomy or penectomy
2. Loss of internal organs, such as prostatectomy or hysterectomy
3. Loss of body function, such as surgery that would result in impotence
4. Relocation of a body orifice, such as colostomy or ileostomy

Changes in sexuality, regardless of the precipitating factor, may mean changes in sexual patterns and behaviors. The role of the professional nurse includes assisting and counseling patients to understand their feelings, explore their options, and facilitate their adaptive adjustment.

■ **THE AGING PROCESS.** Although many researchers throughout the years have documented decreased sexual activity with aging, more recent studies indicate that patterns of sexual activity actually remain relatively stable over middle and late adulthood years with only a modest decline appearing in most individuals. There is nothing in the biology of aging that automatically shuts down sexual functioning; however, specific physiological changes do occur.

In postmenopausal women there is little to no increase in breast size and less muscle tension during sexual arousal. Vaginal functioning changes in two ways; there is reduced elasticity in the walls of the vagina and slower vaginal lubrication. The decrease in vaginal lubrication is the result of decreased blood flow to the vagina, which is caused by low estrogen levels.[18]

In men over the age of 55, several physiological changes occur in the sexual response. A longer time and more direct stimulation are often needed for the penis to become erect, and erections tend to be less firm. The amount of semen is reduced and there is less intensity of ejaculation along with less physical need to ejaculate. The refractory period also becomes longer with age.[18]

In Western culture the myth of the older adult as asexual still prevails. Westerners tend to regard the older adult as one who has no interest in sexual feelings or behavior. Many personality theorists have participated in and encouraged the myth of the older adult as an asexual or childlike being. Psychoanalytical theory describes the sexuality of the aging person as a regression to oral and anal levels of gratification. Since many theories about development have had their roots in psychoanalytical theory, it is not surprising that the stereotypical myth of sexless old age is perpetuated.

People have been taught that older adults have little interest in sex and that it is normal for them to have no interest. Therefore, when health professionals encounter older individuals who do indicate an interest in sex or who are sexually active, the professional often judges the older adult as perverted or "oversexed." Older adults themselves are not exempt from society's false beliefs about sexuality and aging. Many deny sexual attractions and feelings because they also have been socialized to believe that sexual behavior in older people is abnormal or perverted. Older adults are influenced by cultural values of Western society that currently prize youth and vitality and often look with disgust at an elderly person doing anything other than sitting in a rocking chair.

An extremely important variable affecting altered sexuality because of aging is attrition by disuse: "use it or lose it." Prolonged abstinence from sexual activity causes more physiological problems in the older adult. For example, the older female who abstains from sexual activity will have greater shrinkage in vaginal size than a sexually active female of the same age. The older male who abstains from sexual activity may experience difficulty having erections when attempting to return to sexual activity. Most researchers at present agree with the original Kinsey studies, which indicated that persons who enjoy an active sex life as young adults will probably continue their usual pattern in older adulthood with some modifications, rather than experiencing a sudden decrease or cessation of sexual activity and interest in older adulthood.[14]

■ **Behaviors**

There are many modes of sexual expression. In 1948, Kinsey used a seven-point rating scale in examining sexual preference (Fig. 20-3), in which a 0 represented exclusively heterosexual experiences, a 6 represented exclusively homosexual experiences, and a bisexual would rate a 2, 3, or 4 on the scale. He suggested that most individuals are not exclusively heterosexual or homosexual. His studies indicated that a substantial percentage of men and women had experienced both heterosexual and homosexual activity. Specifically, the Kinsey study reported that 25% of U.S. males and 6% to 14% of females have had more than incidental homosexual experiences.[14]

■ **HOMOSEXUALITY.** Marmor defined the homosexual person as "one who is motivated in adult life by a definite attraction to members of the same sex and who usually (but not necessarily) engages in overt sexual relations with them."[15] Marmor's definition excludes transitory homosexual activity in adolescence and in primarily heterosexual persons. Persons who believe in or participate in sexual practices that differ

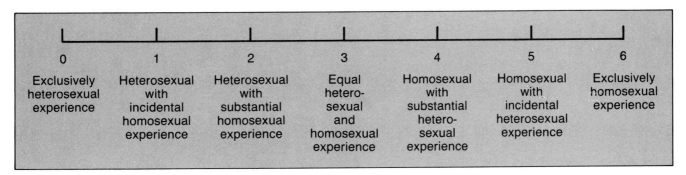

Fig. 20-3. Kinsey's rating scale of sexual preference.

from society's norm are often termed sexual minorities. Homosexuals are the largest sexual minority. The incidence of more or less exclusively homosexual behavior in Western culture conservatively ranges from 3% to 5% in adult females and 5% to 10% in adult males. This estimate does not include bisexual behavior.[15]

For many years the medical profession, including psychiatry, has searched for causes of homosexuality. The message in looking for the cause of a condition is that it is a maladaptive state that can be treated or cured. Many theories of the cause of homosexuality have been formulated; however, none has ever been established. Today emphasis is on learning more about homosexuality and viewing it as a sexual preference or mode of sexual expression. Recent research findings indicate that gay men and lesbian women generally function at least as well psychologically, emotionally, and sexually as nongay persons and in some cases may even function better.[3]

If current estimates of homosexuality are accurate, nurses come into contact with homosexuals daily, but they know little about homosexuality and almost always assume that all patients are heterosexual.

■ **BISEXUALITY.** Bisexuality, sometimes called ambisexuality, is defined as sexual attraction to persons of both sexes and engagement in both homosexual and heterosexual activity.[28] Determining the precise points on the Kinsey scale that would indicate bisexual behavior is controversial. It can be argued that only individuals who are rated as 3 (equal homosexual and heterosexual experiences) are considered bisexual. However, a more flexible interpretation could include all the individuals who are rated from 1 through 5, suggesting that bisexuals constitute a large segment of the population.[20] If bisexuality is defined in terms of sexual activity with male and female partners within the past year, Masters, Johnson, and Kolodny suspect that less than 5% of our society are actively bisexual.[18] Others believe there is no clear way to define bisexuality and that a bisexual orientation is an ambiguous term. Bisexual individuals may prefer one gender over another or they may have no preference at all. They may have several partners of both sexes or may be sexually exclusive with one sex but have more than one partner of another.[23] The difficulty in specifically defining bisexuality has probably influenced the lack of documentation regarding the incidence of bisexuality.

There has been little research on bisexual individuals. They are sometimes included in research samples with homosexual populations, which makes it difficult to examine the bisexual person specifically. Society often labels anyone who has had a homosexual experience as a homosexual; however, the few studies that have been done on bisexuality indicate that bisexuals differ significantly from both the homosexual and the heterosexual populations. It therefore seems important to conduct further research on bisexuals alone, and the practice of combining bisexuals in samples with homosexuals should be discontinued.

■ **TRANSVESTISM.** Transvestism is defined as cross-dressing, or dressing in the clothes of the opposite sex. Clinically defined, "Transvestism is a condition in which a male has a sexual obsession for or addiction to women's clothes, such that he periodically experiences intolerable psychic stress if he does not dress up."[22] Most often the transvestite that seeks treatment is a male; very little is known about female transvestism. No reliable statistics concerning the incidence of transvestism are available; however, many professionals believe it is more common than generally assumed.

Transvestites tend to be married men who report heterosexual behavior. Although they occasionally or frequently dress in female garb, they do not wish hormonal or surgical sex change, as does the transsexual. Many transvestites try to find willing partners, and typically their activities of cross-dressing do not prevent sexual relationships with others.[15]

■ **TRANSSEXUALISM.** The word transsexual simply implies going from one sex to another. A more specific definition specifies a transsexual to be a person who is anatomically a male or female but who expresses, with strong conviction, that he or she (1) has the mind of the opposite sex, (2) lives as a member of the opposite sex part time or full time, and (3) seeks to change his or her original sex legally and through hormonal and surgical sex reassignment.[22] Many times the transsexual client will describe himself as "feeling trapped in the wrong body." Transsexuals genuinely believe they belong to the other sex. Many experience intense emotional turmoil because of stigma from society. There are no accurate estimates of the incidence of transsexualism. However, postoperative transsexuals in the United States now number in the thousands.[22]

Transsexuality is very different from homosexuality in that homosexuals are comfortable with their anatomical identity and do not want to change their sex. Many transsexuals are heterosexual and express distaste for homosexual activity. Transsexuals are essentially heterosexual, not homosexual, but are often mistaken by others or themselves as homosexual.

In Clinical example 20-2, the transsexual's attraction to others of the same sex is understood in the context of his inner identification with the opposite sex. The transsexual does not want a sexual relationship with a person of the same sex, but wishes to have his or her own genitals changed to that of the opposite sex. Thus the attraction is heterosexual.

■ **THE SEXUAL RESPONSE CYCLE.** In addition to modes of sexual expression or sexual preference, one can describe the physiological and psychological behaviors that characterize response to sexual stimulation. Masters and Johnson were the first to describe the physiological changes that occur when men and women engage in sexual activity. According to them, the sexual response cycle consists of four phases[18]:

1. Excitement Phase

    This phase occurs as a result of sexual stimulation (either physical or psychic).

    The excitement phase in the female is characterized by vaginal lubrication, expansion of the inner two thirds of the vaginal barrel, elevation of the cervix and the body of the uterus, and flattening and elevation of the labia majora. The clitoris increases in size, and erection of the nipples occurs.

    The excitement phase in the male is characterized by penile erection. Skin ridges on the scrotal sac smooth out, and the scrotum flattens. The testes are partially elevated toward the perineum. In some but not all men, nipple erection occurs during the excitement phase.

2. Plateau Phase

    This phase describes a high state of sexual arousal that occurs before reaching orgasm. The duration of the plateau may vary greatly with different individuals.

    In the female, prominent vasocongestion occurs in the outer third of the vagina (orgasmic platform), and the opening of the vagina narrows. The inner two thirds of the vagina undergoes minimal expansion, and the elevation of the uterus increases. Vaginal lubrication usually decreases in this phase. The shaft and the glans of the clitoris retract against the pubic bone.

    In males, there is a minimal increase in the diameter of the proximal portion of the glans penis and a deepening in color resulting from venostasis. Testes increase in size. Small amounts of fluid from the urethra may appear.

3. Orgasm

    The orgasm phase is a total body response. In females, rhythmic contractions of the uterus, orgasmic platform, and rectal sphincter occur. In males, rhythmic contractions of the prostate, perineal muscles, and penile shaft combine to assist the propulsion of ejaculation.

4. Resolution Phase

    In the resolution phase the anatomical and physiological changes of the excitement and plateau phases are reversed.

    In females the orgasmic platform disappears, the uterus moves back in to the true pelvis, the vagina shortens, and the clitoris returns to its normal position.

CLINICAL EXAMPLE 20-2

Mr. L is a 21-year-old biological male who was admitted to the psychiatric unit for evaluation after a serious suicide attempt. Mr. L was interviewed by Mr. W, the charge nurse on the unit. Mr. L told the nurse that he tried to kill himself because he has been "sexually mixed up for years" and is tired of feeling like a freak of nature. He said that his friends make fun of him and tell him he is a homosexual, but that he does feel sexually attracted to other men and does not see himself as a homosexual. "I guess I don't feel like a man, I feel like a woman inside a man's body, and as a woman I am attracted to men."

In males the erection diminishes, and the testes decrease in size and descend into the scrotum.

Helen Singer Kaplan[13] has proposed an alternative view of the sexual response cycle, addressing the psychological responses along with the physiological. According to Kaplan, the sexual response cycle consists of a complex series of autonomically mediated visceral reflexes, which can work successfully only if the person is in a calm state and if the process is not impaired by conscious monitoring. To function well sexually, the person must be able to abandon himself to the erotic experience. He must be able to temporarily give up control and, to some degree, decrease his contact with the environment.

Kaplan identifies three categories or stages of the sexual response cycle: **desire, excitement,** and **orgasm.** One of the most significant features of Kaplan's model is her inclusion of desire as a separate phase. She describes desire as the prelude to physical sexual response. Sexual desire is an appetite or drive produced by activation of the brain, whereas the excitement and orgasm phases involve genital orgasms.[13]

Impairment in one's sexual response may occur in any one of these three phases or stages. For example, when the orgasm phase of the human sexual response cycle is disrupted, clinical syndromes such as premature or retarded ejaculation in males and orgastic inhibition in females may result. If the excitement phase is inhibited, it may produce erectile dysfunction in males and a general sexual dysfunction in females. If the desire phase is inhibited, it may be evidenced by low libido in both the male and the female.[13]

■ Coping mechanisms

Numerous coping mechanisms may be used in one's sexual response. These mechanisms may be adaptive or maladaptive, depending on how and why they are being employed. **Fantasy** is a coping mechanism used by individuals who wish to enhance their sexual experiences. Men and women may escape to erotic fantasies with unknown lovers during sex with their husband or wife. Although many people fear that fantasies about individuals other than their sexual partner indicate they are unsatisfied or unattracted to their partner, this is typically not the case. Fantasies are often a creative way to increase sexual excitement and enjoyment and are not usually indicative of dissatisfaction with one's current partner. However, excessive fantasy can be maladaptive when used as replacement for actual sexual expression or the development of intimate relationships with others.

Maladaptive coping mechanisms may result from problems with self-concept. Often one member of a sexually dysfunctional couple may use **projection** in blaming his partner for the total problem, absolving himself of any participation, "I never had a sex problem with any of my previous lovers. I think you are the problem." Projection is also the coping mechanism used when a person's thoughts and feelings are unacceptable and anxiety producing. For example, a wife constantly accuses her husband of wanting to have an affair when actually the wife is contemplating an affair. Because her feelings are unacceptable to her, she projects them onto her husband and accuses him.

Denial and **rationalization** are also common coping mechanisms. Both allow the individual to avoid dealing with sexual issues. The following are maladaptive examples:

DENIAL: **"I don't have a problem with sex" or "I never feel sexual."**
RATIONALIZATION: **"I don't need sex; I'm fine without it. Besides, a good marriage is a lot more than just sex."**

To cope with unacceptable feelings about becoming vulnerable and the resulting ambivalent feelings about intimacy, some individuals **withdraw** from any form of sexual behavior. Others may engage in increased sexual behavior with multiple partners to protect themselves from one intimate relationship.

 ## Nursing diagnosis

When developing a nursing diagnosis for variations in sexual response, the nurse should consider all the information gathered in the assessment phase and the components of the nursing model of health-illness phenomena (Fig. 20-4). The identified nursing diagnosis serves as a foundation for future problem solving. The primary NANDA nursing diagnoses are sexuality patterns, altered, which include lack of sexual satisfaction, alterations in perceived sex role, and conflicts involving values; and sexual dysfunction, which includes actual physical limitations. The primary NANDA diagnoses and examples of complete nursing diagnoses are presented in the box on page 645.

Other related nursing diagnoses that address additional behavioral problems may also need to be included. For example, a patient may be confused regarding his sexual identity while remaining sexually functional. Nursing diagnoses related to the range of possible maladaptive responses and related medical diagnoses are identified in Table 20-1.

■ Related medical diagnoses

Many people who experience transient variations in sexual response will have no medically diagnosed

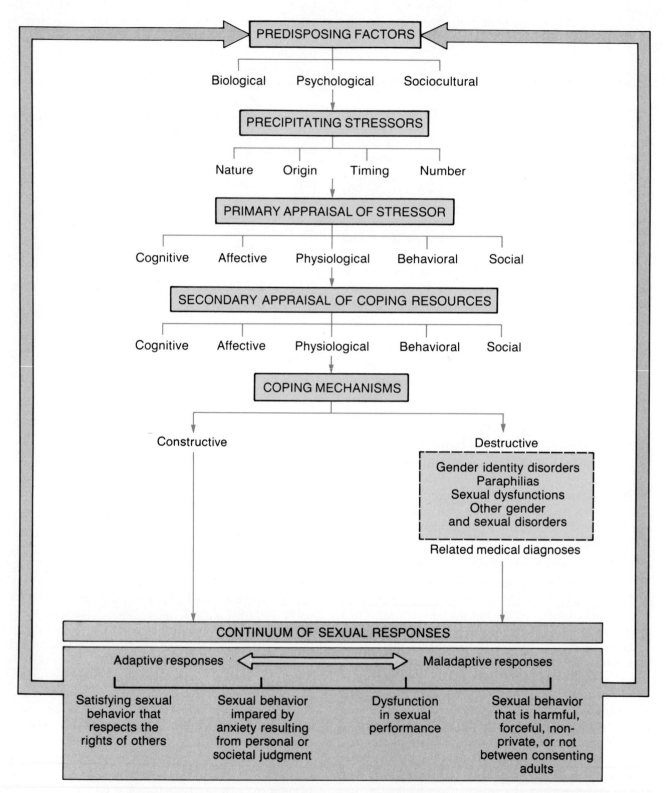

Fig. 20-4. Nursing model of health-illness phenomena related to variations in sexual response.

Nursing Diagnoses Related to Variations in Sexual Response

Primary NANDA diagnoses

Sexuality patterns, altered
Sexual dysfunction

Examples of complete nursing diagnoses

Altered sexuality patterns related to embarrassment about one's body after a mastectomy, evidenced by lack of desire for sex

Altered sexuality patterns related to inability to achieve orgasm, evidenced by lack of sexual satisfaction

Altered sexuality patterns related to marital conflict, evidenced by lack of arousal during foreplay/intercourse

Sexual dysfunction related to excessive alcohol ingestion, evidenced by inability to attain an erection

Sexual dysfunction related to fear of penetration, evidenced by pain with intercourse

TABLE 20-1

MEDICAL AND NURSING DIAGNOSES RELATED TO VARIATIONS IN SEXUAL RESPONSE

Medical Diagnostic Class	Psychiatric Nursing Diagnostic Class
Gender identity disorders	Variations in sexual response
Sexual disorders	
Sexual dysfunctions	
Related Medical Diagnoses (DSM-III-R*)	**Related Nursing Diagnoses (NANDA)**
Gender identity disorder of childhood, adolescence, or adulthood	Anxiety
Transsexualism	Body image disturbance
Exhibitionism	Fear
Fetishism	Grieving, dysfunctional
Frotteurism	Health maintenance, altered
Pedophilia	Knowledge deficit
Sexual masochism	Mobility, impaired physical
Sexual sadism	Pain
Transvestic fetishism	Powerlessness
Voyeurism	Self-care deficit
Hypoactive sexual desire disorder	Self-esteem disturbance
Sexual aversion disorder	Sensory/perceptual alterations
Female/male sexual arousal disorder	†Sexual dysfunction
Inhibited female/male orgasm	†Sexuality patterns, altered
Premature ejaculation	Sleep pattern disturbance
Dyspareunia	Social isolation
Vaginismus	Spiritual distress (distress of the human spirit)
	Violence, potential for: self-directed or directed at others

*From American Psychiatric Association: Diagnostic and statistical manual, Third edition–Revised, Washington, D.C., 1987, Author.
†Indicates primary nursing diagnosis for variations in sexual response.

health problem. Those with more severe or persistent problems will be classified into one of three categories of variations in sexual response according to the DSM-III-R[1]: gender identity disorders, sexual disorders, and sexual dysfunctions. The medical diagnoses that fall under each of these diagnostic classes according to the DSM-III-R[1] are now briefly described.

■ **GENDER IDENTITY DISORDER**

Childhood—female. The essential features are persistent and intense distress about being a girl and a stated desire to be a boy (not merely a desire for any perceived cultural advantages from being a boy) or insistence that she is a boy. There is either (1) a persistent extreme aversion to normative feminine clothing and insistence on wearing stereotypical masculine clothing (e.g., boy's underwear and other accessories) or (2) a persistent repudiation of her anatomical structures, as manifested by at least one of the following:

1. An assertion that she has, or will grow, a penis
2. Rejection of urinating in a sitting position
3. Assertion that she does not want to grow breasts or menstruate

Childhood—male. The essential features are persistent and intense distress about being a boy and an intense desire to be a girl. There is either (1) a preoccupation with stereotypical female activities (as manifested by a preference for cross-dressing or simulating female attire, or by a compelling desire to participate in girls' games and pasttimes) and rejection of stereotypical male toys, games, and activities or (2) a persistent repudiation of his male anatomical structures, as manifested by at least one of the following repeated assertions:

1. That he will grow up to become a woman (not merely in role)
2. That his penis or testes are disgusting or will disappear
3. That it would be better not to have a penis or testes

Adolescence or adulthood. The essential features are persistent or recurrent discomfort and sense of inappropriateness about one's assigned sex. There is also persistent or recurrent cross dressing in the role of the other sex either in fantasy or actuality but not for the purpose of sexual excitement. There is no persistent preoccupation (for at least 2 years) with getting rid of one's primary and secondary sex characteristics and acquiring the sex characteristics of the other sex (as in transsexualism). It is diagnosed only once puberty has been reached.

■ **TRANSSEXUALISM.** The essential features of transsexualism are persistent discomfort, sense of inappropriateness about one's assigned sex, and preoccupation for at least 2 years with eliminating one's primary and secondary sex characteristics and acquiring those of the other sex. (This occurs in a person who has reached puberty.)

■ **EXHIBITIONISM.** The essential feature of this disorder is recurrent, intense, sexual urges and sexually arousing fantasies (lasting a total of at least 6 months) that involve the exposure of one's genitals to an unsuspecting stranger.

■ **FETISHISM.** The essential feature of fetishism is recurrent, intense, sexual urges and fantasies lasting a total of at least 6 months that involve the use of nonliving objects by themselves (e.g., women's underpants, stockings, boots, shoes, or other wearing apparel). Fetishes are not limited to articles of female clothing used in cross-dressing (transvestic fetishism) or to objects used for sexual stimulation (e.g., vibrator).

■ **FROTTEURISM.** The essential feature of frotteurism is recurrent, intense, sexual urges and fantasies lasting at least 6 months in duration that involve touching and rubbing against a nonconsenting person.

■ **PEDOPHILIA.** The essential feature of pedophilia includes recurrent, intense, sexual urges and fantasies that involve sexual activity with a prepubescent child or children age 13 or younger. The individual is age 16 years or older and at least 5 years older than the involved child or children. This does not include a late adolescent in an ongoing sexual relation with a 12- or 13-year-old.

■ **SEXUAL MASOCHISM.** The essential feature of sexual masochism is recurrent, intense, sexual urges and fantasies lasting a total of at least 6 months that involve the act of being humiliated, beaten, bound, or otherwise made to suffer (real or simulated).

■ **SEXUAL SADISM.** The essential feature of sexual sadism is recurrent, intense, sexual urges and fantasies lasting a total of at least 6 months that involve acts in which the psychological or physical suffering (including humiliation) of a victim is sexually exciting.

■ **TRANSVESTIC FETISHISM.** The essential feature of transvestic fetishism is a persistent association in a heterosexual male, lasting a total of at least 6 months, between intense sexual arousal or desire and acts, fantasies, or other stimuli involving cross-dressing. (This does not meet the criteria for transsexualism).

■ **VOYEURISM.** The essential feature of voyeurism is a persistent association, lasting at least 6 months, between intense sexual arousal or desire and acts, fantasies, or other stimuli involving observing unsuspecting people who are either naked, in the act of disrobing, or engaged in sexual activity.

■ **HYPOACTIVE SEXUAL DESIRE DISORDER.** This disorder is a persistent or recurrent deficit or absence of sexual fantasies and desire for sexual activity. The judgment of deficiency or absence is made by a clinician analyzing factors that affect sexual function, such as age, sex, and the context of the individual's life.

■ **SEXUAL AVERSION DISORDER.** This disorder is a persistent or recurrent extreme aversion to and avoidance of all or almost all genital contact with a sexual partner.

■ **SEXUAL AROUSAL DISORDER**

Female. The essential feature of female arousal disorder is either a persistent or recurrent partial or complete failure to attain or maintain the lubrication-swelling response of sexual activity or a persistent or recurrent lack of a subjective sense of sexual excitement and pleasure during sexual activity.

Male. The essential feature of male arousal disorder is either a persistent or recurrent partial or complete failure to attain or maintain erection until completion of sexual activity or a persistent or recurrent lack of a subjective sense of sexual excitement and pleasure during sexual activity.

■ **INHIBITED ORGASM**

Female. The essential features are persistent or recurrent delay in or absence of orgasm in a female following a normal sexual excitement phase judged by the clinician to be adequate in focus, intensity, and duration. Some women experience orgasm during noncoital clitoral stimulation but are unable to experience it during coitus without manual clitoral stimulation. In most of these women, this represents a normal variation of the female sexual response and does not justify this diagnosis. In some, however, this does represent a psychological inhibition justifying the diagnosis. This difficult judgment is assisted by a thorough sexual evaluation, which may even require a trial treatment.

Male. The essential features are persistent or recurrent delay in or absence of ejaculation in a male following a normal sexual excitement phase judged by the clinician to be adequate in focus, intensity, and duration, taking into account the individual's age.

■ **PREMATURE EJACULATION.** In this disorder, persistently or recurrently, ejaculation occurs with minimal sexual stimulation or before, on, or shortly after penetration and before the individual wishes it. The clinician must take into account factors affecting duration of the excitement phase, such as age, novelty of the sexual partner or situation, and frequency.

■ **DYSPAREUNIA.** The essential feature of dyspareunia is a recurrent or persistent genital pain in a male or a female, occurring before, during, or after sexual intercourse. This disturbance is not caused exclusively by lack of lubrication or vaginismus.

■ **VAGINISMUS.** The essential feature of vaginismity is a recurrent or persistent involuntary muscle spasm in the outer third of the vagina that interferes with coitus. This disturbance is not caused exclusively by a physical disorder.

✿ Planning and implementation

■ Goal setting

After assessment, which often includes a complete physical examination, the nurse plans the nursing process. The nurse and patient review the data, define problems, and establish goals that the patient wants to achieve. The nurse should not identify his or her goals, but rather help the patient identify his goals and develop a realistic plan.

The planning phase can simply involve reviewing assessment data, exploring options, and making referral sources known and available. A psychiatric nursing care plan is not included in this chapter since patients with primary diagnoses of maladaptive sexual responses are usually treated in an outpatient setting and do not require hospitalization. The nurse's level of expertise determines the degree of planning done with a patient. This phase can also include a plan of sexual teaching for the patient or the patient and partner together. The nurse and patient can discuss a specific sexual issue and approaches that will provide the needed information. A mental health plan for a patient recovering from an organic illness is presented in Table 20-2.

Goals must be formulated realistically, remembering the uniqueness of each person. The nurse and the patient will need to prioritize goals and the motivation for achieving them. Goals should be written in behavioral terms so that changes can be measured.

■ Intervening with health education

Primary prevention strives to promote health and prevent problems through specific methods, such as teaching and planning. Before engaging in health education or counseling, however, the nurse must examine his or her own values and beliefs about patients with unusual sexual behavior. This can be facilitated by exploring commonly held myths regarding human sexuality.[17] Table 20-3 lists some of these sexual myths, the results of believing them, and the corresponding facts.

Education is the most frequent method of primary prevention for sexual problems. The question of where sex education belongs stimulates much debate among

TABLE 20-2

MENTAL HEALTH EDUCATION PLAN—SEXUAL RESPONSE FOLLOWING AN ORGANIC ILLNESS

Content	Instructional activities	Evaluation
Describe the variety of human sexual response patterns	Discuss the range of sexual desires, modes of expression, and techniques	Patient identifies his preferences and typical level of sexual functioning
Define the patient's primary organic problem	Provide accurate information regarding the disruption caused by the organic impairment	Patient understands his organic illness
Clarify relationship between the organic problem and one's level of sexual functioning	Reframe distorted or confused perceptions regarding the impact of the illness on one's sexual functioning	Patient accurately describes the impact of the illness on his sexual functioning
Identify ways to enhance one's sexual functioning and improve interpersonal communication	Describe additional experiences that would add to the sexual satisfaction and the relationship between the patient and one's partner	Patient and partner report reduced anxiety and greater satisfaction with their sexual responses

TABLE 20-3

MYTHS AND FACTS ON HUMAN SEXUALITY

Myth	Result of myth	Fact
Most individuals who Dsuffer from sexual dysfunctions are deeply psychologically disturbed	Individuals who experience sexual dysfunctions are embarrassed and ashamed, often try to hide their problem, and do not seek professional help	According to Masters and Johnson, "sociocultural deprivation and ignorance constitute the etiologic background for most sexual dysfunctions, not psychiatric illness"[16]
Excessive masturbation is harmful	Individuals often feel guilty or ashamed about masturbating; some individuals deny themselves this experience because of uncomfortable feelings society perpetuates	There is no evidence that masturbation causes physical problems. No medical definition for excessive masturbation exists; masturbation seems to be a self-limiting practice; once the body has reached the point of overload, it temporarily shuts down and does not respond to further stimulation. If masturbation leads to satisfaction and pleasure, it is unlikely to be a problem[18]
Sexual fantasies about having sex with a different partner (other than lover or spouse) indicate relationship difficulties	Individuals may become uncomfortable about having a fantasy with a different partner. They may experience guilt feelings and view the fantasy as a sign of infidelity	Imagining sex with a different partner is one of the most common sexual fantasies and does not necessarily indicate any desire on the part of the individual to act out the fantasized behavior[18]

TABLE 20-3—cont'd

MYTHS AND FACTS ON HUMAN SEXUALITY

Myth	Result of myth	Fact
Sex during menstruation is unclean and harmful	Women often view their bodies as unclean and even unfit or inferior during menstruation; women use menstruation as an excuse to avoid intercourse rather than simply saying no without a "good reason"	Medically, menstrual flow is in no way harmful or dirty; if women desire, there is no reason to abstain from intercourse during menstrual flow[17]
Oral and anal intercourse are perverted and dangerous	Many individuals refrain from these behaviors or indulge in them only to feel ashamed and guilty afterward	According to Masters and Johnson, "nothing could be further from the truth"; they suggest certain precautions when performing anal intercourse, such as avoiding contamination of vaginal tract and wearing a condom to prevent bacteria from entering penile passage[17]
Teenagers are sexually promiscuous because they all learn sex education in school	Parents who believe this myth fight against comprehensive sex education programs in public education; many parents believe their children have sex education in school, when in fact, most do not	The literature has demonstrated that adolescents' knowledge of sex and reproduction is limited.[24] Lack of knowledge does not prevent sexual activity but may promote undesirable consequences[2]
Most homosexuals molest children	Known homosexuals are often fired from teaching jobs, and many parents will not allow their children to spend any time with anyone who is homosexual; children learn from an early age that homosexuals are "bad people," that they should stay away from them	Research data has not supported the myth that homosexuals are particularly attracted to children. The adult heterosexual male poses a greater risk to the under age child than does the adult homosexual male[9]
Homosexuals are sick and cannot control their sexual behavior	Homosexuals are denied jobs and are sometimes jailed for their homosexuality; homosexual parents may have their children taken away by courts	According to Bell and Weinberg, who studied 979 homosexual men and women in a study conducted by the Institute for Sex Research in 1978: (1) most homosexuals' social and psychological adjustment is indistinguishable from the heterosexual majority and (2) objectionable sexual advances are far more likely to be made by a heterosexual (usually male to female) than a homosexual[3]
All homosexuals are alike; men, limp wristed, speak with lisp; women, unattractive, masculine, "butch," short hair, deep voice	Society considers any individual who does not conform to the correct "macho male" and "fluffy female" stereotypes to be homosexual	Bell and Weinberg's study indicates that relatively few homosexual men and women conform to hideous stereotypes[3]
Advancing age means end of sex	Many older adults become victims of this myth not because their bodies have lost the ability to perform, but because *they* believe that they have lost the ability to perform	Sexually men and women can function effectively into their 80s if they understand the physiological changes that occur with aging and do not let these changes frighten them[17]
Alcohol ingestion reduces inhibitions and therefore enhances sexual enjoyment	Many individuals use alcohol in the hope that it will increase their sexual pleasure and performance; alcohol ingestion can also provide an excuse for engaging in sexual behaviors—"I would never have gone to bed with him if I hadn't had all that wine"	According to Wilsnack, empirical data does not support the belief that alcohol ingestion reduces inhibitions and enhances sexual enjoyment[29]

educational and religious groups.[25] Some groups believe that sex education should be censored in public schools and that sexuality should never be publicly discussed. If a professional nurse believes in primary prevention, however, sex education is vitally important.

According to Hacker,[10] sex education needs to be incorporated from kindergarten throughout one's entire educational career. When individuals are not properly educated about human sexuality, they are denied the opportunity to explore their own values and beliefs and to know themselves as sexual beings. Lack of knowledge breeds ignorance that can adversely affect sexual counseling. When individuals are not aware of facts and do not understand their own feelings, important decisions that they may later regret are made on limited information. Sex education can help people know themselves better when the curriculum allows for expression of thoughts, feelings, and examination of behavior while learning factual information.

Concepts that must underlie sex education include: (1) we are sexual from birth, and sexuality is an inseparable part of our identity; and (2) all sexual thoughts and feelings are considered normal, but our behavior needs to be appropriate. The key principle in sex education is teaching individuals when and where to act and not to act on feelings. Finally, sexuality must be viewed as more than genital. It encompasses one's total sense of self.[10]

Nurses have a professional responsibility to become educated about human sexuality so that holistic care becomes a reality. Education can be accomplished in nursing curricula and continuing education programs. Some nurses pursue additional education and a clinical practice in human sexuality. They may become sex educators in schools, outpatient clinics, and planned parenthood agencies. Nurses prepared at the master and doctorate levels may become therapists through postgraduate work in human sexuality and extensive clinical supervision from sex therapists.

■ **Intervening in sexual responses within the nurse-patient relationship**

■ **SEXUAL RESPONSES OF NURSES TO PATIENTS.** A clinical situation in which a nurse feels sexual attraction to a patient can be a problem. Although this does occur, it has received little attention in the nursing literature. One major reason is that nurses often deny sexual feelings for their patients. However, sexual attraction and sexual fantasies are part of the human experience. If the nurse does not explore these feelings, they can interfere with the quality of care by focusing on the nurse's rather than the patient's needs.

First, the nurse must acknowledge her own feelings without judging them. Often nurses try to ignore or deny these feelings because they are uncomfortable and frightening. They make judgments about themselves, such as, "What's wrong with me? I shouldn't feel this way about my patients. I must be really weird" and "I'm sure I'm the only nurse who ever had these feelings." The nurse who admits these feelings without judging them is able to deal with them. Edelwich and Brodsky[5] offer several suggestions:

1. Do not share personal information with patients.
2. Do not become overly involved in patients' problems.
3. Do not discuss with the patient feelings of sexual attraction to him or her.
4. Seek consultation.

Asking for consultation from a more experienced nurse or a supervisor often helps the nurse sort out feelings and, most important, maintain a professional therapeutic relationship with the patient. These interventions are summarized in Table 20-4.

■ **SEXUAL RESPONSES OF PATIENTS TO NURSES.** One of the most common sexual behaviors of hospitalized patients is acting out or displaying seductive behaviors toward the nurse. Nurses are often extremely uncomfortable when they are the recipients of such behavior. Patients making passes at nurses, making sexual comments, asking for their phone numbers, and requesting a date are typical examples of sexual acting out behavior.

The first step in intervening is to let the patient know his behavior is unacceptable. The nurse needs to respond in a firm, matter-of-fact manner that clearly states what limits are being set. For example, "Mr. Moore, I am uncomfortable when you suggest that I get into bed with you. Please stop saying that." or "Mr. Dean, take your hand off my breast."

Nurses are sometimes embarrassed or afraid to confront patients and attempt to laugh it off or ignore it with a "boys will be boys" attitude. Providing health care to patients does not give them permission to be verbally offensive or touch nurses' bodies without permission. Nurses are taught to be accepting of patients' behavior, and this principle is difficult to dispute. However, when the behavior does not respect the rights of the nurse, limits need to be set.

Nurses have a responsibility as professionals to attempt to understand sexual behaviors and to analyze their possible meanings. Patients may show seductive behaviors for various reasons. These may or may not include a serious desire for sex with the nurse. Seduc-

TABLE 20-4

SUMMARY OF NURSING INTERVENTIONS IN SEXUAL RESPONSES OF NURSES TO PATIENTS

Goal—Maintain a professional nurse-patient relationship that will enable the nurse to provide therapeutic nursing care

Principle	Rationale	Nursing intervention
Acknowledge nurse's own sexual feelings	The nurse needs to acknowledge sexual feelings toward the patient, remembering that feelings cannot be judged as right or wrong, but behavior can be evaluated as therapeutic or nontherapeutic for the patient	Be open to one's own feelings Accept one's feelings Explore the course of feelings
Examine nurse's behavior with patient	If the nurse works toward increasing awareness of feelings and thoughts, he or she will be able to more effectively change any nontherapeutic behavior to a more therapeutic approach	Keep the relationship patient focused Do not become overly involved in patients' problems (to the point it would impair one's clinical judgment) Do not share personal information about oneself with the patient Do not discuss feelings of sexual attraction with the patient
Seek consultation	After the nurse has acknowledged feelings and examined behavior, consultation from a more experienced nurse may prove helpful in developing ways to resolve this issue appropriately and feel more comfortable in approaching the patient	Confide in a nurse, experienced colleague, or supervisor Request help in exploring this issue in terms of gaining insight into the factors influencing one's feelings Explore possible ways to resolve one's feelings and maintain a professional relationship with the patient

tive behavior is often a way of getting the nurse's attention. Hospitalized patients can also feel unattractive or insecure about themselves sexually; thus seductive behaviors may be a request for reassurance. Sometimes patients confuse gratitude and appreciation for the nurse with sexual attraction. These feelings may in turn generate thoughts such as, "Wouldn't my nurse make a wonderful wife. She's so giving and understanding all the time." In this case the patient views professional behavior and concern as self-sacrificing and altruistic.

Finally, patients may have difficulty understanding the difference between a professional and a social relationship. In many ways, the nurse-patient relationship is idealized for the patient. All the attention and caring is given to him, and he is not expected to give anything in return. It is easy to see how the patient could be confused about his relationship with the nurse.

Clinical example 20-3 illustrates this point. The nurse helps the patient clear up his confusion regarding his relationship with her. She defines the purpose of the professional therapeutic relationship to aid the patient in understanding why it is impossible to compare that relationship to the one with his wife. As stated previously, many reasons exist why the patient might behave sexually or romantically with the nurse (manipulation, altered self-concept, attention seeking, anxiety related to altered health status). Nursing intervention should be determined by the underlying needs the patient is expressing. Table 20-5 summarizes nursing interventions in sexual responses of patients to nurses.

■ **Intervening in maladaptive homosexual and bisexual responses**

Many people accept their homosexual or bisexual orientations, whereas others have difficulties and seek professional help. Because of the homosexual element of bisexuality, bisexuals often encounter many of the same difficulties stemming from societal attitudes as homosexuals do. Another factor that may present a problem for the bisexual is isolation from a support group. Because bisexuals are frequently accused of "fence sitting," they can be rejected by both heterosex-

---

CLINICAL EXAMPLE 20-3

Mr. P has been hospitalized for an exacerbation of a chronic illness for the past 3 weeks. Ms. S has been his primary nurse during this hospitalization. The following is a conversation between the nurse and patient the day before his discharge.

MR. P: I wish my wife were more like you, Ms. S.

MS. S: Mr. P, I'm not sure I understand what you are saying.

MR. P: Well, it's just that you are always so concerned about me. You always try to make me feel good and want to help me all the time. Sometimes my wife's a grouch; she's so wrapped up in her job and the kids she doesn't always pay as much attention to me as you do.

MS. S: I'm glad you feel taken care of, Mr. P, but I think it's impossible to compare my role as your nurse with your wife's role.

MR. P: I'm not sure I follow you . . . .

MS. S: They are very different types of relationships. It's nice to have someone take care of us when we can't take care of ourselves, but when we are healthy, we don't need someone to take care of us all the time. Your relationship with your wife is more of a sharing one with mutual benefits. You take care of her needs, and she takes care of your needs in return.

CLINICAL EXAMPLE 20-4

Ms. A, a 25-year-old single female, came to the mental health clinic with the complaint of a "sexual problem." Her history revealed that she had been sexually inactive for the past 5 years. At the age of 20, Ms. A had a brief sexual encounter with a man she had been dating for 2 years. She ended the relationship shortly afterward because she had no interest in maintaining a sexual relationship with the man. Recently, she became involved in a relationship with a woman that was very satisfying to her. She felt she had to end the relationship because she would not tolerate thinking of herself as a homosexual. During one of the initial counseling sessions, Ms. A told the nurse that she must end the relationship before "it" happens again.

NURSE: What are you afraid will happen?

MS. A: I'm afraid I'll feel attracted to her again.

NURSE: What about that frightens you?

MS. A: (becoming upset) That will mean I'm homosexual!

NURSE: What does being homosexual mean for you?

MS. A: It means I'm sick. It's a sin, I couldn't go to church anymore.

NURSE: Are all homosexuals sick?

MS. A: Yes.

NURSE: How do you know this?

MS. A: Everybody knows that homosexuals hang out in sleazy bars and don't work and are on welfare. They all have emotional problems, need therapy, and eventually wind up in mental institutions.

NURSE: Do you know any homosexual people?

MS. A: Well, not exactly. . . .

NURSE: What have you read about homosexuality?

MS. A: Nothing.

NURSE: Then it looks to me like you are basing all of your conclusions on hearsay and not real knowledge. I think that you and I need to explore your beliefs in more detail, then you can do some reading to find out the facts.

---

ual and homosexual groups. Bisexuals may complain about lack of support; friends and family may pressure them to decide on one sexual orientation (usually heterosexual) so they will fit into society.

The first step in counseling the homosexual or bisexual who views his or her sexual response as maladaptive is the nurse's acceptance. Most patients are extremely perceptive of their therapist's values and attitudes toward them. The nurse who believes she is hiding her prejudices is fooling only herself. Because she has grown up in a society that believes homosexuals are sick and perverted, it is often difficult to examine myths and search for facts. The patient has grown up in the same society and goes through the same growth experience about homosexuality as anyone else.

Often an important step in counseling the homosexual is to aid him or her in exploring values and beliefs about homosexual people. The person may have internalized some of society's prejudices, such as, "Homosexuals are sick, evil people who should not be allowed to live homosexual life-styles." Therefore, "because I am homosexual, I am sick and should not act on my sexual feelings because they are evil and bad." Common responses include denial, confusion, and sexual promiscuity, which is especially prominent among those trying to prove to themselves that they are not gay.

It is helpful to have patients list their beliefs about homosexuality and bisexuality and to discuss each one.

TABLE 20-5

**SUMMARY OF NURSING INTERVENTIONS IN SEXUAL RESPONSES
OF PATIENTS TO NURSES**

Goal—Maintain a professional nurse-patient relationship that will enable the nurse to provide therapeutic nursing care

Principle	Rationale	Nursing intervention
Establish a trusting relationship	An atmosphere of trust allows for open, honest communication between patient and nurse; when this occurs, the nurse can aid the patient in discovering the underlying issues related to his sexual feelings and behavior	Express nonsexual caring and concern for the patient Be a responsive listener, especially to feelings and needs that the patient may not be able to directly express Reinforce the purpose of the professional, therapeutic nurse-patient relationship
Awareness of nurse's own feelings and thoughts	When the nurse is aware of her feelings and thoughts, he or she will begin to understand how they influence her behavior; with increased self-awareness the nurse will be able to increase the effectiveness of her interactions with patients	Recognize own feelings and thoughts Identify any specific patient interaction or behavior that influences the nurse's feelings and thoughts Identify the influence of the nurse's feelings and thoughts on one's behavior in an attempt to increase the effectiveness of nursing interventions
Decrease patient's expressions of sexual feelings and behavior	If the nurse is able to help the patient see that his sexual interactions and behavior are being expressed to an inappropriate partner (the nurse), the sexual acting out will usually decrease; this allows the nurse to help the patient begin to identify the reasons for his behavior	Set limits on patient's sexual behavior Use a calm, matter-of-fact approach without implying judgment Reaffirm nonsexual caring for the patient Explore the meaning of the patient's feelings and behaviors
Expand patient's insight into his sexual feelings and behavior	Once the patient begins to identify the reasons for his sexual feelings and behaviors, he is able to see that the nurse is not an appropriate outlet for these feelings and behaviors and can move toward a more appropriate and therapeutic relationship with the nurse	Clarify misconceptions regarding any feeling patient may have about the nurse as a possible sexual partner Point out the futile nature of his romantic or sexual interest in the nurse Redirect patient's energies toward appropriate health care issues

However, a review of beliefs about homosexuality may not be sufficient. Although the nurse and patient work to dispel myths, society powerfully reinforces them. Having the person read about homosexuality and bisexuality is also helpful. Throughout this process the patient will be extremely sensitive to the therapist and will test her acceptance or rejection.

In Clinical example 20-4, the nurse and Ms. A developed a plan often used in sexual counseling to explore homosexuality over the next several sessions. Two goals included the following:

1. Understand the facts versus the myths about homosexuals and their life-styles.
2. Understand the patient's feelings about her own sexual identity.

Some of the actions to implement the plan included:

1. Ms. A listed all her beliefs about homosexuality and homosexuals.
2. The nurse encouraged Ms. A to explore the literature on homosexuality and suggested readings to help dispel the myths.
3. The nurse then discussed these with Ms. A and suggested that she attend a social gathering for gay people to test out her new-found knowledge. (The nurse suggested the social gathering because many people struggling with a homosexual identity are frightened to test out situations that would dispel the myths.)

■ **Intervening in transsexual responses**

Treatment of the transsexual person has been a controversial topic in recent years. Recommendations range from long-term psychotherapy to surgical reassignment. Recently, standards of care were developed by the Harry Benjamin International Gender Dysphoria Association.[4] These standards set guidelines for those who are to receive psychotherapy and thorough assessment by a trained professional (including qualifications of therapists), hormonal therapy, and surgical reassignment (not all transsexuals choose surgical reassignment). The standards help professionals who treat transsexual patients give quality care. Criteria include the following:

1. The person must demonstrate discomfort with self and the wish to live in the genetically opposite sex role.
2. Along with criterion one, the person must be known to a professional therapist (who is an expert in sexuality) for 3 to 6 months.

If the person meets these criteria, the therapist then endorses him or her for hormonal therapy. A male changing to a female receives estrogen; a female changing to a male receives testosterone. Before starting hormonal therapy, the patient receives a complete physical examination with specific blood work serum glutamic pyruvic transaminase (SGPT) levels in females changing to males; SGPT, bilirubin, triglyceride, and fasting glucose levels in males changing to females. If the person desires surgical reassignment (penectomy, castration, or vaginaplasty for a male changing to a female; hysterectomy, vaginectomy, or phalloplasty for a female changing to a male), he or she must be known to the professional therapist for at least 6 months. The individual must have been successful in living as the genetically opposite sex role for at least 1 year and up to 2 years. Before the transsexual receives surgical alteration, the original therapist's endorsement must be agreed on by a second therapist who has evaluated the person.

Professionals who care for transsexual patients must be educated in sexuality. The assessment phase of treatment is especially important. The patient and therapist must be certain that implementing the treatment plan is the best approach, because the surgery is not reversible.

■ **Intervening in dysfunctions of the sexual response cycle**

Conducting sexual therapy is beyond the scope of the nurse generalist. However, she should be aware of the principles involved and should also know of creditable sex therapists in the community so she can refer patients.

Although patients are treated from many modalities, two common models of sex therapy are discussed here: the Masters and Johnson and the Helen Singer Kaplan models.

■ **MASTERS AND JOHNSON MODEL.** Masters and Johnson began pioneering research in sexuality in the 1950s. Their book, *Human Sexual Inadequacy,*[16] describes their research and their counseling methods.

Before the work of William Masters and Virginia Johnson, patients who experienced problems in sexuality were generally referred to a psychiatrist for psychotherapy or psychoanalysis. Health professionals assumed that anyone who had a problem with sexuality was emotionally disturbed. Problems with dysfunction of sexual response are usually not psychiatric problems, but the result of sociocultural deprivation and ignorance of sexual physiology.[16] Masters' and Johnson's treatment includes short-term education with step-by-step instructions regarding the physical aspects of sexual activity and supportive psychotherapy. The researchers believe that attitudes and ignorance are responsible for most sexual dysfunctions, contrary to the general belief that dysfunctions of sexual response indicate a severe psychiatric illness.

Masters' and Johnson's approach to patients begins with obtaining a detailed sexual and background history. They recommend a male-female therapeutic team, a dual-therapist approach. On day one of the treatment, therapists meet with the couple in a round-table discussion to review and clarify their histories taken the previous day. Then the couple is instructed to carry out the sensate focus exercise. This requires each partner to instruct the other in specific ways of caressing for sensual pleasure without involving the breasts or genitals. The activity is done first by one partner and then the other. The next day the exercise is repeated, including breasts and genital areas, but without performing coitus. The exercise's purpose is to alleviate performance anxiety and to enhance warm, comfortable feelings between partners. The exercises are done in comfortable, private surroundings with both partners in the nude. After the sensate focus exercises are completed, the therapy is directed to the sexual dysfunction. The Masters and Johnson model emphasizes education, communication, and cooperation between partners.

■ **HELEN SINGER KAPLAN MODEL.** Kaplan's method[12] of treating sexual dysfunctions integrates psychodynamic behavioral principles into conjoint therapy. Kaplan combines specific tasks with psychodynamic insights, dream interpretations, and gestalt and transactional techniques. She differs from Masters and Johnson in that she believes the single therapist is as effective as cotherapists of opposite sexes. According to her, the primary objective of sex therapy is symptomatic relief, achievable by treating the patient without a partner in some cases.

Kaplan's treatment begins with an extensive evaluation, including marital, psychiatric, sexual, medical, and family history from both partners. If profound intrapsychic or interpersonal difficulties are found, the couple may be referred to individual or conjoint therapy and not accepted for sex therapy at that time. According to Kaplan, sex therapy is usually contraindicated in couples who are severely disturbed.

As with Masters and Johnson, Kaplan employs sensate focus exercises and variations, such as showering together, to begin sex therapy or further evaluate a client's suitability for sex therapy. Therapy itself consists of erotic tasks performed at home plus weekly or semiweekly meetings with the therapist. Clients and the therapist explore feelings experienced during the erotic exercises. The Kaplan method prescribes a unique series of home or private exercises for the couple and the dysfunction. The exercises take into account the motivations and dynamics of the relationship. The integration of experiential and dynamic modes is a major feature of Kaplan's approach. The role of the therapist includes education, clarification, and support.

Both Kaplan and Masters and Johnson emphasize communication between partners and exploration of the relationship and emotional concerns. The reader is referred to original works of these therapists for more information.

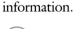 **Evaluation**

In the evaluation phase of nursing, the nurse works with the patient to evaluate effectiveness of the sexual counseling or intervention used. Factors to consider include the following:

1. Sense of well-being. How does the person feel about himself or herself? Have his or her feelings improved during the treatment?
2. Functioning ability. If the individual was dysfunctional, is functional ability restored? Somewhat improved? What about the person's ability to function within primary relations at work? With friends?
3. Satisfaction with treatment. Does the patient believe that treatment was helpful? Were his or her goals adequately met?

CLINICAL EXAMPLE 20-5

Mr. and Mrs. S sought sex therapy because they had been experiencing sexual difficulties since their marriage 2 years ago. Mr. S had been suffering from premature ejaculation, and Mrs. S claimed that she had lost any interest in a sexual relationship with her husband and refused to discuss the problem of premature ejaculation with him.

The couple were seen by a nurse clinician who was an experienced sex therapist. At the onset of therapy, both couple and therapist established the following goals:

1. Improve communication between the couple.
2. Discuss the premature ejaculation problem and explore options of improving the sexual relationship that would prove satisfying to both partners.

During therapy the nurse worked with the couple to discuss openly important issues with each other and improve the patterns of communication. Behavioral sex therapy techniques were employed for Mr. S's problem with premature ejaculation. After 10 weekly sessions the couple and the therapist evaluated the course of treatment together. The following factors for evaluating treatment effectiveness were explored:

1. *Sense of well-being.* Both Mr. and Mrs. S felt better about themselves as individuals and their relationship. They were better able to discuss and solve issues of concern. They felt a renewed affection for each other and a desire to problem solve rather than ignore problematic issues.
2. *Functioning ability.* With the use of behavioral sex therapy techniques, Mr. S's premature ejaculation problem had significantly decreased, and both members began to enjoy a satisfying sexual relationship.
3. *Satisfaction with treatment.* Both Mr. and Mrs. S thought that the goals of treatment had been accomplished and that there was a general improvement in the quality of their relationship.

After the evaluation, the couple, with the therapist's agreement, decided to terminate therapy, since the presenting problem was resolved and the goals of treatment were accomplished. By maintaining a facilitative position, the nurse helped the couple make their own choices in problem solving, and the responsibility for their choices remained solely with the couple. Thus their autonomy and sense of self were affirmed by the nurse, and the goals of high-level wellness and holistic health care were promoted.

DIRECTIONS FOR FUTURE RESEARCH

The following are some of the nursing research problems raised in Chapter 20 that merit further study by psychiatric nurses:

1. The specific nursing behaviors that promote or inhibit the expression of sexual concerns by patients
2. The effectiveness of nursing interventions in the sexual acting out behaviors of patients
3. The validity of various sexual assessment tools in sexual history taking
4. The effects of nurses' feelings, attitudes, and values on therapeutic interventions with patients with sexual concerns
5. The ability of psychiatric nurses to diagnose maladaptive sexual responses in physical and emotional illness
6. The long-term effects of alcohol abuse on male and female sexual functioning
7. The relationship between levels of self-esteem and healthy sexual behavior
8. Effective strategies for sensitizing nurses to the sexual needs of the institutionalized elderly
9. Variations in sexual responses in patients experiencing illness or surgery
10. The impact of AIDS and other STDs on sexual behavior

Evaluation of any form of sexual counseling or intervention should be ongoing. The nurse and patient should work together on goals, problems, and alternatives. Clinical example 20-5 illustrates the evaluation process in a nurse-patient situation.

◼ SUGGESTED CROSS-REFERENCES ◼

Therapeutic relationship skills and self-awareness of the nurse are discussed in Chapter 4. Alterations in self-concept and personal identity are discussed in Chapter 13. Nursing interventions with sexual assault and rape victims are discussed in Chapter 32.

◼ SUMMARY ◼

1. Nurses need to have a knowledge of human sexuality. Information important to the nursing role includes self-awareness, value clarification, and counseling and communication skills.
2. Sexuality is defined as a desire for contact, warmth, tenderness, and love. Criteria for adaptive sexual behavior are identified as (a) consensual, (b) free of force, (c) per-

formed in private, (d) neither physically nor psychologically harmful, and (e) mutually satisfying.

3. Assessment of the nursing process includes two major responsibilities: (a) self-awareness in relation to sexuality and (b) knowledge of the patient's situation and problem. Phases of positive growth include cognitive dissonance, anxiety, anger, and action.

4. Predisposing factors for variations in sexual response are described from biological, psychoanalytical, and behavioral perspectives. Precipitating stressors that may change sexuality include physical and emotional illness, therapeutic and nontherapeutic drugs, surgical intervention, hospitalization, and aging.

5. Data collection includes behavioral responses such as homosexuality, bisexuality, transvestism, and transsexualism. Two models of the human sexual response cycle are (1) Masters and Johnson's four phases: excitement, plateau, orgasm, and resolution; (2) Kaplan's three phases: desire, excitement, and orgasm.

6. A variety of coping mechanisms are used with expressions of sexuality: fantasy, projection, denial, and rationalization. Coping mechanisms may be adaptive or maladaptive, depending on how and why they are used. Ambivalent feelings may lead individuals to withdraw from any form of sexual expression, or they may pursue multiple partners to avoid sexual closeness.

7. Related nursing and medical diagnoses according to NANDA and the DSM-III-R[1] are listed.

8. Planning the nursing process requires the patient's active involvement. The nurse must be careful not to develop a plan and establish goals that *he or she* believes the patient should follow. Rather, the nurse should help individuals identify their own goals and a plan toward achieving them.

9. Interventions depend on the patient's situation and individual needs. Primary prevention, which includes sex education and preventive counseling, is discussed along with interventions for (a) expressions of sexual feelings and behaviors within the nurse-patient relationship, (b) potentially maladaptive modes of sexual expression (homosexuality, bisexuality, etc.), and (c) dysfunctions of the sexual response cycle.

10. The nurse and patient must consider the following factors in assessing the effectiveness of nursing care: the patient's sense of well-being, functioning ability, and satisfaction with treatment.

◼ REFERENCES ◼

1. American Psychiatric Association: Diagnostic and statistical manual of mental disorders, third edition, revised, Washington DC, 1987, The Association.
2. Amonker RG: What do teens know about the facts of life? J School Health 50:4, 1980, 572.
3. Bell AP and Weinberg MS: Homosexualities: a study of diversity among men and women, New York, 1978, Simon & Schuster, Inc.
4. Berger et al: Standard of care, 1981, The Harry Benjamin International Gender Dysphoria Association, Inc.

5. Edelwich J and Brodsky A: Sexual dilemmas for the helping professional, New York, 1982, Brunner/Mazel, Inc.

6. Foley T and Davies M: Rape: nursing care of victims, St Louis, 1982, Mosby–Year Book, Inc.

7. Freud S: Three essays of the theory of sexuality, ed 3, London, 1962, Hogarth Press (originally published 1905).

8. Goldstein B: Human sexuality, New York, 1976, McGraw-Hill, Inc.

9. Groth AN and Birnbaum NJ: Adult sexual orientation and attraction to under age persons, Arch Sex Behavior 7(3):3, 1978.

10. Hacker SS: It isn't sex education unless. . . . J Sch Health 5:209, 1981.

11. Hyde JS: Understanding human sexuality, ed 3, New York, 1986, McGraw-Hill, Inc.

12. Kaplan HS: The illustrated manual of sex therapy, New York, 1975, The New York Times Book Co.

13. Kaplan HS: Disorders of sexual desire and other new concepts and techniques in sex therapy, New York, 1979, Brunner/Mazel, Inc.

14. Kinsey AC, Pomeroy WB, and Martin EC: Sexual behavior in the human female, Philadelphia, 1953, WB Saunders Co.

15. Marmor J, editor: Homosexual behavior: a modern reappraisal, New York, 1980, Basic Books, Inc, Publishers.

16. Masters WH and Johnson VE: Human sexual inadequacy, Boston, 1970, Little, Brown & Co.

17. Masters WH and Johnson VE: Ten sex myths exploded. In Barbour JR editor: Human sexuality 79/80, Guilford, Conn, 1979, The Dushkin Publishing Group, Inc.

18. Masters WH, Johnson VE, and Kolodny RC: Masters and Johnson on sex and human loving, Boston, 1986, Little, Brown & Co.

19. May R: The meanings of anxiety, New York, 1950, Ronald Press.

20. McDonald AP: A little bit of lavender goes a long way: a critique of research on sexual orientation, J Sex Res 19:95, 1983.

21. Mims FH and Swenson M: Sexuality: a nursing perspective, New York, 1980, McGraw-Hill, Inc.

22. Money J and Wiedeking C: Gender identity role: normal differentiation and its transpositions. In Wolman BB and Money J, editors: Handbook of human sexuality, Englewood Cliffs, NJ, 1980, Prentice-Hall, Inc.

23. Nass GD, Libby RW, and Fisher MP: Sexual choices: an introduction to human sexuality, ed 2, Monterey, CA, 1984, Wadsworth Health Science Division.

24. Poorman SG: Human sexuality and the nursing process, Norwalk, CT, 1988, Appleton & Lange.

25. Scales P: Barriers to sex education, J Sch Health 50(6):337, 1980.

26. Sherfey MJ: The nature and evaluation of female sexuality, New York, 1972, Random House.

27. Siegel K and Glassman M: Individual and aggregate level changes in sexual behavior among gay men at risk for AIDS, Arch Sex Behavior 18:(335), 1989.

28. Thomas SP: Bisexuality: a sexual orientation of great diversity, J Psychosoc Nurs Ment Health Serv 18(4):19, 1980.

29. Wilsnack SC: Alcohol abuse and alcoholism in women. In Pattison EM and Kaufman E, editors: Encyclopedia handbook of alcoholism, New York, 1982, Gardner Press.

■ ANNOTATED SUGGESTED READINGS ■

*Adams G: The sexual history as an integral part of the patient history, Am J Maternal Child Nurs 1:170, 1976.

Convincingly and thoroughly presents the importance of the sexual history in the patient's total health history. Gives the what, why, and how of sexual history taking. Highly recommended for all nurses.

*Anderson ML: Talking about sex with less anxiety, J Psychosoc Nurs Ment Health Serv 18(6):10, 1980.

Helps the professional nurse examine the anxiety often involved in discussing clients' sexual concerns. Discusses anxiety from both client's and nurse's perspective, the causes, and how to reduce it.

Bancroft J: Human sexuality and its problems, New York, 1989, Churchhill Livingstone.

Written for health professionals who are interested in working with people with sexual problems. Excellent review of the field including sexual development, behavior, problems, and treatments.

Bell A, Weinberg M, and Hammersmith S: Sexual preference, Bloomington, Ind, 1981, Indiana University Press.

Asks why some people become homosexuals, whereas others become heterosexuals. Dispels many cherished ideas and suggests that sexual identity is impervious to the influence of parents and psychotherapy. Controversial and important research based on data from interviews with approximately 1,500 individuals.

*deChesnay M: Father-daughter incest: issues in treatment and research, J Psychosoc Nurs Ment Health Serv 22(9):8,16, 1984.

Discusses the practical and legal definitions of incest. Presents the incestuous family as a system that acts to maintain the status quo, and suggests that family therapy can be an effective mode of treatment.

*Deevey S: When mom or dad comes out: helping adolescents cope with homophobia, J Psycho Nurs 27(10):33, 1989.

Uses the nursing process in working with families, particularly adolescents, when parents disclose a gay sexual orientation. Clearly and practically written.

Edelwich J and Brodsky A: Sexual dilemmas for the helping professional, New York, 1982, Brunner/Mazel, Inc.

Provides nurses with many helpful suggestions for intervening in sexual situations with clients. Presents a comprehensive analysis of the sexual feelings between client and therapist.

---

*Asterisk indicated nursing reference.

Covers such rarely discussed topics as client seduction of thera-pist and vice versa; referring clients who arouse sexual feelings in the therapist; and ethical responses to feelings of attraction and seductive behavior. Important reading for any health pro-fessional.

Fromer MJ: Ethical issues in sexuality and reproduction, St Louis, 1983, Mosby—Year Book, Inc.

Examines important ethical issues in sexuality and repro-duction. Discusses ethical theory and such controversial issues as abortion, fetal research, homosexuality, and contraception.

*Hacker SS: Students' questions about sexuality: implica-tions for nurse educators, Nurse Educator 10(4):28, 1984.

Identifies major areas of concern for graduate and student nurses in regard to human sexuality, based on the responses of 350 nurses. Also addresses critical need for sex education in the nursing curriculum.

*Krozy R: Becoming comfortable with sexual assessment, Am J Nurs 78(4):1036, 1980.

Offers practical suggestions for initiating a sexual assess-ment with clients. Discusses nurse's need to be comfortable with human sexuality and gives specific characteristics of the "sexu-ality comfortable person."

Leiblum SR and Rosen RC, editors: Sexual desire disorders, New York, 1988, The Guilford Press.

Contemporary theory, research, and treatment of sexual de-sire disorders are addressed in this comprehensive textbook. It addresses all aspects of the difficulties with sexual desire and in-cludes a variety of treatment approaches. A number of profes-sional viewpoints with case illustrations are included. This text can serve as a valuable resource of the nurse clinician working with clients who experience sexual dysfunction.

Leiblum SR and Rosen RC: Principles and practice of sex therapy, ed 2, New York, 1989, The Guilford Press.

Provides an up-to-date theory and research on the evalua-tion and treatment of sexual disorders and contains contribu-tions by foremost sex therapists. Case examples provide the reader with an understanding of the clinical process of sex ther-apy. Excellent chapters on sexuality and chronic illness and sex therapy in the age of AIDS are included.

*Lion E, editor: Human sexuality in nursing processes, New York, 1982, A Wiley Medical Publication.

In a nursing process format, provides concise case examples of common clinical issues and problems. Discusses sexual devel-opment throughout the life cycle.

Masters WH and Johnson VE: Human sexual response, Bos-ton, 1966, Little, Brown & Co.

Authors' first effort to explore the physiology of sexual re-sponse. Discusses male and female anatomy and physiology and describes research findings regarding sexual response and or-gasm.

Masters WH, Johnson VE, and Kolodny RC: Masters and Johnson on sex and human loving, Boston, 1986, Little, Brown, & Co.

In this comprehensive text the authors present the biological, psychological, and social aspects of sexuality in a highly readable fashion. This book is an excellent resource for the health profes-sional and is also appropriate for the general public. It contains excellent chapters on the areas of sexual development through-out the life cycle, gender roles, sexually transmitted diseases, and sexual disorders and their treatment.

*McCabe S: Male-to-female transsexualism: a case for holis-tic nursing, Arch Psych Nurs 2(1):48, 1988.

Presents overview of the history of sexual reassignment sur-gery with respect to unanticipated psychological and social out-comes. Details problems encountered and implications for the field.

*Moses AE and Hawkins R: Counseling lesbian women and gay men, St Louis, 1982, Mosby—Year Book, Inc.

One of first textbooks to discuss counseling the homosexual client. Addresses such issues as attitudes toward gay people, coming out, and the development of sexual identity. Personal accounts of "gay" clients increases understanding of their spe-cial concerns.

*Poorman SG: Human sexuality and the nursing process, Norwalk, CT, 1988, Appleton & Lange.

Explores concepts of human sexuality from a nursing process perspective. The nursing process is applied to clinical issues, and sample nursing care plans demonstrate the transfer of theoreti-cal knowledge to actual clinical experience. A cognitive self-as-sessment model is included to help nurses understand and eval-uate their own feelings and beliefs and their impact on nursing practice. Sexual acting out behavior and the sexual component of the nurse/patient relationship are also explored.

*Satterfield S and Stayton R: Understanding sexual function and dysfunction, Top Clin Nurs 1:4, 1980.

Discusses the similarities and differences in male and female sexual dysfunction. Helps the reader understand the etiology of sexual dysfunction, disorders of response, and treatment options of the clinician specializing in sex therapy.

*Skeen P, Walters L, and Robinson B: How parents of gays react to their children's homosexuality and to the threat of AIDS, J Psych Nurs 26(12):7, 1988.

Describes the five-stage mourning process experienced by parents who learn of their child's homosexuality and the sup-ports available to them.

*Thomas S: Bisexuality: a sexual orientation of great diver-sity, J Psychosoc Nurs Ment Health Serv 18(4):19, 1980.

One of the few readings devoted to exploring the sexual ori-entation of bisexuality. Very good introduction with reference list for further study.

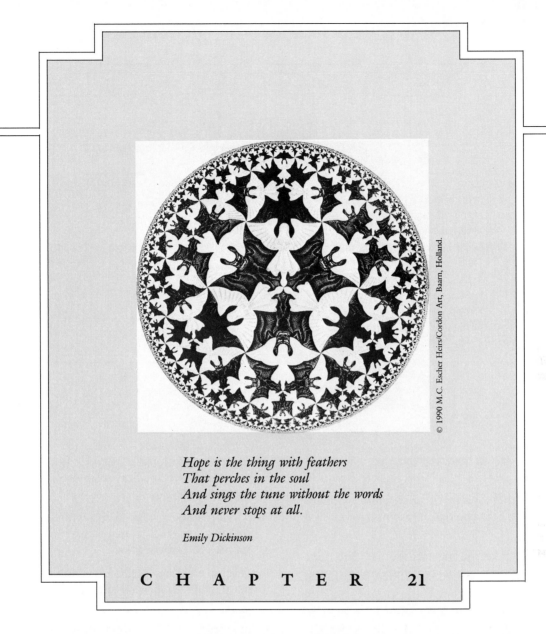

© 1990 M.C. Escher Heirs/Cordon Art, Baarn, Holland.

Hope is the thing with feathers
That perches in the soul
And sings the tune without the words
And never stops at all.

Emily Dickinson

C H A P T E R   21

PSYCHOLOGICAL RESPONSES TO PHYSICAL ILLNESS

DIAGNOSTIC PREVIEW

MEDICAL DIAGNOSES RELATED TO PSYCHOLOGICAL RESPONSES TO PHYSICAL ILLNESS

- Adjustment disorder with
  - Anxious mood
  - Depressed mood
  - Disturbance of conduct
  - Mixed disturbance of emotions and conduct
  - Mixed emotional features
  - Physical complaints
  - Withdrawal
  - Work (or academic) inhibition
- Psychological factors affecting physical condition

LEARNING OBJECTIVES

After studying this chapter, the student should be able to:

- identify characteristics of the experience of illness.

- discuss the concept of uncertainty as it applies to the psychological response to physical illness.

- describe predisposing factors that determine the person's psychological response to physical illness.

- analyze the precipitating stressors related to the nature of the disease that determine the person's psychological response to being physically ill.

- compare and contrast behaviors related to the psychological response to physical illness according to the stage of the illness and the prognosis.

- identify and describe coping behaviors related to the psychological response to physical illness.

- analyze the psychological response to physical illness relative to the nursing model of health-illness phenomena.

- formulate individualized nursing diagnoses for patients that address the psychological response to physical illness.

- assess the relationship between nursing diagnoses and the medical diagnoses of adjustment disorder.

- develop nursing care plans with individualized nursing goals related to psychological responses to physical illness.

- develop a mental health education plan to assist patients to identify and express feelings.

- apply therapeutic nurse-patient relationship principles with an appropriate rationale in planning care to address the psychological needs of a patient with physical illness.

- describe nursing interventions appropriate to the psychological needs of the patient with physical illness.

- assess the importance of the evaluation of the nursing interventions when addressing the psychological needs of patients with physical illness.

- identify directions for future nursing research.

- select appropriate readings for further study.

Illness is an uncommon experience early in the lives of most people. Generally, people develop their ideas about the nature of illness based on their own past experiences. These are usually related to short-term infectious diseases, such as colds or influenza; injuries, such as cuts, burns, sprains, contusions, or fractures; or sometimes relatively minor surgery. Some people have observed more serious or long-term illness in older family members. However, this is not usually believed to have much relevance to oneself. These early experiences lead to expectations about health and illness. Some of these are:

- Physical illness is time limited and usually brief in duration.
- Discomfort can be relieved with medication.
- Most illnesses do not require medical attention.
- Consultation with a health care provider is an extreme measure.
- Physicians can always cure disease and prevent disability.
- Good health is a basic right.
- Good health does not require any particular effort by the person.
- Poor health is the fault of the affected person.
- Disease and infirmity are associated with old age and cannot be prevented.

These beliefs about illness have serious implications for a person who becomes ill. Unless the person perceives himself to be very old, illness is an unexpected event. It is especially hard to adjust to a chronic illness. The person often believes that the problem can be overcome by willpower or that a cure exists; it just needs to be found. Family and friends often share these beliefs. In addition, they may suspect that the person could have prevented the problem by behaving differently, that is, by "taking better care" of himself.

The "blaming the victim" attitude is particularly painful when the illness is, in part, due to the patient's behavior. For instance, infection with the human immunodeficiency virus, type 1 (HIV-1), has been related to sexual relations between gay or bisexual men and to intravenous drug abuse. Both these risk behaviors are considered by many to be socially deviant. In addition, they are believed to be under the control of the person. The occurrence of lung cancer in heavy smokers is another example of an illness that is related to the person's behavior. People with illnesses that are related to life-style carry the burden of responsibility for becoming sick, as well as the impact of the disease

itself. Self-blame and lack of support from others can interfere with coping.

Assumptions about the illness experience are often based on whether it is defined as acute or chronic. Davis[3] has distinguished acute from chronic illness related to the nature of the illness experience, its expected duration, the expected outcomes, the nature and scope of the health services required, and the adaptive tasks of the individual and family. These are summarized in Table 21-1.

Illness differentiated from disease

It is important to differentiate between illness and disease. Benner and Wrubel define illness as the "human experience of loss or dysfunction," whereas disease is the "manifestation of aberration at the tissue, cellular, or organ levels."[2:8] They point out that disease can be present, but the person does not believe himself to be ill unless he is aware of symptoms related to the disease. The severity of illness is not necessarily related to the seriousness of the disease. Some people experience minor injuries as major catastrophes, whereas others ignore serious symptoms and continue to believe that they are well. It is important for nurses to understand this distinction. Much of nursing practice is directed toward assisting the person to cope with the illness. This is the essence of the caring element of nursing. Even when little can be done to change the disease process, nursing intervention can affect the experience of illness.

The psychological response to physical illness should not be confused with psychophysiological disorders, which are diseases that are caused by psychological disruptions. These diseases are discussed in Chapter 12. People with these diseases also experience the psychological responses described in this chapter.

Continuum of psychological responses to physical illness

- **INDIVIDUAL RESPONSES TO ILLNESS.** The nature of the person's response to identifying himself as ill is related to his past experience with illness, his perception of the nature of his illness, and his beliefs about disease and the health care system. At one extreme, the patient responds to illness as an inconvenience, but not a serious threat to his usual functioning. At the other, the patient is overwhelmed by the illness and is unable to carry out his usual activities. These reactions may or may not be related to the actual seriousness of the disease process. Contrast the be-

TABLE 21-1

A COMPARISON OF ASSUMPTIONS ABOUT THE ILLNESS EXPERIENCE AS A CRISIS OR A CHRONIC PHENOMENON

Illness characteristics	Illness as crisis	Illness as chronicity
Nature of illness experience	Acute episodic system disorganization, precipitated by stressful event(s)	Protracted, progressive system dysfunction, often characterized by exacerbation and remission phases
Duration	Short-term, temporary	Long-term, permanent
Expected outcomes	Return to preillness functional levels	Progressive physical loss or functional disability
Nature and scope of health care services	Problem focused Intensive Episodic	Problem and life-style focused Ongoing
Adaptive tasks of individual and family	Cope with stressors Manage anxiety Maintain family stability Mobilize support systems	Monitor/control symptoms Carry out a therapeutic regimen Deal with changes in self-concept and role function Make permanent modifications in life-style Prevent/live with social isolation Maintain/develop strategies to handle episodic crises Maintain personal sense of control

From Davis LL: Image 19:117, 1987.

havior of the patients described in Clinical examples 21-1 and 21-2.

Each of these women reacted in an individual way to the experience of illness. It is important to resist the temptation to place a value on one or the other of their responses. Neither is better or worse than the other. They are just different. Each person eventually recovered from the disease and the illness, returning to a state of wellness.

■ **HOPEFULNESS.** Psychological response to illness is also related to the amount of hope that the person has for recovery. If the person believes that the outlook is hopeful, his psychological response is positive and there is limited need for the use of defense mechanisms. His usual coping responses will be adequate to manage the disequilibrium caused by the illness. On the other hand, if the person believes that his condition is without hope for recovery, there is a major assault on his sense of psychological well-being and ego-defense mechanisms will come into play. In some cases, hopelessness can result in the development of

the mental disorders that are discussed elsewhere in this book. In particular, people with serious physical illnesses are at risk for developing depressive disorders, which can lead to suicidal behavior.

■ **UNCERTAINTY.** Mishel and Braden have applied the concept of uncertainty to the experience of illness. Uncertainty is "the inability to determine the meaning of events."[16:98] This interferes with the person's ability to assess a situation and to predict outcomes. Uncertainty may be related to ambiguity about the illness, complexity of the treatment or the health care system, inadequate information about the diagnosis and its seriousness, or an unpredictable course and prognosis for the illness.

Mishel and Braden[16] have developed a four-stage model of uncertainty in illness. Stage one involves the antecedent events that lead to uncertainty. It includes the pattern of symptoms related to the illness and the person's previous experiences with illness. It also involves "structure providers," such as the credibility of health care providers, the amount of social support

---

CLINICAL EXAMPLE 21-1

Ms. A was a 35-year-old nurse who slipped on an icy sidewalk and twisted her ankle. She immediately applied ice and then an elastic bandage. Although her husband urged her to call her primary physician and arrange for x-ray films, she assured him that it was not serious enough to do this. She borrowed a cane from a friend, which enabled her to walk. Since she was scheduled to attend a continuing education workshop and then had 2 days off, she was confident that she would not miss any work time. Although still limping badly when she did return to work, she negotiated with her head nurse to receive an assignment that minimized the need for her to walk. Within a week, she had resumed her normal activity level, although she continued to limp for the next month.

CLINICAL EXAMPLE 21-2

Ms. B was a 35-year-old nurse who slipped on the ice and twisted her ankle. She called out to her husband and asked him to take her directly to the emergency room, because she feared she had fractured her ankle. Although the intern on duty reviewed the x-ray film and could find no fracture, she insisted that it be reviewed by the orthopedic surgeon on call. No fracture was found again. She was sent home with an elastic bandage and instructions to take an over-the-counter analgesic and resume activity as tolerated. She spent most of the next 5 days in bed and did not return to work for 3 weeks.

---

available, and access to education about the illness. The second stage is appraisal of whether the state of uncertainty is a danger or an opportunity. Uncertainty functions as a danger when the person's inability to determine the meaning of illness-related events leads to pessimism or hopelessness. It may be an opportunity when it allows the person to maintain a positive frame of mind even when the outcome of the illness is likely to be undesirable. Stage three addresses the person's use of coping behaviors to decrease uncertainty appraised as a danger or to maintain it if it is appraised as an opportunity. The last stage represents the adaptation that results from successful coping. Understanding the role that uncertainty plays in a patient's adaptation to an illness can assist the nurse to plan interventions that either support or decrease this response.

Fig. 21-1 illustrates the continuum of psychological responses to physical illness.

 Assessment

■ Predisposing factors

The factors that influence a patient's psychological response to an illness include his knowledge about the disease process, his previous life experience with illness and the health care system, and the support systems that are available to him. Flaskerud[8] has cited the factors that are important to assess concerning a person's psychological response to a diagnosis of acquired immunodeficiency syndrome (AIDS). These include:

- Psychosocial history, including interpersonal relationships, substance abuse, and any previous psychiatric care
- Amount of distress being experienced and crisis response
- Coping skills

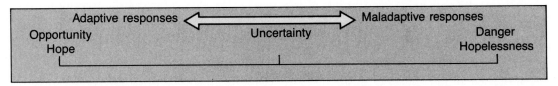

Fig. 21-1. Continuum of psychological responses to physical illness.

- Social support systems, including available resources and the need for additional supports
- Developmental stage
- Phase of illness: immediately postdiagnosis, treatment, posttreatment
- Identity, including self-esteem, valued achievements, goals, and philosophy of life
- Presence of reactions of loss and grief

These factors would be applicable to the assessment of patient's with most illnesses. There is a close relationship to the factors that are assessed during the first phase of crisis intervention. This is because illness is usually experienced as a crisis.

■ **PATIENT'S KNOWLEDGE ABOUT THE DISEASE.** In addition to the factors just listed, it is important to discover the patient's knowledge about his disease. Lack of information or misunderstanding of information can increase the patient's anxiety and interfere with recovery. Sometimes the person's information base is related to his sociocultural background. For instance, some religious belief systems regard disease as punishment for sins. A person with this belief may need to participate in a religious healing experience to recover a sense of wellness. Folk medicine is effective in dealing with many health problems. This may be due in part to characteristics of the treatment that can be explained scientifically. However, it is often also related to the patient's belief that the treatment will be effective and to his trust in the healer.

■ **PAST EXPERIENCE WITH ILLNESS.** The person's past experience with illness, either his own or that of someone close to him, also influences his response to a current illness. If past illnesses were mild and over quickly, the person may become frustrated if he develops a chronic disease requiring long-term treatment. On the other hand, if his experience with illness is that the person never completely recovers, he may be very anxious over even a minor disease. This aspect of the person's response may be related to the specific medical diagnosis with which he has been presented. For instance, most people respond to a diagnosis of cancer with fear and anxiety. This is related to past experiences with the disease, both direct and indirect. Even if the person has not known someone with cancer, he has undoubtedly read or heard about cancer patients. Often the story of someone who has recovered from cancer is described as a stroke of good fortune or even a miracle.

■ **SELF-PERCEPTION AND OUTLOOK ON LIFE.** The patient's response to illness will be affected by his perception of himself and his outlook on life. If he is generally an optimistic person who feels competent

and in control of his life, he will approach illness with more confidence in a positive outcome than a person who is pessimistic and feels out of control. If the person has a well-developed set of coping skills, he will adjust more quickly to the demands of being ill. If he has a firm philosophy of life and if he has confronted his feelings about loss and death, he will be stronger in facing serious illness. In his work with cancer patients, Siegel[19] has recognized the importance of a will to live and a positive mental attitude for recovery. Even patients who eventually die feel better prepared if they have confronted their illness and participated actively in the treatment process.

■ **RESILIENCE.** Resilience is a characteristic that Kadner has described as "an individual's capacity to make a psychosocial comeback in adversity."[10:20] It is defined as "an ability to recover from or adjust easily to misfortune or change" and is conceptualized as an aggregate of ego strength, social intimacy, and resourcefulness. Kadner contrasts resilience to the concept of hardiness. Hardiness consists of commitment, control, and challenge. Commitment involves an ability to involve oneself in an experience. Control is the belief in one's ability to influence the outcome of an experience. Challenge is the belief that change is normal and stimulating. According to Kadner, resilience may be more applicable in cases of serious physical illness when the patient is unable to control the outcome.

■ **Precipitating stressors**

■ **TRANSITION TO ILLNESS.** The primary stressor related to the psychological response to a physical illness is the recognition of a symptom of disease or the diagnosis of the disease. It is at this point that the person becomes the patient and recognizes himself as someone who is ill. Sometimes this transition is quite sudden. For example, a person who is in an automobile accident moves very rapidly into the identity of patient. At other times, the realization that one is ill happens gradually as symptoms accumulate or become hard to ignore. For instance, a person who is developing heart disease may notice shortness of breath on exertion, occasional palpitations, and episodes of lightheadedness. However, he may rationalize these and only seek medical attention when he has chest pain.

The suddenness of the transition from wellness to illness may itself be a stressor. Some people ignore symptoms until they have prepared themselves to be ill. For example, an accountant who has recurrent headaches may treat them with acetylsalicylic acid (aspirin) until after April 15. Some people schedule elective surgery far enough in advance that they can prepare themselves by engaging in health-promoting activities such as exercising and dietary changes. Not only are they better prepared physically, but they approach surgery with a positive attitude and a sense of control over the outcome. If illness occurs without an opportunity to become prepared, the person has more difficulty coping with the change in his life.

■ **PROGNOSIS FOR THE OUTCOME OF THE DISEASE.** The prognosis for the outcome of the disease may be a stressor. People assume that some diseases such as cancer or infection with HIV-1 are always fatal. Being informed of such a diagnosis creates a major crisis for the person. The diagnosis of a disease that is not fatal, but not curable, is also stressful. The amount of stress that is experienced will be related in part to the amount of disability that is expected. For instance, a person is likely to experience greater stress if he becomes paraplegic as the result of an automobile accident than he would if he receives a diagnosis of osteoarthritis resulting in intervals of limited range of motion.

A related factor is the nature of the person's expectations related to convalescence. Davis[3] speaks of the "punctuated progress" of convalescence. By this, she means that the course of recovery from illness is often characterized by progress followed by stabilization at a new functional level and then more progress. This sequence can be frustrating to the patient who evaluates his progress based on an expectation of steady improvement. The impact is similar to the discouragement felt by a dieter who loses several pounds and then reaches a plateau during which no weight is lost even though the diet is still followed faithfully.

■ **INTERVENTIONS REQUIRED FOR TREATMENT.** Stress may also be related to the extent of intervention that is required to treat the disease. If the physician says, "Take two aspirins and call me tomorrow," the patient is likely to feel relieved. However, a recommendation of major surgery, especially if disfigurement or loss of a body part is involved, is very stressful. Interventions may also be perceived as stressful if they continue over a long period of time with little, if any, noticeable progress. An example of this is kidney dialysis for chronic renal failure. Many patients prefer the risk of kidney transplant surgery because of the possibility that they will be able to lead a more normal life.

■ **RESPONSE OF SIGNIFICANT OTHERS.** The responses of significant others can reduce or increase the patient's stress. It is often difficult for a person to tell others about the diagnosis of a serious illness. Repeating the diagnosis may result in reexperiencing all the feelings that were present when it was originally presented to the patient. An emotional response from the other person may cause the patient to cover up his own feelings to spare the other. On the other hand, an unemotional response may make the patient feel isolated and depressed. Telling significant others may be especially difficult for a person with AIDS. It often involves informing them about a life-style as well as a disease. This imposes an additional stress on the patient at a time when his coping resources are likely to be limited.

In a study of the wives of men who had cancer, Kalayjian[11] found four major areas of difficulty for the spouses: emotional, social, family, and financial. Emotional difficulties were related to uncertainty about the future, fear of death, feelings of helplessness and hopelessness, and doubt in previous religious beliefs. Social difficulties were revealed in feelings of loneliness. Family problems were related to changes in routines and childrens' reactions to the father's illness. Financial concerns involved worry over the loss of a substantial part of the family's income.

A supportive response by loved ones can be very helpful to the patient as he tries to adjust to his illness. Sometimes the family has suspected that the person was ill. They may be relieved that he is seeking help. They can help him learn about his disease and assist him with treatment and rehabilitation. The supportive family avoids blaming either the patient or themselves for the disease. Rather, they join forces with the patient to return to wellness.

Behaviors

The behaviors associated with the psychological response to physical illness represent the patient's attempt to cope with a stressful experience. Some of the behaviors that may occur are discussed in detail elsewhere in this book. They include fear and anxiety (Chapter 11), depression and grieving (Chapter 14), self-destructive behavior (Chapter 15), and anger (Chapter 17). Behaviors are discussed here in relationship to the various stages of the illness experience, including diagnosis, treatment, and convalescence.

■ **CRISIS RESPONSE.** At the time of diagnosis, the patient is in a state of crisis. Even for a relatively minor illness such as a cold or influenza, immediate adjustments must be made in planned activities. Appointments must be canceled; child care arrangements must be made or changed; dietary habits may be altered; social roles may need adjustment. The patient reacts to these demands with annoyance. There may also be a sense of relief that obligations are set aside and that one can focus energy on getting well. There may also be a degree of enjoyment if the person is able to avoid or postpone undesirable activities and be taken care of by others. This is the *secondary gain* that is part of the illness experience.

■ **RESPONSE TO THE DIAGNOSIS.** For more serious diseases, the labeling of symptoms with a medical diagnosis can be a psychologically devastating experience. Behaviors will reflect the person's attempt to absorb the information and cope with it. The initial reaction is frequently one of shock and disbelief. The patient may demand additional diagnostic tests or a second opinion. The person is reacting to a serious loss—the loss of his image of himself as a person who is basically well. This change in self-concept is extremely threatening. Some patients respond with the expression of emotions, including sadness and anger. Others seem numb and show no outward feelings. If the disease can be cured or controlled, the person may cling to that information and have many questions about what is to be done next. It is important to remember that the patient is probably very anxious and unable to retain complex information. Any information that is provided at this time should be repeated later. If possible, it should also be given to a significant other.

The treatment phase of the illness may be of short duration. In this case, the patient's behavior will focus on getting well and returning to his usual activities. There is likely to be some regression demonstrated by staying in bed, eating favorite foods associated with being sick, and light activity accompanied by a sense of "playing hookey." Some people become demanding and dependent. Others act like martyrs and persist in their usual activities even though it is obvious that they are miserable.

The psychological responses to serious and long-term physical illness are complex. They are determined in part by the person's personality structure and his

CLINICAL EXAMPLE 21-3

Mr. C is a 42-year-old attorney with a medical diagnosis of AIDS. The diagnosis was made on the basis of a positive blood test for antibodies to HIV-1 and an episode of *Pneumocystis carinii* pneumonia. Mr. C recovered from the pneumonia and receives aerosol pentamidine prophylactically. He lives in a house that he has shared for many years with his lover, Mr. K.

At the time of the diagnosis of AIDS, Mr. C said that he was not surprised. He had had a sexual encounter with a man who had died from the disease and had suspected that he might have contracted it. He decided not to be tested because he was not sure that he wanted to know if he was infected. He did practice safe sex to protect Mr. K, although he did not tell Mr. K that he could be infected. He justified this by saying that all gay men were well informed about the risk and the need to protect themselves. When the diagnosis was made, the clinical nurse specialist offered to assist him to tell Mr. K and any other people who would need or want to know. Mr. C said he was able to tell Mr. K, who was upset but not surprised at the diagnosis. Mr. C did not want anyone else to know his diagnosis. He said that he feared losing his clients and being ostracized by the legal community if his condition was known.

Following discharge from the hospital, Mr. C resumed his work. By pacing himself and cutting back on extra activities, he was able to feel fairly well. He was irritable and tended to avoid other people aside from his clients, co-workers, and Mr. K. He also had dreams about violence or sometimes loss. He felt sad if he thought about his illness, so he tried to keep his mind occupied with other things. He found it helpful to spend time at his hobby of refinishing furniture.

Mr. C's nephew was getting married. He felt compelled to attend the wedding to avoid disappointing his mother. Several family members remarked about how thin he was and asked him if he was well. He denied any illness, but he was tempted to tell his mother the truth. He found that it was a great strain to keep his secret.

When Mr. C returned home from the wedding, he experienced difficulty concentrating. He was obsessed with thoughts that he had failed his family. He had a longing to return to his mother's house and ask her to care for him as she had when he was sick as a child. His inability to do this made him very depressed. When Mr. K expressed concern for him, Mr. C shouted at him and told him to leave him alone. Mr. K went out for several hours. When he returned, he found Mr. C unconscious. There was a note nearby saying that he was too much of a burden to himself and others so he had decided to take his life. He was taken to the hospital, where he recovered from his overdose of sedatives and alcohol. Referral was made to the community mental health center for treatment of his depression and to a peer support group for people with AIDS.

usual response to stress. The physical diseases of cancer and AIDS are used to illustrate these responses. Clinical example 21-3 illustrates some behaviors that might occur in response to a diagnosis of AIDS.

■ **"DOING WELL."** Kendall and colleagues[12] interviewed three patients with AIDS who were identified as "doing well." They identified five dimensions of behavior that contributed to doing well. The first was a feeling of autonomy or mastery over the disease. This could be related to selection of a particular type of treatment or to choosing when to terminate treatment and wait for death. The second theme was the presence of spiritual or existential beliefs. It was important to the patients to feel in touch with the essence of themselves. For some, this was related to a religious belief. For others, it came from an existential experience. The third dimension was self-acceptance. This related to a need to assume responsibility for their own health without blaming themselves for the disease. The fourth need was to stay active and involved. Each man described the importance of participating in life. For one person, this meant taking an active role in directing his treatment. The final dimension was positive thinking. In fact, these patients expressed some reluctance to participate in peer support groups because they were too negative and depressing.

The patients just described represent a positive and hopeful response to their illness. It would be unusual for this to be the response early in the treatment phase of the illness. Feinblum[7] points out that AIDS causes a series of losses for patients. These include the loss of usual activities, both social and vocational; loss of relationships; and the loss of one's perception of oneself as healthy. People respond to loss with grief. People with serious illnesses grieve for their current losses, and if the disease is terminal, for the anticipated loss of their lives and their future plans and hopes.

■ **HOPE AND HOPELESSNESS.** Hopelessness is a behavior that is closely related to grief. Hope has been defined by Dufault and Martocchio as, "a *multidimensional* dynamic life force characterized by a *confident* yet *uncertain* expectation of achieving a future *good* which, to the hoping person, is *realistically* possible and *personally significant*" (authors' emphasis).[4] Lange[15] has identified behaviors that are related to hope and to despair, or hopelessness (Table 21-2). Based on their review of the literature, Farran and Popovich[6] have identified four central attributes of hope:

1. Hope related to some trial, captivity, or suffering
2. Hope involving aspects of transcendence, freedom, and faith
3. Hope as a rational thought process
4. Hope as a relational or interactional process

Each of these attributes has relevance for the response of patients to serious illness.

Hopelessness implies giving up. It is the experience of an uncertain situation as dangerous. Patients who feel hopeless are reluctant to participate in treatment for their illness. They become passive recipients of health care. They may appear to be unmotivated. However, it is more likely that they see no purpose in attempting to treat their condition. This may be especially serious when there is a potentially effective treatment available. For instance, many patients with chronic illnesses such as hypertension and diabetes mellitus fail to comply with their prescribed treatment. Noncompliance with medical treatment is addressed in Chapter 15. Another example of self-destructive behavior related to hopelessness is the case of a patient with cancer who refuses to have surgery even though there is a good chance that he will be cured. This patient is responding to his perception of the prognosis for a person with cancer. Hopelessness may also lead to suicidal behavior. This represents the total absence of hope for an improved life. For some people with terminal illnesses, it may also represent the need to be in control of one's fate.

■ **STIGMA.** The loss of important relationships can be especially difficult for people with serious illnesses. Some diseases, such as AIDS and cancer, are associated with a stigma. This is the same as the stigma attached to serious mental illness. When stigma is present, undesirable characteristics are attributed to the patient. This attribution is irrational and has nothing to do with the person's actual behavior. It leads to retribution toward the sick person. An example of behavior related to stigma is the arson of the home of three hemophiliac brothers who had AIDS. People with AIDS may be portrayed as sexually promiscuous or mentally unstable. This is also related to stigma. Stigma may also affect those who are associated with patients who have these illnesses. O'Donnell and Bernier[18] have addressed the topic of stigma as it is experienced by the parents of people with AIDS. Family members feel isolated because they are reluctant to tell anyone about their child's diagnosis. They are often confronting not only the fact of AIDS, but also the equally stigmatizing fact that their son is homosexual.

Nurses who work in AIDS or oncology settings are often asked why they have chosen such work. Significant others may encourage them to select a different clinical setting. Some nurses are reluctant to tell others where they work because they want to avoid

---

TABLE 21-2

COMPARISON OF HOPE AND DESPAIR BEHAVIORS

Hope	Despair
Activation	**Hypoactivation**
Feeling vitality, vibrancy	Feeling all excitement, vitality gone
Having energy and drive	Feeling empty, drained, heavy
Feeling inner buoyancy	Being understimulated
Seeming to be more alert and wide awake	Feelings seeming to be dulled
Experiencing everything fully	Feeling tired, sleepy
Feeling interest and involvement	Feeling dead inside
Feeling like singing	Feeling mentally dull
Comfort	**Discomfort**
Having a sense of well-being	Having a lump in one's throat
Feeling harmony and peace within	Sensing loss, deprivation
Feeling free of conflict	Heart seeming to ache
Feeling loose, relaxed	Not being able to smile or laugh
Feeling general release, lessening of tension	Having whole body tense, feeling wound up inside
Feeling safe and secure	Feeling trapped, boxed in
Feeling life is worth living	Being easily irritated, hypersensitive
Feeling optimistic about the future	Feeling under a heavy burden
Moving toward people	**Moving away from people**
Having an intense positive relationship with another	Having a sense of unrelatedness
Reaching out	Wanting to withdraw, be alone
Having a sense of being wanted and needed	Lacking involvement
Feeling much respect and interdependence	Not caring about anyone
Wanting to touch, hold, be close	Feeling a certain distance
Sensing empathic harmony with another	Wanting to crawl into oneself
Competence	**Incompetence**
Feeling strong inside	Feeling that nothing one does is right
Having a sense of sureness	Feeling a sense of regret
Feeling taller, stronger, bigger	Feeling vulnerable and totally helpless
Being more confident in oneself	Feeling caught up and overwhelmed
Having a sense of accomplishment, fulfillment	Having no sense of control over situation
Really functioning as a unit	Longing to have things as they were
Being motivated	Feeling unmotivated and afraid to try

Adapted from Lange SP: Hope. In Carlson CE and Blackwell B, editors: Behavioral concepts and nursing intervention, Philadelphia, 1978, JB Lippincott Co.

---

the stigma. The best way to combat stigma is to confront it with factual information. However, since stigma is an irrational response, many will persist in their beliefs.

■ **SOCIAL ISOLATION.** Social isolation is frequently experienced by people with serious illnesses. This is sometimes related to their lack of energy to invest in pursuing continued contact with acquaintances. They may also be uncertain about how their friends feel about them. Fear of rejection may keep them from pursuing relationships. Sometimes these fears are well founded. Many people are frightened or threatened by serious illness. It forces them to confront their own mortality. AIDS and cancer both strike many young people. Their friends may procrastinate about seeing them to avoid their own discomfort. Older people may also be reluctant because they see their own imminent fate. It is important for the patient to know that people are not avoiding him because of dislike or disgust, but that they have not dealt with their own feelings about illness and death.

It is possible to feel isolated even when surrounded by people. Dying is in many ways a solitary experience. Some very ill people prefer to limit their visitors to a few close relatives and friends. They choose people who are sensitive to their feelings and will not need to deny the reality of the seriousness of the illness. The need for interpersonal contact tends to fluctuate during the course of an illness. A person who is angry may appreciate having someone near who can listen to his raging without taking it personally. A person who is depressed may want to spend time alone while he dwells on his situation. A terminally ill person who has accepted his fate may wish to spend time with family and friends to complete unfinished business and say goodbye. Even when the person prefers to be alone, it is always important that he know that close ones are nearby and ready to be with him. That protects him from the loneliness of social isolation.

■ **CONVALESCENCE.** In most cases of illness, the final stage is convalescence, which leads to complete or partial recovery. Norris[17] has identified the expectations that others have of the person who is recuperating. They are that he "be grateful for his recovery, cheerful about joining his loved ones, and eager to begin picking up pieces of his usual way of life."[17:47] These expectations are not usually met. In contrast, the convalescing person is likely to respond to continued helplessness by being easily upset and anxious; responses are apt to be out of proportion to the situation. He will probably have trouble concentrating. He will be frustrated with his continued limitations and his inability to meet the expectations of others and himself. Norris adds that the major work of convalescence is "reassessment of life's goals; modifying one's purposes and values; looking and working toward new meaning; and redirecting one's energy toward the development of one's potential for living, for self-actualization."[17:47] It is no wonder that the patient is sometimes preoccupied or irritable.

During convalescence, the "patient" must make the transition back to "person." This requires giving up behaviors that were learned as part of the sick role. There must be a gradual resumption of independence. The self-concept must shift back to one of wellness and health. This may be reinforced by the assumption of new health-related behaviors, such as dietary changes or exercise regimens. The role structure of the family must also revert to its preillness state. Sometimes it is hard for family members who have temporarily taken on the roles of others to relinquish them. For example, an eldest child who assisted in parenting younger siblings might continue in this behavior and feel in competition with the recovered parent. The convalescent person may feel left out and unappreci-

ated as the family continues to function without his usual contribution.

■ **TERMINAL ILLNESS.** When the patient is terminally ill, the final stage of illness-related psychological behavior is directed toward preparation for death. The classic analysis of behaviors related to dying was done by Kübler-Ross.[14] She identified five stages in the dying process. The first stage is denial. The patient refuses to acknowledge that death is inevitable. The next stage is anger. The patient feels rage at his fate and demands to know why he has been afflicted. This is followed by bargaining. The patient tries to negotiate with a higher power for more time, usually to accomplish an important goal. Next comes depression, when the patient again confronts the inevitability of death. At this point he recognizes the losses that death entails. The final stage is acceptance. The patient has made peace with his life and is prepared to leave it. It should be remembered that all patients do not experience all the stages and that they do not progress through them step by step. Each person has his own unique pattern to preparing for death. By recognizing the stage he is in, the nurse can understand his behavior and assist him to deal with the challenge of dying.

■ **Coping mechanisms**

Denial is a prominent coping mechanism related to physical illness. It serves a protective function by allowing the patient to reach full understanding of his illness gradually. This prevents the overwhelming anxiety that could occur, especially if there is a diagnosis of a serious illness. It is important to support the patient's denial until he communicates that he is ready to give it up.

Regression is another coping mechanism that is usually present with physical illness. This mechanism enables the person to accept the dependence that accompanies the patient role. It also contributes to the secondary gain that may make it difficult to give up the sick role during the period of convalescence.

Compensation is in action when a patient overfunctions to overcome the limitations imposed by illness. For example, a mother who feels guilty because she is unable to clean her house may decide to knit sweaters for every member of the family. She may spend all her time on this project, even though opportunities for other activities are offered.

Aside from defense mechanisms, people with physical illnesses use whatever ways of coping that have worked for them in the past. Some people want to read about their problem and discuss the information that they learn. Others may escape into television, gardening, puzzles, or other hobbies. Sometimes patients cope best if they have time alone so they can think through the meaning of their illness to them. As a part of the nursing assessment, the nurse should find out the person's usual way of coping with stress. If possible, he should be helped to use his favored coping mechanisms.

 ## Nursing diagnosis

The formulation of nursing diagnoses for patients with physical illnesses should always take into account the psychological response. Mental attitude toward being sick and toward the illness itself has a significant impact on the recovery process. Particular attention should be paid to cognitive functioning, mood, and self-concept.

The box below presents primary NANDA diagnoses and complete nursing diagnoses for psychological responses to physical illnesses. Medical and nursing diagnoses for these patients are listed in Table 21-3. The nursing model of health-illness behavior as it relates to psychological response to physical illness is presented in Fig. 21-2.

Nursing Diagnoses Related to Responses to Physical Illness

Primary NANDA nursing diagnoses

Adjustment, impaired
Role performance, altered

Examples of complete nursing diagnoses

Impaired adjustment related to diagnosis of acquired immunodeficiency syndrome (AIDS), evidenced by refusal to get out of bed and angry rejection of help

Impaired adjustment related to exacerbation of sickle cell anemia, evidenced by refusal to arrange for return to school

Altered role performance related to 2-week hospitalization, evidenced by verbalized fear of caring for baby

Altered role performance related to concern about cardiac status after open heart surgery, evidenced by suggesting that wife take over family financial management

---

■ Related medical diagnoses

Patients who are physically ill do not usually have behavioral disruptions that are serious enough to require a psychiatric medical diagnosis. If the person does show evidence of a mental disorder, it is important to request consultation from a psychiatrist or psychiatric liaison nurse. Unless the patient has a history of mental illness, the psychiatric diagnosis is most likely to be one of the adjustment disorders or that of psychological factors affecting physical condition.

■ **ADJUSTMENT DISORDERS.** The diagnostic criteria for adjustment disorder[1] include: (1) the disorder occurs within 3 months of the onset of identifiable psychosocial stressor(s) and lasts no more than 6 months; (2) adaptive problems are indicated by impaired functioning at work or school, problems with social relationships or activities, or symptoms that are out of proportion to the stressor; and (3) it does not represent a pattern of response to stress and is not an exacerbation of another mental disorder. There is not a predictable relationship between the seriousness of the response and the severity of the stressor. Specific anxiety and mood disorders or uncomplicated bereavement should be ruled out.

Types of adjustment disorders[1] include:

a. **with anxious mood:** predominant symptoms are nervousness, worry, and jitteriness

b. **with depressed mood:** predominant symptoms are depressed mood, tearfulness, and feelings of hopelessness

c. **with disturbance of conduct:** predominant behavior is in violation of the rights of others or of age-appropriate norms and rules

d. **with mixed disturbance of emotions and conduct:** combination of behaviors related to b and c

e. **with mixed emotional features:** combination of behaviors related to a and b

f. **with physical complaints:** predominant symptoms are physical and not related to a physical diagnosis

g. **with withdrawal:** predominant behavior is withdrawal without depressed or anxious mood

h. **with work (or academic) inhibition:** predominant behavior is a decline in work or academic functioning when previous performance has been adequate; may be accompanied by anxiety and depression

■ **PSYCHOLOGIC FACTORS AFFECTING PHYSICAL ILLNESS.** This disorder occurs when psychologically environmental stimuli are temporarily related to the initiation or exacerbation of a specific physical condition or disorder that involves either organic pathology or a known pathophysiologic process.

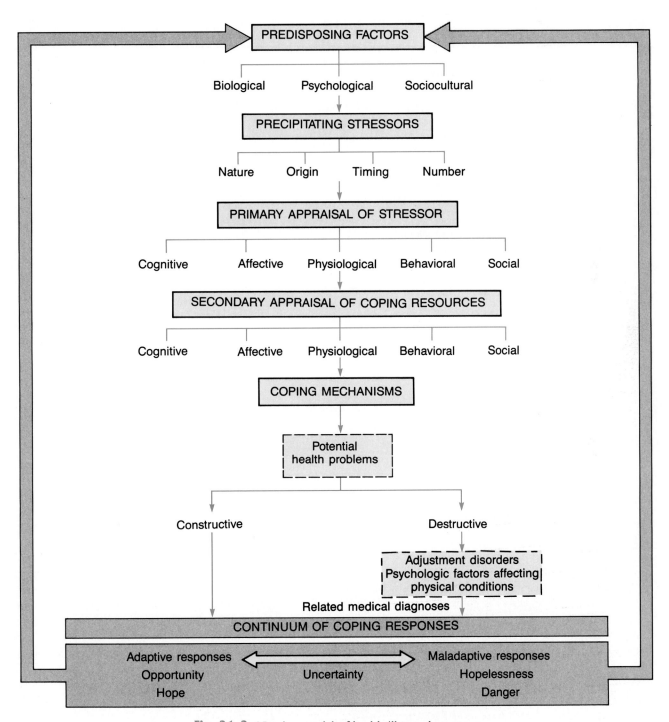

Fig. 21-2. Nursing model of health-illness phenomena.

Planning

■ Goal setting

The main goal for a patient who has difficulty adjusting to a physical illness is to assist him to develop an attitude of hopefulness by realistically confronting his illness and reassuming control of his life. Short-term goals related to this overall goal will address the specific issues causing the adjustment problem. In most cases, these will include goals related to the expression of feelings, changes in self-concept, and mobilization of social support systems. In addition, patients will usually need to be taught about the nature of the illness and related self-care activities.

The nursing care plan builds on the goals for nursing intervention. A sample nursing care plan is presented in Fig 21-3. This plan is based on Clinical example 21-3, the case of Mr. C, the person with AIDS who attempted suicide. The plan is meant to provide an example. It does not address his physiological needs and is only a partial plan for his psychosocial needs. Planning also involves addressing the learning needs of the patient and family. Table 21-4 presents a mental health education plan for a group of patients with problems related to the psychological responses to physical illness. This plan is designed to assist patients to experience and label feelings without requiring them to share their own feelings with the group. Personal feelings may be revealed during the discussion, but this is not an expected outcome.

Implementation

Most people are aware that they have symptoms of a physical illness before a diagnostic label is given.

PSYCHIATRIC NURSING CARE PLAN

Precautions:
  Suicide precautions 1:1

Special nursing needs:

Visitors: {x} No restrictions
  { } Family only
  { } Restricted to:

  { } No visitors

Telephone: { } Limited
  {x } Unlimited

Privileges: {x} Restricted to unit
  { } Off unit accompanied by staff
  { } Off unit accompanied by family/visitor
  { } Off unit unaccompanied
  { } Out of hospital leave (dates)

Assessment data summary: Recently hospitalized with *Pneumocystis carinii* pneumonia; uses pentamidine aerosol; partner knows of AIDS diagnosis and is committed to relationship; family does not know diagnosis; has continued to work; isolated self from friends; dreams of violence/loss; overdose of drugs/alcohol; left note

Nursing diagnoses: 1. Impaired adjustment related to AIDS diagnosis, evidenced by nightmares and inability to tell family.
2. Potential for self-directed violence related to feelings about illness, evidenced by overdose of drugs and alcohol.

Treatment goal: Acceptance of feelings related to diagnosis

Date	Problem/need	Expected outcome (objective)	Target Date	Nursing Intervention
8/2	Suicide attempt	To express feelings in words, not actions	8/9	Provide safe environment; establish trust; use nondirective communication
8/2	Social isolation	To accept visits from family and friends	8/9	Offer to spend time with him during visits; help to talk with visitors about illness and his feelings

Room	Patient's name	Age	Doctor	Primary nurse	Admit date
45	Mr. C	42	Dr. O	Ms. Z	8/2/90

Fig. 21-3. Psychiatric nursing care plan for a patient with an adjustment disorder related to AIDS. (This nursing care plan includes examples of the elements of a total plan as it might appear at a particular time in the patient's course of treatment. It should not be considered all inclusive.)   *Continued.*

Date	Medications	Date	P.R.N. Medications	Diagnostic & psychiatric tests	Req.	Done
8/2	Pentamidine			Routine CBC	8/2	8/2
	aerosol self-					
	administered					
		Date	Treatments	Special orders and concerns		
				Avoid exposure to infectious illness		

Allergies:	Medical diagnosis: (axis I-III)	Diet:
None	Adjustment disorder with depressed mood Acquired immunodeficiency syndrome	Regular

Fig. 21-3, cont'd. Psychiatric nursing care plan for a patient with an adjustment disorder related to AIDS.

The nurse who interacts with the patient at the time of diagnosis should explore the patient's expectations. The patient is likely to be worried about the meaning of his symptoms. Understanding his fears will assist the nurse to provide support in adapting to the diagnosis. Common patient fears include loss of function, disfigurement, and death. The patient is not likely to express a fear directly, especially if the nurse is a stranger. The nurse needs to be alert to indirect communications of fear and anxiety. For instance, the person who fears loss of function may express an urgent need to return to work soon; the person who fears death may ask if the nurse has seen anyone else with the same symptoms and ask if they recovered. Nonverbal communications are also significant. Signs of anxiety should be expected. The person may fidget, pace, turn pages of a book without seeming to read, or sigh frequently. The nurse may offer to talk with the patient, but some people will prefer not to engage in conversation.

■ **CARING.** The most important nursing intervention at every phase of the patient's illness experience is the communication of caring. According to Benner and Wrubel,[2] caring means that "persons, events,

projects, and things matter to people." They have provided several reasons for why caring comes first.

1. "Because caring sets up what matters to a person, it also sets up what counts as stressful, and what options are available for coping. Caring creates possibility."
2. There is an enabling condition of connection and concern. This means that the one who cares focuses attention on the care recipient and his needs.
3. Caring "sets up the possibility of giving help and receiving help."[2]

The nurse communicates caring by accepting the patient as a valued person and respecting his thoughts, feelings, and needs. Acceptance does not always mean agreement with the patient's beliefs or decisions; it does mean that he has a right to these. Nurses should be aware that a person with a physical illness is vulnerable. Arguing with a patient about his decisions is coercive rather than caring. A caring nurse does help the patient identify health care alternatives and assists him to evaluate the choices that are available to him. However, the final choice belongs to the patient.

TABLE 21-4

MENTAL HEALTH EDUCATION PLAN: NONVERBAL EXPRESSION OF FEELINGS

Content	Instructional activities	Evaluation
List feelings associated with physical illness	Ask group members to name feelings that might be associated with having a physical illness Write feelings on blackboard	Members each name one feeling
Describe ways of expressing feelings	Ask for examples of behavior that communicates a feeling	Members each describe a behavior
Differentiate between verbal and nonverbal behaviors	Identify verbal and nonverbal behaviors from list	
Express one feeling nonverbally	Pass out slips of paper with a feeling named on each Ask each person in turn to communicate that feeling to the group without talking Group members are to name the feeling	Each member acts out a feeling; other members guess what feeling is portrayed
Discuss level of comfort with expressing feelings	Using the group experience, lead discussion of usual behavior related to communicating feelings to others	Members share responses to revealing feelings

This process can be difficult when the patient and the nurse have different value systems. Issues such as refusal of treatment and termination of life support often create conflict for nurses. If a nurse feels uncomfortable with a patient's belief system, it is best to refer him to another staff member for discussions about that issue. She can acknowledge to the patient that she views things differently, but she respects his right to his beliefs.

Caring also implies accessibility. Busy nurses sometimes seem uninterested in patients. Even if there are only a few minutes available for the patient, the nurse can concentrate completely on him and his needs during that time. When that happens, the patient feels important and the nurse obtains a clear picture of the patient's status.

Touch communicates caring. The use of touch can range from a handshake to a hug. The appropriate type of touch to use depends on the situation. Much of physical nursing care involves touching the patient. The nurse needs to be aware of where and how she is touching the patient. Gentle touch tends to be soothing. Necessary infliction of pain should be explained and followed by gentle touch. Touch has been found to have healing properties.[13] With special training, some nurses practice healing touch therapy. The nurse also needs to understand the sociocultural meaning of touch to herself and the patient. Some cultures teach

that touching another is unacceptable, particularly if the people are strangers. Other cultures encourage touching. Nurses who are uncomfortable with touch may need to seek help in becoming desensitized.

■ **THERAPEUTIC COMMUNICATION.** Communication skills are as important in the care of physically ill patients as they are with the mentally ill. Physical symptoms may represent an effort to communicate feelings about the illness. For example, pain is increased when the patient is anxious, fearful, or depressed. In addition to giving a prescribed analgesic, the nurse can be helpful by assisting the patient to cope with his feelings.

Listening is essential; not only listening to the words that are spoken and their meanings, but also listening for what is implied, denied, or left unsaid. This type of listening requires the nurse's full attention. Although it may be difficult to find the time to listen attentively to a troubled patient, time can be saved because the patient will be more comfortable and make fewer demands.

Patients shield themselves from the anxiety caused by a physical diagnosis by using coping mechanisms. Some of these behaviors may appear destructive. For example, an executive who has been told that he needs coronary bypass surgery spends hours on the telephone with his office. Although the business activity may appear to be stressful, it is evidence of his use of the defense mechanism of denial. Denial is protecting him from the anxiety that his impending surgery causes. If his telephone were to be removed and he was forced to rest in bed, his anxiety would likely increase. This could be even more stressful than calling the office. The nurse who cares for this patient needs to be available to talk with him about his illness. As surgery nears, he will probably reach a point when he is ready to talk. The nurse who has been supportive will be trusted enough to be allowed to hear his feelings. If a patient insists on performing a particular activity or talks repetitively about an apparently unrelated subject, it is likely that the behavior is a coping mechanism.

Patients may also need to develop new, more effective coping behaviors. If the patient is exhibiting behaviors that are potentially destructive to him or to others, the nurse will need to assist him to find substitutes. Some behaviors that are not effective ways of coping include severe or prolonged depression, crippling anxiety or fear, extreme anger, withdrawal, and substance abuse. Nursing interventions related to these behavioral patterns are described in other chapters of this book.

■ **RELAXATION AND GUIDED IMAGERY.** This intervention is described in Chapter 11. Relaxation therapy and guided imagery are especially helpful for patients who have illnesses that are related to stress or are anxiety provoking. Zahourek has written that relaxation and imagery are "believed to interrupt the disease process and to foster health by dramatically reducing stress and discomfort, enhancing positive feeling states, and enriching perceptions; all of these effects subsequently encourage healing."[20:4] Simple relaxation techniques are easily learned. They have the additional benefit of being within the patient's control at a time when he may feel out of control of much of his life. Siegel[19] reports that the use of these techniques has been very helpful to many of his patients who have cancer.

■ **PATIENT EDUCATION.** The moment of diagnosis is a stressful one. The diagnostician usually provides information about the illness, further diagnostic studies if needed, and an initial treatment plan. It is very important for the nurse to review this information with the patient to be sure that it has been understood. If possible, the patient should be provided with written materials to keep with him. Written materials should also be reviewed to be sure that they are relevant to the patient. Patients vary in their desire for information about their illness. Some go directly to the public library to seek books about their problem. Others are confused if they try to absorb too much infor-

mation too quickly. The nurse can help by offering to teach the patient about the diagnosis, but allowing the patient to decide when he is ready to learn.

■ **MOBILIZING SUPPORT SYSTEMS.** Social support systems become very important to people when they have physical illnesses. Their significant others become their link with "normal life." They also reassure the patient that he is still lovable and important. This is especially important if the person has a stigmatizing illness such as AIDS. The nurse can assist the patient by being available to answer the questions of friends and family members. He or she can also let them know that their visits are important and encourage them to continue to be involved.

Sometimes families and friends become overinvolved. It may be difficult for the patient to tell his visitors that he needs to rest. The nurse can do this in a tactful manner, relieving the patient of the worry that visitors will not return if he sends them away. The nurse can also intervene if there are visitors who are distressing to the patient. The impression that visitors are unwelcome must be validated with the patient. What is apparently upsetting may be a normal relationship in the patient's sociocultural world.

Another source of social support is the peer support group. These groups exist for most major illnesses. It can be very helpful for a patient to talk with someone who has been through similar experiences. Even the most sensitive nurse or physician cannot completely understand the experience of the illness. Peers know about the apparently minor details of treatment and recovery that worry patients. They also provide reassurance that people either recover or function well with the particular illness. Social workers are good resources regarding peer support groups.

■ **THE DYING PATIENT.** Nursing interventions with patients who are dying are related to the stage that the person is experiencing. During denial, the nurse must resist the temptation to force the patient to admit that he will die. The patient is gathering his resources to be able to cope with that overwhelming idea. During anger, the nurse must be careful not to personalize the patient's behavior. The patient may use the nurse as a target for his anger. A care provider is a less threatening target than a family member whom the patient does not want to alienate. Anger can be tolerated as long as one remembers that the patient is angry about his situation. During bargaining, the nurse should support the patient as he tries to take care of unfinished business in his life. During depression, the nurse may need to just be with the patient, demonstrating caring nonverbally. The patient may be quiet and withdrawn or may cry. The patient is letting go of everything that is important to him and needs sensitivity and understanding. If the patient agrees, a visit from a spiritual adviser may be helpful. During acceptance, the patient may wish to reminisce about his life. He may also want quiet time alone. The nurse should respect the patient's wishes and follow his lead.

After the patient dies, the survivors will also need help. Gifford and Cleary[9] have identified four tasks associated with grieving and related nursing interventions:

1. *Task:* Confront the reality of the loss.
   Nursing interventions: Encourage the survivor to talk about the person who has died; share memories of the deceased; call the deceased by name; listen; foster family communication.
2. *Task:* Experience the pain of grief.
   Nursing interventions: Help survivors express feelings; recognize normal feelings and offer reassurance; stress that each survivor will have an individual way of grieving.
3. *Task:* Adjust to the environment without the deceased.
   Nursing interventions: Assist the person to handle tasks, establish a routine, and set goals; help the survivor sort out necessary changes from those that can be postponed; discourage major changes.
4. *Task:* Withdraw emotional energy and invest it in another relationship.
   Nursing interventions: Help the survivor withdraw the emotional attachment by assisting

with activities such as disposing of the deceased's belongings; help the person to anticipate that difficult times will occur; identify maladaptive responses and refer the person for help if needed.

Work with dying people and their survivors can be emotionally draining for the nurse. Eakes[5] has identified coping strategies that have been helpful to nurses who work in hospice settings. It is important to establish collaborative relationships with the patient and family. The nurse may to set limits on the level of involvement with them. Nursing care goals should focus on comfort measures. The nurse needs to ventilate his or her feelings. This could include sharing feelings with the patient or family. However, the nurse also needs to have support systems. It is important to bring closure to the relationships after the patient's death. This can be accomplished by a visit to the family or by going to the funeral home during viewing hours.

Attending to the psychological needs of a patient with physical illness and his significant others is an essential component of nursing care. Patients often form their impressions of their health care experiences on the basis of interpersonal contacts. Positive interactions with nurses will create an atmosphere of collaboration that will assist the patient to make the necessary adjustments in his life-style. A successful experience in coping with illness will also enable him to be more confident when he becomes ill in the future. Nursing interventions with these patients are summarized in Table 21-5.

TABLE 21-5

SUMMARY OF NURSING INTERVENTIONS FOR PSYCHOLOGICAL RESPONSES TO PHYSICAL ILLNESS

Principle	Rationale	Nursing interventions
Establish a caring relationship	Caring enables the patient to feel trust and allows him to make choices	Accept the patient as he is; spend time with patient; use touch
Assist the patient to cope with illness-related stress	Ineffective coping interferes with the healing process by causing a high level of anxiety	Support coping behaviors; use therapeutic communication skills; listen; promote relaxation and guided imagery
Mobilize social support systems	Significant others make the patient feel cared about and provide a link with normal life; peers can provide reassurance	Ensure availability to visitors; serve as an intermediary with visitors; refer to peer support group
Assist the terminally ill patient to have a peaceful death	Interpersonal support offers comfort to a dying person	Accept the person's way of dying; offer support to significant others

⬆ Evaluation

Evaluation of nursing care is based on an analysis of the patient care goals that were recorded in the nursing care plan. If the goals have not been accomplished, the nurse should ask the following questions:

1. Have threats to the patient's physical integrity or self-system been reduced in nature, number, origin, or timing?
2. Do the patient's behaviors reflect greater self-awareness and acceptance of emotional experiences?
3. Have the patient's coping resources been adequately assessed and mobilized?

DIRECTIONS FOR FUTURE RESEARCH

The following are some of the nursing research problems raised in Chapter 21 that merit further study by psychiatric nurses:

1. Correlation of patient satisfaction with nursing care with nurses' awareness of patient's psychological needs
2. Effectiveness of peer support groups for nurses who work with terminally ill patients
3. Cost-effectiveness of consultation services provided by psychiatric liaison nurses
4. Comparison of the amount of time spent on psychological support by nurses who work with terminally ill patients in hospital, home care, and hospice settings
5. Identification of nursing interventions that assist people with AIDS to cope with the psychosocial implications of the diagnosis
6. Identification of nursing interventions that foster an attitude of hopefulness in physically ill patients
7. Evaluation of the effects of relaxation and guided imagery therapy on the outcomes of various physical illnesses.
8. Identification of nursing interventions that assist family members to provide emotional support to physically ill people
9. Analysis of nursing interventions that assist families and patients to manage the role transitions that take place during a physical illness
10. Comparison of patients' and nurses' assumptions about patients' needs for information about the psychological aspect of their illness

---

4. Does the patient recognize his level of stress, and does he have insight into his feelings?
5. Is the patient using adaptive coping responses?
6. Has the patient learned new adaptive strategies to cope effectively with life stressors?
7. Is the patient using greater self-understanding to promote personal change and growth?

■ SUGGESTED CROSS-REFERENCES ■

The nursing model of health-illness phenomena is discussed in Chapter 3. Therapeutic nurse-patient relationships are discussed in Chapter 4. Implementation of the nursing process is covered in Chapter 5, and crisis intervention in Chapter 9. Anxiety is discussed in Chapter 11. Psychophysiological illness is covered in Chapter 12; alterations in self-concept are discussed in Chapter 13; and depression is discussed in Chapter 14. Self-destructive behavior is discussed in Chapter 15. Anger is covered in Chapter 16. Psychiatric liaison nursing is discussed in Chapter 26.

■ SUMMARY ■

1. Common expectations about health and illness were presented.
2. Psychological responses to physical illness were differentiated from psychophysiological disorder.
3. The concept of uncertainty was presented and related to the person's response to a physical illness.
4. Predisposing factors include the person's psychological history, crisis response, coping skills, social support, developmental stage, phase of illness, identity, and grief reaction. In addition, knowledge about the disease, past experience with illness, attitude toward life, and resilience contribute to determining the patient's response to illness.
5. Precipitating stressors include the nature of the transition to the patient role, prognosis for the outcome of the disease, the person's expectations about convalescence, the nature of the intervention that the disease requires, and the response of significant others.
6. Behaviors represent the patient's effort to cope. They are closely related to the nature and duration of the illness. They may include anxiety, depression, anger, dependency, hopelessness, and withdrawal. The patient may be responding to multiple losses, including the loss of important relationships. Behaviors were described related to convalescence and to terminal illness.
7. Common coping mechanisms include denial, regression, and compensation.
8. Nursing and medical diagnoses related to psychological responses to physical illness were presented.
9. Examples were provided of a nursing care plan and a mental health education plan.
10. Nursing interventions were discussed related to car-

ing, therapeutic communication, relaxation/guided imagery, patient education, mobilizing social support systems, and the dying patient.

    11. Suggestions were made regarding questions to ask during the evaluation of nursing care.

■ REFERENCES ■

1. American Psychiatric Association: Diagnostic and statistical manual of mental disorders, ed 3, (revised), Washington, DC, 1987, The Association.
2. Benner P and Wrubel J: The primacy of caring: stress and coping in health and illness, Menlo Park, Calif, 1989, Addison-Wesley Publishing Co, Inc.
3. Davis LL: Convalescence and implications for nursing research, Image 19:117, 1987.
4. Dufault K and Martocchio BC: Hope: its spheres and dimensions, Nurs Clin North Am 20:379, 1985.
5. Eakes GG: Grief resolution in hospice nurses: an exploration of effective methods, Nurs Health Care 11:243, 1990.
6. Farran CJ and Popovich JM: Hope: a relevant concept for geriatric psychiatry, Arch Psychiatr Nurs 4:124, 1990.
7. Feinblum S: Pinning down the psychosocial dimensions of AIDS, Nurs Health Care 7:255, 1986.
8. Flaskerud JH: AIDS: psychosocial aspects, J Psychosoc Nurs Ment Health Serv 25:9, 1987.
9. Gifford BJ and Cleary BB: Supporting the bereaved, Am J Nurs 90:49, 1990.
10. Kadner KD: Resilience: responding to adversity, J Psychosoc Nurs Ment Health Serv 27:20, 1989.
11. Kalayjian AS: Coping with cancer: the spouse's perspective, Arch Psychiatr Nurs 3:166, 1989.
12. Kendall J et al: Doing well with AIDS: three case illustrations, Arch Psychiatr Nurs 3:159, 1989.
13. Krieger D: Therapeutic touch: how to use your hands to help or to heal, Englewood Cliffs, NJ, 1979, Prentice-Hall, Inc.
14. Kübler-Ross, E.: On death and dying, New York, 1969, The MacMillan Co.
15. Lange SP: Hope. In Carlson CE and Blackwell B, editors: Behavioral concepts and nursing intervention, Philadelphia, 1978, J.B. Lippincott Co.
16. Mishel MH and Braden CJ: Finding meaning: antecedents of uncertainty in illness, Nurs Res 37:98, 1988.
17. Norris CM: The work of getting well, Am J Nurs 90:47, 1990.
18. O'Donnell TG and Bernier SL: Parents as caregivers: when a son has AIDS, J Psychosoc Nurs Ment Health Serv 28:14, 1990.
19. Siegel BS: Love, medicine and miracles, New York, 1986, Harper & Row, Publishers, Inc.
20. Zahourek RP: Relaxation and imagery: tools for therapeutic communication and intervention, Philadelphia, 1988, WB Saunders Co.

■ ANNOTATED SUGGESTED READINGS ■

*Benner P and Wrubel J: The primacy of caring: stress and coping in health and illness, Menlo Park, Calif, 1989, Addison-Wesley Publishing Co, Inc.

    All nurses should read this thought-provoking work on one of nursing's central values. Many clinical examples illustrate theoretical discussion.

Cousins N: Anatomy of an illness, New York, 1979, WW Norton & Co.

    Describes author's experience with a physical illness and poor prognosis. Emphasizes the importance of a positive mental state for recovery.

*Davis T and Jensen L: Identifying depression in medical patients, Image 20:191, 1988.

    Discusses that patients often have depressive symptoms but rarely depressive syndromes.

*Henderson, KJ: Dying, God, and anger, J Psychosoc Nurs Ment Health Serv 27:17, 1989.

    Describes how scripture readings can help patients validate their feelings and how religious beliefs can inhibit expression of anger by imposing guilt. Suggests interventions using several psalms.

*Icenhour ML and Calvert, H.: EBV: managing the physiological and psychological implications of the Epstein-Barr virus, J Psychosoc Nurs Ment Health Serv 27:23, 1989.

    Analyzes psychosocial behaviors and nursing interventions related to patients with EBV. Many issues also relevant to patients with other chronic illnesses.

*Morrow BR, Maier GJ, and Kelley W: Dying with dignity: hospice care on the unit, J Psychosoc Nurs Ment Health Serv 27:10, 1989.

    Describes providing hospice-supported care to a terminally ill patient in a forensic psychiatric unit. Discusses reactions of patients and staff; provides recommendations for successful implementation.

*Pheifer WG and Houseman C: Bereavement and AIDS: a framework for intervention, J Psychosoc Nurs Ment Health Serv 26:21, 1988.

    Describes the feelings of survivors of people with AIDS; suggests nursing interventions.

*Richards G: Curtains, Am J Nurs 87:1587, 1987.

    Demonstrates that each person dies in a personal way. Describes a nurse-patient relationship in which this was used to assist the patient to die with dignity.

*Ross SM and MacKay RC: Postoperative stress: do nurses accurately assess their patients? J Psychosoc Nurs Ment Health Serv 24:17, 1986.

    Reports on study that compared psychosocial stress levels in postoperative patients as assessed by patients and nurses.

*Stephany TM: A death in the family, Am J Nurs 90:55, 1990.

    Demonstrates the value of adjusting nursing care to meet the patient's wishes.

---

*Asterisk indicates nursing reference.

*van Servellen G, Nyamathi AM, and Mannion W: Coping with a crisis: evaluating psychological risks of patients with AIDS, J Psychosoc Nurs Ment Health Serv 27:16, 1989.

Describes a Coping Assessment Profile that includes components to be completed by patient and nurse.

*Zahourek RP: Relaxation and imagery: tools for therapeutic communication and intervention. Philadelphia, 1988, WB Saunders Co.

Excellent resource for nurses interested in using these approaches with specific patient populations.

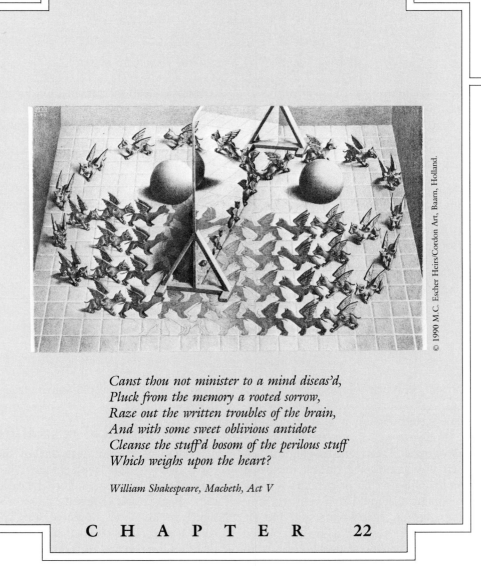

Canst thou not minister to a mind diseas'd,
Pluck from the memory a rooted sorrow,
Raze out the written troubles of the brain,
And with some sweet oblivious antidote
Cleanse the stuff'd bosom of the perilous stuff
Which weighs upon the heart?

William Shakespeare, Macbeth, Act V

CHAPTER 22

SOMATIC THERAPIES AND PSYCHIATRIC NURSING

After studying this chapter, the student should be able to:

- state reasons for the use of physical restraint of patients, including mechanical restraints and seclusion.

- discuss the nursing care of a patient who is in restraints or seclusion.

- identify issues associated with psychosurgical treatment.

- describe the nursing care of a patient receiving electroconvulsive therapy, including pa-

- tient education, patient care during the treatment and recovery period, and assessment of the patient's response to the treatment.

- analyze legal and ethical issues related to the use of restraint, seclusion, psychosurgery, and electroconvulsive therapy.

- identify directions for future nursing research.

- select appropriate readings for further study.

Many somatic treatments have been used in psychiatric settings. As research into the pathophysiology of mental illness continues, it is likely that more and increasingly sophisticated somatic treatment modalities will be developed. Treatment modalities such as restraint, which was among the earliest means of providing nursing care for psychiatric patients, are still used. Psychiatric nursing therapy, like psychiatry, is in transition; old therapies are being reassessed and reconsidered, and new therapies are being discovered and investigated. Nurses will be important contributors to the growth of knowledge in this area and need to scientifically study the effectiveness of the various somatic therapies.

Treatment modalities as described in this chapter will provide some historical perspective on the progression of knowledge in somatic therapies. Although several treatment forms may have been used by clinicians at a given time, generally one form was most frequently used. Few therapies of the past have been totally abandoned; relatively unused treatments sometimes become popular again. Therefore some treatments that are rarely used today, such as insulin coma therapy, are presented briefly. The emphasis in all cases will be on the nursing implications for the treatment described. However, since some treatments are viewed as specific to certain psychiatric diagnostic categories, there will be reference to these diagnoses. These discussions will, therefore, incorporate the medical model more heavily than do other portions of this book. Psy-

chopharmacology, also a somatic therapy, is discussed in Chapter 23.

Use of physical restraints

Physical restraint was one of the earliest means used to try to cope with people who were unable to control their behavior. Before the early nineteenth century, shackles and fetters were used to control the "insane" in "asylums." Some persons spent years bound hand and foot or chained to the wall. Small wonder that families tried to keep disturbed members at home. Modifications in these practices took place after Philippe Pinel campaigned for humane treatment of the mentally ill in France. Similar objectives were pursued in England by Tuke and in the United States by Benjamin Rush and Dorothea Lynde Dix. Gradually the chains fell into disuse. However, other forms of physical restraint were commonly used until the advent of the convulsive therapies and psychopharmacotherapy. These forms of restraint included camisoles ("straitjackets"), sheet restraints, wrist and ankle restraints, sheet packs, and seclusion. Good psychiatric nursing care was essential to humanize what could be a dehumanizing experience.

It is still necessary at times to physically restrain patients. Restraint should be used with great discretion. Civil liberties and the rights of the individual must be considered. Two court decisions have been influential in clarifying this issue. *Rogers v. Okin*,[17] 1975, prohibited the use of seclusion or restraint for treatment purposes. It was the court's opinion that these measures could be used only for control of a behavioral emergency. The 1982 Supreme Court decision in *Youngberg v. Romeo*[21] supported the exercise of professional judgment in the use of seclusion or restraint. The standard to be applied is that of usual and customary professional practice. Wexler[20] notes that "professional" was defined very broadly in this case and could really apply to any direct care provider. Soloff, Gutheil, and Wexler[18] point out that there are issues still unresolved by this decision. For instance, it is unclear whether the use of physical restraint to protect property or to preserve a therapeutic environment would be acceptable. Likewise, the decision did not address the use of seclusion or mechanical restraints as consequences in behavior modification programs. The legal and ethical aspects of psychiatric care presented in Chapter 7 will assist the nurse to analyze the consequences of the use of restrictive or intrusive approaches to patient care.

■ **Related research**

Although the use of physical restraint has led to controversy in psychiatry, there is little research to guide the practitioner. Thirteen reports of research studies of physical restraint were published between 1976 and 1983. These were difficult to compare because of variation in treatment programs and patient characteristics. Soloff, Gutheil, and Wexler[18] were able to make several generalizations. In acute settings, schizophrenic and manic patients were secluded most frequently. In chronic settings, mentally retarded and nonpsychotic patients were secluded or restrained more often. As compared with patients who did not require restraint, physically restrained patients were younger, more chronically ill, and more frequently involuntarily hospitalized. An interesting finding was that in most cases seclusion or restraint was initiated based on nonviolent behavior patterns. The length of time spent in restraints or seclusion was related to age, sex, and diagnosis, but not to the precipitating behavior. Nonpsychotic males under 35 years of age were restricted for a longer period of time than other groups.

Okin[15] reported on a study of the frequency and rationale for the use of seclusion and restraint in seven public mental hospitals. These hospitals were in the same state and were operating within the same set of policies and regulations. The purpose of the study was to determine whether there were differences in the use of these procedures. Differences were found, and the investigator concluded that these variations were influenced by such hospital-related factors as the following[15]:

1. Differences in staff perceptions of patient behaviors
2. More frequent use of alternative interventions in some settings
3. Failure to prevent violence and sometimes even promotion of violent behavior at some hospitals
4. Variation in quality and quantity of staff
5. Different levels of staff competence in prevention and management of violent behavior
6. Varying approaches to the medication of disturbed patients
7. Differences in the characteristics of the milieu
8. More clarity and firmness in limit setting at some of the hospitals
9. Variations in ward organization and physical characteristics

Such studies provide useful clues about factors that may enable nurses to avoid unnecessary use of restrictive treatment approaches. The box on p. 684 illustrates Gutheil's analysis[7] of factors related to increased rates of seclusion and restraint. When it is necessary to limit a patient's freedom and mobility, good nursing care is a necessity and a great challenge. Nursing interventions with the mechanically restrained or the secluded patient are summarized in Table 22-1.

■ **Mechanical restraints**

Mechanical restraints include camisoles, wrist restraints, ankle restraints, sheet restraints, and sheet packs. Any of these measures require a physician's order. The patient should be released from restraints as soon as any dangerous behavior has subsided or other less drastic means of restraint, such as medication, become effective. Release from restraints should be gradual with intervals out of restraints increased over time. Nursing care of patients with restraints other than sheet packs will be discussed first. Care of patients in packs differs slightly and will be discussed separately.

The use of mechanical restraints should be prevented whenever possible. This can be done through timely intervention when a patient begins to appear agitated. A thorough nursing assessment will address the patient's past history of physically assaultive behavior. If the patient is reasonably calm, this is also a good time to ask what is helpful to him when he becomes upset. Some people prefer medication. Some may find relief in talking to someone, while others can regain control if they are allowed to be alone in a quiet place. Nursing care planning can be more effective if the patient's preferences are taken into account.

It is also important to find out what triggers disturbed behavior and how the patient acts when he is

Factors Related to Increased Rates of Seclusion and Restraint

Increase in:
- Violence of patient population
- Number/proportion of involuntary patients, perpetrators of violent crimes
- Attack on the facility from legal, political, professional, economic quarters
- Interstaff tensions, resentments, disagreements
- Legal or departmental intrusiveness, regulation, undermining of on-site decisions

Decrease in:
- Number of staff
- Number of senior, experienced staff
- Number of male staff
- Public support of facility
- Staff morale and sense of security
- Available alternatives through regulation, policy, change, legal interdiction

Increase in rates of seclusion, restraint, forced medication, administrative discharge, transfer to security setting (*Note:* Prohibition of one of these interventions may lead to increases in rates of the others.)

From Gutheil TG: Review of individual quantitative studies. In Tardiff K, editor: The psychiatric uses of seclusion and restraint, Washington, DC, 1984, American Psychiatric Press, Inc.

TABLE 22-1

NURSING INTERVENTIONS WITH THE SECLUDED OR MECHANICALLY RESTRAINED PATIENT

Principle	Rationale	Nursing intervention
Right to least restrictive treatment	Constitutional right of all patients	Identify precipitating events; observe patient for agitated behavior; attempt alternative interventions; document patient behavior and nursing interventions
Protect patient from physical injury	An individual who is not in control of his behavior is at risk of injury and needs safely applied external limits	Provide adequate staff resources to control the patient; be sure staff is trained to manage violent behavior; plan the approach to the patient; use safe physical restraint techniques
Provide a safe environment	The judgment of an individual who is not in control of his behavior may be impaired and he may harm himself accidentally or purposefully	Observe the patient constantly or very frequently, depending on his condition; remove dangerous objects from the area
Maintain biological integrity	Physically restrained patients are not able to attend to their own biological needs and are at risk for complications related to immobility	Check vital signs; bathe the patient and provide skin care; take to the bathroom or provide a bedpan or urinal; regulate the room temperature; position the patient anatomically; pad restraints; offer food and fluids; release restraints at least every 2 hours
Maintain dignity and self-esteem	Loss of control and the imposition of physical restraint may be embarrassing to the patient	Provide privacy; explain the situation to other patients without revealing confidential patient information; maintain verbal contact with the patient at regular intervals while awake; assign a consistent staff member to work with the patient; assign a staff member of the same sex to provide personal care; involve the patient in plans to terminate physical restraint; wean the patient from the protected setting

becoming upset. This information allows the nursing staff to intervene before the patient is on the verge of losing control. Staff must be sensitive to the milieu of the patient care unit. Sometimes initiating a group activity will relieve tension and assist patients to maintain self-control. If a particularly stressful event has occurred, a group discussion may be therapeutic. This is illustrated in Clinical example 22-1.

Patients may be restrained for a number of reasons, including: (1) the risk of injuring themselves or others if allowed free movement of their limbs; (2) an inability to tolerate, or unresponsiveness to, medication that would decrease assaultive behavior; (3) confusion that results in wandering and the risk of falls; (4) the need for decreased stimuli or rest; or (5) a patient's request to provide a sense of security and control. It

---

CLINICAL EXAMPLE 22-1

Mr. T. was a 36-year-old man, who was admitted for the third time to an acute care unit at a state psychiatric hospital. His medical diagnosis was bipolar disorder, manic. The nursing staff was apprehensive because the patient had a history of assaultive behavior on earlier admissions. At the time of this admission, the unit atmosphere was tense because one of the other patients had made a suicide attempt requiring emergency room treatment.

Mr. I. was Mr. T's primary nurse from his previous admission. He was working when the patient arrived on the unit. During the nursing assessment, Mr. I discussed the nursing interventions that had seemed to be helpful in the past. He validated with Mr. T that he had usually been able to maintain control of his behavior by participating in a structured physical activity when he was feeling upset. In addition, he recalled that the patient would begin to pace rapidly and sing when he was losing control. Mr. T agreed with these observations.

Mr. T responded very quickly to the tension on the unit. He began to pace up and down the hall and sing in a moderately loud tone of voice. Other patients also began to show signs of increased agitation. The nursing staff held a brief consultation. They decided that the charge nurse would gather the patients for a community meeting to discuss their feelings about the suicide attempt. Meanwhile, Mr. I would take Mr. T to the nearby gym with one of the nurse's aides. They would perform structured calisthenic exercises. The interventions were successful. None of the patients needed to be restrained.

---

should not be used as a punishment or for the convenience of the staff.

The patient in mechanical restraint may be confused or delirious and will probably be frightened at the limitation of movement. The nurse should not assume that the patient understands the need for restraint. Support and reassurance are essential. Restraints should be applied efficiently and with care not to injure a combative patient. Adequate personnel need to be assembled before the patient is approached. Each staff member should be assigned responsibility for controlling specific body parts. Restraints should be available and in working order. Padding of cuff restraints helps to prevent skin breakdown. For the same reason, the patient should be positioned in anatomical alignment. Provision of privacy is important. If visitors are allowed, the nurse should explain the treatment and the reason for it before they see the patient; this may help them accept the situation. Physical needs must be included in the nursing care plan. Vital signs should be checked, and regular observation of circulation in the extremities is necessary. Fluids should be offered regularly and opportunities for elimination provided. Skin care is also essential. Restraints must be released at least every 2 hours to allow exercise of the extremities.

Camisole restraints are canvas jackets that fasten in the back. The arms are elongated and the ends are also fastened behind the patient's back. When the patient is in the restraint, his arms are folded across his body with limited ability to move them. Some patients feel more secure in a camisole restraint because it prevents them from striking out at themselves or others. It also enables them to discharge anxiety by walking or pacing. Close nursing observation is required to protect the patient from self-injury or attacks by other patients.

Sheet restraints are canvas bedsheets that are fastened to the bedframe with straps. There is a hole in the sheet for the patient's head. Wrist and ankle restraints may be built into the sheet or separate ones may be used in conjunction with it. These are usually necessary to immobilize the patient adequately. This type of restraint should only be used for extremely agitated patients and for short periods of time. Continuous nursing observation should be provided.

On some occasions, restrained patients may be located in general use areas of the unit such as day room hallways or dining areas. If this is the case, constant staff observation is recommended in order to protect them from assault by other patients. Good nursing care and the communication of concern for the patient will contribute to better behavioral control.

Cold, wet sheet packs may be ordered occasionally for extremely disturbed patients who are resistant to treatment with medication. In this procedure the patient is immobilized by being wrapped mummy fashion in several layers of linens. The innermost layer is soaked in ice water. The patient is in a bed with a waterproof mattress and dressed in a hospital nightgown. The sheets are wrapped so that no skin surfaces are in contact, since this could cause chafing and perhaps skin breakdown. The wet sheets are covered by layers of blankets, preferably wool. Although the pack is initially experienced as very cold, it quickly becomes warmed by the patient's body heat, which is retained in the pack. The combination of the transition from cold to warmth, wetness, and swaddling are very soothing and can have a calming effect on even extremely agitated patients. A patient in a pack needs constant nursing observation. Temperature, pulse, and respirations should be monitored. The pack should be discontinued with any significant change in vital signs. The patient will perspire, and fluids should be offered frequently. Soothing verbal contact may be helpful, but the environment should be quiet and conducive to rest. In general, maximum calming does not usually occur in less than 2 hours. Hazards of immobility, however, increase with the duration of the treatment. When the pack is removed, the skin should be thoroughly towel dried and skin care given. Privacy should, of course, be provided throughout the procedure.

■ Seclusion or isolation

A patient who is restrained by the use of seclusion is confined alone in a single room. Degrees of seclusion vary: The patient may be confined in a room with a closed but unlocked door, or a locked room with a mattress without linens on the floor and with limited opportunity for communication. The patient may be dressed in a hospital nightgown or a heavy canvas coverall. A mattress, sheet, or blanket, and the above clothing are minimally acceptable conditions for seclusion, which is to be used only when essential for the protection of the patient or others.

Seclusion is prescribed for a number of reasons. It may be used as a means of controlling the behavior of a patient who has been acting destructively and cannot be controlled by physical or verbal contact. Seclusion is often helpful to patients who are hyperactive and extremely responsive to environmental stimuli. Sometimes these patients will ask to be isolated for a period of time, and this should be allowed. Behavior modification protocols sometimes include seclusion as a negative reinforcer. This use of seclusion borders on punishment and should be used judiciously.

■ THEORETICAL BASES.

Gutheil[6] has identified three theoretical bases for the use of seclusion. The first is containment. This implies that the patient is at immediate risk for causing harm to himself or others. Seclusion protects him from this danger until his internal behavioral controls have been reestablished. He is also protected from the guilt that might be experienced as a result of loss of control. The second theoretical base is isolation. The patient is relieved of the need to relate interpersonally. He is allowed to master a reasonable, limited area before being confronted with the need to relate appropriately in the setting of the whole ward. The third concept is decreased sensory input. Seclusion may be calming to a person who is hyperalert and feeling bombarded by the many sensory stimuli in the hospital environment.[6]

Gutheil and Tardiff[8] have described several contraindications for the use of seclusion. A patient who is medically unstable requires close observation. Mechanical restraints may be more appropriate for such a patient. The patient at high risk for self-harm also requires close observation and must be readily accessible to the staff. No seclusion room is totally safe. A self-destructive patient can hurt himself in a totally empty room by banging his head against the wall. If the seclusion room environment does not meet minimal safety standards, other means of restraint must be used. For instance, a very warm room may be dangerous for agitated patients whose temperature-regulating mechanisms have been impaired by phenothiazine medications. Lion and Soloff[14] caution that secluded patients may become exhausted if agitated behavior continues in seclusion. They also warn that sensory deprivation may actually result in an intensification of psychosis. Socially deviant behavior, such as fecal smearing, may lead to reluctance by staff to have contact with the patient. The nurse, as the leader of the direct care staff, must be aware of these potential risks. It has been documented that patients are at greatest risk for seclusion during the first 24 hours after admission.[13] Continuous nursing assessment and revision of the patient care plan will assist the nurse to anticipate hazardous conditions and take appropriate preventive nursing actions.

Several negative effects of the injudicious use of seclusion have been identified.[6] One is the jealousy other patients might feel over the attention given to the secluded patient. This has been termed *seclusion envy.* Another potential problem is the creation of a lasting rift between the staff and the patient who was secluded; this will occur if the patient does not understand or agree with the reason for the procedure. The use of seclusion for the wrong reasons can also lead to negative consequences. Seclusion should not be used as a punishment or as a way to relieve the staff of the care of a demanding patient. Secluded patients require frequent and intensive nursing care.

■ **PROCEDURE.** The procedure should be carried out quickly and in a manner that demonstrates concern for the patient's dignity. The room should be prepared before the patient is approached.

Lion and Soloff[14] have described the following specific techniques for secluding an agitated patient:

1. Designate a staff member to be the leader.
2. Amass enough staff to provide a "show of force."
3. Assign a monitor to clear the area, observe the implementation of the procedure, and provide feedback after it is completed.
4. Communicate clearly and unambiguously with the patient.
5. Proceed without hesitation.
6. Control aggressive behavior in a safe manner, avoiding pain or injury.
7. Move the patient to the seclusion room.
8. Remove clothing and dangerous objects.
9. Staff should leave the room in a planned and organized way.
10. A debriefing session should be held.

Legal requirements for the care of the secluded patient vary from state to state and are minimal at best. Good nursing care includes optimum fulfillment of basic human needs and concern for personal dignity. The nurse must assist the patient to meet biological needs by providing food and fluids, a comfortable environment, and opportunity for use of the bathroom. Frequent observation is essential. The room must be constructed so the patient can be observed without being unnecessarily exposed to those who are not involved in his care. Staff should be able to communicate with the patient. Careful records should include all nursing care and observation of the isolated patient. The need for continued isolation should be assessed on a regular basis. It may be necessary for the nurse to initiate this review of the patient's condition with other health team members.

The nursing staff should always review the events that led up to the decision to isolate a patient. In particular, staff should be encouraged to give each other feedback about interpersonal relationships involving the secluded patient. Preventive measures that may assist the patient to gain control in the future without requiring seclusion should be identified. It is also useful for staff to ventilate their own feelings following an episode of seclusion. Management of violent behavior is physically and emotionally stressful.

Timely nursing intervention can often avert the need for seclusion of an agitated patient. Spending time with the patient may be helpful. Sometimes the energy of agitation can be channeled into nondestructive physical activity. If a patient is angry and feels misunderstood, an effort to understand may avoid an explosion. Medication may also be useful in calming a patient if it is given in time. Allowing a patient to be alone without being forcibly isolated may also be helpful. Careful nursing assessment and the establishment of a trusting nurse-patient relationship are a good foundation for planning effective action when a patient becomes upset. Any form of physical restraint should be used as a last resort when other nursing interventions have failed.

Psychosurgery

The American Psychiatric Association[3] has defined psychosurgery as:

> . . . surgical intervention to sever fibers connecting one part of the brain with another, or to remove, destroy or stimulate brain tissue with the intent of modifying or altering disturbances of behavior, thought content, or mood for which no organic pathological cause can be demonstrated by established tests and techniques. Such surgery may also be undertaken for the relief of intractible pain.[3:251]

It does not include surgery to treat an organic brain disease.

First introduced in 1936, the early operations were referred to as *lobotomies*. The focus of the surgical intervention was the pathway from the thalamus to the frontal lobes of the cerebral cortex. These surgical procedures were nonspecific because of the limited knowledge at that time of brain functioning. Extensive personality change almost inevitably followed surgery. A nursing article from that era describes vividly the deterioration in social skills that resulted from psychosurgery and the retraining that became an integral part of the nursing care for these patients.[4] Because of the resulting impact on the individual's ability to function adequately, the procedure was usually a last resort. After the introduction of new psychopharmacological agents, it was rarely used.

Knowledge of neuroanatomy and physiology has become increasingly more sophisticated, resulting in the recent increase in interest in psychosurgery. Progress has been made in "mapping" the cortex. This information may help the surgeon to isolate and sever tracts that relate more directly to the patient's individual behavioral problem. Sophisticated surgical tools, such as lasers, which cause far less generalized tissue damage, have been developed. Proponents of this approach now claim that psychosurgery can benefit patients who are unresponsive to other forms of therapy.

They maintain that current techniques minimize damage to the personality and to social functioning. Patients with chronic intractable depression and obsessional conditions accompanied by high anxiety benefit from various types of psychosurgery. Contrary to the practice of the past, schizophrenic patients are not good candidates because of their basically inadequate personality structure.[9]

The nursing care of the psychosurgical patient will not be discussed in detail here, because it is more pertinent to the specialty of neurosurgical nursing. However, the nurse should be aware that the major effect of surgery is on the *emotional* component of the patient's behavior. Intelligence is not affected. Also, the patient may continue to have some preoperative symptoms, such as hallucinations, but will not have the same emotional response. This results in improved functioning in activities of daily living. Henn[9] reports that over 60% of patients improve significantly after psychosurgery whereas only 3% get worse. This form of therapy has raised moral and ethical questions for many professionals on the issue of mind control. Other somatic therapies, such as pharmacotherapy and the convulsive therapies, undoubtedly exert some degree of control over the person's thought process. However, psychosurgery seems to many to be more drastic because it is permanent and irreversible. Nervous tissue, once damaged, does not regenerate. These questions arise particularly when psychosurgery is suggested as a possible treatment for antisocial and violent behavior, such as murder and rape. The responsible professional nurse must form independent opinions about such issues, collecting facts and objective data. Because knowledge of brain functioning is rapidly growing, therapies such as psychosurgery will be changing and improving. An open mind is an asset in evaluating varied approaches to the treatment of psychiatric disorders.

Electroconvulsive therapy

Electroconvulsive therapy (ECT) is also referred to as electric shock therapy (EST). It was first described by Cerletti and Bini in 1938 as a treatment for schizophrenia. At that time it was believed that epileptics were rarely schizophrenic. It was therefore hypothesized that convulsions would cure schizophrenia. Later research did not support this hypothesis. Further experience with ECT demonstrated that it is much more effective as a treatment for affective disturbances than it is for schizophrenia. It has also been noted that epilepsy and schizophrenia do sometimes occur concurrently. ECT is now most frequently used as a treatment for severe depression.

ECT is a treatment in which a grand mal seizure is artificially induced in an anesthetized patient by passing an electrical current through electrodes applied to the temples. In the past the electrodes were generally applied bilaterally. More recently, unilateral electrodes have been used. It has been observed that patients experience less confusion with this method.[19] For the treatment to be effective, a grand mal seizure must occur. The voltage is generally adjusted to the minimum level that will produce the therapeutic effect. The number of treatments in a series varies according to the patient's presenting problem and therapeutic response. For affective disorders, 6 to 10 treatments are normally administered. As many as 20 to 30 may be given for schizophrenia. ECT is most commonly given three times a week on alternate days, although it can be given daily or more than once a day. Some therapists have used multiple ECT in which several convulsions are induced immediately following each other. The proponents of this approach claim greater therapeutic effectiveness with no increase in confusion or untoward responses. However, the American Psychiatric Association has refused to endorse this practice.[1]

◼ Nursing intervention

Nursing intervention begins as soon as the individual and family are presented with this treatment alternative. Most people respond emotionally when told that they or a loved one needs "shock therapy." The nurse should use the term "treatment" and avoid unnecessary use of the term "shock." This places the emphasis on the therapeutic value of the procedure. However, people also need an opportunity to express their feelings about ECT. Many people have heard or read about or seen movies portraying ECT. Many of these emphasize the frightening aspect of the experience. Also, the very idea of an electric current passing through their head causes fear in most people. The nurse must assess the patient's response and provide opportunity for communication. As the patient reveals feelings and concerns, the nurse can clarify misconceptions. The act of discussing ECT openly and directly communicates the attitude that it is a usual method of treatment, without undue risk. However, as with any procedure requiring general anesthesia, there is a degree of risk. Therefore the patient is asked to sign a consent form indicating that he has been fully informed about the procedure and the risks involved.

After the patient has had an opportunity to express his feelings, the nurse should teach him about the procedure. When the patient's anxiety is slightly increased but not overwhelming, he is ready to learn. Some information will probably have been given to the patient by the physician at the time informed consent was obtained. However, a thorough review by the nurse is recommended. The nurse should reinforce what the patient already knows, remind him of anything he has forgotten, and provide an opportunity for questions. Enough time should be provided to encourage free communication. The nurse should also be alert to nonverbal cues of the patient's response to the teaching. Asking the patient to repeat what has been explained helps identify areas of confusion.

Much of the nursing procedure related to ECT is similar to the care of any surgical patient. The patient is not given anything orally after midnight when ECT is scheduled for the morning. In some cases a patient who has difficulty sleeping may be given prescribed sedation with a small amount of water. Before the treatment the patient is asked to remove jewelry, hairpins, eyeglasses, and hearing aids. Full dentures may also be removed. Partial plates should be left in the mouth to provide even pressure on the teeth and jaw during the tonic phase of the convulsion. Dress should be loose and comfortable, usually bed clothing. The bladder should be emptied. The patient awaiting ECT should be accompanied by a trusted, understanding staff member. Under no circumstances should a patient waiting for ECT see another patient receiving treatment or immediately after a treatment.

In the early days of ECT no medication was given before the administration of the shock. Therefore the individual experienced a full-blown, and frequently violent, grand mal convulsion. Although the patient did not remember the convulsive episode, it was a frightening experience. Some complications, particularly fractures and dislocations, resulted from the unmedicated procedure. Current American Psychiatric Association standards unequivocally state that ECT should be given under general anesthesia with the use of a muscle relaxant drug.[1] The patient therefore has no memory of the entire procedure, and the convulsion occurs in an attenuated form. An anesthesiologist is now a member of the treatment team.

■ **MEDICATIONS.** The following medications are commonly given before ECT[5]:

1. Methscopolamine or atropine sulfate is administered for its vagolytic effect. It is frequently given subcutaneously or intramuscularly 30 minutes before treatment. It is most effective, however, when given intravenously with the other premedications immediately before the treatment. This prevents the bradycardia that occurs with the onset of the seizure activity. Enough medication is given to increase the pulse rate by about 10%. This titration is not possible if the medication is given subcutaneously or intramuscularly.

2. A short-acting barbiturate such as sodium methohexital (Brevital Sodium) is administered intravenously to induce anesthesia.

3. Succinylcholine chloride (Anectine), a muscle relaxant, is administered intravenously after the anesthetic. If it is given before the anesthetic, the patient will feel paralyzed. The inability to breathe resulting from paralysis of the respiratory muscles can be very frightening and may be remembered after the treatment. The face and extremities are observed for muscle twitches, which indicate that the muscle relaxant has taken effect. Some authorities recommend isolating one extremity from the general circulation by the use of a tourniquet or blood pressure cuff before administration of the muscle relaxant. This limb can then be observed for unmodified seizure activity when the ECT is given.

These medications may be injected directly into the vein or through the tubing of an intravenous (IV) infusion. The advantage of the latter route is that the IV line is in place should complications arise during the procedure.

Coffey and Weiner[2] recommend discontinuation of psychotropic medications before ECT. Lithium may prolong the effect of the succinylcholine. Benzodiazepines may make it difficult to induce a seizure. Many psychotropic drugs act synergistically with anticholinergics.

ECT may be given in the operating room or in a specially equipped room in the inpatient or outpatient psychiatric setting. The nurse is responsible for checking all emergency equipment, including oxygen, suction, and cardiac resuscitation equipment before ECT. The ECT machine and IV equipment, if used, should also be ready.

Frankel[5] has recommended that specific drugs and equipment be available when ECT is given. These are listed in the box on page 690.

■ **ADMINISTRATION.** The patient lies supine on a bed or cot. Usually, 100% oxygen is administered for 1 to 2 minutes while an IV infusion is being started. This hyperoxygenation prepares the patient for the period of apnea that will result from the muscle relaxant and the convulsion. The patient will also need reassurance while these preparations take place. The medications are then administered. As soon as muscle paralysis has occurred, the treatment is given. Electrodes are placed on both temples for bilateral ECT or on the

Drugs and Equipment to Accompany ECT

Drugs

It is recommended that the following drugs and solutions be available with dose instructions for immediate administration:

1. Atropine sulfate, 0.4 mg/ml
2. Calcium chloride, 10% solution, 10% ml vial (emergency syringe)
3. Dexamethasone (Decadron), 4 mg/ml and/or 24 mg/ml
4. Dextrose, 5% in water, 250 ml units
5. Diazepam, 5 mg/ml, 2 and 10 ml (emergency syringe)
6. Epinephrine, 1:10,000 solution, 10 ml vials
7. Lidocaine (Xylocaine): special preparation for use in cardiac dysrhythmias - 2% solution = 5 ml = 100 mg in emergency syringe
8. Metaraminol (Aramine), 1% solution, 10 ml vial
9. Methylprednisolone (Solu-Medrol), 125 and 1,000 mg/vial
10. Sodium bicarbonate, 7.5% solution = 44.6 mEq, 50 ml (emergency syringe)
11. L-norepinephrine (Levophed), 2 mg/ml, 4 ml ampuls.

Equipment

Equipment to be available for immediate use:
1. Suction—tested for proper function
2. Needles
3. Infusion sets
4. Electrocardiograph
5. Defibrillator. While rare cases of cardiac arrest occurring with ECT can usually be managed by a blow to the precordium, the adjunctive use of a defibrillator may occasionally be necessary. This apparatus should be reasonably accessible for this contingency.

When ECT is administered in a hospital, the emergency (crash) cart should be readily available. In other facilities, a comparably equipped unit should be available.

From the American Psychiatric Association Commission of Psychiatric Therapies: The Psychiatric Therapies: Part I, The Somatic Therapies. Chaired by Karasu TB, Washington, DC, The American Psychiatric Association, 1984, p. 218. Used by permission.

nondominant side temple for unilateral ECT. A mouth gag is inserted between the teeth, and the jaw is gently supported. There is no need to restrain the limbs. The shock is administered. The fingers and toes are watched carefully for a rhythmic twitching, which is the only visible evidence that a grand mal convulsion has occurred. When the twitching has stopped, oxygen is given by bag-breathing the patient through a mask until spontaneous respiration resumes.

Immediately after ECT the patient requires close nursing observation in a recovery area. Emergency equipment should be readily available, although adverse reactions are rare. While unconscious, the patient should receive the same nursing care as is required by any comatose patient. A patent airway must be maintained. Occasionally, suctioning may be required to remove excessive secretions from the mouth and throat. The patient should be positioned on the side to prevent aspiration of secretions or in the event of vomit-

ing. Blood pressure, pulse, and respirations should be monitored closely until the patient has fully awakened.

The patient will generally begin to respond after 10 to 15 minutes. Some drowsiness will be experienced even after the anesthesia wears off. When the patient responds to his name, the nurse should provide orientation to time, place, and situation. Most patients are confused immediately after a treatment and become frightened if they are not oriented. Since ECT is frequently given in the morning, the patient may not remember getting out of bed and preparing for the treatment. He may assume that something happened to him during the night while he was asleep. Following is an example of this type of disorientation:

One patient, who had received ECT in the operating room, began to talk about people "cutting on" him and suspected that one of his fingers had been removed and another sewn on in its place. This was viewed as his attempt to make sense of a situation that confused him. He responded well to an explanation that he did indeed go to the operating room but received a treatment other than surgery. It was further explained that the treatment was for his depression.

Orientation may need to be repeated several times after ECT. It must also be repeated every time the patient has a treatment, because confusion may occur each time. For some persons confusion increases with additional treatments. This is particularly true for older persons, who may have some organic brain changes associated with aging.

When vital signs are stable, the patient should be assisted to ambulate. Postural hypotension sometimes occurs. It is, therefore, wise to check the blood pressure and pulse with the patient in sitting and standing positions before allowing him to walk.

On occasion, a patient may become quite agitated as consciousness returns. The patient should be restrained gently to prevent injury; forceful restraint increases the agitation by frightening him. Although the period of agitation is usually brief, it does tend to recur after each treatment. An injection of an antianxiety agent such as hydroxyzine hydrochloride (Vistaril) 30 minutes before ECT may alleviate this problem. Before the first treatment there is no way to predict how a patient will respond during the recovery phase.

When the patient is ambulatory, he may be returned to his own bed and allowed to sleep for about an hour if he wishes. A light breakfast with others who have had ECT is often reassuring and helps orient the patient to the beginning of the day. Patients should then be included in the usual hospital routine. Resumption of normal activity soon after treatment places it in proper perspective as part of the patient's therapy.

Nurses must be sensitive to the confusion that may follow the treatment and must provide needed orientation. There may also be some amnesia for the period just before the treatment series began. This amnesia usually subsides gradually after the course of treatment is completed. This may also be frightening to the patient who may fear that he is "losing his mind." Reassurance can be very helpful to these people. Observations about the degree of confusion the patient exhibits should also be reported to the physician. Decreasing the frequency or modifying the technique of administering the ECT can sometimes minimize the problem.

Some physical discomfort is frequently experienced after ECT. Most patients have a headache ranging from mild to severe. An analgesic should be included in routine ECT orders. Nursing assessment of the patient should include an inquiry about headache, because the patient may be confused about who to ask for medication. There is no need to be concerned about creating a headache when there is none, because the majority of patients do develop one. Analgesia after ECT also helps relieve any muscle soreness. Occasionally, patients also complain of nausea. This is readily relieved by the administration of an antiemetic medication such as trimethobenzamide (Tigan) or prochlorperazine (Compazine).

■ **PATIENT TEACHING.** The amount of information about the treatment that is shared with the patient should be individualized. The nurse assesses the patient's ability to understand, his anxiety level, and coping mechanisms. Some people become less anxious when they know and understand a great deal about an anxiety-provoking situation; others want to know only generalities. It is the nurse's responsibility to assess individual needs before patient teaching.

The family should also be included in teaching. When the patient is incapable of decision making, they may be asked to give informed consent for ECT. This is an extremely difficult decision to make for someone else, because the treatment is frightening and surrounded by myth. The nurse can help the family by providing time to discuss their concerns and answering their questions honestly and directly. Frequently the family can be supportive to the patient, which can alleviate the patient's anxiety. Family members also need to be informed about what to expect of the patient after ECT. Confusion, particularly, may be distressing to them unless they understand that it is expected and temporary. Hospitalized patients are usually completely recovered from the treatment, dressed, and engaged in their usual activities by the time the family visits. This is reassuring to the family. Family members should never be left alone to watch a patient who is recovering from ECT. Predischarge teaching should include both the patient and the family. They need to know that some lingering confusion may exist. Therefore the nurse should explain medication dosages and schedules to both the patient and a responsible family member. Outpatient appointments should also be communicated to both the patient and a family member. The nursing care of the person who is receiving ECT is summarized in Table 22-2.

If a patient is receiving ECT on an outpatient basis, it is important that the family understand the expected posttreatment behavior. Usually, these patients arrive at the treatment facility in the morning, receive ECT, and remain there until fully awake and ambulatory. They may receive a light breakfast before leaving. The patient must be accompanied by someone who can escort him home after ECT because of the likely

---

TABLE 22-2

NURSING INTERVENTIONS FOR THE PATIENT RECEIVING ELECTROCONVULSIVE THERAPY

Principle	Rationale	Nursing intervention
Informed participation in the procedure	A patient who understands his treatment plan will be more cooperative and experience less stress than one who does not; an informed family is able to provide the patient with emotional support	Educate regarding ECT, including the procedure and expected effects; teach family about the treatment; encourage expression of feelings by patient and family; reinforce teaching after each treatment
Maintain biological integrity	General anesthesia and an electrically induced seizure are physiological stressors and require supportive nursing care	Check emergency equipment prior to procedure; keep NPO several hours before treatment; remove potentially harmful objects, such as jewelry, dentures; check vital signs; maintain patent airway; position on side until reactive; assist to ambulate; offer analgesia or antiemetic as needed
Maintain dignity and self-esteem	Patients are usually fearful preceding the treatment; amnesia and confusion may lead to fear of becoming insane; patient will need assistance to function appropriately in the milieu	Remain with the patient and offer support before and during treatment; maintain the patient's privacy during and following the treatment; reorient the patient; assist family members and other patients to understand behavior related to amnesia and confusion

---

presence of confusion and because there will probably be some aftereffects of the anesthesia. The accompanying person should be instructed in how to orient the patient and what to do for headache or nausea. A telephone number should be provided in case any questions arise after the patient has returned home. Outpatient ECT is generally done about once a month as a maintenance treatment for a person who has recovered from a severe depression. The procedure usually goes smoothly, without complications. Outpatient ECT is less frequently given to patients who are acutely ill or who have not had this treatment previously. These patients are usually hospitalized because of the severity of their conditions.

■ Indications

Although ECT was originally considered as a treatment for schizophrenia, it did not prove to be particularly helpful to most schizophrenic patients. Affective disturbances, however, were frequently alleviated by treatment with ECT. Until the development of antidepressant medications and the discovery of lithium therapy, ECT was a treatment of choice for affective disorders. It is still useful for patients who cannot tolerate or who fail to respond to treatment with medica-

tion. ECT may also be used as an emergency therapy for a patient who is extremely suicidal or so hyperactive that he is in danger physically. ECT is given in these cases because of the lag time between initiation of pharmacotherapy and the establishment of a therapeutic level of medication for the individual. For some older persons who tend to be very sensitive to side effects from medication, ECT may be a safer therapeutic modality.[22]

On occasion, ECT may be used for conditions other than affective disorders. It has been effective in the treatment of catatonic stupor or catatonic excitement. It is sometimes still given to paranoid schizophrenic patients, but generally with little success. A survey conducted by the American Psychiatric Association revealed that most psychiatrists who use ECT recommend it for patients with diagnoses of affective disorders or schizophrenia. A few practitioners use it with other patients, including neurotics and those with organic mental disorders. Very few use it with children and adolescents. The American Psychiatric Association strongly recommends that research be conducted to validate these less common applications of ECT. It does endorse the helpfulness of ECT for affective disorders and some schizophrenic disorders, particularly those with an affective component.[1] Although some patients may view ECT as punishment, it should never be used for this purpose; nor should a patient ever be threatened with punishment by ECT.

Mechanism of action

The specific way in which ECT works is the subject of a great deal of research, but it has not yet been identified. It used to be believed that ECT alleviated depression because the patient viewed it as punishment. The depressed person was supposed to feel better because the self-directed anger that caused the depression was expressed through the "punishment" of ECT. This punishment consisted of the electric shock and the frightening experience of the treatment. This point of view is no longer widely accepted. It is now believed that the electric current passing through the brain causes a biochemical response. The observable behavior that indicates that this response has occurred is the convulsion. Several possible mechanisms of action have been identified. The most promising of these is that the seizure activity in the brain produces changes in neurotransmitters and receptor sites similar to those induced by antidepressant medications.[19] This and other hypotheses require further research. It is also believed that the mechanism of action that is effective with schizophrenia differs from that which occurs with depression.[1]

The American Psychiatric Association Task Force on ECT[1] ruled out several possible modes of action. Stress or fear caused by anticipation of the procedure has been disproven as a therapeutic effect, because simulated ECT is not as effective as actual ECT. Because patients are now usually well oxygenated during the procedure, anoxia does not seem to be involved in ECT's effectiveness. Amount of memory loss is unrelated to success of the treatment. Unilateral ECT results in less amnesia, yet seems as effective as bilateral. It may, however, take longer for the therapeutic effect to occur.

Systemic effects of ECT have been identified. They may provide clues to the mechanism of action, as well as providing guidance for safe administration of the treatment. After the administration of the shock, there is a transient drop in blood pressure and sinus tachycardia. This is followed by sympathetic hyperactivity, resulting in increased blood pressure, increased intracranial pressure, and, less frequently, cardiac dysrhythmias.[5]

Complications

Complications associated with the administration of ECT are infrequent. ECT is used only rarely and with great caution in the presence of an intracranial mass. This is because of the risk of dangerously increased intracranial pressure during ECT.[19] Before the use of muscle relaxants, spontaneous fractures, especially of the spine, occasionally occurred. Cardiac complications, when they do occur, are more likely to result from the anesthesia than the ECT. However, care must be taken if ECT is to be given to a patient with fragile cardiovascular status or aneurysm.[2] Anesthesia is generally given and tonic and clonic seizure activity may occur even with the use of muscle relaxants. Therefore the pre-ECT workup usually includes an ECG and x-ray films of the spine, skull, and chest. Potential problems can then be averted.

Ethical considerations

The legitimacy of ECT as a form of treatment continues to be debated in psychiatric circles. Many professionals regard ECT as a punishment rather than a treatment; they believe that administering a shock to a person is inhumane. Others feel that it is more inhumane to allow a person to suffer a severe emotional disturbance when ECT frequently provides prompt relief. Some are concerned that permanent brain damage could result. Others say that ECT should be given prophylactically to prevent recurrence of problems. It is up to each professional to reach a personal resolution of this debate. These decisions should be based on objective data, including experience with patients who have been treated both with and without the use of ECT. Kalayam and Steinhart[11] conducted an attitude survey of a group of patients, professionals, and members of the general public concerning their perceptions of ECT. There was general agreement that ECT is an appropriate treatment for certain conditions and that it does cause clinical improvement.

Janicak et al[10] have reported a study of the knowledge and attitudes of mental health professionals regarding ECT. They found that as physicians' and nurses' knowledge increased with professional experience, there was a significant positive change in attitude about ECT. This trend was less pronounced with social workers and not characteristic of psychologists. The investigators concluded that education about ECT should lead to higher levels of acceptance by professionals. The nurse should take advantage of any opportunity to observe ECT being administered. The reality of the treatment experience is usually quite different from what has been imagined. Also, nurses who are unable to accept the use of ECT should try not to communicate negative attitudes to the patient. ECT continues to be used because it has been found to be helpful to many patients.

Insulin coma treatment

Before the use of medication as a treatment for serious emotional disorders, insulin coma treatment was frequently used. Use of insulin therapy was first reported by Sakel in 1933. It is not used in contemporary psychiatric facilities.[12] This is primarily because equally good results can be achieved by pharmacotherapy and because of the risk involved. Insulin coma treatment required a large, specialized nursing staff who could provide intensive nursing care to a small group of patients for several hours. The usual course of therapy was 50 treatments, given at a rate of one per day 5 days a week. These factors made insulin coma an expensive form of therapy. It was also dangerous: If a coma was allowed to continue too long, it became irreversible.[16]

Insulin treatment was induced by the administration of a large intramuscular dose of insulin. The exact dose needed to cause a coma varied. The dose needed for each individual was determined by starting with a low dose and increasing it over several days until coma resulted. The patient would usually begin to have hypoglycemic symptoms about 1 hour after the injection. He would progress through a stage of disorientation and restlessness to coma after about 3 hours. The length of the coma was then gradually increased to a maximum of 1 hour. The coma was terminated by administration of glucose solution by nasogastric tube or intravenously or by administration of glucagon intramuscularly or intravenously. Close observation of the patient was required for the rest of the treatment day, because repeat comas sometimes occurred.

Future directions

Somatic therapies have always been and will undoubtedly continue to be important psychiatric nursing skills. The rapid growth of knowledge today makes it mandatory that nurses keep up with current practice through continuing education. Public education is also essential. The consumerism movement has stimulated interest in mental health and psychiatric treatment. Because abuses have occurred in the past, professionals are being held accountable for their actions. Consumer education will be a more and more important priority for the nurse.

Nurses must examine and resolve their own feelings about the treatments that have been presented in this chapter. Many intrude to some extent on the person's exercise of free will and personal decision making. Some seem barbaric and unscientific, because the reason for effectiveness is vaguely understood, if at all. Yet the consequences of treatment may be vastly preferable to the continuing pain and disability of a serious

mental illness. Each nurse must arrive at a personal answer to the questions raised through experience with these treatment modalities. Each nurse has a contribution to make in adding to the growing store of knowledge about the biological aspects of psychiatric disorders. As knowledge grows, so will satisfaction with the treatment that is given.

DIRECTIONS FOR FUTURE RESEARCH

The following are some of the nursing research problems raised in Chapter 22 that merit further study by psychiatric nurses:
1. Nursing interventions that are effective alternatives to the use of mechanical restraints or seclusion
2. Correlation of the relationship between nurse attitudes concerning the use of restraints and the effective use of this therapeutic intervention
3. Indicator behaviors that can be used as guidelines for terminating the use of mechanical restraints, cold wet sheet packs, or seclusion
4. Nurses' awareness of the legal and ethical issues related to the use of somatic therapies
5. Evaluation of the psychosocial functioning of patients who have had psychosurgery
6. Nurses' perceptions of the effectiveness of ECT
7. Information about ECT that is helpful to patients who are deciding whether to agree to this treatment
8. Identification of patterns of cognitive responses to ECT and exploration of pretreatment predictors of cognitive response
9. Predictors of the occurrence of agitation during the early recovery period after ECT
10. Description of patient responses to memory loss and identification of therapeutic nursing interventions

■ SUMMARY ■

1. Physical restraint has been used for centuries and is still appropriate at times for treatment of psychiatric patients. Civil liberties must be considered when physical restraint is used.

a. Mechanical restraints include camisoles, wrist and ankle restraints, sheet restraints, and cold wet sheet packs. The nurse should be familiar with the procedure of applying restraints. Good nursing care includes attention to the patient's biological integrity, interpersonal needs, and right to dignity.

b. Seclusion or isolation involves the confinement of a patient alone in a room. This procedure should be used infrequently for a short time and with a specific rationale. Good nursing care includes frequent observation of the patient, provision for biological needs, and concern for the patient's dignity and privacy. Communication with the patient must be maintained.

2. Psychosurgery refers to the surgical interruption of selected neural pathways. These pathways govern transmission of emotion between the frontal lobes of the cerebral cortex and the thalamus. Nursing care focuses on postoperative needs that include any necessary social retraining.

3. Electroconvulsive therapy is the passage of an electrical current through the brain to induce a grand mal seizure. On average, 6 to 10 treatments are given in a series. Nurses help to support patients who are receiving this frightening treatment by providing patient teaching and reassurance. Later, orientation and supervision are necessary if confusion occurs. The patient may also need help meeting physiological needs.

■ SUGGESTED CROSS-REFERENCES ■

Legal issues and ethical decision-making are discussed in Chapter 7. Care of suicidal patients is discussed in Chapter 16 and interventions with violent patients is in Chapter 18. Psychopharmacology is covered in Chapter 23.

■ REFERENCES ■

1. American Psychiatric Association: Task force report 14: electroconvulsive therapy, Washington, DC, 1978, The Association.
2. Coffey CE and Weiner RD: Electroconvulsive therapy: an update, Hosp Community Psychiatry 41:515, 1990.
3. Donnelly J: Psychosurgery. In Karasu TB, editor: The somatic therapies, Washington, DC, 1984, American Psychiatric Association.
4. Ewald FR, Freeman W, and Watts JW: Psychosurgery: the nursing problem, Am J Nurs 47:210, 1947.
5. Frankel FH: Electroconvulsive therapy. In Karasu TB, editor: The somatic therapies, Washington, DC, 1984, American Psychiatric Association.
6. Gutheil TG: Observations on the theoretical bases for seclusion of the psychiatric inpatient, Am J Psychiatry 135:325, 1978.
7. Gutheil TG: Review of individual quantitative studies. In Tardiff K, editor: The psychiatric uses of seclusion and restraint, Washington, DC, 1984, American Psychiatric Press, Inc.
8. Gutheil TG and Tardiff K: Indications and contraindications for seclusion and restraint. In Tardiff K, editor: The psychiatric uses of seclusion and restraint, Washington, DC, 1984, American Psychiatric Press, Inc.
9. Henn FA: Psychosurgery. In Kaplan HI and Sadock BJ, editors: Comprehensive textbook of psychiatry, ed 5, Baltimore, 1989, Williams & Wilkins.
10. Janicak PG et al: ECT: an assessment of mental health professionals' knowledge and attitudes, J Clin Psychiatry, 46:262, 1985.
11. Kalayam B and Steinhart MJ: A survey of attitudes on the use of electroconvulsive therapy, Hosp Community Psychiatry 32:185, 1981.
12. Kaplan PM and Boggiano WE: Anticonvulsants, noradrenergic drugs and other organic therapies. In Kaplan HI and Sadock BJ, editors: Comprehensive textbook of psychiatry, ed 5, Baltimore, 1989, Williams & Wilkins.
13. Kirkpatrick H: A descriptive study of seclusion: the unit environment, patient behavior, and nursing interventions, Arch Psych Nurs 3:3, 1989.
14. Lion JR and Soloff PH: Implementation of seclusion and restraint. In Tardiff K, editor: The psychiatric uses of seclusion and restraint, Washington, DC, 1984, American Psychiatric Press, Inc.
15. Okin RL: Variation among state hospitals in use of seclusion and restraint, Hosp Community Psychiatry 36:649, 1985.
16. Peasley EL: The patient having coma shock treatment, Am J Nurs 49:623, 1949.
17. *Rogers v Okin*, 478, Fed Supp 1342, 1979.
18. Soloff PH, Gutheil TG, and Wexler DB: Seclusion and restraint in 1985: a review and update, Hosp Community Psychiatry 36:652, 1985.
19. Weiner RD: Electroconvulsive therapy. In Kaplan HI and Sadock BJ, editors: Comprehensive textbook of psychiatry, ed 5, Baltimore, 1989, Williams & Wilkins.
20. Wexler DB: Legal aspects of seclusion and restraint. In Tardiff K, editor: The psychiatric uses of seclusion and restraint, Washington, DC, 1984, American Psychiatric Press, Inc.
21. *Youngberg v Romeo*, 102 Supreme Ct 2452 (1982).
22. Zorumski CF, Rubin EH, and Burke WJ: Electroconvulsive therapy for the elderly: a review, Hosp Comm Psychiatry 39:643, 1988.

■ ANNOTATED SUGGESTED READINGS ■

American Psychiatric Association: Task force report 14: electroconvulsive therapy, Washington, DC, 1978, The Association.

This is a comprehensive report of a task force that was formed by the APA to study the use of ECT. The report is based on an extensive survey of psychiatrists and a thorough review of the literature. It is an excellent source, including recommendations for policies and procedures relative to ECT. There is also a good model for obtaining informed consent.

*Blakeslee JA: Untie the elderly, Am J Nurs 88:833, 1988.

Challenges the usual reasons given for restraining elderly patients. Provides many suggestions for alternative approaches.

Coffey CE and Weiner RD: Electroconvulsive therapy: an update, Hosp Community Psychiatry, 41:515, 1990.

---

* Asterisk indicates nursing reference.

Complete overview of the use of ECT. Addresses the major issues of indications, contraindications, risks, and procedure. Recent research is cited.

Craig C, Ray F, and Hix C: Seclusion and restraint: decreasing the discomfort, J Psychosoc Nurs Ment Health Serv 27:16, 1989.

Describes the development of an "intensive care" approach to the use of seclusion and restraint. Use of seclusion and restraint was lowered dramatically by increasing staffing, improving staff training, and increasing the involvement of other disciplines.

Crowe RR: Electroconvulsive therapy: a current perspective, N Engl J Med 311:163, 1984.

Excellent survey of research on ECT is presented in this article. The author addresses indications and effectiveness, contraindications, mortality, adverse effects, modifications in procedure, and patient acceptance. The conclusion is that ECT is a safe, effective treatment for mental disorders with an affective component, with relatively few complications and side effects.

*Grigson JW: Beyond patient management: the therapeutic use of seclusion and restraint, Perspect Psychiatr Care 22:137, 1984.

Demonstrates the use of theoretical constructs as a basis for nursing care planning. Author describes her theoretical framework, based on psychodynamic theories of behavior. Case examples are provided to demonstrate the model.

Gutheil TG: Observations on the theoretical bases for seclusion of the psychiatric inpatient, Am J Psychiatry 135:325, 1978.

Identifies appropriate and inappropriate conditions for secluding a patient. Author conveys the belief that this can be a helpful treatment for some patients. However, he also presents drawbacks and contraindications for its use. A good overview of some of the debatable issues relative to seclusion.

Karasu TB, editor: The somatic therapies, Washington, DC, 1984, American Psychiatric Association.

Provides an excellent review of current theory and research in somatic approaches to psychiatric care. It is the somatic therapy component of the report of the American Psychiatric Association Commission on Psychiatric Therapies.

*Kendrick DW and Wilber G: When in seclusion..., Am J Nurs 86:1117, 1986.

Provides a brief example of a documentation form used for patients who are in seclusion.

*Mulaik JS: Nurses' questions about electroconvulsive therapy, J Psychiatr Nurs 17:15, 1979.

Comprehensively and concisely describes the nursing considerations related to ECT. An excellent resource for nurses before their first experience with patients receiving ECT and very helpful to nurses who are planning nursing care with ECT patients.

Runck B: Consensus panel backs cautious use of ECT for severe disorders, Hosp Community Psychiatry 36:943, 1985.

Summarizes the findings of an NIMH consensus panel on ECT. The panel members received testimony from health care providers and consumers and reviewed research. This summary of their findings provides a complete overview of current information about ECT.

Strome TM: Restraining the elderly, J Psychosoc Nurs Ment Health Serv 26:18, 1988.

Describes a method of restraint for elderly patients that is a substitute for wrist and ankle restraints and continuous seclusion.

Tardiff K, editor: The psychiatric uses of seclusion and restraint, Washington, DC, 1984, American Psychiatric Press, Inc.

Collection of articles written by many of the most knowledgeable authorities on the uses of seclusion and restraint in psychiatric settings. Contents are comprehensive and include references to research.

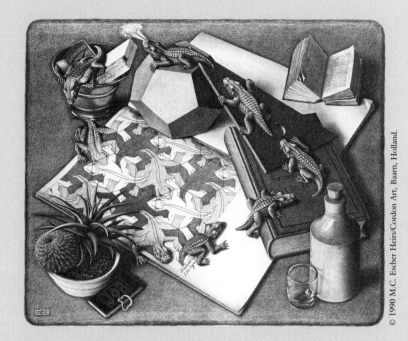

© 1990 M.C. Escher Heirs/Cordon Art, Baarn, Holland.

We must recollect that all our provisional ideas in psychology will some day be based on an organic substructure. This makes it probable that special substances and special chemical processes control the operation . . . .

Sigmund Freud

C H A P T E R   23

PSYCHOPHARMACOLOGY

MICHELE T. LARAIA

LEARNING OBJECTIVES

After studying this chapter, the student should be able to:

- identify the role of the nurse in psychopharmacological treatments.

- describe aspects of patient assessment before beginning pharmacotherapy.

- discuss the problems associated with polypharmacy and drug interactions.

- identify reasons for patient noncompliance with pharmacotherapy and related needs for patient education.

- describe "neurotransmission," including three possible effects of psychotropic drugs on neurotransmission.

- explain the mechanism of action for each of the four major classes of psychotropic drugs described in this chapter.

- list the clinical indications and target symptoms for each of the four major classes of psychotropic drugs described in this chapter.

- identify the related side effects and nursing considerations for each of the four major classes of psychotropic drugs described in this chapter.

- discuss guidelines for administering drugs from each psychotropic category, including acute and long-term use.

- identify directions for future nursing research.

- select appropriate readings for further study.

The past 30 years have produced a revolution in the treatment of psychiatric disorders and in the theories about the pathogenesis of these disorders. This revolution was sparked by the introduction of neuropsychopharmacology: drugs that treat the symptoms of mental illness and whose actions in the brain provide models to understand better the mechanisms of mental disorders. This sense of "revolution" continues as new theories are debated by experts in drug research and as more centers around the world are funded for clinical research drug studies.

Amid the growth and controversy involving new scientific information, the nurse frequently is the one professional to integrate these treatment drugs with the wide range of nonpharmacological treatments in a manner that is knowledgeable, safe, effective, and acceptable to the patient. Regardless of the nurse's theoretical framework, the reality of drug treatment of psychiatric illness must be recognized. Nurses should continue to incorporate psychopharmacology into the knowledge base of nursing theory, the arena of nursing research, and the art and science of nursing care. Nurses should also continue to do what nurses do best—lead the patient through the maze of medical care possibilities in a holistic manner, incorporating these possibilities into an individualized and effective treatment plan.

This chapter is designed to introduce the nurse to psychopharmacology in a basic way and to describe some of the important principles of drug treatment in psychiatry. The theoretical framework suggested here is one of integration: drug therapy can complement problem-solving procedures and the wide range of psychodynamic, psychosocial, and interpersonal interventions. Drug therapy should never be viewed as "an easy way out," "a quick fix," or "a miracle pill." Currently drug therapy treats symptoms of mental illness with some success, but drugs do not treat the patients' personal, social, or environmental responses to the mental illness. In addition, side effects and adverse reactions of drug therapy add another level of concern and need for expertise and judgment in the care of people receiving these treatments. Thus this is a very exciting time in psychiatric treatment, and nurses are in an excellent position to add new dimensions to their role from this expanding aspect of patient care.

Role of the nurse

Psychopharmacological treatment is intended to be integrated with the principles of psychiatric nursing practice presented throughout this text. Although it is important that the nurse be knowledgeable about the psychopharmacological strategies available, this tool must be put in the proper context of a holistic approach to patient care. The psychiatric nurse has a wealth of knowledge and techniques that make nursing unique in the care of people with psychiatric disorders. Following are some examples of the nurse's role in psychopharmacological treatment regimens.

■ **COLLECTION OF PRETREATMENT DATA.** The nurse is well equipped for the important task of establishing a baseline view of each patient. The nurse brings to this role a background in the biological and behavioral sciences, an understanding of the impact of mental illness on the patient's life, and the ability to integrate an interdisciplinary approach to data collection in a way that maintains the patient's integrity. These are necessary elements in designing a psychopharmacological drug trial and treatment plan.

■ **COORDINATION OF TREATMENT MODALITIES.** Based on his or her knowledge and relationship with the patient, the nurse has an important role in designing a viable treatment program for the patient. The most appropriate treatment choices, integrated in a holistic manner and individualized for each patient, should be reflected in the care plan designed by the nurse. The strength of the therapeutic alliance is the single most important factor in a successful treatment program, particularly when psychopharmacology is a part of that program.

■ **PATIENT EDUCATION.** The nurse is in a pivotal position to educate the patient about medications. This includes conveying complex information to the patient so that it is understandable, acceptable, achievable, and often critical for his health and safety.

■ **MONITORING DRUG EFFECTS.** The nurse is the most available professional to the patient and has the critical role of consistently monitoring the effects of psychopharmacological drugs, including their effects on target symptoms of illness, side effects, and adverse reactions and the overall yet often subtle effects on the patient's self-concept and sense of trust.

■ **PRINCIPLES OF PSYCHOPHARMACOLOGICAL DRUG ADMINISTRATION.** No one on the health care team has a greater daily impact on the patient's experience with psychopharmacological agents than the nurse. The nurse administers each medication dose, works out a dosing schedule based on drug requirements and the patient's preferences, and is continually alert for drug effects. This role defines the nurse as a key professional in working to maximize therapeutic effects of drug treatment and to minimize drug side effects in such a way that the patient is included as a true collaborator in his medication regimen.

■ **VIABLE DRUG MAINTENANCE PROGRAM.** The nurse is in a position to be the patient's contact with the mental health care system during maintenance drug treatment. For some patients the maintenance program could last many years. Whether the nurse has a formal therapeutic contract or is the designated contact for the patient regarding maintenance pharmacotherapy, the nurse can assume the important role of maintaining a therapeutic alliance with a patient on drug maintenance in the aftercare setting.

■ **CONCOMITANT NONPHARMACOLOGICAL TREATMENTS.** If the nurse has advanced clinical preparation, his or her role can extend to clinical therapist. The nurse would then choose from a wide range of therapeutic options for the patient, integrate the treatment plan with the patient's pharmacotherapy regimen, and work with the patient in a formalized, ongoing, psychotherapeutic alliance.

■ **INTERDISCIPLINARY CLINICAL RESEARCH DRUG TRIALS.** As a member of the interdisciplinary research team, the nurse can contribute to the body of scientific knowledge, often adding a nursing perspective to team research efforts. The nurse can be included on several levels, from data collector to coinvestigator to principal investigator. The nurse's roles in interdisciplinary clinical research drug trials in the clinical setting are just beginning to be appreciated and defined.

Patient assessment

Psychoactive drugs treat symptoms of mental disorders. However, not all behaviors are treated by drug therapy, and not every identified personality trait is a symptom of illness targeted for treatment with drugs. It thus is essential to obtain baseline information about each patient before drug treatment. This information helps describe aspects of the patient's psychiatric illness as compared to his pre-illness personality. As a result, a list of psychiatric symptoms can be identified as appropriate targets for drug treatment. Residual symptoms of the illness and personality characteristics not related to the illness then can be addressed by nonpharmacological treatments. In addition, drug side effects can be identified and appropriately treated as they appear. Symptoms of organ system dysfunction caused by drug treatment can also be identified and treated. Finally, careful assessment of each patient can help identify medical illnesses the patient may have that are concurrent with psychiatric illness or that possibly cause psychiatric symptoms.

Before beginning psychopharmacological treatment, a patient needs a thorough psychiatric evaluation. Such an evaluation must include the following:

1. Thorough physical examination
2. Laboratory studies
3. Mental status evaluation
4. Medical and psychiatric history
5. Medication and drug history
6. Family history

Various tools can be used in the evaluation process. Specifically, the clinician may use a variety of psychological assessment tools and behavioral rating scales[6] (see Appendix F) that can help define current pretreatment aspects of the patient's illness and can also be valuable in ongoing assessment to document both the patient's progress over time and the efficacy of a treatment regimen. These tools are also useful for comparing a patient's test results to the average results of groups of people with the same illness. This information can help formulate treatment plans and goals. Behavioral rating scales are also used as objective data-gathering tools in psychopharmacological research studies and are heavily relied on as objective outcome measures to document the efficacy of drug treatment. It is always important to include clinical notes with standardized tools. Rating scales are also useful before discharge or after the discontinuation of medication as posttreatment assessments.

In addition, specialized diagnostic procedures such as electroencephalograms (EEGs) and neurological studies can provide important information about effective treatments. More recently, brain visual imaging techniques are showing great promise in increasing knowledge of the pathophysiology of mental illness, in enhancing diagnostic assessment, and in playing a role in the choice of more specific treatments for individual patients. A thorough discussion of the range of psychiatric evaluation procedures is presented in Chapter 6. Knowledge of these procedures is necessary for both prescribing and evaluating psychopharmacological interventions.

Among other elements of baseline patient assessment is a longitudinal description of major illnesses, particularly psychiatric illness. These data should include when the illness began, symptoms, progression, treatments, and treatment outcomes. A family history of illness, particularly psychiatric illness, is also important information. Psychiatric illnesses have been correlated in biological family members, and drug treatments tend to have similar outcomes in family mem-

bers. For example, if schizophrenia has occurred in a patient's genetic family member, he is more likely to get schizophrenia than a person who has no history of this illness in his genetic line; and the former individual is also more likely to get schizophrenia than an affective disorder. Furthermore, a drug that successfully treated a family member with the same illness frequently is the first drug of choice to treat the patient. The box on page 701 provides a medication assessment tool for the nurse to use in taking a drug history.

The family history should include a social support assessment. The family should be integrated into the treatment process and in the aftercare planning. Family support contributes to patient compliance with treatment regimens and is an important component of holistic nursing care. Family and support system status is essential information in helping the nurse organize the patient's resources and other treatment considerations.

When initially assessing the patient, the nurse should remember that hospitalization removes the patient from the stresses in his environment and often results in decreased symptomatology. If the person's behavior is not overtly disruptive, he can be carefully observed during an initial drug-free diagnostic, psychological, and psychosocial evaluation period. Treatment with psychoactive drugs should be instituted without delay for the following reasons: if the patient had been taking drugs before hospitalization that cannot be precipitously stopped; if the symptoms or the patient's behavior is severe; if the patient has a long history of exacerbations of psychiatric illness; or if the patient is a threat to himself or others. Hollister[11] provides a succinct guide describing when to use psychopharmacological drugs.

Pharmacokinetics

Drugs are chemicals with specific properties that affect treatment. For example, it is often useful to know a drug's half-life. The half-life determines how long it takes to achieve a "steady state" concentration. Steady state means that the amount of drug excreted equals the amount ingested, and it occurs in approximately four to six half-lives. Until steady state is reached, the drug level continues to build, and it changes after each dosing. This accounts for some acute side effects in some patients. It also means that until steady state is reached, the optimum dose for a particular patient cannot be determined nor is a blood level accurate in determining a proper dose range. It may take longer to reach steady state in the elderly because of slower gastrointestinal activity and liver metabolism.

Another significance of half-life is in the frequency

Medication Assessment Tool

1. **Psychiatric medications** (for each medication ever taken by the patient obtain the following information):
   A. Name of drug
   B. Why prescribed
   C. Date started
   D. Length of time taken
   E. Highest daily dose
   F. Who prescribed it
   G. Was it effective?
   H. Side effects or adverse reactions
   I. Was it taken as prescribed? If not, explain.
   J. Has anyone else in family been prescribed this drug?
   K. If so, why prescribed and was it effective?
2. **Prescription (nonpsychiatric) medications** (for each medication taken by the patient in the past 6 months and for major medical illnesses if more than 6 months ago, obtain the following information):
   A. Name of drug
   B. Why prescribed
   C. Date started
   D. Highest daily dose
   E. Who prescribed it
   F. Was it effective?
   G. Side effects or adverse reactions
   H. Was it taken as prescribed? If not, explain.
3. **Over-the-counter (nonprescribed) medications** (for each medication taken by the patient in the past 6 months, obtain the following information):
   A. Name of drug
   B. Reason taken
   C. Date started
   D. Frequency of use
   E. Was it effective?
   F. Side effects or adverse reactions
4. **Alcohol, caffeine, and street drugs** (see Appendix E for common street names of abused substances)
   A. Name of substance
   B. Date of first use
   C. Frequency of use
   D. Summarize effects
   E. Adverse reactions
   F. Withdrawal symptoms

---

of dosing. Usually a drug with a half-life of 24 hours or more can be administered once a day when steady state is reached; a drug with a shorter half-life should be administered more often to achieve constant clinical effects. Termination of drug treatment is also affected by half-life. In general, the effects of drugs with a long half-life can last a long time (sometimes weeks) after the last dose. Drugs with a short half-life usually must be tapered (discontinued gradually over several days or weeks). In general, all psychoactive drugs should be discontinued by a tapering period.

This chapter focuses on the adult patient, although children and the elderly are frequently given psychoactive drugs. Generally, adults and children metabolize drugs similarly, although children exhibit a variable response to these drugs. Children must receive lower drug doses because of their lower body weight. (See Chapter 30 of this text and Koplan[14] for further discussion.) The elderly and newborns are particularly sensitive to psychotropic drugs. For the elderly, drug distribution, hepatic metabolism, and renal clearance are all affected by age.[22] If a pregnant woman takes psychoactive drugs before delivery, the infant may experience withdrawal symptoms unless the baby is detoxified from the drug. The infant whose mother takes psychoactive drugs generally should not be breast-fed.[4,15] Patients with liver disease are extremely sensitive to most psychoactive drugs, and patients with renal impairment are particularly sensitive to lithium.

■ Drug interactions

Drugs can interact with each other on two levels:

1. *Pharmacokinetic level*—one drug interferes with the absorption, metabolism, distribution, and excretion of another drug, thus raising or lowering the levels of the drug in the blood and tissue
2. *Pharmacodynamic level*—one drug combines with another to increase or decrease the drugs' effects in an organ system

Concurrent use of drugs, or polypharmacy, can enhance a specific therapeutic action, may be necessary to treat concurrent illnesses, and can counteract unwanted effects of one of the drugs. Unfortunately, a number of problems have been associated with concurrent drug use; confusion over therapeutic efficacy and side effects and development of drug interactions are just two. In general, polypharmacy in psychiatry should be used only when necessary and with caution. The accompanying boxes list guidelines for polypharmacy and alert the nurse to patients at a higher risk for drug interactions. Table 23-1 is a reference list for the more common drug interactions of psychotropic drugs.

This chapter refers to drugs by their generic names. There is a strong movement in practice to use generic names instead of trade names to be more accurate, to take advantage of price differences, and to avoid confusion when a drug becomes generic (when the patent runs out and the drug can be made by any company). A patent secures a drug for the company that owns it for 18 years from the time the drug is discovered. After the patent expires, other companies can market the drug and the price decreases, sometimes drastically. Many drugs that have been in regular use in psychiatry became generic in the 1980s. Once a drug becomes generic, the patient should be taught to use the same brand of a drug, as the bioavailability of psychoactive drugs may vary significantly from one brand to another, thus affecting drug dose and steady state. The patient can use one pharmacy regularly and can ask the pharmacist to use the same company when filling generic prescriptions of a particular drug.

■ **Patient education**

Patients taking psychotropic drugs must be knowledgeable about those drugs. Serious consequences can result from what appear to be minor changes in some of the instructions for drug use, such as skipping medication one day, eating cheese, or failing to recognize certain side effects. Patients and their families need thorough and ongoing instruction on psychotropic drug treatment. Patient education programs run by

---

Guidelines for Polypharmacy

1. Identify specific target symptoms for each drug.
2. If possible, start with one drug and evaluate effectiveness and side effects before adding a second drug.
3. Be alert for adverse drug interactions.
4. Consider the effects of a second drug on the absorption and metabolism of the first drug.
5. Consider the possibility of additive side effects.
6. Change the dose of only one drug at a time and evaluate results.
7. Be aware of increased risk of medication errors.
8. Be aware of increased cost of treatment.
9. Be aware of decreased patient compliance in the aftercare setting when medication regimen is complex.
10. In follow-up treatment, eliminate as many drugs as possible and establish the minimum effective dose of the drugs utilized.
11. Patient education programs regarding concomitant drug regimens must be particularly clear, organized, and effective.
12. Patient follow-up contacts should be more frequent.

Increased Risk Factors for Development of Drug Interactions

Polypharmacy
High doses
Geriatric patients
Debilitated/dehydrated patients
Concurrent illness

Compromised organ system function
Inadequate patient education
History of noncompliance
Failure to include patient in treatment planning

TABLE 23-1

INTERACTIONS OF PSYCHOTROPIC DRUGS AND OTHER SUBSTANCES

Drug/category	Interacting drug/class	Possible consequences
Antipsychotic agents		
	Antacids, oral	Antacids may inhibit absorption of orally administered phenothiazines
	Central nervous system depressants: alcohol barbiturates antianxiety agents antihistamines narcotic analgesics	Additive central nervous system depression, increasing the risk of mental or physical impairment of performance
	Anticholinergic agents: levodopa* (Bendopa, Larodopa, Levopa)	Additive atropine-like side effects; antiparkinson effects of levodopa may be antagonized by antipsychotic agents
Antianxiety agents		
Benzodiazepines	Central nervous system depressants: alcohol barbiturates antipsychotics antihistamines	Potential additive central nervous system effects, especially sedation and decreased daytime performance
	cimetidine	Interferes with metabolism of long-acting benzodiazepines
Antidepressant agents		
Tricyclics	MAO inhibitors*	May cause hypertensive crisis if tricyclic is added to MAO inhibitors
	Alcohol, other central nervous system depressants	*Acute:* additive CNS depression. *Chronic:* may increase tricyclic metabolism.
	Antihypertensives* guanethidine (Ismelin) methyldopa (Aldomet) clonidine (Catapres)	Antagonism of antihypertensive effects with loss of control of blood pressure
	Antipsychotics Anticholinergics	Additive atropinelike effects
	Antiarrhythmics quinidine procainamide	Additive antiarrhythmic effects, prolongation of QRS complex
Mood stabilizer		
Lithium	Diuretics* hydrochlorothiazide	Diuretic-induced sodium depletion can increase lithium levels; may cause toxicity
	Nonsteroidal anti-inflammatory agents* ibuprofen indomethacin phenylbutarone	Increases lithium blood levels; may cause toxicity
Sedative hypnotic agents		
	Alcohol—acutely Analgesics—narcotics Antihistamines Antidepressants Antipsychotics	Combined use of sedative-hypnotics with other central nervous system depressants may impair mental and physical performance (e.g., motor vehicle operation) and result in lethargy, respiratory depression, coma, or death. These drugs may enhance the sedative effects of barbiturates and nonbarbiturates.
	Anticoagulants*—oral	Increased rate of coumarin anticoagulant metabolism, decreasing plasma levels of coumarin and reducing its ability to prevent blood coagulations; higher dose of coumarin required; when barbiturate withdrawn and dose of courmarin not reduced, bleeding episode may occur.

*Potentially clinically significant.

Increased Risk Factors for Patient Noncompliance

Failure to form a therapeutic alliance with the patient

Devaluation of pharmacotherapy by treatment staff

Inadequate patient and family education regarding treatment

Poorly controlled side effects

Insensitivity to patient complaints or wishes

Multiple daily dosing schedule

Polypharmacy

History of noncompliance

Social isolation

Expense of drugs

Failure to appreciate patient's role in drug treatment plan

Lack of continuity of care

Increased restrictions on patient's life-style

Unsupportive significant others

Remission of target symptoms

Increased suicidal ideation

Increased suspiciousness

Unrealistic expectations of drug effects

Failure to target residual symptoms for nonpharmacological therapies

Relapse or exacerbation of clinical syndrome

Failure to alleviate intrafamilial and environmental stressors that precipitate symptoms

---

nurses have been shown to be an effective part of drug treatment programs for psychiatric patients.[16,24,28]

In addition to normal charting practices, the nurse should be sensitive to the importance of documenting the following issues in the pharmacological treatment of mental illness:

1. Drugs administered above daily recommended levels
2. Rationale for medication changes
3. Drugs used for other than the indications approved by the Food and Drug Administration
4. Continued use of a drug that is causing clinically significant side effects
5. Polypharmacy rationale

Patients who do not take their drugs as prescribed or who do not recognize warning signs of drug problems are at risk for unsuccessful results. The box shown above lists common risk factors for patient noncompliance with drug treatment regimens.

Based on current trends in psychoactive drug research, the nurse can expect to see new drugs approved for use in mental disorders on a regular basis. It is important to evaluate new drugs with a great deal of scrutiny as they come into clinical use. The nurse should determine the advantages and disadvantages of a new drug as compared to the standard drugs in that class and in relationship to the patient's reactions and preferences. The following list is a partial guide to help evaluate a new drug and separate the pertinent facts from a drug company's merchandising descriptions.

The nurse should be able to answer questions concerning whether the new drug has:

1. A different mechanism of action more specific to desired biological actions
2. Quicker onset of action
3. Fewer drug interactions
4. A lower side effect profile
5. No addictive or abuse potential
6. No long-term adverse effects
7. No suicide potential
8. Permanent or curative effects on neurotransmitter regulation
9. Several routes of administration, at least PO and IM
10. A wide therapeutic index
11. Fewer discontinuation problems
12. Advantage in cost effectiveness

Finally, the administration of psychotherapeutic drugs places the nurse in a position of power and control over the patient. The nurse should be aware of this issue and should not use the administration of medications to punish or manipulate the patient. The nurse should never withhold a drug that a patient needs. It is also the nurse's obligation to be aware of counter-transference issues and personal attitudes toward the patient, the prescribing physician, the patient's diagnosis, and his psychotropic drug treatment regimen. Effective and safe drug treatment in psychiatry depends on many factors, including the nurse's self-awareness.

Biological basis for psychopharmacology

All communication in the brain involves neurons "talking" to each other at synapses. These nerve cells are the basic functional unit of the nervous system, and the study of this communication process forms the basis of much of the neurosciences.[26] The following description is simplified to present a very basic frame of reference from which to view the rather overwhelming complexity of neuropharmacological mechanisms.

The synapse is a narrow gap separating two neurons (the presynaptic cell and the postsynaptic cell) at a transmission site (Fig. 23-1). During neurotransmission the chemical neurotransmitter is released from a storage vesicle in the presynaptic cell, crosses the synapse, and is recognized by the receptor on the postsynaptic cell membrane (this recognition is called binding). Receptors are the cellular recognition sites for specific molecular structures such as neurotransmitters, hormones, and many drugs. Thus their action is selective for specific chemicals. Neurotransmitters, the "chemical messengers" that travel from one brain cell to another, are synthesized by enzymes from certain dietary amino acids, or precursors. At the synapse, neurotransmitters act as receptor activators (agonists) or inhibitors (antagonists) and trigger complex biological responses within the cell. The chemical remaining in the synapse is either reabsorbed and stored by the presynaptic cell or is metabolized (inactivated) by synaptic enzymes, one of which is monoamine oxidase.

Many of the psychiatric disorders are thought to be caused by an overresponse or an underresponse somewhere along the complex process of neurotransmission. For instance, psychosis is thought to involve excessive dopamine neurotransmission. Depression and mania are thought to result from disruption of

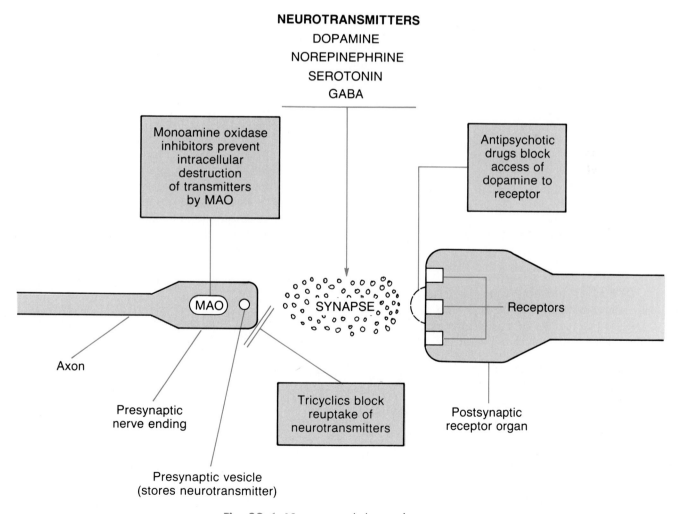

Fig. 23-1. Neurotransmission at the synapse.

normal patterns of neurotransmission of norepinephrine, serotonin, and other neurotransmitters. Anxiety is thought to be a dysregulation of gamma-aminobutyric acid (GABA) and endogenous antianxiety chemicals.

If one understands whether a particular psychiatric illness seems to be the result of "too much" or "too little" neurotransmission in a particular neurotransmitter system and also understands the mechanism of action of the psychiatric drugs, one begins to recognize some order in the various pharmacological strategies used in psychiatry. This process of cell-to-cell communication at the synapse can be affected by drugs in several important ways:

1. Release: More neurotransmitter is released into the synapse from the storage vesicles in the presynaptic cell.
2. Blockade: The neurotransmitter is prevented from binding to the postsynaptic receptor.
3. Receptor sensitivity changes: The receptor becomes more or less responsive to the neurotransmitter.
4. Blocked reuptake: The presynaptic cell does not reabsorb the neurotransmitter well, leaving more neurotransmitter in the synapse and therefore enhancing or prolonging its action.
5. Interference with storage vesicles: The neurotransmitter is either released again into the synapse (more neurotransmitter) or is released to metabolizing enzymes (less neurotransmitter).
6. Precursor chain interference: The process that "makes" the neurotransmitter is either facilitated (more neurotransmitter is synthesized) or disrupted (less neurotransmitter is synthesized).
7. Synaptic enzyme interference: Less neurotransmitter is metabolized, so more remains available in the synapse.

Not all of the above strategies have yielded clinically relevant treatments. Several have, however, and these are emphasized in this chapter (see Fig. 23-1): antipsychotic drugs block dopamine from the receptor site; tricyclic antidepressants block the reuptake of norepinephrine and serotonin and regulate the areas of the brain that manufacture these chemicals; monoamine oxidase inhibitors (MAO inhibitors or MAOIs) prevent enzymatic metabolism of norepinephrine and serotonin; and benzodiazepines potentiate GABA.

Understanding this process has led to the variety of treatment approaches in pharmacotherapy that attempt to change or modify one or more of the steps in neurotransmission. Unfortunately, to date the actions of psychopharmacological drugs are not confined to the specific brain areas that are thought to be associated with psychiatric symptoms. These drugs spread out in the body, causing unwanted drug reactions or side effects and undesirable drug interactions during concomitant drug therapy. Current psychopharmacological research attempts to better understand the cause of psychiatric illness at the neurotransmission level and the increased specificity of psychopharmacological drugs.

Antianxiety and sedative-hypnotic drugs

The diagnosis of anxiety is based on the patient's description and the nurse's observation of behaviors and on the process of elimination of alternative diagnoses. The possibility of a medical cause must be considered. Hyperthyroidism, hypoglycemia, and severe pulmonary disease are characteristic illnesses associated with high levels of anxiety. In addition to a careful physical assessment and a review of laboratory tests, the patient should be asked about use of over-the-counter drugs, "recreational" substances, alcohol, and caffeine. Anxiety also accompanies many psychiatric disorders. In general, the primary disorder should be treated with the appropriate medication. Anxiety may be associated with psychosis or an affective disorder and often goes away when the target symptoms for the primary disorder subside with appropriate treatment.

This section divides antianxiety and sedative-hypnotic drugs into two categories: the benzodiazepines and non-benzodiazepines; the latter group includes several classes of drugs. The benzodiazepines are the most widely prescribed drugs in the world, and within the last two decades they have almost entirely replaced the barbiturates in the treatment of anxiety and sleep disorders. Their popularity is related to their effectiveness and wide margin of safety, and they are the principal drugs used in the treatment of anxiety and insomnia.

■ Benzodiazepines

■ **MECHANISM OF ACTION.** The benzodiazepines are thought to reduce anxiety because they are powerful potentiators of the inhibitory neurotransmitter GABA, although the role of GABA in anxiety is not yet clear. A postsynaptic receptor site specific for the exogenous benzodiazepine molecule has been discovered. The search for a naturally occurring "antianxiety" chemical has recently resulted in the discovery of an endogenous benzodiazepine-binding inhibitor (DBI). The benzodiazepine molecule and GABA do not compete for the same receptor site. However, the benzodiazepines do compete with DBI for a role in neurotransmission, indicating that DBI may be the antianxiety neurotransmitter. Research in this field promises to provide a great deal of information in the future.

■ **CLINICAL USE.** The benzodiazepines are the drug treatment of choice in the management of anxiety, insomnia, and stress-related conditions. The target symptoms for use of these drugs are listed in the accompanying box. The major indications for their use are generalized anxiety disorder, anxiety associated with other psychiatric diagnoses, sleep disorders, anxiety associated with phobic disorders, posttraumatic stress disorder, alcohol and drug withdrawal, anxiety associated with medical disease, skeletal muscle relaxation, seizure disorders, and the anxiety and apprehension experienced before surgery. Major studies are beginning to show that higher-dose benzodiazepines, particularly alprazolam, a triazolobenzodiazepine, appear to have specific antipanic effects in the treatment of panic disorder.

The specific types of benzodiazepines have no sig-

nificant clinical advantages over each other. Some of the differences suggested for the use of these drugs can be attributed more to marketing strategies than clinical efficacy. Prescribing decisions can be made based on whether or not the drug breaks down into active metabolites that extend drug half-life (Table 23-2). Duration of action after a single dose can be relatively brief, depending on how rapidly the drug is metabolized and how extensively it is distributed to body tissues (in turn, this is based on lipid solubility). Duration of action at steady state can be much longer. Differences in half-life can be clinically useful. For example, patients with persistent high levels of anxiety should take a drug with a long half-life. Patients with fluctuating anxiety might be better off with short-acting drugs. When used as hypnotics the benzodiazepines ideally should induce sleep rapidly, and their effect should be gone by morning. The rate of absorption of the different benzodiazepines from the gastrointestinal tract varies considerably, thus affecting the rapidity and intensity of onset of their acute effects. Diazepam and chlorazepate are absorbed fastest, whereas prazepam and oxazepam are slowest. Antacids or food in the stomach slow this process.

Because the benzodiazepines are in the same pharmacological class as alcohol, they can be used to suppress the alcohol withdrawal syndrome. The concomitant use of these two substances can be dangerous, because it produces extreme sedation. Any of the benzodiazepines can be an effective sedative-hypnotic when administered at bedtime.[29]

Although some patients may need to take antianxiety drugs for extended periods of time, the drugs have their drawbacks and should always be used with nonpharmacological treatments for the patient who experiences chronic anxiety. Psychotherapy, behavioral techniques, environmental changes, stress management, and an ongoing therapeutic relationship continue to be important in the treatment of anxiety disorders.

Most experts feel that medication treatment with benzodiazepines should be brief, used during a time of specific stress. Those drugs with a long half-life (longer than 18 to 24 hours) can be given once a day. Drugs with a short half-life (8 to 15 hours) need to be given more frequently; they can be taken as needed for increased symptoms of anxiety as such symptoms occur. The patient should be observed frequently during the early days of treatment to assess target symptom response and to monitor side effects so that the dose can be adjusted. Some patients require long-term antianxiety medication treatment.

Concentrations of benzodiazepine drugs in the blood have not yet been firmly correlated to clinical ef-

---

Target Symptoms for Antianxiety and Sedative-Hypnotic Benzodiazepines

Psychological
Vague sense of irritability and uneasiness
Sense of impending doom or panic
Insomnia

Physical
Flushed skin
Hot or cold flashes
Sweating
Dilated pupils
Dry mouth
Nausea or vomiting
Diarrhea
Tachycardia, palpitations
Dizziness, light-headedness
Shortness of breath
Hyperventilation, with paresthesias
Tremor
Restlessness
Headache
Urinary frequency

TABLE 23-2

ANTIANXIETY AND SEDATIVE-HYPNOTIC DRUGS: THE BENZODIAZEPINE CLASS

Drug family				Drug dosage		
Chemical class generic name (trade name)	Active metabolites	Half-life (hr)	Days to steady state	Equivalence (mg)	Usual dosage range (mg/day)	Available forms (mg)
Antianxiety drugs						
Benzodiazepines						
alprazolam (Xanax)	Yes (Not significant)	6-20	3	0.5	0.5-4	tabs: 0.25, 0.5, 1.0
chlordiazepoxide (Librium)	Yes	5-200	1-3	10	20-100	tabs: 5, 10, 25 inj: 100
chlorazepate (Tranxene)	Yes	30-200	5-16	7.5	7.5-60	tabs: 3.75, 7.50, 15
clonazepam (Klonopin)	No	18-50	3-8	—	1.5-2	tabs: 0.5, 1, 2
diazepam (Valium)	Yes	20-200	4-8	5	10-40	tabs: 2, 5, 10, sustained release 15 inj: 5/ml
halazepam (Paxipam)	Yes	20-100	4	20	80-160	tabs: 20, 40
lorazepam (Ativan)	No	10-20	2-3	1	2-6	tabs: 0.5, 1, 2 inj: 2/ml, 4/ml
oxazepam (Serax)	No	5-15	1-2	15	15-90	tabs: 10, 15, 30
prazepam (Centrax)	Yes	30-200	5-32	10	10-60	tabs: 5, 10, 20
Sedative-hypnotic drugs						
Benzodiazepines						
flurazepam (Dalmane)	Yes	30-250	4-8	15	15-60	caps: 15, 30
temazepam (Restoril)	No	10-20	2-3	15	15-30	caps: 15, 30
triazolam (Halcion)	No	1.5-4	1	0.25	0.25-0.5	tabs: 0.25, 0.50
lorazepam (Ativan)	No	10-20	2-3	1	2-6	tabs: 0.5, 1, 2 inj: 2/ml, 4/ml

fects. All benzodiazepines are rapidly absorbed by mouth. The injectable benzodiazepines have been proven reliable when administered in the deltoid muscle and lead to rapid and predictable rises in the blood level when used intravenously. When given intravenously, administration should be slow (over 1 minute) and direct, not mixed in an IV infusion, because plastic tubing absorbs the drug and the drug can precipitate when mixed with saline or dextrose.

Another clinical indication for the use of benzodiazepines is as a sedative-hypnotic to improve sleep. In-somnia (poor sleep) includes difficulty falling asleep, difficulty staying asleep, or awakening too early. It is a symptom with many causes and often responds to nonpharmacological strategies such as talking about problems, increased daytime exercise, and physical comfort measures at night. Drugs to induce sleep have their place but should be used with discretion and are never a substitute for good nursing care.

■ **ADVERSE REACTIONS.** Because the benzodiazepines have a very high therapeutic index, overdoses of benzodiazepines alone almost never cause fatalities.

TABLE 23-3

BENZODIAZEPINE SIDE EFFECTS AND NURSING CONSIDERATIONS

Side effects	Nursing considerations
Acute/common	
Drowsiness, sedation	Activity helps; caution when using machinery
Ataxia, dizziness	Caution with activity, prevent falls
Feelings of detachment	Discourage social isolation
Increased irritability or hostility	Observe carefully, offer support, be alert for disinhibition of control over socially unacceptable impulses
Anterograde amnesia	Inability to recall events that occur while the drug is active; desirable in preoperative use
Long-term/common	
Minor tolerance to some effects	Short-term use if possible; discontinue, using a slow taper; not recommended for use with people with history of drug or alcohol abuse
Dependency	
Rebound insomnia/anxiety	
Rare (causal relationship uncertain)	
Increased appetite and weight gain	Weight control measures
Cutaneous reactions	Usually not clinically significant
Nausea	Dose with meals, decrease dose
Headache	Usually responds to mild analgesic
Confusion	Decrease dose
Gross psychomotor impairment	Dose related, decrease dose
Depression	Decrease dose; may require antidepressant treatment
Paradoxical rage reaction	Discontinue drug

Side effects are common, dose related, and almost always harmless. Table 23-3 summarizes these reactions and nursing considerations. The benzodiazepines generally do not live up to their reputation of being strongly addictive if they are discontinued gradually, if they have been used for appropriate purposes, and if their use has not been complicated by other factors such as chronic use of barbiturates or alcohol.

Tolerance does develop to the sedative effects of benzodiazepines, but it is unclear whether induced sleep or antianxiety effects develop tolerance. These drugs should be discontinued relatively slowly to minimize withdrawal symptoms and rebound symptoms of insomnia or anxiety. The general rule is a decrease by 5% of the dose each 1 to 3 days, although this varies. All benzodiazepines, regardless of half-life, should be discontinued by tapering. When these drugs are discontinued too rapidly or are stopped precipitously, especially with prolonged use of high doses, a benzodiazepine withdrawal syndrome can occur as described in the accompanying box. If this occurs, the dose must

Benzodiazepine Withdrawal Syndrome

Usually worsens several days after taper begins, increases over several weeks, then subsides. Minimize by slowing taper.

Mild symptoms	Severe symptoms
Tremulousness	Diarrhea
Insomnia	Hypotension
Dizziness	Hyperthermia
Headaches	Neuromuscular irritability
Tinnitus	Psychosis
Anorexia	Seizures
Vertigo	
Blurred vision	
Agitation	
Anxiety	

be raised until symptoms are gone and then tapering is resumed at a slower rate.[25]

An elderly patient is more vulnerable to side effects, because the aging brain is more sensitive to sedatives. The benzodiazepines with no active metabolites (see Table 23-2) are less affected by liver disease, the age of the patient, or drug interactions. Use of benzodiazepines during pregnancy has been associated with infant cleft lip/cleft palate, multiple congenital deformities, and intrauterine growth retardation, especially when used during the first trimester. When used late in pregnancy or during breast-feeding, these drugs have been associated with "floppy infant syndrome," neonatal withdrawal symptoms, poor sucking, and hypotonia.

■ Non-benzodiazepines

The advantages of the benzodiazepines compared to most other antianxiety and sedative-hypnotic agents have led to greatly decreased use of non-benzodiazepines. Non-benzodiazepine anxiolytics and sedative-hypnotics, listed in Table 23-4, are used when alternatives to benzodiazepines are sought or when preferred by physicians or patients.

The barbiturates have been largely replaced by the benzodiazepines, although the former are used occasionally. Barbiturates have numerous disadvantages: tolerance develops to their antianxiety effects; they are more addictive; they cause serious, even lethal withdrawal reactions; they are dangerous in overdose and cause central nervous system (CNS) depression; and they can cause a variety of dangerous drug interactions.

The propanediol drug, meprobamate, has also dropped in popularity. Its adverse effects, drug interactions, potential for abuse, and withdrawal syndromes are similar to those observed with barbiturates. Also, many studies show meprobamate to be no more effective than a placebo.

Ethychlorvynol, an acetylinic alcohol, has a variety of side effects: confusion, hangover, ataxia, hypotension, and gastrointestinal distress. Physical dependence occurs, tolerance develops, abuse is possible, and discontinuation can cause withdrawal reactions.

TABLE 23-4

THE ANTIANXIETY, SEDATIVE-HYPNOTIC DRUGS: NON-BENZODIAZEPINES

Chemical class generic name (Trade name)	Dose (mg)	Half-life (hr)
Barbiturates		
secobarbital (Seconal)	100-200	19-34
pentobarbital (Nembutal)	100-200	15-48
amobarbital (Amytal)	100-200	8-42
butabarbital (Butisol)	100-200	34-42
phenobarbital (Luminal)	100-200	24-140
Propanediols		
meprobamate (Equanil, Miltown)	800	10
Acetylinic alcohols		
ethychlorvynol (Placidyl)	500-1000	10-25
Piperidinediones		
glutethimide (Doriden)	250-500	5-22
methyprylon (Noludar)	200-400	4
Chloral derivative		
chloral hydrate (Noctec, Somnos)	500-2000	4-10
Antihistamines		
diphenhydramine (Benadryl)	50	unknown
hydroxyzine (Atarax)	100 tid	unknown
Beta-adrenergic blocker		
propranolol (Inderal)	10 qid	3
Anxiolytic		
buspirone (Buspar)	10-40	2-5

The piperidinedione derivatives have all the drawbacks of the barbiturates without any added advantages. They have remained in use despite their low therapeutic index, high lethality, and addiction potential because they produce relatively few unwanted effects at therapeutic doses.

Chloral hydrate can cause gastrointestinal irritation and causes a variety of drug interactions. Tolerance, physical dependence, addiction, and a withdrawal syndrome are all problems.

Antihistamines, especially hydroxyzine, are usually not as effective as the benzodiazepines; they cause sedation but do not cause physical dependence or abuse. A disadvantage of the antihistamines is that they lower the seizure threshold.

Propranolol blocks beta-noradrenergic receptors centrally and in the peripheral cardiac and pulmonary systems. This drug probably decreases certain physiological symptoms of anxiety, especially tachycardia, rather than centrally acting on anxiety. More research is needed to define a proper role for propranolol in the treatment of anxiety.[9]

Buspirone, a non-benzodiazepine anxiolytic drug, has been the subject of much discussion. It appears to be a potent antianxiety agent with no addictive potential. Buspirone is effective in the treatment of anxiety and does not exhibit muscle-relaxant or anticonvulsant activity, interaction with CNS depressants, or sedative-hypnotic properties. It is not effective in the management of drugs or alcohol abuse.

Antidepressant drugs

The 1950s were an important time in the history of psychopharmacology with the discovery of drugs that were effective in treating depression. Early in the 1950s dramatic improvements in mood and well-being were noted in tuberculosis patients being treated with iproniazid before improvement in the tuberculosis lesion was noted. This led to the use of monoamine oxidase inhibitors (MAOIs) as primary drug treatments for depression. At this same time, the first tricyclic antidepressant (TCA), imipramine, was tested for potential antipsychotic activity. It was found to be an ineffective antipsychotic, but depression improved. Imipramine was marketed in 1958 for its significant antidepressant properties. These two types of drugs, the MAO inhibitors and the tricyclic antidepressants, remain the major antidepressant medications at present.

Research on the biology of depression has led to many new discoveries and even more questions. It has been proposed that either serotonin or norepinephrine or both are reduced in depression and that an excess of norepinephrine is produced in mania. The biological understanding of antidepressant drugs supports this theory: MAO inhibitors "inhibit" the metabolism of these neurotransmitters, and tricyclic antidepressants block their reuptake at the presynaptic neuron. Both these mechanisms allow more neurotransmitter to remain in the synapse, thereby solving the functional "deficit" in depression. Several problems challenge the simplicity of this theory: 25% to 30% of people who are depressed do not respond to antidepressant drugs, and several new drugs that seem to be effective antidepressants do not appear to affect norepinephrine or serotonin levels. There is also evidence that antidepressants regulate the locus ceruleus, the part of the brain that makes most of the norepinephrine.

The integrative model of depression proposed by Akiskal and McKinney[1] continues to support the holistic approach to patient care so important to psychiatric nursing (see Chapter 14). This model suggests that many factors contribute to a functional impairment of central nervous system centers that help maintain mood, motor activity, appetite, sleep, and libido. Among the list of predisposing and precipitating stressors for depression are biological vulnerability, developmental deficits, and physiological, psychological, and social factors.

The primary clinical indication for use of antidepressant drugs is major depressive illness. These drugs are also useful in the treatment of panic disorder and enuresis in children. A variety of preliminary research studies suggest that they are useful in attention deficit disorders in children and in narcolepsy. Fluoxetine (Prozac) is receiving attention for its effectiveness in treating bulimia and its low side effect profile. Clomipramine (Anafranil), still experimental in the United States, has been shown to be effective in obsessive-compulsive disorder.

Table 23-5 lists predictors of antidepressant response to guide the clinician in the appropriate choice of the type of antidepressant drug.

The current treatment of depression has been greatly improved by a variety of effective drugs, yet depressive illness remains frequently misdiagnosed and often undertreated. It is estimated that 20 million Americans suffer from a serious depressive disorder each year, and suicide is the most frequent complication of depression. Suicide is the tenth greatest cause of death for all ages and the leading cause of death in adults under 25 years of age and in young adolescents. The suicide rate in people with unrecognized or inadequately treated depression is 60 times the rate of suicide in patients who are not depressed. These statistics are alarming and make vigorous and thorough treatment of depressive illness a mandate for ethical care.

TABLE 23-5

PREDICTORS OF ANTIDEPRESSANT RESPONSE

Tricyclics	MAOI
Positive predictors	
Anorexia	Hypochondriasis
Weight loss	Somatic anxiety
Insomnia (middle and late)	Irritability
Diurnal mood swing	Agoraphobia
Psychomotor retardation	Social phobias
Agitation	Anergia
Decreased functioning	Hysterical traits
Acute onset	Bipolar disorder
Family history of depression	Unresponsive to other
Self and family history of	antidepressants
drug responsiveness	
Therapeutic blood levels of	
antidepressants	
Agoraphobia	
Negative predictors	
Presence of other psychiatric	Depressed mood
disturbances	Guilt
Chronic symptoms	Ideas of reference
Psychotic features	Nihilistic delusions
Predominant somatic symp-	Affective personality
toms	disorders
Previous unsuccessful drug	
trials	
Previous sensitivity or ad-	
verse reactions	

Modified from Schoonover SC: In Bassuk EL, Schoonover SC, and Gelenberg AJ, editors: The practitioner's guide to psychoactive drugs, ed 2. New York & London, 1984, Plenum Medical Books Co and Nardil: Parke-Davis Product Monograph, ed 4. Morris Plains, NJ, 1982, Park-Davis, Medical Affairs Department.

When pharmacotherapy is a component of the treatment regimen for a depressed patient, the nurse can help minimize side effects, assess drug effectiveness, and maximize patient safety and drug efficacy. Stimmel[27] and Hayes and Bloom[8] provide guides for nurses treating patients with antidepressants.

■ Biological markers

Perhaps more than in any other diagnostic category, investigators have identified biological markers of clinical usefulness in the diagnosis and treatment of depression. However, these tests are not 100% accurate, research results are often contradictory, the tests are new and expensive, and they uphold the biological psychiatry frame of reference. Thus they are controversial. They merit recognition by nurses because of their increasing popularity and because biological markers are an important research area with implications for the future understanding of exogenous "chemical" treatments in mental illness.

■ **URINARY MHPG.** Norepinephrine, when metabolized, is broken down into several other chemicals. A main metabolite of norepinephrine is 3-methoxy-4-hydroxy-phenylglycol (MHPG). Because this metabolite crosses the blood-brain barrier, its CNS activity can be estimated by measuring MHPG elimination in urine. This measurement is complicated by the fact that peripheral MHPG is also excreted in the urine, although many investigators believe that urinary MHPG gives accurate clues about levels of brain norepinephrine. An aliquot is taken from a 24-hour urine collection on a day (it is hoped) that is average for the individual patient in terms of activity, anxiety, and dietary tyramine ingestion. Serotonin, on the other hand, can be validly measured only in cerebrospinal fluid, since its main metabolite, 5-HIAA, does not cross the blood-brain barrier. Investigators have proposed that patients with low MHPG have less norepinephrine to metabolize and thus theoretically would respond to an antidepressant that blocks the reuptake of norepinephrine. Some evidence suggests that patients with normal or high MHPG have a serotonin-deficient depression (since their norepinephrine levels are not low) and would respond to a drug that blocks serotonin reuptake.

Table 23-6 lists the degree to which each of the antidepressant drugs is thought to potentiate these neurotransmitters. The clinical implication here is that if an adequate trial of desipramine (4+ norepinephrine) is unsuccessful, the next antidepressant of choice should be a serotonin potentiator such as amitriptyline or trazodone. If this drug is also unsuccessful, the third drug trial might be with a MAO inhibitor, which has a completely different mechanism of action. Although it is still highly theoretical, this type of system takes the choice of antidepressant drugs from a "grab-bag" to a scientifically based decision-making process. The hope for the future is that a simple urine or blood test will reliably indicate which antidepressant drug to use for each individual patient, saving what could be several months of frustrating, expensive, and dangerous (if the patient is suicidal) unsuccessful drug trials.

■ **DEXAMETHASONE SUPPRESSION TEST.** Another biological marker for depression in current use is the dexamethasone suppression test (DST). Researchers have established that most depressed people have

TABLE 23-6

PHARMACOLOGICAL PROFILES OF THE ANTIDEPRESSANTS

| Antidepressant drug | Acute side effects | | | Potentiation of neurotransmitter | | | Antianxiety effect |
	Anti-cholinergic	Cardio-vascular	Sedative	5-HT	NE	DA	
Tricyclic agents							
amitriptyline	4	4	4	3	1	0	4
desipramine	1	2	1	0	4	0	1
doxepin	4	2	4	2	1	0	3
imipramine	4	3	3	2	3	0	2
nortriptyline	3	3	2	2	3	0	1
protriptyline	2	3	1	2	4	0	0
trimipramine	4	3	4	2	3	0	3
Nontricyclic agents							
amoxapine	3	2	3	1	4	0	2
bupropion	1	1	0	0	0	0	0
maprotiline	3	2	3	0	4	0	3
trazodone	0	1	4	4	0	0	4
fluoxetine	2	1	2	3	1	0	0

4 = high; 3 = moderate; 2 = low; 1 = slight; 0 = none.
5-HT = serotonin NE = norepinephrine DA = dopamine.

cortisol secretion that does not follow the usual biological rhythm documented in nondepressed people. Normal cortisol levels are relatively flat from late afternoon until about 3 A.M., when they begin to spike at regular intervals until about noon. They then begin to level out again. Biologically depressed people have been found to have erratic spikes over a 24-hour period. The DST involves giving a small dose of the synthetic steroid dexamethasone at 11 P.M. and drawing plasma cortisol at 4 P.M. the next day. The dexamethasone usually suppresses pituitary adrenocorticotropic hormone (ACTH) and circulating adrenal steroids for at least 24 hours with no ill effects to the patient. Researchers report that between 40% and 70% of depressed people "escape" the cortisol suppression. That is, at some time in the next 24 hours, their cortisol levels return to erratic, above-normal spikes. If the post-dexamethasone cortisol level is ≥5 ng/ml, then it "escaped" suppression, and support is added for a diagnosis of biological depression.

The most consistent and currently helpful use for the DST is to repeat this test after depressive symptoms have remitted. If the DST was abnormal previously and has not yet normalized, continued antidepressant drug treatment is indicated. If a depressed patient's initial DST is normal, assuming it is accurate, it means the DST is not helpful in confirming a diagnosis of biological depression. In either case it is important to include nonpharmacological assessments and interventions when treating most people with depression, considering the impact this illness has on the well-being of the individual and society as a whole.

■ **REM LATENCY MEASUREMENT.** Using electroencephalographic tracings during sleep, researchers have identified five patterns, or stages, of sleep. The sleep cycle begins with stage one, the lightest sleep stage, which is followed by successively deeper stages two, three, and four. Stages three and four are characterized by increasing quantities of slow (delta) waves and probably have a restorative effect on body metabolic functions. After this initial cycle of the four stages of sleep, about 60 to 90 minutes in the normal person, the fifth cycle, or rapid eye movement (REM) sleep begins. REM is associated with dreaming, decreased muscle tone, and fast-frequency, low-amplitude EEG waves. This sleep cycle repeats itself approximately four to six times each night, at intervals of approximately 90 minutes. Depressed patients have been shown to spend less time in the more refreshing slow-wave phases of sleep, may have increased periods of REM sleep, and typically have a shorter than normal period before their first REM phase; this is called decreased REM latency, and it suggests another biological marker for depression. Sleep studies done on depressed patients have shown that these patients frequently attain REM sleep within minutes to a half hour after falling asleep, rather than in the normal 90 minutes, thus adding another indication for a diagnosis of depression.

■ Tricyclic antidepressants

■ **MECHANISM OF ACTION.** As new antidepressants were discovered and researched, their actions at the synapse went far beyond the simple reuptake blockade theory. Most experts now believe that depression can have several different biological mechanisms. It remains the task of future research to expand current knowledge and to further refine drugs with specific mechanisms of action to treat depressions with specific biological abnormalities.

Although the class of tricyclic antidepressants includes some drugs that are structurally dissimilar, the drugs in this class are quite similar to one another in their clinical effects and adverse reactions. They are divided into several categories: tertiary tricyclics (or parent drugs), secondary tricyclics (or metabolites), and a newer nontricyclic (or heterocyclic) group of drugs.

■ **CLINICAL USE.** The antidepressant drugs are listed in Table 23-7. Elderly patients and patients with a concomitant medical illness may require lower doses

---

TABLE 23-7

ANTIDEPRESSANT DRUGS

Chemical class generic name (trade name)	Usual dosage range (mg/day)	Available forms (mg)
Tricyclic drugs		
Tertiary (parent drug)		
amitriptyline (Elavil, Endep)	50-300	tabs: 10, 25, 50, 75, 100, 150 inj: 10/ml
doxepin (Adapin, Sinequan)	50-300	caps: 10, 25, 50, 75, 100, 125, 150 oral conc: 10/ml
imipramine (SK-Pramine, Tofranil)	50-300	tabs: 10, 25, 50 caps: 75, 100, 125, 150 inj. 25/2 ml
trimipramine (Surmontil)	50-300	caps: 25, 50, 100
chlomipramine (Anafranil)	50-250	tabs: 25, 50, 75
Secondary (metabolite)		
desipramine (Norpramin, Pertofrane)	50-300	tabs: 25, 50, 75, 100, 150
nortriptyline (Aventyl, Pamelor)	50-150	caps: 10, 25, 75 solution: 10/5 ml
protriptyline (Vivactil)	15-60	tabs: 5, 10
Nontricyclic drugs		
amoxapine (Asendin)	50-600	tabs: 25, 50, 100, 150
maprotiline (Ludiomil)	50-225*	tabs: 25, 50, 75
trazodone (Desyrel)	50-600	tabs: 50, 100, 150
buproprion (Wellbutrin)	50-600*	tabs: 50
fluoxetine (Prozac)	20-80	caps: 20
Monoamine oxidase inhibitors		
isocarboxazid (Marplan)	30-70	tabs: 10
phenelzine (Nardil)	45-90	tabs: 15
tranylcypromine (Parnate)	20-60	tabs: 10

*Antidepressants with a ceiling dose due to dose-related seizures.

of these drugs than healthy adults, and these patients require careful assessments for side effects while they are taking the drugs. For patients with an acceptable cardiac history and an ECG within normal limits, particularly for patients over 40 years of age, tricyclic antidepressants are safe and effective in the treatment of acute and long-term depressive illness.

Two of the tricyclic antidepressants, imipramine and nortriptyline, have rigorously studied blood plasma levels that have been correlated with clinical response. Plasma levels for most other antidepressants, although less extensively researched, are also widely used.[19] Plasma level guidelines are helpful, since each patient metabolizes drugs at a different rate. A plasma level can help keep the dose within the therapeutic range (listed in Table 23-8). It also assures that enough drug is in the patient's system to be effective. Some drugs, particularly nortriptyline, have a "therapeutic window"(the range within which the drug is considered to be therapeutic), and a plasma level below or above the range limits results in a decrease in antidepressant effectiveness. Blood for a plasma level should be drawn 8 to 12 hours after a single (usually bedtime) dose. Measuring the level soon after drug ingestion results in an artificially high level, representing the peak of the drug metabolism rather than the steady-state level.

It is estimated that at least 15% to 20% of patients with depressive illness have chronic or recurrent symptoms. These patients may benefit from a maintenance regimen of antidepressant drugs.[23] A tricyclic that has been successful in the past for a particular patient may be continued indefinitely, usually at a much lower dose

TABLE 23-8

THERAPEUTIC PLASMA LEVELS FOR ANTIDEPRESSANT DRUGS

Drug	Therapeutic range (ng/l)
imipramine and desipramine	150-250
desipramine	125-300
amitriptyline and nortriptyline	80-250
nortriptyline	50-150
protriptyline	70-260
doxepin and desmethyldoxepin	150-250
maprotiline	200-600
amoxapine and 8-hydroxyamoxapine	200-600
trazodone	800-1600

than was successful during an acute episode. These patients need to be followed and assessed regularly, and the drug must be discontinued gradually after a long period of stability to determine whether continued maintenance pharmacotherapy is needed.

■ **ADVERSE REACTIONS.** The nurse should know the common side effects of the antidepressants and their nursing treatments, as described in Table 23-9. Most of these side effects cause minor discomfort, but some can produce serious illness. These drugs have no known long-term adverse effects, tolerance to therapeutic effects does not develop, and persistent side effects often can be minimized by a small decrease in dose. Because antidepressants do not cause physical addiction, psychological dependence, or euphoria, they have no abuse potential. Their long half-life (24 hours or longer) allows them to be conveniently administered once a day, at night for most people. If the bedtime dose interferes with sleeping or causes nightmares, the dose should be given in the morning or divided into several doses throughout the day. Patients with bipolar illness may be switched into mania by these drugs; they should be watched closely for increased activity, greater difficulty concentrating and eating, and decreased sleeping patterns.

Unfortunately, all antidepressants must be taken for 3 to 4 weeks or longer before a therapeutic response is evident. Table 23-10 describes the target symptoms for these drugs in the approximate order of the time it takes for each symptom to begin to improve. When caring for suicidally depressed patients, it is important to remember that they become more motivated and begin to look better long before their subjective depressive feelings and suicidal thoughts are relieved. The nursing care plan must include suicide assessments and suicide precautions for weeks after these patients begin to look less depressed.

Because these drugs are among the most dangerous substances available when taken in excessive amounts, overdoses and suicide attempts using antidepressants are extremely serious and require emergency medical attention. Ingestion of 1,000 to 3,000 mg can be lethal. This may represent barely a 1-week supply of medication. For inpatients, mouth checks may be necessary. Even for outpatients who are not suicidal, antidepressants should be prescribed in small amounts and frequent assessments should be made. Accidental overdoses in children whose parents are taking an antidepressant are unfortunately common and often lethal. The health teaching and care of these patients should include an assessment of household members, and patients should be cautioned to keep these drugs in the childproof bottles received from the pharmacy, to keep

TABLE 23-9

TRICYCLIC ANTIDEPRESSANT SIDE EFFECTS AND NURSING CONSIDERATIONS

Side effects	Nursing considerations
Gastrointestinal	
Heartburn, nausea, vomiting	Administer drug with meals or at bedtime
Decrease in intestinal motility, paralytic ileus	Occurs in half of all patients; elderly are particularly susceptible; bran, bulk laxatives, high-fiber foods, stool softeners, decrease dose, change to a less anticholinergic drug
Dry mouth	Common, tolerance can develop; encourage adequate hydration, sugar-free products, mouth lubricants, try bethanecol (cholinergic agent—25 mg tid), lower dose, change to a less anticholinergic drug
Hematological	
Leukopenia and thrombocytopenia	Monitor; rarely clinically significant
Agranulocytosis: Allergic response of sudden onset; appears 40 to 70 days after initiation of drug (low WBC, normal RBC, infection of the pharynx, fatigue, malaise)	Very rare; discontinue drug and place patient in reverse isolation immediately; never administer drug again; try antidepressant with a different chemical structure and follow patient closely
Hepatic	
Liver toxicity within first 8 weeks of treatment: abdominal pain, anorexia, fever, mild transient jaundice, abnormal liver function tests	Rare hypersensitivity response; discontinue drug; switch to another type of antidepressant
Endocrine	
Amenorrhea, galactorrhea	Due to increased prolactin caused by amoxapine; rare with other tricyclics
Menstrual irregularities	Rare and reversible; decrease dose; change to a different tricyclic
Opthalmological	
Blurred vision caused by ciliary muscle relaxation	Tolerance can develop over the first few weeks of treatment; distant vision is usually intact; do not use with patients with narrow-angle glaucoma
Cardiovascular	
Postural hypotension: lightheadedness or dizziness on rising due to decrease in blood pressure on rising	Occurs frequently; take vital signs sitting and then standing ½ hour after dose; rise slowly, dangle feet, tolerance can develop in first few weeks; not dose related, can continue to raise dose
Tachycardia: rapid heart beat	Occurs frequently; tolerance usually develops; can increase symptoms of angina in patients with coronary artery disease; very frightening to panic disorder patients; in other patients, not clinically significant
EKG changes	QRS and QT interval prolongation; worsening of intraventricular conduction problems; take a careful cardiac history and do a pretreatment EKG, especially with patients over 40 years of age
Sudden death	Rare; patients at risk for cardiac heart block; over 50 years of age, family history of heart disease, preexisting cardiac disease or recent myocardial infarction, or bundle-branch block

TABLE 23-9—cont'd

TRICYCLIC ANTIDEPRESSANT SIDE EFFECTS AND NURSING CONSIDERATIONS

Side effects	Nursing considerations
Neurological	
Sedation, psychomotor slowing, difficulty concentrating and planning	Inform the patient, especially if he operates machinery or must perform mental tasks; tolerance can develop
Muscle weakness, fatigue, nervousness, headaches, vertigo, neuropathies, tremors, ataxia, paresthesias, twitching	Not common; tolerance can develop; lower dose
Lowered seizure threshold	Start drugs at lower dose and increase more gradually with seizure disorder patients
Extrapyramidal side effects (EPS): acute dystonic reactions, akathisia, Parkinson's syndrome, tardive dyskinesia	Rare, since they do not block dopamine; *amoxapine*, the exception, can cause all the common EPS reactions, possibly tardive dyskinesia with long-term use
Psychiatric symptoms: increased anxiety, depression, insomnia, nightmares, psychotic reactions, or confusional states with delusions, hallucinations, and disorientation; mania	Uncommon, may have to discontinue drug; mania may be precipitated if patient has prior history of mania in self or family (avoid tricyclics if possible in patients predisposed to mania)
Cutaneous	
Maculopapular rashes, petechiae, photosensitivity	Rare; can give an antihistamine; may have to discontinue antidepressant
Genitourinary	
Increased or decreased sexual desire, delayed ejaculation	Decrease dose, change to a less anticholinergic drug; take daily dose after sexual intercourse, not immediately before, for delayed ejaculation
Urinary retention	Lower dose, change to a less anticholinergic drug, try bethanecol; rare: acute renal failure following an atonic bladder
Miscellaneous	
Tinnitus, weight loss, increased appetite and weight gain, psychomotor stimulation, parotid swelling, alopecia, allergic response: edema, generalized on face, tongue, and orbits	Very rare; weight control; decrease dose; may have to discontinue drug and try an antidepressant that is structurally different
Pathological sweating	Occurs in 25% of patients; head, neck, and upper extremities; episodic, or occurs only at night
Withdrawal syndrome	
Mild withdrawal after sudden discontinuation: malaise, muscle aches, coryzia, chills, nausea, dizziness, anxiety	Taper patient off drug gradually (one to several weeks)
Intoxication syndromes	
Poisoning: usually seen in overdose with CNS depression and/or cardiotoxicity: hallucinations, delirium, agitation, sensitivity to sounds, dilated pupils, hypothermia, hyperpyrexia, seizures, coma, arrhythmias, respiratory arrest	Treat aggressively; recovery can be slow; induce emesis, gastric lavage, cardiac monitoring, respiratory support, blood chemistry, arterial blood gases, tricyclic plasma levels monitored, carefully administer physostigmine, valium, mannitol, lidocaine, and other symptomatic treatments
Anticholinergic syndromes	
Confusion, delirium, disorientation, agitation, hallucinations, anxiety, motor restlessness, seizures, delusions, constipation, urinary retention, decreased sweating, increased pupillary size, dry mouth, increased temperature, motor incoordination, flushing, tachycardia	Usually occurs with high doses of several psychoactive drugs with anticholinergic effects; physostigmine, cardiac monitoring, respiratory support; in sensitive or aged patients, may occur at normal, therapeutic levels

TABLE 23-10

ANTIDEPRESSANT DRUG TARGET SYMPTOMS

Onset of drug effect	Symptom
Week 1	Middle and terminal insomnia
	Appetite disturbances
	Anxiety
Week 2	Fatigue
	Poor motivation
	Somatic complaints
	Agitation
	Retardation
Week 3	Dysphoric mood
	Subjective depressive feelings (anhedonia, poor self-esteem, pessimism, hopelessness, self-reproach, guilt, helplessness, sadness)
	Suicidal thoughts

Signs and Treatment of Hypertensive Crisis on MAOI

Warning signs

Increased blood pressure, palpitations, frequent headaches

Symptoms of hypertensive crisis

Sudden elevation of blood pressure
Explosive headache, occipital that may radiate frontally
Head and face are flushed and feel "full"
Palpitations, chest pain
Sweating, fever
Nausea, vomiting
Dilated pupils
Photophobia
Intracranial bleeding

Treatment

Hold next MAOI dose
Do not lie patient down (elevates blood pressure in head)
IM chlorpromazine 100 mg, repeat if necessary (*Mechanism of action:* blocks norepinephrine)
IV phentolamine, administered slowly in doses of 5 mg (*Mechanism of action:* binds with norepinephrine receptor sites, blocking norepinephrine)
Fever: Manage by external cooling techniques

the drugs out of the reach of children, and to discard leftover drugs when pharmacotherapy is completed.

Most patients develop tolerance to side effects, and most side effects are dose related; thus they can be minimized by increasing the dose gradually when the drug is first prescribed. This gives the patient time to physiologically adjust to the drug. This is especially true when these drugs are used to treat panic disorder. Patients with panic disorder are particularly sensitized to any drug side effects that remind them of symptoms of anxiety or panic attacks (e.g., rapid heart beat, dizziness, nausea, blurred vision). In the case of severely depressed patients or those who are suicidal, doses are generally increased more rapidly to minimize the time it takes to reach steady state and therapeutic effectiveness.

Tricyclic antidepressants, like all psychiatric drugs, should be avoided if possible during pregnancy, especially in the first trimester. However, these drugs have been given throughout pregnancy without harmful effects on the fetus and should be considered if a pregnant woman is severely depressed, especially if suicide is a risk.

■ Monoamine oxidase inhibitors (MAOIs)

The monoamine oxidase inhibitors are very effective antidepressant/antipanic drugs that have been underused and overly feared. The MAOIs currently used in psychiatry are listed in Table 23-7.[30] Because of the potential for a hypertensive crisis when tyramine-containing foods and certain medicines are taken along with these drugs, careful health teaching of a reliable patient is quite important. The patient must avoid certain foods, drinks, and medicines (Table 23-11), must know the warning signs, symptoms, and even treatment of a hypertensive crisis (box), and must be taught the more common side effects of MAOIs (Table 23-12). For various indications (Table 23-5) these drugs are effective and are safe when used as prescribed. They generally cause fewer anticholinergic, sedative, and cardiovascular effects than tricyclics. They are nonaddicting, and tolerance does not develop toward therapeutic effects; however, safety in pregnancy has not been established. The patient should be

TABLE 23-11

DIETARY RESTRICTIONS 1 DAY BEFORE, DURING, AND 2 WEEKS AFTER TAKING MAOIs

Food and beverages to avoid

Cheese, especially aged or matured
Fermented or age protein
Pickled or smoked fish
Beer, red wine, sherry, liqueurs, cognac
Yeast or protein extracts
Fava or broad bean pods
Beef or chicken liver
Spoiled or overripe fruit
Banana peel
Yogurt

Food and beverages to be consumed in moderation

Chocolate
Yogurt and sour cream
Clear spirits and white wine
Avocado
New Zealand spinach
Soy sauce
Caffeine drinks

Medications to avoid

Cold medications
Nasal and sinus decongestants
Allergy and hay fever remedies
Narcotics, especially meperidine
Inhalants for asthma
Local anesthetics with epinephrine
Weight-reducing pills, pep pills, stimulants
Other medications without first checking with a physician

Illicit drugs to avoid

Cocaine
Amphetamine

Safe food and beverages

Fresh cottage cheese
Cream cheese
Fresh fruits
Bread products raised with yeast (bread)

Safe medications

Aspirin, Tylenol
Pure steroid asthma inhalants
Codeine
Plain Robitusin or terpin-hydrate with codeine
Local anesthetics without epinephrine
All laxatives
All antibiotics
Antihistamines

Medications that may need dose decreased

Insulin and oral hypoglycemics
Oral anticoagulants
Thiazide diuretics
Anticholinergic agent
Muscle relaxants

Modified from Zisook S: Psychosomatics 26(3):240, 1985 and Moreines R and Gold MS: In Gold MS, Lydiard RB, and Carman JS, editors: Advances in psychopharmacology: predicting and improving treatment response, pp 157-177. Boca Raton, Fla, 1984, CRC Press.

on the restricted diet several days before beginning the medication, while on the medication, and for 2 weeks after stopping the medication. No more than one MAOI should be given at a time. Neither should these drugs be used along with tricyclics except in limited cases and under expert supervision.

Tyramine is an amino acid released from proteins in food when they undergo hydrolysis by fermenting, aging, pickling, smoking, and spoiling. It is deactivated by monoamine oxidase in the gut wall and liver. When monoamine oxidase is inhibited, tyramine may reach adrenergic nerve endings, causing the release of large amounts of norepinephrine and producing a hypertensive reaction. Also, sympathomimetic drugs act on the neurotransmission process by releasing norepinephrine from the storage vesicles in the presynaptic

TABLE 23-12

MAOI SIDE EFFECTS AND NURSING CONSIDERATIONS

Side effects	Nursing considerations
Postural lightheadedness	Get up slowly, dangle feet, wear elastic hose, increase salt intake, reduce dose
Constipation	Bran, bulk laxatives, stool softeners, fiber, exercise, reduce dose
Delay in ejaculation or orgasm	Separate last dose and sexual intercourse by as many hours as possible (e.g., 8 A.M. and 12 noon dose, evening sexual intercourse), reduce dose
Muscle twitching	300 mg/day vitamin B₆ often helps; reduce dose
Drowsiness	Encourage activity, avoid using machinery, take short daytime naps
Dry mouth	Lemon/glycerin swabs, sugarless gum and candies, fluids
Fluid retention	Low-dose thiazide diuretics
Insomnia	Last dose should be as early in the day as possible; encourage patient not to remain physically active all evening but to start relaxing several hours before bedtime; reduce dose
Urinary hesitancy	Urecholine may help; reduce dose

nerve ends. Because monoamine oxidase has been inhibited when MAOIs are used, large amounts of norepinephrine are released and a severe hypertensive reaction can occur. Thorazine, an antipsychotic drug, and the alpha-adrenergic blocking agent phentolamine bind to the norepinephrine receptor sites, preventing norepinephrine stimulation and resolving the hypertensive crisis. It remains to be seen if the MAO inhibitors will continue to be used for certain patient populations or if they will be used less frequently for depression and other disorders.

Mood stabilizing drugs

■ Lithium

Lithium, a naturally occurring salt, was noted to have medicinal properties during the nineteenth century, when it was found to be present in the waters of some European mineral springs. It was described as having antimanic properties in 1949 but was not accepted for use in the United States until 1970 because of reports of its toxic effects. Today it is readily and safely administered under careful clinical guidelines and has an important clinical role as a mood stabilizer in the treatment of cyclical affective disorders.

■ **MECHANISM OF ACTION.** The exact mechanism of action of lithium is not fully understood, but many neurotransmitter functions are altered by the drug. It has been suggested that lithium corrects an ion exchange abnormality; alters sodium transport in nerves and muscle cells; normalizes synaptic neurotransmission of norepinephrine, serotonin, and dopamine; increases the reuptake and metabolism of norepinephrine; and changes receptor sensitivity for sero-

TABLE 23-13

TARGET SYMPTOMS FOR LITHIUM THERAPY

Mania	Depression
Irritable	Irritable
Expansive	Sadness
Euphoric	Pessimistic
Manipulative	Anhedonia
Labile with depression	Self-reproach
Sleep disturbance (decreased sleep)	Guilt
Pressured speech	Hopelessness
Flight of ideas	Somatic complaints
Motor hyperactivity	Suicidal ideation
Assaultive/threatening	Motor retardation
Distractibility	Slowed thinking
Hypergraphia	Poor concentration and memory
Hypersexual	Fatigue
Persecutory and religious delusions	Constipation
Grandiose	Decreased libido
Hallucinations	Anorexia or increased appetite
Ideas of reference	Weight change
Catatonia	Helplessness
	Sleep disturbance (insomnia or hypersomia)

Pre-Lithium Work-up

Renal: Urinalysis, BUN, creatinine, electrolytes, 24-hour creatinine clearance; history of renal disease in self or family; diabetes mellitus, hypertension, diuretic use, analgesic abuse

Thyroid: TSH (thyroid-stimulating hormone), T_4 (thyroxine), T_3 RU (resin up-take), T_4 I (free thyroxine index); history of thyroid disease in self or family

Other: Complete physical, history; ECG, fasting blood sugar, CBC

Maintenance lithium considerations

Every 3 months: Li level (for the first 6 months)

Every 6 months: reassess renal status, lithium level, TSH

Every 12 months: reassess thyroid function, ECG

Assess more often if patient is symptomatic

Factors Predicting Lithium Responsiveness

Positive response

Family history of mania or bipolar illness

Positive response of family member to lithium

Prior manic episode

Onset of illness with mania

Alcohol abuse

Cyclothymic personality features (numerous periods of mood disturbances but lack symptom severity and duration to meet DMS-III-R bipolar diagnostic criteria)

Euphoria and grandiosity

Diagnosis of primary affective disorder

History of treatment compliance with pharmacotherapy

Negative response

Rapid cycling (more than 2 episodes/year)

Thought disorder with depression and paranoia

Anxiety

Obsessive features

Onset after age 40

tonin. Its clinical effectiveness is likely the result of several of these complex actions.

■ **CLINICAL USE.** Acute episodes of mania and hypomania and recurrent bipolar illness are the most frequent indications for lithium treatment. Other disorders with an affective component, such as recurrent unipolar depressions, schizoaffective disorder, catatonia, and alcoholism, are sometimes effectively treated with lithium, especially when they are periodic or cyclical. In addition, lithium has been reported to be effective in treating non-affective disorders such as aggressive conduct disorder, borderline personality disorder, and eating disorders. In general, lithium is not as helpful in the initial treatment of an acute depressive episode but can be given with antidepressant drug treatment. Table 23-13 lists the target symptoms of mania and depression for lithium therapy.

Before treatment with lithium, a complete history and physical examination are required, with special attention to the kidneys (lithium is excreted by the kidneys) and the thyroid. Regular medical checkups (see accompanying box) are essential while the patient is on maintenance lithium treatment.

In acute episodes lithium is effective in 1 to 2 weeks, but it may take up to 4 weeks or even a few

months to treat the symptoms fully. Sometimes an antipsychotic agent is used during the first few days or weeks of an acute episode to manage severe behavioral excitement and acute psychotic symptoms. In a maintenance regimen lithium decreases the number of affective episodes, their severity, and the frequency of occurrence. However, mild mood swings or the recurrence of affective symptoms are not uncommon while on lithium maintenance. These problems usually respond to a temporary increase in lithium dose or short-term psychotherapeutic support. The maintenance dose for each patient must be individualized and may vary from time to time. The accompanying box lists factors predictive of a lithium response.

Lithium therapy usually is started with 300 mg t.i.d. until steady state is reached, usually in 7 days. Then a blood level is drawn in the morning, 12 hours after the last dose. Even though the half-life of lithium is 18 to 36 hours, it cannot be given in a single daily dose because of toxic effects of high doses at its peak (3 hours after dosing). Thus b.i.d. or t.i.d. dosing is necessary. Lithium maintenance can be switched to

TABLE 23-14

LITHIUM PREPARATIONS

Lithium salts (trade name)	Available forms (mg)
Lithium carbonate (generic)	150, 300
Lithium carbonate (Eskalith) (Lithotabs) (Lithane) (Lithonate)	300
Lithium carbonate sustained release (Eskalith C-R) (Lithobid)	450 300
Lithium citrate concentrate (Cibalith-S)	5 ml/300

sustained-release capsules for once daily dosing. Table 23-14 lists lithium preparations. Because of the low therapeutic index of lithium, toxic blood levels can be reached quickly. Also, because lithium is a salt, the sodium and fluid balance of the body affects lithium regulation. It is essential clinical practice to monitor serum blood levels regularly (every week for the first month, then every 3 to 6 months) to regulate the dose based on these levels and to teach the patient about lithium toxicity symptoms and issues regarding salt and fluid intake.

The dose is increased until bipolar symptoms are reduced, until side effects are too great, or until the upper limit of the therapeutic blood level is reached. The therapeutic range is considered between 0.6 and 1.4 mEq/l for adults. After the patient has had a good response to lithium, the maintenance lithium dose usually is set much lower to maintain a therapeutic blood level. Raising a daily dose by 300 mg usually increases the level by 0.2 mEq/l.

In geriatric patients or those with medical illness, a serum lithium level of 0.6 to 0.8 mEq/l is recommended. Use of lithium in pregnancy is not recommended. Various congenital abnormalities have been reported in babies exposed to lithium in utero, particularly during the first trimester.

■ **ADVERSE REACTIONS.** Although lithium is used often, it is a challenge to patient education for nurses and other clinicians. Usually patients are on lithium therapy for several years, and various physio-

Lithium Side Effects

Acute/common/usually harmless

CNS: Fine hand tremor (50% of patients), fatigue, headache, mental dullness, lethargy

Renal: Polyuria (60% of patients), polydipsia, edema

Gastrointestinal: Gastric irritation, anorexia, abdominal cramps, mild nausea, vomiting, diarrhea (dose with food or milk; further divide dose)

Dermatologic: Acne, pruritic maculopapular rash

Cardiac: ECG changes, usually not clinically significant, may be persistent

Body image: Weight gain (60% of patients); can be persistent

Long-term/adverse/usually not dose related (patient usually can remain on lithium)

Endocrine: a) Thyroid dysfunction—hypothyroidism (5% of patients); replacement hormone may be necessary

b) Mild diabetes mellitus—may need diet control or insulin therapy

Renal: a) Nephrogenic diabetes insipidus—decreasing dose can help; patient must drink plenty of fluids; thiazide diuretics paradoxically reduce polyuria and may be helpful

b) Microscopic structural kidney changes: (10% to 20%) of patients on lithium for 1 year); usually does not cause significant clinical morbidity

Lithium toxicity/usually dose related

Prodrome of intoxication (lithium level ≥ 2.0 mEq/l)

Anorexia, nausea, vomiting, diarrhea, coarse hand tremor, muscle fasciculations, twitching, lethargy, dysarthria, hyperactive deep tendon reflexes, ataxia, tinnitus, vertigo, weakness, drowsiness

Lithium intoxication (lithium level ≥ 2.5 mEq/l)

Fever, decreased urine output, decreased BP, irregular pulse, ECG changes, impaired consciousness, seizures, coma, death

Stabilizing Lithium Levels

Common causes for an increase in lithium levels

1. Decreased sodium intake
2. Diuretic therapy
3. Decreased renal functioning
4. Fluid and electrolyte loss: sweating, diarrhea, dehydration, fever, vomiting
5. Medical illness
6. Overdose
7. Nonsteroidal antiinflamatory drug therapy

Ways to maintain a stable lithium level

1. Stable dosing schedule by dividing doses or use of sustained-release capsules
2. Adequate dietary sodium and fluid intake (2 to 3 liters/day)
3. Replace fluid and electrolytes during exercise or GI illness
4. Monitor signs and symptoms of lithium side effects and toxicity
5. If patient forgets a dose, he may take it if he missed dosing time by 2 hours; if longer than 2 hours, skip that dose and take the next dose; never double up on doses

Management of Serious Lithium Toxicity

1. Rapid assessment of clinical signs and symptoms of lithium toxicity; if possible, obtain rapid history of incident, especially dosing, from patient; explain procedures to patient and offer support throughout
2. Hold all lithium doses
3. Check blood pressure, pulse, rectal temperature, respirations, level of consciousness. Be prepared to: initiate stabilization procedures, protect airway, provide supplemental oxygen
4. Obtain lithium blood level immediately; obtain electrolytes, BUN, creatinine, urinalysis, CBC when possible
5. Electrocardiogram; monitor cardiac status
6. Limit lithium absorption; if acute overdose, provide an emetic; nasogastric suctioning may help since lithium levels in gastric fluid may remain high for days
7. Vigorously hydrate: 5 to 6 liters/day; keep electrolytes balanced; IV line and indwelling urinary catheter
8. Patient will be bedridden: range of motion, frequent turning, pulmonary toilet
9. In moderately severe cases:
   a. Implement osmotic diuresis with urea, 20 g IV two to five times per day, or mannitol, 50 to 100 g IV per day
   b. Increase lithium clearance with aminophylline, 0.5 g up to every 6 hr and alkalinize the urine with IV sodium lactate
   c. Ensure adequate intake of NaCl to promote excretion of lithium
   d. Implement peritoneal or hemodialysis in the most severe cases. These are characterized by serum levels between 2.0 and 4.0 mEq/l with severe clinical signs and symptoms (particularly decreasing urinary output and deepening CNS depression).
10. When appropriate: interview patient; ascertain reasons for lithium toxicity; increase health teaching efforts; mobilize post-discharge support system; arrange for more frequent clinical visits and blood levels; assess for depression and/or suicidal intent; consider concomitant antidepressant drug treatment and supportive nonpharmacological therapy

logical and environmental factors can rapidly raise their blood levels of lithium above the therapeutic limit. Patients must be taught the difference between acute and long-term side effects and signs of lithium toxicity (see accompanying box). Patients must also be taught the common causes for an increase in the lithium level and ways to stabilize a therapeutic level as described in the box above. Lithium toxicity is an emergency. Management of serious toxic states is outlined in the box at right. Bohn[3] and Prien[20] provide educational pamphlets about lithium for patients.

Treatment failures are unfortunately common, even at therapeutic blood levels of lithium. Several alternatives to lithium alone include the addition of some anticonvulsants for manic breakthroughs or the addition of antidepressant drugs for depression breakthroughs. Electroconvulsive therapy (ECT) for either mania or depression is also effective and should be considered, particularly when the suicide risk seems high. Most importantly, there is no psychopharmacological substitute for a strong therapeutic relationship, patient education, psychodynamic intervention, and regular maintenance evaluations.

■ **Anticonvulsants**

Carbamazepine (Tegretol), marketed since the 1950s as an anticonvulsant, was also seen to have mood stabilizing effects on patients with temporal lobe epilepsy. Research has demonstrated that carbamazepine is helpful in the treatment of acute mania and in the long-term prevention of manic episodes when lithium is ineffective or contraindicated.[13] Carbamazepine has its peak effects within 10 days of administration. Other psychiatric applications of carbamazepine, although still experimental, include the treatment of borderline personality disorder, schizophrenia, and schizoaffective disorder. Side effects include skin rash, sore throat, mucosal ulceration, low-grade fever, drowsiness, vertigo, ataxia, diplopia, blurred vision, nausea, vomiting, hepatotoxicity, and a temporary and benign 25% decrease in the white blood cell count. A rare but serious problem is carbamazepine-induced agranulocytosis, a significant decrease in the white blood cell count that does not return to normal. Thus blood levels and complete blood counts are monitored regularly.

Carbamazepine is administered initially at 200 mg/day and can be gradually increased to as much as 1,600 mg/day. In some rare cases patients may even receive higher doses. Maintenance doses range from 200 to 1,600 mg/day. Therapeutic serum levels range from 6 to 12 µg/l with neurotoxic side effects more common above 10 µg/l. Caution is advised when carbamazepine is used along with haloperidol for the control of excited psychosis (since plasma levels of haloperidol may be reduced) and with lithium (since neurotoxicity may be potentiated).

Another anticonvulsant medicine used in psychiatry is valproate. This drug has been shown to be effective in the manic phase of bibolar disorder and schizoaffective disorder, even in patients who failed to respond to or were unable to tolerate conventional drug therapy.[10,18] This drug is well tolerated in general. The most common side effects include gastrointestinal complaints such as anorexia, nausea, vomiting, and diarrhea; neurological symptoms of tremor, sedation, and ataxia; increased appetite; and weight gain. Very rare but serious side effects include pancreatitis and severe hepatic dysfunction. Liver function and hematology levels are checked monthly during the first 6 months of therapy, and then every 3 to 6 months.

Valproate is begun at 500 to 1,000 mg/day in two to four divided doses until a serum level of 50 to 125 µg/l is achieved. Response usually occurs in 1 to 2 weeks. Valproate is not safe for use during pregnancy. It can be used in long-term maintenance alone or with other drugs such as lithium, antipsychotics, or antipressants.

Antipsychotic drugs

The antipsychotic pharmacological family has become a mainstay in the treatment of psychotic disorders and some nonpsychotic conditions. Although they do not offer a cure for psychosis, these drugs are effective in reducing psychotic symptoms. The discovery in 1952 that chlorpromazine produced significant behavioral changes in psychiatric patients revolutionized psychiatric care. Despite the potential for severe side effects, antipsychotic drugs are widely prescribed and offer an alternative for some patients who might otherwise face a lifetime of institutionalization.

■ **MECHANISM OF ACTION.** The antipsychotic drugs are dopamine antagonists and block dopamine receptors in various pathways in the brain. Their effectiveness is thought to be the result of their ability to block dopamine receptors in the limbic system, which is the emotional part of the brain. Unfortunately, they also block dopamine receptors in other parts of the brain. This explains their side effects and the differences in tolerance to desired and undesired drug effects. A thorough discussion of the biology of the antipsychotic drugs can be found in Richelson.[21] Most recently an atypical antipsychotic drug, clozapine, offers an alternative to the traditional antipsychotic drugs for the treatment of refractory schizophrenia (see box).[17]

■ **CLINICAL USE.** The most frequently prescribed antipsychotic drugs are listed in Table 23-15. Despite the variety of chemical classes, these drugs are not different from each other in terms of overall clinical response at equivalent doses; they all have an equal chance of treating the target of psychosis. What distinguishes the chemical classes of the antipsychotic drugs is the extent, type, and severity of side effects produced. Thus an understanding of the side effects of each class of drug becomes a major nursing focus when caring for patients receiving antipsychotic medications. Black, Richelson, and Richardson[2] provide a good discussion of which drug to choose according to anticipated side effects.

Past success with a psychiatric drug in a patient or his first-degree relative may be the first reason to select a particular antipsychotic drug. The most common

TABLE 23-15

DRUG FAMILY (CATEGORY): ANTIPSYCHOTIC DRUGS

Chemical class Subtype generic name (trade name)	Drug dosage: equivalence (mg)	Usual maintenance dosage range (mg/day)	Available forms (mg)
Phenothiazines			
Aliphatic type chlorpromazine (thorazine)	100	300-1400	tabs: 10, 25, 50, 100, 200 time released: 30, 75, 150, 200 caps: 300 syrup: 10/5 ml conc: 30/ml; 100/ml supp: 25, 100 inj: 25/ml
Piperidine type thioridazine (Mellaril)	100	300-800*	tabs: 10, 15, 25, 50, 100, 150, 200 conc: 30/ml, 100/ml susp: 25/5 ml, 100/5 ml
mesoridazine (Serentil)	50	100-500	tabs: 10, 25, 50, 100 conc: 25/ml inj: 25/ml
Piperazine type perphenazine (Trilafon)	10	8-64	tabs: 2, 4, 8, 16 conc: 16/5 ml inj: 5/ml
trifluoperazine (Stelazine)	5	10-80	tabs: 1, 2, 5, 10 conc: 10/ml inj: 2/ml
fluphenazine (Prolixin)	2	5-40	tabs: 0.25, 1, 2.5, 5, 10 conc: 5/ml elix: 0.5/5 ml
Thioxanthene			
thiothixene (Navane)	4-5	10-60	caps: 1, 2, 5, 10, 20 conc: 5/ml inj: 2/ml, powder 5/ml
Butyrophenone			
haloperidol (Haldol)	2	5-100	tabs: 0.5, 1, 2, 5, 10, 20 conc: 2/ml inj: 50/ml
Dibenzoxazepine			
loxapine (loxitane)	15	50-250	caps: 5, 10, 25, 50 conc: 25/ml inj: 50/ml
Dihydroindolone			
molindone (Moban)	10-15	25-250	tabs: 5, 10, 25, 50, 100 conc: 20/ml
Dibenzodiazepine (Atypical)			
clozapine (Clozaril)	100	300-600	tabs: 25, 100, 7-day pack

*Upper limit to avoid retinopathy.

Clozapine Update

The recent interest in clozapine (Clozaril), which has a more specific action in the brain than the standard antipsychotics, has provided new help for some people with refractory schizophrenia. Although clozapine has increased efficacy and a decreased side effect profile, particularly for EPS, it can cause agranulocytosis in 1% to 2% of patients. This usually is reversible if detected within a week or two of onset. Thus the use of clozapine is restricted to patients who can be entered into a tightly controlled nationwide program developed by the manufacturer, Sandoz Pharmaceuticals. This program, the Clozaril Patient Management System (CPMS), is expensive (approximately $700 per a month) and is designed to provide weekly white blood cell monitoring during treatment by making drug availability dependent upon weekly blood tests. More information is available by calling 1-800-237-CPMS(2767).

Antipsychotic Drug Target Symptoms

Appearance
  Bizarre or disheveled
  Poor hygiene, poor nutrition
Behavior
  Hyperactivity
  Bizarre actions
  Hostility, assaultiveness
  Insomnia
  *Motivation—poor
  *Social functioning—poor
Mood and affect
  Flat affect
  Agitation
  Anxiety and tension
Intellectual functioning—poor
  *Unrealistic planning
  *Lack of insight
  *Poor judgment
Thought processes
  Loose associations
  Delusional ideas
  Hallucinations
  Suspiciousness
  Negativism

---

*Residual symptoms: Not highly responsive to pharmacotherapy.

---

cause of treatment failure in acute psychosis is an inadequate dose. The most common cause of relapse seems to be patient noncompliance with maintenance drug therapy.

The major uses for antipsychotic drugs are in the management of schizophrenia, organic brain syndrome with psychosis, and the manic phase of manic-depressive illness. Their occasional use may be indicated in severe depression with psychotic features or in severe anxiety, particularly when the patient may have a tendency toward drug or alcohol dependency. Nonpsychiatric uses for antipsychotic drugs include treatment of vomiting, vertigo, and the increased effects of analgesics for pain relief.

The clinical symptoms of psychosis that are considered the major target symptoms for pharmacotherapy with the antipsychotic drugs are listed in the accompanying box. The initial nursing care plan should address drug dose, target symptom response, and observed side effects and their treatment, along with patient safety, education, and reassurance. Although the relationship the nurse establishes with the patient who is very psychotic forms the basis for an ongoing therapeutic alliance, active nonpharmacological treatment of the residual symptoms of psychosis is more successful when the patient's behavior, mood, and thought processes begin to show improvement with pharmacotherapy. Hyman and Arana provide a good review of antipsychotic drugs.[12]

General pharmacological principles. Dosage requirements for individual patients vary considerably and must be adjusted as the target symptom changes and side effects are monitored. Initially the patient is dosed several times a day, and the daily dose can be raised every 1 to 4 days until symptom improvement occurs. Some patients respond in 2 to 3 days, some take as long as 2 weeks. Full benefits may take 6 weeks or more. Parenteral high doses can be used initially to control a highly excited or dangerous patient.

When the patient has been stabilized for several weeks, the daily dose can be lowered to the lowest effective dose. The half-life of antipsychotic drugs is over 24 hours, so the patient can be dosed once a day after steady state is reached (approximately 4 days). Bedtime dosing allows the patient to sleep through side effects when they are at their peak. After approximately 6 to 12 months of stable maintenance drug therapy, the patient can be slowly tapered from medication to assess the need for continued drug treatment. Some schizophrenic patients require a lifetime of continuous medication management. A patient who is unresponsive to an adequate trial (6 weeks at a proper dose) frequently responds to another chemical class of antipsychotic drug, so a second drug trial usually is given.

Most antipsychotic drugs can be administered by oral and intramuscular routes. Fluphenazine comes in two depot injectable forms that can be given every 7 to 28 days. Haloperidol decanote is an injectable form of haloperidol that has a 4-week duration of action. It is not appropriate to treat an acute psychotic episode with haloperidol decanote alone, because it takes 3 months to reach steady-state drug levels. Thus this drug is more of a long-term maintenance medication. Acute psychotic episodes require a shorter-acting drug. The patient's ability to take these drugs should be tested by first administering the oral form for several days. Long-acting injectables have been important in treating the outpatient who requires supervision of medication intake because of noncompliance. With the exception of thioridazine, antipsychotic drugs also have antinausea effects. Harris[7] provides an excellent guide for the use of antipsychotic drugs.

Contrary to package inserts, there are no ceiling doses for these medicines with the exception of thioridazine, which can cause pigmentary retinopathy when given in amounts over 800 mg/day. Abruptly stopping antipsychotic drugs can cause dyskinetic reactions and some rebound side effects. The drugs should be tapered slowly over several days to weeks.

Antipsychotic drugs do not cause chemical dependency nor is there tolerance to their antipsychotic effects over time. Because of their wide therapeutic index, overdoses of these drugs ordinarily do not result in death; thus they have a very low suicide potential. Because they do not produce euphoria, they also have a very low abuse potential. Antipsychotic drugs are not respiratory depressants but produce an added depressant effect when combined with drugs that produce respiratory depression. Therefore patients who also may be taking drugs such as benzodiazepines must be

carefully observed. The effects of antipsychotics on the fetus are inconclusive. It is always best to avoid any drug during the first trimester, although what is best for a psychotic pregnant mother must be carefully considered.

■ **ADVERSE REACTIONS.** The side effects of antipsychotic drugs are many and varied and demand a great deal of attention from the nurse. Table 23-16 is a comprehensive list that includes risk factors and treatment considerations. Some side effects are merely uncomfortable for the patient and most are easily treated, but some are life threatening. The nurse should refer to this list frequently but should pay particular attention to the extrapyramidal syndromes (EPS), both short-term and long-term. These are discussed in detail in Gelenberg.[5] It is important to minimize the patient's fears, increased sense of stigmatization, and possible noncompliance with drug treatment by effective patient education and support. Acute EPS side effects are common, effectively treated, and not dangerous consequences of drug treatment. Drug strategies to treat EPS include lowering the dose of the antipsychotic drug, changing to an antipsychotic drug with a lower profile for that side effect (Table 23-17), or administering one of the drugs listed in Table 23-18. These drugs are administered with antipsychotic drugs if acute symptoms of EPS occur. Since tolerance to these symptoms usually occurs in the first 3 months of antipsychotic drug treatment, drugs to treat EPS are used only during the first 3 months and then discontinued. Long-term use usually is not necessary.

Unfortunately, the long-term common extrapyramidal syndrome, tardive dyskinesia, has no effective treatment to date. Thus primary preventive measures are important (Fig. 23-2). The Abnormal Involuntary Movement Scale (AIMS) should be a part of every patient's treatment (see the box on 734). Most patients and their families consider the possible side effects of antipsychotic drugs better than a life of psychosis, but they should be presented with all the choices available to them.

Currently, the correlation between plasma blood levels of antipsychotic drugs or serum dopamine receptor binding and clinical response has yet to be determined, but these tests hold promise for refining drug selection and dosing regimens. Psychopharmacological research has just begun to discover chemical classes of antipsychotic drugs that have mechanisms of action highly specific for the target symptoms of psychosis and yet that do not produce a variety of unwanted side effects.

TABLE 23-16

SIDE EFFECTS AND ADVERSE REACTIONS OF ANTIPSYCHOTIC DRUGS

Side effects/adverse reactions	Mechanism of action	Risk factors	Treatment and nursing considerations
Acute/common/side effects			
Neurological	Dopamine blockade: Acetylcholine/ dopamine balance is disturbed	Extra Pyramidal Symptoms: 40% of all patients get EPS; differs between neuroleptics, highest with high potency drugs	*General EPS Treatment Principles* 1. Tolerance usually develops by the third month 2. Decrease dose of antipsychotic drug if possible 3. Add an anticholinergic drug for 3 months then taper 4. Change to an antipsychotic with lower EPS profile 5. Patient education and supportive care
Extrapyramidal Symptoms (EPS) 1. Acute dystonic reactions: Occur suddenly and are very frightening to the patient; spasms of major muscle groups of the neck, back, and eyes; catatonia; respiratory compromise.		1. 10% of all EPS; occurs within the first 5 days; nongeriatric patients, especially children; males twice as often as females; high potency antipsychotics	*Acute dystonic reactions* Administer a drug from Table 23-17; parenteral routes work more rapidly than PO; have respiratory support equipment available.
2. Akathisia Patient cannot remain still; pacing, inner restlessness; leg aches which are relieved by movement		2. 50% of all EPS; high potency antipsychotic drugs	*Akathisia* Rule out anxiety or agitation (difficult but important distinction)
3. Parkinson's Syndrome a. Akinesia—absence or slowness of motion; patient turns like one solid block of wood; gait is inclined forward with small, rapid steps; masklike facies b. Cogwheel rigidity and muscle stiffness on physical exam c. Bilateral fine tremor, anywhere in body; "pill-rolling" motion of the fingers		3. 40% of all EPS; females twice as often as males; geriatric patients; occurs within weeks to several months or longer after drug treatment begins	*Parkinson's Syndrome* Tolerance does not develop in all patients; the dopamine agonist, amantadine, is sometimes effective (patient must have good renal function to avoid amantadine toxicity); use step 3 (above) early and vigorously.
Behavioral *Sedation* Sleepy, groggy, fatigued		Peaks 2 to 3 hours after dosing	Tolerance occurs within days to several weeks; rule out over-medication; dose once daily at h.s.; change to an antipsychotic drug with a lower sedation profile
Autonomic *Anticholinergic Side Effects* Blurred vision, constipation, tachycardia, urinary etention, decreased gastric secretion, decreased sweating and salivation (dry mouth), heat stroke, nasal congestion, decreased pulmonary secretion; *"atropine psychosis"* in geriatric patients: hyperactivity, agitation, confusion, flushed skin, dilated pupils that are slow to react, bowel hypomotility, dysarthria, tachycardia	Cholinergic receptor blockade at some central and peripheral sites	Concurrent use of anticholinergic drugs; geriatric patients; patients with tachycardia; low-potency antipsychotic drugs; can return as rebound symptoms during antipsychotic drug withdrawal; men with prostatic hypertrophy may have particular difficulty with urinary retention	Tolerance develops in days to weeks; change to drug with a lower anticholinergic profile; treat symptomatically: frequently moisten dry mouth, use sugarless candy and gum; bulk diets, stool softeners, fluids, and exercise for constipation; avoid operating machinery if vision is blurred; cholinergic agonist (bethanecol) for urinary retention; IM physostigmine for severe atropine psychosis; avoid polypharmacy if possible; avoid getting overheated

TABLE 23-16—cont'd

SIDE EFFECTS AND ADVERSE REACTIONS OF ANTIPSYCHOTIC DRUGS

Side effects/adverse reactions	Mechanism of action	Risk factors	Treatment and nursing considerations
Cardiac (autonomic) *Orthostatic Hypotension* Dizziness, tachycardia, drop in diastolic BP by >40 mm/H with a change of position from lying to sitting or sitting to standing	Alpha-adrenergic blockade producing vascular dilation and pooling of blood	Concurrent administration of antihypertensives, diuretics, antidepressants; geriatric patients; worse with injectable low-potency drugs	Tolerance develops in several weeks; lower dose; change to an antipsychotic with a lower hypotension profile, monitor BP; increase fluid intake to expand vascular volume; have patient rise slowly and dangle feet while sitting; have patient wear support hose; use a pure alpha-adrenergic pressor agent (metaraminol) for hypotensive crisis
Acute/rare adverse reactions **Allergic Reactions**	Hypersensitivity reaction		
Hematologic Agranulocytosis: develops abruptly; fever, malaise, ulcerative sore throat, leukopenia (WBC below 500)		Occurs within 3 to 8 weeks of treatment; very rare; clozapine and phenothiazines, especially chlorpromazine; thiothixene; geriatric females; 30% mortality rate	This is an *extreme emergency;* be alert for high fever and ulcerative sore throat with patients on these drugs, particularly geriatric females; monitor WBC with this risk group; if this occurs, discontinue drug immediately and initiate reverse isolation; antibiotics when appropriate
Dermatologic 1. Systemic Dermatosis: maculopapular, erythematous, itchy rash on face, neck, chest, extremities; contact dermatitis when touching drug		Occurs 2 to 8 weeks after treatment; chlorpromazine	Non-dose related; discontinue drug and start again cautiously when rash disappears; change to a drug in another chemical class; topical steroids if necessary
2. Photosensitivity: severe sunburn		Low-potency drugs; brief exposure to direct sunlight	Lower dose; change to a high-potency drug; use sunscreen and wear clothing over exposed areas; topical relief of sunburn
Hepatic Jaundice: fever, nausea, abdominal pain, malaise, pruritus, jaundice; abnormal liver function tests		Rare; was more common in the 1950s and 1960s due to impurities in the drugs; phenothiazines, especially chlorpromazine; occurs in first month of treatment	Discontinue drug, reversible and self-limiting; bedrest; high-protein/carbohydrate diet
Cardiovascular *EKG abnormalities*	Effects in the hypothalamus and the heart	Preexisting cardiac conditions; geriatric patients; low-potency drugs, especially when combined with tricyclic antidepressants (thioridazine and amitriptyline are worst)	Baseline and follow-up EKG and vital sign monitoring for patients with preexisting cardiac disease; change to high-potency drug
Neurological *Seizures* Usually grand mal, no warning aura	These drugs lower the seizure threshold	Patients with preexisting seizure disorder; patients who are poorly controlled psychiatrically; low-potency drugs; during sedative-hypnotic or alcohol withdrawal	Decrease dose; change to a high-potency drug; anticonvulsants don't protect non-seizure disorder patients.

Continued.

TABLE 23-16—cont'd

SIDE EFFECTS AND ADVERSE REACTIONS OF ANTIPSYCHOTIC DRUGS

Side effects/adverse reactions	Mechanism of action	Risk factors	Treatment and nursing considerations
Long-term/common adverse reactions			
Neurological *Extrapyramidal Symptom (EPS)* Tardive Dyskinesia: tongue protrusion, lip smacking, puckering, sucking, chewing, blinking, lateral jaw movements, grimacing; choreiform movements of the limbs and trunk, shoulder shrugging, pelvic thrusting, wrist and ankle flexion or rotation, foot tapping, toe movements	After prolonged blockade from dopamine, post-synaptic receptor site becomes over-active, supersensitive	Estimated that between 15% and 50% of all people receiving antipsychotics, particularly high doses for long-term use (occurs usually after years, but can occur as early as 4 months); geriatric patients; especially females; brain-damaged patients; anticholinergic drugs given for EPS may increase risk	These are stereotyped, involuntary movements which may be mild or become severely crippling; employ primary preventive measures (see Fig. 23-2); patients with severe tardive dyskinesia can become very distressed; may need soft foods, and soft shoes for feet movements. There is no treatment for tardive dyskinesia, though several drugs are in the experimental stages; may be irreversible, especially if not discovered early and if antipsychotic drugs cannot be stopped.
Endocrine Galactorrhea, amenorrhea, breast enlargement and engorgement, decreased libido, ejaculatory incompetence, appetite increase and weight gain, hypothermia or hyperthermia, false positive pregnancy test	Effects on the hypothalamus and pituitary causing an increase in prolactin and leuteotropic hormone secretion	Low-potency drugs, especially thioridazine *mellaril*	Partial tolerance over many months or years may develop; decrease dose or change to high-potency drug, especially with persistent symptoms; be sure that female patients are not actually pregnant; for weight gain—diet and exercise regimen (molindone has less appetite stimulant effects); women should have periodic breast exams especially with a personal or family history of breast cancer, although there is no clear evidence that the risk of breast cancer is increased
Long-term/rare/adverse reactions			
Ophthalmologic problems *Toxic Pigmentary Retinopathy* Patient notices brownish discoloration of vision, loss of visual accuity, possible blindness	Doses of thioridazine above 800 mg/day, even for brief periods of time	Degenerative and irreversible; completely avoidable; never give thioridazine above 800 mg/day; change to another drug if 800 mg/day of thioridazine does not treat target symptoms of psychosis	
Skin/Eye Syndrome Sunlight-exposed skin turns slate gray to metallic blue or purple in color. Color changes are also noted in eyes, without vision impairment.	Deposits of drug substance and pigment in the cornea, lens, and the skin	Prolonged use of chlorpromazine or thiothixene and exposure to sunlight	Change to another drug class; deposits disappear over many months after drug is discontinued

TABLE 23-16—cont'd

SIDE EFFECTS AND ADVERSE REACTIONS OF ANTIPSYCHOTIC DRUGS

Side effects/adverse reactions	Mechanism of action	Risk factors	Treatment and nursing considerations
Short-term or long-term/rare/life threatening			
Neuroleptic malignant syndrome High fever, tachycardia, muscle rigidity, stupor, tremor, incontinence, leukocytosis, elevated serum CPK, hyperkalemia, renal failure, increased pulse, respirations, and sweating	Presumably extreme dopamine receptor blockade is at least part of mechanism	50 cases have been reported in the literature between 1980 and 1985. This develops explosively over 1 to 3 days, from hours to many months after drug treatment begins; high-potency drugs are worse, but other psychiatric drugs have been implicated also; patients with marked dehydration; patients with organic brain disease; 20% mortality rate *Speculative:* young adult men, polypharmacy, haloperidol, fluphenazine, parenteral, long-term drug use	This is an *extreme emergency*—early recognition is critical; avoid marked dehydration in all patients; discontinue all drugs immediately; supportive symptomatic care: nutrition, hydration, renal dialysis for renal failure, ventilation for acute respiratory failure, reduction of fever *Speculative:* dantrolene, bromocriptine. Antipsychotic drugs can be cautiously reintroduced.

TABLE 23-17

ACUTE SIDE EFFECTS PROFILE: ANTIPSYCHOTIC DRUGS

Drugs	Sedation	EPS	Anticholinergic	Postural hypotension
Low potency				
chlorpromazine	4	2	3	4
thioridazine	4	1	4	4
High potency				
trifluoperazine	2	3	2	2
thiothixene	2	3	2	1
loxapine	2	3	2	2
molindone	2	3	2	2
mesoridazine	3	2	3	3
perphenazine	2	3	2	2
fluphenazine	1	4	2	1
haloperidol	1	4	1	1

1 = lowest incidence; 4 = highest incidence.

TABLE 23-18

DRUGS TO TREAT EPS (EXTRAPYRAMIDAL SIDE EFFECTS): NEUROTRANSMITTER SPECIFICITY

Chemical class generic name (trade name)	Equivalence (mg)	Usual dosage range (mg/day)	Available forms (mg)
Anticholinergic			
benztropine (Cogentin)	2	1-6	tabs: 0.5, 1,2 inj: 1/ml
trihexyphenidyl (Artane)	5	1-10	tabs: 2, 5; 5 sustained release; elix: 2/5 ml
biperiden (Akineton)	4	2-6	tabs: 2 inj: 5/ml
procyclidine (Kemadrin)	5	6-20	tabs: 5
diphenhydramine (benadryl)	50	25-150	tabs: 50 caps: 25, 50 elix: 12.5/5 ml; inj: 10/ml, 50/ml
Dopaminergic			
amantadine (Symmetrel)	100	100-300	caps: 100 mg syrup: 50/5ml
Gabaminergic			
diazepam (Valium)	10		(See Table 23-2)
lorazepam (Ativan)	2		

Treatment considerations of anticholinergic drug therapy
1. Geriatric patients are particularly sensitive to these drugs.
2. They can produce a euphoria and have abuse potential.

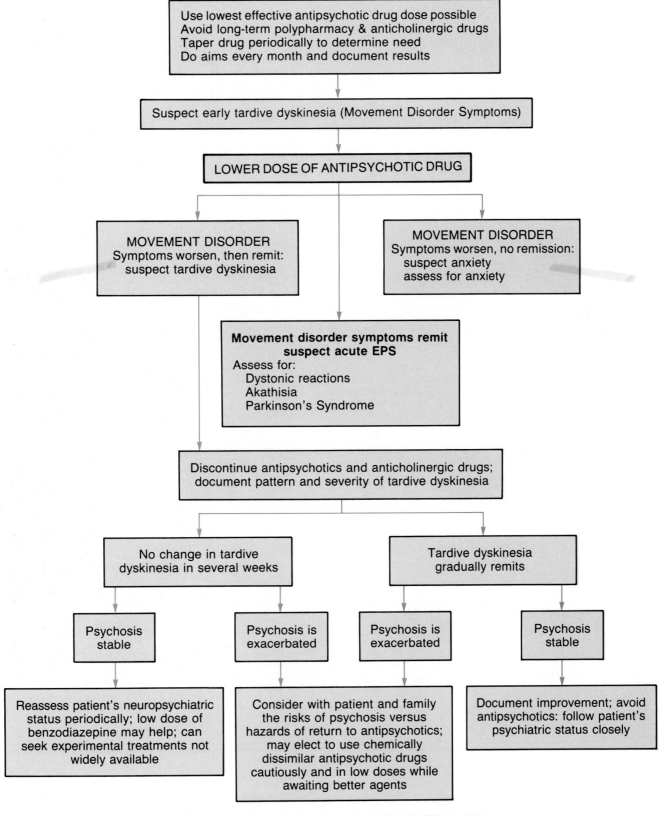

Use lowest effective antipsychotic drug dose possible
Avoid long-term polypharmacy & anticholinergic drugs
Taper drug periodically to determine need
Do aims every month and document results

Suspect early tardive dyskinesia (Movement Disorder Symptoms)

LOWER DOSE OF ANTIPSYCHOTIC DRUG

MOVEMENT DISORDER
Symptoms worsen, then remit:
suspect tardive dyskinesia

MOVEMENT DISORDER
Symptoms worsen, no remission:
suspect anxiety
assess for anxiety

**Movement disorder symptoms remit
suspect acute EPS**
Assess for:
   Dystonic reactions
   Akathisia
   Parkinson's Syndrome

Discontinue antipsychotics and anticholinergic drugs;
document pattern and severity of tardive dyskinesia

No change in tardive
dyskinesia in several weeks

Tardive dyskinesia
gradually remits

Psychosis
stable

Psychosis is
exacerbated

Psychosis is
exacerbated

Psychosis
stable

Reassess patient's neuropsychiatric
status periodically; low dose of
benzodiazepine may help; can
seek experimental treatments not
widely available

Consider with patient and family
the risks of psychosis versus
hazards of return to antipsychotics;
may elect to use chemically
dissimilar antipsychotic drugs
cautiously and in low doses while
awaiting better agents

Document improvement; avoid
antipsychotics: follow patient's
psychiatric status closely

Fig. 23-2. Preventive measures for tardive dyskinesia (TD).

Abnormal Involuntary Movement Scale: AIMS

A Simple Method to Determine Tardive Dyskinesia Symptoms—
Total Score Equals the Sum of the Items

Patient Identification: _____ Date: _____

Rated by: _____ Treatment period: _____

Either before or after completing the examination procedure, observe the patient unobtrusively at rest (e.g., in waiting room).

The chair to be used in this examination should be a hard, firm one without arms.

After the patient is observed, he may be rated on a scale of 0 (none), 1 (minimal), 2 (mild), 3 (moderate), and 4 (severe) according to the severity of symptoms at time of interview.

Ask the patient whether there is anything in his mouth (e.g., gum, candy) and if there is, ask him to remove it.

Ask the patient about the *current* condition of his teeth. Ask if he wears dentures. Do his teeth or dentures bother him *now?*

Ask the patient whether he notices any movement in mouth, face, hands, or feet. If yes, ask him to describe such movement and to what extent it *currently* bothers him or interferes with his activities.

0 1 2 3 4   Have the patient sit in a chair with hands on knees, legs slightly apart and feet flat on floor. (Look at entire body for movements while in this position.)

0 1 2 3 4   Ask the patient to sit with hands hanging unsupported. If male, between legs; if female and wearing a dress, hanging over knees. (Observe hands and other body areas.)

0 1 2 3 4   Ask the patient to open mouth. (Observe tongue at rest within mouth.) Have him do this twice.

0 1 2 3 4   Ask the patient to protrude tongue. (Observe abnormalities of tongue movement.) Have him do this twice.

0 1 2 3 4   Ask the patient to tap thumb with each finger as rapidly as possible for 10 to 15 seconds separately with right hand then with left hand. (Observe facial and leg movements.)

0 1 2 3 4   Flex and extend patient's left and right arms (one at a time).

0 1 2 3 4   Ask the patient to stand up. (Observe in profile. Observe all body areas again, hips included.)

0 1 2 3 4   *Ask the patient to extend both arms outstretched in front with palms down. (Observe trunk, legs, and mouth.)

0 1 2 3 4   *Have the patient walk a few paces turn and walk back to chair. (Observe hands and gait.) Do this twice.

*Activated movements

DIRECTIONS FOR FUTURE RESEARCH

The following are some of the nursing research problems raised in Chapter 23 that merit further study by psychiatric nurses.

1. Identification of people at risk for particular side effects and adverse reactions to psychopharmacological drugs
2. Predictors of factors related to patient noncompliance with medication treatment regimens
3. Effective nursing interventions that maximize patient compliance with medication treatment regimens
4. Nonpharmacological interventions that enhance drug effectiveness and treat residual target symptoms
5. Development of behavioral rating scales that are specific in assessing nursing care effectiveness in the psychopharmacological treatment of mental disorders
6. Outcomes associated with the nurse's role in the long-term psychiatric treatment of patients on drug maintenance regimens
7. Patient education strategies associated with drug therapy effectiveness, compliance, and safety
8. Ways to maximize nurse-patient collaboration in medication treatment regimens and related outcomes
9. Evaluation of the effectiveness of involving the patient's social support system in short-term and long-term medication regimens
10. Knowledge level of nurses of the biological basis, mechanisms of action, clinical uses, and adverse effects of psychopharmacological drugs and its correlation with the effectiveness of nursing care

SUGGESTED CROSS-REFERENCES

The elements of a psychiatric evaluation are discussed in Chapter 6. Legal and ethical issues in psychiatric care are discussed in Chapter 7. Care of suicidal and noncompliant patients is discussed in Chapter 16. Nursing interventions with suspicious and dependent patients are discussed in Chapter 17. Supplemental somatic therapies are discussed in Chapter 22. Psychopharmacology with children is discussed in Chapter 30.

SUMMARY

1. Psychopharmacology is the fastest growing treatment in the current practice of psychiatry.
2. Data gathering, patient education, and knowledge of drug administration and treatment are essential aspects of psychiatric nursing care.
3. Patient assessment includes evaluation of the patient's physical status, mental status, medical and psychiatric history, medication history, and family history.
4. Various aspects of pharmacokinetics were presented, including half-life, steady state, polypharmacy, drug interactions, and aspects of patient noncompliance with related implications for patient education. The biological basis for psychopharmacology was also briefly described.
5. Benzodiazepines, the most widely prescribed class of drugs in the world, have almost completely replaced other classes of antianxiety and sedative-hypnotic agents. Benzodiazepines are therapeutically effective and have a wide margin of safety when taken alone. They can be mildly addictive, especially when taken in high doses over long periods of time or when used concomitantly with other addictive agents such as barbiturates or alcohol. The most common side effects include drowsiness, dizziness, slurred speech, and blurred vision.
6. Antidepressant drugs are frequently used, usually effective, nonaddicting, and can be lethal in overdoses. Tricyclic (and several other nontricyclic) antidepressants are used more commonly than MAO inhibitors because they are safer in combination with other substances. MAO inhibitors, although generally more effective than tricyclics, are not commonly used because they require restrictions on tyramine-containing foods and a variety of other medications. Side effects of antidepressants are usually mild.
7. The mood stabilizer lithium is effective in the treatment of bipolar illness in acute phases and in long-term maintenance regimens. Lithium is not addictive but can be toxic. The therapeutic dosage range is narrow and must be monitored by regularly assessing serum lithium levels. Patients must be taught the differences between common side effects and signs of toxicity and ways to stabilize lithium levels.
8. Antipsychotic agents have made a major difference in the treatment of people with psychotic disorders. The various classes have similar therapeutic effects but are dissimilar in side effect profiles. Side effects are varied and can be disabling and life threatening. Thus a major focus in learning about antipsychotic drugs is learning to prevent, recognize, and treat their related side effects.

REFERENCES

1. Akiskal HS and McKinney WI Jr: Overview of recent research in depression; integration of ten conceptual models into a comprehensive clinical frame, Arch Gen Psychiatry 32:285, 1975.
2. Black JL, Richelson E, and Richardson JW: Antipsy-

chotic agents: a clinical update, Mayo Clin Proc 60:777, 1985.

3. Bohn J and Jefferson JW: Lithium and manic depression: a guide, Madison, Wis, 1982, Publishing Board of Regents, University of Wisconsin System, Lithium Information Center.

4. Cohen LS: Psychotropic drug use in pregnancy, Hosp Community Psychiatry 40(6):566, 1989.

5. Gelenberg AJ: Psychoses. In Bassuk EL, Schoonover SC, and Gelenberg AJ, editors: The practitioner's guide to psychoactive drugs, ed 2, New York and London, 1984, Plenum Medical Books Co.

6. Guy W: ECDEU assessment manual for psychopharmacology, revised. Rockville, Md, 1976, US Department of Health, Education, and Welfare, National Institute of Mental Health, Psychopharmacology Research Branch, Division of Extramural Research Program.

7. Harris E: The antipsychotics, Am J Nurs 11:1508, 1988.

8. Hayes PE and Bloom VL: A nurse's guide to psychotherapeutic drugs: recognition and treatment of depressive illness, PRN learning systems, pharmacology for nurses by home study 2(5):1, 1982.

9. Hayes PE and Schulz SC: Beta blockers in anxiety disorders, Psychiatr Med 3:41, 1985.

10. Hayes SG: Long-term use of valproate in primary psychiatric disorders, J Clin Psychiatry 50(3 suppl):35, 1989.

11. Hollister LE: When to use psychotherapeutic agents, Drug Ther 213, 1982.

12. Hyman SE and Arana GW: Handbook of psychiatric drug therapy, Boston, 1987, Little, Brown & Co.

13. Israel M and Beaudry P: Carbamazepine in psychiatry: a review, Can J Psychiatry 33(7):577, 1988.

14. Koplan CR: Pediatric psychopharmacology. In Bassuk EL, Schoonover SC, and Gelenberg AJ, editors: The practitioner's guide to psychoactive drugs, ed 2, New York and London, 1984, Plenum Medical Books Co.

15. Koplan CR: The use of psychotropic drugs during pregnancy and nursing. In Bassuk EL, Schoonover SC, and Gelenberg AJ, editors: The practitioner's guide to psychoactive drugs, ed 2, New York and London, 1984, Plenum Medical Books Co.

16. Larkin AR: What's a medication group? J Psychosoc Nurs Ment Health Serv 20(2):35, 1982.

17. Mattes J: Clozapine for refractory schizophrenia: an open study of 14 patients treated up to two years, J Clin Psychiatry 50(10):389, 1989.

18. McElroy SL, Keck PE, Pope HG, and Hudson JI: Valproate in psychiatric disorders: literature review and clinical guidelines, J Clin Psychiatry 50(3 suppl):23, 1989.

19. Orsulak PJ: Therapeutic monitoring of antidepressant drugs, Diagnostic Update: Mental Illness and Neurological Disorders 3(1):1, 1989.

20. Prien RF: Information on . . . Lithium (DHHS Pub No[ADM] 81-1078). National Institute of Mental Health, US Department of Health and Human Services, 1981.

21. Richelson E: Pharmacology of neuroleptics in use in the United States, J Clin Psychiatry 46(8):8, (sec 2), 1985.

22. Salzman C, Hoffman SA, and Schoonover SC: Geriatric psychopharmacology. In Bassuk EL, Schoonover SC, and Gelenberg AJ, editors: The practitioner's guide to psychoactive drugs, ed 2, New York and London, 1984, Plenum Medical Books Co.

23. Schoonover SC: Depression. In Bassuk EL, Schoonover SC, and Gelenberg AJ, editors: The practitioner's guide to psychoactive drugs, ed 2, New York and London, 1984, Plenum Medical Books Co.

24. Selander JJ and Miller WC: Prolixin group, J Psychosoc Nurs Mental Health Serv 23(11):17, 1985.

25. Smith DE and Wesson DR: Benzodiazepine dependency syndromes, J Psychoactive Drugs 15(1-2):85, 1983.

26. Snyder SH: Neurosciences: an integrative discipline, Science 225(4668):1255, 1984.

27. Stimmel GL: Affective disorders. In Herfindal ET and Hirschman JL, editors: Clinical pharmacy and therapeutics, ed 3, Baltimore, 1984, Williams & Wilkins.

28. Whiteside SE: Patient education: effectiveness of medication programs for psychiatric patients, J Psychosoc Nurs Ment Health Serv 21(10):17, 1983.

29. Wincor MA: Benzodiazepines drug review: insomnia and the new benzodiazepines, Clin Pharm 1:425, 1982.

30. Zisook S: A clinical overview of monoamine oxidase inhibitors, Psychosomatics 26(3):240, 1985.

■ ANNOTATED SUGGESTED READINGS ■

Ancill RJ, Embury GD, MacEwan GW, and Kennedy JS: The use and misuse of psychotropic prescribing for elderly psychiatric patients, Can J Psychiatry 33:585, 1988.

Evaluates the presenting problems and preadmission diagnoses of 100 consecutive admissions to a geriatric psychiatry inpatient assessment unit. A significant incidence of inappropriate preadmission prescribing of psychotropic drugs was noted, as well as previously undiagnosed major depression, which responded well to appropriate treatment.

*Barrett N, Ormiston S, and Molyneux V: Clozapine: a new drug for schizophrenia, J Psychosoc Nurs Ment Health Serv 29(2):24, 1990.

This article reviews a new neuroleptic drug that was released by the FDA in January 1990 for the treatment of schizophrenia. It describes the psychopharmacodynamics, side effects, and related nursing care. Two case examples are also included.

Gelenberg AJ et al: Treating extrapyramidal reaction, *Massachusetts General Hospital Newsletter,* Biological Therapies in Psychiatry 6(4):13, 1983. PSG Inc, 545 Great Road, Littleton, Mass 01460.

---

*Asterisk indicates nursing reference.

Discusses the treatment of acute dystonic reactions, akathisia, drug-induced Parkinson's syndrome, and tardive dyskinesia. States that since treatment is far from perfect, future research must find antipsychotic drugs without neuroleptic properties. Until then, attention to diagnosis and optimum use of available therapies is necessary for greater patient comfort, enhanced clinical effectiveness, and improved compliance.

*Hooper JF, Herren CK, and Goldwasser H: Neuroleptic malignant syndrome: recognizing an unrecognized killer, J Psychosoc Nurs Ment Health Serv 27(7):13, 1989.

Approximately 1% of all patients treated with psychiatric drugs develop neuroleptic malignant syndrome, a serious complication that can lead to death if untreated. Nurses should be aware of the early symptoms and the treatment of this potentially serious side effect.

Hyman SE and Arana GW: Handbook of psychiatric drug therapy, Boston/Toronto, 1987, Little, Brown & Co.

A handbook that will be helpful to the clinician. Pocket-sized, cross-referenced, user-friendly, inexpensive, up to date, and written with an interdisciplinary perspective.

Hyman SE and Cassem NH: Managing the person with major psychiatric illness, Scientific American, PAM, R-21:1, 1988.

The prevalence of anxiety disorders, depression, and schizophrenia makes it likely that most health care professionals will at some time be involved with major psychiatric drugs. Gives a good overview of these treatments for the general medical community.

*Jackson RT and Haynes-Johnson V: Nutritional management of patients undergoing long-term antipsychotic and antidepressant therapies, Archives of Psychiatric Nursing II (3):146, 1988.

The management of many mental health disorders requires long-term psychiatric, nursing, and nutritional care. This report discusses the relationship between psychotropic drugs, the symptoms they produce, and appropriate nutritional management by nursing and dietetic staff members.

Kutcher SP and Blackwood DHR: Pharmacotherapy of the borderline patient: a critical review and clinical guidelines, Can J Psychiatry 34:347, 1989.

Critically reviews the literature on the pharmacotherapy of borderline personality disorder and suggests guidelines for the appropriate clinical use of psychotropic agents, as well as directions for future research.

Meador-Woodruff JH: Psychiatric side effects of tricyclic antidepressants, Hosp Community Psychiatry 41(1):84, 1990.

Psychiatric toxicity refers to a group of side effects not usually mentioned in the literature. Affecting as many as 5% to 15% of patients treated with tricyclics, this toxicity includes delirium and can be associated with considerable morbidity.

*Michaels RA and Mumford K: Identifying akinesia and akathisia: the relationship between patient's self-report and nurse's assessment, Archives of Psychiatric Nursing III 2:97, 1989.

This study found that generally the patient's self-report and the nurse's assessment were in agreement. This seems to indicate that specific subjective responses, as well as systematic clinical examination, should be included when assessing for drug-induced akinesia and akathisia.

O'Hare TF: Legal issues in prescribing psychoactive medications. In Bassuk EL, Schoonover SC, and Gelenberg AJ, editors: The practitioner's guide to psychoactive drugs, ed 2, New York and London, 1984, Plenum Medical Book Co.

Focuses on the conflicts in psychiatry and patient advocacy regarding the legal issues that must be considered when prescribing and administering psychoactive medications. Covers torts, civil rights, informed consent, and right to withdraw consent and gives suggestions for avoiding litigation.

*Scrak BM and Greenstein RA: Tardive dyskinesia, J Psychosoc Nurs Ment Health Serv 25(9):24, 1987.

Reports the occurrence of tardive dyskinesia (TD) in a nurse-managed Prolixin clinic. The prevalence of TD is estimated by the Task Force Report of the American Psychiatric Association to be 10% to 20%, but some reports estimate up to 57%.

Simeon JG: Pediatric psychopharmacology, Can J Psychiatry 34:115, 1989.

Summarizes current knowledge and advances related to the indications, effects, limitations, and research issues of psychostimulants, antidepressants, antipsychotics, antianxiety drugs, anticonvulsants and diet in the treatment of child and adolescent psychiatric disorders.

Sloboda W and Currier C: Free communications-session B, FDA's monitoring of clinical trials, Psychopharmacol Bull 21(1):105, 1985.

As part of the Bioresearch Monitoring Program of the U.S. Food and Drug Administration (FDA), clinical studies are inspected to monitor research methods used for investigational drugs. Inspections generally focus on which team member did what, where the study was performed, and how the drug was accounted for.

Stanley B et al: Psychopharmacologic treatment and informed consent: empirical research, Psychopharmacol Bull 21(1):110, 1985.

This study investigated the effect of psychotropic medication on the ability to give informed consent to research. The results indicate that medication status does not substantially alter competency, that comprehension of consent information improves over the course of the hospitalization, and that schizophrenic patients tend to have more difficulty in the consent process than patients with major affective disorders.

PART TWO

PRACTICE
OF PSYCHIATRIC NURSING

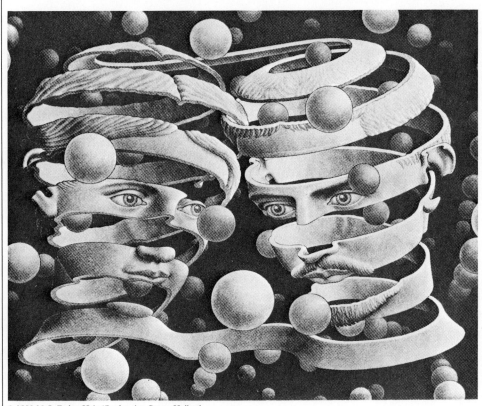

© 1990 M.C. Escher Heirs/Cordon Art, Baarn, Holland.

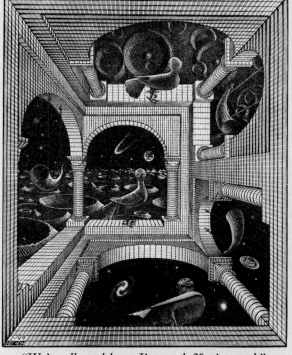

"We're all mad here. I'm mad. You're mad."
"How do you know I'm mad?" said Alice.
"You must be," said the Cat, "or you wouldn't have come here."
Alice didn't think that proved it at all.

Lewis Carroll, *Alice's Adventures in Wonderland*

© 1990 M.C. Escher Heirs/Cordon Art, Baarn, Holland.

CHAPTER 24

INPATIENT PSYCHIATRIC NURSING IN A MENTAL HEALTH SERVICE CONTINUUM

KAY SIENKILEWSKI

After studying this chapter, the student should be able to:

- describe the historical events that have influenced the role of the psychiatric nurse in an inpatient setting.

- discuss the advantages and disadvantages of the use of a primary nursing model for delivering psychiatric nursing care.

- discuss the role of the clinical nurse specialist in an inpatient unit.

- identify the two levels of patient education and discuss the nursing implications.

- analyze and compare the concepts of milieu therapy as described by Cumming and Cumming applied to long-term inpatient treatment and those modifications used in short-term treatment.

- identify the role of individual, group, and

- family therapy programs in the inpatient setting.

- describe psychodrama in terms of major concepts and the therapeutic process.

- discuss the uses of the various occupational and activity therapies in the inpatient setting.

- discusses the current major trends affecting inpatient psychiatric nursing.

- compare the characteristics of acute intensive and long-term custodial inpatient psychiatric units and discuss the nursing implications of the differences in the settings.

- identify directions for future nursing research.

- select appropriate readings for further study.

The practice of inpatient psychiatric nursing is rich in history and tradition. It is impossible to separate the evolution of modern psychiatric nursing from the developmental stages of medical practices in psychiatry, mental health concepts, and the growth of nursing as a profession. Years of progress and successful attainment of knowledge and skills in the areas of psychiatric treatment and nursing care delivery systems have given rise to inpatient psychiatric nursing practice that is exciting, innovative, and challenging. Recently, we have seen major changes in the focus of treatment for patients and families with psychiatric disorders. Where once the inpatient psychiatric hospital was the hub of services for mental health care, there now exists a variety of treatment settings and options in a rapidly advancing mental health service continuum. Thus the mission of the psychiatric hospital must change to reflect recent treatment philosophy, new laws governing patients' rights and admissions to inpatient facilities, and the current environment of cost containment in health care.

Today's inpatient psychiatric nurses must use all of their knowledge of this rich history and tradition in the development of new practice models that will meet the challenge of shortening length of inpatient stays, the increasing acuity of inpatient populations, and the rising trend of readmissions and intermittent short-term inpatient hospitalizations.

Inpatient psychiatric nurse as a caretaker

Early inpatient psychiatric nursing was characterized by custodial care, which ranged from humanistic to neglectful and cruel. Seventeenth century writings reveal that treatment of the "insane," particularly those "subject to melancholy," bore close resemblance to some practices followed in the mental hospital of the late 1930s and early 1940s.[21] Frequent baths, a wholesome diet, and "suitable exhilaration" of the mind were the primary modes of treatment for the depressed patient. The more severely disturbed were also provided these forms of therapy but were restrained in their beds to prevent them from injuring themselves or others. In the early Middle Ages the mentally ill were admitted into general hospitals and treated with kindness. In the three centuries following the Reformation, the system of "appalling neglect and revolting cruelty" developed in the treatment of the mentally ill. This lasted until the drastic reforms of the nineteenth century.

The nurse's role was primarily to oversee patient care and to ensure smooth ward operation. Housekeeping, dietary management, and laundry care commonly became the nurse's responsibility. Thus the early inpatient psychiatric nurse was more the manager of a unit than a provider of direct patient care.[9]

The reforms of the nineteenth century had great impact on inpatient psychiatric nursing. The care of patients once again became humane, and the scientific understanding of the nature, causes, and treatment of mental illness was of primary concern. The increase in this scientific body of knowledge gave rise to a great demand for advancement in psychiatric nursing to ensure that psychiatric treatment kept pace with rapid growth in other branches of medicine and nursing.

Despite this "new era," the role of the inpatient nurse remained primarily custodial. Much of the emphasis was placed on performing tasks and administering somatic therapies. However, the seed had been planted, and the future of psychiatric nursing as a viable specialty was taking root.

Inpatient psychiatric nurse as a member of the team

With the development of social psychiatry, the role of the inpatient psychiatric nurse began to change. Nurses became key figures in milieu therapy and therapeutic communities. The nurse was used as a role model for the patients and their families. The emphasis shifted from performing tasks to establishing interpersonal relationships. Nursing was given "almost free rein" to involve the patient in activities of daily living. Together the nurse and the patient would problem solve important issues centered around self-care and interactions with others within the community.

In 1949 nursing entered yet another "hallowed hall."[24] For the most part, individual psychotherapy had been limited to physicians. Nurses were often instructed to observe and record the patient's behavior but not to make any type of interpretation. With the advent of the health team concept, nurses were encouraged to learn more about the psychodynamics of mental illness and to engage in individual nursing therapy. A physician might supervise a "promising nurse therapist" who was providing individual therapy to a patient.

By the mid-1950s nurses were recognized as being capable of functioning as group leaders and therapists.

This was a major breakthrough, since nursing was no longer limited to custodial care and unit management. Nurses finally had collegial relationships with psychiatric social workers, occupational and recreational therapists, psychologists, and physicians.

In 1949 Dr. Robert H. Felix, director of the National Institute of Mental Health, U.S. Public Health Service, spoke of the importance of a team approach to psychiatric care. At this time teamwork was still in an early experimental stage, and in some institutions the concept had not yet even been accepted, let alone practiced.[22]

In these early days of the team concept the psychiatric team consisted of the psychiatrist, clinical psychologist, psychiatric social worker, and psychiatric nurse. According to Robinson,[22] professional rivalries were often evident and territoriality blocked progress. The psychiatrist saw himself as "the sole dispenser of psychotherapy rather than the captain of a therapeutic team." Psychiatric social workers and psychiatric nurses were often more concerned about "delineating their separate areas of professional responsibility than about cooperating for the total welfare of the patient."[22] To overcome these early stumbling blocks, team concept advocates were pressed to clarify the purpose and to demonstrate the desirability of this approach.

The purpose of the psychiatric team is to provide a forum in which the psychiatrist, psychiatric social worker, clinical psychologist, and psychiatric nurse democratically share professional knowledge and together evolve a therapeutic plan of action.[19]

Many implications arise from this definition of the psychiatric team. It implies that all members have an equal opportunity to share what they have learned about the patient and that these contributions will be welcomed in developing a definite goal-directed plan of action. Implicit to the clinical team approach is the need for a team leader. The psychiatrist most frequently functions in this capacity. According to Mereness, it is the responsibility of the leader to "help mold into an understandable unity the specialized information which is brought to the group by other team members." A final implication is the mutual respect for and understanding of the contributions of each team member.[19]

In the early stages of the team approach most nurses were receptive to the concept and grateful for the opportunity to contribute to patient care. However, old stereotypes of the nurse's subordinate role and inadequate communication skills placed nurses at a disadvantage. It became apparent that "the nurse's academic and professional background must be equivalent to that of her colleagues if she is to feel secure and be accepted as a fully participating member of the team."[19]

Nursing educators responded to the challenge by making needed changes. Curriculum changes included adding scientific psychiatric nursing education, with special emphasis on psychodynamics and interpersonal theory, communication skills, and skills in understanding and working with other disciplines. A new breed of psychiatric nurses began to develop who viewed themselves as professionally and academically competent to be fully participating members of the psychiatric clinical team.

The joint endeavor of a team approach promoted mutual respect among the various disciplines, and nursing benefitted. However, nursing may have lost some of its autonomy. Nagging doubts about nursing being a "true profession" remained as many nurses adopted the role of "junior psychiatrist."

Inpatient psychiatric nursing and the nursing process

Once nurses had been accepted as members of the mental health team and had developed sophistication, skills, and knowledge of psychiatry and psychiatric treatment, it was necessary to reassess and clarify nursing's purpose and identity. Psychiatric nursing returned to the nursing process.

If anything is unique to nursing, it is the nursing process. Sundeen and coworkers[25] describe the nursing process as an "interactive, problem-solving process used by the nurse as a systematic and individualized way to fulfill the goal of nursing care." They distinguish problem solving, which is used by many disciplines, and the nursing process as follows:

Many disciplines incorporate aspects of the problem-solving process. The nursing process, however, is distinguished from the problem-solving process in its purpose and method. The purpose of the problem-solving process is the development of new knowledge. The purpose of the nursing process is to maximize a client's positive interactions with his environment, his level of wellness, and his degree of self-actualization. The methods also differ. With the scientific process one can problem solve in isolation, manipulating objects and ideas without interacting with other people. The nursing process, however, is founded on the helping, interpersonal relationship; the nurse interacts with a client to analyze and meet his biopsychosocial needs.[25:5]

Today's inpatient psychiatric nurses use the nursing process to provide care to individuals, families, and groups. The nurse tries to help the patient find more effective ways of handling the stress that led to his im-

mobilization. The nurse's goal is to participate with the patient in planning the nursing care. By capitalizing on the patient's strengths, the nurse may help him establish more harmonious interpersonal relationships and function more independently. These accomplishments lead to a more positive self-concept and a sense of well-being.

The way in which the nursing process is implemented may vary from institution to institution or from nurse to nurse. However, several factors remain constant. The collection of a data base is the initial step. An individual interview is usually conducted by the nurse within 24 to 48 hours after the patient is admitted to the unit. The nurse also may choose to use family members or friends as sources of information. Once a data base is gathered, the nurse develops a diagnostic impression and plans the appropriate nursing actions. The results of these nursing actions are evaluated as frequently as necessary with appropriate changes and modifications. (See Chapter 5 and Appendices B, C, and D for tools of assessment.)

■ **TEAM RELATIONSHIPS.** It is important to stress that the nursing process does not exist in a vacuum. Each discipline on the health team must work toward common goals and objectives. However, each discipline has a variety of dependent, independent, and interdependent functions. The most familiar dependent nursing functions involve carrying out the physician's orders. The nurse is responsible for giving treatments and medications accurately and on time. The nurse assures that the patient receives all the prescribed laboratory tests, psychological tests, and other appropriate consultations. Despite the fact that these are dependent functions, the nurse has the right and the obligation to question any physician's orders that are unclear or possibly unsafe. The nurse's interdependent functions may range from sharing information with the health team to acting as cotherapist with members of other disciplines in family or group therapy, providing the nurse has appropriate preparation for these roles.

Independent nursing functions often give rise to the greatest sense of job satisfaction for the inpatient psychiatric nurse. Independent nursing actions can range from taking vital signs to carrying out special types of nursing observations and supervision. Together the nurse and the patient develop goals and determine the course that seems most likely to lead to accomplishing those goals. Along the way the nurse must decide what teaching is necessary for the patient, his family, and significant others. The nurse must judge how much can be learned from the patient's milieu and what needs must be met within the patient's home environment, community, or employment situation. The inpatient psychiatric nurse often provides the vital link in bridging the gap between inpatient hospitalization and successful reintegration into the community.

■ **PATIENT INVOLVEMENT.** It is difficult if not impossible to accomplish the nursing objectives without the patient's active participation. Nursing rounds are one method of encouraging the patient to participate. The patient is interviewed by a nurse consultant in front of members of the nursing staff who are working directly with him. The nurse consultant encourages the patient to discuss both useful and nonproductive experiences in his hospitalization. The patient is asked how he believes the nursing staff can best help him reach his goals. He is urged to identify his internal and external resources and to capitalize on these strengths during his hospitalization and when he returns to the community.

Patient response to this format has been favorable. Many patients have said they have been treated as intelligent adults during nursing rounds. They believe that they are given the right, as consumers of health care, to demand to be informed participants.

Clinical example 24-1 demonstrates the nursing process in an inpatient psychiatric unit.

Today's psychiatric nursing practice is founded in behavioral science theories, biopsychological aspects of stress, and sound effective interpersonal relationships. This body of knowledge is translated into action by the nursing process. The question now becomes, What method of care delivery is best suited for implementing the nursing process?

■ **Primary nursing and the nursing process**

This portion of the chapter discusses primary nursing as a method of care delivery on an inpatient psychiatric unit and the experiences of inpatient psychiatric nurses who, in becoming primary nurses, "rediscovered" the nursing process.

■ **CHARACTERISTICS.** Primary nursing is characterized by the assignment of one nurse to coordinate the total nursing care of a patient, from admission to discharge. This provides highly individualized, comprehensive care with a degree of continuity that other nursing care delivery models cannot provide. The assumption of 24-hour responsibility sets the primary nurse apart from other nurses. The primary nurse assesses the patient's nursing needs, develops an around-the-clock plan of care, and evaluates the results. Primary nurses may delegate the responsibility of implementing the care plan, but they are accountable for

---

CLINICAL EXAMPLE 24-1

Ms. R was a 17-year-old, single, high school student who was admitted to an inpatient psychiatric unit with the diagnosis of bipolar disorder. She was admitted for uncontrollable behavior (i.e., sexual promiscuity, running away from home, hyperverbalization, extreme irritability).

The initial nursing assessment provided a data base that revealed a chaotic family system with a long history of mental illness on both sides of the family, a social and cultural environment in which drug and alcohol abuse were prevalent, and a community that, because of its low socioeconomic status, possessed limited mental health resources. However, the patient was very bright, cooperative, and motivated to benefit from her hospitalization.

The initial nursing actions were to carry out the dependent functions of administering the prescribed medications including lithium carbonate, and assuring that blood levels were checked three times a week until a therapeutic level was reached. The nurse assessed that there was an immediate need to protect the patient from her impulsive uncontrollable behavior. The patient was placed under close nursing observation at all times until she was able to be in control of her own behavior.

Once the patient's mood had stabilized, she was presented in nursing rounds. During this time the patient was able to identify a great need for the nurse to teach her and her family about bipolar disorder and the importance of continued lithium treatment. The patient and staff agreed that a home visit would reveal the pressures that the family placed on the patient to function as surrogate mother to her eight siblings. The patient also believed that it was important that her illness not be viewed in exactly the same manner as that of her sister, who was diagnosed as schizophrenic. The patient viewed her intellectual ability and the "love" that existed in her family system as her best resources. She thought that, with the assistance of the nursing staff, she and her family could develop more understanding of her illness and decrease the chaos within the family system.

After discharge the patient was treated in outpatient therapy by a nurse therapist. The family was being seen by a psychiatric social worker.

providing written and verbal directions. Marram, Barrett, and Bevis[18] view the primary nurse as a "triple A" nurse who has "three basic characteristics: autonomy, authority, and accountability."

These three characteristics, more than any others, differentiate a professionally oriented nursing practice from one that is task oriented. A primary nurse with autonomy collaborates with other disciplines. Other health professionals are used by the primary nurse as resources and consultants. However, the nursing care plan is developed by the primary nurse and the patient. Primary nurses must have the authority to develop and implement a total comprehensive nursing care plan on a 24-hour basis. A true test of a professional primary nurse is a willingness to stand accountable for all of his or her decisions and actions.

The departments of nursing of several inpatient psychiatric facilities across the United States have chosen primary nursing as their care delivery system. In these facilities primary nursing has led to increased job satisfaction among the professional nursing staff and increased satisfaction among patients. On the surface it appears that a transition to primary nursing in an inpatient psychiatric setting could be accomplished with ease, because psychiatric nursing lends itself to the establishment of one-to-one relationships. However, many institutions have encountered numerous difficulties in implementing primary nursing.

■ **PROBLEMS.** Two types of problems often arise during the transition to primary nursing care. First are problems that are internal to nursing. Second are the problems that result from the impact that changes in one discipline have on other disciplines. Internal problems center around the redefinition of all nursing positions, from the director of psychiatric nursing to the psychiatric aides and unit clerks. Including nonprofessional nursing staff in primary nursing remains an unsolved problem in need of further exploration. The primary nurses themselves seem to encounter the most difficulty in accepting accountability for their decision making and practice.

To successfully implement primary nursing, both the administration and staff must support and accept this care delivery system. Unfortunately, nursing is characterized by hierarchical authority and bureaucracy. Hospital and nursing administrators are reluctant to provide staffing patterns and the decentralized decision making necessary for primary nursing.[18]

Thus nursing administrators must view themselves as facilitators of change and must be willing to delegate certain authority to make decisions about patient care to the nurses at the clinical levels. Administrators must also be committed to providing adequate staffing

patterns and resource people for clinical supervision, staff development, and inservice education. Once nursing administration has made this commitment, it must realize that organizational change alone will not lead to successful implementation of primary nursing.[15] However, by lending support and leadership through active participation, nursing administration can foster an enthusiasm toward viewing change as a challenge and as an opportunity for personal and professional growth.

Can all psychiatric nurses be primary nurses? This is perhaps the most difficult of the internal problems encountered in the transitional period. In their study on the use of psychiatric nurses, Anderson and Apostoles[2] found that all 26 nurses in their research program were able to successfully complete their rotation through the 18-month project. It was only after the completion of the program that two of the 26 nurses resigned.

A closer look reveals that in this study population, associate degree and baccalaureate graduates were overrepresented, and diploma and master's degree graduates were underrepresented. The project nurses generally agreed (75%) that "any new graduate has the basic skills to function as a primary care nurse." However, these nurses qualified this statement with the provision that the guidance of a clinical specialist, support from the physician, and team cooperation were essential.[2]

In their study on primary nursing, Coates, Falck, and Sienkilewski[3] observed that the essential ingredients of a successful primary nurse on an inpatient psychiatric unit were innovation, motivation, and a patient-centered orientation. They further observed that, with few exceptions, the primary nurses who had these characteristics but who did not already have their baccalaureate degrees soon began working toward them.

It is obvious that not all psychiatric nurses can be primary nurses. No one care delivery system can satisfy the needs of all. There is some evidence that, given a supportive nursing administration, most nurses who are willing to stand accountable and are motivated to accept the challenge will experience some success as primary nurses.

The transition to primary nursing has an impact on other health care providers, and the responses vary from humorous to serious. An initial response from the resident physician group is often to become territorial about their patients. This phase may be referred to as the "not with my patients, you don't" phase. In a similar manner, psychiatric social workers may respond to the threat of boundary encroachment by countering, "Not with my families, you don't." Occupational and recreational therapists, who are often involved in their own search for autonomy, may be heard to say, "Here we go again."

After many of these problems are resolved, the multidisciplinary team enters into the second phase of transition. This phase is frequently characterized by the beginning development of mutual sharing, respect, and trust. "Not with my patient" becomes "What can nursing offer the patient?" "Not with my family" is replaced by "Would you like to sit in on a family assessment?" or "Shall we do a joint home visit?" It is at this stage that the "here we go again" truth tellers may ask, "Have we really made it this time?"

The benefactor of a collaborative approach to care is the patient. When the psychiatric team works in a collegial fashion, energy is not wasted on protecting boundaries and territories and the team's attention is focused on the patient's needs. Clinical example 24-2 is an actual patient's account of her experience as a primary patient in an inpatient psychiatric unit.*

Problems related to psychiatric settings. The three major characteristics of the primary nursing modality (autonomy, authority, and accountability) are the same in inpatient psychiatric nursing as in any other clinical specialty. However, unique complications do arise because of the nature of psychiatry. More than in other areas of medicine, psychiatric care providers share an almost universal ingredient—the therapeutic use of self. Frequently, clinical territory is shared and skills are equalized, and "gender and character style rather than strict professional discipline lines are drawn."[27] Psychiatric nurses are often asked to expand their roles to include psychotherapy and social work. If this occurs too frequently and if primary nurses are supervised exclusively by other disciplines, they can lose their identity with their own profession. At this point they can no longer be considered primary nurses.

Thus primary nursing in psychiatric settings must be clearly defined in relation to other professionals and paraprofessionals. Primary nurses must maintain their involvement in the milieu. They must participate in experiences with patients "because they are part of patients' everyday lives."[27] The primary nurse teaches the patient how to use all his social, interpersonal, and environmental experiences within the hospital system. From these experiences the patient can often learn more effective ways of dealing with those real-life stresses which can lead to the need for hospitalization.

This involvement in the patient's everyday life al-

---

*Excerpt from an interview I conducted for nursing rounds.

CLINICAL EXAMPLE 24-2

When I came here I was completely immobilized. I was afraid of everything. The fears started as small silly things that my family and I tried to laugh off. But soon the little fears became bigger and bigger, and soon I wasn't able to function as a wife, a mother, or a human being.

Do you know that I hadn't been able to do any shopping for 2 years. I hadn't been out of my house at all for the past 6 months—except to come to the hospital. I had often thought of killing myself, but I was even too afraid to do that.

I can't tell you what being here has meant to me. Everyone has been understanding and supportive. My psychiatrist saw me three times a week in therapy and helped me learn about my illness and what caused my fears. The more I understood, the less frightening things seemed.

But I give most of the credit for my recovery to my primary nurse. She was the person who helped me to function again. She made me feel less ashamed and helped me to realize that I wasn't a total, no good weakling.

Together we planned strategies of how to get me moving. We started very slowly with short trips off the ward. The next step was to go to the market to buy cake mix for the ward bake sale. The big step happened just a few weeks ago when my nurse and I went all the way downtown to Christmas shop for my family. My family and I cried together when I gave them their gifts on Christmas Day. It was the first time in 2 years that I was able to buy them anything. I'm preparing for discharge with my primary nurse. Last weekend I went home, and I was able to shop alone. I am still apprehensive, but my nurse says that this is not unusual.

I'm being discharged next week and the plans are for me to see my doctor on an outpatient basis for awhile. My primary nurse is going to make a follow-up home visit in 2 weeks to see how things are going. I really feel comfortable with this arrangement.

Are all the other wards going to start primary nursing? I think that all the patients here should have the opportunity to have a primary nurse.

lows the primary nurse to provide and integrate data from many sources. It is also this involvement that best differentiates the role of the primary nurse from other psychiatric professionals.

Recent legislative changes and budgetary constraints have had great impact on mental health care and the use of professional personnel. As previously mentioned, psychiatric nurses are being asked to expand their roles to include such functions as psychotherapist and case manager. Nursing administrators must be responsive to these current trends and creative in meeting these additional service demands. Lack of responsiveness could result in a professional loss of identity for psychiatric nurses and a decrease in the quality of nursing care.

■ **MODELS OF PRIMARY NURSING.** It is possible to combine the concepts of primary nursing and primary care in psychiatric settings. This combination encourages nurses to expand their roles and to continue their primary nursing activities and milieu involvement. The amalgamation of these two concepts should be tailored to meet the organizational, treatment, and fiscal policies of the institution. However, the integrity of the modalities must be maintained. Two models of a primary nursing–primary care system are presented.

Model A was developed for a small psychiatric department in a general hospital. The department housed one 20-bed inpatient unit and an active outpatient clinic. The nurses functioned exclusively as primary nurses on the inpatient unit. Each primary nurse spent approximately half a day in the outpatient clinic functioning as a psychotherapist. Thus the primary nurse's caseload consisted of three or four primary nursing patients and two or three psychotherapy outpatients.

In this model the head nurse was responsible for assigning the nursing caseloads. Supervision for nursing care was provided by clinical nurse specialists with graduate education in psychiatric nursing and in peer groups with other primary nurses. Outpatient assignments were made by the treatment team responsible for planning the follow-up care for the inpatient unit. Outpatient supervision was provided by the same clinical specialists (who were also qualified therapists) with regular consultations from assigned medical-psychiatric backups. The primary nurses had direct input into the selection process of both the inpatient and outpatient caseloads.

Model B was developed for a large state psychiatric hospital. Here the primary nurse functioned as both case manager and primary nurse on an inpatient admissions unit. As in Model A the head nurse was responsible for assigning the primary nursing patient caseload, and supervision for these patients was pro-

vided by clinical nurse specialists with graduate education.

The patients for whom the nurse functioned as case manager and therapist were assigned by the psychiatrist in charge of the treatment team. Patient supervision was provided by the psychiatrists and the clinical specialists. The average caseload for these nurses was five or six primary nursing patients and two or three case management patients. The primary nurses were involved in the selection of both caseloads.

A comprehensive inservice educational program and qualified clinical nurse specialists were essential to the success of both models. If primary nurses are to expand their roles, they must have an adequate theoretical and clinical base. An indepth inservice program that is balanced in didactic theory and related clinical experience should be required for all primary nurses who are expanding their roles. These program models should be designed, implemented, evaluated, and controlled by nursing. In this way primary nurses are given the support they need to maintain the integrity of the nursing model and their professional identity.

The immediate future of primary nursing in inpatient psychiatric settings will more likely be influenced by political, legislative, and financial factors than by therapeutic objectives or philosophies. Cost containment has become a major focus of public and private hospitals. Hospitals must use their financial resources and personnel to provide timely patient evaluations, family involvement, relevant treatment methods, and appropriate dispositions. The long-term future of primary nursing depends on psychiatric nurses' ability to demonstrate that this type of care provides quality therapeutic interventions in a cost-effective manner.

The clinical nurse specialist in the inpatient setting

The concept of a "specialist" who provides nursing care to a patient or group of clients first took the form of the private duty nurse. It was not until the mid-1960s that the role of the master's level clinical nurse specialist was developed to improve the quality of nursing care. Those first nursing visionaries realized that they would need to justify having master's prepared nurses at the patient's bedside. Consequently, early writings contained broad definitions of educational qualifications and role functions.[8]

Although the role of the clinical nurse specialist may differ from one inpatient facility to another, Clinical example 24-3 and Table 24-1 suggest a model that may be modified to meet many inpatient settings.

Unfortunately, use of clinical nurse specialists has not lived up to the high expectations of the nursing

CLINICAL EXAMPLE 24-3

In 1980 the nursing department of a large state psychiatric hospital made a commitment to the introduction of the role of the clinical nurse specialist as a vital part of its integrated organizational structure. These nursing leaders believed that quality nursing care can be accomplished only when nursing administrators, clinical nurse experts, nursing educators, and nursing researchers work in unison toward a common goal of excellence. The director of nursing, along with the three associate directors, designed an organizational plan based on ANA standards of practice (see Chapter 5 and Appendix A) and Joint Commission on Accreditation of Healthcare Organizations (JCAHO) standards. The plan called for

1. Nursing administration to appoint a task force to develop a protocol for all registered nurses to be privileged in basic nursing care and expanded role functions
2. Nursing inservice to develop the appropriate educational modules to provide the didactic and theoretical basis needed by staff nurses for expanded role functions
3. Clinical nurse specialists to provide formal clinical supervision, role modeling, and consultation to staff nurses
4. Nursing researchers to provide program evaluation to identify quality and cost issues

Fourteen clinical nurse specialists were recruited and placed strategically in the clinical areas. Their job descriptions called for them to

1. Provide direct patient care
2. Provide formal clinical supervision to staff nurses
3. Act as expert nursing consultants to the interdisciplinary team
4. Provide formal and informal inservice education to nursing staff
5. Participate in nursing research

The clinical nurse specialists were given the autonomy to determine which aspect of their job needed to take priority. Along with this autonomy, they were given the authority to arrange their work schedules to meet patient and staff needs. After ten years, the clinical nurse specialist has been accepted and has become a valued member of the nursing team. The impact of their efforts on the organization has not been limited to direct patient care. Much of the success in recruiting professional nurses and much of the credibility the department of nursing has gained are a result of the presence of these nursing experts. This experience has convinced the nursing leaders of this hospital that the risks they took and the initial resistance they had to face were well worth their efforts. They believe that the clinical nurse specialist is a necessity in an inpatient psychiatric setting.

leaders who developed the role. Nursing now more than ever needs to demonstrate that quality care and cost containment are not mutually exclusive. Otherwise the role of the clinical nurse specialist may not survive.

Patient education on an inpatient unit

The consumer movement in mental health has led to requests for information by patients and their families. Mental health care providers are recognizing that informed patients are more likely to participate actively and productively in the treatment process. Families who are knowledgeable about the patient's illness can work with nurses to assist the patient toward wellness.

Because of their frequent and intimate contact with patients, nurses should be actively involved in formal and informal patient education. The education process begins with the orientation of the patient and significant others to the inpatient setting. Written materials often are used to describe the policies, procedures, and activities that take place in the hospital. The nurse must consider the learner's reading ability and level of comprehension. Important points should always be presented verbally as well as in writing.

Although the physician may initiate the patient's education about the medical diagnosis, the nurse needs to reinforce the teaching. In addition, nurses are usually the best sources of information about practical management of illness-related behaviors, including symptoms and expected responses to treatments. The basic patient services provided by the nurse in the hospital may need to be continued by the family at home. Therefore the family must understand the treatment plan. Both the patient and the family must be aware of such information as side effects of medications and signs of a relapse.

Aside from personalized, individual, or family-oriented patient education, nurses frequently initiate group education programs for patients and/or significant others. Some types of groups that might be led by nurses include medication groups, assertiveness training groups, sexuality groups, community living skills groups, health education groups, and stress management groups. Education in a group setting may be enhanced by the feedback and peer support from other members. Further information on patient education in groups may be found in Chapter 28.

Aside from the primary goal of developing an informed consumer, there are also legal implications related to patient education. Consumers are beginning to bring suit against providers who have not given them adequate information to practice self-care safely.

TABLE 24-1

MODEL FOR ROLE OF INPATIENT PSYCHIATRIC CLINICAL NURSE SPECIALIST

Direct patient care	Clinical supervision	Consultation	Education	Research
Individual therapy	Individual supervision of staff	Serve as nurse expert to treatment team	Assist inservice faculty in developing and teaching education modules	Conduct clinical studies to identify effective nursing intervention for specific diagnostic groups
Family theapy	Group supervision of staff	Provide link between hospital and community		
Group therapy	Conduct staff meetings	Conduct transition groups in placement homes	Serve as guest speakers at schools of nursing	Participate in program evaluation to determine the impact and cost-effectiveness of the clinical nurse specialist
Patient education groups	Peer supervision			
a) Medication	Cross-discipline supervision		Serve as guest speakers to community and patient advocacy groups	
b) Sex education				Identify effective methods for clinical supervision
c) Activities of daily living group				Identify effective intervention for the chronically mentally ill
Milieu group meetings				
Community living transitional groups				
Nursing rounds				
Case management				
Program coordinator				
Home visiting				

The nurse is obligated to provide necessary information in an understandable manner. Careful documentation of the material presented and the method of evaluating patient comprehension is also required. Of course, it is important for the nurse to coordinate all patient education activities with the rest of the health care team.

In addition to health-related educational programs, many long-term hospitals also provide academic and prevocational education programs for patients. These are usually under the auspices of the vocational rehabilitation department, frequently in conjunction with the local school system. Patients enrolled in this type of program need the support and encouragement of nurses. Successful vocational training may make the difference in a patient's ability to survive in the community.

Design of an inpatient psychiatric unit

The design of an inpatient psychiatric unit is important to the patients, their families and friends, and to the members of the health care team. The facility's design should reflect the departments' philosophy, the methods of care provided, and the types of patients to be served.

Despite changing tastes in architectural and interior design, several principles continue to hold true. Adequate space is of utmost importance. Patients need an environment that promotes socialization but allows privacy. The unit should be flexible. Day areas and dining rooms can be designed to easily convert into group meeting rooms. Adequate storage space should be provided to prevent a cluttered, unkempt look.

Offices should be provided for individual sessions, charting, and dictating. An adequate treatment room facility is essential for providing quality medical treatment. In the more modern inpatient units the nurses station is replaced by a reception desk with work areas that are open and accessible to patients.

In addition to a day area, dining room, and lounge facilities, space should be provided for a kitchen and a laundry and linen area. The bedrooms should be furnished with comfortable, attractive, sturdy beds and chairs. There should be a combination of single and semiprivate rooms. Small dormitory rooms of three or four patients may be desirable in some hospital settings.

Room for occupational and recreational activities is provided either on the unit or in separate adjacent activities wings. These activities wings may include an arts and crafts room, music room, and areas for indoor exercise and sports such as yoga, table tennis, and basketball.

Occasionally psychiatric patients need to be secluded or isolated. Isolation rooms can be designed to maintain the privacy and dignity of the isolated patient but still allow for free flow of traffic. This is accomplished with a vestibule between the door of the isolation room and a door that opens onto the main corridor. Often private bathrooms are located in these vestibules. Patient safety is of primary importance in the design of isolation rooms.

The use of color, furniture, plants, paintings, graphics, and decorator pieces is very important. The walls of the rooms are usually painted with subtle, quiet hues. Colorful accents are added with graphics, paintings, and furniture. Materials that withstand long-term use and maintenance and that meet safety requirements enable architects and interior designers to create noninstitutionalized inpatient units at reasonable costs.

Modalities of therapy on an inpatient psychiatric unit

Inpatient psychiatric care is currently undergoing major changes. The hospital has become a part of a continuum of mental health services available to patients and their families.

Many inpatient psychiatric facilities continue to offer a variety of therapies in the treatment of psychiatric and behavioral disorders. However, the number of short-term hospitalizations is rapidly growing. This trend requires a rethinking of the hospital's mission and purpose, and an evaluation of the effectiveness of treatment programming.

Some patients will continue to need the more traditional intensive inpatient psychiatric care. But, for that growing number whose hospital stays are brief, inpatient clinicians must develop new practice models that provide effective and timely evaluation, diagnostic workups, stabilization, and referral services.

These recent changes in inpatient psychiatric care have also led to a need to assess the use of clinical resources. In many hospitals psychiatric nurses are being utilized to provide a variety of therapeutic services. This use will depend on the nurse's preparation and the philosophy of the use.

■ Milieu therapy

Milieu therapy is a "scientific manipulation of the environment aimed at producing changes in the personality of the patient."[4] The word "milieu" was first used to mean a scientifically planned environment by Bettleheim and Sylvester in the late 1930s and early 1940s.

■ **CONCEPTS.** Early research and experiments in milieu therapy almost exclusively used psychological or psychiatric theories of illness to determine the kinds of environments that would be most therapeutic. Attempts were made to "prescribe" minutely detailed interpersonal environments based on the psychodynamic needs of a "carefully diagnosed" patient. This ambitious undertaking included attempts to prescribe and program staff attitudes and responses as well as patient activities.

In 1954 Stanton and Schwartz suggested that the environment can be the primary treatment as well as a supporting or complementary influence to other forms of treatment. They noted that the environment may frequently have components that are irrelevant to the psychodynamics of the patient but may be important to his general welfare. Later Caudell described the effect that culture, organized values, norms, and customs have on patient care. In 1958 Freeman, Cameron, and McGhie developed the relationship between ego psychology and specific characteristics of the environment. Despite all this accumulated information, until the work of Cumming and Cumming in 1962 there had been a reluctance to consider the possibility that "the milieu might itself bring about specific changes in the behavior of patients and thus specific changes in their personalities."[4]

Milieu programs may differ widely from system to system. However, several basic assumptions appear to be common to all therapeutic milieu approaches to inpatient psychiatric treatment. The first assumption is that patients have strengths and conflict-free portions of their personalities. These strengths are optimally used by the scientific manipulation of the institutional environment. Second, patients have abilities to constructively influence their own treatment, the treatment of others, and to some degree the organizational structure of the hospital. The third assumption is that successful treatment of seriously disturbed patients depends heavily on a pervasive, therapeutic staff involvement. The final assumption is that all levels of hospital personnel have the potential for exercising a therapeutic influence.[26]

■ Therapeutic community

According to Kraft, "The therapeutic community is a very special kind of milieu therapy in which the total social structure of the treatment unit is involved as part of the helping process."[13:543] How does this differ from the concept of milieu therapy, and what are the implications of those differences? Perhaps the clearest distinction is that in the therapeutic community, it is believed that all social and interpersonal interactions in the hospital are the main therapeutic tools used to bring about specific changes in the patient. As previously mentioned, in milieu therapy the emphasis is on the manipulation of the environment to bring about changes in the patient's behavior, with efforts to keep all interpersonal discussions in the context of a goal-directed activity.[4]

■ **CONCEPTS.** It is impossible to discuss the treatment modality of the therapeutic community without exploring the original concept as set forth by Maxwell Jones. According to Jones,[10] a therapeutic community is distinguished from other comparable treatment programs by the way in which the total resources of the staff, the patients, their relatives, and the institution are pooled for the purpose of treatment. Thus the patient must undergo a change in status. The staff must encourage his active participation in his care planning. This would be a marked contrast to the conventional passive recipient role.[11]

In the structuring of a therapeutic community, Jones suggested that the emphasis should be placed on free communication both within and between staff and patient groups. The end results of free communication were hoped to be the examination of roles, the clarification of what behavior is regarded as appropriate, some loss of apparent distinctiveness of particular roles, and attempts to modify some overall cultural attitudes and beliefs that are antitherapeutic. Thus the therapeutic community would be democratic as opposed to hierarchical, rehabilitative rather than custodial, permissive instead of limited and controlled, and, finally, communal as opposed to emphasizing the specialized therapeutic role of the physician. In the early Jones model of a therapeutic community, the environment was essentially permissive and flexible.

The roles of the participants were purposely unspecified, the patients' activities were highly individualized, and participation was completely voluntary. The one exception was a daily community meeting that all staff members had to attend and all patients were encouraged to attend. Group responsibility was emphasized, and opportunities for corrective learning experiences were deliberately provided. The primary role of the staff was to help the patients gain new insights and test new behavioral patterns.

Jones believed that each treatment unit ideally should be free to operate in the manner best suited to its own particular style and approach. However, he offered several components that he believed were characteristic of a therapeutic community. The daily community meeting was used as a format for discussing day-to-day life on the unit. Since these gatherings were often composed of 80 or 90 patients, many of the tensions and concerns of the individual patients were "worked through" in small group therapy sessions that followed the community meeting.

Another component of the therapeutic community is patient government. The purpose of the patient government or ward council is to deal with practical unit details such as privileges and housekeeping rosters. Jones suggested that a staff member be available to the patient government and that all decisions be fed back to the community through the community meetings.

Jones viewed the staff meeting or review as essential to on-the-ward training. He saw these meetings as taking place for at least 30 minutes after each community meeting. In this meeting the staff members would examine their own responses, expectations, and prejudices. Another important characteristic of the therapeutic community is the living-learning opportunities provided to the patient within the social milieu. Thus the therapeutic community is like a "school for living" in which the patients learn to meet the demands of everyday life.

According to Jones, "Feedback is one of the fundamental concepts in therapeutic community practice."[11] It is of great importance that all decisions, disputes, progress, and accomplishments be conveyed to the community as a whole. Very little, if anything, is purely confidential in a therapeutic community. The staff members must be sensitive in their role of demonstrating how and when to feed back information to the community.

Although Jones' original concept of the therapeutic community has been added to and modified, it is still considered a viable model. The Marlborough Hospital in London has used the Jones model of therapeutic community and has added some creative and innovative activities. Included in this program are the typical community meetings, staff meetings, small psychotherapy groups, work groups, admission meetings, badminton groups, and pottery groups. In addition this therapeutic community offers individual reviews, encounter groups, projective art sessions, gestalt groups, occupational therapy workshop sessions, patient meetings, and a dream group. Three other groups also have been created for this particular community. The "Leavers group" is designed to look at the feelings and problems related to leaving the community. In this group the need for further treatment is discussed. The "Concern group" is composed of patients the community believes cannot make use of their therapy. The purpose of this group is to clarify the aim and purpose of the hospital and the individual's role within it. "The committee" is composed of five patients, one from each small psychotherapy group, and a number of staff members. It functions as a feedback source to the community meetings and to the business and patients' meetings.[16]

■ **MILIEU TREATMENT IN SHORT-TERM ACUTE INPATIENT CARE.** Several of the original principles of the therapeutic community and milieu therapy remain relevant in current acute inpatient care. There is little doubt that: environment influences cognition, behavior, and emotion; group dynamics are always operant; focusing on responsibility and rehabilitation encourages growth; and integrated treatment is extremely effective.[12]

What have become less applicable are some of the specific models and frameworks that were originally developed to implement these principles. Many of these models depended upon having the time in the hospital setting to socialize patients to community norms. Current inpatient stays of fourteen to twenty-one days are disruptive to the development of a therapeutic culture. Inpatients with high acuity of illness, impaired cognition, and tenuous control may be overstimulated by confrontational group encounters, blurring of roles, and immediate therapeutic responsibility for others. "Treatment outcome research shows little measurable benefit for patients, and sometimes harm, when classic milieu techniques are applied in short-term, acute treatment settings."[12]

Kahn and White[12] outlined three principles necessary to the successful integration of milieu treatment in short-term inpatient care: establish a holding environment; provide graduated therapy; and emphasize commonality. The focus of a "holding environment" is consistency and caring. In this environment, three provisions of safety, structure, and support are immediate priorities. As patients reach a higher level of need, socialization and self-understanding are added to the environment's essential elements.

The concept of graduated therapy embraces the belief that a treatment program must provide the flexibility to respond to a patient's individual capacities, resources, and support systems. Patients may enter the program at different levels and may progress or "graduate" at their own rate according to their goals. Kahn and White suggest the following scheme for graduated therapy: orientation, engagement, education, and understanding. Each level of treatment in a graduated model requires a patient to utilize greater organization of thinking and an increased tolerance to stress.

The principle of "emphasized commonality" is key to effective milieu treatment in short-term inpatient

hospitalizations. Recent studies indicate that patients most value treatment that assists them in gaining a sense of mastery over crises and aids them in social connectedness. These patients indicated that these skills were achieved by attending support groups that were focused on common issues and the sharing of common response to crises situations.[12]

■ **ROLE OF THE NURSE.** If milieu therapy is to remain a viable treatment for inpatient psychiatric care, it must be modified to meet the changing mission of the psychiatric hospital as a part of a mental health care continuum. Today's milieu models must be integrated with new findings from biological and psychosocial research.

There is little question that the advent of milieu therapy helped change the course of psychiatric nursing. Before 1946, psychiatric nursing literature stressed the importance of the management of a safe and secure environment. With milieu therapy the nurse's role in the environment began to change from custodial to therapeutic and rehabilitative. According to Wolf,[26] Sills recommends a "social learning model" as an appropriate guide for nurses' interventions in a therapeutic milieu. This would shift the emphasis away from "caring for the patient" to teaching the patient social skills. This model complements and supports the two basic goals of milieu therapy: limit setting and learning the basic social skills of orientation, assertion, occupation, and recreation.[26]

Recent research by Kathleen Emrich reconfirms that "patient-staff interactions that are confirming, open, and emphasize dignity and responsibility are significantly correlated with positive treatment outcomes."[6] She goes on to elaborate on the fact that nurses continue to bear the primary therapeutic responsibility for the effectiveness of the milieu.

However, the results of this study indicate that many nurse-patient interactions do not regularly promote responses associated with healthy adjustment. Thus, it is imperative that nurses expand their knowledge and understanding of the effects of spontaneous interactions and unstructured aspects of the milieu. This expanding knowledge may be used to develop more effective models for future nursing roles in milieu treatment.

■ **Individual psychotherapy**

Traditionally, individual inpatient psychotherapy is conducted by the psychiatrist, who sees the patient on the average of one to three times weekly. Individual psychotherapy offers the patient an opportunity to develop insight into the sources of his thoughts, feelings, perceptions, and behavior. By developing these insights, the patient can improve his skills in establishing and maintaining interpersonal relationships and can use more effective behaviors in dealing with stress. Despite the fact that individual psychotherapy has come under attack as an ineffective method of treatment, most acute psychiatric facilities continue to view it as a viable and desirable practice.

In a multidisciplinary approach to patient care, other health care providers may function as psychotherapists. For example, a nurse may function as primary nurse for a selected number of patients and as psychotherapist for others. However, the expanded role of the nurse as a psychotherapist must not be confused with primary nursing. Although primary nursing is purely a method of nursing care delivery, the expanded role of psychotherapist requires additional training in the fields of human growth and development, psychodynamics of human behavior, and the art and science of psychotherapy.

■ Family therapy

The focus of family therapy is to treat a social system as the primary unit, rather than an individual member who has been defined as a "patient." A variety of techniques and practices may be used in the process of family therapy. There may be any combination of pairing or grouping in each session or a series of sessions. For example, Ackerman recommends that the entire family unit be seen for therapy, but for the diagnostic phase he conducts sessions with various individuals, pairs, or triads. Wynne varies the member composition to discover which family members should be included in treatment. Bowen will see the entire family in what he calls "family group therapy" for brief periods. He views the optimum approach as starting with the husband and wife together and continuing with both for the entire period of family therapy. Bowen will often see a single family member to help that person achieve a higher level of differentiation.[23]

The goals of family therapy are to reduce conflict and anxiety, to make the family members more aware of each other's needs, to increase the family's ability to deal with external and internal crises, to develop more appropriate role relationships, to help individual family members cope with destructive forces within and outside the family, and to promote health and growth.

The psychiatric nurse should have special training in family systems and conjoint family therapy before attempting to function as a family therapist. The role of the therapist is to penetrate family secrets and myths, to counteract the process of scapegoating, and to pick up nonverbal communication and make it explicit. At other times the therapist may serve as a parent figure or a personal instrument for reality testing. The family therapist must be sensitive to the needs of the individual members and the family unit as a whole and respond appropriately.

A more comprehensive discussion of family therapy is presented in Chapter 29.

■ Group therapy

There are various types of group therapy. Traditionally the term "group therapy" describes a form of psychiatric treatment in which six to eight patients attend a specified number of meetings that are conducted by a therapist. The advantages of group therapy lie in the fact that most people's problems involve their feelings and behavior toward others. In a group setting the patient can develop an awareness of how his thoughts, feelings, and behavior affect others. Through group feedback and support the patient can change his behavior and establish more effective interpersonal relationships.

Too often groups are established as a time-saving device or because there are not enough therapists to care for individual patients. There are times when unskilled personnel are made "group leaders." This is a grave misuse of an effective therapeutic modality. Nurses who become group leaders or therapists should ensure that their group is being offered because it is the most appropriate form of treatment for those patients involved. The nurse should be skilled in group dynamics and behavior and have a thorough understanding of individual psychodynamics and psychopathology.

The types of group psychotherapy used on inpatient psychiatric units vary in aim, purpose, and intensity. The selection of specific groups will be determined by the philosophy of the unit, the skills of the staff, and the capacities of the patients. Some of the more common inpatient group therapies are personality reconstruction groups, insight without reconstruction groups, problem-solving groups, remotivation and reeducation groups, and supportive groups.[17]

Recently assertiveness training has become a popular form of group therapy. The goal of assertiveness training is to help the patient differentiate between passive, assertive, and aggressive behavior. Opportunities are provided for the patient to practice using assertive behavior. As a result, the patient has a choice of how he will approach a situation. The payoff is that he develops more self-confidence and can make his views and needs known without infringing on the rights of others.

"Specialty groups" are used on many inpatient psychiatric units. These groups are often composed of patients within a specific age range (e.g., young adult groups), patients with common problems or needs (e.g., predischarge groups), or patients of the same sex (e.g., women's sex education groups). These groups may be open-ended discussion groups or highly structured didactic groups. They may be offered on a continuing basis or be time limited. The important factors are that all groups should serve some purpose and meet some therapeutic need and the therapist should be skilled in group process and group dynamics.

Recent research proposes that changes in health care financing and decreasing hospital stays may place group psychotherapy in a position of being viewed as an efficient use of resources. Thus, it becomes vital for sound clinical research to establish the efficacy of short-term group therapy in acute inpatient treatment.[14]

The role of the psychiatric nurse in group therapy is explored in Chapter 28.

■ Psychodrama

Psychodrama uses structured, directed dramatizations of a patient's emotional problems and experiences. These "dramas" provide the patient with the opportunity to develop greater awareness of his thoughts, feelings, and actions and of how they affect others. Psychodrama was devised by Dr. Jacob L. Moreno in 1914.

Moreno established psychodrama on several theoretical principles. The **action principle** is that just as life is not limited to a single verbal dimension, so psychodramatic action overcomes the linguistic restrictions placed on understanding oneself. Moreno believed that action is "the most integrative vehicle for social learning and has the most cathartic impact."[23]

The principle of the **social atom** states that each person is the center of his "structure of primary interpersonal relationships." This interpersonal network is filled with incomplete perceptions and distortions. Psychodrama allows for the recreation of the social atom and the exploration of role function in an immediate feedback system that is conducive to learning.[20]

An important goal or outcome of psychodrama is spontaneity. Moreno[20] defined spontaneity as an ability to respond to a new situation with some "degree of adequacy" and to an old situation with a "degree of novelty."

Moreno believed that the human being was not overdetermined by his past. He thought that at any moment in time the human is in "a state of great growth-potential."[20] In psychodrama, **catharsis** is used to mean a bursting through of a personal or cultural conserve. **Tele** is a word used to describe a two-way feeling that cements and holds a relationship together. **Surplus reality** refers to the act of going beyond reality. An example of this may be having a dead person, as represented by a group member, speak.

Psychodrama has several important elements. Although a stage is not an absolute necessity, it provides a flexible, multidimensional living space. The stage should be round and should have two or three steplike levels. Since psychodrama is primarily a group process, the psychodramatist's effort is to mobilize the group to work together. The response to the action on the stage may be greater in the group than it is with the people on the stage. The protagonist is the star. At the moment he best typifies the concern of the group. The auxiliary egos are people in the group who take roles on stage in relationship to the protagonist and his action. Psychodramatic techniques are used to help the star and the group achieve spontaneity. Two important techniques are role reversal, in which the star exchanges his role for that of a significant other, and the use of the double, which is an auxiliary ego who gets behind the protagonist and attempts to express thoughts and feelings with which the protagonist is having difficulty.

There are three phases of psychodrama. The first phase is the warmup. During the warmup the psychodramatist involves the group in a discussion of issues deemed important to explore for that session. Once a group concern emerges, a protagonist is supported and encouraged to come forth. The second phase is composed of the shaping and presentation of the drama. If this stage is conducted properly, the entire group may benefit from the action. The final phase is the postaction group sharing. In this phase the group members express what events in their own lives were touched on by the action. The psychodramatist attempts to draw from the group some identification with the protagonist.

What are the indications for psychodrama? Advocates of this method have reported success with treating individual patients, groups of patients with marital discord, and groups of alcoholics. Psychodrama is used in milieu therapy as a form of group therapy and as a diagnostic tool in dealing with problems within the social system of the therapeutic community.

Psychodrama seems to have a valid place among the group treatments on an inpatient psychiatric unit. Clinical example 24-4 is an account of an actual psychodrama.

■ Rehabilitation therapies

A number of vital programs fall under the general classification of rehabilitation therapies. These pro-

CLINICAL EXAMPLE 24-4

A member of a psychodrama group came to each session with his mattress strapped on his back. He would enter a closet, close the door behind him, and remain there until the session was finished.

During one session the group decided during the warm-up phase that they wanted to deal with rejection. They believed that the group member in the closet best typified rejection. The patient was invited to be the star and to everyone's astonishment he accepted.

The psychodramatic action centered on the death of the patient's father. During the drama the patient was able to express all the anger that he had kept inside. He screamed and yelled at his father (who was described as being in hell but could hear him) for abandoning his family. Finally, he was able to say good-bye without anger.

During the group sharing phase many of the group members were in tears. Many shared their own experiences of the loss of someone close to them. The patient from that time on came to the sessions without his mattress and was able to sit on the fringe of the group.

grams are used on an active inpatient psychiatric unit as either adjunctive or primary treatment modalities. Occupational therapy, recreational therapy, art therapy, horticultural therapy, and dance and music therapy constitute this general classification while functioning as specialties in and of themselves.

Occupational therapy was formally established on March 15, 1917. This profession has grown into a highly complex specialty with a specific body of knowledge and several conceptual frameworks of its own. Occupational therapy is defined as the art and science of directing a person's participation in selected activity to diminish or correct pathological problems and promote and maintain health.[7]

On an inpatient unit the occupational therapy program usually consists of a wide range of both individual and group experiences designed to meet the patient's social, emotional, and occupational needs. After an initial assessment, the occupational therapist helps the patient select group and individual activities, depending on his skill levels. Traditional crafts groups teach patients to sew, make leather projects, work in ceramics and wood, and weave. Beyond this these programs offer assertiveness training, daily living skills groups, and current events groups. The occupational

therapist is frequently involved in adjunctive treatments such as plant therapy and pet therapy. In the absence of an educational therapist, occupational therapists often work with psychiatric nurses to provide patients with needed tutoring or intellectual stimulation.

Recreational therapy may be offered by a certified recreational therapist or by an occupational therapist who has special training in this area. These programs are usually geared toward physical or gamelike activities. The theory holds that the relationship of one's physical self to the immediate environment is important to the individual's total health. Organized tournaments in volleyball, basketball, table tennis, cards, dominoes, or checkers provide the patients with useful leisure activities and help them develop skills in engaging in healthy, competitive interactions. Recreational therapists may also develop programs using community resources to help patients identify socialization activities that they can become involved with after discharge from the hospital. Movement or dance therapy is a specific example of how the body can be used as a medium for change. Since body and mind cannot be separated, the dance therapist works toward integrating the muscular and cognitive expressions of the patient's feelings and thoughts.

Art therapy is used as both a diagnostic tool and a treatment modality. The art therapist's goals are to help the patient express his thoughts and emotions through his drawings, to help the patient gain relief from anxiety by graphically representing conflicts and aggressive and traumatic material without guilt, to provide a socially acceptable outlet for fantasy and wish fulfillment, and to help the patient develop more dexterity.

The general goal of pet and horticultural therapy is to allow the patient to express tender, loving, and nurturing feelings without great fear of rejection. Plants and pets respond well to care but make fewer demands than families and friends. Through this form of therapy patients become alerted to the needs of other living organisms and may develop a sensitivity and sense of responsibility to respond to these needs in an appropriate manner.

Rehabilitation therapies help patients develop occupational and leisure skills that provide a smoother transition back into the community. These programs have become an important and highly respected part of active treatment facilities throughout the country.

■ Somatic therapies and psychopharmacology

The somatic therapies and psychopharmacology are discussed in detail in Chapters 22 and 23. However, it is important to emphasize the nurse's role in these vital treatment methods.

On the modern inpatient psychiatric unit for acutely ill patients, chemotherapy and ECT are the most frequently used of all the somatic treatments. The inpatient psychiatric nurse must develop an indepth knowledge of these therapies to provide quality nursing care. The two most important functions of the nurse in relationship to these somatic therapies are observing the patient's responses to his treatment and teaching and preparing the patient and his family.

Other forms of somatic therapies are used infrequently on an inpatient unit. Psychosurgery is used so rarely that a nurse may never encounter this particular treatment. However, recent research indicates that new and innovative technologies may lead to safe and effective procedures that may be used as "last resort" treatment. Insulin shock has all but become a treatment of the past. Cold, wet sheet packs are used occasionally but are still more of historical interest, since their use is diminishing.

Long-term custodial facilities

Many long-term custodial care facilities still exist. These institutions house patients who (1) have not responded to treatment in an acute treatment facility, (2) will not seek treatment on a voluntary basis, (3) have been committed by the courts, (4) do not have the financial resources to seek treatment elsewhere, (5) are chronically ill and cannot function in society, or (6) are homeless and forgotten.

These facilities generally share several characteristics. There is usually a severe shortage of staff members, particularly qualified registered nurses. Conditions are often crowded, and the physical environment frequently is drab and depressing. Patients' personal possessions may be kept locked up and access to them may be limited to rigid routine schedules created for staff convenience. The design of the units is routinely stark. Beds may be lined up in dormitory fashion, with little or no privacy. It is not uncommon for each unit to have a large, sparsely furnished day area in which the patients watch television, play games, or congregate to have a cigarette if smoking is allowed.

The quality of care provided by these long-term facilities is extremely inconsistent. Federal, state, and local legislation has made some attempts to ensure improvements and standardization. Some of the dedicated and caring staff members of these institutions have made heroic efforts to develop quality treatment and rehabilitation programs. However, lack of funding and incredible bureaucratic snags and snarls make it painfully difficult if not impossible to implement change in a system that is invested in maintaining a status quo.

Consequently, patients in chronic long-term custodial care facilities are more often subjected to a program of therapeutic routine than of therapeutic design. Some of the most common methods of therapy are group therapy, occupational and recreational therapy, chemotherapy, and work therapy. Most of the group therapies are remotivational groups. Since long-term hospitalization often produces apathy and social isolation, detachment, and impoverishment, activities may be used to stimulate group interactions. Activities such as games, sports, artwork, and music can be used to prepare the patients for verbal interaction. Once the patients are ready to talk, the activities are gradually decreased.[17]

Work therapy describes various employment situations. In some institutions patients are used as part of the work force in housekeeping, food preparation, and maintenance of the grounds. Most institutions pay the patients for this work. In some institutions patients are involved in a planned vocational rehabilitation program, including sheltered workshops, and may be employed in the community.

For a number of reasons chemotherapy is frequently the primary treatment prescribed in a long-term custodial care facility. The nature of the patient's illness often dictates an aggressive, long-term drug regimen. Shortage of staff and limited psychotherapy programs greatly influence the physician's decision about the types of chemotherapy programs for his or her patients. In many of these institutions one of the most noticeable elements is the staff's need to be in control. Thus chemotherapy may be used to control patient behavior that is viewed as antagonistic, rebellious, or disruptive to the system.

In recent years deinstitutionalization programs have been established to help chronically hospitalized patients move back to community settings. Case management and community support programs provide the necessary services. The nursing care of the chronically mentally ill patient is discussed in greater depth in Chapter 33.

Future of inpatient psychiatric nursing

The treatment of hospitalized psychiatric patients is undergoing major change. Clinicians and researchers are testing new approaches or modifying classic principles in an effort to develop more effective inpatient treatment.

The psychiatric nurse is in an excellent position of

being able to integrate new psychobiological information with current findings in psychosocial, developmental, and learning theory. No other discipline is better able to manage patient care across the mental health service continuum.

The role of the mental health team in a primary care system has been a topic of discussion by leaders in the mental health field. They view involvement in primary care as an absolute necessity, and they include psychiatric nurses as a vital part of the mental health team of tomorrow.

Despite changes in the future, one may assume that nursing care will be delivered through the nursing process. Individual assessment, nursing diagnosis, planning, implementation, and evaluation may all deliver treatment. Nursing will probably continue to emphasize the importance of using the patient's strengths to assist him in reaching an optimum level of functioning. Hopefully, nursing will never lose sight of the patient as an individual needing respect for his privacy and human dignity.

DIRECTIONS FOR FUTURE RESEARCH

The following are some of the nursing research problems raised in Chapter 24 that merit further study by psychiatric nurses:
1. Description of effective nursing interventions that increase patient compliance with medication regimens
2. Description of patient outcomes that are directly related to nursing intervention
3. Evaluation of the role of the clinical nurse specialist in cost containment
4. Effective methods of clinical supervision to enhance role expansion of psychiatric nurses
5. Patient education techniques that result in greater patient participation in treatment
6. Description of factors that influence the nurse's effective participation as a member of the treatment team
7. The nurse's role in the deinstitutionalization of the chronically mentally ill
8. The effectiveness of nurse-led transitional groups in keeping chronic mental patients out of hospitals longer
9. The impact of primary nursing on the "revolving door" syndrome
10. Comparison of various staffing patterns and methods of utilization of nursing resources in an inpatient psychiatric setting

A health care provider once said with great disgust that the problem with "all this individual assessment" is that it "makes a person a snowflake." How sad that he cannot see that just as the beauty of a snowflake lies in the uniqueness of its pattern, so does the key to wellness and recovery lie in the uniqueness of the individual's strengths and desires. That is the beauty of the human spirit.

■ SUGGESTED CROSS-REFERENCES ■

The roles and functions of the psychiatric nurse and the mental health team are discussed in Chapter 1. The phases of the nursing process are discussed in Chapter 5. Rehabilitation of psychiatric patients is discussed in Chapter 10. Somatic therapies are discussed in Chapter 22. Family therapy is discussed in Chapter 29. Deinstitutionalization of the chronically mentally ill is discussed in Chapter 33.

■ SUMMARY ■

1. Inpatient psychiatric treatment is part of a mental health service continuum.

2. The history of inpatient psychiatric nursing practice reflects an evolutionary process from that of custodial caretaker to active member of the mental health team. The reforms of the nineteenth century were the first major influences to have an impact on the role of the psychiatric nurse.

3. The development of social psychiatry opened the door for nursing involvement in the areas of group and milieu therapy. By 1949 nurses were functioning as individual therapists, and by the mid-1950s the role of group therapist had become a recognized and accepted part of nursing practice.

4. The concept of the health team led to needed changes in the educational preparation of psychiatric nurses. This new breed of psychiatric nurses viewed themselves as professionally and academically competent to be fully participating members of the health team.

5. The implementation of the nursing process is vital to inpatient psychiatric nursing. The steps of the nursing process include the collection of a data base, development of a diagnostic impression, planning and implementation of appropriate nursing actions, and evaluation and modification of those actions.

6. Various modalities of nursing care delivery may be used on an inpatient psychiatric unit. Primary nursing is a care delivery system that has recently gained much support and recognition from many professional nurses throughout the country.

7. The necessity of the clinical nurse specialist in inpatient psychiatric nursing may be debated. Budgets, fiscal constraints, and pressures for cost containment make it difficult for nursing administrators to justify a role that originally was developed solely to improve the quality of nursing care. However, when given the opportunity, the clinical nurse

specialist can demonstrate that quality care is worth the investment.

8. Inpatient psychiatric units should be designed to reflect the philosophy of the department, methods of care provided, and types of patients to be served.

9. Many active psychiatric treatment facilities use concepts of milieu therapy in their inpatient programs.

10. Maxwell Jones coined the term "therapeutic community." He believed that all social and interpersonal interactions in the hospital are therapeutic tools that should be used to bring about specific changes in the patient. Jones stressed that the patient must be an active participant in planning his care.

11. The focus of family therapy is to treat a primary social system, rather than one individual who has been defined as a "patient." The goals of family therapy are to reduce conflict and anxiety, make the family more aware of each other's needs, increase the family's ability to deal with internal and external crisis, develop more appropriate role relationships, help individual family members cope with destructive forces within and outside of the family, and promote health and growth.

12. Individual psychotherapy continues to be a method of treatment offered on active inpatient psychiatric units. The purpose of individual therapy is to offer the patient an opportunity to develop insights into the sources of his thoughts, feelings, perceptions, and behavior, as well as to learn about his illness.

13. Many active treatment facilities offer group therapy either as a primary treatment modality or as an adjunctive treatment to individual psychotherapy. Group therapy should never be used as a time-saving device. Some of the more common inpatient groups are the supportive groups, remotivation groups, personality reconstruction groups, problem-solving groups, and insight groups.

14. Psychodrama was devised by Dr. Jacob L. Moreno in 1914. The purpose of psychodrama is to allow the patient to express himself in both words and action. Psychodrama is considered a special form of group therapy. It is frequently used in milieu therapy to deal with problems within the social system of the therapeutic community.

15. Rehabilitation therapies are used on inpatient units to help patients develop occupational and leisure skills that will help provide a smoother transition back into the community. Occupational, recreational, art, dance, and pet and plant therapies are all highly respected parts of active treatment facilities throughout the country.

16. Somatic therapies play a vital role in psychiatric treatment. Some of the common somatic therapies are chemotherapy, ECT, and psychosurgery.

17. To this day some psychiatric facilities still offer little more than custodial care. Some patients do not respond to active treatment and must be hospitalized for long-term care. Others, because of the nature of their illness, will not voluntarily admit themselves to active treatment facilities. Efforts are being made to improve the treatment provided by these long-term hospitals.

18. The future of psychiatric nursing appears bright for those willing to accept the challenge. Primary care, day care, partial hospitalizations, and community support for chronically mentally ill patients appear to be the subjects of many future-oriented discussions.

■   REFERENCES   ■

1. American Nurses' Association, Congress of Nursing Practice, Description of practice. Clinical nurse specialist: the scope of nursing practice, Kansas City, Mo, 1976, The Association.

2. Anderson C and Apostoles F: Primary care nursing: an exploratory project in psychiatric nurse utilization. In Kneisl C and Wilson H, editors: Current perspectives in psychiatric nursing: issues and trends, vol 2, St Louis, 1978, Mosby–Year Book, Inc.

3. Coates D, Falck A, and Sienkilewski K: Primary nursing: one giant step toward professionalism, 1974. (Unpublished)

4. Cumming J and Cumming E: Ego and milieu, Chicago, 1962, Atherton Press.

5. Detre T and Jarecki H: Modern psychiatric treatment, Philadelphia, 1971, JB Lippincott Co.

6. Emrich K: J Psychosoc Nurs 27:26, Dec 1989.

7. Engelhardt HT: Defining occupational therapy: the meaning of therapy and the virtues of occupation, Am J Occup Ther 31:666, 1977.

8. Hamric A and Spross J: The clinical nurse specialist in theory and practice, Orlando, Fla, 1983, Grune & Stratton Inc.

9. Jamieson E and Sewall M: Trends in nursing history, Philadelphia, 1941, WB Saunders Co.

10. Jones M: Towards a clarification of the therapeutic community concept, Br J Med Psychol 32:200, 1959.

11. Jones M: Social psychiatry in practice, Harmondsworth, England, 1968, Penguin Books, Ltd.

12. Kahn EM and White EM: Adapting milieu approaches to acute inpatient care for schizophrenic patients, Hosp Community Psychiatry 39:609, 1989.

13. Kraft A: The therapeutic community. In Arieti S, editor: American handbook of psychiatry, vol 2, New York, 1966, Basic Books, Inc.

14. Lettieri-Marks D: Research in short-term inpatient group psychotherapy: a critical review, Arch Psych Nurs 1:407, 1987.

15. Manthey M: Primary nursing is alive and well in the hospital, Am J Nurs 73:83, 1973.

16. Marlborough Hospital: Therapeutic community, 1976. (Unpublished; available from Marlborough Hospital, 38 Marlborough Place, St John's Wood, London, England.)

17. Marram G: The group approach in nursing practice, ed 2, St Louis, 1978, Mosby–Year Book, Inc.

18. Marram G, Barrett MW, and Bevis E: Primary nursing: a model for individualized care, ed 2, St Louis, 1979, Mosby–Year Book, Inc.

19. Mereness D: Preparation of the nurse for the psychiatric team, Am J Nurs 51:320, 1951.
20. Moreno J: Psychodrama, New York, 1959, Beacon House.
21. Pavey A: The story of the growth of nursing, Philadelphia, 1937, JB Lippincott Co.
22. Robinson A: Changing of the guard, Am J Nurs 50:152, 1950.
23. Saklas C: Psychosocial group therapies, The Practice of Medicine and Psychotherapy 10:41.
24. Santos E and Stanbrook E: Nursing and modern psychiatry, Am J Nurs 49:107, 1949.
25. Sundeen S et al: Nurse-client interaction: implementing the nursing process, ed 4, St Louis, 1989, Mosby–Year Book, Inc.
26. Wolf MS: A review of literature on milieu therapy, J Psychiatr Nurs 15:7, 1977.
27. Zander K: Primary nursing: development and management, Germantown, Md, 1980, Aspen Systems Corp.

■ ANNOTATED SUGGESTED READINGS ■

*Carser DL: Primary nursing in the milieu, J Psychiatr Nurs 19:35, 1978.

Examines the interaction between primary nursing and the therapeutic milieu. The author uses case examples to illustrate the impact at the individual patient level. She also discusses the effect of the introduction of primary nursing on the treatment team and recommends interventions with the staff that are helpful during the transitional period.

Engelhardt HT: Defining occupational therapy: the meaning of therapy and the virtues of occupation, Am J Occup Ther 31:666, 1979.

This volume marks the sixtieth anniversary of the occupational therapy journal. Each article presents an informative historical overview as well as current conceptual frameworks. Will give the nurse an appreciation of the struggles that another discipline has encountered in its search for professional recognition and autonomy.

*Asterisk indicates nursing reference.

Jones M: Social psychiatry in practice, Harmondsworth, England, 1968, Penguin Books, Ltd.

Packed full of information. A large section is devoted to the concept of therapeutic community, but Jones also elaborates on the concept of social psychiatry in general. The author is outspoken in his opinions about the preparation and participation of nurses and other health team members.

Kahn E and White M: Adapting milieu approaches to acute inpatient care for schizophrenic patients, Hosp Community Psych 39:609, 1989.

An exceptionally informative and useful article. The authors clearly articulate how to modify classic milieu principles to fit short-term inpatient treatment.

*Marram G, Barrett MW, and Bevis E: Primary nursing: a model for individualized care, ed 2, St Louis, 1979, Mosby–Year Book, Inc.

Although it contains no discussion of primary nursing as it relates to inpatient psychiatric nursing, this book should be considered a must. It was the only text in this field for a long time. The reader may enjoy the introductory comparison of the growth of the women's movement and the growth of nursing as a profession.

*Mereness D: Preparation of the nurse for the psychiatric team, Am J Nurs 51:320, 1951.

Despite the era in which it was written, this article is ageless. There will always be a need for changes in educational curricula as the role of the professional nurse grows and expands.

*Sundeen S et al: Nurse-client interaction: implementing the nursing process, ed 4, St Louis, 1989, Mosby–Year Book, Inc.

A consistently excellent text. The use of clinical illustrations is particularly valuable to both experienced nurses and beginners. Although much of the literature "talks" about the nursing process, this work puts it into "action."

*Templin H: The system and the patient, Am J Nurs 82:108, 1982

A thought-provoking article that looks at three aspects of psychiatric hospitals from both the patient's point of view and that of organizational theory—the hospital as a hierarchical system, mutual adaptation, and modes of transaction. Demonstrates the benefits of viewing hospitals as social systems.

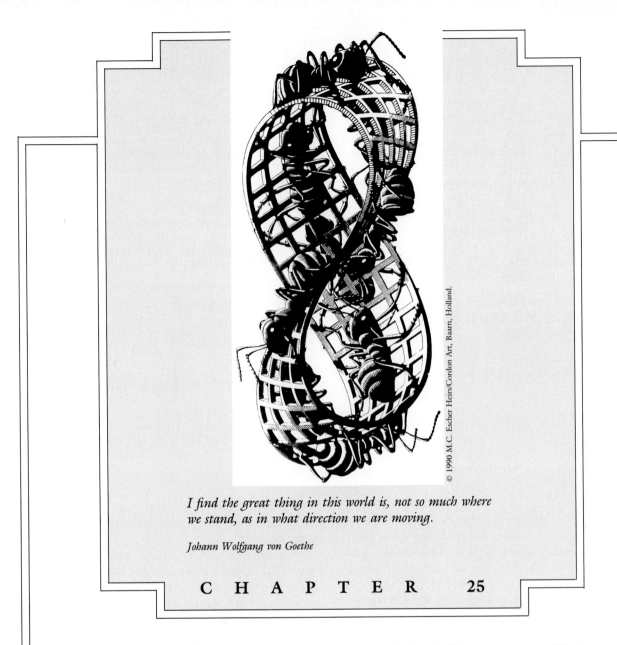

I find the great thing in this world is, not so much where we stand, as in what direction we are moving.

Johann Wolfgang von Goethe

C H A P T E R   25

COMMUNITY PSYCHIATRIC CARE

JEANETTE LANCASTER
DIANE E. BOYER

LEARNING OBJECTIVES

After studying this chapter, the student should be able to:

- describe the history of the community mental health movement in the United States and the role of the government as reflected in the Community Mental Health Center Acts of 1963 and 1975, the 1978 President's Commission on Mental Health, the Mental Health Systems Act of 1980, and the block grant and community support systems programs of the 1980s.

- critique the goals, staffing, services, and effectiveness of the community mental health movement.

- contrast a community orientation to mental health with an individual orientation.

- relate the role of the community mental health nurse in case management and target marketing.

- analyze the impact of deinstitutionalization and its implications for nursing care.

- assess the importance of interdisciplinary collaboration in community mental health.

- describe three methodologies for program evaluation and issues that must be considered in their use.

- identify directions for future nursing research.

- select appropriate readings for further study.

The mental health system is part of a rapidly changing health care environment. An increasing aging population, new financing mechanisms and pressures, and a growing population of under and uninsured affect the demand for mental health services. For the past three decades, concerted efforts have been made to move mental health care out of the institution and back into the community.

Historical development of community mental health nursing

The community mental health movement represents the fourth revolution in psychiatry. The first occurred in 1793 when Pinel, a psychiatrist, removed the chains from the mentally ill people confined in Bicêtre, a hospital near Paris. Before 1840, people diagnosed as mentally ill were housed in jails and county homes. The conditions barely allowed existence and, because mental illness was considered permanent, offered no treatment. For the affluent, a few private and public hospitals were available.

Benjamin Rush, "the father of American psychiatry," pioneered humanitarian methods in psychiatry in America. Although Rush encouraged humane treatment, he continued to use remedies such as blood let-

ting, purgatives, and a torture-like device called "the tranquilizer."

An energetic New England school teacher, Dorothea Dix, carried on the work of Rush. In 1841 Miss Dix appointed herself inspector of institutions for the mentally ill and began crusading for more humane treatment. She recommended that each state assume responsibility for its mentally ill. The result was the establishment of 32 mental hospitals in the United States. During this late 19th century period most mental hospitals were built in rural areas, which offered inexpensive land, the removal of troublesome people from the mainstream of society, and fresh air and quiet for the patients.

The accompanying box chronicles the development of the community mental health movement.

Governmental involvement in mental health

The federal government entered the health field in 1935 with the passage of the Social Security Act. During the Great Depression the public's view was that if the community could not care for its sick, the government should. World War II had a significant impact on the community mental health movement, when an

Milestones in the Development of the Community Mental Health Movement

1841 Dorothea Dix appointed herself inspector of institutions for the mentally ill

1935 Passage of Social Security Act

1946 Enactment of the Mental Health Act

1949 Creation of NIMH under the Mental Health Act

1955 Congress enacted the Mental Health Study Act creating the Joint Commission on Mental Illness and Health

1960 Joint Commission on Mental Illness and Health submitted its report to Congress

1961 Report of the Joint Commission on Mental Illness and Health published as *Action for Mental Health*

1963 First Presidential message on behalf of the mentally ill; enactment of Public Law 88-164, the Mental Retardation Facilities and Community Mental Health Centers Construction Act

1975 The Community Mental Health Centers Amendments of 1975, Title III of Public Law 94-63, was enacted

1977 President Jimmy Carter organized the President's Commission on Mental Health

1978 Report of the President's Commission published

1980 Mental Health Systems Act

1981 Omnibus Budget Reconciliation Act (PL97-35) passed

1982-3 States began to distribute mental health funds via block grants

1984 Funding for community mental health terminated under terms of 1981 Budget Act

1987 NIMH sponsored Community Support Program.

---

estimated 875,000 draftees out of 15 million were rejected for mental or neurological impairment.[35] After the war the federal government began funding mental health endeavors. In 1946 Congress enacted the National Mental Health Act, which made grants available to states to develop mental health programs outside state hospitals.

The Mental Health Act radically altered the care of the mentally ill. Shocked at the number of young men rejected from military service for mental illness, embarrassed by inhumane treatment, and tempted by the vision of an enlightened system, citizens, professionals, and legislators banded together to support a national program. These efforts were intended to apply a public health approach to mental illness.[30] Although the intent was prevention, in actuality individual psychotherapy was supported.

Under the act the National Institute of Mental Health (NIMH) was organized in 1949 as headquarters for the federal mental health program. Initially NIMH emphasized research into the cause and treatment of mental illness. The institute also assumed responsibility for training programs and for assistance to states that were trying to develop treatment programs.

The 1940s saw the widespread development of two important types of treatment facilities: outpatient clinics and psychiatric units in general hospitals. In contrast, advances in research had little effect on state hospitals. Meanwhile, psychiatry continued to prefer to provide private care for those who could afford it, and serious inequities between private and public treatment developed.

In 1955 the Mental Health Study Act created the Joint Commission on Mental Illness and Health, consisting of representatives from 36 organizations and agencies selected by the NIMH. The agencies represented were largely medical and allied medical.[35] In 1960 the Joint Commission submitted its report to Congress and in 1961 published it as *Action for Mental Health*. The 338-page report emphasized the need for training, education, early and intensive treatment of acutely disturbed patients, and research. The report further recommended that additional clinics and psychiatric units in general hospitals be established and that regional state hospitals of not more than 1000 beds be supported. It suggested the creation of aftercare and rehabilitation programs; and mental health education.[12]

After the publication of this report, President John F. Kennedy appointed a cabinet-level committee to review it and to recommend action. This report and that of a presidential panel on mental retardation formed the basis for President Kennedy's message to Congress in 1963 on mental illness and retardation. This first presidential message on behalf of the mentally ill called for a "bold new approach to bring psychiatry back into the mainstream of medicine and community life."[32] The president further stated that a new type of facility, the community mental health center, was needed to provide a complete range of care with an emphasis on prevention.

■ **COMMUNITY MENTAL HEALTH CENTERS ACT.** Eight months later, on October 31, 1963, Congress enacted Public Law 88-164, the Mental Retardation Facilities and Community Mental Health Centers Construction Act of 1963. The act authorized $150 million over 3 years to match states' spending on construction of community mental health centers. Congress believed that community-based centers would be able to treat mentally ill people more effectively than the large residential hospitals. Each center was to serve an area with a population of 75,000 to 200,000. The centers were to provide mental health services in new or renovated buildings.

To qualify for federal funds, a program had to offer five services[14]:

1. Short-term inpatient care
2. Partial hospitalization, including day hospital care for patients who could return home at night and night hospital care for patients who could work but needed some care each day
3. Outpatient treatment, allowing patients to live at home and go to the center at regular intervals
4. Around-the-clock emergency care
5. Consultation and education for community members

The original community mental health legislation included five additional services. Centers applying for federal support were looked on favorably if they documented a plan for:

1. Diagnostic services, including treatment recommendations when possible
2. Rehabilitation and vocational counseling
3. Precare and aftercare, with screening before admission and evaluation after discharge
4. Training for mental health personnel
5. Research and evaluation

The original legislation provided federal funding for a center for 8 years on a decreasing formula. At the end of the eighth year the federal grants ceased, and centers were to operate on state and local funds as well as revenue from services.[14]

The fiscal arrangement failed because many centers were unable to get enough revenue to meet costs. State and local funds were not consistently available. Centers were often forced to cut services, especially those that did not produce revenue, such as consultation and educational services.

The money provided through the 1963 Act was to encourage states to develop or expand community-based mental health centers. This aim to promote deinstitutionalization reflected the social and political tone of the 1960s—President Kennedy's "bold new approach." The MHC Act, along with the Medicare/Medicaid bill of 1965, led to a 75% reduction in the population of state mental hospitals.[21] Although the reduction succeeded in limiting the size of institutions, it "dumped" mentally ill people into the community before strategies and facilities were fully developed. Deinstitutionalization, while a victory in theory, fell far short of its goal: humanistic care and treatment in the least restrictive way. The outcome of the early community mental health legislation has been to create a revolving door for the chronically mentally ill.

By 1970 deinstitutionalization and community mental health were a disaster. To deal with the crisis, the federal government provided a nominal amount of money for community support systems. Mentally ill patients began to file lawsuits stating that they got neither humane care nor adequate treatment while hospitalized. Between 1972 and 1977, a series of judicial decisions led to revolutionary changes in community mental care. The decisions were intended to ensure that patients were held in the least restrictive alternative, protected from harm, and given safeguards in the civil commitment process, and that monitoring of restraint, psychotropic drugs, electroconvulsive therapy, and psychosurgery was increased.

■ **COMMUNITY MENTAL HEALTH CENTERS AMENDMENTS OF 1975.** The Community Mental Health Centers Amendments of 1975, Title III of Public Law 94-63, was enacted on July 22, 1975. This amendment extended the flow of funds to community mental health centers and set forth specific guidelines for services.[23] Congress reiterated the original intent of the Community Mental Health Centers Act: to provide construction and operation funds to centers on a declining basis with the goal of independence from federal support.

Specifically, centers were to provide the five essential services mandated in 1963 and add:

1. On-going follow-up programs for discharged patients
2. Diagnostic treatment, liaison, and follow-up services for children, adolescents, and the elderly

3. Screening services to residents of the catchment area
4. Prevention, treatment, and follow-up of alcohol and drug abuse
5. Transitional living arrangements for discharged patients unable to live on their own

Unfortunately, the 1975 amendments limited flexibility and were complex to implement.

■ **REPORT OF THE PRESIDENT'S COMMISSION ON MENTAL HEALTH—1978.** Early in 1977 President Jimmy Carter organized the President's Commission on Mental Health; of the five professionals on the commission, one was a nurse. The principal recommendation called for a "new federal grant program for community mental health services to encourage the creation of necessary services where they are inadequate and increase the flexibility of communities in planning a comprehensive network of services.[18]

The purpose of the Commission was to review and make recommendations on the mental health needs of the nation. After a year of study, the 20 commission members issued its final report containing 117 recommendations. Although the commission found that significant progress had been made in treating mentally ill people since the enactment of the MHC Act of 1963, they noted that certain populations including the chronically mentally ill, children and youth, the elderly, racial and ethnic minorities, the poor, and rural residents remained underserved.

The report made recommendations in eight broad areas: community support, services provided, insurance, personnel, patients' rights, research, prevention of mental illness, and public understanding.[18] In general, the report called for: (1) strengthening linkages among parts of the community mental health system so patients could receive better coordinated services; (2) focussing attention on helping high-risk populations such as minorities and the chronically mentally ill; and (3) greater flexibility in planning services to meet the needs of a community.[26]

The report led Senator Edward Kennedy to introduce a bill, P.L. 96-398, called the Community Mental Health Centers Act of 1980. The intent of this legislation was to coordinate the existing two-tiered system of mental health that had evolved since 1963: the severely mentally ill were treated in state hospitals and the acutely ill were managed in community mental health centers.

Before the programs authorized by the 1980 legislation could get started, the political and fiscal climate changed. The 1980 Community Mental Health Centers Act was essentially repealed in 1981 when the Ninety-seventh Congress passed the Omnibus Budget Reconciliation Act (P.L. 97-35 and known as OBRA). The intent of OBRA was to reduce federal spending on health care and give states more flexibility in health care decision making by way of block grants. The decreased federal funding placed more decision making on states and moved a variety of mental health programs formerly administered by NIMH to the states.

Decreased federal funding has and will continue to have far-reaching effects on community mental health. Funds to community mental health centers have been dramatically reduced and mandated services are now down to the following five:

1. Outpatient care
2. Partial hospitalization
3. 24-hour hospitalization and emergency care
4. Consultation and education
5. Screening services

The availability and quality of services for centers depends on state support, private funds, and fees collected.

Title VI in the Social Security Amendments of 1983 introduced prospective payment to the federal Medicare program. Although psychiatric hospitals were deemed exempt for this payment scheme, all of health care was affected. The premise of prospective payment is that money can be saved if hospitals are paid a set amount for each type of diagnosis, rather than paying for services retrospectively, or after the hospitalization and based on the accumulated charges incurred during the hospital stay. Prospective payment is based on a belief that a fixed payment schedule will motivate hospitals to be more efficient and cost-effective. This system fails to take into account the variations in patients' needs for nursing care that cannot be predicted by diagnosis alone.

Criticism of the community mental health movement

The enthusiasm of the 1960s for community mental health has been overshadowed by criticism. Former enthusiasts are dissatisfied, because the original goals are unmet. Critics contend that the most obvious shortcoming of community mental health has been a tendency to move treatment into the community without changes in techniques. There has been a reluctance to view the community itself—the macrosystem—as the patient. Instead, the focus continues to be on the individual—the microsystem.[44]

The community mental health system gave minimal attention to population dynamics that have led to an increasing adolescent, young adult, and older population who use considerable amounts of service.[17]

There is a great need in community mental health for forming coalitions with people in the welfare, housing, vocational rehabilitation, general medical, and criminal justice systems so that organized, comprehensive care can be delivered. Developing service networks for seriously mentally ill people is not easy because their needs are often extensive and the providers represent different cultures, levels of government, and varying philosophies.[17]

■ Financing mental health care

Mental health care increased dramatically in the 1980s and has also been heavily influenced by the political climate and influential policy decisions. Compared to other types of health services, mental health care historically has had distinct public and private providers, patients, and funding sources.

There has been an increasing movement toward privatization of mental health care as the federal government has reduced its role in this area. As mental health care continues to be increasingly provided for in the private sector, the chronically mentally ill will become more disenfranchised. With fewer services available at the federal or state levels, under or uninsured people will have limited access to mental health services.

Mental health care is no longer the priority for federal funding that it was in the 1960s. Education, roads, the war on drugs and crime, and the maintenance of a sound national defense program are higher on the funding priority list than mental health care.[6] Politics and social policy have joined hands with economics, and increasingly mental health care has become a private not a public service. Private psychiatric facilities are mushrooming; public facilities are closing due to lack of funds; and the competition for patients with insurance or other third party coverage is growing. Alternative health service programs such as health maintenance organizations (HMOs), preferred provider organizations (PPOs), and independent practice associations are showing rising enrollments of patients who can pay.

Unfortunately, many of the patients who need psychiatric care cannot pay. To survive, public hospitals are changing their patient mix to also attract patients who can pay. The current transformation of mental health services is being driven more by social and economic pressures than by clinical judgment. As a result of price reduction (funds decreased) and growing price competition, as many as 40% of U.S. hospitals will close by the year 2000.[11]

The most vulnerable groups will be hospitals (and mental health centers) that are publicly owned facilities (by city, county, or state governments). They typically treat a disproportionately high percentage of people who cannot pay thus reducing the agency's overall revenues. Rural facilities are at risk because they are typically small and cannot easily increase their paying service users.

Mental health expenditures have grown rapidly during the 1980s.[36] Approximately 70% of mental health dollars are spent on inpatient care.[34] The 53% of mental health costs paid by governmental sources is more than the percentage (43%) of total health costs covered by governmental sources. Funds are disproportionally used by the chronically mentally ill. Approximately 5% of the nation's mentally ill (1.7 million chronically mentally ill) consume 37% of overall spending for the mentally ill.[8]

If costs are to be controlled, people must seek mental health intervention early and use outpatient facilities as much as possible. Options that could reduce costs, if funded adequately, include intensive mental health center or other ambulatory care; 24-hour walk-in services; mobile outreach and residential crisis interventions; home health care; transitional and supported living facilities; residential care (especially for adolescent and substance abuse treatment); and partial hospitalization.

Case management by psychiatric nurses and social workers will continue to be used to maintain patients outside the hospital. Nearly 30% of the nation's chronically mentally ill reside in hospitals. Yet Public Law 99-600 (1987) requires all states to develop comprehensive community based services that include case management, crisis intervention, mental health care, family support services, social and vocational rehabilitation, protection and advocacy, income maintenance, and housing.[36] Preliminary data indicate that case management of chronically mentally ill people costs $15,000 per year per patient versus $45,000 to $80,000 in a public hospital.[10]

Community mental health in the 1990s

With the advantage of hindsight it is possible to see that the community mental health movement was ushered in with much naivete and many simplistic notions about what would become of the severely and long-term mentally ill. The significance of psychoactive medication and a stable source of financial support was recognized, but the necessity of developing fundamental resources such as adequate and supportive living arrangements and case management was not effectively handled.[16] Nor was the deinstitionalization movement able to anticipate the problems that would arise for the young chronically mentally ill person growing up outside of the hospital in an era of substance abuse.

Dysfunctional characteristics of community mental health care systems

In 1980, Tarail[41] summarized problems of service delivery in the community mental health system. These problems are listed below.

1. Mental health care is fragmented.
2. Not only is there no one single system of service, but there is no *coordinated* system of service.
3. Each mental health system has a built-in self-survival goal with different characteristics.
4. Emphasis is placed on the preservation of private systems instead of the creation of a network of public and private nonprofit facilities.
5. There is no reimbursement and very limited funds for outreach, prevention, and community education.
6. Third-party reimbursement agencies have varying and limited benefits.
7. Mental health is not a right in the United States.
8. A conservative finding is that 20% of the population need professional mental health intervention.
9. Mental health services have a low priority.
10. Mental illness has a stigma.
11. Schizophrenic patients who live in communities are visible because of their sometimes bizarre bahavior.
12. State mental health facilities often are the largest employers in communities.

Many of these problems still exist. But despite its failures, the community mental health movement continues to improve the living options for mentally ill patients, and many patients lead more satisfying lives than they did in the past.[16] Most of the dysfunctional characteristics mentioned by Tarail are being addressed by the government, the mental health system, and consumers. For example, in 1985 the Robert Wood Johnson Foundation, in collaboration with the U.S. Department of Housing and Urban Development, announced a $100 million program for community-wide projects aimed at consolidating and expanding services for the long-term mentally ill. As part of the program the Social Security Administration (SSA) brought workers into mental health settings to help grantees

improve the disability determination process. The program has funded projects in eight of the 60 largest urban centers. It has allowed for the development of community mental health authorities, as well as projects that are coordinating and providing a wide spectrum of services including health, social services, and housing for large mentally ill populations that have not had access to these services.

Although there is compelling evidence supporting the need to develop comprehensive community support systems (CSSs) for the treatment of the long-term mentally ill, states have been reluctant to make the transition from a primarily institutional system to one that emphasizes community-based services. The reasons for this reluctance are multiple and complex.[16,19] When examining the potential for service system change, there are two critical factors associated with the difficulty of this transition. First, most federal funding for mental health services has been allocated for medically oriented, facility-based hospital and community services. This has resulted in a large percentage of states' resources being directed toward hospital rather than community based services. It also has limited the funding necessary for the development of more innovative programs that support individuals in obtaining their own housing, developing educational and vocational opportunities, and using paraprofessional and peer supports and services. Without these types of resources to assist individuals in the community, the demand for institutional services increases, thus creating a vicious circle that continues the dependence on hospital care as the central focus of the service delivery system.[43]

The second reason it has been difficult for many state governments to develop effective community-based service systems is more endemic. Despite the fact that the effectiveness of community based mental health care is supported by research, state governments still experience uncertainty as to whether community services should actually replace most hospital programs on a long-term basis.[43] The relative youth of the community mental health system and the lack of resources to develop innovative service and support options have led to both a mistrust of the community system and a dearth of actual experiences with truly comprehensive community systems of care. Institutional care, on the other hand, is a familiar resource that is much easier to understand and trust. Despite some advances in community mental health care, the development of comprehensive community service systems in many states has been hampered by lack of support on a political level for the risk taking necessary for innovative systems development.

■ Discharged patients

Community mental health centers have suffered from serving two masters—the federal regulations and a local board often inexperienced in mental health and pressured by local politics.[3]

Initially, most state mental hospitals served three primary purposes: (1) to protect the public from insane people, (2) to provide an asylum and humane care for mentally ill people, and (3) to provide a place for "deviant" members of society who were not candidates for jails.[9] In the enthusiasm to overcome the syndrome of "institutionalism," characterized by lack of initiative, apathy, withdrawal, and submissiveness to authority, mental health providers forgot that these characteristics can be caused by schizophrenia itself, not just by long tenure in a hospital. That chronic mentally ill patients need structure, medical care, and a social network was forgotten in the rush to free them from the "shackles of hospitalization." The pressure during the earliest days of deinstitutionalization to provide patients with the least restrictive alternative (LRA) led to hasty actions.

In an effort to provide patients' with the greatest freedom from restrictions, major changes in commitment procedures occurred. This resulted in changes in interpretation of commitment procedures by the psychiatric community and by many judges. As a result of these changes it became more difficult to protect patients and the community during serious psychiatric episodes. Many seriously mentally ill patients unsuitable for civil commitment but involved in law violations were then, and are now, increasingly dealt with through the criminal justice system.[16] The chronic mentally ill patient with a criminal history often ends up cycling through the criminal justice system because of lack of extensive and conclusive research on how best to treat these clients in the community.

In the midst of deinstitutionalization many discharged patients have no place to live because of poor follow-up or non-compliance with the few disorganized services available. The problem of homelessness is closely linked with deinstitutionalization in the sense that three decades ago most of the long-term mentally ill had a home in the state psychiatric hospital.[16] It is likely that without deinstitutionalization there would not be large numbers of homeless mentally ill. But that does not mean that homelessness can simply be explained as a result of deinstitutionalization. Instead it is necessary to consider what conditions these persons must face in the community, what needed resources are lacking, and the nature of mental illness itself.

As a result of continued efforts to provide the least restrictive alternative of treatment to the long-term mentally ill, a whole generation of mental health consumers has grown up outside of the hospital. This group of clients has come to be known as the young adult chronic patient.[27] These clients are extremely vulnerable to chemical dependence. The difficulty in treating these individuals and of finding suitable programs for them has heightened criticism of the deinstitutionalization movement and contributed to a growing belief that deinstitutionalization has failed.[19] Young adult chronic patients have a serious mental illness and enormous needs. They may be unable to meet the expectations of society, yet they may not choose to accept the identity of patient. Therefore, even though they need a great deal of help, they may not be willing to accept help from a system that insists on people voluntarily defining themselves as mentally ill. During adolescence all young people begin to face the tasks of becoming adults through achieving a measure of independence, choosing a vocation, establishing satisfying interpersonal relationships, and acquiring some sense of identity. Because mental illness tends to begin in adolescence, young mentally ill patients are often faced with a major conflict: to become passive, dependent, resigned, and with limited goals, or to become "adults," where they must become independent, risk-taking, adventurous, and intimate.[13] The emergence of the young adult chronic patient, and the understanding of their struggles and treatment needs, may be viewed as the inevitable result of the success of deinstitutionalization.[19]

Postinstitutional clinical ideology

Since 1960, in the postinstitutional era, understanding the importance and difficulty of the patient's adaptational process has led to change in mental health ideology. Community mental health ideology has evolved from an orientation of deinstitutionalization to a postinstitutional clinical ideology. The ideology of deinstitutionalization is described by Minkoff[19] as follows: institutions are bad for chronic mentally ill patients, and community care is good for them. Therefore deinstitutionalization should be the major programmatic goal and will make patients better and happier. The key concept in postinstitutional clinical ideology is not locus of care but adaptation to long-term mental illness in the community. With the "remedicalization" of long-term mental illness it is recognized that schizophrenia, bipolar disorder, and related psychoses are in fact medical illnesses that have primarily biologic etiologies, with resultant psychological and social consequences.[28] Treatment, therefore, involves both psychopharmacologic interventions to control the primary symptoms and psychosocial interventions to assist the person with severe, disabling mental illness to function at optimal levels in the community.[20]

Community orientation to mental health

A community orientation requires a change of focus. A premise basic to community mental health is that all people experience stress and have problems coping, but some have fewer support systems and react in a dysfunctional way.[22] The community approach to mental illness focuses on prevention by identifying high-risk populations and providing services before mental health is disrupted. The aim is to balance the stressors with support. Community mental health can be approached in a number of ways. Intervening in poverty, crowding, discrimination, and crime decreases stressors, whereas health care, police, social service, and educational resources increase support. On an individual or small-group level, crisis intervention, guidance, consultation, and education also decrease stressors and provide support.

The treatment area is the community in which the client is experiencing stress. Dealing with the client's internal dysfunction is not enough. Treatment requires attention to sociocultural background, adaptive ability, support systems, and family interaction.[44] Most emotional disorders are rooted in a network of systems.[15] A person's mental health depends on internal and external factors. A systems approach is used in community mental health nursing to provide a holistic view of a person as he relates to both inner and external environments. Reactions to environments are ever changing. A person's responses are attempts to maintain a steady state, or homeostasis. The human system, like all living systems, is in continuous interaction with the environment. Each individual's personality develops out of this interaction with the subsystems that make up his daily life. For example, interactions with family, significant groups, work, and school play a crucial part in psychological development. Problems or stresses in one system affect others.

The effort to adapt is complicated by the fact that one responds to all the stressors at once. One cannot sort out components but must respond to the total environmental impact. Furthermore, each human system strives to achieve homeostasis. Symptoms of emotional disturbance indicate distress and disequilibrium. Community mental health assumes that relieving stress in one part of the system will affect others. Poor housing, lack of sanitation, unemployment, crowding, and other effects of poverty affect mental health.

■ Community ideology

Continuity of care is a basic principle of community mental health. If programs are to be effective, some staff member must maintain contact with and responsibility for each discharged patient as the patient moves from one system to another.[33] Although this principle is widely accepted, it is infrequently practiced. Few community mental health agencies provide systematic assistance in locating housing, obtaining employment, managing finances, developing a social system for interaction, and, of primary importance, mastering skills essential to functioning outside the hospital.[35] Many patients discharged from public mental hospitals lack abilities to meet the demands of life outside.

Rachlin[29] contended that the major reason for failure of deinstitutionalization is that the needs of patients and the directions of programs have been disjointed. Deinstitutionalization has frequently served only to decrease the population in mental hospitals. Substitute domiciles and coordinated programs for discharged patients have been lacking in both quality and quantity. Even when unique model programs work, it has been hard to sustain enthusiasm because dealing with chronically ill patients is difficult and does not always provide visible and immediate results.

Dickey et al[5] documented the success of a deinstitutionalization program by studying 27 patients 4 years after discharge. These patients had been hospitalized for an average of 24 years. The authors interviewed both patients and caretakers to gather data on place of residence, mental status, time spent in the hospital since discharge, level of functioning, and quality of life. They found that the best predictor of success at remaining in the community was age at hospital admission. Those who entered the hospital at an early age had more difficulty readjusting to community life. The authors also found that all but two patients preferred their present living situation to the hospital. Also, patients living in the community had a better average mental status and level of functioning than patients who were hospitalized. This study supported the belief that organized and systematic aftercare is a prerequisite for maintaining chronically ill patients in the community.

Personnel deployment is a problem when large numbers of patients are discharged into community-care programs. A question in deployment planning is whether personnel familiar with one role can work with a new concept of mental health care. Inpatient psychiatric care has been accused of rigidity, lack of interest in the individual, and limited creativity. Each of these criticisms must be reversed if community care is to enhance mental health. For a community to establish a comprehensive program for discharged patients, inpatient services must be available. Some patients experience an exacerbation of symptoms and require short-term hospitalization.

■ **Community support systems model**

Research over the past 30 years about the treatment, needs, and capabilities of individuals with long-term mental illness supports a progressive movement away from the exclusive use of institutional care to an emphasis on the development of services and supports that assist people to remain in their home communities.[39] This movement was dramatically enhanced in 1987 by the initiation of the National Institute of Mental Health (NIMH) Community Support Program (CSP), that provided much needed conceptual guidance and resources to states and communities to enhance community mental health systems.[2,25] States continue to struggle with the financial implications of operating dual service systems, the increasing numbers of people being identified as needing mental health services, and the lack of a clear consensus about the role and function of public mental hospitals.[31] All of these factors contribute to the recognition that mental health systems cannot continue to allocate a majority of their resources into facility-based care and also effectively serve all people in need.[43]

For individuals with serious mental illness who are living in the community, it is clear that mental health treatment is not enough. Among mental health professionals, there is general agreement that persons with long-term mental illness require a wide range of basic community services and supports to function effectively outside the hospital. What has evolved from the development of these services and supports has come to be known as the Community Support System (CSS). The CSS concept was developed by NIMH's Community Support Program (CSP) with the assistance of state mental health officials, family groups, consumer groups, researchers, citizen advocates, and others.[24] The CSS ideology, is described by Stroul[38] as one that embraces the notion that services should maintain the dignity of clients and respect the individual needs of each person. She goes on to say that individuals with mental illness are seen, first and foremost, as persons with basic human needs and ambitions and as citizens with all the rights, privileges, opportunities, and responsibilities granted other citizens. In addition to mental health services, they should have access to the supports and opportunities needed by all persons. The CSS philosophy is based on creating opportunities for individuals to develop their capacities for growth, improvement, and movement toward independence rather than promoting a life of dependency, disability, and "chronic patienthood."

Another value inherent in the CSS philosophy is that the community is the best place for providing long-term care. Inpatient care is considered one of the necessary services to support community-based services and should be used both for short-term evaluation and stabilization and for small percentages of individuals who may require long-term hospitalization.[38] Another concept that is important to consider in the CSS is continuity of care. This is defined as a single, continuous treatment team that is responsible for the client in both inpatient and outpatient settings.[42] In sum, the essential components of the CSS that are needed to assist persons with severe, disabling mental illness to function at optimal levels within the community include: client identification and outreach; mental health treatment; crisis response services; health and dental care; housing; income support; entitlements; peer support; family and community support; rehabilitation services; protection and advocacy; and case management. Nurses coordinating any combination of these services must have the ability to work effectively in the areas of networking, client advocacy, interfacing of systems, and the vertical and horizontal integration of services.

■ **Successful centers**

In thinking about the progress of the mental health movement it is important to mention that many excellent model programs have been developed to provide community support to persons with long-term mental illness.[37] For example, many psychosocial rehabilitation programs have been designed from the Fountain House in New York City, which provides a model comprehensive psychosocial rehabilitation center. The Training in Community Living Model, which originated in Madison, Wisconsin, concentrates on teaching the basic coping skills necessary to live as autonomously as possible in the community through an aggressive outreach method. In Sydney, Australia, a special care program was designed to help seriously mentally ill clients avoid hospitalization whenever possible. The success of this program seems related to the 24-hour availability of comprehensive care.[42] In 1955 a program was begun to train community living and support skills to seriously mentally ill clients in a Vermont State Hospital. These skills were taught by a treatment team consisting of a psychiatrist, psychologist, nurse, and vocational counselor that continued following these clients once they were out in the community. In a 1985 follow-up study it was found that three-quarters of these clients were leading full lives in the community. Once again the clients reported that the continuity of caregivers had been important to their successful adjustment to the community.

Although the community mental health system has flaws, some centers have worked well. These centers are often in communities whose populations and resources are compatible with the community mental health movement's view and the prevalent model of care. Other effective centers have developed slowly, continually responding to the community and in concert with available funds. Successful centers have tended to construct strong community links and to focus on local needs rather than solely on federal guidelines.[3]

The Committee on Psychiatry and Community of the Group for Advancement of Psychiatry lists ingredients of a successful center[3]:

1. Consistent and adequate funding
2. Assignment of top priority to the most seriously ill
3. Accessibility
4. Availability of a full range of treatment and rehabilitation for individuals
5. Responsiveness to expressed local needs rather than categorical needs
6. Interagency communication and planning
7. Maximum use of community resources and development of new resources to fill gaps
8. Involvement of psychiatrists as caregivers and planners
9. Use of well-trained professionals for services and supervision
10. Harmony among the staff
11. Pursuit of staff development and "antiburn-out" strategies
12. Encouragement of participation of the private psychiatric sector in care
13. Objective assessments of needs and well-designed program evaluations

The nurse's role

■ Case manager

Nurses working in the field of community mental health must have the knowledge and skills to implement all components of the Community Support System. The function of case management in the CSS concept is to guarantee continuous availability of appropriate support and services to patients.[43] One role that involves nurses in all components of the CSP is that of case management. This role has evolved as a solution to problems in treating the long-term mentally ill primarily in the community. Baier[1] describes case management as a brokerage of services for seriously mentally ill patients who would otherwise be unable to live successfully in the community. A case manager must be talented in the following skills:

- Assessment
- Coordination
- Advocacy
- Discharge planning
- Referral
- Teaching
- Rehabilitation
- Psychotherapy
- Home visiting
- Crisis intervention
- Medication monitoring
- Physical assessment

While a variety of professionals do serve as coordinators of client treatment in the community, nurses are uniquely prepared through their education and training to work both as case managers and supervisors of teams of case managers.

Case management requires a working knowledge of both the client's 24-hour functioning in all aspects of life and interventions for assisting clients to function at their maximum potential. A concept that is central to the success of all functions of the CSS, and especially case management, is client advocacy. In case management an advocate consistently coordinates care and provides assistance in clarifying expectations as well as providing the encouragement to meet those expectations. A basic nursing function has traditionally been to coordinate and integrate patient care.[4] The presence of a nurse as a client advocate promotes the interpretation and reinforcement of a client's functioning successfully in the community.

Another aspect of the philosophy of nursing that lends itself to case management is that of holistic care. Knowledge of holistic care includes having the assessment skills to evaluate the community in which the client lives, and the ability to assist the client in obtaining social supports and maintaining the most appropriate living arrangement. The interaction of man with environment as well as the interaction of mind and body is an established theory guiding both assessment and intervention processes of community mental health care.[40] The influence of the body on the mind is most evident when medical problems present with psychiatric symptoms. Many long-term mentally ill patients have very poor health care practices and are subject to the misdiagnosis of their physical disorders. There is a need for more extensive health care and illness documentation, including the use of Axis III diagnosis. There is also a need for health care plans to be included in regular treatment planning of patients. The plans need to include interventions by psychiatric nurses for high-risk patients, and oversight responsibilities by nursing when non-nursing staff are assigned to these patients.

Interdisciplinary collaboration in community mental health

Interdisciplinary interaction is a basic tenet of community mental health. In the community mental health movement, professionals seem to perform tasks using strikingly similar skills. Rapid societal change has demanded new services to meet the mental health needs of consumers. Health professionals are attempting to adapt, change, and expand skills to provide a relevant service to consumers. The subsequent "identity crisis" in what belongs uniquely to each profession has added stress to the effectiveness of service. Nursing is changing rapidly, as is every other health profession. Each nurse should have a clear concept of nursing's unique role and contribution to the team. To interpret the nurse's role and maintain accountability, the nurse must know his or her responsibilities and where those responsibilities end.

Interprofessional teamwork is subject to the rules of group process. The team should devote considerable time and energy to defining and delegating responsibilities so they will avoid infringing on one another's sense of territoriality. A major team goal is to determine mutually satisfactory modes of interaction and negotiation. Teamwork is an approach both to providing services and determining ways in which members can work together. The team must be clear about goals and individual responsibilities and must establish a mechanism for renegotiation of roles. Just stating the goals of the team in no way ensures agreement. Dialogue is continuous in an interdisciplinary team, and modification of goals and strategies is integral to functioning.

Interprofessional teams typically go through a series of stages: (1) early enthusiasm and lively interest in one another's contributions, (2) insecurity and sense of role threat combined with guarding of one's territory, and (3) role negotiation and effective functioning or abandonment of the team concept. Teams in community mental health are often described as more democratic than those in other settings. The leader is likely to be elected rather than designated by job title. Decisions regarding the tasks of team members are based on competence, interest, availability, and match between client or family needs and provider ability and preference.

Evaluation in community mental health

Community mental health is a new concept in a field characterized by lack of agreement about values, modes of treatment, and standards of practice. Evaluation, although difficult because of the intangibility of community mental health services, is essential for quality control and accountability. Program evaluation must answer questions about both the quantity and quality of services.

■ Quality assessment methods

In general, three methods—structure, process, and outcome—used either singly or in combination, make up the foundation of quality assessment in health care. In the **structural** approach to quality assessment, standards and criteria are designed to determine the impact of organizational patterns on the delivery of quality health care services. Two basic assumptions underlie the use of a structural approach: It is possible to assess what is "good" by identifying staff, physical, and organizational structure, and care is improved as staff qualifications are upgraded, physical facilities are improved, and sounder fiscal and administrative procedures are applied.[24] Structural standards are widely used in assessment because the data assessed are quantifiable. The government traditionally uses this method, because it is the easiest to apply.

In the **process** approach to assessing quality of care the activities of health professionals are evaluated in terms of what is determined to be "good care." The assumption underlying this approach is that health care providers can agree on what constitutes high-quality care. Process standards are of two types: normative, which are derived from the formulations of recognized leaders, and empirical, which are based on actual patterns of care. Both approaches entail observation and experimentation and change over time. Providers use this approach largely to pinpoint problem areas.

The **outcome** approach assesses care on the basis of the result of treatment. These standards measure survival, recovery, and the patient's satisfaction with treatment. Both government and health care providers use outcome measures. Many consider these to be the most useful forms of evaluation, albeit the hardest to obtain.

■ National standards

The National Standards for Community Mental Health Centers developed by the NIMH describe three major areas for evaluation. One is administration and direction of the center, which includes organizational patterns, staffing, facilities, use review, and provision of requested information. The second category is accessibility, specifically community orientation, visibility, prevention, including consultation and education, and coordination and collaboration with other agencies. The third area is specific service activities and includes the five major modes of treatment (inpatient, outpatient, partial hospitalization, emergency care, and consultation and education), as well as individualized treatment plans, a range of treatment modalities, and continuity of care. As a public agency NIMH evaluates programs to ensure that grant recipients are using their funds according to guidelines. NIMH's monitoring is carried out through site visits, applications for future support, and an annual inventory completed by each center.[7]

■ Issues in evaluation

Each community mental health program must decide on a mode of evaluation. The major choice is between a structural approach, which relies largely on enumeration, and an outcome method, which is more difficult to carry out but may be more useful in providing relevant services to consumers. Although quantity of services (i.e., the number of individuals who partake of any service) is far easier to measure than quality, relevant evaluation demands attention to effectiveness of services. Client outcomes after treatment are a major criterion for evaluation. Outcome is measured against predetermined goals, often stated as behavioral objectives. A disadvantage to outcome evaluation is that few follow-up data are collected in community mental health programs.

An outcome evaluation program begins with stated goals determined at the onset of treatment. The client and nurse decide what they expect to accomplish. Many call this a contract. The items on the contract are stated in behavioral terms, such as "the client will return to work with less than a 10% absentee rate due to 'nervousness.' " The major problem in outcome evaluation is determining what kinds of information or change constitute effective treatment. Outcome measures should be simple, concrete, readily observable or measurable, and not readily open to interpretation based on opinion. Client reports and nurse observation make up a component of evaluation. Although such indicators as number of hours expended in services, number of patients seen, and scope of services offered constitute data for evaluation, these measures are insufficient. Outcome and service effectiveness measures must be included, even though they are difficult to establish.

■ SUGGESTED CROSS-REFERENCES ■

Evolutionary perspectives of psychiatric nursing are discussed in Chapter 1. A nursing model of health-illness phenomena is discussed in Chapter 3. Evaluation of the nursing process is discussed in Chapter 5. Defining mental health, high-risk populations, and primary prevention activities are

DIRECTIONS FOR FUTURE RESEARCH

The following are some of the nursing research problems raised in Chapter 25 that merit further study by psychiatric nurses:

1. Exploration of factors present in successful community mental health programs
2. The role of nurses in community mental health
3. Specific benefits associated with patients' use of community mental health services
4. Identification of successful primary prevention programs
5. The cost-effectiveness of treating specific patient target groups in the community versus the cost of hospitalization
6. Systematic analysis of the role of case manager in terms of efficiency, effectiveness of coordination, and aspects of cost
7. The differential characteristics of patients who do and do not respond to coordinated social treatment in the community
8. Predictor variables related to patients who do not receive follow-up and benefit from community mental health care
9. Development of an accurate evaluation method for use in community mental health
10. The relationship between early discharge planning and aftercare and readmission of psychiatric patients

discussed in Chapter 8. Crisis intervention is discussed in Chapter 9. Tertiary prevention and rehabilitation activities are discussed in Chapter 10. Liaison psychiatric nursing and consultation are discussed in Chapter 26. Care of the chronic mentally ill patient is discussed in Chapter 33.

■ SUMMARY ■

1. A brief overview of the history of mental health care in the United States was presented, including the work of Benjamin Rush, Dorothea Dix, and Adolf Meyer. A summary was provided of governmental involvement in the mental health field leading up to the legislation enabling the development of community mental health centers.

2. The five essential services described in the 1963 legislation—inpatient, partial hospitalization, outpatient, emergency care, and consultation and education services—were described, as were the additional services of diagnosis, rehabilitation, precare and aftercare, training and research, and evaluation. Modifications of the law included in the 1975 amendments, the 1978 report of the President's Commission on Mental Health, and the 1980 legislation were also described. The Mental Health Systems Act and the initiation of a Block Grant System were discussed.

3. Several criticisms and benefits of community mental health programs were compared.

4. Community support systems and case management were discussed.

5. The impact of deinstitutionalization was described.

6. The concept of the mental health team was described as it pertains to the role of the community mental health nurse.

7. Evaluation is an extremely important facet of community mental health and was presented in terms of both quantity and quality of services. Methods of evaluation are applied to structure, process, or outcome of services.

■ **REFERENCES** ■

1. Baier M: Case management with the chronically mentally ill, J Psych Nurs 25(6):17, 1987.

2. Brown NB and Parrish J: Community support and rehabilitation of the mentally disabled in the United States, Inter J Mental Health 15(4):16, 1987.

3. Committee of Psychiatry and Community, Group for the Advancement of Psychiatry: Community psychiatry: a reappraisal. New York, 1983, Mental Health Materials Center.

4. Crosby RL: Community care of the chronically mentally ill, J Psychosoc Nurs 25(1):33, 1987.

5. Dickey B et al: A follow-up of deinstitutionalized chronic patients four years after discharge, Hosp Community Psychiatry 32:306, 1981.

6. Dorwart RA, Horgan C, Schlesinger M, and Davidson H: The privatization of mental health care and directions for mental health services research. In Tauke CA, Mechanic D, and Hohman AA, editors: The future of mental health services research, Washington DC, 1989, US Government Printing Office, p 139-154.

7. Feldman S and Windle C: The NIMH approach to evaluating the community mental health centers program, Health Serv Report 88:174, 1973.

8. Goldman HH: Financing the mental health system, Psych Annal 14:861, 1984.

9. Hager L and Kincheloe M: The disintegration of a community mental health outpatient program, or off the back wards into the streets, Perspect Psych Care 113:102, 1983.

10. Harris M and Bergman HC: Capitation financing for the chronic mentally ill: a case management approach, Hosp Community Psychiatry 39:68, 1988.

11. Jackson T: Government and private sector initiatives in health care cost containment, Psych Annal 19:412, 1989.

12. Joint Commission for Accreditation of Hospitals: Principles for accreditation of community mental health service program, Chicago, 1979, p 19.

13. Lamb HR: Young adult chronic patients: the new drifters, Hosp Community Psychiatry 33:465, 1982.

14. Landsberg G and Hammer R: Possible programmatic consequences of Community Mental Health Center funding arrangements: illustrations based on inpatient utilization data, Community Ment Health J 13:63, 1977.

15. Marmor J: The relationship between theory and community psychiatry, Hosp Community Psychiatry 26:807, 1975.

16. Mechanic D: The challenge of chronic mental illness: a retrospective and prospective view, Hosp Community Psychiatry 37(9):891, 1986.

17. Mechanic D: The evolution of mental health services and mental health services research. In Tauke CA, Mechanic D, and Hohman AA, editors: The future of mental health services research, Washington, DC, 1989, US Government Printing Office.

18. MH-MR Report: A Morris Associates report from Washington DC 15:1, May 5, 1978.

19. Minkoff K: Beyond deinstitutionalization: a new ideology for the postinstitutional era, Hosp Community Psychiatry 38(9):945, 1987.

20. Minkoff D and Stern R: Paradoxes faced by residents being trained in the psychosocial treatment of people with chronic schizophrenia, Hosp Community Psychiatry 36:859, 1985.

21. Morrissey JP and Goldman HH: Cycles of reform in the care of the chronically mentally ill, Hosp Community Psychiatry 35(89):785, 1984.

22. Murray J: Failure of the community mental health movement, Am J Nurs 75:2034, 1975.

23. National Council of Community Mental Health Centers: Renewal of CMHC Act: amendments to PL 94-63, Washington DC, 1977.

24. National Institute of Mental Health: National standards for community mental health centers: report to Congress, Rockville, MD, 1977, The Institute.

25. National Institutes of Mental Health: Toward a model plan for a comprehensive community based mental health system, Rockville, Md, 1987, US Department of Health and Human Services, Alcohol, Drug Abuse, and Mental Health Administration.

26. Nation's health. Mental health bill signed into law, Washington DC, Am Public Health Assoc 10(11):1, 1980.

27. Pepper B and Ryglewicz H: The developmental residence: a 'missing link' for young adult chronic patients, Tie Lines 2(3):1, 1985.

28. Peplau H: Future directions in psychiatric nursing from the perspective of history, J Psychosoc Nurs 27(2):19, 1989.

29. Rachlin S: When schizophrenia comes marching home, Psychiatric Q 50(3):202, 1978.

30. Ramshorn MT: The major thrust in American psychiatry: past, present, and future, Perspect Psychiatr Care 9(4):144, 1971.

31. Rodenhauser P and Greenblatt M: Transformations in mental health system management: an overview, Psych Annals 19:408, 1989.

32. Rubins J: The community mental health movement in the United States circa 1970, Am J Psychoanal 31:68, Jan 1971.

33. Ruybal S: Community health planning, Fam Commun Health 1:9, Spring 1978.
34. Sharfstein SS and Beigel A: Less is more? Today's economics and its challenge to psychiatry, Am J Psychiatry 141:1403, 1984.
35. Snow D and Newton P: Task, social structure, and social process in the community mental health center movement, Am J Psychol 31:582, 1976.
36. Staton D: Mental health care economics and the future of psychiatric practice, Psych Annals 19:421. 1989.
37. Stroul BA: Introduction to the special issue: the community support systems concept, Psychosocial Rehabilitation Journal 12(3):5, 1989.
38. Stroul BA: Community support systems for persons with long-term mental illness: a conceptual framework, Psychosoc Rehab J 12(3):9, 1989.
39. Talbot JA: The chronically mentally ill: a look at the past five years with an eye to the future, Psychosoc Rehab J 6(3):12, 1983.
40. Talley S: Basic health care needs of the mentally ill: issues for psychiatric nursing, Issues Mental Health Nurs 9,409, 1988.
41. Tarail M: Current and future issues in community mental health, Psychiatry Q 52(1):27, 1980.
42. Torrey FE: Continuous treatment teams in the care of the chronically mentally ill, Hosp Community Psychiatry 37(12):1243, 1986.
43. Wilson SF: Implementation of the community support system concept statewide: the Vermont experience, Psychosoc Rehab J 12(3):27, 1989.
44. Zusman J and Lamb JR: In defense of community mental health, Am J Psychiatry 134:887, 1977.

■ ANNOTATED SUGGESTED READINGS ■

Bachrach LL: Young adult chronic patients: an analytical review of the literature, Hosp Community Psychiatry 33:189, 1982.

Analyzes the impact of an emerging new psychiatric service group, young adult chronic patients. This population presents a highly variable clinical picture constituting neither a uniform diagnostic category nor a population with fixed or predictable symptom pictures. They typically use psychiatric facilities in a "revolving door" fashion, requiring considerable linkage among facilities if care is to be beneficial.

Belcher A and Toomey BG: Relationship between the deinstitutionalization model, psychiatric disability, and homelessness, Health Social Work 13(2):145-153, 1988.

According to a follow-up study, 35% of 133 people released from a state mental hospital became homeless within 3 months of their release. This supports the theory that deinstitutionalization contributes to homelessness. Describes key characteristics of the homeless person and the process of homelessness with implications for solutions for improved care.

Belcher R: Mothers alone and supporting chronically ill adult children: a greater vulnerability to illness, Women and Health 14(2):61-80.

Qualitative methodology captures the problems and strug-

gles of caretaking mothers of severely mentally ill patients. Mothers were at greater risk for vulnerability of illness because of increased stress. Suggests interventions to reduce the burden and to contribute to a more healthy environment.

*Boondas J: The despair of the homeless aged, J Gerontol Nurs 11(4):9, 1984.

The homeless elderly, suffering from the effects of poor health, poverty, and social isolation, are in desperate circumstances. At least 1% of the nation's population (approximately 2.2 million people) lack shelter. The increased homeless population is attributed to a variety of factors including deinstitutionalization and urban redevelopment.

Dorwalt RA: A ten year follow-up study of the effects of deinstitutionalization, Hosp Community Psychiatry 39(3):287-291, 1988.

Between 1977 and 1987, the Cambridge-Somerville unit of the Massachusetts state hospital system resurveyed the patient population. Findings indicate that the number of patients remained the same, but there were increases in the number of male patients, patients on involuntary legal status, and patients with hospitalizations of between 1 and 12 months. The number of patients who had hospital stays of 30 days or less, or more than 5 years, decreased. Concludes that the effect of deinstitutionalization continues even though the census reduction trend has been stabilized.

Dworkin RJ, Adams GL, and Telschow RL: Cues of disability and treatment continuation of chronic schizophrenics, Social Science Med 22(5):521-526, 1986.

Investigates the concern of maintaining chronically ill patients in outpatient community mental health centers (CMHC). Tested the economic, social, and medical cues facilitating disability self-definition that contributes to treatment continuation. Data were collected from 879 charts of chronic schizophrenic patients in five CMHCs. The multiple and logistic regression analyses indicate that the level of functioning is an important explanatory variable and the efficacy of the medical model in treatment continuation.

Echeper-Hughes N: "Mental" in "Southie": individual, family, and community responses to psychosis in South Boston, Culture Med Psychiatry 11(1):53-78, 1987.

Explores the meanings of "going mental" and "being mental" in the white, working class, ethnic neighborhood of South Boston. Data were collected in a study of the impact of deinstitutionalization on a cohort of middle-aged, psychiatric patients from the Boston State Hospital returning to the community. Responses and interpretations of symptoms of mental distress from the individual, family, and the community indicate that even seriously disturbed individuals are sensitive to cultural meanings and social cues.

Goodman AB and Siegel C: Elderly schizophrenic inpatients in the wake of deinstitutionalization, Am J Psychiatry 143(2):204-207, 1986.

Investigating the observed age-related increase in the ratio of patients with paranoid schizophrenia to those with nonparanoid schizophrenia, the authors tested 1518 elderly patients

---

*Asterisk indicates nursing reference.

during a 5 year period for the numbers of late onset paranoid conditions, length of stay for recently admitted paranoid patients, and changing diagnosis over time. The data did not support their observation but did suggest that paranoid conditions were related to those patients admitted before age 54. The reasons for the poor prognosis of this group is discussed.

Grella CE and Grusky O: Families of the seriously mentally ill and their satisfaction with services, Hosp Community Psychiatry 40(8):831-835, 1989.

Fifty-six family members were interviewed to determine their satisfaction with community support programs (CSPs). The results indicate that the majority were dissatisfied with various aspects. Multiple regression analysis indicated that sex of the respondent, type of family member relationship, and illness onset time were significant contributors to family dissatisfaction. Emotional support interaction with case managers was the strongest factor in family interaction.

Kurtz LF, Bagarozzi DA and Pollane LP: Case management in mental health, Health Social Work 9(3):201, 1984.

Report on a survey of 403 case managers in community mental health centers in Georgia to identify their educational level, professional identification, and demographic characteristics influencing their performance. Findings indicated that workers with higher educational levels performed a greater number of case management activities and required less supervision.

Lamb HR: What did we really expect from deinstitutionalization? Hosp Community Psychiatry 32(2):105, 1981.

Author asks "what went wrong with deinstitutionalization?" He suggests that severely disabled psychiatric patients have remained a marginal population with few continuity of care programs helping them to assimilate into the community. He contends that the goal of making it possible for these patients to live with dignity in a comfortable low-energy but satisfying life-style is a great step toward achieving the initial goals of deinstitutionalization.

Lehman AF: Strategies for improving services for the chronic mentally ill, (review), Hosp Community Psychiatry 40(9):916-920, 1989.

Four current policies are examined—continuous care teams, local mental health authorities, integrated entitlement programs, and capitation payment systems—and discussed in terms of four model programs of integrated services. Success of these strategies depends on the systems ability to regulate services and to ensure incentives for cost effective services at the staff level.

*Lowery BJ and Janulis D: Community mental health and the unanswered questions, Perspect Psychiatr Care 21(4):156, 1983.

Examines the nature of conflicts inherent in the community mental health movement. Authors contend that complex issues exist and revolve around a series of fundamental questions, including: Who is the patient? Who is the therapist? What is the process? What is the goal? What is the theory? and What is the role? Authors offer alternative responses to these questions, acknowledging that there is no one right or wrong answer to each one.

*Mackenzie JA: Order out of chaos: changes in community health and home care, Nurs Health Care 6:37, 1985.

The nature of community health, especially home health care, is changing dramatically. The community health nurse is ideally suited to serve as a case manager. To maintain the viability of agencies, administrators must look to new models of practice. One successful model is a corporate organizational structure in which the corporation is a tool for achieving tighter networks, for creating partnerships and mergers, and for achieving surpluses.

Pardes MD and Stockdill MA: Survival strategies for community mental health services in the 1980s, Hosp Community Psychiatry 35(2):127, 1984.

According to these authors, widespread reduction of financial resources has created a growing concern about the survival of community mental health services and their inherent values and ideals. A variety of survival strategies has become essential, including incorporation, alternative services, innovative funding, and political activities. Authors urge the use of business techniques to make mental health services more efficient and cost effective.

President's Commission on Mental Health: Report to the president, vol 1, Washington, DC, 1978.

Government report of a 1-year study commissioned by President Carter to review the mental health needs in the United States. It is strongly recommended that psychiatric nurses be familiar with the content of this report, although its impact on legislation and funding was diminished with the Reagan administration.

Prindaville GM, Sidwell LH and Milner DE: Integrating primary health care and mental health services—a successful rural linkage, Public Health Reports 98(1):67, 1983.

Describes one successful linkage between a small primary health care center and a non-federally-funded, multicounty mental health center. The services of the linkage project included direct clinical mental health services delivered at the primary health care site, consultation and education activities, and coordination of interagency services. Authors analyzed the key elements in the successful linkage and the subsequent attainment of goals.

Shadish WR Jr: Private-sector care for chronically mentally ill individuals: the more things change, the more they stay the same, (review), Am Psychol 44(8):1142-1147, 1989.

Profit-making nursing homes and board-and-care homes provide primarily custodial care for the approximately one million chronic mentally ill; this is not much different from the care received prior to deinstitutionalization. Problems exist because these patients are not informed consumers and because care is not publically regulated. The fundamental problem, however, is in the overall social policy that reflects a reluctance to care for chronically indigent individuals.

Sommers I: Geographic location and mental health services utilization among the chronically mentally ill, Community Mental Health J 25(2):132-144, 1989.

Data was collected from 1053 Community Support Programs (CSPs) to investigate the relationship between geographic location (urban, suburban, rural) and use of mental health services. Controlling for the availablilty and accessibility of services, socio-demographic, and need factors, analyses indicate that location of the CSPs influenced their use. Rural CSPs were more likely to be utilized for crisis and housing services than those in urban locations; the suburban-urban CSPs were more likely to be used for psychosocial services. Concludes that models of service use must be specified according to the geographic location.

Thompson JW, Burns BJ, and Taube CA: The severely mentally ill in general hospital psychiatric units, General Hosp Psychiatry 19(1):1-9, 1988.

The NIMH Survey of Discharges from Non-Federal General Hospitals Study conducted between 1970-1980 found that severely mentally ill patients became an increasingly larger proportion of general hospital discharges. This number had also increased between 1975 and 1980. This trend seems to confirm that State mental hospital care is being replaced by nongovernmental-owned general hospital care. Discharge referrals from governmental general hospitals became rare in 1980 compared to 1970 when referral predominated.

Wilk RJ: Implications of involuntary outpatient commitment for community mental health agencies, Am J Orthopsychiatry 58(4):580-591, 1988.

Reviews the empirical evidence for the proposal to use direct involuntary commitment to outpatient treatment rather than hospitalization or preventive detention. Discusses the administrative policy implications.

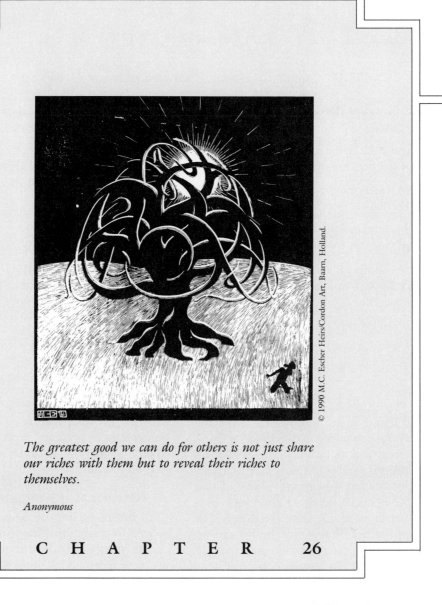

The greatest good we can do for others is not just share our riches with them but to reveal their riches to themselves.

Anonymous

C H A P T E R   26

PSYCHIATRIC LIAISON NURSING: A CONSULTATION MODEL

FRANCES G. LEHMANN

779

LEARNING OBJECTIVES

After studying this chapter, the student should be able to:

- relate the historical development of the liaison nursing role.

- identify the role characteristics and practice settings of the liaison nurse.

- state three categories of problems encountered by the liaison nurse.

- analyze the implications of the present economic environment for liaison nurses.

- describe a conceptual model and theoretical framework for liaison nursing practice.

- discuss the three phases of the liaison process, including the four steps that comprise the working phase.

- compare and contrast direct and indirect care functions of the liaison nursing role.

- discuss future trends and challenges for liaison nursing practice.

- identify directions for future nursing research.

- select appropriate readings for further study.

H istorically many forces have helped shape the role, need, and use of liaison nursing. Liaison nursing is a model for nursing practice that has developed from the consultative process, and is considered a psychiatric nursing subspecialty.[7] It was generated out of two needs: (1) the psychosocial needs of the client in a general hospital setting and (2) the ethical needs of nursing to deliver holistic professional health care to the client in the most practical and economical method available. The liaison nurse has expertise in psychiatric nursing and a special ability to integrate these skills with knowledge in medical-surgical nursing to provide comprehensive nursing service.

The psychiatric liaison nursing role

There are various models of psychiatric liaison nursing. A review of the literature on consultation points out the diversity, complexity, and widespread use of the role.[11,12] The model used in this chapter is based on a consultation process developed and used in community mental health by Caplan. In this model, an identified expert relates by request with a consultee in order to solve the consultee's work-related problem.[3]

The term *liaison nursing* describes a particular professional process between two systems. One system (the user/consultee) has a current work-related problem and voluntarily requests help from an outside system (the provider/consultant). Liaison nursing is further viewed as a learned process that promotes planned change by the use of interpersonal skills and specialized knowledge.[13]

■ Historical development

Liaison nursing becomes more meaningful when viewed from the broader historical perspective of psychiatric nursing. A major influence on psychiatric nursing was federal legislation (Public Law 88-164, the Community Mental Health Centers Act) passed in 1963. This legislation authorized the establishment of a comprehensive mental health delivery system in the United States to meet the psychiatric needs of all socioeconomic classes of Americans. This major mental health movement created a lack of qualified people to staff the centers. To help solve this problem, several professions, including psychology, sociology, social service, and nursing, designed and implemented educational and training programs to prepare mental health workers. The significance of the legislation on nursing education is seen by the number of schools of nursing that took advantage of federal training grant money and by the number of psychiatric/community mental health nurses prepared at the graduate level in the last three decades. Psychiatric nurse specialists have thus taken their place alongside other mental health specialists in the health care delivery system.

Along with the increased demand for professional

and competent psychiatric nurses to serve as program staff members, another force within the comprehensive mental health center movement made psychiatric nurses more visible. Mental health centers and many other health facilities provide mental health consultation. As a result, psychiatric nurse specialists have regular contact with other human service agencies and institutions. Through this contact, many disciplines have recognized the unique viewpoint of nursing in treating individuals in relation to one another and to their environment.

The thrust toward holistic health care has become popular within the last 25 years. In nursing, however, total patient care is documented as far back as Florence Nightingale's time. At present, nurses continue to care for human beings in a holistic manner. Nursing activities are concerned with those factors that influence both the client and his environment. Traditionally, interventions have focused on the client's mental, psychosocial, spiritual, and physical needs, regardless of the setting.

The title "liaison nurse" became popular in the 1970s when primary care nursing demonstrated nursing's commitment to providing comprehensive, individualized care. In general hospitals the liaison nurse became a part of the nursing services department and consulted with staff and clients in all nursing units.[2,7]

Not limited to hospitals, however, nurses have a long history of caring for a client in his own environment. This is evidenced by community health nurses going into the home, occupational nurses being available in work places, and school nurses being staff members of educational institutions.

By the 1980s the title "mental health nurse consultant" had come into use. This umbrella title usually indicates that the person is professionally prepared to deal not only with the effects of disease on human beings but also with health promotion, human relations, and process consultation involved in organizational management and development. Now, in the 1990s, a major concern in health care settings is effective and efficient delivery of services with the issue of cost containment being critical to the organization. As a facilitator of interpersonal relationships and clear communication, the psychiatric nurse consultant can be a key to the success and growth of any work setting in which people interact to achieve organizational goals. Today consultation is seen as an integral part of the psychiatric nurse specialist role, and a large number of specialists are available for both direct and indirect mental health services. Their visibility, accessibility, and clinical competence should help to assure their future survival.[4,8] Thus the capacity of psychiatric nurses to provide on-the-scene consultation services in various settings is a natural unfolding of another chapter in the evolution of nursing.

■ Role characteristics

The psychiatric nurse specialist functions in many professional roles and applies the knowledge and theory of mental health concepts. These roles may resemble each other, but they have different goals, outcomes, strategies, and methods. The liaison nurse works closely with other members of a health team in promoting effective problem management. Liaison nursing refers to an expert who provides problem-centered consultation service in a coordinate relationship; the mutually shared goal of both partners is problem resolution.

Problem solving is a function of any nurse, regardless of educational preparation or defined roles. Many essential qualities, however, contribute to the specialized problem-solving activity of liaison nursing. It is important to differentiate commonly blurred activities, such as supervision and education, from liaison nursing. The liaison nurse should distinguish between these various activities to define his or her own role, responsibilities, performance, and outcome.

Essential differences between the liaison role and supervisor role are the authority base and administrative responsibility for outcome. The liaison nurse should have a coordinate professional relationship with the user. This means she should have no administrative authority or coercive power over the user. The liaison nurse is not responsible for implementing recommended changes, and the user is free to accept or reject any or all parts of the recommendation.

Organizationally, a liaison nurse position should be a staff rather than a line position. This differs from a supervisory role, in which authority is based on hierarchy rank. By definition, the liaison nurse is outside the user system. This means she is outside the regular chain of command within the user organization. This aspect also provides the liaison nurse with the necessary freedom to work with people at any level within any needed time frame rather than in a full-time line position that fills a slot within the organizational structure.

The power of the liaison nurse rests in her own authority of ideas based on a specialized area of expertise. The user explicitly and voluntarily asks for help. The liaison nurse respects the user as a professional partner in problem-solving activities. While dealing with the current problem, the liaison nurse works to add to the user's knowledge, allowing him to deal more effectively with similar situations in the future.

Thus the liaison nurse facilitates the user's potential by asking for and using his input.

The liaison process emphasizes the idea that the provider and user deal with aspects of the problem that are unclear and confusing rather than with inadequate or incompetent people. The liaison nurse should project the attitude that the user is an active, interdependent partner who is ultimately responsible for implementing the proposed interventions.

Although the liaison nurse may provide new information and knowledge to the user, the liaison process differs from an educational activity. The stated goal is not to teach a specific body of knowledge to the user. Rather, the liaison nurse provides support and guidance while helping the user to enhance his own understanding of the issues. The user can then develop more effective ways to handle the current problem and future similar situations.

Liaison nursing practice

■ Settings and functions

There are several ways of practicing liaison nursing. Some nurses are independent private practitioners who are employed for a specific assignment by the consultee organization on a fee-for-services basis. Other clinicians are staff members of an organization.

The liaison nurse can provide either direct or indirect service. In both categories the liaison nurse acts as an outside consultant, on a time-limited basis. She facilitates and enhances a person's, family's, group's, or organization's knowledge and skills. In direct service the liaison nurse provides direct care and intervenes so that her activity has a measurable effect on the health status of a person, group, or family. In indirect service the liaison nurse functions as a resource, supporting key people directly responsible for the operation of the consultee system.

Nurse practice acts in each state dictate a registered nurse's scope of practice and the educational preparation required to function in a specialty role. A psychiatric liaison nurse requires a master's degree in psychiatric–mental health nursing with knowledge and clinical skills in specific areas of psychosocial nursing.[5]

The setting in which a liaison nurse may function is limited only by imagination and demand. Her services may be used in acute or rehabilitative inpatient units of general hospitals, ambulatory health services, home health care organizations, community agencies, educational institutions, employee health components of industry or business, and special population settings such as extended care facilities, retirement communities, summer camp programs, and church-sponsored social support programs.

■ Types of problems

The liaison nurse intervenes in various types of problems. The identified problem can focus on one client (**case problem**), a series of related problems (**program problem**), or a particular administrative problem (**organization problem**). In practice, these artificial categories generally overlap. However, the liaison nurse's awareness of the identified problem and the target system with which she is interacting helps in working through the entire liaison process.

The **case** category relates to helping the user become more effective as a human being. The liaison nurse focuses on ways to increase the user's skill and knowledge. The spotlight is on the client and alternative ways of problem resolution. The **program** category relates to helping the user define or meet particular professional goals. The liaison nurse focuses on ways to improve the user's professional functioning in dealing with more than one client. The **organization** category relates to developing new programs or improving existing ones that affect the organization. The liaison focuses on the administrative system and on organizational change to produce a desired outcome.

Clinical example 26-1 illustrates each category of problems encountered by the liaison nurse.

Economic considerations

As the largest health care provider, nursing is becoming more complex, specialized, and technical. Its latest challenge in the wave of cost containment is to provide nursing services to (1) sicker hospitalized clients who stay a shorter time, (2) clients with complex health problems in ambulatory settings, (3) clients in home settings with limited resources, and (4) increasing numbers of chronically ill, poor, and older Americans.

The need for cost-effective and efficient quality care has resulted in the increasing demand for skilled and professional nursing services. Decreased inpatient days and increased complex outpatient procedures demand accurate nursing assessments, diagnoses, and interventions. Quality, comprehensive nursing care affects the clients' welfare and the financial base of the health care delivery system. Nursing leaders across the country are required to allocate resources to improve health care efficiency and reduce costs.[6] Nursing managers in all settings are results oriented and business minded.

As a result of cost containment, all specialized nursing positions must be justified on a cost-benefit ra-

CASE PROBLEM

Mr. C, a 68-year-old widower who had been living in a retirement home for about 6 months, began withdrawing from all social activities. Formerly he had been active and an initiator of planned outings for other members of the home community and generally appeared to be adjusting to the move after the death of his wife some 9 months previously. The staff of the home had vast experience in helping other clients work through similar life situations, but they believed that all the interventions implemented on Mr. C's behalf had minimum effect. The director of activities therapy and the director of nursing services requested a case consultation with Mrs. L, a clinical nurse specialist working as an independent practitioner. Mrs. L entered the user system at middle-management level and was asked to focus on Mr. C by working with the nursing staff to help it develop a more effective nursing care plan.

PROGRAM PROBLEM

The teaching staff in a private preschool facility went to the director of the program and requested more help. Mrs. B, the director of the program and a capable administrator, believed the present staffing pattern was adequate but also recognized that the faculty as a whole was experiencing more and more frustration in providing high-quality care for the children enrolled in the program. She requested Mr. G, a clinical nurse specialist working in a community mental health center, to consult with the faculty regarding the problem.

ORGANIZATION PROBLEM

A small manufacturing plant was in the process of expanding its product line and corporate structure. The organization had legally been a partnership with two principals of equal salary and stature. With the expansion, the organization became a legal corporation with a board of directors, major officers, and department managers. The growth and development of the organization had created a tremendous strain on the newly appointed officers, and their interpersonal relationships were dysfunctional.

The president recently had successfully completed family therapy with a clinical nurse specialist and decided that the company officers might profit from mental health counseling. He contacted the nurse therapist who agreed to serve as liaison nurse and consult with the company officers regarding their transition problems.

tio basis. Logic suggests that liaison nursing has important economic and clinical benefits. As an advanced practitioner, the liaison nurse (1) integrates a biopsychosocial perspective to client care, (2) provides a holistic rather than dualistic approach to care, and (3) serves in both direct and indirect ways to produce desired outcomes. Economy results when experts are used on a time-limited, consultative basis.[9] On an economies-of-scale principle, the liaison nurse can provide reduced labor-intensive indirect service. Resource sharing can be applied to offer psychosocial nursing expertise to a wider range of participants. The bottom line is cost-effective use of nursing hours to produce holistic quality care and individualization of services.

Liaison nurse positions, previously carried as line items in organizational budgets, are losing their institutional support. The paradox is that holistic interventions produce less relative costs. Everyone agrees, for example, that too much anxiety interferes with the healing process. What better way to justify the actual cost savings of the liaison nurse who provides expert direct service to decrease the client's stress, diminish the degree of anxiety, and promote the healing process. This outcome would be cost-effective on a relative basis by shortening the client's recovery period.

Two other developments have created a ripple effect. The government and private prospective payment systems are emphasizing prevention. Industry and business also are becoming aware that health promotion for the employee is cost-effective and results in higher productivity and decreased costs for insurance and illness care. The aggressive approach to health promotion and wellness provides an opportunity to use liaison nurses' skills and knowledge. In any setting the liaison nurse can intervene to reduce stress and increase personal functioning. Employing liaison nurses in non–health care settings is on the rise as employers begin to measure improved employee efficiency in terms of greater profit margins.

Community programming also should be considered in light of current economic attitudes. Use of the liaison nurse in this nontraditional setting can provide mental health services as community needs arise. Service recipients can have greater access to the expertise of a wellness-oriented health care provider. For example, in church-sponsored social programs for retired people, liaison nursing could play an active part in maximizing the health of the participating citizens.[14]

Given the present financial situation, it is essential that the liaison nursing role demonstrate its economic value. Through nursing research, the outcomes associated with the psychiatric nurse specialist need to be documented. In addition to quality of care measures, nurses need to justify the cost-effectiveness of their care as it impacts on the client, health care organizations, and governmental and private reimbursers. Such documentation is needed for the growth of this nursing role and for its survival.

The liaison process

■ Conceptual model

The liaison nurse should have a conceptual model and a theoretical framework for practice. This combination of style and method (structure and function) helps the liaison nurse provide maximum return for her efforts and time and makes the work exciting and rewarding. The conceptual model used in this chapter is a coordinate, nonhierarchical relationship between a provider and a user. This model sets the tone of the interactive relationship. Within this model, both provider and user bring distinct contributions to the problem-solving tasks, as depicted in Fig. 26-1.

■ Theoretical framework

The liaison nurse is responsible for: (1) using sound principles, (2) applying concepts to the information available, and (3) providing practical and easy-to-understand interventions based on carefully thought out theory.[5] The practitioner therefore needs to develop a framework under which she functions in her role. The liaison nurse uses sound knowledge and organizes theory from a variety of disciplines to formulate her own model for nursing. The theory base should include knowledge of systems theory, change theory, staff management, organizational behavior, problem-solving theory, growth and development, cultural and ethnic norms, stress and stress reduction theory, and crisis theory, as well as environmental, interpersonal, and intrapersonal psychiatric dynamics. In one situation organizational theory may become the primary focus, another time interpersonal relationships may be the frame of reference, and yet another situation will deal directly with an intrapersonal problem.

The theoretical framework allows flexibility for the nurse as she adapts to both the expected and unexpected parts of any liaison situation. The particular methods chosen come from her own sense of purpose and professional identity. Within a defined framework she can shift the focus of the problem to meet the needs of the users, based on their organizational structure, institutional policies, and her own perceptions. This framework becomes a guide and a practical reference for the liaison process.

■ Phases of the process

Although liaison nursing is a specialized type of nursing, it can be compared to the traditional nursing process. Both liaison nursing and the nursing process (1) are orderly, mutual, problem-solving activities; (2) relate to at least two people interacting to cause change; and (3) hold the partners responsible for participation. The nursing process involves five steps: assessment, diagnosis, planning, implementation, and evaluation. Four of these steps comprise the working phase of the actual liaison process, with an orientation and termination phase marking the beginning and end of the formal liaison activity. As with any "process," liaison nursing is an ongoing activity and all steps are interrelated.

■ **ORIENTATION PHASE.** As defined earlier, liaison nursing refers to a nonhierarchical relationship in which the provider, as an outside expert, joins the user in problem solving. The relationship requires that certain issues in addition to the task at hand be attended to so that both systems will find it mutually satisfying and beneficial.

It is important for the liaison nurse to immediately contact the appropriate authority personnel in the system to make her purpose and presence known. This contact also serves as a way to gather data about the organizational structure and the communication network operating there. It is also important for the liaison nurse to understand the services provided by the

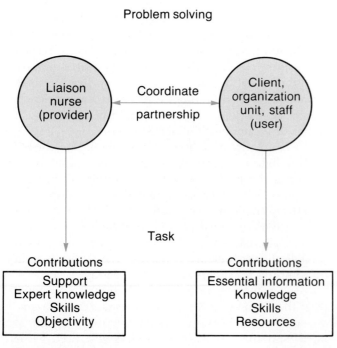

Fig. 26-1. Conceptual role model used by the liaison nurse.

organization, the philosophy, and any operating policies relevant to the target unit.

Any role is defined in relation to the social system of which it is a functioning part. The entire liaison process is affected by the type of setting and the professional background of the personnel involved in the relationship. Settings could include health care settings, such as acute care general hospitals, ambulatory care facilities, and nursing homes; non–health care settings would be industries, schools, churches, self-help groups, and human services agencies, such as welfare departments, judicial systems, penal systems, and child care services. Each setting will have its own unique philosophy, organizational structure, established protocol, and expectations of how the liaison nurse will function in that particular setting. The liaison nurse's knowledge of and experience with organizational theory will benefit her intrapersonally and interpersonally as she functions within any setting.

The effectiveness of the liaison process is influenced by the user's concept of the liaison nurse's role. It is important for both sides to clarify the liaison's role. This avoids two common causes of failure of a liaison process: (1) the staff has unrealistic expectations or (2) they distort the purpose for which the consultation was requested. The liaison nurse should also evaluate the accuracy of the user's perception of the present liaison nurse on the basis of past experience with other personnel in a similar role.

The liaison nurse will have the opportunity to work with intraprofessionals (fellow nurses), interprofessionals (other disciplines), and nonprofessional (technical) personnel. Thus the liaison nurse will have to maintain the strength of her own identity, as well as an awareness of the identities of others. The liaison nurse should interact with other people under the assumption that they have a sense of accountability, responsibility, and competency in their own area of work. This respect for others transcends educational background or professional experiences.

Effective communication. The liaison nurse's ability to communicate effectively is a skill that makes the process much smoother. The communication process depends on the liaison nurse, setting, and user of services. Developing communication channels involves identifying key formal and informal networks. It is important for the success of the liaison process that both sides have a working arrangement for giving and receiving information.

Basic conceptual differences will become apparent as people work together in the task of problem solving. Finding a common language in which both partners are comfortable and feel productive will minimize differences. It is helpful for the liaison nurse to use words that are familiar to other people. This will help prevent the nurse from talking on an inappropriate level or skirting the subject. Using abstract approaches or focusing on what seem to the user to be impractical or irrelevant issues will not promote their self-confidence. The liaison nurse should not give advice or use declarative sentences when communicating with staff. It is preferable to use questions that guide the user to alternative ways of viewing the problem. Helping the user to reduce the complexities to relevant facts promotes clarity and mutual understanding of the situation.

It is important for the user to know that liaison discussions are confidential. This means that the liaison nurse guards against being a "switchboard" or carrier for messages that should be delivered directly within the organization. Also a liaison nurse should not take sides in differences of opinion among staff members. It is important to demonstrate that any information gathered will not be used to purposely harm any person or the reputation of the organization. The focus of any interaction should be work difficulties and not the private personal needs of staff members. If personal issues are hindering a staff member's performance and interventions are needed, this recommendation is not transmitted within the official liaison process. The liaison nurse restrains from gathering personal information that could turn the liaison session into a therapy session. Instead, she can tactfully encourage the troubled staff member to seek out an impartial skilled listener.

Contract. Although liaison nursing is an ongoing process, the formal liaison process is guided and evaluated by a written agreement between the liaison nurse and the user. This agreement is simply called a contract. The contract represents an exchange between the partners of the specific services to be provided and the nature of the complementary activity. If the request for services comes through informal channels (via telephone or face-to-face contact), the liaison nurse needs to verify with the appropriate authority that permission is given for the liaison activity. The purpose behind requesting a letter of contract therefore is to prevent misunderstandings between the parties.

To avoid possible misrepresentation or ambiguity, a letter or memorandum from an authority person in the user organization should be directed to the liaison nurse. This document can describe the various aspects of the user's expectations. It eventually serves as a tool for outcome evaluation.

The contract is not so much a legal document as an agreement between professionals of two systems. It can be kept simple. It should be dated and signed by both user and provider. The main points to cover include the following:

1. A brief description of the problem situation
2. Expected goals
3. Estimated time to be used on the project
4. Means of compensation for the time
5. The key department and personnel involved, including the contact person

The liaison nurse can also use the contract to better understand the informal relationship. By expanding and examining the statement of problem in point 1, she can decide if it is a case, problem, or program consultation process. She can gather more background information about what action has been taken so far to resolve the problem and what personnel have been involved in the activity to date. The stated goals in point 2 may end up as part of the original problem. Viewing both the expected goals and stated problem in context will show how the user perceives the entire situation.

Points 3 and 4 help the liaison nurse learn about the organization's perception of both quality and quantity regarding time. Point 4 clarifies whether the organization sees the compensation as an hourly rate or a job rate. If the consultant is in-house, it should be clear to which department the time is to be charged. Point 5 includes the communication network to be used, the names of staff and their jobs, a list of people who are available for discussion, the scope of confidentiality expected, the kinds of information appropriate for discussion with whom, and who the authority source is for permission.

■ **WORK PHASE.** After the orientation phase in which the initial contact and contract are completed, the actual liaison process begins. Fig. 26-2 is a representation of the process model, which depicts the four steps of assessment, planning, implementation, and evaluation. This same model is used on case, program, and organization problems. A more detailed discussion of the various steps follows. The model can be applied to both the direct and indirect care functions.

Assessment. This step actually begins when the contract is formulated. It continues with the two participants collecting data, clarifying the information available, and assessing it in a conceptual manner. The liaison nurse can ask questions to stimulate the staff's thinking and show them that they are capable. The liaison nurse can guide the discussion to a deeper level by asking herself aloud, questions about the complexities of the situation. By speculating aloud, she promotes new understanding among the staff. She also demonstrates a willingness to risk and act as a role

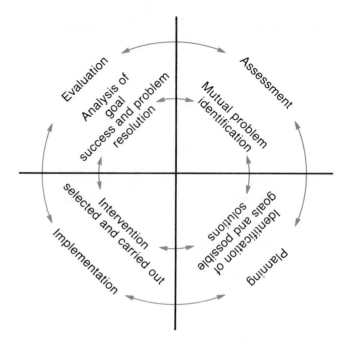

Fig. 26-2. Stages of the liaison process.

model for the problem-solving process. Beginning sentences with "I wonder if . . ." facilitates a feeling of joint endeavor. During this stage the liaison nurse should (1) assess the strengths and weaknesses of the user, (2) identify the real and potential barriers to action, (3) determine what impediments have kept the user from resolving the problem, and (4) assess the general problem-solving ability of the partners.

This step ends when an identified problem is agreed on by the user and the nurse. The activity in this stage is most critical to the rest of the liaison process. It may be repeated a number of times until the identified problem is manageable and realistic enough to be resolved by the user organization. A concise conclusion derived from the assessment stage makes the rest of the process easier.

Planning. This step starts with the liaison nurse reframing the problem so the user can view the situation objectively and without feeling threatened. The liaison nurse uses theoretical concepts that promote learning and can be generalized to similar situations. She listens to and values the staff's ideas. She may modify them by expanding the proposed intervention or by suggesting unusual but theoretically sound ways to implement them. All interventions should be feasible, practical, and in line with the skills and abilities of those responsible for implementation. This avoids upsetting the existing lines of communication and authority. The suggestions should also be sensitive to the rights and well-being of those affected by the potential change. The planning should reflect what presently exists and not what should be. It is unethical to propose interventions based on an idealist level of problem management.

This step ends when the liaison nurse and the user arrive at possible solutions to the problem. Goals should be stated based on the desired outcome. These goals provide a framework for interpreting, planning, and evaluating ongoing activities.

Implementation. This step begins with the user selecting the interventions to be tried. This stage may take place after the liaison nurse has left the physical environment and the actual liaison process is terminated. This stage includes testing alternative suggestions that came out of the planning step. The step ends when the interventions have been in effect long enough to assess observable change.

Evaluation. This step begins with asking to what extent the interventions met their stated goals. This step may also take place after the liaison nurse has left, but it is still important that she help the user find specific ways to measure the expected outcome or the interventions. The evidence used to evaluate should include obvious data, although implied data are used occasionally. The evaluation focuses on the effects of the planned interventions and not on the staff who implemented the plan. This is an important difference in that the total situation is examined, not how individual people are functioning. Another aspect of evaluation is identifying that gaps of knowledge or lack of skill exist on the part of the staff. These needs may be met through an educational approach to the problem.

This step ends when the user determines whether the defined problem has been resolved, to what degree of success the solution worked, and what additional problems, if any, were uncovered during the process.

■ **TERMINATION PHASE.** Termination involves both physical and psychological closure. Tasks such as writing reports and leaving are needed. Much of the work involved in this phase depends on the liaison nurse's basic personality, the setting, and the formal contract. If the liaison nurse is a staff member of the user organization, her visibility will continue. If she has a one-time relationship, leaving will be more formal.

Liaison report. Progress may have been verbally discussed throughout the liaison process but at the end of the consultation activity, a formal written report is required. This allows all members of the organization to have access to relevant information.

The format of the report will vary with the type of consultation, the setting, the level of organization involved, and the issues under focus. The following areas should be included:

1. The purpose, dates, and activities during the process
2. A statement of the identified problem
3. An assessment of the situation
4. Alternative plans for problem resolution
5. Specific interventions
6. Suggestions on how to evaluate the interventions

This formal report can be brief but explicit regarding what the liaison nurse believed happened in the total process. The report should be consistent with the theoretical framework on which she bases her practice.

Professional development. The liaison nurse uses the contract and summary report to evaluate her own performance in the process and to make revisions in using the process on the next occasion. The liaison nurse is constantly changing and growing in her own professional development as a consultant. Self-evaluation is a necessary part of the liaison process. Areas that need evaluation are goal setting, problem solving, communication skills, and theory application.

Performance evaluation is easier if criterion-referenced measurements are used. This is preferable over norm-referenced evaluation, since comparing oneself to others in the field is almost impossible. The liaison nurse can attend professional meetings and conferences. This allows her to keep in contact with other professionals and helps to assess her own growth and development. Reading professional literature and textbooks is another way to increase one's theory base and scope of knowledge.

Direct care provider

■ Role characteristics

As a direct service provider the liaison nurse acts autonomously as a psychosocial therapist to provide mental status assessment, nursing diagnosis, treatment, and evaluation services. She may use individual, family, or group therapy, crisis intervention, and stress reduction counseling. The liaison nurse intervenes on an interpersonal level to expand the health services available to clients in nonpsychiatric settings. Her direct services may be requested by the attending physician, the client, or a member of the nursing staff.

In direct service the types of problems that may arise are considered client-centered case problems. Most of the liaison nurse's time is spent with the client, and the interaction is primarily client-supportive

CLINICAL EXAMPLE 26-2

Mrs. W, a 68-year-old widow, was admitted to a surgical unit of a general hospital for a colostomy after x-ray examination and biopsy revealed colorectal cancer. She had a history of three previous admissions for various somatic complaints over the last year since the death of her husband. During the presurgery workup, the attending physician requested a liaison nurse consultation to establish a therapeutic relationship with Mrs. W in anticipation of the colostomy, and to obtain an evaluation of Mrs. W's coping abilities.

ASSESSMENT

Mrs. H, the liaison nurse, reviewed the client's charts from the present and previous hospitalizations and talked with the family physician and the surgeon. She also talked with the ostomy service nurse and with Mrs. W's primary nurse. Mrs. H then met with Mrs. W in her private room for almost an hour.

After a thorough assessment of Mrs. W's physical, social, mental, emotional, and spiritual health, the nurse explored with her the meaning Mrs. W gave to the situation she was experiencing. The nurse also talked with her about her family and social support network and received permission to talk with her adult daughter. Rapport was established between Mrs. W and Mrs. H, and they mutually decided subsequent visits would be in order.

The nurse made the following nursing diagnoses:
1. Severe level of anxiety related to medical diagnosis of cancer
2. Disturbed body image related to the impending colostomy
3. Anticipatory grieving related to the loss of body functioning

PLANNING

The nurse conferred with the family physician and together they decided that Mrs. W, because of her high-risk stress factors, would benefit from six to eight psychosocial therapy sessions to be provided by the nurse, Mrs. H. The sessions were to be held in Mrs. W's hospital room at a mutually agreed-upon time. The scheduled surgery and Mrs. W's recuperation would be primary factors in the immediate treatment plan. The nurse charted her assessment, diagnoses, treatment recommendations, and therapeutic goals in Mrs. W's chart. She also talked with Mrs. W's primary nurse, and then stopped by Mrs. W's room to arrange another visit with her the next afternoon, the day before surgery.

IMPLEMENTATION

In this phase of the liaison nursing process, strategies would be based on a continuous evaluation of Mrs. W's changing health status and surgical intervention. Theoretical considerations shaping the therapeutic relationship would be life developmental stage, stress management, and the process of grieving for body changes. The strategies would include (1) decreasing Mrs. W's level of anxiety; (2) providing therapeutic support for the grief and mourning process; and (3) reducing present and potential problems in the areas of self-esteem, body image, and personal control. The rationale for liaison nursing participation is preventive intervention to reduce the negative effects of stress, while improving Mrs. W's coping abilities at a time when she is dealing with a major health problem.

EVALUATION

Evaluation of the client's changing health status and how she is functioning is a shared responsibility of all health care team members. Specifically, the liaison nurse, functioning as a therapist, monitors the effectiveness of the psychosocial interventions and Mrs. W's mental, emotional, and social health status.

The following are a few of the liaison techniques used in this clinical example:
1. Focus on time-limited interventions and well-defined goals.
2. In promoting stress management, recognize the reality of the health-threatening situation and Mrs. W's compromised health status.
3. Build on the strengths of the client, her support network, and the team so that synergism enhances the healing process.
4. Use the liaison process as one component of the team's commitment to comprehensive care by participating in team conferences and communicating with the team members in an ongoing manner.

and goal-directed. The identified case problem may be to

1. Establish the client's mental status
2. Assist the client through a crisis
3. Counsel and support the client who has impaired body functions; has loss of self-esteem; is grieving; has suffered family abuse, violence, or rape; demonstrates impaired mental or emotional functioning; or needs guidance in coping with a personal life situation that presently or in the future could interfere with optimal functioning

In direct service the client and liaison nurse are the primary participants. The nurse uses advanced nursing skills and knowledge to provide direct care that causes predictable and measurable changes in the client's psychosocial welfare. The liaison nurse is directly responsible for implementing, evaluating, and documenting her liaison services. The liaison nurse must also provide other team members with any information that may contribute to the client's total welfare.

Clinical example 26-2 illustrates the role of the liaison nurse as a direct care provider.

Indirect care provider

■ Role characteristics

When the liaison nurse functions in an indirect manner, the consultee is responsible for resolving the identified problem. The liaison nurse assists the consultees in improving their problem-solving skills in the specific presenting situation and in handling similar work problems that might arise in the future. The liaison nurse is not expected to be an expert in the consultee-organization's specific operations. She is acknowledged as an expert in maximizing human resources to resolve the current problem and to enhance the consultee's own abilities and efforts.

Her indirect services are used by a wide variety of consultees from nurses to other health professionals, schools, industries, business corporations, civic and community organizations, or church-sponsored social groups. Problems can range from employee-assistance brokerage service programs to interpersonal relationship enhancement among members of a corporate board of directors. The content of the identified problem is secondary to the human relationship dynamics surrounding the problem.

The indirect care functions can be applied in any setting in which the liaison nurse feels comfortable. The consultee maintains full coordinate partnership.

Clinical example 26-3 illustrates the role of the liaison nurse as an indirect care provider.

A forward look

Psychiatric liaison nursing will continue to evolve and be influenced by movements within the general practice of nursing, as well as forces within psychiatry and the comprehensive health care delivery system. Cost considerations in health care dictate allocation of resources.

Incentives from the federal government's pricing system and the private sector's initiatives to reduce hospital use have shifted the locale of health care services, including nursing. In fiscally constrained eras, psychosocial aspects of health care are most vulnerable and yet greatly needed. Psychiatric liaison nursing must continue to make itself visible, accessible, and cost-effective in both health care and community systems. Special emphasis should be placed on health promotion, wellness, and human resource enhancement.

Basic changes are taking place in how nursing services are allocated and reimbursed. Direct reimbursement through third-party and self-pay measures is increasing through state and federal legislation, expanded nurse practice acts, and demonstrated cost savings. Continued political activity at the policy-making level is needed to change the shortcomings of government, commercial, and prospective payor systems. Liaison nursing must continue to strengthen its position as a necessary component of client care, especially in the general hospital and intermediate care facility. Cost-offset studies are imperative to specifically show the reduction of overall cost of health care by inclusion of a liaison nurse on the health team and the cost-benefit ratio of liaison intervention with medically sick clients.

Marketing is a required skill of every liaison nurse. Because of the scarcity of the health care dollar and the various providers competing for the same clients, it is mandatory for all of nursing to guard its service area. It is even more important for psychiatric nursing to promote and document its contribution toward quality, cost-effective care. Acceptance and use of mental health nurse consultants in traditional health care settings and nontraditional community and commercial settings depend on active political endeavors, especially on the part of independent practitioners. It also takes recognition and acknowledgment by nurse colleagues through client referral to provide support to the role and validation of its contribution to health care.

As the consultation role continues to grow and nurses develop expertise and recognition in specialty

CLINICAL EXAMPLE 26-3

ASSESSMENT

Mrs. L responds to a telephone call from Mrs. K, director of nursing of the retirement home. Mrs. L, Mrs. K, and Mrs. P, director of activities, meet. After informal conversation regarding the case problem, a contract letter is drawn up by Mrs. K: "Whereas our home has a resident whose lack of participation in planned activities keeps him isolated from other residents, we would appreciate your help in developing a treatment plan that provides opportunity for Mr. C to increase his involvement in group activity. As mutually agreed, this project should entail approximately 3 hours of joint effort. Our standard pay rate for nurse consultants is $35 per hour with no employee fringe benefits. Please feel free to talk with any staff or residents at their discretion. Mrs. P or I will arrange our time to meet your schedule." Both Mrs. K and Mrs. L sign the contract and an appointment is set for the next day with Mrs. K and Mrs. P.

The next day Mrs. L meets with Mrs. K and Mrs. P in the latter's office. A report is given regarding Mr. C's current status. Mr. C's physician prescribed a tricyclic antidepressant the previous week. No therapeutic effects had been noted. Mrs. L encourages both Mrs. K and Mrs. P to recount past interventions that were tried. Mrs. L uses nonthreatening questions to ascertain how both staff members see Mr. C in relation to his environment, life stage, grief phase, and physical and mental capacities. By speculating aloud to herself, she brings out different aspects of the same information in such a way as to increase the complexities and broaden the focus of the stated problem. By elaborating on certain points, she increases the staff's knowledge base. She is able to assess the collaborative relationship between nursing and activity therapy. She reflects her thoughts to the other two professionals in such a way that all three professionals engage in data gathering, investigating, and organizing the various information.

Mrs. K arranges for Mrs. L to talk with Mr. C during one of the structured activities held in the recreation room. During this time Mrs. L also talks informally with other residents and staff members in the same social setting. On returning to Mrs. K's office, Mrs. L encourages the staff to ask meaningful questions to increase their own knowledge regarding the total situation. After about 45 minutes of dialogue the three participants arrive at a concise conclusion. Mr. C is having an anniversary grief reaction to his wife's death. They mutually agree upon the nursing diagnoses of (1) delayed grief reaction related to his wife's death and (2) social isolation related to the grieving process. These diagnoses describe the response of the client and reflect the hypothesis on which the treatment plan will be based. This identification of the problem makes it easier for the staff to focus objectively on the client and not be threatened by feelings of guilt or inefficiency in not meeting his social needs.

PLANNING

The grief process is the theoretical concept Mrs. L uses to help the staff reframe Mr. C's situation. The emphasis is shifted from engaging Mr. C in more activity to evaluating his behavior in terms of the stages of grief as outlined by Kübler-Ross. The goal of problem resolution is to facilitate Mr. C's grief work. Although the aim is to provide individualized care for Mr. C, the staff benefits from learning about theoretical aspects of grief that can be generalized to other clients. The liaison nurse uses leading questions such as "Do you suppose Mr. C was in a state of denial when he first came here? That might explain how he got so busily involved in so many activities." Mrs. L provides information for discussing the various stages of grief and draws out examples of behaviors or attitudes that help assess which stages Mr. C has worked through. By increasing the staff's understanding of a specific need or reason for a particular behavior, approaches can be planned to help Mr. C relate to the emotional reactions manifested by his behavior.

At one point the discussion focuses on alternative housing for Mr. C. It is suggested he might live temporarily with his daughter. On closer evaluation it is ascertained that the daughter is unable

CLINICAL EXAMPLE 26-3—cont'd

to provide for her father at this time, since she recently changed jobs, moved to another city, and is living in an efficiency apartment until she decides if she likes the job and location. This alternative is discarded, since any recommendation should be sensitive to the rights of others. The treatment plan is written specific to actions of the patient with the underlying assumption that present behaviors are meaningful in helping him work through the loss of his wife, his home, his daughter, and his life-style. The liaison nurse uses the conference to have the staff look at Mr. C's behaviors as goal directed and to generate interventions that facilitate his emotional release. Mrs. K and Mrs. P mutually agree to reduce Mr. C's expected involvement in activities and to provide a psychologically appropriate environment for the various stages of grief.

Several strategies were discussed, and it was agreed that Mr. C should be included in the planning stage of his treatment program. Mr. C's participation in the planning and implementing stages recognizes his strengths and allows him to remain self-reliant.

IMPLEMENTATION

Without describing specific interventions used in this case, a few guidelines are offered regarding this phase of liaison nursing. Short-term objectives can be used as selected steps toward reaching a long-range goal. In Mr. C's case "facilitating client's grief work" is one step toward helping him adjust to his life stage and life-style. The interventions should focus on specific, expected actions of the client and not nursing care provided by staff. The interventions should be written in short concise statements (e.g., "introduce Mr. C to Mr. O, who has successfully completed grieving for his wife"). Expected measurable outcomes are established and a time frame is placed on each suggested intervention. Mrs. L negotiates with the directors to be available as a resource for 2 months as the planned interventions are tried and the results are measured.

EVALUATION

Mrs. K receives a report from staff members in an ongoing manner regarding Mr. C's progress. A few minor revisions were made in the original plan. According to the evaluation of both Mrs. K and Mrs. P, the client profited, the interdepartment staff became more cohesive because of the cooperative effort at problem solving, and the staff's increased knowledge would benefit all residents of the home.

Mrs. L spent a total of 2 hours at the actual consultation site. The liaison project ended when she sent a summary letter to the retirement home at the end of the 2 months. The established relationship continued from time to time with other projects.

The following are a few of the liaison techniques used in this clinical example:
1. Keep the focus on the client's situation and away from the staff's handling of the situation so that the users recognize their work performance is not under investigation.
2. Avoid personal issues. If a staff member talks about personal or private material, gently and purposefully direct the discussion back on focus by asking a client-related question.
3. As information is reviewed, raise questions to discover additional details and enrich the staff's awareness.
4. Use inquiry in such a way as to show the staff's wealth of valuable information.
5. Avoid asking for information that the staff would perceive as testing its knowledge base.
6. Allow the staff to know when you are confused. Being open to your own confusion allows the staff to recognize that clarifying is one of the steps in problem solving and when the pieces are put together, the patterns and meanings become clear.
7. Whenever possible, interview the referred client and the staff members who provide direct service to that client.

areas in expanded practice settings, accountability becomes even more important. Accountability is especially critical for independent practitioners who are more vulnerable to potential lawsuits.[10] Professional liability insurance protection is an issue the liaison nurse needs to consider because of society's increased emphasis on litigation.

Challenges from other professions and the current liability environment in a cost-conscious health care system have also influenced the development of a national policy on peer review within nursing.[1] Various state nursing associations have implemented peer review committees. Peer review is an organized procedure carried out by registered nurses who systematically review and make judgments about the quality of nursing care provided by peers as measured against professional standards of practice. It is meant to be a formal, systematic, objective, focused, and noncritical exchange between and among professional colleagues. It is important that the individual nurse consultant use such a structured process in carrying out her legal responsibilities for quality assurance.

Liaison nurses can influence their own professional future in three major dimensions. These dimensions and the tasks involved in each follow.

■ Accountability

1. Attain ANA certification as clinical specialists in psychiatric nursing.
2. Develop instruments for self-evaluation, since most clinicians work independently and can learn from retrospective audit.
3. Document liaison services in an official manner to validate and justify needs, as well as to promote referrals.
4. Work within guidelines of peer review as proposed by the American Nurses' Association.

■ Accessibility

1. Participate in as many interprofessional and community activities as possible to provide role identity, visibility, and leadership.
2. Initiate liaison services to outreach agencies and rural and smaller consultees, even at the sacrifice of time or money, to promote improved and newly developed client care practices.
3. Use effective and creative marketing strategies to promote the consultation services. Competition for the declining health care dollar is a realistic component to consider in a cost-effective health care delivery system.

■ Application

1. Identify and practice within a sound theoretical framework.
2. Devise and implement research projects that test clinical theory and cost-effectiveness.
3. Use creative and flexible ways to effect change.
4. Be well prepared by keeping up with new developments through formal or continuing education.

■ SUGGESTED CROSS-REFERENCES ■

Roles of psychiatric nurses are discussed in Chapter 1. Therapeutic relationship skills are discussed in Chapter 4. The phases of the nursing process are discussed in Chapter 5. Elements of the psychiatric evaluation are discussed in Chapter 6. Strategies for promoting health are discussed in Chapter 8. Psychological responses to physical illness are discussed in Chapter 21.

DIRECTIONS FOR FUTURE RESEARCH

The following are some of the nursing research problems raised in Chapter 26 that merit further study by psychiatric nurses:

1. Cost analysis studies, especially in the area of the cost-effectiveness of liaison nursing services.
2. Whether liaison nursing direct care interventions promote shorter hospital stays or fewer nursing care hours for certain diagnostic-related groups in the general hospital.
3. The use of the liaison nurse role in health promotion in a nontraditional setting, such as a retirement center, particularly one in which nursing care is part of the self-contained health maintenance package.
4. Whether employee access to a liaison nurse within an organization has any effect on employee absenteeism or illness.
5. Ways in which liaison nurses are marketing their skills and knowledge.
6. Business strategies used by liaison nurses in clinical practice, in the documentation of direct and indirect service productivity.
7. The extent to which psychosocial dimensions are incorporated in the plan of care for medical and surgical clients in general hospitals.
8. Organizational aspects of the liaison nursing role within a health care setting.

SUMMARY

1. Liaison nursing is a model for nursing practice that has developed from the consultative process. The liaison nurse has a master's degree, expertise in psychiatric nursing, and an ability to integrate these skills with knowledge in medical surgical nursing to provide expanded services.

2. Liaison nurses practice in a variety of settings, and they may be either private practitioners, employees on a fee-for-service basis, or employed staff of an organization.

3. Three categories of problems are encountered by the liaison nurse:

a. Case problems that focus on the problems of one particular client.

b. Program problems that focus on a series of problems related to the user's professional functioning.

c. Organization problems that focus on developing new programs or improving existing ones within the organization.

4. The liaison nurse has no administrative authority within the consultee organization. She is not necessarily responsible for implementing recommended changes, and the user is free to accept or reject any or all parts of the recommendation. The provider-user relationship is voluntary and time-limited. The goal of the liaison nurse is to assist the user in increasing his ability to handle similar problems in the future.

5. The liaison process is based on the nursing process and consists of three phases: orientation, work, and termination.

a. A written agreement or contract should be obtained during the orientation phase.

b. The work phase consists of the four steps of assessment, planning, implementation, and evaluation.

c. Termination involves both physical and psychological closure. Self-evaluation is another important activity at this time to further the nurse's professional growth.

6. The liaison nurse can be either a direct or indirect care provider. Either function can be carried out in case problems. Indirect service is generally involved in program or organization problems.

7. Research is necessary in the liaison nursing role. Cost analysis studies involving both cost-offset and cost-benefit of liaison nursing practice are needed to demonstrate the relative cost-effectiveness of this role and ensure its survival.

REFERENCES

1. American Nurses' Association: Peer review guidelines, Kansas City, Mo, The Association, 1988.
2. Beraducci M, Blandfor K, and Grant CA: The psychiatric liaison nurse in the general hospital, Gen Hosp Psychiatry 1:66, 1979.
3. Caplan G: The theory and practice of mental health consultation, New York, 1970, Basic Books, Inc, Publishers.
4. Collins BA: Do you need an external consultant? A model for decision making, Clin Nurse Specialist 3(2):91, 1989.
5. Lewis A and Levy JS: Psychiatric liaison nursing: the theory and clinical practice, Reston, Va, 1982, Reston Publishing.
6. McKibbin RC et al: Nursing costs and DRG payments, Am J Nurs 85(12):1353, 1985.
7. Nelson JK and Schilke DA: The evolution of psychiatric liaison nursing, Perspect Psychiatr Care 14(2):60, 1976.
8. Noble J and Harvey K: Selecting and using nursing consultants, Nursing Economics, March-April, 83, 1988.
9. Pincus HA: Making the case for consultation-liaison psychiatry, Gen Hosp Psychiatry 6:173, 1984.
10. Reinert BR and Buck EA: Issues in liability insurance and the nursing consultant, Clin Nurse Specialist 3(1):42, 1989.
11. Rogers M and Trimnell J: Maximizing the use of the clinical nurse specialist as consultant, Nurs Admin Q 12(1):53, 1987.
12. Rutherford DE: Consultation: a review and analysis of the literature, J Professional Nurs 4(5):339, 1988.
13. Soda D: Consultation: an expectation of leadership, Nurs Leadership 5(1):7, 1982.
14. Tobin SS: Embracing community mental health center and church collaboration for the elderly, Community Ment Health J 21(1): 58, 1985.

ANNOTATED SUGGESTED READINGS

*American Nurses' Association: Peer review guidelines, Kansas City, Mo, 1988, The Association.

Various state nursing organizations have implemented, or are in the process of implementing, peer review systems to demonstrate to the public and the professional community that nurses are self-regulating. The guidelines set out in this booklet are a framework for understanding and setting in place a mechanism for quality assurance in keeping with standards of nursing practice. A must reading for all nurses, especially those in independent practice who receive third party payment.

*Badger T: Mental health consultation with a surgical unit nursing staff, Clin Nurse Specialist 2(3):144, 1988.

Describes the effectiveness of collaboration among a psychiatric nurse specialist, nursing administration, and nursing staff in dealing with work-related stress, including burnout and the nursing shortage. Uses author's five-step consulation process in a clinical example to show how staff benefit from incorporating mental health principles in their work setting.

Caplan G: The theory and practice of mental health consultation, New York, 1970, Basic Books, Inc, Publishers.

The acknowledged prototype for both consultation theory and practice. Many principles discussed are applicable to liaison nursing as a consultation process. An excellent resource book for a practitioner or student of liaison nursing.

---

*Asterisk indicates nursing reference.

*Critchley D and Maurin J: The clinical specialist in psychiatric–mental health nursing, New York, 1985, John Wiley & Sons.

Explores the various ways in which psychiatric–mental health clinical nurse specialists use their education, experience, knowledge, and skills. Discusses the liaison nurse role, as well as many other advanced practitioner roles. A wealth of information from which masters' prepared nurses can learn.

Dychtwald K: Age wave, Los Angeles, 1989, Jeremy P Tarcher, Inc.

Offers insight into some interesting opportunities (related to the senior boom) for nursing consultation services today and into the twenty-first century.

*Hough A: The nursing consultant role, Nursing Management 18:65, 1987.

An appropriate resource for the consultant to have available in justifying costs for consultant fees in this time of cost containment.

*Lewis A and Levy J: Psychiatric liaison nursing: the theory and clinical practice, Reston, Va, 1982, Reston Publishing.

Devoted to the liaison nursing role. A classic and excellent resource for developments in the field.

Mason D and Talbott SW: Political action handbook for nurses, Menlo Park, Calif, 1985, Addison-Wesley Publishing Co.

Practical and useful to the nurse who wants to be an effective agent of change through political activities.

*Robinson L: Psychiatric consultation liaison nursing and psychiatric consultation liaison doctoring: similarities and differences, Arch Psychiatric Nurs 1(2):73, 1987.

Explores similarities and differences in perception and intervention into psychiatric and psychological problems of patients in the general hospital, as viewed by medicine and nursing. Describes evolution of each specialty, which gives the reader both a historical perspective and a clearer idea of the separate and complementary nature of medicine and nursing in relation to psychiatric liaison activities.

UNIT II
SPECIALIZED TREATMENT APPROACHES

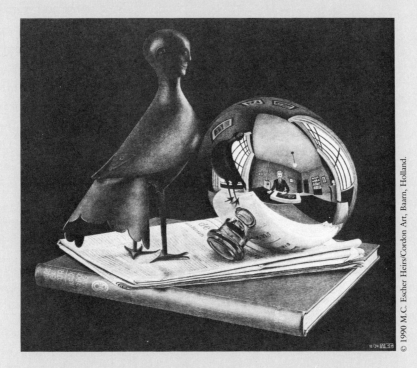

© 1990 M.C. Escher Heirs/Cordon Art, Baarn, Holland.

But humanism stands for the whole person, the whole individual striving to become as conscious and responsible as possible about everything in the universe. But now you sit there quite calmly and as a humanist you say that due to the complexity of scientific achievement the human being must never expect to be whole, he must always be frightened.

Doris Lessing, The Golden Notebook*

CHAPTER 27

BEHAVIOR MODIFICATION

HELEN R. PEDDICORD

After studying this chapter, the student should be able to:

- define behavior in specific terms.

- define behavior modification.

- analyze the application of operant conditioning principles to behavior modification.

- describe behavior modification techniques, including positive and negative reinforcement and positive and negative punishment.

- compare and contrast fixed interval, variable interval, fixed rate, and variable rate reinforcement schedules.

- discuss the ethical issues relative to the practice of behavior modification.

- identify directions for future nursing research.

- select appropriate readings for further study.

The principles described in this chapter are derived from psychology, particularly B.F. Skinner's work. In 1953, *Science and Human Behavior*[9] by B.F. Skinner was published. This work presented the findings of animal behavior experiments and discussed their application to human behavior. This was an attempt to move toward a science of human behavior. Later studies during the 1950s applied the principles to profoundly retarded and psychotic institutionalized persons and indicated their effectiveness. By 1958 the *Journal of the Experimental Analysis of Behavior* was published. This journal, although largely concerned with laboratory experiments with animals, printed some articles about applied behavior therapy with humans. In 1965 this journal published the results of the first experiment with the token economy.[1] The authors, Ayllon and Azrin, had developed and evaluated an environment for psychotic patients that consistently and systematically reinforced adaptive behavior. The motivating environment and operant conditioning principles they described were effectively applied later to populations such as the mentally ill, mentally retarded, juvenile delinquents, preschoolers, and slow learners.[2]

The late 1960s saw applied research in operant conditioning expand into the areas of education, classroom management, parenting, community work, and self-control. During the 1970s operant conditioning principles were used by most of the helping professionals, including nurses, physicians, social workers, teachers, and psychologists. Textbooks on behavior modification appeared in the professions of medicine, social work, nursing, education, psychiatry, and rehabilitative medicine.

The 1980s brought an emphasis on cognitive behavior therapies. This recognizes the value of both self-regulation and thought processes, as well as human behavior and experience being strongly influenced by internal phenomena. Much current research explores the internal (cognitive) antecedents and reinforcers that debilitate or habilitate.

Definition

Behavior modification involves the application of operant conditioning principles and procedures to human affairs. Operant conditioning, according to Reynolds, "refers to a process in which the frequency of occurrence of a bit of behavior is modified by consequences of the behavior."[8:1] Careful reading of this definition may lead one to assume it is a simplistic approach to the complexities of human behavior; however, its application breaks the complexities down to a manageable level and clarifies many events that affect behavior.

The terms "behavior modification" and "behavior therapy" have some distinct meanings but are often used interchangeably. This chapter uses the term "behavior modification." A primary focus of behavior modification is the effect of the environment on human behavior. Cognitive behavior therapies emphasize the effect of thought patterns on human behavior.

These therapies are therefore helpful to self-improvement efforts. One application of cognitive behavior therapy is in the treatment of fear.[4,5]

Behavior modification techniques, such as relaxation, are treatment strategies to reduce anxiety and foster more healthful physiological reactions. Progressive relaxation, the sequential tensing and releasing of large muscle groups, is used to decrease anxiety. Biofeedback, the procedure of learned control of involuntary body reactions using electronic devices, is taught to alter physiology. Biofeedback techniques are best learned and practiced experientially. The nurse should be alert to a paradoxical relaxation-induced anxiety in some clients.[3] Chapter 11 discusses these interventions in detail.

This chapter introduces behavior modification principles. It is not written with the expectation that the reader will be able to design, implement, and evaluate a behavioral treatment program without supervision. Appropriate application of behavioral techniques can be made in any setting in which psychiatric nurses work.

Describing behavior

Behavior is any observable, recordable, and measurable act, movement, or response of the individual. It refers to everything a person does. It may only be observable to the person who performs the behavior. When affect, cognition, sensation, and imagery are treated behaviorally, the treatment largely depends on self-observation. This chapter focuses only on behaviors that are observed by others and subject to quantitative measurement.

Before a behavior can be measured, it must be defined or accurately described. In defining behavior, one can break it into microscopic or macroscopic elements. For example, fire setting done by a child can be defined microscopically as gathering flammable objects, striking the match, lighting the objects, fanning the lit objects, and watching the resultant blaze. Macroscopically, this action is described as lighting a fire that blazes. This shows that there are several different and accurate definitions of what appears to be a simply defined behavior. Behavior definition can be a difficult task. One starts by describing what is seen and/or heard and then clarifies this until observers can agree that the behavior occurs.

Consider defining the behavior of fighting. It can be described as disagreement, with raised voices, exchanged insults, and a physical struggle of reciprocal blows and kicks. In the process of clarifying this description, questions such as the following arise: Is it fighting if there is no yelling? Is it fighting if each person hits the other only once? Is it fighting if there is a physical struggle (similar to wrestling) with no hitting or kicking? As these questions are answered, a definition that is both clear and related to the purpose of the definition unfolds. If one is establishing rules and consequences for aggressive adolescents, it may be decided that there is a consequence imposed simply for one student hitting and/or kicking another student. This is likely to prevent a fight. If one is developing a treatment plan for a child who is said to "fight all the time" in a classroom, the clinician, teacher, and child together may arrive at a different definition. They may decide that the significant behavior is pulling classmates' hair or pushing them out of their seats.

These examples show that a behavior is what is observed—not conclusions, inferences, or interpretations drawn from observation. Hyperactivity is not a behavior. It is a conclusion about a set of behaviors. One cannot measure hyperactivity; one can measure the number of times a child looks away from an assignment within a specified time, how many times he interrupts a conversation in a given period, the number of toys he displaces, the pages of classwork completed, and the length of time he remains in one body posture. The behavioral treatment would not focus on hyperactivity; it would focus on those specified behaviors that interfere with the child's success in the school, home, or community.

Other examples of conclusions instead of behaviors are psychiatric diagnoses and descriptions such as uncooperative, aggressive, compliant, depressed, hostile, and withdrawn. When using a particular adjective or label to describe a specific individual, one can identify the behaviors that were the basis for the description. The behaviors underlying the adjectives will vary from person to person. Little chance exists that the behaviors will be the same for more than one person. A clear definition of a behavior decreases various interpretations from person to person. A clear behavior definition is a statement of what the person does, is accessible to measurement, and is not subject to interpretation.

Once a behavior is defined, one expects that behavior to increase, decrease, or remain the same. Those procedures that increase, maintain, or decrease behaviors are given in Table 27-1. Each of these operant conditioning procedures are now briefly described.

Increasing or maintaining behavior

A behavior may increase in frequency, complexity, or duration. For example, when one is learning to walk a step occurs more often; the complexity of the step increases (forward, backward, sideways, turning,

TABLE 27-1

OPERANT CONDITIONING PROCEDURES

Maintain or increase behavior	Decrease behavior
Positive reinforcement: Addition of an environmental event as a consequence of operant, increasing probability of operant's recurrence Operant → Consequence → Operant ↑	**Positive punishment:** Presentation of aversive stimulus following operant, decreasing probability of operant's recurrence Operant → Aversive event → Operant ↓
Negative reinforcement: Removal of part of an aversive stimulus as a consequence of operant, increasing probability of operant's recurrence Aversive stimulus → Operant → Removalof aversive stimulus → Operant ↑	**Negative punishment:** Removal of something following operant, decreasing probability of operant's recurrence **Response cost:** Negative punishment in which a reinforcer is lost or withdrawn following an operant Operant → Reinforcer withdrawn → Operant ↓ **Timeout from reinforcement:** Negative punishment in which no reinforcement is available following an operant Operant → No reinforcement available → Operant ↓
	Extinction: Withholding reinforcement following an operant that was previously reinforced Operant → No reinforcement → Operant ↓

becoming longer); and the amount of time walking increases. One can observe an increase in at least these three ways in the acquisition of most skills.

Operant behavior is that behavior maintained, increased, or decreased according to the environmental events that follow it. For clarity, the word "operant" instead of "behavior" is used throughout this chapter. **When the environmental events following an operant increase the probability that the operant will recur, the process is reinforcement.** Both positive and negative reinforcement increase the chances of an operant occurring again.

The addition of an environmental event (consequence) contingent on the operant is **positive reinforcement.** An example of positive reinforcement is the response of a smile to a greeting. The operant, greeting, is followed by a smile from the person addressed. The chances that the greeting will happen in the future are increased by the smile given in response. The smile is a positive addition of an environmental event.

$$\text{Operant} \xrightarrow{\text{Positive reinforcer}} \xrightarrow{\text{Probability of operant recurring}} \uparrow$$

Greeting → Smile → Greeting in future ↑

Sometimes the person responding to an operant intends to **decrease** the frequency of the operant, but the operant actually increases in frequency or remains the same. A parent may yell at a young child whenever he climbs on the table; the process in operation is positive reinforcement if he continues to climb on the table or does so more often in the future.

$$\underset{\text{on table}}{\text{Child}} \xrightarrow{\underset{\text{yells}}{\text{Parent}}} \underset{\text{on table}}{\text{Child}} \uparrow = \underset{\text{reinforcement}}{\text{Positive}}$$

In this example the process is defined as positive reinforcement because the child climbs on the table more often. If the child decreased his climbing on the table as a result of his mother's yelling, the process would not be positive reinforcement. Many factors may possibly explain why the mother's correction did not result in a decrease in table climbing. The important point is that the intent of the person providing a consequence does not determine what process is in operation. The effect of the consequence on the behavior's future occurrence determines the process.

When the reinforcer removes an aversive stimulus contingent on the operant, the procedure is **negative reinforcement.** An example of negative reinforcement is putting on sunglasses in glaring sunlight. The sunlight is an aversive stimulus; the placing of the sunglasses over the eyes is the operant; the removal of, or escape from, the sunlight's glare is the negative reinforcer. It is a reinforcer because the glare's removal **increases** the probability that the person will use sunglasses when exposed to bright sunlight in the future. A reinforcer increases the probability that an operant will recur. It is negative when the reinforcer was the removal, or **subtraction,** of something from the environment.

> Aversive stimulus→   Operant   →
> Glare of sun   →Use of sunglasses in bright sun→
> **Escape from   Probability of**
> **aversive stimulus→ operant recurring ↑**
> Escape from   →   Probable use of ↑
> sun's glare   sunglasses in future

The example just given is one of **escaping** the glare of the sun. Putting on the sunglasses before going out into the sun would be an example of **avoiding** the sun.

Negative reinforcement is the procedure by which one learns to escape or avoid unpleasant situations. This is evident in the following examples.

EXAMPLE 1

A mother is scolding a young child; the child goes to his mother and kisses her, and her scolding stops.

> **Chance of child**
> **Scolding kissing mother**
> Scolding→Kiss→ **stops** → **when again**
> **scolded ↑**

EXAMPLE 2

Nurse A tells nurse B she wants to discuss the conflicts in their work relationship. Nurse B becomes too busy to talk, thus avoiding the discussion. As a result, nurse B is likely in the future to be busy whenever she sees nurse A.

> **Busyness**
> **Sees   Discussion   whenever**
> Nurse A →Busyness→ **avoided** → **sees Nurse A ↑**

EXAMPLE 3

An adolescent's parents are displeased with their son's misbehavior in school. The adolescent runs away, thereby escaping the direct experience of his parents' displeasure. In the future he may run away again.

> **Running away**
> **Parental   Run Escape from when parents**
> displeasure→away→displeasure→ **displeased ↑**

Negative reinforcement may also maintain some work habits. Employees in a work situation arrive on time for work to avoid a supervisor's reprimand or loss of wages.

Decreasing behavior

Negative reinforcement is not to be confused with punishment. **Punishment decreases the probability that the operant will recur.** Negative and positive describe punishing procedures. **Positive punishment,** as Reynolds describes it, is "the presentation of an aversive stimulus following and dependent upon the occurrence of an operant."[8:111] In other words, an operant occurs and is immediately followed by an aversive environmental event. Occurrence of the operant decreases. A person wearing sunglasses on a bright day removes them. Removing the glasses is the operant. Immediately the glaring light hurts the person's eyes; this is the aversive event. Subsequently the person removes the sunglasses less often in glaring sunlight. This is an example of positive punishment.

> **Operant** →Aversive stimulus→ **Operant** ↓
> Sunglasses off→   Glare in eyes   →Sunglasses off ↓

The procedure may also occur when the parent yells at a child immediately after he climbs on a table. If the child climbs on the table less often, the procedure in operation serves as punishment, the operant being climbing on the table and the aversive stimulus being the yelling.

> Child on table→Parent yells→Child on table ↓

As pointed out in the explanation of positive reinforcement, the process at work is not necessarily the one intended by the person who is responding to another's operant. One might praise a noncompliant adolescent for a particular operant whenever it occurs, but the operant may occur less and less often. The process then is not positive reinforcement but positive punishment.

Negative punishment, according to Mikulas, is "a contingent event whose offset or decrease results in a decrease in the behavior it is contingent upon. This generally consists of taking away something that is reinforcing from a person when he misbehaves."[6:97] The major forms of negative punishment are response cost and timeout.

Response cost is the loss of a previously available reinforcer following an operant. After hitting her young brother, the child is deprived of her allowance. An adolescent may lose the opportunity to use the family car after coming home beyond her curfew. A consumer pays the bank a fee after overdrawing his checking account.

> **Operant**   →   **Reinforcer**   →Operant ↓
> **withdrawn**
> Child hits   →Loses allowance→Hitting ↓
> Late coming in→Loss of car   →Late coming in ↓
> privileges
> Overdraw   → Loss of money →Overdrawing ↓
> account

Timeout (or timeout from reinforcement), according to Mikulas, is "the punishment procedure in which the punishment is a period of time during which reinforcement is not available."[6:99]

A young child throws toys at the wall. His mother places

him on a chair in the corner. When he plays again, he is less likely to throw toys at the wall.

$$\text{Operant} \rightarrow \begin{array}{c} \textbf{Loss of all} \\ \textbf{environmental} \\ \textbf{reinforcement} \end{array} \rightarrow \text{Operant} \downarrow$$

$$\text{Throwing toys} \rightarrow \begin{array}{c} \text{No reinforcement} \\ \text{while in chair} \end{array} \rightarrow \text{Throwing toys} \downarrow$$

Extinction is the final behavior-decreasing procedure to be discussed. Extinction is the withholding or removal of a reinforcer that was previously maintaining or increasing an operant. A fairly typical example of extinction involves temper tantrums.

A child has a temper tantrum. The mother tells the child to stop, and because she is concerned that he will injure himself, hovers about the child. She then decides to no longer pay attention to future tantrums. When the next tantrum occurs, she completely ignores it. The previous reinforcer, mother's attention, is no longer presented. It is predictable that the tantrum will become louder and more intense, then gradually taper off. As the mother continues to ignore all tantrum behaviors, they will gradually decrease. The mother is employing the extinction process.

$$\text{Operant} \rightarrow \textbf{Previous reinforcer withheld} \rightarrow \text{Operant} \downarrow$$
$$\text{Tantrum} \rightarrow \text{Mother's attention withheld} \rightarrow \text{Tantrum} \downarrow$$

Extinction does not usually result in an immediate decrease in the operant. After an initial increase in rate, intensity, or duration, the operant gradually decreases.

An example, taken from group therapy, of several procedures in action follows. In human interactions there is an interplay of operants, reinforcers, punishers, and aversive stimuli. When one observes a given behavior, it may be an operant of the person observed, a reinforcer to an operant of a second person, and an aversive stimulus to a third person. This example, for simplicity's sake, does not relate the content of the group's interaction. It deals only with a narrow aspect of the process to exemplify four operant procedures: positive reinforcement, negative reinforcement, positive punishment, and extinction.

Abraham, usually silent in the group, speaks. Zelda laughs while Abraham is speaking. Abraham is then silent, and Zelda speaks. While she does so, all group members look at her. Zelda verbalizes more frequently than the other group members. Each time she speaks, most group members look at her. Later, Abraham speaks again; again Zelda laughs, and again Abraham stops speaking. He does not speak again in this session.

At least three operant procedures are in action. Zelda's laughter when Abraham speaks and Zelda's speaking are both reinforced; the former is negatively reinforced, the latter positively reinforced. The operant, laughter, is followed by Abraham's cessation of speech. Abraham's speaking is an aversive stimulus to Zelda, who removes it by the operant laughter. Her laughing when he speaks will increase. This is **negative reinforcement.** Zelda's operant of speaking is **positively reinforced.** The reinforcer is the eye contact of the other members. The frequency of her speaking increases. Abraham's operant of speaking decreases in frequency. Zelda's laughter is an aversive stimulus or punisher to his verbalizing. His speaking is punished by her laughter. This is **positive punishment.**

It is important to note that these processes are defined by what happens. The processes are not defined before they occur. The eye contact of others (added positive event) is defined as a **positive reinforcer** to Zelda's speaking because this is what happens when she speaks. Her speaking is maintained or increased in frequency. Zelda's laughter (added positive event) when Abraham speaks is defined as a **punisher** to Abraham's operant of speaking because this happens when he speaks. His speaking decreases in frequency (punishment). Abraham's silence (removed or terminated event—negative) after Zelda's operant laughter is a **negative reinforcer** to the laughter. The probability that Zelda will laugh when the aversive stimulus (Abraham's speaking) recurs increases. The laughter will remove the aversive stimulus.

In the next group session Zelda monopolizes the group during the first 10 minutes. All group members are looking at her at least occasionally during these 10 minutes. Gradually, one person stares out the window, another gazes at a picture, two others look at one another, and the last looks from one member to another but not at Zelda. As this starts to happen, Zelda's speech rate initially increases, then gradually decreases; finally, she pauses, then is silent.

This is **extinction.** The eye contact that had been reinforcing Zelda's verbalization is withheld, and her talking eventually ceases.

As mentioned earlier, this example indicates a narrow aspect of the behaviors in question for the sake of simplicity. There are many reinforcers and punishers relative to any operant. When assessing an operant, one begins with what is most obviously thought to be a reinforcer. If the operant is maladaptive and is to be altered, one identifies the reinforcer that is maintaining the maladaptive operant, removes the reinforcer, and provides reinforcement for an alternate adaptive operant. Schedules of reinforcements are considered in the following discussion of applications of behavior modification.

Applications of behavior modification

■ Increasing behavior

The simplest form of behavioral treatment is rearranging the environmental reinforcers. Sometimes this is not simple. A pediatric nurse consults with the psychiatric liaison nurse about an 8-year-old girl, Carole, whose treatment requires bed rest. The child is constantly out of bed playing despite the following interventions: the need for bed rest has been explained to the child and parents, parents have been cooperative, the child life worker has provided abundant activities for the child in bed, and there are other children in the room requiring bed rest who provide companionship. Carole's noncompliance with the bed rest requirement is now imitated by the other children. They also are frequently out of bed. All involved adults are now scolding Carole.

Initially, one must define bed rest. Does it mean simply remaining on the bed? If so, is jumping on the bed within limits? In this situation bed rest means remaining in the bed and includes only those activities that can be done in a sitting or lying position. The second step is obtaining information about what happens when Carole is found out of bed (the undesirable operant) and when she is found in bed (the desirable operant). Staff members will be able to describe these events. The third step is designing a data collection system and obtaining a baseline, that is, how often the behavior occurs before intervention. During waking hours Carole will be checked every 30 minutes. It will be noted whether she is or is not in bed.

After a half day of baseline data collection, it is observed that Carole was in bed only twice, at mealtime. The staff reports that this is worse than usual. Each time Carole was observed out of bed, staff scolded her. This suggests that the scolding may be reinforcing the behavior, since the staff reports that she now seems to be out of bed more often, is being checked more often, and is therefore scolded more often. A current baseline is established.

The fourth step is to establish the goal of intervention. Although it might be assumed that the goal is that Carole remain in bed 100% of the time, it is always desirable to state the intervention goal or terminal behavior clearly. The intervention goal should also include the time during which it is to be accomplished. The intervention goal in this situation might state, "Carole will remain in bed 100% of the time within a week of treatment."

Now intervention can begin. Staff is instructed to continue checking every 30 minutes but to say nothing, maintain a blank expression, and simply place Carole in bed if she is not already there. A second staff person is to enter the room before Carole can get out of bed, congratulate her about being in bed, and present the designated reinforcer. If two staff persons cannot be involved, both roles can be accomplished by one person.

Data collection and constant evaluation should continue throughout the week. Once Carole is remaining in bed more often, she may be checked less often. All staff and family must be informed of the treatment. This increases cooperation and prevents the inadvertent positive reinforcement of scolding. In this situation the environmental reinforcer, staff attention, is rearranged. Staff no longer give Carole attention for being out of bed. The attention is given for being in bed.

Let us take the same initial situation. Perhaps the initial data indicate that it is not staff attention but the gleeful laughter of her roommates that is reinforcing Carole's getting out of bed. This may be noted by Carole's increase in remaining in bed when a particularly lively roommate is not present or Carole's looking at her giggling roommates even when being corrected. One cannot suppress the children's spontaneous laughter, but one could devise a way for Carole to engage their laughter even while in bed. For example, Carole may use a drawing pad large enough for the others to see on which she draws funny faces. One could also ask the children to help by explaining the situation. This is not likely to help unless one provides a group reinforcement contingent on Carole being in bed a certain number of times a day. The group reinforcement could be a staff person playing a game with all of them, an extra snack, parents staying some time past the end of visiting hours, or being the last group to be awakened in the morning.

The group in the room, including Carole, could easily be told that they will receive a specific reinforcer if Carole is in bed at least half the times that she is checked. They can also be told that it is hard for Carole to stay in bed when they laugh each time she gets up. In this way the group is involved in rearranging the reinforcement they provide Carole. The only way to know whether the reinforcer has been correctly identified or effectively altered is by the results: does Carole stay in bed more often?

Social attention is probably the most pervasive and readily available reinforcer for human beings. At times, however, primary reinforcers, such as food or activity, are the reinforcers of choice. A client may not observe or respond to social attention. Sometimes the client and the potentially reinforcing person have such an angry or rejecting relationship that attention from that person would not be reinforcing. In these situations a primary reinforcer such as food, or a material reinforcer such as money, would be more effective. At other times social reinforcers may be so multiply endowed that a primary reinforcer may be necessary to gain an immediate response from the client.

The first situation, that of nonobservance or nonresponse to social attention, is seen in a client who has been institutionalized for several years and gives no sign that he is aware of others. A piece of sugarless chewing gum contingently delivered for eye contact will be more effective than social attention. A goal of treatment for such a client is the development of social attention as a reinforcer. This is done by pairing the primary reinforcer, chewing gum, with social attention, then occasionally reinforcing with only social attention, and finally reinforcing with social attention and infrequently with a primary reinforcer.

The second situation, mutual anger and rejection, can be seen between an adolescent with a long history of behavior problems and his parents, whose many interventions have failed. In other words, the parents have received little reinforcement for parenting from the child. The child has received little reinforcement for being their child. Reinforcers of choice may be money, privileges, or activities.

Multiply endowed reinforcers are constantly occurring, as in a young child who has many persons laughing at his misdeeds. The child will probably not be aware of a change in the quality of attention of one person if many are laughing, but he will notice if he receives a favorite treat when he behaves differently.

In each of the situations just described, primary reinforcers should be accompanied by social reinforcers. Eventually the social reinforcers alone will maintain appropriate behaviors as the primary reinforcers are gradually decreased.

■ **REINFORCEMENT SCHEDULES.** Another consideration is the timing of the data collection and the schedule of reinforcement. In the example of the child prescribed to have bed rest, the data were collected and the reinforcement was delivered (if Carole was in bed) every 30 minutes. Reinforcement can be delivered according to a time schedule, as in this example, or according to a performance schedule. The time schedule is called **interval schedule reinforcement;** the performance schedule is called **ratio schedule reinforcement** (see accompanying box on p. 803, which describes simple reinforcement schedules). Each type can be delivered on a fixed or variable schedule. An in-

terval schedule refers to reinforcement being presented for the first designated behavior after a given period. If it is a fixed interval (FI) schedule, the time period is stable (e.g., every 5 minutes or, as in the example of Carole, 30 minutes). If a variable interval (VI) schedule is used, an average time lapse is designated (e.g., 30 minutes), as well as a minimum and maximum interval.

Behavior performance varies according to the reinforcement schedule (see box). On an FI schedule the operant increases just before the end of the interval and then, after reinforcement, decreases. One could predict that if Carole is checked and reinforced every 30 minutes, she will get out of bed soon after being checked and given staff attention. She will then get into bed shortly before she thinks she will be checked again. If a VI schedule is employed, behavior is more consistent. If Carole cannot predict when she will be reinforced, she is more likely to remain in bed.

A fixed ratio (FR) schedule refers to reinforcement being provided after an operant is performed a designated number of times. A variable ratio (VR) schedule refers to reinforcement of the performance of an operant a predetermined average number of times. The minimum and maximum number of times is established.

FR and VR schedules result in higher rates of responding and greater resistance to extinction than either FI or VI schedules. If this fact is overlooked in clinical practice, treatment effectiveness is short lived. Consider a child in residential treatment whose major problem is hitting peers in response to being teased. The child is taught an alternative response to being teased and is heavily praised every hour if he has engaged in the alternative response. This treatment is effective and the child is discharged. Suddenly the child is receiving no praise for his relatively new skill. He quickly resorts to his previous immediate feedback system of hitting.

While the child was in treatment, the reinforcement schedule could easily have been altered to a variable ratio. The average ratio would gradually increase until the reinforcement was being received at a rate closely approximating that in the natural environment. The child would thereafter have a greater chance at permanently incorporating his new skill.

■ **SELECTING A REINFORCEMENT SCHEDULE.** The choice of reinforcement schedules during clinical intervention depends on the severity of the presenting problem, the intended duration of the operant to be learned, the age of the client, the number of available persons, and many other factors. If the presenting problem behavior is life threatening, one pref-

Simple Reinforcement Schedules

Type of schedule

Time or interval: Time lapse between behaviors before reinforcement

Fixed interval: Specific lapse of time required for reinforcement (e.g., every 5 minutes, every month, every hour, paychecks)

Variable interval: Various amounts of time elapse between possible reinforcement (e.g., 1 minute, 32 minutes, 3 hours, 5 minutes)

Performance or ratio: Number of times an operant is performed between reinforcement

Fixed ratio: Same number of responses required for each reinforcement (e.g., for every fifth performance of operant, piecework in factory)

Variable ratio: Various numbers of responses required for each reinforcement (e.g., after 3, 10, 11, 19, 29, 33, 35 performances of operant; slot machines)

Characteristics of schedule

Fixed interval (FI)

High rate of performance before interval ends; low rate after reinforcement, the rate gradually accelerating until interval ends

Response to extinction: Responding ceases abruptly, recurs at a high rate, ceases, and recurs, with pauses increasing until rate is zero; relatively susceptible to extinction

Variable interval (VI)

Stable high rate of performance, rate lower than VR schedule

Response to extinction: Steadily decreasing rate until response is zero; of all simple schedules, most susceptible to extinction

Fixed ratio (FR)

Quickly developed high rate of performance; rate stable; especially if ratio is small

Response to extinction: Alternating pauses and high performance rate, the pause increasing until ratio is zero; relatively resistant to extinction

Variable ratio (VR)

High rate of performance, developing less quickly than FR; high rate stable even if average ratio is relatively high, except when average ratio is increased too quickly

Response to extinction: Responses continue at high sustained rate with alternating pauses until pauses lengthen and rate gradually reaches zero; of the simple schedules, most resistant to extinction

---

erably designs an FR schedule with a very small ratio, graduates slowly to a VR schedule with a small average ratio, and then slowly increases the average of VR reinforcement. For example, a child with poor judgment runs away from a residential treatment center several times a day. While away, he engages in such behaviors as fire setting, theft, and running into heavy traffic. The initial FR schedule might reinforce him every time he walked by, instead of running out of, an exit door. The schedule is altered to every second time he walks by an exit door, then every third, then gradually a VR schedule is introduced.

The intended duration of the operant influences the choice of schedule. In Carole's case there is a time limit on her bed rest requirement; a small-interval FI schedule is likely to result in Carole rapidly learning to be in bed as the interval end approaches, although after reinforcement she is likely to get out of bed. The advantage is that Carole is receiving reinforcement for appropriate behavior. As the reinforcement becomes more important to her, a VI schedule is introduced, ensuring her remaining in bed more constantly. The VI schedule is appropriate, since one need not be concerned with the operant of staying in bed as necessary for a long period. Operants reinforced on a VI schedule cease quickly when reinforcement is withheld (extinction). Also, busy staff in a hospital setting seem more likely to provide reinforcement on the VI schedules.

On the other hand, if the treatment goal is a child's learning appropriate classroom behavior, the ratio schedules seem more desirable. These are operants that will prove helpful to the child for many years. The reinforcement schedule should be one that will result in the operant's resistance to extinction, as well as its maintenance by the reinforcers that will occur in the natural environment.

The age of the child affects the rapidity with

which the fixed schedules can be increased in ratio and interval length and with which they can be changed to variable schedules. A 2-year-old learns operants rapidly. The new behavior may be maintained simply by reinforcers as they occur in the natural environment in a few days. By the time a child is 4 years old, it seems to take longer. By adolescence, the reinforcement history is so long and complex that months of intervention may be necessary before reinforcers in the natural environment can maintain newly learned operants.

The number of persons available to apply reinforcement schedules and the number of persons in treatment affect the schedule chosen. In general, ratio schedules require more persons because behaviors must be counted. Token economies in psychiatric hospitals and residential treatment centers are an approach in which the patient receives a token for the operant. Tokens can be spent for privileges or goods. Token economies usually are designed on FI and VI schedules. The number of staff needed to provide reinforcers on an FR or VR schedule to 20 to 50 clients would be exorbitant. Although the general reinforcement design of token economies is interval schedules, some provision is usually made for ratio schedules.

■ **Decreasing behavior**

Punishment and extinction are the operant procedures used to decrease behaviors. Most behaviorists do not recommend punishment except in situations in which the behavior is physically dangerous. There is no question about the effectiveness of punishment. There is question about the concomitant effects of punishment, and ethical considerations do not make punishment a desirable treatment. A behaviorist is not likely to recommend hitting a child, except in situations in which his behavior must be immediately altered for his safety. If a young child, for example, runs into a busy street or picks up a sharp knife, the parent wants the child to immediately alter this behavior.

Extinction, withholding what was previously reinforcing an operant, is recommended while positive reinforcement is provided for an incompatible behavior. For example, a patient may express many nonsequential and nonsense remarks that make conversation impossible. The psychiatric nurse may note that typically when this happens, the staff person comments on this to the patient and talks to him about the irrelevant material. She observes that this may be reinforcing the nonsense talk. She instructs all staff to ignore such statements, bring the conversation back to the topic at hand, and give the patient attention for attending to the topic. Extinction is being used for the irrelevant material, and positive reinforcement for relevant con-

CLINICAL EXAMPLE 27-1

Joe, a 7-year-old child, was in serious jeopardy of being removed from his home because of his playing with matches and setting fires. It was agreed that treatment would be limited to 5 days from 9:30 AM to 12 PM and from 1 to 3 PM while the child continued to live at home. Within the 2 years preceding treatment, he set three fires that caused damage, the last fire precipitating the referral. The mother and family were frightened but did not reject the child.

Prior consultation and experience with a satiation procedure treatment suggested that intensive use of the procedure might be more effective than daily 1-hour sessions. The satiation procedure for fire setting involved the client lighting and blowing out matches one by one in a well-ventilated room in the presence of the therapist. The therapist supervised the activity, maintaining minimum verbal interaction, neither reinforcing nor punishing the child as he lit the matches. Records were kept of the endeavor.

On the first treatment day, Joe lit matches during two sessions for a total of 4 hours. More than a thousand matches were lit and blown out during this time. The child's initial response to being allowed to light matches was surprise and some confusion. It was explained that it was all right for him to light the matches only in this particular room. His rate of lighting matches remained relatively constant. The mean number lit during intervals of 5 minutes was 34, the range from 22 to 45, the mode 34, and the median 33.

Observation of Joe outside the satiation sessions revealed how much he enjoyed being praised and hugged, as well as his affinity for all social contact. Joe initiated interpersonal interactions frequently, laughed and talked while playing with peers, and often sought physical affection from staff. These observations supplied data useful in Joe's subsequent treatment sessions.

On the second day Joe lit matches for only 55 minutes; the mean rate for a 5-minute interval dropped to 21, the range being 15 to 27, the mode 20, and the median 22. During this session Joe tried avoidance maneuvers, wanting to practice throwing matches away, and stating at least five times, "I don't want to strike more." Each time he made the statement, he was told quietly, "Keep doing it." Finally, he stated firmly, "I ain't gonna strike no more" and walked away from the matches.

CLINICAL EXAMPLE 27-1—cont'd

This was greeted with a hug and praise from the nurse and a discussion with him about alternative treatment. Joe then identified, in response to questions, several areas in his home where he found matches. A book of matches was placed on the window, and Joe then rehearsed, both physically and verbally, finding the matches in a specific place at home. Initially he was not instructed what to do with the book of matches. After picking it up, he opened the book and the therapist immediately yelled, "No!" Joe replaced the matches, went through the rehearsal a second time, and the same sequence occurred. At the third rehearsal he was instructed to say aloud, "I'm not going to open up the matches," when he approached them. When he did so, he did not pick up the matches and was given a hug. Joe looked elated. His pleasure with himself increased as the rehearsals went on for over an hour and covered in his own imagery every place in his house where he could find matches.

Throughout the rehearsals several changes relating to his self-cueing and the reinforcers were gradually and progressively introduced. By the session's close, the self-cueing was inaudible and the reinforcing hug was being imagined each time he picked up and replaced a book of matches. Joe's facial expressions were so spontaneous and revealing that they left no doubt about his repeating the cue to himself and fantasizing the hugs.

These alterations were developed to increase the likelihood of Joe's continuing the behavior when not in the therapist's presence. The change from not picking up the book of matches to picking it up and replacing it was introduced to break the behavior chain of picking up matches, pulling out a match, and lighting it. It seemed important for Joe to realize that he could see and pick up matches without lighting them. Although not of major concern in comparison to fire setting, consideration was given to the possibility of the child developing a phobia of matches. A phobic response seemed more likely if he learned not to touch a book of matches. Being able to hold the matches and replace them made matches simply another object in his environment over which he had control.

On the following day, when Joe entered the room, the equipment for the satiation procedure was still in the room. Since Joe spent a few minutes looking at it, it was suggested to him that he again light the matches. Because the environmental conditions were vastly different from the previous day's rehearsal and because Joe's expression indicated a curiosity about lighting the matches, it was appropriate to continue the satiation.

The satiation session was 55 minutes long, 158 matches were lit. The 5-minute mean was 15, the range 0 to 25, the mode 20, and the median 15. During the last 10 minutes no matches were lit. There was also a qualitative difference in this session. After the first 5 minutes, during which Joe lit 25 matches, he was increasingly bored and disinterested.

The rehearsals were then started and Joe was again lively, spontaneous, and happy in his endeavor. The rehearsals were broadened to include areas outside his home where he might find matches. Joe and the therapist then went throughout the building, where he found and replaced many books of matches after the activity was explained to the occupant of each office. The social contacts, needless to say, were reinforcing to Joe, and he was lavished with encouragement and praise (perhaps too much) for his efforts.

During these rehearsals, Joe was instructed to imagine his mother giving him a hug when he replaced the matches. Since it was his mother who would be giving him real hugs in the future, it would be easier over time for him to fantasize a hug from her. His image of the therapist would dim as the actual contact became a progressively distant memory.

On the final treatment day, Joe showed no interest in the satiation equipment. Some time was spent on the rehearsals, but the major portion of the day Joe devoted to good-byes and playing with peers. The mother, who could not attend any of the sessions, was informed of the treatment and instructed to give Joe affection and praise periodically for not playing with matches. Phone contact with her was continued for 3 weeks. Follow-up contacts over 2 years indicate that Joe has neither played with matches nor set fires since treatment.

versation. Whenever extinction is used, one should be careful to ensure that reinforcement is given for a behavior that is incompatible with the one being treated by extinction.

Clinical case analysis

Clinical example 27-1 describes behavioral treatment initiated and carried out by a nurse.

The procedures used in this treatment were behavioral and included punishment, satiation behavior rehearsal, overt differential reinforcement, and covert positive reinforcement. The punishment was the "no" yelled at Joe as he opened the book of matches when the behavior rehearsal started. This punishment was almost immediately effective, having to be used only twice.

We experience satiation when overdoing a good thing. We may frequent a favorite restaurant so often that we are tired of it or overindulge in a food until we do not want to see it again. This is satiation. Some theorists assert that the effects of satiation are temporary. Satiation was certain to inhibit Joe's current interests in matches. The possibility that satiation's effects are temporary necessitated the development of the behavior rehearsal. In the behavior rehearsal Joe practiced an alternative response to matches, which could be reinforced. The practice response was incompatible with lighting a match; the reinforcement of this response was gradually altered from overt to covert so that it would not be dependent on others. The covert reinforcement was also important because Joe had played with matches and set the fires when he was alone. Future interest in match play and fire lighting would probably occur when Joe was alone. Having experienced covert reinforcement would probably help him resist returning to his former play with matches.

Ethical issues

Behavior modification intervention has raised many ethical issues, mostly because of behavior therapists' assertion that they can change behavior. In addition, behavior modification techniques can be applied to the environment and result in behavior change. All psychiatric treatments have at least a component of behavior change as their goal. Therefore it is not behavior change itself that has resulted in behavior modification being questioned on ethical grounds. It is that the behavior change can be caused by alterations of environmental responses to the behavior. Other psychotherapies seem to do so by working directly with the client, not the environment. Therefore it seems that they alter nothing for a client without his direct cooperation and knowledge. The possibility of using behavioral techniques without such involvement requires special consideration.

The techniques that have been presented in this chapter are indeed effective, not always, not everywhere, but they are effective. The most basic issues related to them at present are the following: Does one human being have the right to control another? Who decides the goals of treatment? Other issues arise as well, such as obtaining client consent, guaranteeing basic human rights, weighing potential risks and benefits of treatment, evaluating treatment, and being accountable for treatment.

The two major issues of control and goals of treatment are explored here. Control is a strong word; it arouses fear in most people when they think they are being controlled by others. It arouses anger when people in power are seen to be abusing their power by controlling others. This word carries a connotation of totality, a totality that allows no escape.

In a society, people seem to expect that certain human behaviors be controlled. Some of these behaviors are murder, theft, assault, and property destruction. Laws are established to ensure compliance, and a judicial system is responsible for punishing the violators of the laws. Basically these laws state that a person may not abuse others or their property.

Beyond these behaviors, the issues become less clear. What about emotional abuse: the way in which one slowly or quickly pecks away at another through ridicule, sarcasm, disapproval, or bitterness? Should this be controlled? Would a society in which people are encouraged, supported, openly disagreed with, and congratulated be preferred? Many people would prefer such a society, but few would want such behaviors legislated or designed into the judicial system and controlled by a behavioral engineer. This is not desired because it would increase the government's power. History documents how easily power is abused.

Although most behavior therapists have a treatment goal of specific and limited behavioral change, this does not alter the fear that behavioral technology could, in the wrong hands, be abused. Such is the case in every scientific advance. Does this mean that it should not be used at all? No, it means that one must use knowledge carefully and spread information about the technology as widely as possible so that use and abuse of the knowledge can be readily recognized. This is particularly helpful, since all people are affected by the reinforcers and punishments in the environment. As behavioral technology has become more widely understood, this fear of control by others has decreased. This is because familiarity with it and with its ensuing application increases each person's control of himself. It is also becoming more evident that behavioral techniques indicate how one is influenced, not controlled, by the environment. Influence allows for a wide range of choices.

The specification of goals can be complex. Ideally the goals of treatment are the client's goals. In reality a client's goals may be at odds with those of the therapist. The therapist must establish goals that please both client and therapist. An extreme example of conflicting goals would be a parent's request that a behavioral therapist design a program with the goal that a 4-year-old child would sit silently in a chair 4 hours a day. No competent therapist could agree to such a goal. The therapist in such a situation may spend much time helping the parent establish more reasonable goals. The goal of the therapist during this time is the development of reasonable parental goals. However, is this use of time unethical because it is clearly not the parent's goal? This question is nonsensical; however, it points out that recommending client input into goals is not as simple as it may appear. The client who is actively hallucinating or contentedly masturbating for hours on end may want only to remain in such a state. It is most unlikely that a therapist could share

this same goal. Pesut suggests outcome specification as an alternative to goal setting.[7]

With these and other issues in mind, it is possible to offer general guidelines for the ethical use of behavioral modification:

1. Treatment is to be preceded by informed consent; specification of procedure, goals, and measures to be taken; and client input.
2. Once begun, treatment should include an ongoing assessment of progress.
3. Before and during treatment the therapist should recognize that the treatment should be relevant to the client's adjustment to his natural environment.

These guidelines are not complete answers. However, they may help to prevent potential abuses of therapy and contribute to client growth. These are worthwhile pursuits for all therapy modalities used by psychiatric nurses.

■ SUGGESTED CROSS-REFERENCES ■

Ethical decision making is discussed in Chapter 7. Child psychiatric nursing is discussed in Chapter 30. Adolescent psychiatric nursing is discussed in Chapter 31.

■ SUMMARY ■

1. Behavior modification is the application of operant conditioning principles and procedures to human affairs. Operant conditioning is modification of the frequency of occurrence of a bit of behavior by the consequences of that behavior.

2. Behavior modification is an effective treatment modality for alleviating many human problems, and it can be used by psychiatric nurses in many areas of their practice.

3. Behavior refers to everything a person does and is observable. Behavior may be defined in specific or general terms. Specific measurable definition facilitates behavior modification.

4. Behavior modification techniques may be applied to increase or decrease the occurrence of behavior. Positive reinforcement and negative reinforcement both maintain and increase behavior. Positive punishment, negative punishment, and extinction decrease behavior. Negative punishment includes response costs and timeout from reinforcement.

5. Reinforcement schedules may be based on fixed or variable intervals or fixed or variable ratios of reinforcement. Fixed and variable rate (FR and VR) schedules result in higher rates of responding and greater resistance to extinction than either fixed or variable interval (FI or VI) schedules.

6. An example is given of the use of behavior modifica-

DIRECTIONS FOR FUTURE RESEARCH

The following are some of the nursing research problems raised in Chapter 27 that merit further study by psychiatric nurses:
1. Validate composites of behavior amenable to behavior treatment
2. Identify long-term outcomes of behaviorally oriented milieus versus psychodynamically oriented milieus
3. Compare outcomes of patient-determined reinforcers versus staff-determined reinforcers
4. Describe outcomes associated with teaching patients behavioral principles
5. Correlate noncontingent nursing behaviors with improved treatment effectiveness
6. Describe reinforcers that staff inadvertently provide for maladaptive behaviors
7. Explore effective change mechanisms used by staff for eliminating inadvertent reinforcement of maladaptive patient behaviors
8. Report effects of nurse-monitored, but patient-initiated and patient-implemented behavioral self-treatment
9. Examine mother/child relationships in which prenatal teaching includes behavioral principles

tion techniques by a nurse in therapy with a fire-setting child.

7. The techniques of behavior modification have raised many ethical issues. The two major issues of control and goals of treatment are explored. General guidelines for the ethical use of behavior modification are presented.

■ REFERENCES ■

1. Ayllon T and Azrin N: The measurement and reinforcement of behavior of psychotics, J Exp Anal Behav 8:35, 1965.
2. Ayllon T and Azrin N: The token economy, New York, 1968, Appleton-Century-Crofts.
3. Heide F and Borhovec TD: Relaxation-induced anxiety: mechanisms and theoretical implications, Behav Res Ther 22:1, 1984.
4. Mathews SJ: Nothing to fear but fear, Nurs Times 84:28, July 13, 1988.
5. Moones A: Frightened of fear, Nurs Times 83:13, April 1, 1987.
6. Mikulas WL: Behavior modification, New York, 1978, Harper and Row, Publishers, Inc.
7. Pesut DJ: Aim versus blame, J Psychosoc Nurs Ment Health Serv 27:5, 1989.
8. Reynolds GS: A primer of operant condition, Glenview, Ill, 1968, Scott, Foresman and Co.
9. Skinner BF: Science and human behavior, New York, 1953, The Free Press.

■ ANNOTATED SUGGESTED READINGS ■

Arkin AM et al: Behavior modification: present status in psychiatry, NY State J Med 76:190, 1976.

Provides a comprehensive overview of the many issues related to behavior modification. Introduces the types of behavior modification approaches. Discusses ethical issues related to this therapeutic modality, particularly when aversive techniques are used.

Behavioral Disorders, Lancaster, Pa. Quarterly journal of the Council for Children with Behavioral Disorders.

Oriented toward special education teachers. Helpful for psychiatric nurses working with children and adolescents.

Behavior Modification, Beverly Hills, Calif, Sage Publication.

Interdisciplinary journal published four times a year on research and clinical studies of applied behavior modification in a broad scope of settings.

Behavior Research and Therapy, Great Britain, Pergamon Press, Ltd.

Bimonthly, international, interdisciplinary journal relates the application of behavior theory to maladaptive behaviors.

*Berni R and Fordyce WE: Behavior modification and the nursing process, ed 2, St Louis, 1977, Mosby–Year Book, Inc.

Particularly recommended is the chapter on ethical issues. Appropriate for all levels of nursing students.

Dobson KS, editor: Handbook of cognitive-behavioral therapies, New York, 1988, The Guilford Press.

Excellent text for graduate students and practicing clinical nurse specialists.

*Hauser MJ: Cognition commands change, J Psychiatr Nurs 19:19, 1981.

Discusses cognitive models of behavioral change as they relate to work with disturbed children. Models include cognitive restructuring, as exemplified by rational-emotive therapy, self-instruction, and problem solving. Advocates teaching the treatment approach to parents. Cognitive restructuring and self-instruction are rather sophisticated methodologies that should only be implemented by nurses with advanced training in child psychiatric nursing.

Journal of Applied Behavior Analysis, Lawrence, Kan, Society for the Experimental Analysis of Behavior, Inc.

Quarterly journal primarily covering experimental research.

Journal of Behavior Therapy and Experimental Psychiatry, Great Britain, Pergamon Press, Ltd.

Quarterly journal on behavior therapy and experimental psychiatry.Also relevant for nonbehaviorally educated clinicians.

Lazarus AA: Multimodel behavior therapy: treating the "basic id." In Franks M and Wilson GT, editors: Annual review of behavior therapy theory and practice, New York, 1974, Brunner/Mazel, Inc.

Appropriate for graduate students. Assumes basic knowledge of behavioral principles and their application.

Mikulas WL: Behavior modification, New York, 1976, Harper and Row, Publishers, Inc.

Provides overview of the field of behavior treatment. Recommended for both undergraduate and graduate students.

*Peterson KA and Erickson EA: Use of reinforcement principles to reinstate self-care activities in a deaf and blind psychiatric patient, J Psychiatr Nurs 15:15, 1977.

Illustrates the application of behavior modification principles to the care of one patient withchallenging nursing care problems. A detailed discussion of nursing intervention and patient response.

*Asterisk indicates nursing reference.

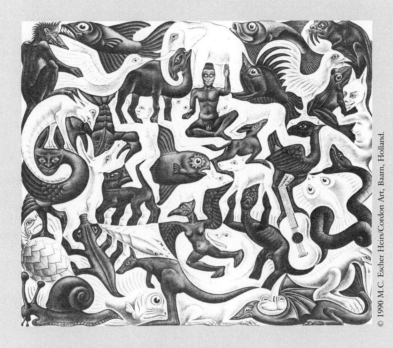

*Self and world are correlated, and so are
individualization and participation. . .
Participation means: being a part of something from
which one is, at the same time, separated.*

Paul Tillich, The Courage To Be

C H A P T E R   28

SMALL GROUPS AND THEIR THERAPEUTIC FORCES

PAULA C. LASALLE
ARTHUR J. LASALLE

LEARNING OBJECTIVES

After studying this chapter, the student should be able to:

- define a group.

- compare and contrast the various types of groups, including identification of the nurse's role with each.

- identify and describe the two basic functions of groups.

- analyze group process in terms of the dynamic dimensions of communication, roles, norms, cohesion, and power.

- identify the four stages of group development.

- discuss the therapeutic aspects of group experiences.

- compare and contrast informal, therapeutic, and psychotherapeutic groups, describing indications for each and differentiating leadership roles.

- describe a variety of group psychotherapy models and theoretical frameworks.

- discuss the phases of development of a psychotherapy group, including therapist responsibilities and typically encountered group behaviors.

- identify the need for nursing research relative to the therapeutic use of groups.

- identify directions for future nursing research.

- select appropriate readings for further study.

"There seems to be no agent more effective than another person in bringing a world for oneself alive, or, by a glance, a gesture, or a remark, shriveling up the reality in which one is lodged."[10]

Likewise, Lewin[13] observed in 1947 that individuals under certain conditions are influenced more easily in group rather than individual settings. Groups have been increasingly studied and used, and today they are an essential part of a nurse's repertoire of therapeutic skills. Health professionals, administrators, and the public have accepted groups as an effective, efficient methodology for the treatment of a wide range of problems. To lead a group requires an understanding of its component parts and its developmental processes. Also, the nurse needs supervised practice in group leadership to become skilled and comfortable in handling the group's complex nature.

Definition

A basic definition of a group is a collection of individuals who have a relationship with one another, are interdependent, and may have common norms.

Therapeutic groups have a shared purpose, for example, to help members who consistently put themselves into destructive relationships to identify and change codependent behaviors. Each group has its own structure and identity. The power of the group lies in the contributions of each member and the leader to the shared purpose of the group. These contributions are content and process oriented. Content functions of the groups are fulfilled when each member shares his or her own experiences and explanations to help another member. When members share the methods they used to solve a common problem, they are assisting each other with the group's content functions.

Process functions allow the individual member to receive feedback from other members and the leader as to how the member operates and is perceived within the group. The group is used as a practice laboratory or an arena to see, experiment, and define relationships and behaviors. For example, a member who complains that his or her spouse is always accusing the member of being domineering may receive feedback from the group as to whether other members see that person acting in similar ways in the group. The person then has the opportunity to work on changing his or her behavior in the group and then risking the change in the outside world.

The group has primary and secondary tasks. The primary task is necessary for the group's survival or existence; secondary, or ancillary, tasks may enhance the group but are not basic to its survival.[17] An example of a primary task for a group of mothers might be to gain further mothering skills; a secondary task might be to improve the mother's social network. The psychosocial aspect of the group may either impede or enhance the group's willingness to share concerns regarding mothering.

Groups as a potential therapeutic tool

To be effective in therapeutic group work, one must understand the complex processes that occur in small groups and be able to use various approaches to increase the therapeutic potential of the group for its members. This chapter focuses on these processes and approaches only as they relate to small groups. The study of large groups, such as ward or community meetings, is beyond the scope of this chapter.

■ Group structure

Group structure refers to the group's underlying order. It describes the boundaries, communication and decision-making processes, and authority relationships within the group. The structure offers the group stability and helps to regulate behavioral and interactional patterns.

■ Group size

The size of an interpersonally oriented group is seven to 10 members. The group must have enough people to give members the opportunity for consensual validation, as well as the expression of different viewpoints. If the group has too many people, all members will not be given enough time to speak and some will feel excluded. There will also be insufficient time to analyze and discuss interactions. If the group has too few members, not enough sharing and interaction can occur.

■ Length of sessions

The optimum length of a session is 45 to 60 minutes for fragile, or lower-functioning, groups and 90 to 120 minutes for higher-functioning ones. For 15 to 30 minutes the group warms to the task of working, then spends approximately an hour of work time, and finally summarizes and takes care of "unfinished business" from that session for 10 to 15 minutes

■ Communication

One of the group leader's primary tasks is to observe and analyze the communication patterns within the group. Using feedback, the leader helps members become aware of the group dynamics and communication patterns so that they may realize the significance of these patterns for the group and for them individually. The group or individual members may then experiment and may change these patterns if they choose to do so.

Observable verbal and nonverbal elements of the group's communication include (1) individual member communications, (2) spatial and seating arrangements, (3) common themes expressed by the group, (4) how frequently and to whom members communicate, (5) how members are listened to in the group, and (6) what problem-solving processes occur in the group. These aspects help the leader assess resistance within the group, interpersonal conflict, the roles assumed by some of the members, the level of competition, and the degree to which the members understand and are working on the task.

■ Roles

In studying groups, it is important to observe what roles members assume in the group. Each role has certain expected behaviors and responsibilities.

The role a member assumes can be determined by observing the communication and behavioral patterns of that member while in the group. The following factors influence role selection: the member's personality, the group's tasks and their significance to a member, the interaction in the group, and the individual's position in the group. Benne and Sheats[2] catalogued three major types of roles individuals can play in groups: (1) building or maintenance roles, which involve the group processes and functions; (2) task roles, which deal with completing the group's task; and (3) individual roles, which are not related to the group's tasks or maintenance and may be self-centered and distracting for the group. These roles are summarized in Table 28-1. A person in a maintenance role, for example, would act as a harmonizer and peacemaker. A person in a task role might clarify and seek new information. The importance of group maintenance and task roles has been observed by Bales and Slater,[1] whose studies demonstrate evidence that groups encourage members to specialize in one of these two role functions.

Persons may experience a conflict when a discrepancy exists between the role they seek or assume and the role ascribed to them by the group. For example, a member may be expected to be a peacemaker because that is what he did in the past. Now, however, this member may be under additional stress or angry with someone in the group and may choose to start rather than resolve conflict. The group will often be confused and upset by this new role.

TABLE 28-1

GROUP ROLES AND FUNCTIONS

Maintenance Roles	Function in Group
Encourager	To be positive influence on the group
Harmonizer	To make/keep peace
Compromiser	To minimize conflict by seeking alternatives
Gatekeeper	To determine level of group acceptance of individual members
Follower	To serve as interested audience
Rule maker	To set standards for group behaviors (e.g., time, dress)
Problem solver	To solve problems to allow group to continue its work

Task Roles	Function in Group
Leader	To set direction
Questioner	To clarify issues and information
Facilitator	To keep group focused
Summarizer	To state current position of the group
Evaluator	To assess performance of the group
Initiator	To begin group discussion

Individual Roles	Function for Individual
Victim	To deflect responsibility from self
Monopolizer	To actively seek control by incessant talking
Seducer	To maintain distance and gain personal attention
Mute	To seek control passively through silence
Complainer	To discourage positive work and ventilate anger
Truant/late comer	To invalidate significance of the group
Moralist	To serve as judge of right and wrong

Chart is extrapolated from structure provided by Benne KD and Sheats P: J Soc Issues 4(2):41, 1948.

■ Power

Power is the member's ability to influence the group and its other members. The power structure in the group is usually resolved in its initial stages. To determine the power of various members, it is helpful to assess which member(s) receive the most attention, which are listened to most, and which make decisions for the group.

Resolution of the power struggle does not necessarily mean, however, that everyone will be satisfied with the arrangement. Sometimes a continual struggle for power occurs within the group. Such a struggle may be functional if the members are trying to attain new leadership that is more conducive to their therapeutic goals. It can also be dysfunctional in that it takes the group's energy and attention away from other tasks.

■ Norms

Norms are standards of behavior adhered to by the group. They are expectations of how the group will act in the future based on its past and present experiences. It is important to understand norms because they influence the quality of communication and interaction within the group. The observance of norms results in conforming. The member who does not follow the norms may be considered rebellious or resistant by the other group members. Conforming to group norms is considered essential to being a fully accepted member. A member who continuously comes late to meetings that the group has decided will start on time is nonconforming to group norms. The group will decide to what extent it will tolerate this behavior.

Norms are created to facilitate accomplishment of the group's goal(s) or tasks, control interpersonal conflict, interpret social reality, and foster group interdependence.

Norms may be communicated overtly or covertly. Overt expression of norms may be written or clearly stated. For example, members may tell a new member that smoking is not allowed in the group. Covert expression of norms may be implied through members' behaviors. For example, a member who uses foul language may be ignored by the other members. It must be noted that a highly cohesive group may have appropriate or inappropriate norms. For example, a group of patients may unite to help a patient sneak a cigarette when such behavior is contraindicated because of that patient's health problems. The group may also unite to do what it can to prevent that patient from smoking.

■ Cohesion

Cohesiveness is the strength of the members' desire to work together toward common goals. It acts on members to remain in the group. It is related to the attraction to and the satisfaction derived from the group by each member. Cohesiveness is a basic fiber of any group because it affects its life span and success.[5]

Many factors contribute to the level of cohesiveness, including agreement of members on group goals, interpersonal attractiveness between the members, degree to which the group satisfies individual needs, similarities among members, and satisfaction of members with the leadership style. Since cohesion is such an important dimension, some group leader interventions are aimed toward promoting cohesiveness. Methods used to foster cohesion include encouraging members to talk directly with each other, discussing the group in "we" terms, and encouraging all members to be in similar spatial arrangements, for example, not permitting some members to move their chairs away from the group. A leader can also promote cohesion by pointing out similarities among group members, assisting members in listening to each other, and encouraging cooperation among the members.

The group leader continually monitors the level of cohesiveness in the group. Group leaders might observe to what degree members express interest in each other and recognize each other for their individuality. Another way to measure cohesion is to determine the degree of member identity with the group as a whole and the expression of members' desire to remain in the group.

Group development

Groups, as with individuals, have an innate capacity for growth and development. Likewise, they have an ability to regress and to resist working effectively. Small groups are recognized as having various definable stages of group development. Bennis and Sheppard[3] studied these phases in sensitivity groups and theorized that central concepts of group development are dependent and interdependent issues. The authors relied heavily on Freudian theory and viewed the issues of power, authority, and intimacy as important to the group's life.

Martin and Hill[16] studied the various phases of psychotherapy groups. They described six phases of group development, ranging from the individual's unshared behaviors to the individual's use of a group as an effective and creative problem-solving agent. Schutz[22] stated that every group developed according to three sequential interpersonal states: inclusion, or being "in or out"; control, or being "top or bottom"; and affection, or being "near or far." Each stage is characterized by members expressing various aspects of the same interpersonal issue or conflict.

Tuckman[25] believed that any group is concerned with the completion of the task. He referred to the group structure as the interpersonal relationships among the members and task activity as the interactions directly related to the task. Tuckman summarized the various phases of group development as forming, storming, norming, and performing. These phases have been confirmed in at least one research study that observed groups in a classroom setting.[21] Table 28-2

TABLE 28-2

DEVELOPMENTAL PHASES IN SMALL GROUPS

Phases	Definition	Task activity	Interpersonal activity
Forming	Group members concerned with orientation	To identify task and boundaries regarding it	Relationships tested; interpersonal boundaries identified; dependent relationship with leaders, other group members, or preexisting standards established
Storming	Group members resistive to task and group influence	To respond emotionally to task	Intragroup conflict
Norming	Resistance to group overcome by members	To express intimate personal opinions around task	New roles adopted; new standards evolved in group feelings; cohesiveness developed
Performing	Creative problem solving done; solutions emerge	To direct group energy toward completion of task	Interpersonal structure of group becomes tool to achieve its task; roles become flexible and functional

Modified from Tuckman B: Psychol Bull 63:384, 1965.

summarizes Tuckman's categories and model.

Tuckman did not mention the termination phase. In a reclassification of Tuckman's theory of development, Lacoursiere (as cited by Dolgoff[7]) proposed that a mourning phase be added and combined in the norming stage with the performing and storming phases. Termination occurs when the group dissolves because the task is accomplished. It may also occur when interpersonal issues prevent the group from accomplishing its task.

Group development does not occur in distinct phases. Phases may overlap each other, and a group may regress to a previous phase. For example, group regression can occur with the addition of a new member. Phases of group development can be thought of as a path that a group takes to form and accomplish its objectives. The leader's task is to understand and assist the group as it moves along its growth path.

Group stages

■ Pregroup phase

An important factor to consider in starting a group is its goal or goals. The group's purpose will greatly influence many of the leadership behaviors. There may be more than one group goal; if so, the primary goal should be clearly identified. To guarantee success, the group's goals must be clearly understood by all persons involved, including the members and sponsoring agencies. An essential task of the leader is to clarify and assist the group in achieving its purpose. An example of a group goal would be to provide support for each member, all of whom share a similar characteristic, such as victims of spousal abuse.

Once the purpose is established, the leader must be certain that the group has administrative permission. A written group proposal is one effective way to discuss the group with the administration. The box below lists information to include in a group proposal. To avoid possible problems, the therapist should determine if any administrative limitations exist. For example, an agency may not permit a group to meet beyond its physical facilities or may prefer that the therapist not use certain techniques in the group. Also, any financial cost factors to the agency should be clearly identified.

The leader is also responsible for securing the physical space for the group. In choosing a room, the leader identifies the room requirements needed by the group. For example, in a therapeutic group where teaching will take place, educational resources such as a blackboard or movie projector may be needed. Likewise, a psychotherapy group may need space for comfortable chairs to be placed in a circle without a table. In a group that plans to use human relations exercises, a more spacious room will probably be needed. In all

---

Group Proposal Guideline

1. List the group goal(s).
   a. Primary goal
   b. Secondary goal
2. List group leader(s) and their related expertise.
3. List theoretical framework(s) utilized by the leader(s) to meet the group goals.
4. List criteria for membership.
5. Describe the referral and screening process.
6. Describe the structure of the group.
   a. Meeting place _____
   b. Meeting time _____
   c. Length of each meeting _____
   d. Number of members _____
   e. Length of group _____
   f. Expected member behaviors _____
   g. Expected leader behaviors _____
7. Describe the evaluation process for members and the group.
8. Describe resources needed for the group, such as coffee, a movie projector, or audiovisual equipment.
9. If pertinent, describe the expected cost and financial benefits incurred by the group.

cases the room in which the group meets should be comfortable, private, and free from intrusive noises and interruptions. The same room should be used for each meeting. Leaders often have to adapt inadequate space to fit the needs of the group. The session itself is more important than where it is conducted.

The next step usually undertaken by the group therapist is to select members. The selection is based on the purposes of the group, referrals to the group, and interviews with potential members. In screening individuals, the therapist and/or the agencies must provide information about the group to selected persons or groups. All information should clearly identify the group's purpose and state the criteria for membership eligibility and the time, place, and duration. The therapists' names and the appropriate professional credentials should be provided.

The group's composition will greatly influence its outcome. In selecting members, the leader should determine which variables will foster group cohesion and therapeutic problem solving. Generally, selection criteria should be based on both heterogeneous and homogeneous variables. Selection criteria include problem areas, motivation, age, sex, cultural factors, educational level, socioeconomic level, ability to communicate, intelligence, and coping and defensive styles. Homogeneous groups will share preselected criteria; for example, all members will be women who suffered incest as a child. Heterogeneous groups will include a mixture of individuals based on selected variables, such as a group for men and women who want to build their self-esteem.

In a mixed (homogeneous and heterogeneous) group, members share an essential feature of their clinical diagnosis (e.g., depression), but their age, sex, and educational and family backgrounds vary. Yalom and Vinogradov[32] advocated that cohesiveness should serve as a primary guide for selection of patients for therapy groups and that heterogeneous factors be chosen from demographic variation.

If possible, the therapist should decide whether the membership of the group will be closed or open before screening members. A group is closed if no new members are added once the group is started. In an open group, members leave and new members are added throughout the duration of the group. Open groups may maintain the same purpose, with both members and leaders changing. They usually continue indefinitely with no termination date. The closed group offers the advantage of consistency of leadership, norms, and expectations. The open group, on the other hand, continually brings fresh ideas and opportunities for learning to its members.

The screening interview's primary purpose is to determine the appropriateness of the potential member to the group. Secondary purposes accomplished during the screening interview include:

1. Beginning to develop a relationship between the therapist and the member
2. Determining the motivation of the possible member
3. Determining if the candidate's goals are in agreement with the group goals
4. Educating the candidate about the nature of the group
5. Determining the type of group experience the individual has had
6. If appropriate, beginning to review the group contract

In addition to or instead of the screening interview, some clinicians use a "group intake." Several new members meet in a group for one to three sessions to learn about the group psychotherapy process and identify some possible treatment goals. This approach is less costly and has the same objectives as the screening interview.

As soon as possible a decision should be made about group membership. Candidates not selected should be provided with other treatment options. The reasons for not being selected should be explained to the individual and if appropriate, to the referring person.

■ **Initial phase**

The initial phase includes meetings in which the group's members begin to "settle down" to work. This phase is characterized by anxiety regarding being accepted by the group, the setting of norms, and the casting of various roles. Curative factors such as catharsis and universality begin to operate. This phase has been subdivided into three stages by Yalom[31]: the orientation, conflict, and cohesive stages. The stages correspond to Tuckman's first three stages of group development.[25]

■ **ORIENTATION STAGE.** During the first stage of this phase the therapist is more directive and active than in other stages. The therapist orients the group to its primary task and assists the group in arriving at a group contract. Some common factors that therapists may include in the group contract are goals, confidentiality, meeting times, honesty, structure, and communication rules (e.g., only one person may talk at a time). Since an important part of this phase is norm setting, the therapist should ensure that the norms will facilitate the group's achieving its primary and secondary goals. Another task of the therapist in this stage is to foster attractiveness or cohesion among the members. In fulfilling this task, the therapist encourages interaction among members and maintains the group at a working level of anxiety. For example, the therapist could refer to the group as "our" group and suggest how members can help each other. One method would encourage members to state what they hope to learn from the group. The therapist would then reinforce the realistic expectations and give examples of how the group might meet these expectations.

During the first stage the members are evaluating each other, the group, and the therapist. They are deciding if they are going to be a part of the group and are determining what their level of participation will be. Some common conscious or unconscious concerns of members during this stage are the fear of being rejected, fear of self-disclosure, and fear of not being seen as an individual. Social amenities are important, and the members are attempting to develop their social roles. The roles members assume during this stage are often renegotiated during other stages. The group at this time is dependent, and frequently members will test out their dependency needs and wishes on the leader. Members look to the leader for structure, approval, and acceptance, and they may try to please the leader with reward-seeking behaviors. The leader must not gratify all the dependency wishes of the members but must encourage members to interact more with one another. This supports members in becoming more interdependent on each other and less dependent on the leader. The dependency issue between the leader and the members may lead the group into conflict and thus into the second stage.

■ **CONFLICT STAGE.** This stage of the group corresponds to Tuckman's storming stage of group development. Issues related to control, power, and authority become of prime importance. Members are concerned about the "pecking order" or determination of who is "top or bottom" in regard to issues of control and decision making. The dependency conflict may be openly or covertly expressed, with members polarized between independent and dependent issues. Bennis and Sheppard[3] describe this stage as a struggle between the counterdependent and dependent members, with the counterdependent members waiting to assume the leader's role. For example, a group may be divided over the issue of whether members can telephone each other. Some members may want the leader to decide, whereas others may think that the leader's statements are irrelevant. During this phase the counterdependent members might sit in the leader's chair and let the leader know the directions have been un-

successful or unheard. The dependent members might ask the leader for more directions. Other members who are neutral (neither dependent nor counterdependent) eventually may assist the group in resolving this conflict.

Subgroups usually form within the group, and hostility may be expressed. Often the hostility is directed toward the leader, but it may also be expressed toward other members. The therapist's tasks are to allow for the expression of both negative and positive feelings, to help the group to understand the underlying conflict, and to prevent and/or examine nonproductive behaviors such as scapegoating. This phase is usually the most difficult for the new therapist, because some members may lead the therapist to believe he or she has failed the group by not living up to its unrealistic expectations. Yalom[31] described some reasons that typically lead certain members to express resentment toward the leader: the member's awareness of the therapist's limitations, the therapist not fulfilling a "traditional leader" role, and awareness that the therapist will not give each member a favorite standing.

The therapist must be careful not to avoid or suppress the group members' anxiety and, at times, should encourage the expression of hostility. If hostility toward the therapist is expressed indirectly, such as anger toward other authority figures (e.g., staff members, teachers, parents), the therapist should assist the group in expressing its anger more directly. A useful technique is for the therapist to give the group permission to discuss its anger by acknowledging that the group may be disappointed or angry at the leader.

By the end of the conflict stage the therapist may be dethroned, and his or her omnipotent role, with its "magical" solutions, may be discarded. Slowly the therapist becomes humanized. Members learn that responsibilities for the group are shared. Members may also learn that expressions of anger and disappointment do not destroy the leader and may assist the group to assess its resources and limitations more accurately. The group's resources can then be used to achieve its primary and secondary tasks. Members may realize that conflicts need not be avoided; instead, through discussion, conflicts may increase the group's maturity and usefulness.

■ **COHESIVE STAGE.** Tuckman's norming phase[25] is closely related to the cohesive stage. Group members, after resolving the second stage, feel a strong attractiveness toward one another and a strong attachment to the group. Expressions of positive feelings toward one another and toward the group are frequently verbalized, and expressions of negative feelings are usually suppressed.

At this stage, members feel free to give self-disclosing information and share more intimate concerns with one another. However, the group's problem-solving ability is restricted because negative communication is usually avoided in order to maintain the high group morale. The therapist's task is to facilitate further exploring of the members' disclosures in relationship to the group's primary task. The therapist should not hinder the group's basic cohesiveness but should encourage the group eventually to use its problem-solving ability. Through this behavior the therapist models how a group member can have individual concerns and values and still be productive within the group. In other words, the therapist demonstrates that differing and opposite opinions may not destroy the group identity.

At the resolution of this stage, members may learn that self-discoveries and differences should not be feared. They also learn that similarities and differences between the members may help the group to achieve its tasks. At the end of the cohesive stage the group begins to see task achievement as a reality. The members gain a more realistic and honest view of their ability to work together and accomplish their primary and secondary tasks.

■ Working phase

The working phase of a group can be compared with Tuckman's performing stage of group development.[25] During this stage the group becomes a team. It directs its energy mainly toward completion of its tasks. Although they are hard at work, this phase is an enjoyable one for both the leader and the members. Responsibility for the group is more equally shared, anxiety is usually decreased and is tolerated better than in the previous phases, and the group is more stable and realistic.

In a psychotherapy group, members begin seriously to work through their concerns related to their therapeutic goals. They begin a more in-depth exploration of the various goals related to their group's tasks. For example, in a psychotherapeutic group for mothers with chronically ill children, the members may discuss their various reactions to the children, their ambivalent feelings, some of their thoughts regarding the reason for their feelings, and various alternative ways to cope with their present daily realities.

The leader's major role is to facilitate the group's completing its task or tasks by maximizing the group's effective use of its curative properties. Because the members are fully participating in the group's work, the therapist's activity level decreases in this phase. The leader now acts more as a consultant to the group. The

leader helps to keep the group on its proper course and, if possible, tries to decrease the impact of any factors that may regress or retard the group.

Because this phase is mainly characterized as the group's creative problem-solving and resolution phase, there are few, if any, specific guidelines for the leader. The leader's interventions are primarily based on his or her theoretical frameworks, experiences, personality, and intuition and the needs of the group and its members. In addition to fostering group cohesion, maintaining its boundaries, and encouraging the group to work on its tasks, the leader's interventions may be directed toward helping the group solve specific problems. Because these problems are unique to the group, many are not universally predictable. Some of the more common problems identified by Yalom[31] are the formation of subgroups, the management of conflict, and determination of the optimum level of self-disclosure.

Subgroups that conflict with the group's goals and are not acknowledged by the group can restrict its work. Other members may feel excluded, and loyalties will be divided between the subgroup and the group as a whole. For example, in a women's group, two of the members may become close friends, keeping secrets from the group and engaging in private conversations during the session. Other members may feel excluded from this pair and may be ineffective in working with them. To decrease the negative impact of a subgroup, its consequences and the group's reactions should be openly discussed.

Conflict is unavoidable and can be used to foster group and individual growth. However, the expressions of conflict may need to be controlled so that their intensity does not exceed the group's tolerance. Examples of conflict are competition among members for leader's attention and a disagreement between two members. A leader may manage conflicts by acknowledging that the conflict does exist, explaining that conflicts are natural occurrences and can be growth producing, and encouraging members to discuss the reasons behind the conflict. The tolerance for successful conflict resolution is related to the amount of group cohesiveness, trust, and acceptance experienced by the members.

The amount of self-disclosure is usually related to the amount of acceptance and trust the discloser feels. Self-disclosure is always risky. If persons give pertinent or private information too quickly, they will feel vulnerable. Likewise, during the working phase if persons disclose too little, they may be ineffective in forming interpersonal relationships. Their growth potential in the group may consequently be decreased.

Resistance, or the forestalling of the therapeutic process, is one form of behavior that can be expected in therapy groups. Resistance to working on the therapeutic goal can occur at both an individual and a group level. It is one matter to agree on the therapeutic goals and another to work on obtaining the actual therapeutic outcomes. Resistance by individual members may take many forms, such as avoiding discussion of a conflict area, frequent or prolonged silences, attempting to become an assistant therapist, absence of members, pairing between two members, and prolonged expression of hostility. Resistance by the group or a majority of its members may be expressed in ways similar to those used by individuals. Other examples of group resistance include shared silence among the members, unusual amounts of dependency on the leader, an unusual amount of hostility, scapegoating, subgroup formations, and the wish for magical solutions to resolve the group conflict. Resistance may occur because of individuals' or the group's increased anxiety, which is experienced around conflict or change. The management of resistance depends on the type of psychotherapy group, the group contract, and the therapist's theoretical framework. Some methods of decreasing resistance are to make observations regarding the group process or individual behaviors, offer interpretations, counteract the resistant behavior, and demonstrate more adaptive behavioral patterns.

By the end of the second phase, members have begun to achieve their goals, and it is hoped they have a sense of their own productiveness and accomplishments. The need for the group or their involvement in the group has become less apparent. The group or its members of the group must begin to deal more actively with its final task—separation.

■ **Termination phase**

The work of termination begins during the first phase of every group. However, as the group or its members approach termination, certain processes are more likely to occur. The termination phase is not always discussed as a definite phase in the literature. It is discussed as a separate phase here because of the significance that termination may have for the members.

There are two types of termination: termination of the group as a whole and termination of individual members. A closed group usually terminates as an entire group; in an open group, members (and perhaps the therapist) terminate separately. Members and groups may terminate prematurely, unsuccessfully, or successfully.

Termination is a highly individualized process. Individuals and groups will terminate in ways that are unique to themselves. If the group has been successful, termination is a painful process and involves grieving or a sense of loss. Termination may cause the group to experience increased anxiety, regression, or a feeling of accomplishment. To permit members to avoid this subject would be the same as preventing individuals from having a possible successful growth experience. Behaviors used by therapists include encouraging an evaluation of the group or its terminating members, reminiscing about important events that occurred in the group's history, and encouraging members to give feedback to each other. An evaluation usually is restricted to the achievement or lack of achievement of the group's or the individual's goals. Therapists must be careful not to collude with members in denying termination; rather, they must encourage termination to be fully discussed. Termination should be talked about several sessions before the final session to allow members time to work through issues that surface. Termination may lead to the discussion of many related topics, such as other separations, death, aging, and the use and passage of time. If terminated successfully, members may eventually feel a sense of resolution about the group experience and may use these experiences in many other encounters in life.

Premature termination is the group ending before its tasks are completed and/or a member leaving the group before his or her work is finished. Premature termination may occur for appropriate and inappropriate reasons. Appropriate reasons include moving to another city before the group is terminated. Inappropriate reasons might include a member's unwillingness to discuss an issue central to the group but painful to that member.

Evaluation of the group

Evaluation of the group and the progress of individual members in the group is an ongoing process that begins in the selection interview. Most clinicians keep records to remember the critical events in the group. Such records are subject to the ethical guidelines for group notes. These records can later be used to evaluate the group from a descriptive point of view. To make record keeping easy, it is usually helpful to have a "group notebook." In this notebook, leaders can write pertinent data on individual members, such as their group's goals, their telephone numbers, their addresses, the screening note, any individual comments, and a termination summary note. In another section of the group notebook the leaders can describe each group meeting. One format for quickly recording each group meeting is provided in the box that follows.

In addition to these measures, it is sometimes

Group Session Note Outline

Date _____ Group Meeting No. _____
1. Membership:
   a. List members attending (state if new member).
   b. List members who were late.
   c. List absent members.
2. List individual members' pertinent issues or behaviors discussed in the group.
3. List group themes.
4. Identify important group process issues (e.g., developmental stage, roles, norms).
5. Identify any critical leadership strategy used.
6. List proposed future leadership strategies.
7. Predict member and group responses for the next session.

helpful to determine each member's goal attainment. This can be done using subjective ratings by the group leaders or obtaining individual members' perceptions on how they are meeting their goals. For a slightly more objective evaluation, members are asked to rate their goal achievement on a Likert scale (one that al-lows members to rate their response along a contin-uum, e.g., 1 being low, 5 being high). The evaluation of members' goal achievement should always be done at termination. Depending on the nature and duration of the group, it may also be done on a regular inter-view basis.

In addition to the descriptive evaluation, the clini-cian may decide to administer a before- and after-group written test(s). The tests selected should be con-gruent with the expected changes in the group. For ex-ample, an anxiety scale could administered to members attending a group whose major goal is to reduce anxi-ety. If this type of evaluation is used, it is critical that the clinician use the most appropriate scale available and that the agency's and the members' permissions are obtained. It is paramount that all parties involved know the intent of using such tests and the disposition of test results.

Therapeutic aspects of groups

Nurses and other health providers need to under-stand how a group can exert influences on its members so that they may consciously use these forces to en-hance or modify the effects on individuals in the group.

Yalom[31] has clearly described some of the positive forces that occur in group therapy. He listed 11 cura-tive factors that may occur in every type of therapy group (Table 28-3). Yalom's curative factors do not occur in isolation. Although these factors may be more

TABLE 28-3

YALOM'S CURATIVE FACTORS

Factor	Definition
Imparting information	Receiving didactic information and advice
Instillation of hope	Increasing hopefulness of group members
Universality	Realization that others experience same thoughts, feelings, and problems
Altruism	Experience of sharing part of oneself to help another
Corrective reenactment of primary family group	Ability of members to alter learning experience previously obtained in their families
Development of social interaction techniques	Opportunity to increase one's awareness of social interactions and develop social skills
Imitative behaviors	Opportunities to increase skills by imitating behaviors of others in group
Interpersonal learning	Ability to engage in wider range of interpersonal exchanges, thereby increasing each member's understanding of responsibility and complexity of interpersonal relationships and decreasing member's interpersonal distortions
Existential factors	Ability of group to help members deal with meaning of their own existence
Catharsis	Opportunity to express feelings previously unexpressed
Group cohesion	Attraction of member for group and other members

Modified from Yalom I: The theory and practice of group psychotherapy, ed 3, New York, 1985, Basic Books, Inc.

pertinent to therapy groups, they are important factors to consider in all groups. Several studies indicate that cohesiveness, catharsis, and interpersonal learning are rated by group therapy practitioners as the most important curative factors in their groups.[15]

In a study by Lieberman, Yalom, and Miles[14] on encounter groups, cognitive learning appeared to be the most important factor in differentiating those who learned from those who did not learn from the group experience. Cognitive learning is gaining and applying information or insight that is useful to oneself. Examples of this are found in groups that learn about a condition or disease as a primary task. In this same study on encounter groups, four major leadership dimensions were identified: caring, emotional stimulation, meaning attribution, and executive functioning. Caring included warmth, affection, acceptance, encouragement, and communication of positive regard. Emotional stimulation occurred when the leader challenged and encouraged the revelation of feelings and personal values. Meaning attribution involved increasing cognitive dimensions, and executive functioning included limit setting and managing activities. In this study the leaders who were rated most effective were high on caring and meaning attribution and moderate in emotional stimulation and executive functioning. Although these leadership dimensions have not been adequately studied to be conclusive, they do offer a group leader a different way to think about leadership skills.

Theoretical frameworks of group psychotherapy

In leading a psychotherapy group, the therapist should act from a theoretical framework. The theoretical framework serves as a guide to assess the group, determine the therapist's behaviors and interventions in the group, and evaluate the effectiveness of the therapeutic techniques employed. The theoretical frameworks of group therapy are mainly derived from various theories in psychiatry, such as psychoanalytical, interpersonal, and behavioral theory, and from social psychology. Differences in theoretical frameworks may range from emphasizing the individual in the group to emphasizing the group as a whole.

A few theories are discussed here briefly. However, to obtain a working knowledge of group psychotherapy theory, the reader must consult other sources.

■ Focal conflict model

One theoretical framework that nurse therapists have found useful is Whitaker's and Lieberman's Focal Conflict Model.[27] This model is based on the assumption that the therapist's primary interventions are at the group rather than the individual level. This theory is based on the principle that therapy groups will develop unconscious conflicts that have meaning to all members. The conflict arises from the group experiencing simultaneously a wish (a disturbing motive) and a fear (a reactive motive). When confronted with such a conflict, the group seeks resolution that may alleviate the fear and/or, at the same time, gratify the wish. The therapist's task is to help the group to understand the conflict and to arrive at a successful solution. Successful solutions will be shared by all members, will reduce reactive fears, and may also partly satisfy the wish.

An example of how this model may be used can be shown through the issue of a therapist's vacation. The disturbing motive or wish is to express anger at the therapist for taking a vacation; the fear or reactive motive is fear of retaliation if anger is expressed. For example, the group may fear the therapist will not return to the group after the vacation. A successful resolution of the wish versus the fear conflict would be for the group to discuss openly their fears and anger regarding the therapist's vacation and the group's wish for the therapist to return to the group. The therapist could facilitate the group by giving the members permission to express their anger and fears and by demonstrating acceptance when members discuss these fears. The therapist may also choose to offer reassurance that he or she will return to the group following the vacation.

■ Communication model

The communication model uses principles of communication theory and therapeutic communication. It assumes that dysfunctional or ineffective communication in groups may lead to members' dissatisfaction, inadequate feedback, and a decrease in group cohesion. Using this model, the leader facilitates efficient communication among group members. Through effective communication, problems of the individual members and the group can be identified and resolved.

The leader teaches the group that (1) it is impossible for members not to communicate; (2) members must take responsibility for what they communicate; (3) communication takes place at many levels (e.g., verbal and nonverbal, overt and covert); (4) for a message to be effective, it must be understood by other members; and (5) members can use communication theory to help each other communicate more effectively. An example of the application of communication theory is a therapy group that has the primary goal of helping members improve their social and interpersonal skills. Communication theory is used to help members realize how they communicate nonverbally and show them how to practice more effective ways of communicating. One member may learn that because she is always looking down, other members think she is disinterested in them. Once they learn to acknowledge her nonverbal communication, their concern can motivate her to describe what her looking down means (she feels anxious about being with new people). The leader in this group, when appropriate, briefly explains some principles of communication and illustrates how these principles can be used in the group. The leader models effective communication and uses Yalom's curative factor of imparting information. The leader also helps the group decide when it is useful to analyze a specific message or communication sequence.

■ Interpersonal model

The interpersonal theory of interactional group theory is derived from Sullivan[24] and the interpersonal school of psychiatry. In this theory, therapists work at both the individual and the group level. Group members learn by examining their transactions and feelings within the group and between themselves and the therapist. Through this process, disturbed perceptions are corrected and socially effective behaviors are learned. Feelings of anxiety and loneliness are especially targeted for identification and change.

For example, the primary goal of a women's therapy group may be to improve members' interpersonal relationships. When an interpersonal conflict occurs, the leader uses the situation to encourage members to discuss their feelings, learn what in the conflict made the members feel anxious or distressed, and determine the behaviors used to avoid or decrease anxiety during the conflict.

■ Psychodrama

Psychodrama, introduced by Moreno,[19] is another form of group therapy that also requires specialized training. In this model, members are encouraged to act out immediate or past life situations. Members are assigned roles, such as the audience, stage, protagonist (the patient selected to be the major subject for the specific enactment), auxiliary egos (the therapeutic actors to whom the protagonist is responding or reacting), director, and producer. Psychodrama is based on spontaneity, reality testing, catharsis, and role reversal and allows members to act out specific situations, conflicts, or problems. For example, a disagreement may occur between a group member and his landlord regarding unsatisfactory repairs that were made. The patient (protagonist) could play himself, and another member (auxiliary ego) would play the landlord. The group leader would direct the scene. As the script is acted out, the patient would gain further understanding of himself and his behavior during the disagree-

ment. This understanding would also increase when other members (the audience) give feedback to the patient. At another time the roles of the patient and the landlord might be reversed. The role reversal would facilitate the patient's understanding of the landlord's predicament and how the patient might communicate more effectively. Additional information about psychodrama is presented in Chapter 24.

Many other theories can be employed in group therapy. Specific theories, such as transactional analysis, behavior therapy, and gestalt therapy, have gained acceptance in group work. These theories use specific techniques, games, and rules. References about these theories can be found in this chapter's annotated suggested readings. Some group therapists use a combination of theoretical approaches and techniques with groups. Most importantly, the therapists must be well versed in the theories and techniques that they use in group work and must choose them appropriately.

Responsibilities of leaders in group psychotherapy

Nurse therapists must be concerned about the many factors regarding the group that were previously discussed. The group leader must be able to study the group and interact in it at the same time. The leader is constantly monitoring the group and, whenever necessary, is ready to help the group toward achieving its goals.

Effective group leaders possess a high degree of **therapeutic empathy.** Generative empathy is the inner experience of "sharing in comprehending the psychological state of another person."[3] It is the basis of altruistic behavior but is also much more. It is an attitude that leads inevitably to helping someone grow. The generative empathic process is based on relating our own experiences to those that someone else is having and assuming their feelings are similar to those we have had. Observing a client's life at any one point, "we tentatively project onto him the feelings we once felt under similar circumstances, and then test this projection by further observation."[4] Therapeutic empathy is the use of generative empathy in trying to understand someone.

Nurturance is another attribute of skilled nurse therapists. "Nurturance is the caring and helping that are fundamental to human relationships and groups. It includes any interactions that build unity and support. It may run the gamut, from exploratory nurturing remarks to intense personal exchanges"[11] regarding behavior that the therapist considers to be self-defeating or destructive.

The therapist needs to understand that nurturance does not mean "feeling sorry" for the client. It means caring in a way that the therapist will take appropriate risks to help the member and the group achieve their desired goals.

An example of empathy would be when a nurse therapist who once smoked truly understands and feels the conflict and anguish of a member who is trying to quit. Nurturance might be expressed by verbal encouragement or by not accepting the member's excuses for needing cigarettes.

A third skill requirement of effective nurse therapists is what Rogers[20] calls **genuineness.** It is the ability to share appropriately with the group the therapist's true feelings at the moment. For example, therapists might share their frustration with the group for its unwillingness to work at its task. The purpose of such sharing is to help the group realize its effects on others and to understand what messages the therapist is sending.

Nurse leadership qualities

The nurse leader of a therapy or support group must be able to tolerate a high level of ambiguity. It is essential that the leader be able to believe in the group and be patient with the process of the group forming itself from a collection of individuals into a cohesive group.

Creativity and opportunism are helpful qualities for leaders to possess. While they are listening to members' words, leaders also need to be aware of the group process. They must be vigilant of opportunities for the group to use members' themes and behaviors and see how these affect individual issues. Leaders may resemble an orchestra leader who seeks to focus on the sound of a particular instrument for the appreciation and reaction of the total orchestra. The leader may encourage examination of the music from different perspectives and look for possible variations that would create a new piece of music.

Group leaders must be prepared to offer themselves as a safe authority figure to challenge. In examining this interplay between the leader and the members, opportunities are offered for members to practice conflict management, confrontation, and assertive communication. The leader needs to accept these confrontations without taking them personally.

Leaders also need to have assertive communication skills that help them maintain a balance between fostering independence in the group and helping the group focus to reach its goals. This requires a blend of skills and judgment that can be best gained with practice in group leadership, supervision by an experienced group facilitator, and study of group process.

The ability to organize a great deal of information and to select themes for the data presented in a session

are necessary skills. It may be helpful for novice leaders to review the group experience for 1 to 2 hours after the session so that they can select the important rather than the final events of the group.

A nurse therapist also needs to possess a sense of humor. Laughter helps reveal the truth and enables participants to share and empathize on serious matters without the high levels of tension that frequently accompany such discussions. In one of our women's codependent groups, we regularly use humor and laughter. The group has adopted this technique to talk about their "rescuing" and controlling behaviors. This group, in the working phase, is composed of a fragile group of individuals who have grown up in abusive families. They work hard at seeing, understanding, and changing their contribution to the destructive relationships they develop. The members bring examples of their "setting themselves up" to the group weekly and laugh as they are able to find humor in recognizing behavior that is similar to their own. The humor also allows the members to give feedback in a less confrontive manner.

Cotherapist-led group

For a group, the presence of cotherapists may have advantages and disadvantages. When two therapists share the leadership, the breadth of observation and the repertoires of therapeutic interventions are much greater than with one therapist. For example, a male and female cotherapist team may represent the family and offer the group members an opportunity to deal with different issues because of the availability of "Dad and Mom" or other significant male and female figures.

A male/female cotherapist team also offers group members opportunities to observe a man and a woman work together with mutual respect and without exploitation, sexualizing, or putting each other down. A variety of transference reactions are provided with mature and experienced cotherapists to assist in the learning and resolution. The full and open exploration of the members' fantasies regarding the relationship between therapists can be used. Differences of opinion between cotherapists can give members the chance to see conflict and resolution. This can contribute significantly to the groups' openness and power.

The disadvantages of the cotherapists team are often the result of difficulties between the therapists. When there is competition, a major philosophical difference, or great variance in strategy or style, the group will not work effectively. Differences in levels of experience are handled if both therapists are comfortable with their roles of apprentice and senior therapist. Conflict between cotherapists could lead to the splitting of the group or the group developing alliances with one of the therapists. This could be very damaging to the group. Splitting needs to be openly interpreted in the group and dealt with by the group members and leaders.

Types of groups

Clark[6] lists three type of groups: task, teaching, and supportive/therapeutic.

Task groups are designed to accomplish a particular task, such as a nursing care conference. The emphasis of these groups is on decision making and problem solving. The goal of **teaching groups** is to impart information. Examples of teaching groups are orientation to a unit, management of a particular disease process, and labor and childbirth preparation. The nurse leader is able to educate more people more efficiently via the group format, and the members themselves become coteachers as they share their information and experiences.

The primary goal of **supportive/therapeutic** groups is to help the members cope with sources of stress in their lives. The focus of these groups is on the thoughts, feelings, and behaviors that are judged dysfunctional. Examples are groups for persons trying to lose weight, for those who have lost a child (Compassionate Friends), and for adolescents with a parent who abuses drugs. These groups strive to provide a safe yet stimulating environment so that members may ventilate their feelings, share their experiences, and gain insights into their behavior. The strength of such groups is the members' shared experience.

A fourth type of group is the **psychotherapy group.** Its goal is the treatment of emotional, cognitive, and/or behavioral dysfunction. Group techniques and processes are used to help members learn how they behave with other people and how this behavior is related to the core personality issues. The intent is for the members to change their behavior, not just understand or seek support for it. Members also learn that they have responsibilities to others and can help other members achieve their goals. An example of a psychotherapy group is a scheduled group of inpatients from a psychiatric unit who focus on the problems that led to their admittance and what they need to do to resolve those problems.

Another group that is being increasingly used by nurses is the **peer support group.** This is designed for the nurses to share the stresses and problems related to their work, such as peer support groups for nurses working with people with AIDS.

Recent research

Several recent research articles are mentioned here to give the reader an appreciation of both the research and the clinical uses of groups. Recent nursing research studies indicate a strong investment in groups as a practical treatment modality used by nurses. Whitman and Gustafson[30] describe how to initiate, lead, and analyze supportive group therapy for families of individuals with cancer. After 12 years of experience with more than 600 groups, these authorities state that "most families can benefit from multiple-family therapy sessions and that highly stressed families can benefit significantly from both multiple- and single-family therapy meetings." They stress the importance of understanding the disease process as well as group dynamics and mental health issues. Such a group may be led by a single therapist with a background in both areas or by a teaming of, for example, an oncology nurse and a psychiatric clinical specialist.

Nurses are researching the use of small groups in working with people who have experienced incest and other sexual abuses. Krach and Zens[12] use group technique to work with court-ordered perpetrators of incest, who attend weekly 2-hour sessions over 12 months. These nurse researchers characterize perpetrators as people with a great need for control and power, which they assert over passive women. The group, facilitated by two female cotherapists, offers opportunities for members to deal with assertive women. It also provides an environment of sharing, caring, and mutual support to reduce the isolation typically experienced by perpetrators. Issues of denial, anger, bargaining, and depression are examined.

Urbancic[26] uses Yalom's curative factors in discussing group work with incest victims. She emphasizes the "secret" nature of the incest experiences and the helpfulness of the group in "instilling hope, universality, imparting of information, altruism, socialization opportunities, imitative behaviors, interpersonal learning, group cohesiveness, catharsis and existential issues." The author states that "psychiatric nurses are in an excellent position to identify the sexually abused woman on the ward and provide effective group therapy that will enable the survivor to resolve her incest trauma and become a survivor rather than a victim."[26]

Gilbert[9] studied sexually abused children who were treated in a group setting. The author includes a clear outline of the structure of the group, giving themes of the 8-week series and the activities she used in working with the seven preadolescent and adolescent members. Gilbert discusses the naturalness of the group approach for this age-group and includes their developmental tasks.

Staples and Schwartz[23] describe a cotherapist-run

group for anorexia nervosa patients. This group originated to assist these patients in the transitional phase between inpatient and outpatient treatment. It specifically was formed to decrease isolation and prevent the recidivism that is so high during this period. These authors discuss the changes of themes as the group progressed and the changing expectations the cotherapists had for the group members. The most remarkable change in group members was a "clear attitudinal shift away from valuing an anorectic identity to investing in meaningful relationships with others as a means of providing a sense of self-worth and identity." These authors observe that a chronic population among their members appeared to be using the group to "create the illusion of treatment" without any evidence of change or understanding and that alternative treatments may be useful.

A psychoeducational group is the modality described by Moores.[18] This study examines a structured group of six to eight clients who had a prerequisite of a relaxation class and had specific teachings assigned to each session. The first segment of the session reviewed progress of the members throughout the previous week. The middle of the session consisted of formal teaching using visual aids and demonstration as appropriate. Topics included the physiological effects of anxiety, the cycle of fear, methods used to interrupt this cycle (e.g., breathing exercises), identification of negative thinking patterns that sparked member's fears, assertiveness skills, and guided imagery. Homework was assigned and members were held accountable. Final evaluation by clients and staff generally showed improvement in the members.

Extensive study is being done by nurse researchers on the configuration and efficacy of short-term inpatient groups, since there is an increasing mandate for short-term hospital stays in psychiatric settings with increasingly acutely ill patients. White[29] studied the leadership skills, including negotiating, collaborating, and confronting, needed to maintain a working group.

Nurse educators are examining group process as a teaching method that offers distinct advantages to the learner over the passive learning of the lecture format. The benefits described by Fontes[8] include:

Interacting with other members through use of the course content

Acquiring factual content relevant to course objectives

Providing a forum to promote understanding, tolerance, respect, and support for diversity among members

Providing a safe environment for members to look at and reveal themselves

The use of small groups with patients with long-term medical or psychosomatic problems is the subject of White's clinical work.[28] The author cites the advantages for those frequently considered "problem patients" to include decreased isolation, opportunities for helping others, interpersonal learning and development of coping skills, decreased dependence and transference with leaders, and ability to listen to other members. White includes a description of the leader's use of patients' physical complaints as metaphors of their believed situation, such as "pain in the neck" and "crying with pain." This technique demonstrates that if it is presented in a gentle empathic manner, the connection between body and feelings may be made.

■ SUGGESTED CROSS-REFERENCES ■

Conceptual models are discussed in Chapter 2. The nurse-patient relationship is discussed in Chapter 4. Psychodrama is discussed in Chapter 24.

DIRECTIONS FOR FUTURE RESEARCH

The following are some of the nursing research problems raised in Chapter 28 that merit further study by psychiatric nurses:

1. The role of nurses as group co-leaders with professionals of other disciplines (e.g., social work, psychiatry, psychology)
2. Role of psychiatric nurse as in-house consultant to general hospital staff and patients
3. Examination of effect of including family members in group psychotherapy
4. Comparison of behavioral, analytical, and cognitive-behavioral treatment methods as short-term modalities
5. Cost-effectiveness of group as a therapeutic technique
6. Effectiveness of groups for medical patients (e.g., post–myocardial infarct patients) in coping with disease process and its implications
7. Training modalities for nurse therapists
8. Utilization of groups for staff team building, skill acquisition, and support
9. Effectiveness of patient/family peer support groups
10. Effects of cross-cultural differences on nurse therapist/group interaction

SUMMARY

1. Groups are a specific social system that can be defined and studied. A group consists of individuals who are interrelated and interdependent and who may share common purposes and norms.

2. All groups have content functions and process functions.

3. Some common dimensions often used to evaluate a group's progress are communication processes, membership roles, norms, power structure, cohesion, and stages of group development.

4. A group psychotherapist has specific responsibilities in leading the group. Some of these responsibilities may be studied in relationship to the phases of group development.

    a. During the pregroup phase, therapists determine the purpose of the group, arrange for a place for the group to meet, determine criteria for membership, and select group members.

    b. In the orientation stage, therapists facilitate the group's arriving at a group contract, orient the group to its task, and promote group cohesion.

    c. In the conflict stage, therapists may encourage members to express their disillusionment and hostility and maintain the group's activity within a working level.

    d. During the cohesive stage, therapists assist the group to improve its problem-solving ability by helping the group to use negative feedback and disagreement.

    e. In the working stage, therapists facilitate the group's accomplishing its tasks by acting as resource persons to the group, assisting the group in handling problems such as subgroup formation, and managing conflict and resistance.

    f. In the termination stage, therapists assist the members in evaluating what they have learned and in separating from one another.

5. Identifiable curative or therapeutic factors may occur in groups.

6. Group psychotherapy is a useful and beneficial treatment modality for alleviating emotional disturbances.

7. There is a wide range of models of group psychotherapy, from supportive therapy to personality reconstruction.

8. Specific theoretical frameworks should be used by group therapists. Theoretical models can be used to assist therapists to assess the group, intervene in the group, and evaluate the effectiveness of their interventions.

9. Nurses can use informal groups to enhance their assessments and to provide a therapeutic experience for the group's members.

10. The leading of therapeutic groups, which prevents or decreases emotional disturbances or stress, should be viewed as being in the realm of nursing practice.

REFERENCES

1. Bales R and Slater P: Role differentiation in small decision-making groups. In Parsons T and Bales RF: Family socialization and interactional process, Glencoe, Ill, 1955, The Free Press.
2. Benne KD and Sheats P: Functional roles and group members, J Soc Issues 4(2):41, 1948.
3. Bennis W and Sheppard H: A theory of group development, Hum Rel 9:415, 1956.
4. Bilodeau CB and Kackett RP: Issues raised in a group setting by patients recovering from myocardial infarction, Am J Psychiatry 128:73, 1971.
5. Cartwright D and Zander A, editors: Group dynamics: research and theory, ed 3, New York, 1968, Harper & Row, Publishers, Inc.
6. Clark CC: Nurse as group leader, New York, 1987, Springer Publishing Co, Inc.
7. Dolgoff T: Small groups and organizations: time, task and sentient boundaries, Gen Systems 10:135, 1975.
8. Fontes HC: Small group work: a strategy to promote active learning, J Nurs Educ 26:212, 1987.
9. Gilbert CM: Sexual abuse and group therapy, J Psychosoc Nurs 26:20, 1988.
10. Goffman E: Encounters: two studies in the sociology of interaction, Indianapolis, 1961, Bobbs-Merril.
11. Greenberg-Edelstein RR: Nurturance phenomenon: roots of group psychotherapy, East Norwalk, Conn, 1986, Appleton-Century-Crofts.
12. Krach P and Zens D: Incest: nursing interventions for group therapy, J Psychosoc Nurs 26:32, 1988.
13. Lewin K: Group decision and social change. In Newcomb TM and Hartley BL, editors: Readings in social psychology, New York, 1947, Holt, Rinehart & Winston, Inc.
14. Lieberman MA, Yalom I, and Miles M: Encounter groups: first facts, New York, 1972, Basic Books, Inc.
15. Long LD and Cope CS: Curative factors in a male felony offender group, Small Group Behav 2:889, 1980.
16. Martin E and Hill W: Forwards a theory of group development: six phases of therapy group development, Int J Group Psychother 7:20, 1957.
17. Miller EJ and Rice AK: Selections from systems of organization. In Colman A and Bexton W: Group relations reader, Sausalito, Calif, 1975, GREX Publishing.
18. Moores A: Facing the fear, Nurs Times 83:44, 1987.
19. Moreno JL: Psychodrama and group psychotherapy, Sociometry 9:249, 1941.
20. Rogers CR: Client-centered therapy, Boston, 1951, Houghton Mifflin Co.
21. Runkel P et al: Stages of group development: an empirical test of Tuckman's hypothesis, J Appl Behav Sci 7:180, 1971.
22. Schutz W: Interpersonal underworld, Harvard Bus Rev 36:123, 1958.
23. Staples NR and Schwartz M: Anorexia nervosa support group: providing transitional support, J Psychosoc Nurs 28:7, 1990.

24. Sullivan HS: Interpersonal theory of psychiatry, New York, 1953, WW Norton and Co, Inc.
25. Tuckman, B: Developmental sequence in small groups, Psychol Bull 63:384, 1965.
26. Urbancic JC: Resolving incest experiences through inpatient group therapy, J Psychosoc Nurs 27:5, 1989.
27. Whitaker D and Lieberman M: Psychotherapy through the group process, Chicago, 1964, Aldine Publishing Co.
28. White EM: Effective inpatient groups: challenges and rewards, Arch Psychiatr Nurs 1:6, 1987.
29. White EM: Use of a medical support group on a medical psychiatric unit, Issues Ment Health Nurs 9:353, 1988.
30. Whitman HH and Gustafson JP: Group therapy for families facing a cancer crisis, Oncol Nurs Forum 16:539, 1989.
31. Yalom I: The theory and practice of group psychotherapy, ed 3, New York, 1985, Basic Books, Inc.
32. Yalom ID and Vinogradov S: Group psychotherapy, Washington, DC, 1987, American Psychiatric Press, Inc.

■ ANNOTATED SUGGESTED READINGS ■

*Affonso DD: Therapeutic support during inpatient group therapy, J Psychosoc Nurs Ment Health Serv 23:11, 1985.
Focuses on nurse-patient interactions and their impact on patient progress. Examines milieu analysis, patient values and responsibility, and empathy as they relate to therapeutic interactions.

*Baier M: Group therapy with parolees in a community mental health center, J Psychosoc Nurs Ment Health Serv 20:26, 1982.
Good example of a nurse's creative use of group intervention. Describes a short-term, modified self-help group established for recently paroled offenders.

*Birckhead LM: The nurse as leader: group psychotherapy with psychotic patients, J Psychosoc Nurs Ment Health Serv 22:6, 1984.
Examines the unique opportunity for psychiatric–mental health nurses to assume leadership roles in group psychotherapy. Focuses on nurses as advocates of the most regressed members of an inpatient population and indicates the nurses' qualifications to lead these groups.

*Clark CC: Nurse as group leader, New York, 1987, Springer Publishing Co, Inc.
Short, practical guide useful for beginning group therapists. Includes phases of development, problems, and specifics of recording.

*Collison CR: Grappling with resistance in group psychotherapy, J Psychosoc Nurs Ment Health Serv 22:8, 1984.
Examines resistance typically seen in groups. Explores types of patient and therapist resistance and suggests interventions.

*Griffin W, Ling I, and Staley D: Stress management groups, J Psychosoc Nurs Ment Health Serv 23:1, 1985.
Excellent practical article on the teaching and the benefits of group relaxation training in a psychiatric outpatient setting.

Kaplan HI and Sadock BJ: Comprehensive group psychotherapy, ed 2, Baltimore, 1983, Williams & Wilkins.
Covers a broad range of subject areas concerned with group psychotherapy: basic principles, specialized techniques, special categories of patients, training and research, and international groups.

*Loomis M: Group process for nurses, St Louis, 1979, The CV Mosby Co.
Discusses small group dynamics to assist a nurse leading or participating in a group.

Tuckman B: Developmental sequence in small groups, Psychol Bull 63:384, 1965.
Summarizes many theories of group development. Multiple readings may be necessary to obtain the material's full benefit.

*Van Servellen GM: Group and family therapy: a model for psychotherapeutic nursing practice, St Louis, 1984, The CV Mosby Co.
For advanced students in psychiatric–mental health nursing, but may also be useful to beginning therapists. Covers conceptual perspective, scope of nursing practice, basic interventions, and special considerations, including techniques, evaluation, and research issues.

Weiner MF: Techniques of group psychotherapy, Washington, DC, 1984, American Psychiatric Press, Inc.
Clearly organized, basic group psychotherapy text on technique. Provides extensive bibliography and listing of teaching and training aids on film and videotape.

*Witt J: Transference and countertransference in group therapy settings, J Psychosoc Nurs 20:31, 1982.
Good overview of the application of these psychoanalytical concepts to group interaction. The illustrative clinical example should be of particular interest to beginning group leaders.

Yalom ID: Inpatient group psychotherapy, New York, 1983, Basic Books, Inc.
Excellent reference for beginning and experienced group therapists. Includes practical suggestions for formation, structure, and leadership of inpatient groups.

Yalom I: The theory and practice of group psychotherapy, ed. 3, New York, 1985, Basic Books, Inc.
Extremely useful for both new and experienced therapists. Cites relevant research and uses many clinical examples to illustrate ideas.

Yalom ID and Vinogradov S: Group psychotherapy, Washington, DC, 1987, American Psychiatric Press, Inc.
Concise guide to using group psychotherapy. Includes methods of starting a group regarding size, goals, cotherapists, and use of other treatments.

*Asterisk indicates nursing reference.

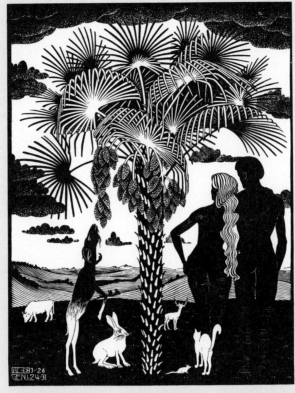

© 1990 M.C. Escher Heirs/Cordon Art, Baarn, Holland.

We are truly heirs of all the ages; but as honest men it behooves us to learn the extent of our inheritance. . . .

John Tyndall, "Matter and Force" in vol. 2, Prayer as a Form of Physical Energy

C H A P T E R   2 9

FAMILY THERAPY

PATRICIA E. HELM

L E A R N I N G   O B J E C T I V E S

After studying this chapter, the student should be able to:

- state the purpose and indications for family therapy.

- identify the role of both the generalist and the specialist in family therapy.

- analyze the family systems model, structural model, and strategic, or brief, model of family therapy with regard to the following elements: theoretical basis, goal, and treatment.

- within the context of a family systems model of therapy, differentiate between self, triangles, nuclear family emotional system, multigenerational transmission process, family projection process, sibling position, and emotional cutoff.

- within the context of a structural model of therapy, describe subsystems, subsystem boundaries, and restructuring operations.

- assess the importance of communication theory to the development of strategic, or brief, family therapy.

- identify directions for future nursing research.

- select appropriate readings for further study.

In the 1950s, if a nurse therapist admitted that she was seeing anyone in the family other than the patient, she risked censure by the entire psychoanalytical community. She could be accused of breaking a confidence and of failing to protect the therapeutic relationship between nurse and patient from contamination. Forty years later, the field of family therapy includes many well-known persons in the field, numerous conferences and workshops, countless books and videotapes, and various training programs.

Family therapy explores the *gestalt,* the context in which an emotional problem occurs and is played out between family members. Rather than viewing one member as sick or one relationship as pathological (such as the much-researched "schizophrenogenic mother" and symbiosed child), the family therapist focuses on the symmetrical process between family members that creates the "sick" behavior of one identified member. All family members are equally involved. For example, the school-phobic boy's overclose relationship to his mother is seen as the solution to her problem. Her husband emotionally withdraws from her into his business for 16 hours of the day. The boy's attention-demanding behavior saves both spouses from confronting their conflicts with each other. No one member of the family is to blame. Rather, a skewed family process has become fixed and requires rebalancing.

Viewing symptoms within this context requires a theoretical reorientation. To view family therapy as a modality of treatment is obsolescent; rather, it is a different way to conceptualize human relationship problems. It broadens the isolating, individual point of view to include the context in which relationships evolve.

This chapter provides a summary of three of the major, current theoretical approaches to family therapy. It delineates some of the main techniques that have evolved from these theories. The best guides to the history of family therapy, highlighting the work of the "first-generation" personalities, are works of Chris Beels and Andy Ferber[3] and Phil Guerin.[18] The chapter goals are to develop an informed interest in the field, to facilitate the pursuit of further reading, and to inspire training in family therapy. For those nurses who work with patients' families in a nonpsychiatric capacity, this chapter provides some helpful theories.

Role of the nurse in family therapy

Nurse therapists have evolved with psychiatry. "Insanity" moved out of the hands of priests who exorcised it, out of prisons that contained it, and into the hands of physicians who cured it. When "insanity" was seen as "mental illness," it became a medically treatable illness. As medicine became more psychologically sophisticated, the intimate connection between the body and the mind was established. Psychiatry has struggled to gain a position of legitimacy in the medical field. Psychosomatic medicine and psychiatric liaison services in medical hospitals are evidence that the emotional and psychological needs of patients must be met to maximize physical healing.

As medicine became more complex, the number of available physicians proved inadequate to perform multiple treatment procedures. Under these circumstances, nurses were asked to assume more and more responsibility for total patient care. Observing emotional stress in patients and patients' families has always been an integral part of this care. Nurses responded intuitively to stress in their patients long before intrapsychic and interpersonal theories of psychiatry were conceived. Public health nurses observed the emotional stress of illness and social deprivation in patients and families in community settings. Just as one goal of psychotherapy is to reduce acute stress in a patient, family therapy is a natural evolution of the nurse's traditional role.

■ **Functional families**

Contact with patients' families is a natural part of patient care. For many years nurses have been making intuitive observations about functional and dysfunctional families. They have been intervening with families without formal training in family therapy. A well-functioning family can shift roles, levels of responsibility, and patterns of interaction as it experiences stressful life changes. A well-functioning family may, under acute or prolonged stress, produce a symptomatic member. This family rebalances in such a way that function of all members is restored and symptoms fade. A functional family has the following characteristics.[1,16,25]

1. It maintains a homeostatic balance and flexibility and adapts to change as it passes through transitional stages of family life and periods of stress.
2. Emotional problems are viewed partly as a function of each person, rather than residing entirely in one family member.
3. Emotional contact is maintained across generations and between family members without blurring necessary levels of authority.
4. Overcloseness or fusion is avoided, and distance is not used to solve problems.
5. Each twosome is expected to resolve the problems between them. Bringing a third person in to settle disputes or to take sides is discouraged.
6. Differences between family members are encouraged to promote personal growth and creativity.
7. Children are expected to assume age-appropriate responsibility and to enjoy age-appropriate privileges negotiated with their parents.
8. The preservation of a positive emotional climate is more highly valued than doing what "should" be done or what is "right."
9. Within each spouse there is a balance of affective expression, careful rational thought, relationship focus, and care taking; each spouse can selectively function in the respective modes.

■ **Dysfunctional families**

Dysfunctional families lack one or more of these characteristics. All nurses, regardless of their area of expertise or practice setting, encounter dysfunctional families. The problem may be overt or covert, and the satisfaction of members may be low. Some of the more common dysfunctional family patterns include (1) the overprotective mother and the distant father (distant at work, in alcohol, or absent from the home) with a timid, whiny child or a destructive, acting-out adolescent; (2) the overfunctioning "superwife" or "superhusband" and the underfunctioning passive, dependent, and compliant spouse; (3) the spouse who maintains "peace at any price" and who whitewashes difficulties in the marriage but who suddenly feels wronged and self-righteous when the mate is discovered to be in legal difficulty or having an affair; (4) the child who evidences poor peer relationships at school while attempting to parent younger siblings to compensate for ineffective and emotionally overwhelmed parents; and (5) the overclose three generations of grandparent, parent, and grandchild in which lines of authority and generational identity are poorly defined and the child is acting out because of a lack of effective limit setting by an agreed-on parental figure.

Deciding when family therapy is appropriate, or indicated over individual or group therapy, is not always easy. Resource availability is a factor; many settings do not have anyone trained in family therapy. When the resources are available, the therapist's bias may have an influence. Some family therapists conceptualize all emotional problems within the family framework. Others recommend certain guidelines in determining which problems should be treated in family therapy. They may suggest that family therapy is indicated in the following situations*:

---

*I am indebted to Behnaz Jalali, MD, for her ideas on this subject.

1. The presenting problem appears in system terms, such as marital conflicts, severe sibling conflicts, or cross-generational conflicts (parents versus offspring; parents versus grandparents).
2. Various types of difficulty and conflict arise between the identified patient and other family members.
3. The family is experiencing a transitional stage of the family life cycle, such as beginning a family, marriage, birth of the first child, entrance of children into adolescence, the first child leaving home, retirement, or the death of one spouse.
4. Individual therapy with one family member results in symptoms developing in another family member.
5. No improvement occurs with adequate individual therapy. Enlarging the conceptual field to include the family in therapy may produce therapeutic movement.
6. The individual in treatment seems unable to use an intrapsychic or interpretive mode of individual therapy but primarily uses therapy sessions to talk about or complain about another member.

In most cases, clinical training programs in family therapy are open to nurse specialists with graduate degrees. Workshops in family therapy are offered across the United States. They vary in duration, theoretical model used, and the level of clinical sophistication required of participants. The nurse therapist doing family therapy should have some formal graduate training or on-the-job education through didactic and clinical seminars. She should obtain individual or group supervision for her clinical work in treating families to refine her clinical skills and deepen her theoretical understanding of family systems.

■ Practice settings

Family therapy is being done in inpatient and outpatient settings. In the home it is used by crisis intervention teams. It is also being used with groups of families of chronically ill patients in aftercare clinics at state psychiatric hospitals. Family therapy is performed by mental health professionals who volunteer their time to private or nonprofit associations, such as the Cancer Foundation. These professionals work with families experiencing a specific disease. Family therapy is used in some intensive care units such as kidney dialysis and coronary care units. In these settings, a severe psychological disturbance may be seen in the patient or family as a result of the acute illness.

The generalist nurse, without a graduate degree, is exposed to family therapy in many areas of practice. This therapy involves families at all levels of functioning. The nurse benefits by understanding theoretical models of family therapy. He or she may apply certain principles of these models in the work done with families of medically hospitalized patients. The nurse must promote their functioning and support their methods of coping with stress and illness. The family's method of coping with a member's illness can affect the outcome of the illness either positively or negatively. Knowledge of family therapy theories can help the nurse make more acute observations. It helps him or her to more readily identify problems within family systems and assists in selecting effective nursing interventions. Evaluation of the accuracy of the assessment by the interactional or functional change evident in the family then takes place. Knowledge of family therapy theories may also assist the nurse in initiating appropriate referrals.

The theoretical views of family therapy presented in this chapter are (1) family systems therapy, (2) structural family therapy, and (3) problem-solving, strategic, or brief therapy. These therapies are distinct and at times conflicting. They define theoretical frameworks developed from clinical research with families. Deciding which treatment approach is most effective depends on the nurse therapist's theoretical orientation. No well-defined criteria or conclusive research exist in this area.

Family systems therapy

Family systems therapy was developed by Bowen[5] in the 1950s and continues to evolve. A premise of this therapy is that a family is a homeostatic system. A change in functioning of one family member results in a compensatory change in the functioning of other family members. It resembles a centerless web in which, when one strand moves, the tensions in the entire web readjust.

Systems therapy explains emotional dysfunction in human relationships, specifically in the family system. Symptoms in any member of the family, whether social (e.g., child abuse, delinquency), physical (e.g., alcoholism, chronic illness), emotional (e.g., depression, schizophrenia), or conflictual (e.g., marital conflict), are viewed as evidence of dysfunction in the family relationship process. Although the family is only one emotional system in which an individual is involved, it is probably the most intense and influential one. Extrafamilial relationships rarely carry the intensity of the family emotional system. One's family system does not totally determine behavior and function. Rather, the family system fosters or inhibits function. The individual's responsibility for his actions is never lost.

The purpose of any theory is to understand, predict, and gain some control of the phenomena being studied. Understanding, as applied to family systems therapy, does not entail uncovering intrapsychic motivations. It identifies the functional facts of a relationship—what happened, when, where, how, and who was involved. These observable facts are more important than the reasons why the problematical behavior occurred. A systems therapist gathers from family members descriptions of behavior rather than feeling states. Conventional psychodynamic jargon is not present in family systems writing. This absence reflects a conscious attempt by Bowen and early systems researchers to remove the cause and effect medical model or "why thinking." Systems therapy uses simple, descriptive words.

Bowen[4-8] has described in detail the team research he conducted in the early 1950s on schizophrenic families in a live-in hospital setting. A new theory of family psychotherapy evolved from this live-in research. This theory, based on clinical observations of the research families' behavior, also applies to relationship patterns in more functional family systems. Bowen believed that "patterns originally thought to be typical of schizophrenia are present in all families some of the time and in some families most of the time."[8:61]

A cornerstone of systems therapy developed from a central pattern observed in research families. Some families failed to distinguish between the intellectual process of thinking and the more subjective process of feeling. It was as if the thinking processes were so flooded with feeling that members were unable to separate intellectual opinion and belief from subjective feelings. Routinely a person would say, "I feel that . . ." when "I think/believe that . . ." would have been more accurate. The families tried to foster feelings of togetherness and agreement in relation to others. They avoided statements of opinion or belief that would establish one member as different or separate from the family "party line."

A key goal of systems therapy, therefore, is to clarify and distinguish thinking and feeling processes in family members. Bowen's belief in the importance of distinguishing between feeling and thought is reflected in his use of the phase "emotional illness or dysfunction" rather than "mental illness." Emotional illness is deeper than a disorder of the mind and the thinking process; rather, it is a disturbance in the basic life processes of a person. The observation of this fusion between thinking and feeling led to the concept of the "undifferentiated family ego mass." People with the

greatest fusion between feeling and thinking function the most poorly. They inherit a high percentage of life's social, psychiatric, and medical problems.[8]

Family systems theory consists of seven interlocking concepts. Three concepts apply to overall characteristics of family systems: differentiation of self, triangles, and the nuclear family emotional system. The remaining four concepts are elaborations of the central family characteristics: the multigenerational transmission process, the family projection process, sibling position, and the emotional cutoff.

All these concepts refer to family processes that inhibit or promote individual family members' rising out of the emotional "we-ness," or fusion. This fusion binds us all to our families. Bowen believes forces toward fusion are as instinctual in a person as opposing forces toward differentiation. A member's movement toward either increased emotional closeness or distance is reflexive and predictable. The higher the level of differentiation in a person, the higher is the level of functioning. Differentiating the self from the "we-ness" is the goal of treatment. Guerin, on the other hand, sees the goal of family systems therapy as attainment of emotional freedom in the context of the family system. He is less militantly opposed to "we-ness" in the system than Bowen. Guerin's goal "leaves room for the ability either to be fused into a period of relationship refuge or to clearly draw one's boundaries and hold a functional position against the weight of the system."[18:19]

■ Differentiation of self

The concept of differentiation of self is Bowen's attempt to measure all human functioning on a continuum. The continuum proceeds from the greatest emotional fusion of self boundaries, to the highest degree of differentiation or autonomy. A concise description of the differentiated person is the person who is less anxious than the family system. This person is able to bring up emotion-laden issues in a nonassaulting way without anxiety. In his earlier work, Bowen refers to the "undifferentiated family ego mass" or the "conglomerate emotional oneness" that exists in varying degrees of intensity in families. The intensity of emotional closeness in a family may enable members to know each other's thoughts, feelings, and fantasies.

There is a cyclical quality to this closeness. As the emotional intensity or fusion between two individuals increases and the self of one is incorporated into the other self, the relationship is perceived to be uncomfortably close. This is usually followed by distance-creating behavior characterized by hostile rejection of the overcloseness. The two individuals actively repel each other.[6] Relationships can cycle through these phases, since anxiety in the relationship ebbs and flows at frequent intervals. Relationships can also become fixed at an angry, repelling standoff. In people who operate at this lower reactive end of the continuum, their intellect and emotions are so fused that they are dominated by the automatic emotional system. These people are less adaptable, less flexible, and more emotionally dependent on those about them. They are easily stressed into dysfunction. People at the upper end of the continuum maintain a degree of separation between thought and emotion. In periods of stress, they can retain a relative amount of intellectual functioning. They are more flexible, adaptable, and more independent of the reactive emotionality around them.[8]

The concept of differentiation eliminates the notion of normalcy. It has no direct connection to presence or absence of symptoms, although Bowen believes people at the lower end of the scale tend to inherit more of life's problems. People at the upper end of the continuum recoup rapidly if they are stressed into dysfunction.

■ Triangles

The concept of triangles is the key to understanding the systems approach to emotional function. Many techniques evolve from this concept. The idea of triangles is not a new one. Freud's theory of the oedipal complex describes a sexual triangle. Bowen has called the triangle the basic "building block of an emotional system." A triangle is a predictable emotional process that takes place in any significant relationship experiencing difficulty. The three corners of the triangle can be composed of three people; two people and a group, such as a religious affiliation or Al-Anon; two people and an issue, such as drinking or success; or two people and an object, such as the house or drugs.[15] The possible list of groups, issues, or objects is endless; it must have an emotional significance equal to that of a person.

All people seek closeness in emotional systems. Emotional closeness but separateness is difficult for two people to maintain; the tendency is to fuse, to lose self, or parts of self, in the other. A natural urge exists to seek completeness of self by accumulating parts of the other. The old adage "opposites attract" reflects this assumption. It is difficult for two people to maintain sufficient emotional closeness without fusion. The inevitable result is emotional distancing. The system is then ripe for the formation of a triangle. For example, the husband wants more expression of affection from an emotionally constricted wife. The more he pursues her, the more she withdraws, most often into preoccu-

pation with her child. The husband starts working longer hours. Husband and wife then start arguing circularly: "You care more about making a new account than you do about your wife and children!" "You expect to have nice things and then blame me for working extra hours!" Triangles stabilize by maintaining the status quo while avoiding tension, conflict, or talking about sensitive emotional areas. The two people can then focus on the new issue (or person or object) and avoid discussing the painful issues between them. Feelings are thus drained off, and the focus is removed from the self and one's own part in the problem. Change in self is avoided.

The reciprocal function of a triangle and the idea of equal responsibility can be difficult to convey to a couple. This is especially true when the distancing mechanism used by one spouse is as emotionally charged as an extramarital affair. Suppose the wife distances from the painful issues in the relationship. By "triangling" an affair, it is difficult for the husband to relinquish his self-righteous position of the "wronged husband." He does not see his behavior of working 14 to 16 hours a day as serving the same distancing function in the relationship. The nature of the distancing mechanism has meaningful content, whether it is overwork, extramarital affairs, homosexuality, psychotic symptoms, religious preoccupation, suicide gestures, depression, or psychoanalysis. All serve the same function as a triangular relationship within the family.[14]

The concept of a family scapegoat originally broadened the individual pathological view to include the part the family played in the symptomatic behavior. The tendency, however, is to view the scapegoat as the helpless victim of a persecuting family. For example, a husband and wife who are unable to settle their differences and wish to avoid their marital discord may focus on the "victim child." This leads to blaming the parents. From a systems view, with the concept of triangles, this process operates with all three twosomes that make up the triangle. A diagram of this triangle is presented in Fig. 29-1. Father and mother avoid conflict by focusing on the son. Mother and son avoid dealing with their overcloseness by having a common enemy in the father. Father and son avoid awareness of their emotional distance by relating through the mother as go-betweens. The "victim" is eliminated. Fogarty stresses, "All members of a triangle participate equally in perpetuating the triangle and no triangle can persist without the active cooperation of all its members."[15]

It is not a problem to be in a triangle; in fact, it is impossible to stay out of all triangles. Triangles form and re-form rapidly and are the daily reflexive way

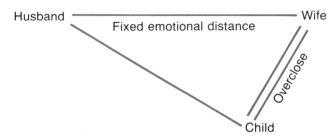

Fig. 29-1. A typical family triangle.

most people handle conflict or tension. Problems will arise if a triangle becomes fixed and when it involves significant relationships of deep friendship, blood ties, or marriage. Triangles are not static but form and re-form around emotion-laden issues, such as money, sex, child rearing, religion, alcohol, and education. A person's position in a triangle alters depending on the issue. A mother and father may be distant on the highly charged issue of how to spend their money. They may be close and in accord about their adolescent daughter's sexual activity. Judgments about these issues are most often based on emotion rather than careful thought.

■ **OPERATING PRINCIPLES.** A person's operating principles are the laws that govern his conduct. To determine what one's operating principles are, they must be inferred from what the person does in regard to an emotion-laden issue rather than what he says. Operating principles vary from intrinsically valuable ones based on conscious conviction to more immature, reactive, impulsive principles. Immature principles are other-focused rather than self-focused. They lead to a loss of freedom of self-determination. Any behavior that is predictable, as in behavior operated by a triangle, is not free. The loss of freedom impairs self-functioning, perpetuates problems, causes a deterioration in family functioning, and promotes symptom development.[14]

Other-focused, triangle-promoting operating principles are reflected in various ways. These include declaring feelings "right" or "wrong"; using plural pronouns "we" or "us" rather than "I"; accusing the other person of "you made me mad/do it"; stepping in to settle, side taking, or blaming in two other people's conflict; telling or holding secrets; telling the other person what to do; and assuming responsibility for the other person's feelings, for example, "I want to make her happy" or "I couldn't tell him because it would hurt him." These statements are typically interpreted as thoughtful or being very responsible. In fact, avoiding one's own feelings by focusing on the other person is

irresponsible. Everyone falls into this pattern, especially in a marriage or parent-child relationship. When a person becomes anxious, it is more comfortable to project the problem onto the other person and then work to change the other. The implicit assumption here is, "I can't help my behavior, but he is behaving that way deliberately."[19]

In more dysfunctional, closed family systems, interaction between family members is determined by fixed interactional patterns. This is observed, for example, in schizophrenic families. These fixed triangles are an effort to maintain a homeostatic balance and to avoid stress. When an additional stress occurs outside or within the family, such as a job change or the birth of a new member, symptoms may arise in a dysfunctional attempt to reduce stress and restore balance. This is evident in Clinical example 29-1.

■ **INTERVENTIONS.** Treatment encourages key figures in key triangles to identify their emotional "triggers." The person identifies the verbal or behavioral cues of the other person, to which he reflexively reacts with a predictable behavior. When the person pinpoints these cues, he can take control of his part in the process. Once one person takes control and changes his part in a triangle, the whole system changes.

An example of this was a mother who was overclose to her 16-year-old daughter. The daughter had become school phobic and stayed home from school

---

CLINICAL EXAMPLE 29-1

Mr. and Mrs. D, whose family consisted of six children, had a seventh unplanned child. The family was financially strained, and Mr. and Mrs. D had a conflictual and distant relationship. When the last child was born, a middle sibling, 13-year-old Andy, developed symptoms and became school phobic. The school insisted the child receive treatment. Late in the treatment the mother finally revealed that one of the reasons for the family's financial strain was the husband's work phobia and his occasional gambling sprees. The wife had covered for him for years, calling his boss to make excuses and taking part-time work herself. Until the birth of the last child, the family was able to maintain a precarious, minimally functional balance. The additional stress, however, produced symptoms sufficiently noticeable to cause an outside agency, the school, to become involved.

for a year before the family sought treatment. The father would come home from work, see the daughter had missed school another day, and angrily attack her with "shape-up speeches." The mother bitterly complained about the daughter being home all day doing nothing. However, when the father began his verbal attacks, she would then become protective of the daughter and launch an attack on the father: "How can you say those things to her; you know how upset she gets." When the mother was able to get a "handle" on her emotional trigger (the mother had always been terrified of her "drill sergeant" father), she was able to control her protective reflex, step back, and permit the father to become more effective with his daughter.

The nurse must identify key triangles in a family and operating principles of its members. She must understand what sets off her own emotional triggers and assume that the family will attempt to triangle her into its own emotional system to reestablish equilibrium. The nurse's job is to maintain sufficient emotional distance to watch the process unfolding between family members. At the same time she maintains emotional contact with each family member.[10] Bowen[34] has enumerated many therapist's reactions that indicate that the therapist is part of a triangle. These include feeling sorry for or pitying the other, feeling angry at the system or member, being overly positive about the system, wanting to correct horrendous behavior, and finding oneself without questions or responses in the session. The nurse must limit the action to the two family members and avoid becoming involved. Once the therapist steps in to take sides, progress stops and status quo is reestablished.[35] Side taking should be a planned strategy in which the nurse maintains the freedom to realign with specific family members.

Systems therapists do not believe they can change family members; change is possible only when it is generated within the self. Family members are encouraged to take responsibility for the self and not try to change the other. The therapist must avoid becoming part of a triangle in the system. To get out of an emotional process she reacts to in the session, the nurse may elicit the member's responses. For example, if she becomes irritated at a critical intrusive husband, the nurse can ask the wife, "What happens to your insides when your husband interrupts with criticism?" This feeds the process back into the system, keeping it between the spouses.

One of the areas of controversy in the field of family therapy is the importance of the therapist's working on his or her own family of origin (referred to as TOF, therapist's own family). Systems therapists contend that it is a major aspect of training as a family

therapist. "Working on" means the nurse differentiates herself in her own family of origin. She identifies the issues in her family that she is reactive to and with whom she is part of a triangle around these issues. She then works to get out of the triangle by gaining control of her reflexive distancing and fusing in her family. This way she has the freedom of emotional closeness and of some emotional distance with each family member (without using geographical distance to create emotional space). Unless a therapist is conscious of the triangles she is a part of in her own family, she will be vulnerable to the same roles and behaviors in the families she is treating.

■ **Nuclear family emotional system**

The nuclear family emotional system refers to patterns of interaction between family members and the degree to which these patterns promote emotional fusion. These patterns of interaction, called operating principles, are the ways the person behaves in most significant relationships. All marriage relationships reflect a balance, or complementarity, of operating principles and reciprocal function.[19] For example, the reasonable, object-oriented, and emotionally distant spouse is married to the affectively expressive, relationship-oriented, emotional pursuer. These differences in operating principles provide the attraction and the balancing stability to the marriage relationship. One spouse is the subject overfunctioner, the other the emotional overfunctioner. Difficulty arises when dependence on attributes of the spouse reduces functional attributes in the self. Self borrows on the functioning of the spouse, and self boundaries are blurred. This is referred to as **ego fusion.** When these reciprocal functions become fixed positions of overfunction-underfunction, emotional dysfunction and symptoms occur, such as chronic depression or physical illness. In such a relationship, to view one spouse as strong and independent and the other as weak and dependent fails to recognize the overfunctioner's dependence on the underfunctioning of the other spouse. The underfunctioner must be one-down for the other to appear one-up.

Emotional fusion operates in all marriages to a lesser or greater extent. When the relationship is unstressed, the reciprocal function works smoothly. When stress occurs, each spouse becomes more as oneself. The distancer seeks space and objects (the job, art, alcohol); the pursuer seeks togetherness and expression of personal feelings. Both are efforts to avoid personal anxiety. The pursuer takes the distancer's withdrawal as personal rejection and reactively withdraws. No longer feeling crowded, the distancer then moves in emotionally, only to be met with, "Where were you when I needed you; get lost." The distancer then pulls back, baffled and angry at the rejection. A fixed emotional distance sets in.[19] These are the relationships nurses see just before the couple decides on a divorce. These relationships are ripe for triangulation with an affair or with an unsuspecting therapist.

People pick spouses who have equivalent levels of differentiation of self.[5] The greater the undifferentiation, the greater is the tendency toward fusion and potential problems. If there is a high degree of ego fusion and intensity in the nuclear family, this intensity can be diffused and reduced through active contact with the family of origin. In periods of stress, contact with the extended family or family of origin can stabilize the nuclear family. Promoting such contact can be an effective therapeutic strategy.

Bowen[6] has identified two patterns in the nuclear family emotional system, which he labels the "explosive family" and the "cohesive family." Family units of a cohesive family are geographically close, in frequent contact and communication. The person who geographically separates from his family of origin because of the fusion or intensity of attachment there may marry a spouse from a cohesive family. The person's unresolved attachments to his own family of origin lie dormant until ritualized contact (at a wedding or funeral) stirs them up. In a nuclear family in which both spouses are detached from their families of origin, the spouses tend to be more dependent on each other. The process between them is more intense. These are the explosive families.

Bowen[5] postulates three mechanisms by which spouses maintain sufficient emotional distance from each other to handle the anxiety associated with fusion. All three mechanisms may be used by the couple, or tension may be focused in one area. If tension is great enough, it will spill over into other social systems, such as mental health centers or school counselors. The three mechanisms used are (1) marital conflict, (2) dysfunction in one spouse, and (3) projection of the problem onto one or more children.

■ **MARITAL CONFLICT.** Conflictual marriages are built on a constant struggle between spouses. They want "their fair share" of needs met, of freedom, of love, of attention, or of control. Neither spouse is willing to compromise. A high percentage of the self is wrapped up in the "happiness" of the other. Functioning of the self is enmeshed in the function of the other. These relationships tend to be stable, whether positive ("Anything to make her happy") or negative ("I sacrificed the best years of my life helping him be a success; I'll never let him go now"). They endure predictable cycles of intense closeness, distance-creating conflict, making up, then renewed closeness. It is commonly believed that this amount of conflict would harm the children of such marriages. Bowen[9] postulates, however, that the children are protected from overinvolvement because tension is focused between parents.

Intervention in conflictual marriages usually involves working with the most motivated spouse at first. If both spouses are seen together, frequently the uproar between them is too great to tolerate. They are very reactive to each other. Limit setting, such as prohibiting interruptions, and strategies such as a "listening chair" or turning one spouse's chair to the wall to listen are ineffective. In such situations spouses must be seen separately initially. The approach is to get the focus on the self and decrease efforts to change the other. The nurse focuses on what part the spouse plays in the situation. This spouse gains some control of his or her own reactive triggers. Once blaming is reduced, the spouse reevaluates his or her own set of beliefs and values without the need to attack the other. Such reevaluation entails contacting one's family of origin by phone, letters, or planned visits. The goal is to understand better the source of the nuclear family conflict and to work to establish more personal relationships with one's family of origin. Bowen calls this "process coaching." Usually, before this point is reached in the treatment, the absent, less-motivated spouse has sought to join the sessions because of the changes that have occurred.

Significant changes in the marriage system occur when one spouse reduces overinvestment in the other and focuses on self. The spouse making changes must be warned of predictable efforts by the other to reestablish status quo. This may occur in the other through an escalation of anger-provoking behavior, threats to leave, and so on. If the spouse making changes can maintain a self-focused position through the resistance, both partners may become active in the treatment. While temporarily working with one spouse, the nurse must guard against becoming part of a triangle. She may emotionally side with the spouse initially in treatment or become his or her only support. This can be especially difficult for the nurse when the unexpressed plan of the unmotivated spouse is to deposit the husband or wife in treatment and obtain a divorce. The nurse may then be expected to "take care of" the spouse.

■ **SPOUSE DYSFUNCTION.** The second mechanism used by spouses to maintain emotional distance is the dysfunction of one spouse. As mentioned earlier, one spouse may be emotionally, socially, or physically disabled to varying degrees. The degree to which the

CLINICAL EXAMPLE 29-2

Mr. and Mrs. S are a couple who sought treatment because the husband was missing so many days at work. The couple would have extensive arguments about the husband not wanting to work and the wife feeling outraged at the financial stress he was creating. It became apparent that Mrs. S. treated Mr. S as one of their adolescent boys. She overfunctioned to the point of cleaning up after her husband's destructive temper tantrums. Over time, with considerable coaching, she was able to pull back in several areas, refusing to wake the husband or clean up after him, leaving it up to him to pay the bills, and generally holding back her critical nagging. The first sign of progress was at the husband's next temper tantrum (he did delicate electrical work and had a low frustration tolerance). He carefully selected which objects he would throw or smash in his workroom, for example, not throwing a box of small nuts and bolts. He cleaned up his own workroom and began going to work regularly. As the husband's functioning improved, the wife became significantly depressed and began addressing unresolved issues in her family of origin. This couple demonstrated the reciprocity in the mechanism of underfunctioning and overfunctioning in a marriage.

one underfunctions is the degree to which the other overfunctions. This ensures that emotional equilibrium is maintained, since both partners are locked into a mutually dependent relationship. Interventions with such a relationship are similar to those used with the conflictual marriage. Bowen suggests working with the overfunctioning spouse by first helping him to pull back. The underfunctioning spouse then moves in to take up the slack. This is evidenced in Clinical example 29-2.

■ **PROJECTION ON CHILD.** The third distancing mechanism used by spouses to control the intensity of fusion between them is the projection of the problem to one or more of the children. Before the development of a family pathology theory, the parents of a symptomatic child would be excluded from therapy. This further reinforced the dysfunction in the family by focusing on the child as "the problem." Child-focused families either view the problem as exclusive to the symptomatic child or deny the existence of a problem entirely. When the school or probation officer recommends treatment, they passively comply but participate reluctantly. When a couple centers on their chil-

dren, it is easier to avoid marital confrontations because there is always something to worry, criticize, or complain about with the children. These families strongly depend on the children's symptoms and resist exploring broader issues in therapy.

How one child becomes a parental concern is a complex process. It may have its roots in several previous generations. Key triangles tend to repeat themselves over generations; thus the parent's natural tendency is to put one child in the parent's past position in the triangle. Nodal events are the normative events that occur in every family life but generate anxiety because change ensues. These include such events as birth, death, sickness, marriage, job changes, school changes, divorce, and family relocation. The amount of stress generated around a nodal event depends on the amount of resultant change. If a significant developmental stage of the child (e.g., in utero, birth, entering school for the first time, adolescence) coincides approximately with the occurrence of a nodal event, this child is vulnerable to the focus of family stress and to impairment. The first-born and last-born children are also particularly vulnerable to family focus.

The primary goal of treatment is to remove the focus from the child and place the conflict between the parents where it belongs. The child's dysfunctions must be placed within the context of the family system by taking a family history and drawing a family genogram. Drawing a three-generation family genogram is a structured method of gathering information and graphically symbolizing much factual and emotional relationship data in the initial interview.[20] A sample genogram is presented in Fig. 29-2. Drawing a family genogram in full view of the family on large easel paper or a blackboard broadens the family's focus. The therapist's questions and comments are geared toward change of self rather than changing the child.

The therapist may identify problematic behavior in other family members to remove blame from the child. Another therapeutic strategy is to discuss how grandparents might handle the problem. With some families the nurse can coach the overinvolved parent, such as the mother, to pull back from the focused child and send a note to her own mother telling her one thing about herself that she does not want her to know. This reveals the three-generational aspect of the presenting problem. Guerin recommends working with the sibling subset at times, separately from the parents. This promotes a more positive support system among sibs. Frequently, sibs mimic their parents' negative behavior toward the focused child. However, they may resent the excessive attention he receives from parents and act aggressively toward him.

Families with an acting-out child and two parents

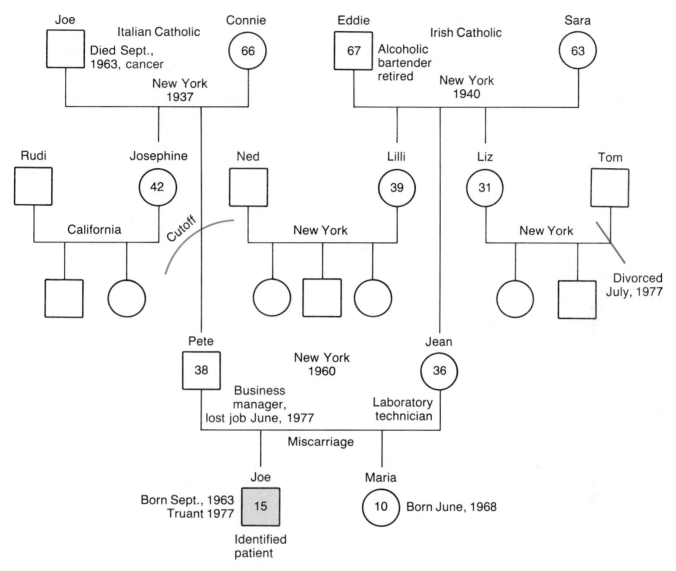

Fig. 29-2. A hypothetical family genogram.

in the ineffective helpless position (or one parent set up as the "heavy" and the other as "the nice guy" saboteur) need a direct approach initially. The parents may relinquish authority to the child. This may be determined by asking them the following extreme questions: "If your child had third-degree burns, could you get her to take the horribly painful treatments?" or "If your child had heart disease, could you limit her activities?" Following are four guidelines for parents locked in a triangle with the acting-out "problem child":

1. The person who sets the rule must be present to enforce it.
2. With two parents in the home, divide the areas of responsibility (e.g., allowance, bedtime, nights out) so that when a dispute comes up, it is clear with whom the child must negotiate.
3. Yelling is ineffective and inhibits thinking. Parents need to control their reactions.
4. Decide the consequences of repeated disobedient behavior and inform the child of them. When the behavior occurs, without yelling, carry out the consequence even if the parent's personal plans must be changed to do so.*

As soon as the child focus is sufficiently reduced, the child is removed from the sessions. The therapist then becomes the third corner of the triangle, actively

---

*I am indebted to Betty Carter for her ideas on this issue.

relating to both spouses without taking sides and thereby keeping conflict between the spouses.

■ Multigenerational transmission process

The roots of the family emotional system extend back through generations. When emotional dysfunction occurs, it can be scattered throughout the family tree. Drawing a three-generation family genogram frequently reveals certain relationship patterns otherwise believed to be peculiar to one nuclear family. For example, suicide of younger brothers, divorce among female siblings, or alcoholism might be a pattern across a family system when four or five generations are mapped out on a genogram. In family therapy, a symptom in one family member in one generation has its origin several generations before. This differentiates it from other forms of family therapy. Families seeking treatment, however, usually present symptoms as a nuclear family problem.

■ Family projection process

The family projection process refers to the way anxiety about specific issues is transmitted through the generations. These are emotionally powerful issues, such as money, sex, child rearing, religion, work or school achievement, alcohol, politics, illness and death, and around which a rigid "party line" develops. Family members polarize around these issues, taking the family position or the direct opposite. Neither position allows freedom or flexibility of thought. Positions are reactive and fixed. Studying the family of origin helps identify a person's predictable position in family triangles involving specific issues. By thinking about the issues he normally reacts to emotionally, the person can plan strategies that will free him from his triangled position.

The family projection process also refers to the process that labels and assigns characteristics to certain family members. These labels may be overpositive ("Mary Sunshine," "The Genius") or overnegative ("the crazy one," "dummy"). They are equally unrealistic and confining. After years of family labeling, the labeled person will come to volunteer for the label and deserve it.

■ Sibling position

The concept of personality profiles based on sibling position is borrowed by family systems theorists from Walter Toman, a Viennese psychiatrist. Toman's basic thesis[37] is that important personality characteristics are determined by the sex of one's siblings and one's birth order. For example, the younger brother of two older sisters will be quite different from the older brother of a brother. The personality profiles Toman developed can suggest marital discord or harmony on issues of rank or sex. A younger brother of brothers would have more difficulty relating to his spouse than a younger brother of sisters. If this younger brother of brothers married a younger sister of sisters, they would both have discomfort with the opposite sex. In addition, they would struggle for juniority rights (who's going to take care of whom). The couple who recognizes sibling rank and sex as a possible source of their conflicts can help each other to cope with their differences.

■ Emotional cutoff

The emotional cutoff is a way to deal with intense unresolved attachment between children and parents. The cutoff may be emotional isolation, although members still live geographically close. It also may be physical distance from the family of origin.[8] The cutoff creates the illusion of separation from one's parents. The more intense the emotional cutoff, the more likely the person will recreate the same problem in his own marriage. Reconnecting emotionally with his cutoff family may prevent the same process from occurring with his own children. Such patterns tend to repeat over the generations.

■ Modes of therapy

Several modes of therapy have been mentioned thus far, including therapy with both spouses. Another mode of family therapy is with one family member. This is most frequently used with the young adult who is single and self-supporting. This method involves learning about the functioning of family systems and triangles. It also involves keeping an active emotional relationship with important family members by planned phone calls, letters, and visits. This therapy requires developing an ability to control emotional reactiveness to avoid becoming part of an emotional triangle during visits with the family.[5] The goal is to achieve more self-differentiation from the family of origin. One must also develop a person-to-person relationship with important family members. This therapy is referred to as coaching. Once the person is knowledgeable about triangles and methods of detriangling within his own family, coaching sessions can be held as needed to supervise ongoing self-differentiation efforts.

The last mode of therapy is multiple family therapy (MFT), developed in its present form in the late 1960s. MFT is to be distinguished from multiple family group therapy. The latter uses role playing and psychodrama and promotes interfamily group process to change family interaction and increase its sensitivity to the family environment.[33] MFT, from a family systems framework, is different. Sessions are structured to ensure against emotional exchange between families. Bowen believes this emotional exchange encourages a fusion of other families into a large, undifferentiated ego mass. The idea behind MFT is (1) to conserve teaching time of families, (2) to provide contact with a greater volume of families, and (3) to allow the opportunity for families to learn from the efforts and experiences of other families. While other families observe, the nurse therapist works with each family as if she were working alone with that family. She asks detailed questions about the family's problem. She defocuses feelings and addresses one spouse while the other spouse listens. Then she asks the silent spouse for thoughts or reactions to what the other spouse has said. The family members observing can talk to the therapist about another family but cannot directly talk to the other family.

Structural family therapy

Structural family therapy is a body of theory and techniques based on the individual within his social context. The assumption is that behavior is a consequence of the family's organization and the interactional patterns between members. Changing the family organization and the feedback processes between members changes the context in which a person functions. Thus the person's inner processes and behavior change. The therapist temporarily becomes part of the context. This approach is clearly conceptualized by Minuchin[25,26] and those associated with the Philadelphia Child Guidance Clinic.

The implicit question of a structural family therapist is, "In what way is this family structure maintaining this dysfunctional symptom?" Family structure is the invisible set of functional demands that organize the way in which family members interact. A family is a system that operates through transactional patterns. Repeated transactions establish patterns of how, when, and to whom to relate, and these patterns determine whether the system is functional or dysfunctional.

■ Components

■ **FAMILY IN TRANSITION.** In this model the family is a social system in transformation. The family system must maintain its continuity so family members can grow. At the same time it must adapt to both internal and external stresses to the system. Normal anxiety occurs during transitional stages to accommodate new circumstances. Traditional therapists call this anx-

---

CLINICAL EXAMPLE 29-3

An elderly widow decided to move from her apartment where she had lived for 25 years because she came home one day and found it had been robbed. Soon after moving, she sought treatment from a psychiatrist. She complained that the people who moved her were trying to control her and had purposely lost precious possessions. They were leaving sinister messages for each other on her furniture, and when she went outside, people followed her and signaled to each other. The psychiatrist diagnosed her as psychotic with paranoid delusions and prescribed tranquilizers. When this did not help, she sought a second psychiatrist, who recommended hospitalization. The third therapist she saw was a context-related therapist. He understood her symptoms as an ecological crisis. It was precipitated by feeling forced to move into an unfamiliar environment. He explained to her that she had lost her shell—the familiarity of objects in her apartment, the neighborhood, the neighbors. As any crustacean who has lost its shell, she felt vulnerable and was experiencing reality differently than before. He instructed her to go home, unpack, and place her familiar objects, books, and pictures in the new apartment. He told her to do her daily chores routinely, go to the same shops and checkout counters, and for 2 weeks make no effort to meet neighbors. She was to visit old friends and family but not discuss her recent experiences. If anyone asked, she was to explain that those had just been the problems of an illogical, fearful old woman.

---

iety pathological. This is described in Clinical example 29-3 by Minuchin.[25]

Structural family therapists change the relationship between a person and the familiar context in which he functions. This changes his subjective experience and enables new, more functional behavior to emerge. In this clinical example, the therapist's interventions protected the woman from the unfamiliar and frightening environment until she could "grow a new shell." He blocked the environmental feedback that confirmed her paranoid fears as friends and family secretly discussed her frightening behavior. As her experience of her environment changed, her symptoms disappeared.

■ **STAGES OF FAMILY DEVELOPMENT.** According to Minuchin's second component of a viable functional family, the family undergoes predictable stages of development over time. These stages require adaptive restructuring. Each stage has appropriate developmental tasks that must be accomplished for the family to pass on to the next stage. One stage is the courtship period, when the young person shifts to membership in the adult community. He establishes status in relation to others and selects a mate. This is one of the major times when professional help is sought. The marriage stage is preceded by negotiation of the spouses' relationship with respective families of origin. The families of origin must adjust to partial separation of one member, inclusion of a new member, and accommodation to a new spouse subsystem in the family system functioning. The new family unit may never succeed if families of origin do not undergo this transformation. Couples who cut themselves off from extended families are equally unsuccessful.

During the marriage stage, many complex rules and transactional patterns must be established between partners. Some ways of relating are reinforced, and others are shed in the process of mutual accommodation. When a child is born, the functioning of the spouse unit must be modified to include parenting functions. It must shift from an intimate unit of two to a system of three. Frequently the new child becomes the excuse for new and previously unresolved conflicts between spouses. Many past battles are fought during child rearing because the couple cannot separate parenting functions from spouse functions.

In the middle years of marriage, a major task is the weaning of parents from children. This is a particularly stressful time for families in which spouses established communication through the children and the children are leaving (or struggling to leave) home. This can be a period of enrichment for spouses. This is true if the husband is enjoying career success and the wife is freer now to pursue career plans or other interests. Finally, a family member enters the stage of retirement and old age. This can be harmonious or problematical as spouses are thrown together 24 hours a day. In time, one of the partners dies. Adult children then face the crisis of caring for an aging parent. These adult children who assume the care provider role (most commonly daughters or daughters-in-law) may have young children or adolescents at home or may themselves be old. The family cycle continues to unfold. As the family is transformed over time, it must adapt and restructure itself to continue functioning. When a family adheres inappropriately to previous structural schemas, stress builds and symptoms develop. See Carter and McGoldrick[11] for in-depth discussion of the family life cycle, therapeutic considerations of each stage, and normative interruptions of the life cycle.

■ **FAMILY STRUCTURE.** A third component of Minuchin's model of a viable functioning family relates to the family structure. The major elements of structure are power and influence, sets of relationships, and boundaries (individual, sexual, generational). Structure can become dysfunctional in any or each of these areas.[31] As in any organization, the family system must have a power hierarchy with different levels of authority to function efficiently. Functions must be complementary; the family functions as a team. Over the years, mutual expectations of particular family members evolve. These expectations may be openly negotiated but more often are implicit, with patterns of behavior developing around minor daily events.

The family system differentiates and functions through subsystems. Subsystems can be made up of individuals or dyads. They are formed by generation, sex, interest, or function. Each person belongs to many subsystems. Each subsystem has different levels of power in which differentiated skills are learned. The boundaries of a subsystem are the rules defining who participates in subsystem functions and how. Boundaries must be free of intrusion. Each subsystem has specific functions and interpersonal developmental tasks to be accomplished. Patterns of mutual accommodation as well as healthy competition cannot develop among siblings if parents or grandparents constantly interfere. Subsystem boundaries must be clear for proper family functioning but must also permit emotional contact among members.

Minuchin[25,26] describes families with extreme boundary problems as either enmeshed or disengaged. Enmeshed boundaries are weak and fluid; personal space and subsystem boundaries rapidly change and impact all subsystems. This diffuseness of boundaries inhibits the development of autonomy and competence. Perceptions of self and others are poorly differentiated. A child in such a family might be so sensitized to conflict between parents that he is unable to perform in school. The parents in such a family can become upset because the child refuses his vegetables at dinnertime. Such families flood with anxiety at times of stress and adapt poorly to change.

Disengaged families have rigid boundaries. Communication between subsystems is poor; supportive or protective contact is minimal. Members of such systems may function autonomously but have a skewed sense of independence. They lack feelings of loyalty and belonging and the capacity for interdependence. Stierlin[32] hypothesizes that the product of a disengaged family is the sociopath. Because of the rigidity of subsystem boundaries, members may fail to respond adequately when one member is stressed. In such a family, a child's reading disorder might go unnoticed or a husband's suicidal behavior be disregarded.

The nurse often functions as a boundary maker. He or she may clarify diffuse boundaries by blocking interruptions, may encourage shutting bedroom doors, or may open overly rigid boundaries by recommending that a distant parent and child spend time together. The nurse may call attention to a member's nuance of feeling that would otherwise go unnoticed by other members. The nurse's assessment of family subsystems and boundary functioning provides a rapid diagnosis of the family. It indicates the direction and goals of therapeutic interventions.

As mentioned earlier, each subsystem has specific functions and interpersonal developmental tasks to be accomplished. The spouse subsystem must develop patterns of mutual support. Couples must make decisions and settle arguments without domination or relinquishing of self by either spouse. Ideally, they will bring out the best in each other, with each promoting personal growth and creativity in their spouse.

Spouses typically engage in an "other-improvement program." They bring into the marriage certain expectations of their spouse and work hard to have the spouse meet them. Interpretations in this area should be directed to both spouses. The part each plays in the destructive process should be pointed out. A mutual interpretation would be to say to the wife, "In your efforts to make contact with your husband, you are driving him away," and to the husband, "Your strong silent style is alluring and elicits nagging." Balanced interpretations emphasize the complementarity of the system. Both positive and negative qualities are recognized in each spouse.

The parental subsystem socializes the children without sacrificing mutual support and accommodation between the spouses. Children must have access to each parent but be excluded from spouse functions. Minuchin advocates parental authority in an era that promotes "pure democracy" between parents and children. He recognizes the difficulty of parenting. Many parents are not satisfied with their own functioning. Parenting processes are different depending on the child's age. Part of promoting differentiation in the family is making the differentiation in ages clear. Adolescents have responsibilities and privileges that 12-year-old siblings do not. Children must learn to negotiate with their parents to live in a world of unequal power relationships.

Children first learn about peer relationships in the sibling subsystem. They learn to make friends, compete, negotiate, cooperate, and gain recognition of their skills. Knowledge of growth and development of children is valuable for the nurse who at times must translate age-appropriate skills, needs, and values to baffled parents. The nurse should support the child's right to autonomy and the parents' authority at the same time.

■ Goals of the initial interview

A vital component to structural family therapy is the process of joining the family.[25,26] The nurse temporarily becomes part of the family system. The nurse adapts his or her behavior to the particular family's rules and manner. This can be done either purposefully or unconsciously. The aim is to accommodate himself or herself to the family to gain experiential entrance into the family system. Unless this is accomplished at the outset, restructuring and change is impossible. Following are methods of joining:

1. Mirroring or mimicking—matching the family's mood, pace, communication patterns, or kinesthetic cues (e.g., becoming jovial or somber, communication becoming terse or punctuated with long pauses, becoming fidgety)
2. Respecting families' values and hierarchies (e.g., if one spouse is the "central switchboard," addressing all communication through that spouse first)
3. Keying in culturally when possible or finding elements of kinship (e.g., "I have an adolescent boy, too")
4. Searching for strength—observing for the smallest positive detail about individual family members that the nurse can use to confirm the individual's sense of self and make contact with him (e.g., appreciating a clever phrase or a preadolescent's poised manner)
5. Supporting family subsystems (e.g., giving smaller children toys to play with while talking to older ones, having parents sit together as they discuss their difficulty with the children)
6. Tracking—asking for elaboration with concrete details and examples of specific content in the family's discussion. This confirms individuals who are speaking and explores family structure (e.g., tracking a mother's mentioning that she and her son are close by asking what time of the day and in which part of the home they are closest, thus learning that the mother and son sleep together while father sleeps in another room)

Another initial task of the nurse is to assume leadership in the session. The nurse must join the family while still retaining the freedom to confront and challenge. He or she can assume leadership by presenting himself or herself as an expert, gaining the family's confidence, and instilling hope. The nurse establishes the rules of the system by determining who attends the session, allowing no one to talk for another, and prohibiting interruptions. The nurse controls the flow and direction of communication.

At the beginning of the session, the nurse contacts each member. The nurse must not spend more than 15 to 20 minutes with an individual or he or she will become part of the system. Very soon the nurse asks two people to interact directly to enact a problem they have been describing. The nurse can now directly observe dysfunctional interactions. Rather than going from content issue to content issue, the nurse therapist can introduce the conflict inherent in small events and make conflictual events from nonevents.

Minuchin is a master of intensifying minute, simple nonevents for therapeutic intervention. For example, in a demonstration videotape, a father is "helping" the identified patient, the adolescent son, adjust his video microphone wire. Minuchin turns this into a therapeutic intervention focusing on the family's infantalization of the son. This occurs in the first 5 minutes of the tape. The amount of knowledge needed about the family to diagnose and begin restructuring dysfunctional interactions is available quickly.[30] Structural family therapy does not explore or interpret the past. It is active and immediate.

Diagnosis in family therapy depends on the nurse's observation of how the family affects his or her behavior. It is also based on the nurse's impact on the family. The interactional diagnosis changes according to the family's acceptance or resistance of the therapist's restructuring interventions. It also varies depending on which family subsystem is active in the therapeutic situation at any one time. In this way, diagnosis and therapy are inseparable.

■ Restructuring interventions

Restructuring intervention transforms the dysfunctional transactional patterns that maintain symptomatic behavior. The nurse is concerned about symptom removal and changes the family's organization to ensure that the symptom is not passed on. However, if an area of organization such as the parents' relationship does not contribute to the symptom, Minuchin does not enter there. He believes that therapy should be limited to the family's presenting symptom.

Minuchin identifies seven categories of restructuring operations: enacting family transactional patterns, marking boundaries, escalating stress, assigning tasks, using symptoms, manipulating mood, and supporting, educating, or guiding.[25]

■ **ENACTING TRANSACTIONAL PATTERNS.** Enacting transactional patterns involves family members actively discussing an event that they might otherwise be describing to the nurse. Instead, the nurse instructs specific members to discuss the matter between themselves. The nurse disengages from the interaction to observe nonverbal confirmation or contradiction of the content, patterned sequences, interruptions, distractions, alliances, and coalitions.

The nurse may find it difficult to stay outside these transactions, permitting the family to drag her back into direct discussion. Going behind a one-way mirror after giving the family directions is a way to avoid this temptation. Manipulating space by rearranging seating or position can be an effective way of encouraging or intensifying dialogue. The seating pattern a family assumes when it first walks into a session provides clues to alliances, coalitions, centrality, and isolation. The nurse's manipulation of seating and space can be a diagnostic probe to see how flexible the family is to such change. It is also a graphic indication to the family of a therapeutic goal. For instance, the nurse may seat the spatially isolated father next to his son where the mother was seated. The wife is placed next to the nurse. This encourages more direct involvement between father and son, with the mother outside that relationship.

■ **MARKING BOUNDARIES.** Boundaries must be marked in both individuals and subsystems. This promotes clarity in the enmeshed families and reduces rigidity in disengaged families. Simple rules promote individual autonomy. These include insisting family members speak *to* each other and not *about* each other. No one speaks for another, no one may interrupt, and no one acts as another's memory bank. The nurse encourages subsystem boundaries by including or excluding various subsystems attending a session. She would ask children to leave or not attend a session in discussing spouses' sex life. The nurse may assign tasks to promote subsystem boundaries. She might instruct the father and daughter to go out for a pizza once a week without the mother or younger siblings. Having the sibling subsystem interact in a session, with the mother behind a one-way mirror, helps the children find alternate ways to resolve conflicts normally interrupted by mother's interventions. At the same time, this lets mother identify more positive interaction among the children. Previously, she could only reflexively react to their anger, rebelliousness, and selfishness by intruding on their boundaries. Rigid triads involving cross-generational interactions can be especially resistant to boundary marking.

■   **ESCALATING STRESS.** Increasing stress in a family forces members to develop more functional ways of resolving stress. In families seeking treatment, dysfunctional patterns have developed around the symptomatic member. To escalate stress, the nurse may block usual transactional patterns and emphasize differences the family ignores. Asking for the silent spouse's opinion following the dominant spouse's statements highlights unspoken family disagreements. Developing implicit conflict involves making covert conflict overt.

Families develop methods for diffusing conflict rapidly. For example, siblings may tease and shove each other noisily just before their parents argue. This prevents the parents' conflict from surfacing. Blocking the sibling conflict forces the parents to contact directly. The nurse can polarize conflict to increase stress. If a couple appear equally concerned about their son's delinquent activities, the nurse may ask the husband if he had ever tried telling his wife she was "messing up" with the son. The positions of the overprotective mother and the "reasonable" distant father develop.

The nurse can also produce stress by temporarily joining one member or subsystem. This operation must be carefully planned and requires the nurse's ability to disengage. She can do this serially to help members take differentiated positions. She can also form a coalition, usually with a spouse, when the system rigidly resists open conflict. Joining a husband's attack on the wife makes the conflict too intense for the wife to diffuse stress onto the son. She is forced to address the conflict between herself and the husband.

■   **ASSIGNING TASKS.** The assigning of tasks structures the setting for alternate interactions and behavior. In designing tasks, the nurse must have a clear idea of the family's structure and dysfunctional patterns. She must have specific interactional goals to accomplish through the task. Tasks can be simple. The nurse may ask a husband and wife to sit next to each other as they discuss an issue. In a family in which the wife disciplines the children, the father is assigned the job. The mother handles only emergencies; otherwise, the father learns of infractions he does not directly observe. The wife may not interfere with her husband's disciplinary tactics. She takes notes. Both parents become active and effective.

In assigning tasks, the nurse should give all critically involved members a portion of the task to complete. This reduces the likelihood of one member sabotaging another's new behavior if each has a focus on himself. This also makes it easier to relinquish a fixed behavior if another behavior is assigned to replace it. Whether the task is completed or not, the family and nurse have new information about family patterns and progress.

■   **USING SYMPTOMS.** Symptoms can be used in restructuring operations in various ways. Symptoms may be focused on, as in a family Minuchin describes in which the daughter was a fire setter. The focus remained on the daughter, but the mother was instructed to spend time daily teaching the daughter how to light matches safely. This promoted a closer mother-daughter relationship, which was previously obstructed. A helpful focus remained on the symptom. Symptoms can be exaggerated to increase their intensity and mobilize family resources. A symptom can be relabeled, as in the case of a mother who continually nagged critically at the son. Redefining her nagging as concern encouraged caring interactions. A new symptom shifts the family's focus onto another family member temporarily. For example, the husband fails to go to work and the wife alternately protects and threatens to leave him. Identifying her behavior as seriously depressed reduces her intense focus on the husband. A symptom's effect can also be changed, thereby altering interactions around it. For example, the mother who interacts positively with her fire setter daughter shows a new effect of the symptom.

■   **MANIPULATING MOOD.** Manipulating the family's mood is another restructuring operation. For example, by exaggerating the common family mood, the family reacts by showing a wide range of expressions. The nurse can also model a more appropriate affect for the family. For example, she may react with strong indignation to a young boy's criticism of his mother. This promotes respect and clarifies the boundaries of a passive, enmeshed parental subsystem.

■   **SUPPORTING, EDUCATING, GUIDING.** Support, education, and guidance can be a restructuring operation. They can take the form of modeling, assigning tasks, or sharing concrete information. Minuchin shows families how they program each other in the circular process of a family system.

The goal of structural family therapy is not a change in behavior but a change in the whole family's organization. This allows individual members a new experience in the family. Using a model of an effectively functioning family, the therapist joins the family in a therapeutic system, hoping to restructure the family. The restructuring either helps to maintain functional subsystems or helps to form new subsystems that will promote healing and growth.

Strategic, problem-solving, or brief family therapy

Communication theory has undergone evolutionary changes. These changes have occurred ever since the double-bind theory was first proposed in Palo Alto, California, in 1956.[2] These changes have revolutionary implications for the practice of psychotherapy. Out of communication theory has developed strategic short-term, or problem-solving, family therapy.

The original communication theorists included Gregory Bateson, John Weakland, and Jay Haley, with Don Jackson and William Fry consulting. The focus of their early study was observable face-to-face communication, verbal and nonverbal. They studied families and other ongoing social groups, noting how face-to-face communication affected actual behavior.[41] The clearest explication of early communication theory is in *Pragmatics of Human Communication* by Watzlawick, Beaven, and Jackson.[39]

■ Assumptions of communication theory

Communication theorists contend that *all* behavior, not only verbal productions, is communication. It is impossible not to communicate.[38] The theorists recognized that most communication consists of many levels between sender and receiver. The verbal and nonverbal levels of a message necessarily modify and qualify each other. That is, the significance of any message depends on how it is reinforced, contradicted, or specially framed by other simultaneous, preceding, or following messages. These, along with the setting and the relationship between sender and receiver, constitute the context that must be considered in interpreting any message.[41]

Another basic tenet of communication theory is that communication is an ongoing process. Originally, for purposes of analysis, communication was broken down into discrete units of "stimulus" and "response" in a linear structure reflecting cause and effect thinking. It later became apparent that this was both inaccurate and inappropriate. There is no beginning point or end point in the stimulus-response-reinforcement pattern of human interaction (referred to later as a positive feedback loop). In most relationships, the behavior of each participant depends on the other's behavior. In families, complex, highly patterned, repetitive interactions become established.

When a two-person (or more) system is dysfunctional in its communication, potential exists for a pathological condition. Studying communication patterns in schizophrenic families, the researchers identified several forms of "pathological communication." Disqualification in communication includes self-contradictions, inconsistencies, subject switches, tangentializations, incomplete sentences, misunderstandings, obscure mannerisms of speech, and literal interpretations of metaphor, and vice versa.[39] An example of disqualification is a question an older brother used to baffle his younger sister: "Do you walk to school or carry your lunch?" Disconfirmation in communication involves ignoring or invalidating essential elements of a significant other's view of himself. It involves telling the person you do not feel the way you feel, need what you need, or experience what you experience.[31]

Incongruent communication is delivering two conflicting messages simultaneously. If the receiver responds to either message, he will be charged with "badness or madness." This is the basis of the double-bind, or paradoxical, injunction. An example is the command "Be spontaneous!" or, from Greenberg's collection of maternal communications, "Give your son Marvin two sport shirts as a present. The first time he wears one of them, look at him sadly and say in your Basic Tone of Voice: 'The other one you didn't like?' "[38:111] Finally, symptoms are means of communication; the symptomatic person is convinced the symptoms are out of his control. The symptoms can serve as a controlling mechanism in the family. Psychosomatic symptoms come under this description.

The treatment goals of family therapy, based on the early communicational view of behavior, were (1) to correct pathological patterns of communication and (2) to promote functional communication between family members. Family members were to express themselves clearly and directly and ask for and receive feedback. Thus behavioral change would occur in the family as a result of direct, clear, unambiguous communication.[31] From their research of schizophrenic families, the Palo Alto group expanded their research and practice to other types of clinical problems. They recognized that the manifestations of schizophrenia included characteristics of other problems. From their observations of here-and-now communication in families, it was a short conceptual leap to the formulation of strategic family therapy.

■ Components of strategic family therapy

In 1966 Fisch proposed the establishment of the Brief Therapy Center of the Mental Research Institute in Palo Alto, California. He was joined by Watzlawick and Weakland. All were previously involved in the communication research under Jackson at the Mental

Research Institute. They were interested in the function (the "what") and not the meaning (the "why") of behavior. They wanted to shorten treatment and facilitate change. Initially the therapeutic interventions that did this appeared gimmicky. However, the researchers gradually evolved a conceptual framework to explain these successful interventions. They focused on how symptoms or human problems arise and how they are resolved, especially through paradoxical intervention.[38] Haley[21] developed the problem-focused family therapy approach through his association with Minuchin, Erikson, and Montalvo. Family therapy is different from structural and systems therapy in its primary goal: the removal of the presenting symptom through directives or tasks in conjunction with the use of paradox.

Whether one speaks of problems or symptoms, they are not an entity in their own right. A problem is only a problem when it is labeled as such by those involved. A problem is behavior between two or more people that one or more persons do not like. It persists despite efforts to change. Strategic therapists make a distinction between difficulties and problems. Difficulties are either (1) undesirable states of affairs that can be removed by a logical solution or (2) undesirable, common life problems that must be lived with.[40] Problems arise from small difficulties that escalate. They are maintained by mishandling attempts to solve them. Mishandling frequently occurs around adaptation to ordinary life events and ranges from (1) ignoring or denying difficulties that require action to (2) attempting to resolve an ordinary life difficulty that is unnecessary (e.g., a husband who would not talk to his wife before breakfast) or impossible to resolve (e.g., the generation gap) to (3) difficulties where action is needed but the wrong kind is taken.[41]

Strategic family therapists are not concerned with the history of the problem or the motivation behind it. They are not interested in characteristics of people (passive, hostile, hysterical). They place no importance on insight. Little distinction is made between acute and chronic problems. Chronic problems are ones that have been mishandled longer. The presenting problem behavior and the problem-maintaining behavior are the primary focus of treatment.

Communication theorists borrowed from cybernetics when they identified a positive feedback loop in human interaction. This is the vicious cycle that develops from efforts by family members, or the identified patient himself, to stop or "help" undesirable behavior. For example, the rebellious teenager, when faced with parental discipline, becomes increasingly rebellious. As discipline becomes harsher, the boy's behavior escalates further. Thus "the action which is meant to alleviate the behavior of the other party aggravates it."[13:610] From this view, the cause and the nature of a problem are essentially the same process. People try to change behavior in the most logical way possible. Common sense suggests prevention or avoidance of undesirable behavior by means of the reciprocal or opposite behavior. If this does not work, they try harder with the same behavior. The resolution of problems therefore requires changing the problem-maintaining behaviors. This interrupts the vicious positive feedback cycles.[41]

■ Problem-solving interventions

Intervention occurs with the patient, the unidentified patient, or both. This depends on who is most concerned with the problem. This is the person most willing to change. Effective intervention can be made through any member of the system to break the positive feeback loop. This is illustrated in Clinical example 29-4.

These examples demonstrate the use of reversal or symptom prescription. They carry the message "do not change" or "more of it," both of which stop the family or patient from trying to stop. Persuading people to

---

CLINICAL EXAMPLE 29-4

A colonel is being militarily strict with his son, and the boy is becoming increasingly defiant. The therapist tells the father his son is "going to the dogs." The therapist suggests that the father hold back on his discipline to get a baseline measurement of how bad the boy's behavior will become. As pressure on the boy is reduced, his behavior improves.

Another example is a woman who suffered from urinary frequency. She was isolated at home, feeling unable to leave the house to socialize. She was also isolated at work because she had her machine set by the bathroom door where there were no co-workers. She worked from 12 to 8 PM. The therapist instructed her to urinate as many times as she felt she had to each morning before going to work but to use the toilet only three times; after that she was to urinate sitting in the tub. She was to make no effort to change her pattern at work. The next week the woman reported she had been in agony the first morning but was unable to urinate sitting in the tub. She then figured that if she could limit herself at home, she could do so at work, and had no further urinary frequency.[6]

change behavior that common sense tells them is correct often requires treatment strategies that appear "weird," illogical, or paradoxical.

The nurse's first task is to obtain a statement from the patient of the presenting complaint in specific, concrete terms. As Haley states, "Problems . . . should be something one can count, observe, measure, or in some way know one is influencing."[21:40] After obtaining this statement, the nurse determines what about the behavior makes it a problem. The nurse asks what solutions the family has tried. This identifies which remedies to avoid and indicates the problem-maintaining behavior.

Next, the nurse asks what the family's or patient's minimum goal of treatment would be—what smallest identifiable change would signify progress or some success. General goals such as "improved communication" are not acceptable. Feeling changes such as "to feel happier" or negative goals such as "to stop certain behavior" are equally unacceptable. Rather, the nurse seeks positive statement-of-action goals. These goals describe behavior that reflects an attitude or feeling change. According to the cybernetic view, if a small but significant change can be made in what appeared to be a hopeless situation, a so-called ripple effect may occur. That is, "once a patient is mobilized and regains confidence in his ability to solve problems, he sometimes finds that he can tackle other difficulties."[29:47]

As soon as possible, the therapist attempts to grasp the patient's "language" and his main ideas and values. "Tuning into" the family's view and then extending that view is a critical step known as *reframing*. It precedes the therapist's strategic intervention. To reframe means to change the conceptual or emotional setting or viewpoint in which a situation is experienced. Using language common to the family's world view, the therapist places the experience in another frame that fits the "facts" of the same concrete situation equally well. The situation's entire meaning changes.[38] An example of reframing includes using hostility when it is present in a woman's frigidity. The therapist may reframe the problem as one produced by her overprotecting the male. Assuming there is hostility and protecting the husband is the last thing the woman would want to do, the new frame to the problem uses hostility as an incentive to release her inhibited sexual feelings. Tom Sawyer reframed whitewashing the picket fence as an artistic, entertaining enterprise rather than a dreary chore. He used his friends' competitiveness to vie for the opportunity to whitewash. Reframing causes an attitudinal change and a change in emphasis of a situation's facts. This changes the situation's meaning to permit new behavior. The concrete facts remain unchanged.

A team of Italian family therapists, led by the psychoanalyst Mara Selvini Palazzoli, has gained increasing recognition in the United States. This team is known for its successful short-term therapy with anorectic families[27] and more recently with schizophrenic families.[28] Two cotherapists work directly with the family while their two colleagues observe and support them behind a one-way mirror. Interventions, designed by the whole team, address each family member's cyclical behavior. Their therapy centers on the use of paradoxical injunctions. Interventions are designed to produce resistance in the family. Resistance produces the desired change in behavior.

Strategic therapists place no importance on the therapist having therapy as psychoanalysis does. The nurse can be trained in this theoretical framework without understanding her own involvement with her family. Structural therapists share this view.[21]

Strategic therapists are attacked for the "manipulative, insincere" nature of their approach. They acknowledge that this is the case. Communication research stresses that it is impossible not to communicate. Likewise, it is impossible not to influence. A nondirective, dynamically oriented therapist influences the patient's communication in hundreds of subtle ways. These ways include body movement, intonation, and leading responses. The "insight" school and the nondirective school of therapy influence patients outside the patient's awareness. Strategic therapists do so openly. The patient's "awareness" of the manipulation itself is irrelevant as long as the strategy is given and followed. The difference between the "insight" school and the strategic school of psychotherapy is conceptual rather than ethical. The "insight" school believes that change in people occurs through the therapeutic relationship with a change in their understanding of themselves. The strategic school persuades a person to change "spontaneously." It arranges a situation so that the person initiates the change in behavior.[21]

The strategic therapist is an active and deliberate change agent. The therapist creates a strategy to bring about the change the patient is paying money to achieve. The responsibility for success or failure therefore rests on the nurse. The nurse never takes the credit for change in the patient's eyes. In this therapy the point at which termination takes place is clear. According to Fisch and co-workers:

If a therapist accepts the patient's complaint as a reason for starting therapy with him, he should, by the same logic, accept his statement of satisfactory improvement as a reason (and time) for terminating treatment.[13:599]

Recent developments in family therapy

The family self-help movement is an important development in the mental health field. Families of schizophrenics have long been blamed by professionals for the family member's illness. Two of the family therapy theories discussed in this chapter, Bowenian and strategic, originated from the study of families of schizophrenics. These families feel guilty, bewildered, angry, frustrated, and ultimately exhausted and hopeless about the catastrophic and chronic illness of their family member. These families mainly live in isolation from their extended families and communities.

In the 1970s some families began forming local self-help and consumer-advocacy groups for families of the mentally ill. In 1979, about 100 such groups together formed the National Alliance for the Mentally Ill, organized with the goal of improving treatment and services for the chronic mentally ill. As a national organization, the Alliance advocates increased funding for research, training, and public education. It advocates more progressive attitudes in public policy affecting services for the mentally ill. As enlightened consumers, its members pressure mental health professionals for information about services needed for their ill member and themselves during the various phases of the illness. For participant families, local self-help groups offer mutual aid, intimacy with others, and involvement beyond the immediate family needs.[22,23,24]

Renewed interest in family treatments of schizophrenia has resulted in the development of psychoeducational programs for families of schizophrenics. These programs are influenced by Brown's and Birley's compelling British studies.[9] Although these programs vary widely, they share certain features. The family intervention programs begin during or just after hospitalization of the schizophrenic member. The program's approach is mainly educational and pragmatic, in a multiple family group setting. Their aim is to improve the course of the illness, reduce relapse rate, and improve the patient's psychosocial functioning. These goals are achieved through educating the family about the illness, using treatment approaches, and helping the family reduce stress on the patient. Families are taught techniques to cope with symptomatic behavior of the ill member and effective communication skills. Not all programs include the ill member, but all programs promote regular contact with other affected families. The effectiveness of these treatment programs has been tested, and favorable outcome results have been published.[12,17,36]

Conclusion

The theoretical models of family therapy presented in this chapter are diverse and at times conflicting. There are, however, similarities in the characteristics of a well-functioning family identified by the various theoretical views. These common characteristics suggest directions any nurse might take when intervening with families. Reducing the intensity of anxiety and stress in a family reduces the likelihood of secondary stress symptoms, such as divorce, exacerbation of disease, death, or accidental injury of a family member, or conflictual interpersonal relationships. In the high-stress setting of the general hospital, anxiety in a family escalates when their questions, feelings, and fears are not openly expressed to medical staff. Their fear escalates when medical staff fail to listen attentively or answer directly. Family and staff mutually try not to "upset" the other person by bringing up emotion-laden subjects. In an atmosphere of mutual avoidance of taboo subjects, a closed communication system develops between medical staff and family. The nurse handles his or her own anxiety about the issues of acute and chronic illness and death, listens and responds empathically but nonreactively to patients and families, and shares factual information clearly, promoting open communication systems. Opening a closed communication system reduces the intensity of a family's emotional reaction to illness and death.

Nurses working in obstetrics and pediatrics are in contact with families at the outset of a normative crisis in family life. This crisis is the addition of another member into a homeostatic family system. Families expect (except when the pregnancy is an unwanted one) the event to be joyful and satisfying. Mothers, however, may become frightened, believing something is wrong with them. This occurs when confronted with feelings of helplessness or inadequacy, severe anxiety or panic, and perhaps almost homicidal rage at the spouse or infant. Mothers may fail to perceive their reactions as predictable in a crisis. As nurses educate families about normative life crises, the family's anxiety diminishes. They are less likely to view their emotional reactions as problems. They are more likely to see them as normal responses to transitional family stress.

For the nurse therapist working with couples or families in treatment, the sense of bewilderment and information overload makes this work exciting and difficult. It is important for the nurse to develop a thorough understanding of one conceptual framework for herself. She can then use treatment strategies and techniques from various models congruent with the theoretical framework developed. The choice of strategy depends on assessment of the specific family and the level at which the nurse decides to intervene.

The essence of family therapy is conceptualizing the nature of human relationship problems or behavioral disorders within the natural context of the family. The family, as a system, seeks to maintain a dynamic equilibrium. Change in any one part of the system shifts the balance, resulting in alterations throughout the system. This is leverage for effective therapeutic change.

DIRECTIONS FOR FUTURE RESEARCH

The following are some of the nursing research problems raised in Chapter 29 that merit further study by psychiatric nurses:

1. Empirical validation of Bowen's self-differentiation scale
2. The relationship between the therapist's level of self-differentiation and the highest level of self-differentiation achieved by the treatment family after completing family therapy
3. The therapist's exploration of the issues into which he or she is most vulnerable to being triangled
4. Comparison of the effectiveness of individual family therapy versus multiple family therapy with a specified presenting problem
5. Comparison of nurse-run multiple family therapy groups to non–nurse-run groups, measuring comparable effectiveness and cost
6. The effectiveness of doing therapy with the single-generation sibling group when the parental dyad or single parent refuses to participate in the target child's treatment
7. Outcomes associated with creating a ritual with a family suffering unresolved grief from loss through death, miscarriage, or abortion, to promote freer affect or grieving
8. The effect of nurse-run multiple family support groups for families suffering from chronic medical illness on measures of quality of life and family coping
9. Outcomes of a group composed of nursing staff and family caregivers (of the chronically medically ill family member) on the quality of care and use of services of respite care in a hospital or nursing home setting
10. The adjustment of new parents when content on the normative crisis aspects of the first child's birth is included in prenatal classes

SUGGESTED CROSS-REFERENCES

Assessment of families is discussed in Chapter 5. Vulnerable families are discussed in Chapter 8. Working with families of psychiatric patients is discussed in Chapters 9 and 10. Intervening in family abuse and violence is discussed in Chapter 32.

SUMMARY

1. Family therapy is not a modality of treatment but rather a way of conceptualizing human relationship problems. It focuses on the context in which an emotional problem is generated. The process between family members that supports and perpetuates symptoms is the focus of treatment rather than the individual member who manifests the family's problems.

2. Characteristics of the well-functioning family, common dysfunctional family patterns, and indications for family therapy are described. The role of both the generalist and the specialist nurse in family therapy is identified.

3. Bowen's family systems therapy conceptualizes all family systems on a continuum ranging from total dysfunction to high levels of functioning. A cornerstone in systems theory is separating the thinking and feeling processes of family members. The goal of systems therapy is for individual members to differentiate themselves from the family emotional "we-ness" system. Seven central interlocking concepts of systems theory follow:

   a. *Differentiation* reflects sufficient separation between intellect and emotions so that one is not dominated by the reactive anxiety of the family's emotional system.
   b. A *triangle* is a predictable emotional process that takes place in any significant relationship when difficulty exists in the relationship.
   c. The *nuclear family emotional system* refers to patterns of interaction between family members and the degree to which these patterns promote emotional fusion.
   d. The *multigenerational transmission process* is the assumption that relationship patterns and symptoms in a family have their origin several generations earlier. A four- or five-generation genogram reveals such patterns.
   e. The *family projection process* is the projection of spouses' problems onto one or more children to avoid the intense emotional fusion between the spouses.
   f. One's *sibling position,* that is, birth order and sex, is a determining factor in a person's personality profile.
   g. The *emotional cutoff* is a dysfunctional way in which some family members deal with intense family conflict by using either emotional isolation or geographical distance.

4. Structural family therapy, as conceptualized by Minuchin, assumes that behavior and the family's level of

function are a consequence of the family's organization and the interactional patterns between members. The major elements of a family structure that enable viable family functioning are (1) a power hierarchy with different levels of authority, (2) differentiated subsystems with different functions and levels of power, and (3) subsystem boundaries sufficiently well defined to prevent intrusion but sufficiently permeable to permit emotional contact between members.

Tasks of the nurse according to this structural model include defining boundaries and supporting the functions of family subsystems. Restructuring interventions serve to transform dysfunctional transactional patterns that maintain symptomatic behavior. These include enacting transactional patterns, marking boundaries, escalating stress, assigning tasks, using symptoms, manipulating the family mood, and family support, education, and guidance.

5. Strategic, or brief, family therapy evolved from the communication theorists' earlier work.

Strategic therapists are concerned with the removal of problematical behavioral patterns or symptoms. Effective therapeutic intervention frequently involves the use of paradox and reverse psychology. The goals of strategic therapy include obtaining a clear statement from the client of the presenting complaint in specific, concrete terms. The therapist reframes the problem, thereby changing the situation's meaning, permitting new behavior to occur.

6. Knowledge of theoretical models of family therapy can help the nurse when intervening in health promotion and illness prevention with families in a variety of settings. The nurse therapist should use a conceptual framework with families and integrate various treatment strategies and techniques.

■ REFERENCES ■

1. Barnhill L: Healthy family systems, Fam Coordinator 94, 1979.
2. Bateson G et al: Toward a theory of schizophrenia, Behav Sci 1:251, 1956.
3. Beels C and Ferber A: Family therapy: a view, Fam Process 8:280, 1969.
4. Bowen M: Family psychotherapy with schizophrenia in the hospital and in private practice. In Bosormenyi-Nagy I and Framo J, editors: Intensive family therapy, New York, 1965, Harper & Row, Publishers, Inc.
5. Bowen M: Family therapy and family group therapy. In Kaplan H and Sadock B, editors: Comprehensive group psychotherapy, Baltimore, 1983, Williams & Wilkins.
6. Bowen M: Multigenerational transmission process. In Haley J, editor: Changing families, New York, 1971, Grune & Stratton, Inc.
7. Bowen M: The use of family therapy in clinical practice. In Haley J, editor: Changing families, New York, 1971, Grune & Stratton, Inc.
8. Bowen M: Theory in the practice of psychotherapy. In Guerin P, editor: Family therapy theory and practice, New York, 1976, Gardner Press, Inc.
9. Brown G and Birley J: Crises and life changes and the onset of schizophrenia, J Health Soc Behav 9:203, 1968.
10. Cain A: The role of the therapist in family systems therapy, Family 3(2):65, 1976.
11. Carter E and McGoldrick M: The changing family life cycle, a framework for family therapy, New York, 1989, Gardner Press, Inc.
12. Faloon I, Boyd J, and McGill C: Family care of schizophrenia, New York, 1984, Guilford Press.
13. Fisch R et al: On unbecoming family therapists. In Ferber A, Mendelson M, and Napier A, editors: The book of family therapy, New York, 1972, Science House, Inc.
14. Fogarty T: Family structure in terms of triangles. In Bradt J and Moynihan C, editors: Systems therapy, Washington, DC, 1971, The Groome Child Guidance Center.
15. Fogarty T: Triangles, Family 2(2):165, 1975.
16. Fogarty T: System concepts and dimensions of self. In Guerin P, editor: Family therapy theory and practice, New York, 1976, Gardner Press, Inc.
17. Glick I and Spencer J: Commentary on D Hunter. On the boundary: family therapy in a long-term patient setting, Fam Process 24:349, 1985.
18. Guerin P: System, system, who's got the system, Family 3(1):13, 1976.
19. Guerin P: Theoretical aspects and clinical relevance of the multigenerational model of family therapy. In Guerin P, editor: Family theory and practice, New York, 1976, Gardner Press, Inc.
20. Guerin P and Pendagast E: Evaluation of family system and genogram. In Guerin P, editor: Family therapy theory and practice, New York, 1976, Gardner Press, Inc.
21. Haley J: Problem solving therapy, San Francisco, 1987, Jossey-Bass, Inc, Publishers.
22. Hatfield A: What families want of family therapists. In McFarlane W, editor: Family therapy in schizophrenia, New York, 1983, Guilford Press.
23. Lamb R et al: Families of schizophrenics: a movement in jeopardy, Hosp Community Psychiatry 37(4):353, 1986.
24. McFarlane W, editor: Family therapy in schizophrenia, New York, 1983, Guilford Press.
25. Minuchin S: Families and family therapy, Cambridge, Mass, 1974, Harvard University Press.
26. Minuchin S and Fishman H: Family therapy techniques, Cambridge, Mass, 1981, Harvard University Press.
27. Palazzoli M: Self-starvation, New York, 1978, Jason Aronson, Inc.
28. Palazzoli M et al: Paradox and counterparadox, New York, 1979, Jason Aronson, Inc.
29. Rabkin R: Strategic psychotherapy, New York, 1977, Basic Books, Inc.
30. Ritterman M: Paradigmatic classification of family therapy theories, Fam Process 16:29, 1977.
31. Steidl J and Wexler J: What's a clinician to do with so many approaches to family therapy? Family 4(2):59, 1977.

32. Stierlin H: The dynamics of owning and disowning: psychoanalytic and family perspectives, Fam Process 15:277, 1976.

33. Strelnick AH: Multiple family group therapy: a review of the literature, Fam Process 16:307, 1977.

34. Terkelsen K: Bowen on triangles—March 1974 workshop. I, Family 1(2):45, 1974.

35. Terkelsen K: Bowen on triangles—March 1974 workshop. II, Family 2:1, 1974.

36. Terkelsen K: Schizophrenia and the family. II. Adverse effects of family therapy, Fam Process 191:204, 1983.

37. Toman W: Family constellation, New York, 1969, Springer Publishing Co, Inc.

38. Watzlawick P: Some basic issues in interaction research. In Framo J, editor: Family interaction, New York, 1972, Springer Publishing Co, Inc.

39. Watzlawick P, Beaven J, and Jackson D: Pragmatics of human communication, New York, 1967, WW Norton & Co.

40. Watzlawick P, Weakland J, and Fisch R: Change, principles of problem formation and problem resolution, New York, 1974, WW Norton & Co.

41. Weakland J: Communication theory and clinical change. [1]In Guerin P, editor: Family therapy theory and practice, New York, 1976, Gardner Press, Inc.

■ ANNOTATED SUGGESTED READINGS ■

Anderson C and Stewart S: Mastering resistance: a practice guide to family therapy, New York, 1983, The Guilford Press.

Offers beginners and advanced students from any of the various "schools" of family therapy accessible strategies for confronting family resistance to treatment.

Anonymous: Toward the differentiation of a self in one's own family. In Framo J, editor: Family interaction: a dialogue between family therapists and family researchers, New York, 1972, Springer Publishing Co, Inc.

Describes Bowen's efforts to differentiate himself from his family of origin. Demonstrates the application of family systems theory with his own family. A classic in systems theory.

Bowen M: Family therapy in clinical practice, New York, 1978, Jason Aronson, Inc.

Recounts development of Bowen's thinking with classic and original articles. Important for any student who wishes to understand systems theory in depth.

*Cain A: Family therapy: one role of the clinical specialist in psychiatric nursing, Nurs Clin North Am 21(3):483.

Discusses the role of the clinical specialist as a family therapist, and applies Bowen's theory to families with depressed members.

*Caroselli-Karinja M: Asthma and adaptation: exploring the family system, J Psych Nurs 28(4):34, 1990.

Uses a family systems approach to explore the physiology, case management, and treatment approaches for the child with asthma. Includes case studies.

Carter E and McGoldrick M: The changing family life cycle, a framework for family therapy, New York, 1989, Gardner Press, Inc.

Contains original contributions from well-known practitioners in the family therapy field. Covers the developmental stages of the family life cycle and disruptive problems. Valuable for both beginning and advanced students.

Fogarty T: Triangles, Family 2(2):11, 1975.

Thoroughly examines the family systems concept of triangles. Important for the advanced student.

Guerin P, editor: Family therapy and practice, New York, 1976, Gardner Press, Inc.

Contains original contributions from the most distinguished leaders in the family therapy field. Excellent reference for beginning and advanced students.

Haley J, editor: Changing families, New York, 1971, Grune & Stratton, Inc.

Well-known authors cover a spectrum of theoretical approaches to family therapy. Includes many classics.

Haley J: Problem solving therapy, San Francisco, 1987, Jossey-Bass, Inc, Publishers.

Clearly presents the problem-focused, strategic approach to family therapy. Supports theory and technique with case examples. Important for beginners and advanced students alike.

Kerr M: Chronic anxiety and defining the self, The Atlantic Monthly September:35, 1988.

Overview of Bowen's family systems theory and its relation to modern day anxiety. Clear and thorough in presentation, written for the lay public.

Kerr M and Bowen M: Family evaluation: an approach based on Bowen theory, New York, 1988, WW Norton & Co.

Excellent reference for describing family work based on Bowen's theory of family therapy. Highly recommended reading.

Lederer W and Jackson D: The mirages of marriage, New York, 1968, WW Norton & Co.

Explodes false myths and assumptions about marriage and offers no-nonsense suggestions for solving marital problems from a communication theory framework. For families and therapists alike.

McFarlane W, editor: Family therapy in schizophrenia, New York, 1983, Guilford Press.

Increasing emphasis on biochemical and genetic factors has revolutionized family therapies of schizophrenia. Recognizes families as the principal caregiver of the schizophrenic patient and working allies of the therapeutic team. Describes the controversy surrounding the two basic approaches: the medical model approach, which includes a "psychoeducational" component, and the communication theory approach. Also attempts to synthesize the various treatment approaches by offering a "decision-tree model." Recommended for any practitioner interested.

McGoldrick M and Gerson R: Genograms and family assessment, New York, 1986, WW Norton & Co.

Presents a standard format for constructing genograms and clearly outlines the principals underlying their interpretation and application. Using genograms of famous people, introduces the beginner to this essential tool in systems therapy.

---

*Asterisk indicates nursing reference.

McGoldrick M, Pearce J, and Giordano J, editors: Ethnicity and family therapy, New York, 1982, Guilford Press.

Describes ethnic and cultural characteristics of specific groups. Examines attendant values and social and religious beliefs that influence individual and family behavior.

Minuchin S: Families and family therapy, Cambridge, Mass, 1974, Harvard University Press.

Contains clear exposition of structural family therapy. Integrates case examples into theoretical discussion. Important for beginning and advanced students.

Minuchin S, et al: A conceptual model of psychosomatic illness in children, Arch Gen Psychiatry 32:1, 1975.

Compares the medical model of psychosomatic illness to a systems, multiple-feedback model within the family structure. Describes the necessary conditions in a family for the development of severe psychosomatic illness in children and the family therapy strategies used to treat it.

Minuchin S and Fishman HC: Family therapy techniques, Cambridge, Mass, 1981, Harvard University Press.

Provides definitive coverage of the techniques and skills used in structural family therapy. Describes techniques, and includes excerpts of sessions to amplify theoretical descriptions. Logical sequal to Families and Family Therapy.

*Smoyak S: Family therapy. In Psychiatric nursing 1946 to 1974: a report on the state of the art, New York, 1975, American Journal of Nursing Co.

Identifies the nurse's evolving role in family therapy. Excellent resource for nursing's involvement with families.

Toman W: Family constellation, New York, 1969, Springer Publishing Co, Inc.

Describes personality profiles based on sibling position. A classic that should be read by all students of family therapy.

Watzlawick P, Beaven J, and Jackson D: Pragmatics of human communication, New York, 1967, WW Norton & Co.

Describes the effects of human communication, with special attention to behavior disorders. Defines general communication theory, presents characteristics of human communication, and offers examples of pathological communication. Basic text for understanding the origins of strategic, or brief, family therapy.

Weitzman J: Engaging the severely dysfunctional family in treatment: basic considerations, Fam Process 24:473, 1985.

Recommends a generic approach toward difficult, severely dysfunctional families. Proposes acceptance of and sensitivity to the family "as is" before initiating more traditional interventions. Recommended for the "overwhelmed" beginning clinician.

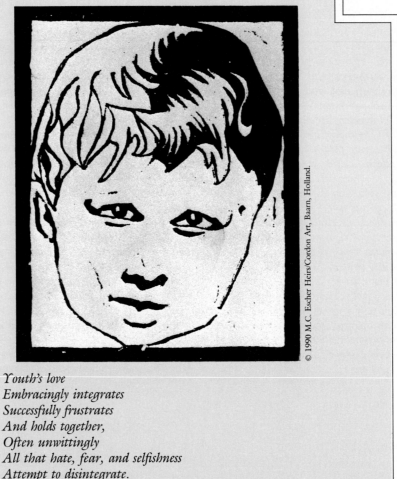

Youth's love
Embracingly integrates
Successfully frustrates
And holds together,
Often unwittingly
All that hate, fear, and selfishness
Attempt to disintegrate.

R. Buckminster Fuller, And It Came to Pass—Not To Stay

C H A P T E R   30

CHILD PSYCHIATRIC NURSING

RITA L. RUBIN

After studying this chapter, the student should be able to:

- describe the major influences on the development of child psychiatry.

- state the levels, scope, and settings of child psychiatric nursing practice.

- assess the purpose and importance of the *Standards of Child and Adolescent Psychiatric and Mental Health Nursing Practice.*

- discuss the elements of the latency period of child development, including Piaget's cognitive processes, the functions of the ego, and the role of Mahler's individuation theory.

- identify the major categories of data that the nurse should collect with regard to the child's health status.

- describe common medical diagnoses used for children with ego deficits.

- compare and contrast the characteristics of

the following diagnostic groups: autistic-presymbiotic, symbiotic-psychotic, and borderline.

- discuss typical areas of conflict and nursing diagnoses for children with ego deficits.

- analyze the usefulness and effectiveness of the various therapeutic modalities that can be included in the plan of care.

- describe the phases, techniques, and components of nursing intervention with disturbed children.

- assess the importance of evaluation of the nursing process when working with children.

- identify directions for future nursing research.

- select appropriate readings for further study.

Historical perspective

Child psychiatry had its beginnings in the early 1900s. It developed from four major bodies of knowledge: psychoanalysis, education, psychology, and an outgrowth of information from work with delinquent youth. Sigmund Freud's major influence on child mental health was his recognition of the role of early childhood experiences in the adult's mental health. He also treated a phobic child, Little Hans, by coaching his father in the technique of analysis.[11] Child psychoanalysis owes its development and practice to two analysts, Melanie Klein, who worked in Berlin in the 1920s and 1930s, and Anna Freud, who worked simultaneously in Vienna. Klein used play in the same way an analyst would use adult free association. Thus the term *play therapy* became the key to treating mentally disturbed children. Anna Freud also used the medium of play but differed from Klein in her approach. Anna Freud's major emphasis was the development of a positive transference with her child patient. Play with toys was a technique of communicating and relating to the child

in a way he could understand. Both child analysts were uprooted by World War II and resumed their work later in the United States and England.

The field of education promoted the idea that children needed both nurturing and learning experiences to become responsible adults. As early as the mid-1800s, students of educational science recognized that children progressed through developmental stages and learned spontaneously by doing. Contributors in the early 1900s included Sully,[24] who recognized the importance of play in children's communication, and the normative studies of Binet and Binet,[2] Catell,[5] and Gisell,[12] who developed the concept of intelligence and set the groundwork for the developmental theory of Erikson.[9]

The educational psychologists Dewey and James furthered the study on the range of normal and also questioned how the child learns. Their work was important in bridging knowledge from education to psychology in teaching and testing children. Influential in the field of psychology were Pavlov, Watson, and

Skinner, who established the behaviorist school. Their descriptions of stimulus-response (S-R) learning have been applied not only to the education of children, but also to modifying troublesome behaviors. In addition, Jean Piaget, a Swiss psychologist, provided child psychiatry with a developmental theory of cognitive growth.[8]

The contribution from concern about juvenile delinquents and orphans came in the early 1900s with the great influx of immigrants and the Industrial Revolution. During this time, almshouses and foster homes were established to keep children off the streets. In 1909, Healy[13] studied the problem of delinquency in Chicago and concluded that aberrant behavior was produced by many factors, including the family. Another important name associated with the treatment of delinquency is Aichhorn, who treated delinquent youths in Vienna in the 1920s using psychoanalytical principles.

A final major influence on the field of child psychiatry was the child guidance movement that began about 1930. The psychiatric treatment of children began in the court system, later becoming community based. This classic team approach is still used widely: a therapist sees the child, a psychologist does the testing, and a social worker works with the family, in addition to coordinating community resources.

The theory base for the practice of child psychiatry remains a "mixed bag," pulling from a variety of frameworks, yet having no unique theory itself. No one method of treatment has been helpful to all children in need of psychiatric intervention. The field of child psychiatry continues to be the product of psychology, education, psychiatry, nursing, and social work.

Child psychiatric nursing practice

Nurses entered the field of psychiatry initially as custodial caretakers. Then, with the advent of the somatic therapies between 1930 and 1940, some effort was placed on educating nurses in psychiatry to improve patient care. Since 1940 nurses have functioned in ever-expanding roles, their advanced training mandated by federal legislation. The National Mental Health Act of 1946 provided funding for advanced training of psychiatric nurses (among other professionals) in undergraduate and graduate nursing programs. This became the steppingstone to recognizing that psychiatric nurses needed specialized training. Within the next decade, Boston University had a graduate program for child psychiatric nurses. In 1955 Mental Health Law 182 charged the Joint Commission on Mental Health and Illness to conduct a study of mental illness and prevention. One of the significant findings was the recommendation that nurses be used more efficiently to provide mental health care because of personnel shortages.

One could argue that since that time little progress has been made in meeting the mental health needs of children. Recent studies suggest that between 17% and 22% (11 to 14 million children) suffer from some type of diagnosable mental disorder. But even the most conservative estimate is that 12% of the 63 million young people in the United States under the age of 18 suffer from clinical maladjustment. Of these 7.5 million youngsters, nearly half are presumed to be severely handicapped by their mental disorder. And even in less severe cases, a child or adolescent may have difficulty coping with the demands of school, family, or community life.[15] Yet only 7% of the children and youth who need mental health services receive them because of the lack of both professional personnel and clinical services.

Child psychiatric nurses are prepared to diagnose and treat mental disorders in children, but a gap exists between the need for services and the numbers and use of child and adolescent psychiatric nurses.[18] Thus preparing sufficient numbers of child psychiatric nurses and gaining access to populations in need of services continue to be major challenges facing nursing.

■ Scope of practice

Child psychiatric nurses practice at two levels: generalist and specialist. Educational preparation differentiates the two levels. The registered nurse is considered a **generalist** and may intervene independently to provide care for nursing problems or dependently, through physicians' orders, for medically diagnosed problems. The **child psychiatric nurse specialist** has a master's degree and the appropriate clinical background. There are approximately 1000 child and adolescent psychiatric nurses with a master's degree; of these about 2% are doctorally prepared. At present, eleven schools offer graduate programs in this field.[17] With successful completion of certification by the American Nurses' Association, the specialist may choose to engage in private practice. When employed by a health care facility, a nurse may assume indirect and direct care specified by the current state nurse practice act.

Another professional organization, Advocates for Child Psychiatric Nursing, Inc., has provided a position statement on the education of a child psychiatric clinical nurse specialist, which concurs with the American Nurses' Association definitions.[7] These two groups specify the need for a nursing framework and a

STANDARDS OF CHILD AND ADOLESCENT PSYCHIATRIC AND MENTAL HEALTH NURSING PRACTICE

The American Nurses' Association, in cooperation with Advocates for Child Psychiatric Nursing, Inc., published standards for child and adolescent psychiatric nursing in 1985. These standards may be applied to inpatient, outpatient, and community practice settings. They are divided into professional and performance practice standards and parallel the generic standards of practice presented in Chapters 1 and 5.

PROFESSIONAL PRACTICE STANDARDS

STANDARD I. THEORY

The nurse applies appropriate, scientifically sound theory as a basis for nursing practice decisions.

Rationale

Child and adolescent psychiatric and mental health nursing is characterized by the application of relevant theories to explain developmental and behavioral phenomena of concern to nursing, and to provide a basis for intervention and subsequent evaluation of that intervention. Primary sources of knowledge for practice are the scholarly conceptualizations of child and adolescent psychiatric and mental health nursing practice and research findings generated from intradisciplinary and cross-disciplinary studies of child and adolescent development, cultural differences, human behavior, and treatment issues. The nurse's use of appropriate theories provides comprehensive, balanced perceptions of client characteristics or presenting conditions and ensures accurate diagnoses. The nurse focusing on children, adolescents, and their families needs to use a broad range of theories, including developmental theory, systems theory, theories of prevention, and nursing theory.

STANDARD II. ASSESSMENT

The nurse systematically collects, records, and analyzes data that are comprehensive and accurate.

Rationale

Effective interviewing, behavioral observation, and developmental and systems assessments enable the nurse to reach objective conclusions and plan appropriate interventions with and for children and adolescents.

STANDARD III. DIAGNOSIS

The nurse, in expressing conclusions supported by recorded assessment data and current scientific premises, uses nursing diagnoses and/or standard classifications of mental disorders for childhood and adolescence.

Rationale

Nursing's logical basis for providing care rests in the recognition and identification of those actual or potential health problems that are within the scope of child and adolescent psychiatric and mental health nursing practice.

STANDARD IV. PLANNING

The nurse develops a nursing care plan with specific goals and interventions delineating nursing actions unique to the needs of each child or adolescent, as well as those of the family and other relevant interactive social systems.

Rationale

The nursing care plan is used to guide therapeutic intervention and move effectively toward the desired outcomes.

STANDARD V. INTERVENTION

The nurse intervenes as guided by the nursing care plan to implement nursing actions that promote, maintain, or restore physical and mental health, prevent illness, effect rehabilitation in childhood and adolescence, and restore developmental progression.

Rationale

Mental health is one aspect of general health and well-being. Nursing actions reflect an appreciation for the hierarchy of human needs and include interventions for all aspects of physical and mental health and illness not only for the child or adolescent but also for the family.

STANDARD V-A. INTERVENTION: THERAPEUTIC ENVIRONMENT

The nurse provides, structures, and maintains a therapeutic environment in collaboration with the child or adolescent, the family, and other health care providers.

Continued.

STANDARDS OF CHILD AND ADOLESCENT PSYCHIATRIC AND MENTAL HEALTH NURSING PRACTICE—cont'd

Rationale

The nurse works with children, adolescents, and families in a variety of environmental settings that can themselves contribute to the movement toward mental health. The nurse can structure the environment in a goal-directed manner to assure that the environment is therapeutic.

STANDARD V-B. INTERVENTION: ACTIVITIES OF DAILY LIVING

The nurse uses the activities of daily living in a goal-directed way to foster the physical and mental well-being of the child or adolescent and family.

Rationale

The nurse is the primary professional health care provider who interacts with young clients on a day-to-day basis around the tasks of daily living. Therefore, the nurse has a unique opportunity to assess and intervene in these activities to encourage constructive changes in behavior so the children or adolescents can realize their potential for growth and health or maintain the level previously achieved.

STANDARD V-C. INTERVENTION: PSYCHOTHERAPEUTIC INTERVENTIONS

The nurse uses psychotherapeutic interventions to assist children or adolescents and families to develop, improve, or regain their adaptive functioning, to promote health, prevent illness, and facilitate rehabilitation.

Rationale

The nurse diagnoses those actual and potential health problems in the child or adolescent that impede or impair the client's normal, healthy development. The nurse assists the child or adolescent and family to become aware of dysfunctional behavior, to modify or eliminate the behavior, and to develop functional behaviors.

STANDARD V-D. INTERVENTION: PSYCHOTHERAPY

The child and adolescent psychiatric and mental health specialist uses advanced clinical expertise to function as a psychotherapist for the child or adolescent and family and accepts professional accountability for nursing practice.

Rationale

Acceptance of the role of psychotherapist entails primary responsibility for the treatment of a child or adolescent and family and entrance into a contractual agreement. A contract includes a commitment to see a child or adolescent and family through the problem presented or to assist them in finding other appropriate assistance. It also includes an explicit definition of the relationship, the respective role of each person in the relationship, and what realistically can be expected of each person.

Treatment modalities are selected based on the developmental and system needs of the child or adolescent and family.

STANDARD V-E. INTERVENTION: HEALTH TEACHING AND ANTICIPATORY GUIDANCE

The nurse assists the child or adolescent and family to achieve more satisfying and productive patterns of living through health teaching and anticipatory guidance.

Rationale

Health teaching and anticipatory guidance are an essential part of the nurse's role with the child or adolescent and family who have actual or potential health problems. Many nursing interactions can be teaching-learning situations. Formal and informal teaching methods can be used in working with children, adolescents, families, and groups. The emphasis of the teaching and guidance is on the principles of mental health, normal development, and developmental needs, and on developing appropriate coping and adaptation patterns.

STANDARD V-F. INTERVENTION: SOMATIC THERAPIES

The nurse uses knowledge of somatic therapies with the child or adolescent and family to enhance therapeutic interventions.

Rationale

Various somatic treatment modalities may be needed by the child or adolescent and family during the course of treatment. Pertinent clinical observations and judgments are made concerning the effect of drugs and other somatic treatments used in the therapeutic program.

STANDARDS OF CHILD AND ADOLESCENT PSYCHIATRIC AND MENTAL HEALTH NURSING PRACTICE—cont'd

STANDARD VI. EVALUATION
The nurse evaluates the response of the child or adolescent and family to nursing actions in order to revise the data base, nursing diagnoses, and nursing care plan.
Rationale
Nursing care is a dynamic process that incorporates ongoing alterations in data, diagnoses, or care plans.

PROFESSIONAL PERFORMANCE STANDARDS

STANDARD VII. QUALITY ASSURANCE
The nurse participates in peer review and other means of evaluation to assure quality of nursing care provided for children and adolescents and their families.
Rationale
Evaluation of the quality of nursing care through examination of the clinical practice of nurses is one way to fulfill the profession's obligation to ensure that consumers are provided excellence in care. Peer review, clinical supervision, consultation, and other quality assurance procedures are used in this endeavor.

STANDARD VIII. CONTINUING EDUCATION
The nurse assumes responsibility for continuing education and professional development and contributes to the professional growth of others studying children's and adolescents' mental health.
Rationale
The scientific, cultural, social, and political changes characterizing contemporary society require the child and adolescent psychiatric and mental health nurse to be committed to the pursuit of knowledge that will enhance professional growth.

STANDARD IX. INTERDISCIPLINARY COLLABORATION
The nurse collaborates with other health care providers in assessing, planning, implementing, and evaluating programs and other activities related to child and adolescent psychiatric and mental health nursing.

Rationale
Child and adolescent psychiatric and mental health nursing practice requires planning and sharing with others to deliver optimal psychiatric and mental health services to children and adolescents and their families. Through the collaborative process, different abilities of health care providers are used to communicate, plan, solve problems, and offer a variety of treatment modalities.

STANDARD X. USE OF COMMUNITY HEALTH SYSTEMS
The nurse participates with other members of the community in assessing, planning, implementing, and evaluating mental health services and community systems that attend to primary, secondary, and tertiary prevention of mental disorders in children and adolescents.
Rationale
The high incidence of mental illness in contemporary society and the increasing incidence of emotional disorders in children and adolescents requires greater effort to provide effective prevention and treatment programs. Child and adolescent psychiatric and mental health nurses must participate in programs that strengthen the existing health potential of children and adolescents in society. Concepts such as primary, secondary, and tertiary prevention and continuity of care can guide nurses in providing services to address a wide range of health needs of children and adolescents in the community. The nurse uses organizational, advisory, and consultative skills, as well as advocacy, to facilitate the development and implementation of such mental health services for children and adolescents.

STANDARD XI. RESEARCH
The nurse contributes to nursing and the child and adolescent psychiatric and mental health field through innovations in theory and practice and participation in research, and communicates these contributions.
Rationale
Each professional has responsibility for the continuing development and refinement of knowledge in the child and adolescent psychiatric and mental health field through research and through testing new and creative approaches to practice.

theory of human behavior to apply to practice. Together, they have developed Standards of Child and Adolescent Psychiatric and Mental Health Nursing Practice (see box on pp. 855-857) to guide generalists and specialists in their clinical work with youth. In addition, they see the specialist as a therapist who demonstrates her competence through the certification procedure and maintains her competency by continued formal and informal education.

■ Practice settings

The child psychiatric nurse may work in primary, secondary, or tertiary prevention settings. In **primary prevention settings** the aim is to prevent emotional problems. Nurses with knowledge in child psychiatry may provide services to prenatal clinics, day-care centers, nursery schools, and other child care programs. Preventive care includes health education in the areas of infant and child development, child rearing and parenting, and counseling for life stresses such as divorce, death, or chronic illnesses. The child psychiatric nurse specialist may consult day care centers, nursery schools, and pediatric floors in hospitals.

Secondary prevention settings are geared toward early intervention in mental illness to minimize its disabling effects. Examples of such settings in child psychiatry include outpatient clinics and partial hospitalization programs. The nurse therapist in this setting may use a variety of therapeutic modalities to help children and their families cope with high stress levels. If learning problems occur, the nurse may consult with schools to provide coordination of services and disseminate information relative to the child experiencing emotional difficulties.

Tertiary prevention settings provide rehabilitation to reduce the severity of mental illness. Typical settings include child psychiatric inpatient units of general hospitals, residential treatment in psychiatric hospitals, transitional care settings, such as day-care and group homes, and outpatient clinics. The child psychiatric nurse serves predominantly as a milieu therapist. He or she provides therapeutic experiences by helping the child deal with daily life occurrences and providing a healthy adult-to-child relationship and role model.

Development of the school-age child

■ The latency period

The school-age child from ages 6 to 12 years has become an independent human being. When com-

pared to earlier stages, he is competent in many areas. He is able to leave his parents for the 6-hour school day and comes under the influence of a complex world of teachers, peers, and other adults. He has established gender identity and is increasingly concerned with measuring up to his peers. Cognitively, he is able to reason, based on the perception of his senses. Emotionally, he has the potential of reaching "latency," which is, according to Sarnoff, ". . . the ability to achieve a state of calm, educability and pliability, using an age-appropriate organization of defenses."[21] The child achieving latency has a sufficiently developed ego to exercise control over his impulses; therefore he is able to behave appropriately to the situation. In the classroom he may sit in a seat for several hours and perform intellectual tasks, provided that he is able to release pent-up energy at intervals on the playground.

Erikson describes the task of latency as achievement of a sense of competency.[9] The 6-year-old is aware of his "inferiority" to adults and sets about with "industry" to learn the many skills and attain the necessary knowledge to achieve a feeling of competency. Freud was the first to describe the latency period and he believed that during this phase of psychosexual development the sexual impulses of the id were quiet or repressed. The ego psychologists concentrated their efforts on explaining the developing ego and less on the role of the id. Consequently, theorists such as Erikson, Mahler, Chess, and others have posed explanations for psychopathological conditions based on deficits in ego strength. Ego disturbances are believed to be caused either by organic defects, as in the case of autism, or by some distortion of the experiential history within the family during the child's development, as in borderline states.[6] It is less clear what is causative of childhood schizophrenia, and both biological and environmental factors are believed to play a role.

■ Functions of the ego

The cognitive domain of the ego is the seat of thought, sensory perception, memory, and language. Piaget, in his cognitive developmental theory, calls the school-age years the **concrete operations stage** and notes that the "age of reason" begins here. A concrete operation is a thought process based on a concrete (as opposed to abstract) point of reference. The ability to perform concrete operations moves the school-age child beyond the magical thinking of preschool years. Learning is enhanced by the cognitive developments in this age range, as is the skill of relating to others. Cognitive growth and its affective correlates that occur during the concrete operations stage, as described by Piaget, are presented in Table 30-1.

TABLE 30-1

COGNITIVE PROCESSES OF THE EGO IN PIAGET'S CONCRETE OPERATIONS STAGE

Ego function	Cognitive process	Affective correlate
Sensory perception	Takes in information more rapidly Organizes perceptions	Perceives reality in organized way
Thought	Demonstrates cause and effect thinking Problem-solves and reasons Can follow rules	Learns and profits from formal education Behaves appropriately to given situation
Language	Knows basic rules of grammar Vocabulary increases Comprehension increases	Engages in meaningful communication and becomes more social
Memory	Mental representations are symbolic of objects, thus has increased ability to store and re- trieve information	Establishes interpersonal relationships based on past events that give relations value

Another function of the ego is that of defending against instinctual drives using defense mechanisms. Sarnoff[21] believes a major defense during latency is reaction formation. The anxiety of the oedipal period is harnessed during latency by converting one's drive to disorder into a desire for order and neatness. An example of this is the enthusiasm with which many children engage in collections of baseball cards, stones, and small toy cars.

Fantasy is important in reducing anxiety for the child achieving latency. Through fantasy, impulses may be eliminated without actually being acted out. Reading fantasy tales performs this function, as does the fantasy that occurs in spontaneous play and enacting imaginary games and characters.

The ego also provides a sense of identity. Mahler developed the theory that the child must separate from the mother and "individuate" to develop a sense of self.[14] Between birth and 6 months of age, the mother and infant are partners in a symbiotic relationship. The infant's awareness of self is limited to physical sensations. He has no external reality, and therefore mother and infant are fused into one unit.

At the end of the first year of life, the infant begins the transition into Mahler's **separation-individuation phase.** His ability to move around allows the external world to broaden under his control. His improved vision and memory help him realize he has one mother. During the following months the infant will continue to grow and experiment with leaving his mother. The crisis occurs between 18 and 24 months, when the walking toddler realizes that he is separate from his mother and, more importantly, has no control over her.

The reality of separating benefits the child by increasing ego strength. Mother's former help in the areas of impulse control, frustration tolerance, and reality testing are now part of the child's ego functions. Mother encourages and supports the child's attempts to achieve autonomy and so cushions him from being overwhelmed by a sense of abandonment. Successful resolution of the rapprochement, or crisis, subphase in the separation-individuation process results in mother and child forming a reciprocal partnership, known as object relations, trading gradual maturity of the child for ego support from the mother.

Implementing the nursing process

The child psychiatric nurse may intervene with children who have insufficient ego strength to function outside the inpatient setting. This may be caused by a lack of differentiation among family members or by a failure of the separation-individuation phase to progress according to Mahler's theory. Consequently, the child is unable to function when he reaches school age and must leave the comfort of his family. The anxiety of separating, along with a fear of abandonment, inhibit the calm period of latency that should allow the child to take his place in school. Signs of this poor sense of identity, or lack of ego strength, are diverse, and many have biological and organic overlays. Examples of psychiatric conditions from the DSM-III-R[1] that may be seen among some children are attention deficit–hyperactivity disorder, conduct disorder, autistic disorder, and disorders of elimination.

 # Assessment

A child may be found in an inpatient child psychiatric setting for several reasons. At times the primary consideration in the decision to admit the child is that an accurate and thorough diagnostic evaluation has not been possible with the child as an outpatient. Other times, outpatient therapy has not been helpful to the child, and his behavior may worsen. Thus hospitalization may minimize regression, as well as rehabilitation time. In addition, the child's behavior may have become bizarre and irrational, making the child difficult to manage in the home setting or at school.

Another criterion for inpatient admission is to protect the child from a severely pathological or abusive family. When this is the case, it might be helpful to admit the child to an inpatient facility to serve as a transition to foster home placement. Finally, "any child lacking the ego strength to control drives and instincts sufficiently enough to engage in the tasks of mastery and growth, and being unable to establish interpersonal relationships in the home, school or community for psychosocial development, is a candidate for inpatient admission."[20]

The assessment phase of nursing care begins as the child is admitted to the unit. It is often useful to bring the child in to visit and become oriented before admission to ease a traumatic separation.

The nurse collects data to formulate a picture of the whole child, including his strengths and weaknesses. The first data obtainable are his response to the admission procedure and his initial symptoms. Does he separate easily from his parent or significant other? If his separation is difficult, does he react by demonstrating feelings of abandonment or by masking his feelings with a violent and aggressive explosion? Lack of affect or a disinterested attitude will also give the nurse data relative to the child's relationship with his parents.

■ **MENTAL STATUS.** The child's psychiatric hospitalization enables the nurse to gather information relative to several areas. The first area is mental status. A mental status examination produces a picture of the child's ego functioning and may be used to document his functioning during a single contact or over a longer period. When focusing on a narrow time frame, however, generalizations and conclusions about the child are limited only to that time. Its greatest value is in comparing the child's behavior and level of functioning from one time to another.

The child's mental status should ideally be assessed over time, with a relaxed atmosphere and minimum stressors. Use of play materials is valuable in displacing focus from the child (which is anxiety provoking) to an imaginary doll or character. Data should be recorded as observable behaviors to maximize the objectivity of the assessment, and impressions, feelings, and opinions should be labeled as such. A list of areas usually covered by the mental status examination with a brief explanation of each part follows:

appearance Description of the physical size, manner of dress, hygiene, posture, and any obvious handicaps

defense mechanisms Description of major defenses the child uses to cope with anxiety

neuromusculature Description of the child's ability to locomote in a coordinated fashion and execute gross and fine motor movements

thought processes Description of the child's thoughts (verbalized). Are they a logical, cohesive, and secondary process, or are flight of ideas, loose associations, and primary process thoughts present? Is the child preoccupied or having hallucinations or delusions?

fantasy Description of the child's ability to fantasize and know the limits of fantasy, which gives data relative to wish fulfillment, dreams, and so on.

concept of self Description of the child's level of self-esteem, self-image, and self-ideal

orientation Description of the child's concept of time and ability to perceive who and where he is

superego Description of the child's value system, ability to discern right and wrong, and ability to respond to limit setting

estimated intelligence quotient (IQ) Description of the child's general fund of information for his age and other age-appropriate tasks.

A more detailed explanation of mental status and children can be found in Simmons.[23]

■ **INTERPERSONAL RELATIONSHIPS.** Observations about how the child relates to peers are important. Knowledge of age-appropriate behaviors for peer relations will help the nurse know what to observe. Following are a few of the many questions one should bear in mind:

- Are the relationships formed with those of the nearest age to the child? With the same or opposite sex?
- What is the child's position in the power structure of the group?
- How good are the child's social skills in ap-

proaching other children and getting along with them?

■ Does the child have a "best friend"?

The child's ability to relate to adults is also important, as are the child's comfort and skill in forming these relationships. Also, the age and sex of the adults sought out reflect his needs for role models and nurturance. Does the child use adults for support or see them as hostile enemies? Is he able to sublimate sexual interest? Is he able to accept limits from adults?

■ **ACTIVITIES.** Observations about the type of activities the child enjoys and in which he or she does well, the energy level and response (bored, excited), and the ability to engage in solitary, as well as group pastimes, should be noted.

■ **PERSONAL AND FAMILY HISTORY.** A thorough history, including the precipitating problem, history of symptoms, growth and development, family life, school adjustment, and medical status, is usually compiled by one or more members of the multidisciplinary team. This information serves as a backdrop against which the child's current functioning appears. It provides the nurse with an understanding of the child's behavior and helps in setting goals for realistic and achievable treatment. For example, the treatment goals of a child who has had several foster home placements would differ with reference to adult relationships from goals for a child growing up in a traditional home environment.

As the picture of the child approaches completion, data are analyzed to make a diagnostic formulation. The diagnostic formulation serves as a basis for planning further treatment. In some instances, inpatient treatment ceases at this point. For the child with severe ego deficits, however, a comprehensive long-term treatment program usually is recommended.

 ## Nursing diagnosis

Children with severe ego deficits fall into a variety of diagnostic categories and make up most of child psychiatric inpatient admissions. There are various ways of conceptualizing the diagnostic categories based on the underlying psychodynamics, etiology of the disorders, and background of the mental health professional.

■ **RELATED MEDICAL DIAGNOSES.** The nurse should be familiar with the major medical classes of disorders to identify related nursing diagnoses. The DSM-III-R[1] classifies disorders usually first evident in infancy, childhood, or adolescence by separating them into nine major groups. These diagnostic categories are listed in Table 30-2. In addition, the DSM-III-R[1]

TABLE 30-2
DSM-III-R* DISORDERS USUALLY FIRST EVIDENT IN INFANCY, CHILDHOOD, OR ADOLESCENCE

Mental retardation
  Mild (50-70 IQ)
  Moderate (35-49 IQ)
  Severe (20-34 IQ)
  Profound (below 20 IQ)
Pervasive developmental disorders
  Autistic disorder
Specific developmental disorders
  Academic skills disorders
  Language and speech disorders
  Motor skills disorders
Disruptive behavior disorders
  Attention deficit–hyperactivity disorder
  Conduct disorder
  Oppositional disorder
Eating disorders
  Anorexia nervosa
  Bulimic disorder
  Pica
  Rumination disorder of infancy
Tic disorders
  Tourette's disorder
  Chronic motor or vocal tic disorder
  Transient tic disorder
Elimination disorders
  Functional encopresis
  Functional enuresis
Speech disorders
  Cluttering
  Stuttering
Other disorders of infancy, childhood, or adolescence
  Elective mutism
  Identity disorder
  Reactive attachment disorder of infancy and early childhood
  Stereotypy—habit disorder
  Separation anxiety disorder

*American Psychiatric Association: Diagnostic and Statistical Manual of Mental Disorders, 3rd edition-revised, Washington, D.C., 1987, Author.

---

notes that a variety of other diagnostic categories are often appropriate for children and adolescents: schizophrenic disorders, substance abuse disorders, mood disorders, and adjustment disorders.

Mental retardation is defined as significantly subaverage general intellectual functioning, resulting in impaired adaptive behavior with onset before age 18. Children in this category are likely to have associated impairment in the areas of emotional, behavioral, neurological, and developmental functioning.

Pervasive developmental disorder and autistic disorder are DSM-III-R[1] correlates of childhood psychosis. School-age children with pervasive developmental disorder are grossly dysfunctional in social relationships, anxiety levels, affect, and response to environmental change and stimulation. They tend to engage in self-mutilation. The disorder often is chronic, with a high degree of impairment and poor outcome.

Attention deficit–hyperactivity disorder (ADHD) is characterized by inattentiveness and impulsity. Children typically are diagnosed about the age of entry into school, when they are unable to maintain concentration and complete tasks. Hyperactivity further disrupts participation in classroom activity, and the child may be labeled as a discipline problem. ADHD is attributed to a neurological deficit, and children often improve with stimulant medication. The disorder is prevalent in 3% of prepubertal children and is 10 times more prevalent in boys than girls. Adolescents may have some residual impairment or show little of the behaviors.

Conduct disorder is demonstrated by a repetitive, persistent pattern of conduct in which others' basic rights are disregarded and societal norms are violated. Behaviors may include running away from home, fighting, cruelty to people or animals, fire setting, lying, and stealing.

Oppositional disorder is characterized by defiance of adult rules, anger, loss of temper, vindictive behavior, obscene language, and blaming others for one's own mistakes.

Eating disorders with onset in childhood include pica, or eating nonnutritive substances, and rumination, or repeated regurgitation without nausea or associated gastrointestinal illness.

Tic disorders include Tourette's disorder, chronic motor or vocal tic disorder, and transient tic disorder. A tic is an involuntary, sudden, rapid, recurrent, nonrhythmic, stereotyped motor movement or vocalization. It cannot be controlled but can often be suppressed for varying lengths of time. All forms of tics are exacerbated by stress and are usually diminished during sleep.

Elimination disorders include functional enuresis, or the repeated voiding of urine during the day or night into bed or clothes, whether voluntary or involuntary, by a child at least 5 years old. Functional encopresis is the repeated passage of feces into places not appropriate, whether voluntary or involuntary, by a child at least 4 years old.

Reactive attachment disorder results from the psychological or physical abuse or neglect of the child or repeated changes in the primary caregiver, as characterized by the child's inadequate or disturbed social relatedness.

Separation anxiety disorder is characterized by the child's excessive anxiety about separating from those to whom he is attached, as evidenced by persistent worry, refusal to go to school, nightmares about separations, social withdrawal, avoidance of being alone, and complaints of physical symptoms or excessive distress when anticipating or experiencing separation from attachment figures.

■ **EGO DEFICITS.** Another way of categorizing childhood disorders has been offered by Rinsley.[20] This classification is based on ego deficits and divides children into the autistic-presymbiotic group, the symbiotic-psychotic group, and the borderline group.

The **autistic-presymbiotic group** constitutes the following medical diagnostic labels: nonremitting schizophrenia, infantile psychosis, pseudoaffective schizophrenia, nuclear or process schizophrenia, and early infantile autism. The onset of symptoms is 3 to 5 months of age, and symptoms are pervasive. The child is considered fixated in the presymbiotic phase of development according to Mahler's theory. The child does not achieve a symbiotic relationship with the mother and does not differentiate self from mother. The symptoms include failure to learn, communicate, and form relationships. Consequently, these children are often mistaken as mentally retarded. Those attributing the cause to emotional or organic disturbances are almost equally divided.

The **symbiotic-psychotic group** is differentiated from the autistic-presymbiotic group by age of onset of symptoms, which usually appear between 3 and 4 years of age. These children are fixated in the symbiotic phase and are poorly individuated from their mothers. This group of disorders is characterized by disrupted and distorted body image and boundaries, pananxiety, fluctuating hyperactivity and withdrawal, delusions, distorted perception, and cognitive, adaptive, and coping failure. In adolescence this group takes on the classic picture of adult-onset schizophrenic thought disorder.

The **borderline group,** as with the autistic-presymbiotic group, has several medical diagnostic labels: character disorder, adjustment reactions of childhood or adolescence, delinquency, and conduct or behavior disorder. Onset of symptoms usually occurs at about 10 to 12 years. In this disorder the child is believed to be fixated in the separation-individuation phase of development according to Mahler. The mother of the borderline child is also fixated in this phase. She is unable to provide the child the support he needs to separate from her. Consequently, he has the biological drive and emotional need to separate from the mother but cannot do so without an overwhelming fear of abandonment and ensuing depression. The depression is characterized by feelings of rage, fear, passivity, helplessness, and emptiness. Clinically the borderline child or adolescent uses acting out as a defense against the abandonment depression.

■ **PSYCHODYNAMICS AND MALADAPTIVE RESPONSES.** The children in all three groups may be characterized as having ego strength deficits. These deficits may be caused by biological factors or developmental arrests during critical periods of early childhood. The period in which the child becomes fixated determines the extent to which his ego functioning is impaired; the earlier the fixation, the more likely the child will appear psychotic.

Fritz Redl and David Wineman[19] were pioneers in the topic of the ego functioning of emotionally disturbed children. Their description of the "ego that cannot perform" was derived from work in a Detroit group home for boys and for the next 20 years was unchallenged in the literature dealing with understanding and treating the aggressive child.

The first problem of a child with a poorly functioning ego is controlling his impulses. The child cannot stand even slight frustration and insists on immediate gratification. When faced with a frustrating situation, panic overwhelms the child, and he becomes aggressive and destructive. The child is extremely susceptible to temptation; mere accessibility lures the child into the forbidden. The excitement of the forbidden then quickly spreads to the whole group of children. This "group intoxication" presents problems in many areas as ego boundaries blur and the atmosphere thickens with the excitation of aggressive impulses. The children show limited ability to use play materials for their intended use and destroy them, unable to see that this prevents the pleasure of future use.

New situations are frightening and overstimulating to the child with a poorly functioning ego. They may be the stimulus for a paranoid distortion, or the newness may be denied to squelch the anxiety of confronting the new experience honestly. Buffoonery and ridicule, as well as overly rough manipulation of materials, are used to master new situations, however maladaptive the results may be.

The child's social savvy is almost nonexistent, and his presence in public places is painfully obvious. He is insensitive to feelings of others and cannot read the code of the informal social structure or abide by its mores. Rules are often seen as persecuting and, without external control, are forgotten by the child.

The child's ability to see his role in problems and bad experiences is severely limited. The few times when guilt feelings predominate, the anxiety-panic-aggression cycle is triggered again. The child does not have the capacity to learn from his or others mistakes, which is taken for granted in the normal child. Normal doses of challenge, success, or failure totally disintegrate the ego's control.

Perhaps the most devastating problem posed by the child with deficits in ego functioning is his resistance to forming relationships with mature, emotionally healthy adults. The very need he has for a nurturant role model sets off feelings of mistrust and fears of rejection. Communication is hampered by the child's secretive, guarded, and aloof nature. The usual social reinforcers an adult uses to show he is willing to form a relationship with a child, such as smiles, praise, or attention, are met with indifference. Consequently, many therapists believe that the classic one-to-one relationship is ineffective and even contraindicated when working with such children initially.

Table 30-3 summarizes some of the psychodynamics and maladaptive responses occurring in children with severe ego deficits. From an understanding of the child, his stressors, and environment, the nurse can arrive at an appropriate nursing diagnosis.

■ **FAMILY PSYCHODYNAMICS.** The child with severe emotional problems is usually considered a "symptom bearer" for the larger family unit. Over the past 30 years attention has been increasingly placed on a systems theory view of psychopathology. In other words, the "problem" does not necessarily lie entirely within the identified patient; rather, the patient is one part of the problem. Certain children seem to be set up for emotional problems, particularly those having special meaning to their parents at birth, such as the first born, the only child, or the child with a chronic illness or handicap. Parenting begins under anxious conditions and the child responds anxiously, eventually manifesting symptoms.

Parents who have been inadequately parented themselves are impaired in their abilities to parent. Winnicot's concept of the "good enough mother" requires that she be able to respond to the child's cues to separate and individuate with support and encouragement. If she experiences the growth process of her child as abandonment, she will be unable to facilitate the process without becoming depressed herself.

A final family phenomenon is the blurring of ego boundaries. This is manifested in several ways. Roles may overlap or be reversed, such as a child being ex-

---

TABLE 30-3

SOME PSYCHODYNAMICS AND MALADAPTIVE RESPONSES APPLICABLE TO CHILDREN WITH SEVERE EGO DEFICITS

Psychodynamics	Maladaptive responses
Failure of normal repression	Sexual acting out
Persistence of primitive defense mechanisms	Extreme use of denial and projection
Pervading anxiety	Severe level of anxiety
Failure of ego to synthesize perceptual, cognitive, and motor functions, thus disrupting child's relationship to environment	Impaired reality testing
Lack of basic trust	Withdrawn and self-isolating behavior
Impaired object relations	Inability to establish intimate relationships
Persistence of narcissism	Lack of insight into own problems
Persistence of primary process thinking	Hallucinations
Failure of sublimation of impulses	Aggressive and destructive behavior
Various degrees of impairment of self-mother differentiation	Negative self-concept

---

pected to parent his parent. Feeling states may be blurred, such as when a mother projects her feelings onto the child. Another example is how the family handles anxiety. High levels of anxiety in one family member may be easily picked up by other members, causing confusion and disorganization.

Perhaps the most interesting family observation was made by Bowen.[3] He found that all these faulty mechanisms occur to some extent in almost every family. The ability to improve family adaptation rests on learning to separate and differentiate from other family members in a nonreactive and emotionally mature way. He believes that the symptomatic child in a family is representative of a family having a poor capacity to tolerate differentiation of family members.

 Planning

Once a thorough assessment is completed and the child's major problems have been identified, a comprehensive treatment plan is made. The nursing responsibility is generally for milieu therapy, but involvement is not confined to that area. The nurse may take an active role in other therapeutic modalities, such as group therapy or family therapy, depending on level of practice and specialized training.

The inpatient setting provides various functions for the child psychiatric patient. First, the inpatient admission may be merely intended for diagnostic and evaluative purposes, and treatment will be carried out elsewhere. A second function is the case finding of children who could most benefit from a residential treatment center. The inpatient setting permits a com-

prehensive treatment plan in which individual, milieu, group, family, drug, occupational, and recreational therapies are all readily available. Finally, it provides a setting and stimulus for family treatment of pathogenic relationships.

■ **GOALS.** Based on the identified problems, goals should be set that are tailored to the child's needs. Treatment goals usually include intervening in one or more of the following areas: modification of intrapsychic processes, altering peer group interactions, altering interfamily functioning, modifying the child's adjustment to school, and changing the child's environment. Some of the following are broad goals for child psychiatric inpatients:

- Meeting the child's needs so anxiety will be decreased and maladaptive coping responses will be minimized
- Helping the child form positive relationships with others
- Promoting the child's sense of self and competency
- Providing the child an opportunity to relive earlier developmental stages that were not successfully resolved
- Helping the child learn to communicate effectively
- Preventing the child from hurting self or others
- Promoting the child's physical health
- Encouraging the child's reality testing
- Helping the child learn more adaptive coping behaviors

In addition, most hospitalized children need to develop some degree of internal impulse control.

Specific objectives for nursing care further specify the treatment approach. For instance, a child with a medical diagnosis of conduct disorder may have a nursing diagnosis of noncompliance to therapeutic milieu. Initially the objective might be to have the patient admit to breaking rules. Later the objective would be modified to have the patient comply to rules and finally to comply to limit setting without arguing or becoming combative. In this way, the treatment plan is individualized and based on the nursing diagnosis. When progress is made, the plan is revised to build on the changes in behavior.

Once goals are set, the appropriate therapeutic modalities are chosen to help the child reach the goal. One must be reminded again of the "mixed bag" nature of child psychiatric treatment and the useful combination of various therapies. The practice of the following psychotherapies are fully explained in other chapters in this text. A few highlights specific to child psychiatry are mentioned here.

■ **FAMILY THERAPY.** Ideally, each child's family should be involved in family therapy (see Chapter 29). From a systems perspective, expecting a young child to assume responsibility for changing when the family system opposes those forces toward change (in hopes of maintaining homeostasis) is absurd. Consequently, parents should be involved from the outset and slowly educated about their role in the problem and their responsibility for change. The family must be dealt with carefully, since they are being asked to give up their symptom bearer (the hospitalized child) and are often overwhelmed by the task of changing their viewpoints. On the other hand, parents who are allowed to view their child as the only problem will be poorly prepared to deal with him when the hospitalization ends. Often they become willing to abandon their problem (the child) after a significant time lapse has occurred. Some families resist adopting a systems perspective, a phenomenon discussed by Bradt and Moynihan.[4] In such cases, special techniques are offered to avoid alienating families from involvement in treatment.

■ **GROUP THERAPY.** Group therapy (see Chapter 28) is often a useful adjunct to inpatient milieu therapy. It may take the form of an activity group or a talking group. It is helpful in promoting reality testing, impulse control, self-esteem, growth, maturity, and social skills. The group therapeutic environment allows members to form relationships and experience a positive social situation in a controlled environment. It is hoped this will be transferred to the outer world environment over time.

■ **PSYCHOPHARMACOLOGY.** Drug therapy (see Chapter 23) is a controversial issue in child psychiatry. However, under a physician's supervision and following appropriate guidelines, drugs often are helpful in decreasing symptoms sufficiently for other therapies to be more effective.[16] Drugs should be chosen based on a target symptom rather than a diagnosis. Dosages are prescribed on the basis of an effective *range,* rather than by body weight, because of the variability of response. Symptoms that have been most successfully treated with drugs to date are hyperactivity, depression, impulsivity, and anxiety.[22] Tables 30-4 and 30-5 list common child psychiatric disorders with the drug of choice and dosage most widely used.

■ **INDIVIDUAL THERAPY.** Individual psychotherapy in the child's latency period usually employs age-appropriate play equipment. A variety of individual therapies exist, including psychoanalytical play therapy, psychoanalytically based psychotherapy, experiential play therapy, and various eclectic approaches. Play therapy provides a controlled, stable environment for the child to work through conflicts and master phase-specific developmental tasks with the aid of an adult therapist. Play serves as a tool for communication with the child's inner self and with the therapist. With play the child can master past experiences that have been problematical to normal adjustment and development. In the older latency-age child, play often serves as a diversion to help the child express anxiety-provoking thoughts and feelings, such as in artwork or board games. The relationship between the child and the therapist provides the opportunity for experiencing a positive adult relationship tempered with judicious amounts of nurturance and reality testing.

■ **PARENT EDUCATION.** Parent education is a vital ingredient to children's preventive mental health as well as the promotion and maintenance of long-term gains from hospitalization. Parent education programs should cover a variety of subjects. Growth and development milestones are taught so parents have age-appropriate expectations of their children's behavior. Values clarification is helpful to parents in identifying what type of person they want their children to become.

Communication skills promote understanding and empathy between parent and child. Appropriate child-rearing techniques are necessary to help children develop self-discipline. Other helpful topics for an effective educational program are family psychodynamics, concepts of mental health, and use of medications.

■ **MILIEU THERAPY.** This occurs in an inpatient setting. The milieu is the actual background of daily events and interactions occurring in the unit or ward.

TABLE 30-4

CHILD PSYCHIATRIC DISORDERS AND DRUG TREATMENTS

Disorder	Drug class	Comments/nursing considerations
Attention deficit–hyperactivity disorder (ADHD)	Stimulants	Used when primary symptoms are manifest in school
		Less reliable in preschooler and adolescent
	Antidepressants	Once-a-day dose and improved monitoring of compliance and toxicity using plasma levels
		Monitor cardiac status and signs of overdose
	Antipsychotics	Sometimes used in combination with stimulants for symptomatic relief.
Conduct disorders	Antipsychotics, stimulants	May improve a child's capacity to benefit from social and educational interventions
Functional enuresis	Antidepressants (imipramine)	Used when an immediate therapeutic effect is necessary due to severe emotional distress
Eating disorders	Antihistamines (cyproheptadine), antipsychotics	Anorexia nervosa
	Antidepressants (imipramine)	Bulimia
Affective disorders: depression	Antidepressants	Careful diagnosis is necessary to differentiate depression from normal feeling states
Tic disorders: Tourette's disorder	Antipsychotics (haloperidol) Alpha-adrenergic agonist (clonidine)	Stimulants are avoided because they worsen symptoms
Pervasive developmental disorders	Antipsychotics	Used to treat agitation, insomnia, stereotypic movements
Mental retardation with psychiatric symptoms and behavioral problems	Antipsychotics	Used to control behavioral and psychiatric complications
	Antidepressants	Treat affective symptoms
	Stimulants	Treat ADHD
	Lithium	Helps control aggression
Separation anxiety disorder	Antidepressants (imipramine)	Effective at high doses
		Speculative: panic disorder symptoms
Schizophrenic disorder	Antipsychotics	As with adults, choice of drug depends on prior efficacy and the spectrum of pharmacological properties
Anxiety, impulse problems, transient insomnia, acute EPS	Antihistamines (Benadryl)	Tolerance to sedative effects may develop

A therapeutic milieu is present when daily life events are exploited to provide learning experiences for the patients. How this is done is the major topic in the following implementation section.

 ## Implementation

Inpatient treatment in child psychiatry usually consists of three major components. The first is the life space interview, a group of techniques used to manage the behavior of children with weak ego strength. The second is some form of token economy that serves as a sanction for positive behavior. The third is the establishment of therapeutic one-to-one relationships.

Treatment is best provided by professionals who have a genuine interest and concern for children. They need to have the capacity to withstand the many moods and emotional outbursts that occur. The nurse's role as a good parent demands that he or she be able to provide an environment with open, honest

TABLE 30-5

DRUGS TYPICALLY USED IN CHILDHOOD PSYCHIATRIC DISORDERS

Drug	Description	Daily dose (mg/kg of body weight)	Side effects
Stimulants: generic (Trade)			
dextroamphetamine (Dexedrine)	short-acting (2-4 hr)	0.3-1.5*; 1-3 doses daily	*Short term:* Decreased appetite, sleep disturbances
methylphenidate (Ritalin)	short-acting (2-4 hr)	0.3-1.5*; 1-3 doses daily	*Long term:* Possible minor effects on growth; associated with onset of Tourette's syndrome in children with family history of tics
pemoline (Cylert)	long-acting (2-4 wk delay in therapeutic effect)	0.5-3*; 1 daily dose	*Abrupt discontinuation:* Behavioral deterioration
Antidepressants			
imipramine (Tofranil)	10-17 hr half-life; immediate response with enuresis or ADHD; 2-4 week delay in response with depression	Usual daily dose should not exceed 5 mg/kg/day	*Short term:* Dry mouth, blurred vision, constipation, electro-cardiogram changes, insomnia *Abrupt discontinuation:* Gastrointestinal (GI) symptoms, drowsiness, headaches
Monoamine oxidase inhibitor (MAOI) and newer drugs: inadequate information on efficacy and toxicity			
Mood stabilizers			
Lithium	12 hr half-life	Maintain plasma level between 0.6 and 1.2 mm/L	*Short term:* GI symptoms, polyuria, polydipsia, tremors, sleepiness, impaired memory *Long term:* Decreased calcium metabolism and thyroid function; possible kidney changes
Antipsychotics			
chlorpromazine (Thorazine)	low potency	3-6	*Short term:* Drowsiness, weight gain, dry mouth, blurred vision, nasal congestion, acute dystonia, parkinsonism, postural hypotension, hyperpyrexia *Abrupt discontinuation:* Withdrawal dyskinesias
thioridazine (Mellaril)	low potency high potency	0.5-3.0 0.1-0.5	
trifluoperazine (Stelazine)	high potency		
perphenazine (Trilafon)	high potency		
haloperidol (Haldol)			
Antianxiety agents			
diphenhydramine (Benadryl)		37.5-50 mg/day, children ≤ 20 lb 37.5-100 mg/day, children > 20 lb	*Short term:* Drowsiness; may cause excitation in young children *Contraindications:* Bronchial asthma; narrow-angle glaucoma; pyloroduodenal and bladder neck obstruction

*Doses are lower for younger children.

communication and clearly delineated adult-child boundaries that is free from pseudointimacy. The therapeutic milieu should provide the child with sanctuary from the pathological family dynamics that were detrimental to growth before hospitalization.

■ **PHASES OF TREATMENT.** A comprehensive treatment plan for the child with weak ego strength can be as long as 3 or 4 years. Treatment usually proceeds in three phases.[20] The first is the testing, or resistance, phase. In this phase the child orients himself to the setting and "cases it" to find out who is in charge and with whom he may align. After this brief "honeymoon," the pseudocompliant front falls away and the child begins to test limits and demonstrate his problem with ego functioning. This entails negativism, reluctance to follow the program or form relationships, and destructiveness. The message is, "There is nothing wrong with me. I don't need to be in this place." The phase may last as long as 1 year.

The second phase is the definitive, or working-through, phase. The child drops his resistance and begins to face his problems. Significant regression may occur during this time, which often scares the child's family enough to withdraw him from treatment. However, the stormy phase gives way to therapeutic work toward separation-individuation, and the child begins to show improved ego functioning. This phase usually lasts 1 or 2 years.

The final phase, resolution or separation, is the child's successful achievement of object relations. The rapprochement crisis is resolved, and the child moves toward age-appropriate relationships with significant others. The child handles extra privileges, visits home, and works through termination with the staff and other patients. This can also last up to a year.

■ **THERAPEUTIC MILIEU.** The concept of a therapeutic milieu is built on daily events in the child's life. In the inpatient setting this comprises a daily routine of meals, school, sports, group and individual activities and pastimes, outings, and bedtime. Trieschman, Whittaker, and Brendtro[25] discuss the ways in which deficient egos are supported by the milieu. One way is through *shared ego,* in which the child behaves appropriately to please persons with whom he has positive relationships. The group of children and adult workers in an inpatient setting makes up a *group ego* to which conformity is exchanged for acceptance and a feeling of belongingness. The institution's culture is made up of rules and routine, as well as tradition, which serves as an *external ego* that guides the children's behavior. Finally, the milieu therapist, through careful assessment, picks out the *ego pieces* or functions the child has and finds ways for him to use them in managing his own behavior.

■ **TYPES OF INTERVENTIONS.** With the daily routine, experiences arise that prove problematical to the child with inadequate ego strength. The nurse, as milieu therapist, focuses on these problematical events and chooses one of two basic types of interventions to manage them: ego supportive or ego interpretive. A *supportive ego intervention* serves as a method of easing the child who is about to lose control, out of his panic-aggressive cycle and back into control, so that he may continue with the daily activity. These interventions serve to maintain the child at his current level of ego function through external control. Over time they set the stage for improving ego function. When conditions are appropriate, the nurse is able to use *interpretive ego interventions.* These help the child gain insight into his problematic behavior and use this insight as a basis for change, thus internalizing ego control.

These two types of interventions were first described by Fritz Redl and are known as **life space interview techniques.**[19] The life space interview is an interaction that takes place outside the context of individual therapy. It occurs between the child and the adult involved in the situation. The focus is on improving the child's sense of self-identity and ego functioning within the developmental process.

Ego supportive techniques. These techniques can also be called "emotional first aid on the spot." When the child inpatient confronts a developmental challenge or a demanding life situation, the milieu therapist may need to assist the child in coping with it. One technique for this is draining off the overwhelming frustration, caused by an interruption in the child's fun or routine, by communicating sympathy for the child's frustration and inconvenience. During periods when the child loses control and slips into his panic-aggressive cycle, it is important that the adult show support by staying with the child. This provides a sense of security and also allows the adult to talk the child back into the daily routine after the stormy period wanes.

Often the child withdraws from relationships during emotional turmoil. To prevent this, Redl advocates dropping the issue that is being confronted in an endeavor to keep the child engaged, however trivial the subject may be. This prevents the phenomenon of "winning the battle, but losing the war."

The milieu therapist also functions as a police officer in regulating and enforcing the children's social behavior. This entails the act of benign and neutral reminding of rules and routines. "Enforcing the law" serves as an external booster to the children's ego when behavior is on the verge of slipping from the established norm. Also, the presence of an umpire is often necessary in settling arguments. A neutral outsider prevents breakdown in fair play or "petty swindling" in the children's transactions.

Ego interpretive techniques. The real therapeutic gains the child makes in ego strength occur as a result of self-examination and learning alternate behaviors to the difficult ones. In working with children prone to distorting and misinterpreting their experiences, insight may never be reached without a "reality rub in." This technique involves repeated confrontation with the reality that the child plays a part in his own self-defeating transactions.

Another intervention strategy is symptom estrangement. This interview situation focuses on having the child see his symptom as problematical, rather than as a tool used to manipulate and control. Symptom estrangement is accomplished by piling up evidence from past life events that provides proof that the symptom costs more than it pays to keep it.

Appealing to a sense of fairness and equality is helpful in awakening a value system in the children. The importance of developing an internalized standard for behavior may begin by this initial adherence to a code of fair play.

The technique Redl calls new-tool salesmanship has been enlarged on by Trieschman, Whittaker, and Brendtro, who call it learning alternate or new behaviors.[25] This new behavior improves the child's coping ability, adaptation, and social acceptability. Selling a new way to handle frustration or guilt takes time and is often a by-product of a child's one-to-one relationship with an adult. Substituting a mature behavior, from the adult model, for the past self-defeating behavior provides a step toward increased ego functioning.

The inclination to group contagion that many child psychiatric inpatients possess must eventually be countered. In this situation the life space interview focuses on increasing the child's boundaries so that he may withstand the group's atmosphere of excitement. In this way the child is taught how the process works and is helped to avoid the lure of misbehavior.

The clinical exploration of life events offers the opportunity to learn new behaviors and gain insight into the futility of previous ones. The process of change takes time, and often the stage must be set first through the use of ego supportive techniques.

Use of natural and logical consequences. Natural and logical consequences are an effective tool for teaching children responsibility for their own behavior. Natural consequences occur in the natural course of events (e.g., one becomes hungry if one does not eat). Logical consequences are formulated by the caregiver and facilitate learning from the reality of social order (e.g., not completing homework will result in falling behind in schoolwork). Nurses can use these concepts in managing a child's behavior and also teach them to parents. The consistent exposure to natural and logical consequences of behavior over time enables the child to eventually see his behavior as self-defeating and avoids many power struggles.

Behavior modification. Many inpatient settings use behavioristic principles (see Chapter 27) to manage the aggressive and limit-testing child. This is usually in the format of a token economy, in which socially acceptable behavior is rewarded or reinforced with points or tokens. The tokens are redeemable for extra privileges, such as an extended bedtime, a favorite food, or a special outing.

Maladaptive behavior is either ignored or punished by the use of timeout. A timeout requires that the child spend a brief period away from the group following acting-out behavior. This serves as a time for the child to gain self-control and talk to an adult about the difficulty. It also inhibits the spread of the child's acting out to other group members.

Another behavioristic program is contingency management. In this system the milieu schedule promotes the use of positive or "on task" behavior with naturally occurring reinforcers, such as meals, free time, and outings. This is simply a variation of "grandma's law," which states, "If you want to eat dessert, you first must eat your peas."

These intervention strategies may be used together or singly with excellent results. One principle, however, should be kept in mind. The focus is on the positive, self-esteem–enhancing aspects of the program. The nurse and co-workers should avoid slipping into a negative or threatening attitude by emphasizing that points are earned by the child rather than taken away by the adult. Target behaviors should be clearly understood by the children and, whenever possible, positive reinforcement used instead of punishment.

A problem encountered in some behavior programs is that the child, after many acting-out episodes in one day, has so few tokens that he gives up and completely decompensates. To provide further incentive to regain control, one can build into each program a way for the child to make up a portion of the points he has not earned. In doing so, he may not be able to reach the highest privilege status, but he will be able to rise above the lowest with some additional effort.

The nurse must also remember that the end point of behavior management is to internalize or learn self-control. Therefore it is hoped that social reinforcers such as praise will be paired with the token or extrinsic reinforcers so that the child eventually will reward himself for good behavior by feeling good about himself.

One-to-one relationships. Children with deficits in ego strength have difficulty forming relationships with adults. They are often distrustful because of their past experiences. Unable to discriminate a trustworthy adult, they withdraw from everyone. Therefore some special effort is usually required on the nurse's behalf to seek out and work toward establishing contact with the child.

In a relationship's early stages, small talk is usually all that can be tolerated. Topics such as the child's reason for admission and other psychotherapeutic issues hinder the child's ability to view the nurse positively in the milieu setting. Instead, the child should be approached casually, with the purpose of becoming acquainted with his interests and reactions to various situations or activities in the milieu. Exchanges should be short to avoid provoking the child's suspicious nature.

The adult working in this setting walks a precarious tightrope between appearing unapproachably "square" and disrespectfully "hip." It is important for the child to view the nurse as an adult to promote his sense of security. Therefore gossip and off-color humor should be avoided, since they are tests of the adult's ability to abide by the rules of socially correct behavior. On the other hand, current fads in music, television, or movies may provide openings for conversations that demonstrate the adult's genuine interest in the child's world.

The adult will maximize his attractiveness to a child if he is able to find a common interest or skill to share with the child. This allows for many hours of diversional activity, which serves as a backdrop for conversation in later stages of the relationship. It is important for the adult to show his inability to be manipulated. Since these children need external control, they will not trust someone they are able to con.

Another important consideration in establishing and maintaining relationships is minimizing adult aversiveness.[25] One way in which this is accomplished is by staying out of power struggles. Sometimes potential altercations may be avoided merely by the adult failing to pick up a challenge. For instance, the child is asked to take a seat and responds by saying, "Make me!" The adult immediately picks up the child's cue and counters with, "All right, I will." Avoiding a power struggle might be the answer here, and the response could be, "For those who are seated, let's begin to clean up for a snack." The child is left to stand if he pleases while the rest of the group moves on with their activity. It is not always possible to avoid power struggles, but a concerted effort should be made, at least in the case of minor squabbles.

The nurse must prove his or her own trustworthiness to the child. One way to do this is by being as open and honest as possible with the child at all times. Admitting mistakes to a child communicates one's humanness. One can show increasing trust of the child by offering him small amounts of responsibility.

Once a positive relationship has been formed with the child, it becomes more natural and the adult does not need to pursue the child so intensely. Topics center around daily activities. The techniques outlined in the life space interview should then be incorporated into the adult-child interaction.

 ## Evaluation

Most treatment facilities for child psychiatric patients have programs designed for specific periods. The brief hospitalization is usually 2 or 4 weeks and is planned for diagnosis and evaluation, crisis intervention, and comprehensive case planning. Therefore, when the presenting symptoms have receded sufficiently, the child's clinical picture is completed, and a long-term plan has been formulated, the child will be discharged.

The success of brief hospitalizations in terms of patient outcome is determined mostly by the patient's follow-up care. Consequently, the multidisciplinary team's ability to formulate a plan mutually agreeable to the child and his family is vital. Early in treatment the family should be engaged as partners with the health care team so that they will assume responsibility for the long-term treatment plan.

Long-term hospitalizations are more complicated in terms of determining readiness for discharge. Generally the nurse's observations focus on basic changes in the child's behavior. The child should demonstrate some insight and understanding of himself through self-reflection and increase his ability to make rational decisions. Behavior should become less impulsive and drive ridden. Instead, the child should begin to live adaptively in his surroundings.

When the child's behavior has become more socially acceptable to the inpatient setting, it is important to begin expanding his environment to the community. The use of the public school system provides an excellent opportunity for the hospitalized child to stay "tuned in" to the outside world and also to demonstrate his ability to handle his environment before discharge. The child should be provided home visits or visits to wherever he will be placed after discharge. This also broadens the child's environment and tests his ability to internalize ego control. Social outings into the community should be ongoing in the course of treatment and should be handled age appropriately before discharge. In this way institutionalization is avoided.

When evaluating the child's overall therapeutic gains, it is important to examine regularly the problems or symptoms, goals, and interventions. The treatment plan should be updated. As problems resolve, the lower priorities may be integrated into the plan. Sometimes the original goals must be reconsidered, or interventions may not work and alternatives must be found. The use of team planning conferences is often helpful in the ongoing process of evaluation. Aspects of the treatment plan that need special scrutiny include the following:

1. Effectiveness of interventions in managing behavior
2. Ability to relate to peers, adults, and parents appropriately
3. Ability to carry out self-care and care of possessions
4. Ability to use program activities in recreation and learning, including school
5. Response to limits, rules, and routines
6. Development of insight into problems and willingness to change
7. Overall mental status, as outlined earlier
8. Discharge coordination and planning

■ **TERMINATION.** Terminating a therapeutic relationship is difficult for many nurses. This is partly because of the universally experienced feeling of emptiness described by Fogarty.[10] Many people "use" relationships, although unconsciously, as a mechanism to avoid the empty feelings of loneliness, abandonment, and incompleteness. Unfortunately, one must acknowledge these feelings to allow the termination to proceed therapeutically with the child.

The child also has problems in leaving. Behavior often regresses as the hospitalization draws to an end and a discharge date has been set. The child seems to want to prove that he still needs the hospital and its staff.

Some guidelines are helpful in terminating therapeutic relationships with children. Introducing the idea that there is an end point should be done early in treatment and stressed again when discharge nears. This allows ample time for the child and staff to talk about their feelings. Positive aspects of the termination process can be pointed out; for example, with discharge into family and community, the child is moving into a new phase of life where new relationships will be established. Listing of the child's gains from hospitalization increase the child's confidence in facing a new environment. Finally, it is a valuable experience for the child to learn that one does not have to be mad or hurt to end a relationship. A successful positive termination will occur when the child is able to grasp this.

The use of ritual is a helpful method of handling "last days." Parties or special activities may be planned. Children sometimes enjoy autographs with special messages written to them from staff and other patients.

■ **FOLLOW-UP AND DISCHARGE.** Discharge should occur only when the health teaching plan has been completed. The child and his family should have information about the nature of the child's illness and his status at discharge, including the family's role in the pathological condition. They should also know how stress relates to emotional illness and ways to cope more effectively with it. In addition, anticipatory guidance is often helpful in forewarning parents and children about future developmental or situational stressors that may negatively affect the child or family's functioning.

If the child will be receiving drug therapy, it is extremely important that the child and family know the reason for the drug's prescription, the dosage, times of day it is given, and side effects that should receive medical attention. This cannot be overemphasized because of the common experience of many nurses with well-meaning parents who do not understand how many psychoactive drugs build up in the body. The layman's perception that the drug works much in the same way as an "aspirin stops a headache" may lead to misuse or abuse.

Follow-up care usually consists of some type of ongoing psychotherapy, whether individual, group, or family. Medication monitoring is carried out according to the specific indications of the prescribed drug. Sometimes vocational and school placements are part of the posthospitalization plan. Dispositions are made to the family of origin whenever possible. If this cannot be accomplished, placements with extended family members, boarding schools, and foster homes or group homes are considered.

Clinical example 30-1 describes the psychiatric nursing care provided to a 6-year-old boy and his family in dealing with his frequent temper tantrums.

■ **EXPANDED SERVICES IN THE COMMUNITY.** Current trends include new services aimed at bridging the gap between inpatient and outpatient therapy. Preschool children may benefit from therapeutic nurseries that provide intensive education for the parents and developmentally appropriate activities for the children. Risk factors such as a history of child abuse, parental depression, developmental delays, and parental substance abuse suggest that a child might benefit from the therapeutic nursery program.

Similarly, after school treatment programs (ASTP)

CLINICAL EXAMPLE 30-1

ASSESSMENT

The following case study involves psychiatric nursing care provided to a 6-year-old male child, Ted, and his family. He was admitted to an inpatient unit for assessment because of temper tantrums and inability to accept limits set by the parents. The mother was also concerned about his dislike of school. The father's perception of his son's problem consisted primarily of his belief that he and his wife had been unable to provide effective discipline.

The temper tantrums would erupt in a variety of situations, but most typically when limits were set on Ted's behavior. He would be verbally abusive toward either parent involved, calling them names and swearing. At times he would hit his sister and threaten to destroy his toys or surroundings. Cruelty to animals was not reported by either parent.

Both parents had tried to avoid spanking and relied on other forms of discipline, such as sending Ted to his room or denying him a privilege (e.g., TV). These techniques of managing Ted's temper outbursts were not helpful, and Ted was successfully making everyone in the family miserable when he was punished. Ted's parents argued over his behavior.

PSYCHOSOCIAL HISTORY

Ted was the first child born to his parents. They had been married 13 years before his birth. Ted's mother had required surgery for infertility so she could bear children. Ted was born by cesarean section 2 weeks before his mother's EDC, without complications. He was bottle-fed and was an easy baby to care for according to both parents. No feeding problems, colic, or other conditions were reported. He was weaned at 10 months with no problems. All development milestones were within normal limits (sat—5 months, crawled—6 months, walked—13 months, 1 word—8½ months, sentences—15 months, toilet trained—3 years).

Ted was reported to have a special interest in natural sciences, particularly animals, from his toddler years. He demonstrated the capability of memorizing names of animals from a picture book, by 6 years of age was attached to a pet cat, and had great knowledge about animal behavior.

Because of their financial situation, Ted's mother returned to work as a secretary for a brief period before the birth of her second child. Ted was taken to a babysitter in the morning by his father and picked up in the afternoon by his mother. He cried when he was left, but his care-taker was considered very capable and he was left with her consistently. Ted's mother did not return to work after the birth of her daughter.

Ted was 18 months of age when his sister E was born. He was somewhat jealous of her and balked at giving up his crib. Consequently, he was allowed to use a porta-crib until he was convinced that he was ready to sleep in a twin bed. He also shook his sister's crib when he was unaware that his parents were watching and reported that she was "bubnoxious." Ted's mother had prepared him for his sister's birth in the later stages of her pregnancy. It seemed that Ted's strong will and intense anger became noticeable around this time and persisted *after* he had accepted his sister's existence.

Ted attended nursery school without problems. Kindergarten presented no problems academically, but his teacher reported that he and another male child distracted the class with their talking.

Ted's sexual behavior presented no problems, and he asked questions and received age-appropriate answers.

Ted's mother sought help with her son's behavior 1 month after he entered first grade. He had resisted going to school the first 2 weeks, and his behavior at home had deteriorated.

FAMILY HISTORY

The father of the patient was born in 1941 in a small midwestern town. He was the third of six children and was raised in the Catholic faith. His father worked in a feed plant in a managerial capacity, and his mother was a housewife. They were described as strict, and they used authoritarian parenting styles. Anger was dealt with openly, and conflict was part of the family atmosphere, along with other warm and loving feelings expressed equally.

Of the six children, the eldest brother had problems with alcohol abuse and had numerous marital separations over his drinking. A younger brother had recently had an extramarital affair and had divorced his wife. The other children were considered to have successful marriages and careers and had achieved varying levels of higher education.

Ted's father identified himself as being the most troublesome child in the family, requiring frequent discipline, including physical punishment. He graduated from a state university in 1963. After 2 years in the army he entered a field of business requiring considerable time and effort.

The mother of the patient was born in 1942 in the same small town that her husband was. She was the second of three daughters and was raised in the Protestant faith. Her father worked for a utilities company, and her mother was a housewife. The family was described as closely knit, and angry feelings were seldom expressed. The parents did not use physical punishment, relying mainly on "talking things out."

Ted's mother described herself as making the most waves in her family. She was closest to her older sister, who was nearest in age to her.

The parents met in high school and dated throughout college. They were married after a courtship of more than 7 years and moved to the east coast shortly thereafter. Ted's father pursued his business career, and his mother worked as a schoolteacher.

Ted's birth followed a long period of infertility, and his parents were ecstatic following the birth of Ted.

MENTAL STATUS

Ted appeared as a well-nourished, white, male child who was neatly groomed and casually dressed. He was very cooperative with the admission procedure and required minimal reassurance to separate from his mother. He was willing to play with toys and talk about nonthreatening topics, but he resisted any attempt to discuss problems. Mental status was assessed over a week's time.

Ted was oriented to person, place, and time and was alert and attentive. His general fund of knowledge was above average as he shared his in-depth knowledge of natural science with the interviewer. He also had some idea of current events and knew his address, phone number, and so on. His judgment was considered to be appropriate to his age. He used a right versus wrong set of values to distinguish moral dilemmas.

Ted was able to express himself verbally. His speech was clear, organized, and grammatically correct. His vocabulary was well developed and he liked to use "big words." His ability to spell was poor, although he knew the first letters of most words.

Ted shied away from fantasy in play except in terms of stereotyped games of cowboys and Indians. His concrete thought processes seemed to block attempts to become more intimate with the nurse. Attempts to ask questions about play themes were firmly resisted by Ted. His response to what his three wishes would be were: a seagull so he could fly; "to have a hood in the back of me like a cobra, so I can scare people when I'm angry"; and to live in "Bubble Gum Land." Ted spontaneously shared his knowledge of different types of fish, butterflies, and so on.

Ted's concept of self was considered to be well developed. His manner of relating was self-assured, and he portrayed a bravado of the tough guy who was able to take care of himself. He confronted the nurse about various injustices, such as not offering him chewing gum when she had some. He asked a few personal questions as well. The self-ideal was expressed in the form of super-heroes with supernatural powers, such as Batman and Popeye.

The common theme in play was the bad guys against the good guys. Ted had issues such as freedom in mind to explain the conflict, and the good guys did win. He refused to use the doll house figures, which were more real, and stuck to monsters, cowboys, and Indians. This could indicate resistance to exposing threatening materials or sex role behavior that would inhibit doll play.

Ted's dominant mood seemed to be bright and cheerful, although he was somewhat concerned about why he was in the hospital. He had considerable self-control in a one-to-one situation. However, he quickly disregarded hospital rules in a less structured setting. No self-destructive behaviors were noted or reported.

NURSING DIAGNOSIS

The Draft of the DSM-III-R in Development[1] diagnosis for Ted was oppositional disorder. The mental status examination revealed no evidence of thought disorder, depression, hyperkinetic behavior, or separation problems. His difficulty seemed to lie in the area of accepting limits and following instructions. Personality features such as his bravado and unwillingness to try things he could not do well were considered to be part of his willful behavior. His perception of self seemed to border on feeling omnipotent in view of the control his temper tantrums held over the family.

The parental histories suggested a moderate degree of family psychopathology. In both families, one or two children functioned at a lower level than the others, and Ted's sister was seen as having no problems. Both parents recognized similar willfulness in themselves as children. In addition, there was a high degree of conflict over the child-rearing practices. Consequently, one nursing diagnosis was identified as altered parenting, related to conflict between parents over parenting styles, with the child responding in an omnipotent and controlling manner. Altered family processes and social isolation were also identified as nursing diagnoses.

CLINICAL EXAMPLE 30-1—cont'd

PLANNING

The nurse proposed that treatment should be focused on learning about effective parenting behavior and discussing their ideas and philosophy of parenting. Treatment goals were as follows:

After completing a parent education program the parents will:

1. Describe three parenting styles—authoritarian, democratic, or inconsistent/laissez-faire and identify the type they use.
2. Describe democratic parenting techniques.
3. Set consistent limits on Ted's behavior.
4. Learn to apply logical consequences of Ted's behavior when he does not accept parental limits.
5. Praise Ted for positive behavior.
6. Allow appropriate ventilation of anger from Ted in the form of verbalization of complaints and sublimation of aggression in play and sports.
7. Conceptualize Ted's problem with temper tantrums in a family context.
8. Examine their own relationship and describe the effects of focusing their emotional energy on Ted and his problems.

A related treatment goal for Ted was that he would:

Accept and respond to limits set by his parents or experience logical consequences of his behavior.

IMPLEMENTATION

The first priority in working with the parents was to have positive or negative attention. Specific guidelines for handling temper outbursts were given. The parents were able to follow these guidelines while Ted was visiting home, and they achieved initial success in that Ted's outbursts were shorter and less frequent and intense, and the parents were less angry at him for throwing tantrums. However, they had to be reminded to keep using the techniques consistently. They had the expectation that their son would learn to control himself in a short period and not slide back into previous habits from time to time.

The success in handling the temper tantrums was encouraging and made them more able to hear and practice effective limit setting. Again, specific guidelines were given. The parents were encouraged to record their efforts at setting limits so that they could be examined and discussed with the nurse. In this way, application of the specific guidelines could be evaluated. They required additional coaching in applying logical consequences.

After achieving some success in handling temper tantrums and setting limits, the parents could turn to more positive aspects of parenting. They were instructed to obtain a copy of *PET: Parent Effectiveness Training* by Thomas Gordon to learn about communicating more effectively. They were reminded of the importance of praising good behavior and also for allowing appropriate ventilation of anger and frustration by talking to Ted and throughout his play.

Later, parent education meetings were used to teach the importance of keeping up interpersonal contacts with one's family of origin to avoid emotional overinvestment in one's own children. In addition, the nurse recommended that the parents continue to carve out time for relating as a marital pair, spending time together as a twosome, and talking about issues that concerned their marriage other than the children. These interventions were geared toward defocusing Ted as the problem child and helping to prevent further development of dysfunctional behavior in the future.

EVALUATION

Ted returned home after 3 weeks of hospitalization. He and his parents had achieved the treatment goals and had obtained symptom relief. On discharge, Ted's behavior had improved, and the parents had more realistic expectations of their son's behavior. They had some conception of the family dynamics and had learned a variety of democratic parenting techniques.

offer added therapeutic services for the school-age child. Structured activities, peer groups, behavior modification programs, and help with homework are some of the services provided. Candidates for the ASTPs are children who are experiencing a moderate to high degree of dysfunction in their roles within the school, family, or community but who do not present a danger to themselves or others that would warrant hospitalization.

Finally, in-home intervention teams are being used to work with families in crisis. These families may be unable to use traditional outpatient therapy due to the lack of awareness of the availability of needed psychiatric services. Mental health professionals in these programs work intensively to stabilize the family and help to connect with appropriate service systems such as supplemental income, social services, or mental health clinics. The length of treatment is usually from 3 to 6 weeks, and the health care workers can spend up to 20 hours per week in the family's home as part of this innovative program.

DIRECTIONS FOR FUTURE RESEARCH

The following are some of the nursing research problems raised in Chapter 30 that merit further study by psychiatric nurses:
1. The number, settings, and scope of practice of child psychiatric nurses throughout the United States
2. Curative factors of the milieu of child psychiatric inpatients
3. Attitude change of parents toward their child following psychiatric nursing intervention
4. Methods for establishing relationships with children who have difficulty trusting adults
5. Prospective studies of child patients to identify factors associated with the development of adult psychiatric disorders
6. Retrospective studies of the childhood environment of adults with psychiatric disorders
7. The use of prn medication for the behavioral management of children
8. Frequency and type of family interventions provided by child psychiatric nurses
9. The effect of locked-door seclusion on child psychiatric patients
10. Types of nursing diagnoses used when working with child psychiatric patients

SUGGESTED CROSS-REFERENCES

Behavior modification is discussed in Chapter 27. Group therapy is discussed in Chapter 28. Family therapy is discussed in Chapter 29. Adolescent psychiatric nursing is presented in Chapter 31. Intervening in family abuse and violence is discussed in Chapter 32.

SUMMARY

1. Child psychiatry evolved from the fields of psychoanalysis, education, psychology, and social welfare.
2. The child psychiatric nurse functions in a therapeutic role as a milieu therapist. The expanded role as an independent practitioner requires advanced study at the master's level. Care settings in child psychiatry are diverse and vary from primary to tertiary prevention.
3. Standards of child and adolescent psychiatric and mental health nursing practice are presented along with rationales for their use.
4. Latency has a potential for growth that the school-age child reaches by sublimating basic instinctual drives to reach a sense of self-competency. Children with ego deficits are believed to have developmental delays in differentiating from their mothers and developing object relations.
5. The data collection phase involves the development of a profile of the child that includes presenting symptoms, mental status, interpersonal relationships, activities and behaviors, and personal and family history. Brief hospitalizations are often used for diagnostic purposes.
6. Nursing diagnoses are formulated from the psychodynamics specific to each child's problems. Common problem areas include faulty impulse control, negative self-concept, impaired reality testing, poor interpersonal relationships, and lack of insight. Major medical diagnoses are described.
7. Helping children with deficits in ego strength requires a comprehensive treatment plan and specific nursing care goals. Residential treatment programs serve as therapeutic milieus in which daily living experiences are used to help children learn more adaptive behaviors and gain a stronger sense of self.
8. Interventions such as the life space interview, behavior modification programs, and one-to-one relationships are helpful in facilitating the child's growth and development. Therapeutic modalities have an impact on the child in residential treatment and include individual, group, family, drug, special education, and recreational therapies.
9. The child hospitalized on a long-term basis should achieve some insight into his problems, impulse control, reality testing, and more adaptive coping responses before discharge. Health teaching and follow-up care are important to the child's outcome after discharge.

REFERENCES

1. American Psychiatric Association: Diagnostic and Statistical Manual, third edition revised, Washington, DC, 1987, The Association.

2. Binet A and Binet S: The development of intelligence in children, Baltimore, 1916, Williams & Wilkins.

3. Bowen M: Theory in the practice of psychotherapy. In Guerin P, editor: Family therapy, New York, 1976, Gardner Press, Inc.

4. Bradt JO and Moynihan CJ: Opening the safe: a study of child-focused families. In Bradt JO and Moynihan CF, editors: Systems therapy, Washington, DC, 1972, Groome Child Guidance Center.

5. Catell JM: Mental tests and measurements, Mind 15:373, 1890.

6. Chess S and Hassibi M: Principles and practice of child psychiatry, New York, 1978, Plenum Publishing Corp.

7. Child psychiatric–mental health nurse clinician, position statement, Chicago, 1980, Advocates for Child Psychiatric Nursing, Inc.

8. Elkind D: Children and adolescents: interpretive essays on Jean Piaget, New York, 1974, Oxford University Press, Inc.

9. Erikson EH: Childhood and society, New York, 1950, WW Norton & Co.

10. Fogarty TF: On emptiness and closeness. I, Family 2(1):22, 1975.

11. Freud S: Sexual enlightenment of children, New York, 1963, Macmillan, Inc.

12. Gisell AL: Infancy and human growth, New York, 1928, Macmillan, Inc.

13. Healy W: Twenty-five years of child guidance, Chicago, 1934, Institute for Juvenile Research.

14. Mahler M: The psychological birth of the human infant, New York, 1975, Basic Books, Inc.

15. National Advisory Mental Health Council: National plan for research on child and adolescent mental disorders, Rockville, Md, 1990, US Department of Health and Human Services.

16. Popper C, editor: Psychiatric pharmacosciences of children and adolescents, Washington DC, 1987, American Psychiatric Press.

17. Pothier P: Graduate preparation in child and adolescent psychiatric and mental health nursing, Arch Psych Nurs II(3):170, 1988.

18. Pothier P, Norbeck J, and Laliberte M: Child psychiatric nursing: the gap between need and utilization, J Psychosoc Nurs Ment Health Serv 23(7):18, 1985.

19. Redl F: Life space interview, AM J Orthopsychiatry 1:1, 1957.

20. Rinsley DB: Principles of therapeutic milieu with children. In Sholevar GP, editor: Emotional disorders in children and adolescents, New York, 1980, Spectrum Books.

21. Sarnoff CA: Latency-age children. In Sholevar P et al, editors: Emotional disorders in children and adolescents, New York, 1980, Spectrum Books.

22. Simeon J: Pediatric psychopharmacology, Can J Psychiatry 34:115, 1989.

23. Simmons JE: Psychiatric examination of children, ed 2, Philadelphia, 1987, Lea & Febiger.

24. Sully J: Studies of childhood, London, 1903, Longman Group.

25. Trieschman AE, Whittaker JK, and Brendtro LK: The other 23 hours: Child care work with emotionally disturbed children in a therapeutic milieu, New York, 1969, Aldine Publishing Co.

■ ANNOTATED SUGGESTED READINGS ■

Axline UM: Play therapy, Boston, 1947, Houghton Mifflin Co.

This classic work describes the author's unique art and style of play therapy.

Dinkmeyer D and McKay GD: The parents' handbook: systematic training for effective parenting, Minnesota, 1989, American Guidance Services.

Essential teaching aid for parents. Provides basic skills for the nurse beginning to work with children. Includes parenting styles, the meaning of a child's misbehavior, communication skills, and natural and logical consequences.

Elkind D: Children and adolescents: interpretive essays on Jean Piaget, New York, 1974, Oxford University Press, Inc.

For the student interested in cognitive developmental theory. Readable interpretation of the extremely technical writing of Jean Piaget.

*Fagin CM, editor: Readings in child and adolescent psychiatric nursing, St Louis, 1974, Mosby–Year Book, Inc.

Examines beginnings of child psychiatric nursing and provides intervention techniques for specific situations.

Garfinkel G, Carlson G, and Weller E: Psychiatric disorders in children and adolescents, Philadelphia, 1990, WB Saunders Co.

Overview of psychiatric disorders in infancy and adolescence. Thorough and up-to-date reference text.

Gordon T: PET: parent effectiveness training, New York, 1988, Wyden Books.

Alternate approach to child-rearing based on communication techniques. Helpful for parents as well as professionals.

*Jones R and O'Brien P: Unique interventions for child inpatient psychiatry, J Psych Nurs 28(7):29, 1990.

Describes three child inpatient treatment techniques and the child's perceptions of these and other milieu treatments and techniques.

*Journal of Child and Adolescent Psychiatric and Mental Health Nursing.

Nursing journal published quarterly that is devoted exclusively to issues related to child and adolescent psychiatric nursing. A required addition to the library of any child psychiatric nurse.

Kestenbaum C and Williams D, editors: Handbook of clinical assessment of children and adolescents, vol 1-2, New York, 1988, New York University Press.

Presents a wealth of information on assessment and treatment issues. Comprehensive in covering diagnostic categories, syndromes, and other problems.

---

*Asterisk indicates nursing reference.

*McBride A: Coming of age: child psychiatric nursing, Arch Psych Nurs 2(2):57, 1988.

Explores developments in nursing in general and in psychiatric nursing in particular. Suggests steps that must be taken if child psychiatric nursing is to become a force in improving health care.

National Advisory Mental Health Council: National plan for research on child and adolescent mental disorders, Rockville, Md, 1990, US Department of Health and Human Services.

Describes a national research incentive to intensify work with children and adolescents with mental illnesses. This plan will influence service delivery and research initiatives for many years to come.

*Pothier P: Child mental health problems and policy, Arch Psych Nurs II(3):165, 1988.

Summarizes and critiques the findings and recommendations of the National Mental Health Association's study on the mental health problems of children and youth. Specific recommendations for advocacy for child mental health service delivery are included.

Rappaport JL: DSM-III training guide for diagnosis of childhood disorders, New York, 1984, Brunner/Mazel, Inc.

Provides specific instructions for diagnosing childhood disorders using the DSM-III manual. Includes information on the adult disorders that appear in childhood and those specific to infancy, childhood, and adolescence.

Redl F: The life space interview, Am J Orthopsychiatry 1:1, 1959.

Presents author's classic work concisely.

Redl F and Wineman D: The aggressive child, Glencoe, Ill, 1957, The Free Press.

Required reading for milieu therapists. Describes aggressive child's ego pathology and delineates life space interview techniques. Replete with clinical examples.

Schulman JL and Irwin M: Psychiatric hospitalization of children, Springfield, Ill, 1982, Charles C Thomas, Publishers.

Comprehensive description of treatment for children requiring acute and chronic levels of care.

Simeon J: Pediatric psychopharmacology, Can J Psychiatry 34:115, 1989.

Brief overview of pediatric psychopharmacology. Summarizes current knowledge of psychostimulants, antidepressants, antipsychotics, anxiolytics, anticonvulsants and diets used in the treatment of child and adolescent psychiatric disorders.

Simmons JE: Psychiatric examination of children, ed 2, Philadelphia, 1987, Lea & Febiger.

Compact, concise manual explaining mental status and psychiatric examination of children. Includes case study and suggested format.

*Special issue: Focus on the child, J Psychosoc Nurs Ment Health Serv 22(3):11, 1984.

Devoted to exploring various aspects of child psychiatric nursing. Recommended to all interested nurses.

Trieschman AE, Whittaker JK, and Brendtro LK: The other 23 hours: child care work with emotionally disturbed children in a therapeutic milieu, New York, 1969, Aldine Publishing Co.

Describes the concept of milieu therapy, therapeutic relationships, program development, and recording. Basic text for beginning practitioners; available in paperback.

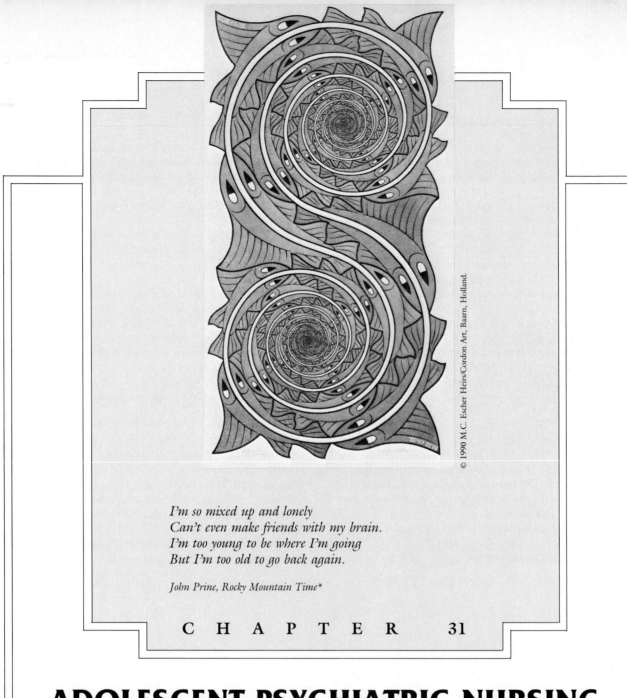

I'm so mixed up and lonely
Can't even make friends with my brain.
I'm too young to be where I'm going
But I'm too old to go back again.

John Prine, Rocky Mountain Time*

CHAPTER 31

ADOLESCENT PSYCHIATRIC NURSING

AUDREY REDSTON-ISELIN

- state the scope and function of adolescent psychiatric nursing practice.

- list the developmental tasks of adolescence.

- compare and contrast the following theoretical views of adolescence: biological, psychoanalytical, intellectual, and cultural and multidimensional.

- identify the major categories of data that the nurse should collect with regard to the adolescent's health status.

- discuss common areas of conflict during adolescence and their implications.

- describe specific problems frequently experienced by adolescents.

- analyze the nurse's use of patient and parent education and family, group, and individual therapies when working with adolescents and their parents.

- assess the importance of evaluating the nursing process when working with adolescents.

- identify directions for future nursing research.

- select appropriate readings for further study.

A dolescence is a time of transition—an age when one is not an adult and not a child. However, the issues reflected in the adolescent experience are central to one's development as a person. The intense feelings during the teenage years are perhaps the most meaningful of any experienced in a lifetime. Assisting adolescents during this complex period of development can be an enlightening and rewarding experience.

Role of the adolescent psychiatric nurse

Adolescent psychiatric nurses are prepared in psychiatric–mental health nursing and have a specific interest in meeting this age groups needs. They focus on adolescents as they develop toward adulthood, considering social, emotional, and physical aspects of their adjustment in their family, school, and peer groups. These nurses concentrate on facilitating the adolescent's successful movement toward adulthood. Adolescent psychiatric nurses become experts in identifying deviations or stalls in the developmental process and work closely with the adolescent's support systems to enhance the growth process.

The scope of adolescent psychiatric nursing practice includes direct and indirect care in the areas of prevention, intervention, and rehabilitation. **Direct nursing functions** focus on actions toward the adolescent and include:

1. Psychotherapy (individual, family, and group)
2. Intake screening and evaluation
3. Home visits
4. Provision of therapeutic milieu
5. Counseling (time limited on a specific problem)
6. Health teaching (role model and didactic teaching, usually on sex and health)
7. Support and medication surveillance
8. Community action (resource person to others dealing with adolescents; help formulate programs needed)
9. Crisis intervention

Indirect nursing functions focus on actions taken to assist another person who carries out the adolescent care. These functions are usually performed by an adolescent psychiatric nurse specialist in the following roles:

1. Educator
2. Administrator
3. Clinical supervisor
4. Consultant
5. Nurse researcher

Developmental stage of adolescence

Adolescence is a unique, distinct stage of development that has great significance in the understanding of human behavior. The common age range for adolescence (11 to 20) indicates that during that time a shift in the developmental and learning process occurs. It is more accurate to view this progression as continuous, with each stage overlapping the next. Various theorists have studied goals and tasks within the specific stage of adolescence and the way each stage of life moves into the next ones.

The new developmental tasks that emerge during adolescence stress the individual's defenses. They can either stimulate growth through new ways of coping or lead to regression and disorganization from failure to cope. Longstanding difficulties may contribute to disorganization, and the current environment may help or hinder the adolescent's attempt to deal with these issues. Beginning at infancy, development is often marked with episodes of disintegration when learning a new skill, then with movement toward integration as the new skill is acquired. The pattern of dealing with developmental stress contributes to how the adolescent copes with current anxieties. Skills established during latency do little to ward off anxieties associated with changing body image and new instinctive feelings. Past coping skills, if integrated successfully, can assist healthy integration of adult functions.

An earlier, although still popular, view of adolescence described it as a time of conflict and upheaval that was seen as necessary for normal personality integration. More recent research suggests that this is not true; the complex changes in biological, social, and emotional development do not necessarily lead to psychological conflicts. Studies show that only 10% to 20% of adolescents have psychological disturbances, which is about the same percentage found in adults.[24]

During adolescence, major events occur and attempts to resolve these events are made. These result in behavior uniquely "adolescent."[25] Havighurst identified tasks that should be accomplished during adolescence[13]:

1. Achieving new and more mature relations with age mates of both sexes
2. Achieving masculine or feminine social roles
3. Accepting one's physique and using the body effectively
4. Achieving emotional independence from parents and other adults
5. Preparing for marriage and family life
6. Preparing for an economic career
7. Acquiring a set of values and an ethical system as a guide to behavior and developing an ideology

Different theoretical concepts describe how these developmental tasks are encountered and resolved to produce an adolescent moving toward adulthood.

Theoretical views of adolescence

■ Biological theory

Gesell, Ilg, and Ames[11] believed that biological influences are the major determinants of adolescent development. They studied humans from birth to age 16, placing great emphasis on behaviors of the child and adolescent and the role of environmental influences on adolescent development. They believed that growth patterns followed certain principles of maturation. Through maturation and environmental influences, a person learns how to adjust. Behavior is therefore a conscious growth experience. Gesell and associates described adolescent development as consisting of intense and dramatic physical growth changes that affect all aspects of the human being. They presented a normative theory, which describes certain behaviors that occur at particular points in the maturational development of most adolescents. The authors' specific normative data consist of feelings, thoughts, and behaviors seen at each age. They indicated differences in equilibrium, ranging from stormy disequilibrium to calm equilibrium. These changes result from maturational states that cause the adolescent to grow.

■ Psychoanalytical theory

Freud also believed that human development was biological and was marked by stages. He put more emphasis on the first year of life, concluding that adolescence and adulthood have their roots in the resolution of childhood developmental stages. These stages originated in the sexual instinct he called the id, which he viewed as a primary factor in determining an individual's successful personality development. The rational, reality-based part of humans he called the ego. The ego helped control and modify the id and created coping mechanisms to deal with the environment. The superego was described as the conscience. It assisted the ego in establishing socially acceptable behaviors and attitudes. Freud constructed five stages of development from birth to adolescence: oral, anal, phallic, latency, and genital.

During puberty (ages 13 to 18), Freud's genital stage, a reawakening of sexual interest occurs. The adolescent with new sexual urges looks for gratification outside the home. This renewal comes from physiological maturing. The genitalia mature, and the release of sex hormones increases. Sexual exploration and maturation often occur. Freud stressed that the first years of life were important in establishing traits that become permanent in adolescence.[8]

The more modern psychoanalytical theories are the most descriptive in defining adolescence. They define it as the stage between childhood and adulthood correlated with the biological changes of puberty. Adolescence is described by Josselyn[15] as the psychological development that attempts to deal with pubescent changes and is therefore initiated by them. The biological changes of puberty upset a balance that existed between the ego and id during latency. Increased drives or impulses initiated by the greater hormonal secretion cause a personality reorganization in adolescents as they attempt to adjust to their new physical status. These increased impulses confront a relatively weak ego. Most evident at this time is a resurgence of the oedipal complex, which brings along with it derivatives of pregenital drives, oral and anal impulses, and aggressive drives. Adolescents therefore return to earlier modes of adaptation in an effort to reevaluate and reestablish mastery over the environment. Many solutions to problems caused by instinctual pressures are tried.

Psychoanalysts believe that sexual development does not begin with puberty but that new avenues for dealing with drives and the growth spurt surface in adolescence. The simple solutions of drive satisfaction that a child used no longer work, and efforts toward new solutions are made. The ability to make these adjustments arises from the ego's capacity to renegotiate between the id, the superego, and the environment. The groundwork for this is laid earlier in development. If there has been inadequate accommodation in earlier stages, difficulties in adolescence occur. Adolescence is a developmental, maturational process in which the individual attempts to work through his life experiences to achieve maturity. Related to the oedipal conflict is the adolescent's task of freeing himself from dependency on parents. This detachment from incestuous objects can be evident in rejection, resentment, and hostility toward parents and authority. For this reason, Blos[6] calls adolescence a "second stage of individuation," the first occurring during the oedipal period.

The classic psychoanalytical description of adolescence has been modified by Erikson, Fromm, Horney, Sullivan, and others, who emphasize the effect of social factors on these developmental processes. Erikson[9] describes ego identity, or the relationship between how a person appears to others and how the person views himself. To Erikson, adolescence represents an attempt to establish an identity within the social environment. This search is described as "normal adolescent identity crisis." Erikson outlines this in the theoretical framework of his eight stages of humans. He calls the stage of adolescence "identity versus identity diffusion," which is followed in young adulthood by the stage of "intimacy versus isolation." He stresses that identity must be established before intimacy can occur.

■ Intellectual development theory

Cognition is most completely described by Piaget.[23] By gradually internalizing actions, one evolves a system of thought processes. A child learns to reason by a process Piaget describes as "concrete operations," based on tangible objects. Adolescence is defined as an advanced stage of cognitive functioning in which one is able to reason beyond concrete objects to symbols or abstractions, or what Piaget calls "formal thought." Piaget believes the adolescent has the ability to deal with propositional logic, to grasp metaphors, and to reason about thought. This develops continuously from the concrete thinking of childhood to (at about age 12) a rapid progression toward free reflection. Piaget calls this the "formal operational period." The concern with realities, tangible objects, and action is transferred to an ideational plane, permitting one to draw conclusions and reflect without the reality or object being present. Piaget calls this ability the "logic of operations."

■ Cultural theory

Anthropologists concluded from studies of adolescents in different cultures that primitive cultures had less stressful periods than those experienced by American teenagers. Mead[19] concluded that adolescent rebellion was culturally determined and not biologically based. Anthropologists view adolescence as a period when the person believes he deserves adult privileges that are not given to him, which ends when society gives him the full power and social status of an adult. Anthropologists see growth as a continuous process and a cultural phenomenon, with individuals reacting to social expectations. The more clearly defined these expectations are, the less stressful and ambiguous the adolescent period. The more the culture has changed, the greater the generation gap.

Adolescents have today's culture to cope with, which can add to conflicts awakened by increased drives and changes in body image. Several issues in

American society directly influence the support an adolescent can obtain from the environment. Blurring sexual roles is one such issue. Women have less traditional attitudes, expectations, and behaviors. Men have become more involved in functions that were previously believed to be women's, and vice versa. The anxiety associated with these role changes has begun to be identified and explored.

The current economic focus on conservation includes economic stability, restraint, and budgeting. There are fewer jobs, particularly for adolescents. The cost of higher education has increased dramatically, which has resulted in prolonged economic dependency. Women are developing careers and entering the work force, which requires a new view on two-parent working families. Divorce rates and single-parent families have also increased. These changes increase the complexity of society and add new pressures to adolescents, who are becoming adults and attempting to define their role in today's cultural milieu.

■ Multidimensional theory

Multidimensional theory proposes that no singular view of adolescent development and mental health exists. Rather, these issues are related to the wide variation in adolescents' social relationships, behaviors, and attitudes and revolve around three main themes.[24] First, profiles of ego and moral development are used to characterize adolescents for rates of progression, regression, and stability in age-related development. Second, attention is given to biological, sociological, psychological, and cultural integration. These variables change rapidly during adolescence, interrelate, and together impact the adolescent's behavior and view of self at any time. Third, the developmental issues of both psychological and biological maturation are viewed as affecting the adolescent's adaptation and functioning. For example, the timing of one's development in relation to a peer group has a direct influence on the teenager's self-esteem. These issues may vary widely not only individually, but also by culture and society.

The multidimensional view of adolescence sees adaptation on a continuum of development. Less emphasis is placed on one's specific age, and more on one's developmental level and the timing of various biological, psychological, and environmental influences. This theory also proposes that severe family conflict need not necessarily occur. Rather, the degree and nature of conflicts change from childhood through the adolescent years and reflect both the diversity and the functional and dysfunctional aspects of family life.

 ## Assessment

Collection of data about the adolescent's health status involves the organized observation and interpretation of behavior patterns. Other disciplines often refer to it as the developmental history. It includes the following information:

1. Growth and development (including developmental milestones)
2. Biophysical status (illnesses, accidents)
3. Emotional status (relatedness; affect; mental status, including evidence of thought disorder and suicidal or homicidal ideation)
4. Cultural, religious, and socioeconomic background
5. Performance of activities of daily living (home, attending school)
6. Patterns of coping (ego defenses such as denial, acting out, withdrawal)
7. Interaction patterns (family, peers)
8. Adolescent's perception of and satisfaction with his health status
9. Adolescent's health goals
10. Environment (physical, emotional, ecological)
11. Available and accessible human and material resources (friends, school and community involvement)

These data are collected from adolescents, their families, and other significant persons, such as school personnel and the physician, through interviews, examinations, observations, and reports. Data collection by the nurse is based on current, as well as past, functioning in all aspects of adolescent life. It helps to give a view of the adolescent experience and aids the nurse in assessing the success of the adolescent's attempts to complete the prescribed tasks.

An examination of typical adolescent behaviors reveals that adolescence is a time of change. The complex issues most often confronting adolescents are body image, identity, independence, sexuality, social role, and sexual behavior. These issues can produce adaptive or maladaptive behaviors in an attempt to master the tasks at hand.

■ Body image

Chronological age is not a true guide for physical maturation, since growth often occurs in spurts and individual differences exist. Because the grouping of adolescents is usually done chronologically, the adolescent must face being with others who vary greatly in physical development and interests. This explains why adolescents often imitate behavior as an effort to keep within the expected range of conduct and be compatible with peers. The greater the divergence from the rest of the group, the greater is the adolescent's anxiety. The lack of uniformity of growth often puts great demands on physical and mental adaptability. Growth being uneven and sudden, rather than smooth and gradual, causes a change in body image.

Adolescents reevaluate themselves in light of these physical changes, particularly the onset of primary and secondary sex characteristics, which are so pronounced. They tend to compare themselves and their physical development to that of their peers. They are very concerned about the normality of their physical status. The absence of clear-cut norms only adds to this uncertainty. The physical changes of puberty cause adolescents to be self-conscious of their changing bodies. Often they are reluctant to have medical examinations because they fear abnormalities will be found. Examinations may intensify masturbatory conflicts, sexual fantasies, and guilt feelings. Extreme concern with body changes may lead to deviant behaviors such as hypochondriasis, in which physical complications are the focus of underlying conflicts.[5] The early and middle phases of puberty may also give rise to increased conflict, distance, and dissatisfaction in parental relationships.

Usually self-esteem increases between early and middle adolescence. However, some girls show a decrease in self-esteem at this time, which is associated with negative feelings about body image and their comparison of themselves to older adolescents. Offer, Ostrov, and Howard[21] present evidence that this vulnerable time for girls may be associated with the onset of differences that begin to appear at this age and that coincide with an increased incidence of depression.

■ Identity

In an attempt to adjust to the physical changes of puberty, adolescents experience excitement and tension. They employ methods of gratification and defenses against these feelings that they used in infancy and childhood. This mixture of previous infantile solutions, plus new adult attempts at mastery, accounts for the often bizarre and regressive nature of adolescent behavior. As they attempt to cope, adolescents sometimes act as adults and other times as children.

They can be seen to be experiencing a second individuation process, similar to the first one noted at about age 2. Blos[6] equates the characteristic "no" in the 2-year-old's effort to differentiate between self and nonself with the adolescent rebellious and oppositional behavior. Adolescents show behavior marked with ex-

---

> ### CLINICAL EXAMPLE 31-1
>
> David, although an avid football fan for several years, suddenly switched his interest to basketball. He quit his local football team despite his father's urgings to continue. His father, also a football fan, could not understand David's sudden negative attitude toward football and newly found interest in basketball.

---

perimentation, testing the self by going to extremes. This is useful to establish self-identity. The rebelliousness or negativism shows a movement toward individuation and autonomy that has greater complexity but also elements similar to the 2-year-old's "no." Adolescents assert themselves in their self-identity by being negative to parents and other authority figures whom they believe are not allowing them to be separate and unique, as illustrated by Clinical example 31-1.

The individuation process is accompanied by feelings of isolation, loneliness, and confusion, since it brings childhood dreams to an end and attributes them to fantasy. This realization of childhood's end can create intense fears or panic. Many adolescents therefore attempt to remain in this transitional stage. The awakening of emotional ties with the family also occurs in the establishment of new, more interdependent relationships. This fearful, yet exciting, entrance into adulthood is a profound personal experience that is not totally resolved in adolescence but dealt with throughout life. Adolescents mourn the loss of childhood, and the feelings of loneliness and isolation that accompany this loss establish an intense need for closeness, love, and understanding. If they are unable to obtain support during this struggle, depression may result.[5]

Parenting styles that encourage individuality and relatedness to families are associated with support and adolescent identity exploration. Adolescents expressing high levels of identity exploration have parents who express mutuality and separateness, encourage member differences, and are aware of clear boundaries between themselves and their teenagers. These adolescents are also more likely to have competent approaches to peer and social relationships and more developed skills in initiating, diversifying, sustaining, and deepening peer friendships.[24]

Independence

Adolescents have an unconscious longing to give in to their dependency needs. It is also a time of profound movement toward independence. Adolescents show this ambivalence by responding to petty annoyances and irritations with outbursts more intense than seem warranted. They see the process toward independence as being free of parental control. They do not see gaining independence as a gradual learning process but as an emancipation accomplished by acting "differently." If one acts adult, then one is adult. Therefore they expose themselves to situations beyond their capabilities and then become overwhelmed and frightened. They seek reassurance in an attempt to alleviate their anxiety by returning to childlike ways and being dependent on those with whom they feel most secure, usually their parents. This accounts for the inconsistency of adolescent behavior.

Well-adjusted adults usually use a problem-solving approach and do not feel as threatened when inexperience requires dependency on others. Adolescents, however, already tempted to give in to dependency needs, feel as if they are regressing to childhood, which deflates their self-esteem. They must deny their need for their parents. Sometimes they will criticize their parents for treating them as a child and not allowing them freedom and then remark that their parents are not helpful enough. When adolescents seem to be rebelling against their parents, they may be rebelling against their own childhood conscience or superego. They project their ambivalence onto their parents, since they were the original source of restrictions. This projection actually reveals a movement toward a more mature standard and also indicates their insecurity about relinquishing childhood standards. By blaming their parents for their childish actions, they can avoid blows to their fragile self-esteem and protest that their actions result from parental demands, not their own.

The interaction between adolescent changes in autonomy and family relationships is an important consideration. Three parenting styles have been described in relation to whether they help or hinder independent functioning in adolescence.[24]

1. Traditional parents tend to value a sense of continuity and order. They accept the patterns of understanding and value judgments that come from previous generations. Adolescents from these families tend to be more attached to their parents, more conforming, and achievement oriented. Often they bypass major conflicts in their teenage years.
2. Authoritarian parents are oriented toward shaping, controlling, and restricting the adolescent to fixed standards set by religious or other secular societies. Obedience is seen as a virtue. Power and responsibility are not shared with the adolescent. Harsh discipline is used to curb autonomous strivings that are viewed as willfulness. The approach here is punitive and it can result in problems with the adolescent's development of autonomy.
3. Democratic parents do not believe that their standards are infallible. They tend to be supportive and committed to responses that are geared to the specific situation. The content of issues and individual differences are reflected in their support of solutions that promote autonomous expression by the adolescent. These parents emphasize "disciplined conformity." The environment fostered is one of stimulation and challenge. This parenting style combines limit setting with negotiation, thus encouraging the teenager's participation in the disciplinary process. It is shown to predict greater independent functioning in adolescents.

Sexuality

Most adolescents accept the sexual norms of our culture, which dictate that sexual feelings be directed toward persons of the opposite sex. The biologically induced sexual feelings that intensify during adolescence accompany intensified emotional feelings. The fusion of sexual impulses with love means that sex is the usual way of expressing feelings of deep affection. The strongest emotional ties are felt toward the parents, but the channeling of these sexual impulses creates a conflict. The adolescent interprets love for the parent of the same sex as suggestive of homosexuality. Feelings of love toward the parent of the opposite sex are equally conflictual, since they are viewed as incestuous.

Rejection of parents, so frequently expressed by adolescents, can thus be seen as a defense to diminish ties to the parents and therefore avoid sexual arousal. Efforts to resolve this conflict can also be seen in experimentation through heterosexual and sometimes homosexual relationships. Ambivalence is apparent, since adolescents are often flirtatious one moment and rejecting the next, and parents may find these flirtations enjoyable. Clinical example 31-2 shows this ambivalence.

Social role

Adolescents respond intensely to persons and events. They may be totally invested in one interest and then suddenly change to something different. These intense feelings and lack of stable identity can account for their extreme sensitivity to the response of

> ## CLINICAL EXAMPLE 31-2
>
> Debbie, at age 13, would not let her father kiss her. She was often distant and aloof when he attempted closeness. In contrast, she was often teasing and flirtatious, often remarking about his muscular body structure.

others. They are easily hurt, disappointed, and fearful of others. There is a tendency toward "hero worship" and "crushes," but with poor discrimination in evaluating the persons to whom these feelings are directed. Adolescent relationships serve many functions. Often adolescents relate to a chum as if neither person were a separate individual. They often mimic each other's dress, speech, language, and thoughts. These relationships help in the development of self-identity and establishment of a social role.

The peer group is extremely important, since within the security of the peer group, adolescents can attempt to resolve conflicts. They can relate to peers in a way they cannot relate to others. With peers they can test out their thoughts and ideas. Their thoughts may differ, but through mutual sharing, they can try to find an answer. The peer group explores more autonomous ways of dealing with problems. A peer group that shares these things offers its members companionship, protection, and security, with acceptable amounts of dependent gratification. In the peer group, adolescents can accept dependency, not as a child but as one of the gang, testing out ideas and trying new values. Within the safety of the peer group, they can observe, comment on, and evaluate the activities of other peer groups. Adolescents usually are very loyal to their group of friends. Sometimes group security is so important that it is necessary at all costs. Then destructive experimentation may occur to preserve acceptance in the group.

Adolescents often test out ideas pertaining to values. They either eventually abandon them or incorporate them into their adult personality. They react to many stimuli and drain off the tension created by new drives and impulses by investment in many interests. They do this with great intensity, which is why adolescents are susceptible to fads. This is often seen in their dress, music, or hobbies.

Close relationships with the opposite sex provide adolescents with security (often by "going steady")

and a person with whom to discuss problems and evaluate solutions. Often the partner may take on similar characteristics. This reciprocal relationship enhances self-esteem by demonstrating sexual attractiveness to the self and to the world, and it indicates that one is lovable. It also allows for bisexual expression, since the girl expresses her partner's feminine parts and her boyfriend represents her masculine parts. It is often observed that people tend to marry someone resembling the parent of the opposite sex. However, adolescents may purposely choose someone different to free themselves of their ties to their parents or may choose someone who is an acceptable substitute for parents.

■ Sexual behavior

Adolescents use fantasy to discharge tension meant for sexual play. Secretly they can be participant and observer and try out means of direct sexual discharge. They may, however, feel guilt and shame about sexual feelings, or they may experience the incompatibility of their fantasies with their ideal of themselves. Fantasies usually are an attempt to find solutions and evaluate consequences. Most adolescent fantasies are a way of problem solving. They may indicate a disturbance if they continually occupy the adolescent's thoughts, are not converted into constructive actions, or are not modified by reality. Then they may disrupt other activities important to adolescent functioning and indicate a withdrawal from reality.

Masturbation is also a frequent mode of discharge of tension for adolescents, particularly when alone, unhappy, or frustrated. It serves to fuse psychological and physical sexuality. It is not always associated with sexual fantasies. The value of masturbation may be lessened by the shame and guilt that accompany it. Male adolescents often fear discovery of evidence of ejaculation, and females often fear changes in their genitalia as a result of masturbation. Fears are not limited to discovery by others. They also are caused by orgasm, with the resulting feelings of loss of ego boundaries. If masturbation is used as a constant source of comfort or with inappropriate exposure (exhibitionism), it indicates a disturbance.

Mutual masturbation can also serve the purposes of tension release and fusing of identity. If mutual masturbation is the primary focus of the relationship, without the enrichment of other aspects of a relationship, it may be maladaptive. Mutual masturbation is often acceptable to adolescents as long as it does not lead to intercourse. It can help to dispel anxieties about sexuality by assuring adolescents that they are sexually adequate.[15]

Nursing diagnosis

Behaviors that impede growth and development may require nursing intervention. The nurse should consider the degree of harm and the nature of the defense and regression that the adolescent experiences. If the difficulty is significant and ongoing, it may mean intervention is needed. These destructive behaviors become the basis for the identification of specific problem areas.

■ Sexually active adolescent

Sexual behavior is often not as much an outlet for sexual passion as a desire to achieve closeness with another individual. The sexual expression seems to fulfill needs of love and security. Adolescents tend to use their sexuality to sublimate other needs. Josselyn[15] mentions some of the common interpretations sexual relations may have:

1. Finding an alternative choice to replace incestuous feelings about the parent of the opposite sex
2. Identifying with the parent of the same sex and trying to do what they do
3. Attempting to camouflage homosexual feelings
4. Expressing anger or hostility toward the parent of the opposite sex

Personal anxiety about sexual adequacy and peer group pressure also add to the possibility of using sexual relations inappropriately. Some adolescents use sexual relations as a means of punishing themselves. Their promiscuity elicits external control and condemnation from others. This is apparent when there is an exhibitionistic quality, and subtle efforts to "get caught" are seen. Periods of extreme prudery may alternate with periods of extreme sexual activity. Adolescents often attempt to have the nurse take a stand against their behavior and thereby avoid the underlying conflictual issues.

Meeks[20] suggests exploring the meaning of sexual behavior in adolescents by asking the following questions:

1. Does the adolescent desire sexual gratification for punishment?
2. Do the adolescent's goals match the situation, or is he deceiving himself?
3. Is he demanding adult privileges while acting irresponsible and dependent?
4. To what extent is the behavior a defense for depression, anger toward others, or exploratory experimentation?

5. Is the behavior to avoid anxiety-producing fantasies?
6. How close is the relationship to a mature one?

Clinical example 31-3 illustrates inappropriate use of sexual activity.

Another example of inappropriate use of sexual activity is a new thrill-seeking experience, based on an old Japanese act of heightening the sexual experience by asphyxiating the adolescent male just at the point of ejaculation. This has accidentally sent several adolescents to an early death.

The additional risk of sexually transmitted diseases, including acquired immunodeficiency syndrome (AIDS) makes sexual experimentation more problematic for its potential short-term and long-term impact on the adolescent.

■ Pseudohomosexuality

Adolescents who are uncertain of their sexual identity often misinterpret certain characteristics as being masculine or feminine. The anxiety that results can cause a fear of homosexuality. This triggers feelings of depression and anxiety that exaggerate the initial ones. This is common in males who see characteristics such as passivity as diminishing their maleness. Their fear of homosexuality increases their anxiety, causing them to withdraw into a cycle of failure. They may then feel dependent, have trouble asserting themselves, and respond by "acting out." It is important to differentiate between deviant behavior and defects in socialization

---

CLINICAL EXAMPLE 31-3

Janet, a 14-year-old adolescent, had apparently been sexually active since age 12. She was brought to the clinic by her parents when they had been told by a neighboring friend of Janet's exploits. Janet had bragged to the neighbor of her sexual ventures. Two years before referral, her parents had placed Janet in a more controlled parochial school because they were concerned she was "acting wild." It became apparent that Janet had wanted her parents to know about and put limits on her behavior. She admitted to not enjoying sexual intercourse very much. She seemed to be trying desperately to get approval from her distant and punitive mother. Her father, who was a policeman, was what she described as "a hopeless case," secretly wishing that he would be a better policeman for her.

skills. Defects in socialization skills causing a pseudohomosexual response may result from the absence of an adequate male figure, the mother or father's expressed fearfulness of aggressiveness, physical disabilities, sexual abuse by an older adult, or a personality temperament of passivity.[20]

■ Overt homosexual activity in adolescence

During adolescence, when identity is unclear and much experimentation occurs, the individual may have homosexual and heterosexual experiences. This does not mean that the adolescent is homosexual or bisexual.[9] If he is not conflicted either in his experimentation or in his regular homosexual relationships, he probably will not reach the nurse therapist. If he does, it may be to appease a conflicted family. Sometimes, however, homosexual relationships may interfere with establishing an adequate sexual identity. In this case, homosexual behavior may indicate anxiety about heterosexuality.

An added dimension to homosexual activity in adolescence is the AIDS epidemic. Anxiety over sexual identity issues are heightened by fears of contracting this fatal illness. It also appears that the epidemic has heightened social stigma about homosexual preference and experimentation, thus further complicating sexual identity issues for the adolescent. This is evident in Clinical example 31-4.

■ Unwed motherhood

Pregnancy in adolescence is a complicated issue because social, as well as intrapsychic, factors are involved. Some adolescent girls fear inadequacy of their femininity. These fears may stem from dependent attachment feelings toward the mother, which often occur during regressive periods and are mistaken as signs of homosexuality.[5] To ease these fears, the adolescent girl may become pregnant. Sometimes pregnancy is an effort to escape a difficult family situation or to force the parents to agree to a marriage that may be inappropriate, as shown in Clinical example 31-5.

Occasionally, emotionally deprived adolescents hope to give their child what they believe they have never received (or, probably more accurately, receive from the child what they have not received).Sometimes pregnancy appears to be a way to allow parents to give up parental responsibility for the adolescent. In some cases the adolescent has lived out a scapegoat role as the bad one in the family, thereby justifying parental neglect and hostility. The pregnancy can then improve family relationships because, with the adulthood the pregnancy implies, parents may be freed of guilt and may then not need to encourage the adolescent to act in ways that make her unlovable.

Pregnancy in adolescence may have other origins. It can occur accidentally after sexual exploration. The adolescent may be unaware of contraceptive methods. Pregnancy in an unmarried adolescent is often associated with sexual promiscuity. If it is, the girl may be ostracized. Sometimes pregnancy occurs from a close interpersonal relationship. Both the circumstances and the adolescent's level of maturity need to be assessed. Peer groups can be supportive to a girl who becomes pregnant as a result of a meaningful relationship but intolerant of one whose pregnancy is the result of promiscuity. In some cultures, out-of-wedlock pregnancies are an accepted part of adolescence.

Decisions involving abortion, placement of the baby, and marriage are difficult. Attitudes and laws in-

---

CLINICAL EXAMPLE 31-4

Joanne, age 16, was engaged in homosexual experiences with an 18-year-old girl. She claimed she enjoyed sexual experiences more with girls than boys. She had poor sexual experiences with boys and believed boys wanted girls for their sexual exploits. Her history revealed that she was sexually abused by her paternal grandfather several times and once by her father at about age 5. She was doing well in school but was very worried about her family finding out about her sexual preference and their response to her.

CLINICAL EXAMPLE 31-5

Susie, a 15-year-old adolescent, had run away for the second time, only to return home to the same chaos. She had tried to run away with her boyfriend. Her alcoholic mother and psychotic 19-year-old brother were making life unbearable. Her mother was surprised to learn about 3 months after her return that Susie was pregnant. Susie was delighted because she had hopes that now she could get out of the house, knowing her mother would now approve of her marriage to her boyfriend Jim.

fluencing these decisions are diverse. Many believe that to force the adolescent to have the baby and then give it up is more traumatic for her than abortion. Others believe that abortion can be more disturbing. Marriage is another alternative. Forcing a marriage to avoid societal stigma usually adds to the adolescent's problems, but a mature couple might do well in marriage. All the alternatives should be presented to the adolescent, with the consequences clearly stated. The adolescent makes her decision with the aid and support of her partner, her family, the nurse, and other involved health care professionals.

■ Adolescent suicide

One of the most common factors in adolescent suicide is lack or loss of a meaningful relationship.[14] Many researchers think suicide is an attempt for attention and does not necessarily represent a true desire to die. Regardless, it is a bid for help that must be recognized. Subtle references, as well as attempts, should always be taken seriously and explored. Suicidal gestures are more often seen in girls, with boys expressing their depression by bravado that results in accidents, as in Clinical example 31-6.

The adolescent may be prevented from acting on suicidal feelings by parental concern and the establishment of new relationships.[22] Adolescents may avoid the depression triggered by separating from their parents through delinquent behavior. This behavior serves as a defense against self-destructive impulses that accompany feelings of low self-esteem. The attempt to manipulate parents, which can motivate the runaway as well as the suicidal adolescent, is less important than the internal conflict causing this manipulation. Feelings of helplessness and worthlessness can be caused by threatened abandonment, being asked to take the adult role, and lack of opportunities to be dependent. Sometimes these adolescents perceive themselves to be expendable because the family unconsciously wishes them dead.

The nurse must make it clear to the adolescent that suicidal behavior is something that is not confidential and that parents must be told. Family involvement is essential to avoid angry, hostile, and hopeless feelings of abandonment and to create support and caring.

In working with suicidal adolescents, the nurse should explore the following areas[16]:

1. The seriousness of the attempt (What were the chances of rescue?)
2. The mental status of the adolescent (Was he psychotic?)
3. The extent of environmental stress, especially family disintegration
4. The adolescent's wider social environment and the strength of his support systems (social isolation, school performance, parental loss, disruption of friendship or romantic alliance)
5. The likelihood of repeated suicidal attempts, especially if conditions remain the same

Clinical examples 31-7 and 31-8 illustrate suicide attempts by adolescents.

The nurse must realize that adolescent suicide is not as prevalent as many believe, and its incidence is the same as that of the adult population. More specifically, suicide is highest among the elderly population, followed by young adults.[7] Suicide is seldom seen before puberty and is the second leading cause of death in adolescence. Unfortunately, the romanticism of suicide, the drama of adolescence, and the media focus contribute to encouraging teenagers at risk to choose this tragic solution.

■ Adolescent runaways

Adolescents trying to free themselves from an unbearable living situation may run away. The exit can indicate unconscious conflicts, and the running away usually points out difficulties between the parents and the adolescent. Parental rejection is often experienced from birth, and the parent may alternate between extreme punitive measures and a "laissez-faire" attitude toward the adolescent. Adolescent runaways are often conflicted, especially regarding dependency-independency, and feel embarrassed, helpless, and defeated by their dependency wishes. This can result in a panic that motivates running away to prove autonomy and escape painful circumstances. They usually run away

---

CLINICAL EXAMPLE 31-6

John, a 12-year-old depressed adolescent, had just gotten a small dirt bike. Six months earlier John's grandfather, his only friend, had died. John's father had died when he was 2 years old, and he had lived with his mother and grandparents ever since. John, feeling hopeless, had ridden his bike into a car. Luckily, after medical treatment for his broken arm and rib and multiple bruises, John was able to come to therapy. He described feeling helpless and lonely, especially without his grandfather.

CLINICAL EXAMPLE 31-7

Maria, a 15-year-old girl, was referred to her local community mental health center from the neighborhood emergency room after ingesting pills. Maria had taken five of her mother's "arthritis pills" after an argument with her father about her 17-year-old boyfriend, José. Her father, who came home only on weekends, told her to stay away from him. After he left, the other family members noticed Maria had become sleepy while playing cards in the living room. Maria admitted to taking the pills and was rushed by her mother to the emergency room. Maria claimed she would never do it again. She had clearly wanted to be rescued, not really wanting to die. She had had poor school performance for the last year since her father had left the family. She had many friends and had been dating José for the past year. Maria had always been her father's favorite. When she reached puberty at age 13, that relationship changed a great deal. Maria's position as her father's favorite was delegated to a younger female sibling, causing Maria to feel angry and rejected. Her father left the family a year later and returned for weekend visits, during which he mainly disciplined the children. Maria's attempt to get close to José as a replacement for her father was sabotaged by her father as well. Her only recourse was to elicit her father's caring and concern through a suicide attempt. Maria and her family later were receiving outpatient treatment.

CLINICAL EXAMPLE 31-8

Donald, age 13, was brought to the emergency room after cutting his wrists one evening when he thought his family was asleep. His mother had awakened and found him bleeding. She rushed him to the local emergency room, where he received medical treatment. It was then revealed that this was Donald's second suicidal attempt. The first attempt occurred a year ago when he had ingested pills. Donald had received therapy for about a month. It was then discontinued because of the family moving to a new location, despite recommendations to continue with a new therapist. Donald was always an isolated child. He was never very close with anyone but had two friends. Since the move he had become more withdrawn. He had done well in school in the past but now had given up and was failing almost every subject. The youngest of nine children, Donald had little relationship with his siblings, who were all older than he and not at home much. Donald's parents, both approaching old age, seemed not to notice that he had become increasingly upset. Donald was hospitalized, since the risk of his attempting suicide again was high. He was an isolated and depressed adolescent, seeking refuge from loneliness and defeat in death. He had not wanted to be rescued. The last year, especially, revealed many unsuccessful attempts to find meaningful relationships.

from disappointment toward something viewed as favorable and supportive. Parents often feel guilty and ashamed and have difficulty acting on practical issues, although some, relieved of their responsibility, are secretly pleased. Often the adolescent becomes involved in dangerous activities after running away. Most runaway adolescents want to return home if they believe their parents really want them.[20] Clinical example 31-9 illustrates home conditions that may lead to an adolescent's running away.

■ Conduct disordered adolescent

Conduct disordered adolescents often have poor parent-child relationships. Antisocial acts enable the adolescent to express anger toward parents, who are punished for the adolescent's acts. Parents are often scapegoated because the child is seen as a helpless victim. The nurse must remember that some parents are not effective with some adolescents. Children are socialized mainly by the parents and, it is hoped, learn from the parents acceptable behaviors that become part of the internalized self or conscience. A good relationship between parent and child facilitates this process.

However, adolescents learn not only from their parents but also from others. The school and peer groups are influencing factors, as are the social, economic, and cultural environments. The self-destructive behaviors seen in conduct disordered adolescents may indicate the need for punishment, anger at the family, peer group pressure, depression, feelings of self-defeat, a search for opportunities to take what they feel emotionally deprived of, and testing omnipotence through exciting experiences. Alignment with delinquents gives a defeated adolescent a feeling of self-respect and companionship through a sense of belonging to a subculture.[15]

Research by Offer, Ostrov, and Howard[21] sup-

CLINICAL EXAMPLE 31-9

Karen, age 14, ran away from home to a friend's house. Her mother had often expressed a desire to leave; in fact, she had once left the family to the charge of Karen's father when Karen was 9 years old. Karen's mother had suddenly told her she could not see her boyfriend for a month because she had come in late the night before. This caused a tremendous scene because Karen had been out late every night the week before without her mother even noticing. Karen's friend's mother was different. She spent a lot of money on her children, talked to them, and never limited their activity; thus the friend's home appeared attractive to Karen.

CLINICAL EXAMPLE 31-10

John, 13 years of age, was referred by the juvenile court for psychotherapy because he had been picked up for the second time after breaking into a store with another boy. John's parents were separated for the past 2 years after John's father had served a sentence in jail for tax evasion. John, very attached to his father, was extremely upset when his parents separated and rarely saw his father. His antisocial acts caused his father to become more involved with him, since his father claimed he did not want John to go through what he had experienced in prison. John gained his father's attention during these times, even though his father was angry. His delinquent actions therefore enabled John to express his anger at his father's leaving, as well as to fantasize about having his father return.

ports the idea that when depression and conduct disorder occur together, the central problem is depression. They identify features that best differentiate depression from conduct disorder. Adolescents who report helplessness, with the expectation that someone should do something for them, and who report fewer sad moods and lethargy, probably have conduct disorders. The authors also found distinct patterns of characteristics in both depressed and conduct disordered adolescents. Although both groups share problems with morals and superego, conduct disordered adolescents had more family problems than depressed adolescents. A similarity is that depressed adolescents with eating disorders and conduct disordered adolescents all had problems with impulse control.

Clinical example 31-10 of an adolescent who steals illustrates the many factors that may lead to adolescent delinquency. John's actions show that adolescents may not differentiate between their stealing and their parent's business dealings. Stealing may also be an effective way to rebel against parents. Adolescents may perpetuate childhood by indulging in immediate gratification through stealing rather than maturely working for things. Sometimes adolescents steal in hopes of getting caught and obtaining help. Parents may consciously or unconsciously condone stealing. Adolescents may act out their anger with the justification that they deserve the stolen items. The reasons for stealing must be established for the individual adolescent, since there may be many causes for this behavior.

The conflict of dependence versus independence can also be expressed in poor school adjustment. Some adolescents view teachers as parental surrogates who do not help or who merely apply rules of attendance and homework. Dependent feelings are sometimes elicited by these rules, and adolescents, in proving their independence, may become negative about learning. They may think that schoolwork is secondary to more important activities they are attempting to master. Daydreaming may interfere with schoolwork as adolescents concentrate on and fantasize about achieving independence.

Adolescents may drop out of school for financial reasons, or they may be rebelling against education laws. The adolescent may be part of a peer group that denounces school attendance and involvement. Parents may overtly or covertly discourage education. This is conveyed through lack of support and approval for education or by their making it difficult for the adolescent to follow through with school expectations, as illustrated by Clinical example 31-11.

■ Violent adolescents

Most adolescents displaying aggression have experienced frustration and have had violent role models during their childhood. Aggression is a human impulse that must be channeled constructively by a learned process that occurs within a supportive, loving relationship. Under favorable conditions, a child learns the healthy expression of aggression by involvement in activities that result in pleasure and active problem-solving attempts. Under less ideal conditions, aggres-

---

CLINICAL EXAMPLE 31-11

Debbie, a 15-year-old adolescent, dropped out of school after several years of poor school performance and truancy. She would occasionally go shopping with her mother on a school day. Her mother never knew the names of her teachers or guidance counselor, and no provisions for a place or time to study were made.

---

sion can occur in destructive activities that are harmful to self and others. In adolescence, when aggressive as well as sexual impulses are increased, the energy that strengthens these impulses also strengthens the adaptive and defensive aspects that accompany aggression.[2]

Much anxiety of adolescents is therefore related to the fear that they may be unable to control their destructive aggression. Adolescents often have violent dreams and fantasies that they express in threats, even though in some the potential for violence is minimal. Pointing out the harmlessness of these thoughts is helpful to adolescents, since it shows them that these thoughts are not as powerful as they fear. Some adolescents, however, are genuinely fearful that they will be unable to stop their thoughts from becoming actions. They require the recognition of their fear and the reassurance of the existence of external limits. Pointing out to the adolescent the necessity of self-responsibility and control is very important. Their defenses against aggressive outbursts should be reinforced and supported. Focus should be on the behavior and feared loss of control, not on the roots of the anger.[20] Clinical example 31-12 is an example of management of a violent adolescent.

Adolescents who have committed extreme acts of violence, or homicide, are often from families in which violence is the norm. These adolescents may have experienced physical or sexual abuse. If not, they may have witnessed violence between their parents. Behavior toward them has often alternated between seductiveness and physical brutality, adding to the adolescent's confusion and arousing intense frustration. Often these adolescents are encouraged to be violent, since their outbursts are not firmly limited. Sometimes parents can predict the adolescent's ability to injure or kill. Often there is a history of dangerous assaults on family members and pets. In severely violent adolescents, violent acts can be followed by a calmness and lack of sorrow or guilt, or they may claim that outside

---

CLINICAL EXAMPLE 31-12

Ricky was a 14-year-old boy referred for treatment for violent outbursts at home. When frustrated, he would break and destroy objects in his path. Ricky was an only child, adopted shortly after birth by a couple in their forties who were unable to have children. Now Ricky's parents, who were about 55 years of age, were increasingly frightened by his aggressive outbursts. They had also felt powerless with his childhood temper tantrums and had consistently responded to outbursts by attempting to limit frustrating situations. They felt guilty and inadequate about his being an adopted child and continually made attempts to reassure Ricky of their love for him. They consequently reinforced his lack of control by assuming these outbursts were results of his fear of being unloved and would offer peace offerings of gifts and rewards. Ricky assumed he was omnipotent, successfully controlling his parents, but was fearful that he could not control his anger. Acknowledging Ricky's fear of loss of control, applying external controls, and pointing out areas of Ricky's ability for responsibility and control resulted in a gradual decrease in outbursts. First the outbursts became more limited as Ricky began breaking specific things that he did not value. Then he progressed to an elimination of violent outbursts.

---

forces provoked them. Many homicidal adolescents will freely discuss their violent plans or fears. These should be explored and homicidal intent evaluated. Does the adolescent have a victim, weapons, or plan? This information, along with the history, shows the level of success or failure in controlling feelings and delaying gratification. Poor rapport with the therapist and evasiveness may indicate disturbing paranoid tendencies, revealing a greater potential for violence.

■ Adolescents and drugs

Adolescents may turn to drugs to relieve tension when pressures are intense. Meeks[20] and other theorists have spoken of the following types of drug users:

1. **Casual users—"the experimenters."** These adolescents use mostly alcohol or marijuana in small quantities to maintain their position in the peer group and to decrease the anxieties experienced by their movement away from the family.

2. **Sociological users—"the seekers."** These adolescents are aware of social realities, and they want to be active participants in the social process. They tend to form separate communities in which they attempt to create a society free of social conventions. Many seek relief from boredom through drugs and membership in this society. They lack the ability to express their inner feelings and tend to deal with their loneliness through mystical revelation and the group connection, with the hope of a conflict-free life with others.

3. **Sick users—"the heads."** These adolescents use drugs to mask or correct maturational problems. This distinction is difficult to make. Those with serious interpersonal difficulties often are in a group that is bonded together by a high frequency of drug use. They turn to drugs in times of stress and prefer drug-induced pleasures to those arising from interpersonal relationships and competitive efforts. This group also includes those who are socially critical and use social injustice as a personal justification by their drug habits.

Social implications connected with drug use must be considered. Our "pill relief" society gives a backdrop for drug abuse. Drug abuse can reflect a general discontent with society's shortcomings in values and organization. The awakened interest in magic and mysticism also adds the potential of drug-induced exploration of life.

The meaning of drug use in adolescence is a difficult, complex question. The adolescent's motivation must be explored. The nurse must keep in mind that it may be an expression of rebelliousness with support of a peer group, as well as a way of obtaining gratification of instinctual needs at a regressed level. It may also indicate an effort to come to grips with feelings of vulnerability and emptiness.

Adolescents often report a wish for closeness that is satisfied by sharing a drug experience with friends. Drug users can experience an illusion of closeness because drugs decrease anxiety and users can share anticipation of drug use. Some adolescents fill the void of isolated loneliness with drugs and would otherwise feel suicidally depressed. Drugs can be crippling and delay healthy maturity by promoting the avoidance of developing an adult identity in a real world, as illustrated in Clinical example 31-13.

Rarely does drug use cause difficulties when the adolescent was previously well adjusted. This is especially true with "soft" drugs such as marijuana. Al-

---

CLINICAL EXAMPLE 31-13

Tommy was a 16-year-old adolescent boy who had been school phobic since age 10. He had been on home instruction since that age and was referred for a yearly assessment to obtain approval for a continuation of home instruction services. Tommy proudly spoke of his drug episodes. He and his small group of friends were close and had many exciting experiences induced by various hallucinogens and amphetamines. Tommy had little support in the real world, since he had been isolated at home and experienced interpersonal relationships primarily in terms of obtaining and experiencing the effects of drugs.

---

though not highly addictive, the long-term side effects of marijuana include visual and spatial distortion, distorted time sequence, and short-term memory loss. The most serious physiological side effect is related to lung damage. In contrast, adolescents have been known to become psychotic, panicked, and assaultive after drug ingestion, especially of "harder" drugs. Phencyclidine hydrochloride (PCP), or "angel dust," has been noted to produce violence and incoherence. Sometimes PCP is mixed with marijuana and other drugs without the adolescent knowing it. Bad trips have been reported with hallucinogens, as well as with belladonna and opiate drugs. Often friends help to deal with upsetting reactions, but occasionally medical care is sought. Amphetamines may produce psychosis. Belladonna can produce acute maniclike psychotic states accompanied by hallucinations.

One of the more frequently abused drugs is cocaine. This drug is snorted, free-based, injected, or smoked, producing euphoria, grandiosity, and increased feelings of confidence and esteem. In addition to emotional euphoria, it produces a sense of physical well-being that exceeds the normal body capacity.

Alcoholism among adolescents is increasing. Addeo and Addeo[1] have suggested some possible origins for alcoholism in adolescents, including parental and social influence, peer pressure, and emotional disturbances. Many people believe that teenagers are currently switching from drugs to alcohol and that alcoholism is the greater social problem.

A final group of drugs often abused by adolescents are called "designer drugs." They are available in abundance and at low cost because they are easily produced by chemists. One designer drug of major concern is steroids, which is often abused by athletes and adolescents who attempt to increase their physical strength, speed, and muscle mass. Steroids can give the adolescent a magical resolution to their lack of physical development, thereby enhancing their body image. Other designer drugs include opiate derivatives, or "knockoffs," which can produce aggressive or paranoid behavior, hallucinations, and euphoria.

■ Hypochondriasis

Adolescents are preoccupied with their bodies and body sensations. Many reasons exist for this concern and preoccupation. Adolescents are uncomfortable with their bodies because of the rapid changes in size, shape, and functioning. To establish their identity, adolescents try to become familiar with their changing bodies. They respond to sensations with increased intensity. When an adolescent appears overly concerned, it may indicate underlying difficulties in formation of self-image.

Hypochondriasis occurs when the adolescent has intense anxiety about his health. This anxiety may be diffuse or directed toward one specific area. Adolescents' concern that their bodies are inadequate, that they will be rejected by others, or that they are unable to reach adulthood may predominate. Hypochondriasis may be a way of avoiding activities that expose these and other stressful fears. Fears such as inadequacy at school, either socially or in schoolwork, may be a projection of general fears of inadequacy. Lack of knowledge of normal body changes may be a simple precipitating factor. This can be tackled by reassurance that these changes are normal. If reassurance does not alleviate anxiety, other more intense fears may be involved.

Reassurance and support can frighten the adolescent who uses body concern to mask an intense conflict. This is important to consider—the adolescent may then have no means to discharge the pressures of the basic anxiety, since the defense is removed. Support may imply to adolescents that the nurse or parents do not care for them. It is important to communicate to adolescents that people are aware something is wrong and that their concerns will be taken seriously until the core problem is alleviated. Intense body concern is a signal that something is wrong and help is needed. Physical status must be assessed first before a psychological basis for concern is assumed. Sometimes body preoccupation is an effort to recreate infantile dependency by eliciting caregiving. This is particularly seen in adolescents who experienced early emotional deprivation.[15] John in Clinical example 31-14 is an interesting example of this.

CLINICAL EXAMPLE 31-14

John, age 12, was referred for treatment from the local hospital after having been seen for chest pains. The physician found no medical problems. John was embarrassed and angry about the episode, insisting that the physician was wrong. The chest pains had disappeared, but he now had injured his arm. He also was often plagued by genuinely uncomfortable attacks of tonsillitis and middle ear infections. John had experienced early emotional deprivation because he was often moved around in his living arrangements. He was born out of wedlock and lived occasionally with his mother, often with his maternal grandmother, and infrequently with his father. He generally had the feeling that no one really cared for him. Further exploration revealed that John's body concerns were to initiate caregiving by those around him, whom he feared really were not there for him. He performed well in school and had friends, but none of these compensated for his feelings of inadequacy.

■ Weight problems

Eating disorders are another group of problems often seen in adolescence. They include anorexia nervosa, bulimia, and obesity. The sociocultural milieu for female adolescents in the United States apparently has precipitated substantial identity and body image confusion in this age group. The emphasis on thinness, athletics, and physical attractiveness suggests that these are highly valued achievements for young women. These traits demonstrate self-control and social success and are culturally rewarded. The result is that fear of fat, restrained eating, binge eating, and body image distortion are typical problems among teenage girls.

Many authors suggest that the underlying conflict in these disorders is sexual. Denying a wish to be sexual is expressed by being unattractively thin or hiding feminine or masculine characteristics with childlike heaviness. Often heaviness is equated with pregnancy, which represents sexuality. Others speculate that anorexia nervosa is a reaction formation to the desire to be gluttonous, whereas excessive eating is the symbolical taking in of love. Extreme restraint of gluttonous wishes or giving in to these wishes represents a desire to return to infantile dependency, often precipitated by emotional deprivation.

More recent understandings suggest that eating disorders represent a complex of issues related to etiology. Psychodynamics, family characteristics, physiol-

CLINICAL EXAMPLE 31-15

Janet, age 15, was admitted to the hospital because it was feared that her extreme loss of weight was endangering her life. Exploration revealed that Janet was afraid of her sexual feelings and the response of others to her budding sexuality. Her father, provocative and teasing toward Janet, was continually kidding her about her oncoming sexual attractiveness and implied that he really preferred her to her mother. This created panic and Janet refused to eat. She liked her thinness, which was a protection from sexual desires. In the hospital, the area of concentration was not the behavior of not eating, but rather the underlying panic feelings about her sexuality and her relationship with her father. This provided freedom for normal sexual growth and development.

CLINICAL EXAMPLE 31-16

Donna, a 13-year-old girl, had always been shy with others. She was referred for therapy after the third week of classes in her new junior high school because she was not attending school on account of illness. Her mother claimed that despite her efforts to get Donna to school, she would return home with an upset stomach or headache. Her mother had taken her to school the 2 days she had attended, only to have her return home 3 hours later. A medical workup provided no medical basis for her stomach and head pains. As the evaluation proceeded, it became clear that Donna had an extraordinarily close relationship with her mother. In the past her mother had worked as a teacher's helper at the elementary school Donna attended. Treatment dealing with the mother-daughter dyad was instituted.

ogy, and biochemical interactions all appear to play a part in the development and treatment of these disorders.[17] Clinical example 31-15 illustrates the development of anorexia nervosa in a young girl.

■ School phobia

School phobia is an example of neurotic anxiety often seen in adolescence. Some school dropouts may be suffering from undiagnosed school phobia. This differs from other disturbed behaviors in that school represents the focus of their fears. The parents (most often the mother), although verbalizing the wish for the adolescent's maturity, often unconsciously want the adolescent to remain at home, limited in opportunities to move toward adult development.[15] Other possible causes may be the adolescent's fears concerning maturing and leaving childhood protection, the meaning of new knowledge, exposure to feelings and wishes stimulated by close relationships with peers and adults, and failure to meet the adolescent's idealized self-image.[4]

Adolescents may use destructive means of obtaining attention, demonstrate their poor self-concept, or hide from dealing socially with the opposite sex by remaining at home. Clinical example 31-16 is an example of school phobia.

■ Occult involvement

Adolescent risk-taking behavior has become evident more recently in the involvement of teenagers in the occult.[10,25] Individuals particularly prone to this involvement tend to be alienated from their family, be socially isolated, and have poor skills for interacting with others. They are cognitively curious and seek attention; they have their own belief system and are attracted to the bizarre. They are often negative, fatalistic, sensation seeking, poor judges of danger, and have low self-esteem. They rely on superstition to deal with their feelings of powerlessness and their fear of making decisions. In this way, their belief system establishes a sense of control for them. These adolescents depend on external rewards to make them feel good, and they conjure up spells to help them make decisions.

Satanism, the worship of Satan, is usually the choice of males and is the dark side of the occult. Satanists do not necessarily believe in a personal devil, but rather that Satan symbolizes evil. Witchcraft, usually the choice of women, is a variety of magic with the goal of manipulating the spirits to do the will of humans. Astrology uses the earth-centered view of the solar system to interpret the influence of the heavenly bodies on human affairs.

Adolescent behaviors that are often associated with involvement in the occult include:

- Sleep disturbances, including insomnia and nightmares
- Suicidal ideation with overwhelming feelings of guilt
- Chemical dependency and drug use
- Voyeurism, nudity, and sexual activity that includes thrill seeking

- Feelings of learned helplessness
- Fantasy role-play, including Dungeons and Dragons and various computer games
- Ritualistic use of objects such as knives and black clothing
- Preference for heavy metal music with hidden messages that ridicule society.[25]

Family systems that predispose adolescents to use the occult may have unresolved conflicts and may use distancing frequently to solve problems. A tolerance for deviance and a disengaged family structure may be present. Families are frequently critical and rejecting, and often the family structure has recently changed because of death or crisis. The families are generally characterized by the lack of nurturing for their members and inadequate support for the child's developmental transition into adolescence. The adolescent's peer relations are often characterized by isolation and peer group rejection. Involvement in the occult therefore provides the teenager with an opportunity for acceptance. Environmental factors may include frequent exposure to the supernatural in movies, books, and games. These suggest magical solutions to life's problems. Finally, the adolescent may experience a disenchantment with formal religion and contempt for social norms and values.

 # Planning and implementation

When dealing with the adolescent, it is advisable for the nurse to have an initial contact directly with the adolescent. Many adolescents are concerned that the nurse therapist is aligned with the parents. Other adolescents take a passive role, letting the adults straighten things out for them. By initiating contact with the adolescent, an alignment is made with his independent, mature aspects. Parents asking for advice on how to present coming to a therapist to the adolescent should be advised to be honest, stating the true nature of the visit and their reasons for requesting it. Many agencies and institutions use a child guidance approach, seeing the parents first to obtain a full developmental history. Family sessions have also been used in diagnostic evaluation, helping to reveal family interaction and later being helpful in establishing family support.

■ The nursing care plan

Knowledge of normal adolescent development is necessary to differentiate between age-expected behavior and maladaptive responses. Most adolescents are well adjusted, have good relationships with family and friends, and generally accept societal values. Studies by Offer, Ostrov, and Howark,[21] however, suggest that professionals view normal adolescents from an analytical perspective as being more disturbed than they really are. Despite new data refuting this view, professionals still persist in describing normal adolescents as having a disturbed self-image based on the "analytical turmoil" theory.

Identifying maladaptive responses and defining the problem in behavioral terms is the first step in planning intervention. The nurse can then explore the underlying conflicts. All adolescents may have conflicts in some areas, but many are able to respond to them in an adaptive manner. It is problematic when conflicts are expressed in a maladaptive or destructive way. Establishment of short-term goals based on the maladaptive responses is done after the adolescent's strengths are recognized. Long-term goals and rationales are also listed. Recommend treatment with appropriate rationale or a recommended referral completes the plan.

Review of nursing care plans is necessary periodically to update situations, note progress, and consider new problem areas. Short- and long-term goals are reassessed at this time and, based on new developments, are revised if indicated. Most important, the nursing process is assessed and reevaluated.

■ Patient and parent education

The psychiatric nurse is in an excellent position to educate the adolescent, the parents, and the community. Basic health information can be given in such areas as drugs, sex and contraception, suicide prevention, and crime prevention. The nurse can also provide information on healthy emotional functioning. By educating parents and the community on normal adolescent behavior and by interpreting the underlying conflicts, parents, teachers, and other community members are better prepared to react supportively to adolescents and encourage healthy independent functioning. Often parents and others become frustrated, angry, and confused by the independent strivings of adolescents. Encouraging independence and lessening power struggles can produce a positive change in adolescents' relationships with adults and in their feelings about themselves. However, adults should still set limits. Limit setting and providing structure can be done in a way to encourage the adolescent's independent functioning. Many parents are conflicted about their children becoming adults. This, together with the adolescent's own ambivalence and fears about independence, can create havoc.

One of the best ways to educate parents on adolescent development is through a parents' group. In this way the nurse can inform parents on normal adolescent functioning, as well as provide them with much needed support from other parents in the same situation. Sharing mutual experiences and searching for solutions in a supportive environment can be extremely helpful to parents. It is important to remember that parents have nurtured children to reach this juncture of adolescence, moving toward adulthood. Many believe that "showing them how" is their primary parental responsibility. It is a difficult change for them to suddenly switch from the "how to" of the child to the "try to" of the budding adult. Parents can learn the process of providing increased responsibilities based on a gradual progression of independent functioning. Despite their fears of their teenagers "getting into trouble," they can be educated to promote self-reliance in their adolescents. Clinical examples 31-17 and 31-18 show the need to educate parents and community members.

■ Family therapy

Recent studies show that conflict and disorganization do not usually occur in most families with adolescents. Although the overall amount of conflict does not appear to increase, the focus of conflict does change with the new developmental stage. Thus the nurse needs to assess carefully the level of family functioning and the diversity present within it to determine how she might best interact with and help the family of the adolescent.

Family therapy is particularly useful to an adolescent when chronically disturbed family interaction is

---

CLINICAL EXAMPLE 31-17

Mr. and Mrs. B came to the attention of the psychiatric nurse by their distressed calls to the community mental health center. Mrs. B tearfully explained that they had lost all control of their 14-year-old daughter. She had become arrogant and hostile, locking herself in her bedroom after an argument they had about her going to the movies with a 14-year-old boy she had met at school. Further exploration revealed that Emily was an honor student at school, maintaining a solid A average. She had many friends at school, was on the volleyball team, and babysat regularly on weekends for the neighbors' two children. She had always been pleasant, happy, and friendly. Suddenly this boy that the parents did not know called her at home. After many phone conversations he asked Emily to join him on a weekend evening at the movies. Mr. and Mrs. B felt Emily was much too young to date, that she could get involved with drugs, sexual promiscuity, and the so on. They were sad and worried that they had lost their little girl who always did what she was told. Emily was hurt and furious. She thought her parents were being totally unreasonable and that they did not trust her. Further exploration revealed that Mrs. B had gotten into trouble sexually as a young girl. She did not want Emily to make the same mistake. Her parents had been very lenient. She blamed their lack of guidelines for her error. Mrs. B became aware of her overreaction. She was able to understand that dating was a normal part of adolescent development after discussion with the psychiatric nurse. A compromise was arranged after she recognized Emily's competent and responsible functioning. After Mr. and Mrs. B met the boy at Emily's house, Emily was able to go to the movies with him and two other friends on a Saturday afternoon.

CLINICAL EXAMPLE 31-18

Barbara, an adolescent girl starting high school, had always functioned adequately. Beginning high school was a totally different experience. She became overwhelmed by the large building, increased academic responsibilities, and complex peer relationships. She began school in September with much anxiety. By October she began having numerous illnesses that prevented her from attending school. This came to the attention of the school guidance counselor, who noticed her increased absences. The guidance counselor saw her and, after no medical etiology was found, offered to have Barbara come to her office whenever she felt sick at school. When this did not help, she suggested Barbara receive some home instruction until she felt less anxious. This suggestion validated Barbara's fears that she could not handle high school and its increased pressures. Her solution of retreat was supported. Fortunately, her parents sought the help of a psychiatric nurse, who encouraged immediate return to school with entry into a peer support group with individual sessions initially as needed. This enabled her to talk out her fears and receive support from her peers. This also strengthened her confidence and fostered healthy functioning. She found she could handle high school after all. The nurse educated the guidance counselor on ways to be supportive while encouraging independent functioning.

seriously interfering with the adolescent's development. Sometimes a series of family sessions may be enough, and the adolescent may benefit from either individual or group approaches to support his effort to separate emotionally from his family. Occasionally, after a few family sessions, it may become clear that the adolescent may not need the intervention directly. Engaging the parents may free the adolescent to progress on the developmental continuum.

The techniques used in family therapy are reviewed in detail in Chapter 29. Whatever modality is selected in working with the adolescent, a family orientation and the adolescent's attempt to separate from his family and become an independent adult should be considered.

■ Group therapy

Group therapy uses adolescents' tendency to gain peer support. The conflict of dependence-independence with adults becomes somewhat diluted by the presence of other adolescents. Conflicts, especially about authority, can be detected by peers rather than adults, making group therapy particularly desirable for adolescents. Many nurses use group therapy as a catalyst and combine it with individual therapy. It is valuable in teaching skills in relating and dealing with others. Group therapy helps fulfill the adolescent's need for a positive, meaningful peer group for ego identity formation.

Adolescent groups, in contrast to other groups, are difficult to manage bacause many adolescents turn to peers in a defensive and tenuous connection. Sibling rivalry often disrupts group cohesion. Many groups suffer from poor attendance, a high dropout rate, antisocial behavior, and a lack of group cohesion. However, group therapy with adolescents has proved to be successful in many community mental health centers, outpatient clinics, and hospital settings.

Berkovitz[3] believes that coed groups decrease homosexual anxiety and anxious disruptiveness. Often, beginning groups with some activity helps to provide a stabilizing factor for young adolescents. The number of members to include in the group depends on the type. For example, it may not be feasible to limit an outpatient "drop-in" group. Because of the age spread among adolescents, it is usually preferable to form at least two groups. A possibility is an early adolescence group consisting of 13- to 15-year-olds who have conflicts of separation from parents as well as homosexual and incestuous anxieties. An older adolescent group, age 15 to 17, would probably consider issues such as the further establishment of identity, the beginning of dating or exploration of relations with the opposite sex, experimentation with drugs, handling money, responsibilities of driving, and vocational plans. Mixing two age groups with varying concerns may not be productive.

The ideal situation is to have male and female cotherapists; however, this is not always possible. If there is a single therapist for an unmixed group of the opposite sex, group members may show anxiety by disruption or flight. Conflict between therapists, if there is an open and honest discussion, can provide a corrective experience because adolescents can see adults disagree without devastating consequences. If therapists are of the opposite sex, a parental similarity is often apparent; members often play on the therapist's feelings and try out tactics as they would with their own parents. Even if both therapists are of the same sex, one is usually more active, and a member may project a good or bad image onto each therapist that corresponds with his view of his parents.

Group process with adolescents is often similar to that with adults, and specific aspects of group therapy are reviewed in Chapter 28. Resistances such as silence, passivity, disruptiveness, and intellectualization are often seen with adolescents, since they tend to act out rather than verbalize anxiety. Differences among various types of groups, such as residential groups versus outpatient groups, must be considered.

■ Individual therapy

Individual therapy done by the psychiatric nurse specialist can consist of brief goal-directed therapy, behavioral therapy, or insight therapy. A description of insight therapy is presented here, since the principles are helpful in other types of individual therapy. Once the decision to engage in individual therapy is made, a pact or contract between the nurse and adolescent is established, depending on the approach and type used.

■ **THERAPEUTIC ALLIANCE.** This contract in insight therapy is described by Meeks[20] as a "therapeutic alliance" in which the nurse aligns herself with the healthy, reality-oriented aspect of the adolescent's ego and moves toward an honest and critical understanding of the adolescent's inner experience. This alliance is created through the orderly interpretation of the adolescent's feeling states and defensive behavior, especially toward the nurse.

Adolescents' alliances are focused toward links between their feelings and behavior in the present. Brief regressions still occur, and focuses usually are aimed at efforts to recover from regressions and at reinforcing and supporting progressive development. The alliance is a central aspect of individual therapy. Once it is established, a feeling of working together is apparent. Meeks[20] mentions specific hints to establish and maintain this alliance:

1. Point out that behavior is motivated by feelings. Often, early in treatment, adolescents may express feelings of impatience, helplessness, and failure at having to see a therapist. Defenses are often seen in rebelliousness, passivity, shyness, negativism, and intellectualization. Adolescents generally have a tendency to act out and avoid feelings.

2. Limit acting out by pointing out how it interferes with the therapeutic process and that it must be controlled to proceed. Maintain a neutral but interested attitude toward all behavior.

3. Point out the adolescent's tendencies to be judgmental and self-critical. This is supportive and helps to encourage the adolescent to look for sources of behaviors, attitudes, and feeling states.

4. Establish that the adolescent's behavior is the end result of many inner feelings. Some of these unknown feelings sabotage freedom. This knowledge strengthens motivation for therapy and maintains an alignment with the adolescent's wishes for autonomy. Encourage therapeutic efforts as a means to alter rebellion into true self-direction and freedom.

5. Point out the adolescent's tendency to see things in extremes; the desire to be complete master opposes the feelings of total helplessness. Reveal areas of strength and competence that are often unrecognized. Avoid focusing exclusively on problems and weaknesses. This shows neutrality and is supportive. Giving the adolescent as much information as possible to be prepared to make his own decision helps the adolescent work toward self-direction.

6. Distinguish between thought and action, discouraging impulsiveness. Encourage open expression of strong feeling but not strong action. For example, anger does not mean killing; sexual feeling does not mean intercourse. Adolescents sometimes confuse discussion with permission to experiment with action, especially with sexual issues.

7. Encourage real emotion in sessions by expressing interest in and acceptance of feelings involving the nurse and events outside the session. Point out the importance of feelings. If, however, the adolescent is psychotic, an effort is made to limit the expression of feelings. In this case, strengthening reality testing is the goal rather than encouraging the open expression of feelings.

8. Be alert to the defenses of denial and reaction formation. Maintain neutrality and encourage objectivity without directly assaulting essential defenses. Adolescents will resort to pathological defenses when threatened by emergencies.

9. Adolescents often act provocatively to force important adults to delegate punishment. This puts the nurse in alignment with the self-hatred aspect of the adolescent's conscience and should be avoided. The nurse is supportive by continuing therapy even during these difficult periods.

The work of the nurse therapist is to recognize the adolescent's anxiety and try to assist him in finding ways to deal with emerging impulses. Defenses suggested by the nurse are rarely useful, but pointing out, supporting, and accepting any healthy defense of the adolescent strengthens his sense of ego mastery. Adolescents often have wishes that they regard as crazy and frightening. Open discussion of fears of homosexuality, incest, or homicide helps adolescents realize these feelings do not lead to psychosis and are uncomfortable but harmless thoughts.

■ **TRANSFERENCE.** Transference is an important aspect of adolescent treatment. The nurse must point that these irrational projections originate in the adolescent's mind and not in reality and that they usually represent a meaningful person such as a parent. It often helps to mention this is a common response. The nurse interpretes transference to diminish its impact on the therapeutic situation. Several common transference patterns have been identified[20]:

1. **Erotic-sexual**—especially if the nurse is young and of the opposite sex. This transference typically is shown by awkward blushing and agitated confusion by the adolescent. It is usually best to emphasize value in the mutual work of emotional growth while establishing, tactfully, the nurse's unavailability as a sexual object. Focusing on origins or encouraging elaboration of these feelings is not helpful and is anxiety provoking.

2. **Omnipotent**—expecting the nurse will have answers to all questions. It is easy for the nurse to drift into this pattern, since often the adolescent appears to be helpless. The adolescent's secret desire for personal omnipotence is some-

what fulfilled by granting it to the nurse. The nurse then serves as a front, hiding the adolescent's fear of confronting reality without magical powers.

3. **Negative transference**—usually intense and pervasive. Negative feelings toward the nurse usually represent a negative attitude toward all adult authority figures. This transference is often defensive to cover feelings of shame, inadequacy, and anxiety, and it disappears as the adolescent respects the nurse's feelings. The adolescent tries to force the therapist to reject him. Open discussion to explore these feelings objectively and establish their origin is beneficial. Sometimes interpretations arouse anger toward the nurse because of the anxiety they create. These are reactions to the realities of therapy and are not to be confused with negative transference.

A true negative transference occurs when situations reactivate early experiences in which negative feelings toward important others predominate. The nurse is seen as a frustrator whenever she, representing reality, opposes gratification of impulses and ego drives. Negative transference tends to appear whenever the nurse refuses to gratify needs that the adolescent thinks are important and legitimate. The nurse unavoidably will frustrate the adolescent, who often has trouble delaying gratification to reach long-range goals. The nurse should point out the true motive behind activities that express anger. Clarifying hidden hostile feelings frees them for expression toward the nurse, and irrational expectations may then be revealed. Negative transference, as with any other resistant behavior, is dealt with through objective exploration, which includes seeking causes of anger and pointing out irrationality. This is often followed by an expected period of regression and depression. Empathic understanding that the adolescent is mourning a loss is helpful, but it should be emphasized that what was lost was an illusion.

Another negative transference occurs when the adolescent sees the nurse as his superego. Projecting his superego onto the nurse may cause all interventions to be seen as superego sanctions. Adolescents have trouble understanding the rationale for foregoing gratification of an impulse. It is important to point out that these are the adolescent's own taboos and to encourage open confrontation with these taboos rather than avoidance. A common occurrence is for an adolescent to rebel against his conscience and then respond to guilt through self-destructive behaviors. Pointing out

this pattern helps the adolescent to eventually become aware of this.

■ **TERMINATION.** Termination of therapy is an important part of the therapeutic process. Often, leaving therapy symbolizes the process of loosening bonds to parental images, giving up accompanying desires to be passive and expectations of the omnipotence of these figures. One therefore expects defensive and regressive behaviors as the adolescent attempts to deal with the anxieties related to the termination process. This can mean the recurrence of emotional crises, symptoms, self-destructive fantasies, and even dependency behavior to provoke rescue.

Termination should be flexible and correctly timed. The decision should be made in line with adolescent norms, not adult ones. Often adolescents will verbalize appropriate interest in termination. When this occurs, it is often helpful to open it to discussion without commitment to a set time. This implies that further work needs to be done in a definite time span, and it maintains a focus on the adolescent's responsibility to finish. Gradually supporting and approving of the adolescent's independence and mature functioning prepares for a positive termination. Some adolescents leave therapy to return later. Some can never leave forever, seeing termination as a rejection rather than a vote of confidence. Gradual reduction of sessions without pressing for final termination may help as long as the overall situation is reviewed occasionally.[12]

Sometimes terminations occur prematurely because either an alliance has not been established or some external event has occurred. Occasionally terminations are forced because of a nurse's change of location, death, or illness. The adolescent will express anger at the new therapist until the feelings about the lost therapist are accepted and resolved. In working out this attachment, a new therapeutic alliance can be established.

■ **Talking with adolescents**

The following discussion focuses on some important considerations in communicating with adolescents.

■ **SILENCE.** Silence is often effective with adults but frightening to the adolescent, especially in the beginning stages of treatment or evaluation. This anxiety often reflects the adolescent's feelings of emptiness and lack of identity. Brief silences can be creative and productive when the adolescent is engaged in treatment; when the adolescent is able to tolerate them without anxiety, it indicates growth in self-confidence and acceptance of inner feelings. More often, however, silence is used defensively by adolescents to avoid discovery of hostile feelings or fantasies. Older adolescents may tolerate interpretive remarks, but with younger adolescents it is usually helpful to suggest an activity to help facilitate discussion and establish a relationship. For some adolescents, silence is a defense of inhibition and withdrawal, since they have never learned to communicate in a positive way. In these cases the therapist must be responsible for dialogue.

■ **CONFIDENTIALITY.** Confidentiality is a concern to many, but especially to the adolescent who is fearful of the nurse reporting to his parents. A blanket promise to tell nothing to the parents is not advised, since the nurse may need to contact the parents if the adolescent reveals suicidal or homicidal behavior or the use of illegal drugs. It is usually best to tell the adolescent that the nurse will not give out any information without informing the adolescent in advance. It is also helpful to explain that feelings are confidential but that actions considered dangerous to the adolescent or others may need to be shared.

■ **NEGATIVISM.** Negative feelings are often expressed by adolescents, especially initially, because they are frightened of the implications of coming for treatment. The young adolescent's lack of objectivity and upsurge of instinctual impulses, as well as the tendency to confuse fantasy and action, make the discussion of feelings threatening. Usually, gently noting in a supportive way defensive techniques the adolescent uses during the session helps to gain cooperation.

■ **RESISTANCE.** Often adolescents begin by testing the nurse to see if she will be another authoritarian figure. The rebellious adolescent may claim he does not need therapy or help. If the adolescent appears anxious, it is best to be supportive and sympathetic, expressing interest in getting to know the adolescent and then discussing a neutral area. A more angry, rebellious adolescent may require a direct approach, with the nurse saying openly that she thinks the adolescent is opposing the visit because he believes no help is needed. This can lead to a further discussion of feelings about the visit (e.g., parental coercion to come to the session) or feelings about authority. Some adolescents are just baiting and testing to see if the nurse is an anxious, defensive adult. If so, it is best to ignore their comments about not wanting treatment and move on. Often adolescents with an angry facade depend on their omnipotent control of the environment and are often successful in manipulating their families. They are angry at attempts to disturb this power, and the anger is expressed in their lack of cooperation in the session.[18]

■ **ARGUING.** Adolescents always argue and, although they do not admit it, learn from arguments.

Often the adolescent goes against the viewpoint of the nurse and then in the next session states the nurse's opinion as his own. It is best not to comment on this and accept it as a harmless defense. If the nurse admits having areas of ignorance, it is productive to the adolescent, who may fear that he must be perfect.

■ **TESTING.** Adolescents often need and want limits. They are confused and cannot set their own limits. They experiment by trial and error to find a self-concept. Often an adolescent will test the nurse to see how firm and consistent she will be. Controls frequently are effective if there is a basic positive relationship with the nurse. Limits should be set only when they are essential for current and future well-being, and the adolescent will value the security they provide. The nurse represents a substitute parental figure allowing independence. Adolescents will dare to be independent if it is conveyed that the nurse will serve as a control against carrying independence too far.

■ **DREAMS AND ARTISTIC CREATIONS.** Adolescents are often creative, and much can be learned from studying their works. As long as the discussion is relevant to achieving ego synthesis, it can be a productive source for exploring inner feelings. Along with dreams, these feelings can reveal valuable information about their real concerns, even when the adolescent attempts to avoid them. The nurse must be careful not to engage in intellectual discussion irrelevant to the adolescent's inner life.

■ **BRINGING FRIENDS.** The adolescent who brings a friend to a session may be attempting to avoid the seriousness of therapy. There is some benefit in sharing the experiences with the peer group, since this lowers anxiety. Telling the adolescent that bringing friends is not allowed may not be successful because the nurse cannot always enforce such a rule. The reason for bringing friends may vary, but the action should be seen as communication to be explored and understood. Sometimes adolescents want to refer friends. This may be positive but may also focus attention away from the original adolescent. The nurse should insist on exploring motives behind the referral before accepting the new patient, since the adolescent may think the nurse's acceptance of another is a betrayal of loyalty. If the friend clearly wants and needs therapy, referral to a colleague is usually best. If a friend is brought late in therapy, it may mean the adolescent is preparing to terminate.

■ **EMBARRASSMENT ABOUT BEING IN THERAPY.** Embarrassment may occur in any age group, but it is prominent in adolescents, especially during the early stages of treatment. It also can become an issue as therapy progresses, since it often reveals the adolescent's embarrassment about his wishes for dependency. Therefore adolescents may become uncomfortable in the therapeutic relationship. This is usually dealt with effectively by indicating that these feelings are normal. Behind the fear of accepting help is the wish for care, and this can be dealt with by pointing out the adolescent's strengths and areas of independence. The nurse can then reveal that the adolescent thinks any wish or thought of care or dependency represents total dependency. This helps the adolescent to be more tolerant of his wishes, seeing them realistically as wishes that all people have.

Some adolescents, by expressing embarrassment about being in therapy, are actually revealing a fear or social stigma that they have heard from their parents. The adolescent who has feelings of inferiority often focuses these on the therapeutic process, blaming therapy for discomfort. It is best to encourage and be supportive to the adolescent, gently refusing to accept blame for this discomfort. The issue of whether to tell friends should be explored dynamically.

■ **REQUESTS FOR SPECIAL ATTENTION.** Some adolescents can develop intense dependency ties to the therapist. They reflect this in requests for additional appointments, extra time in appointments, frequent telephone calls, or social contact outside the therapeutic sessions. Late in therapy there is little advantage to meeting these primitive needs. The regressed adolescent needs an undemanding nurse who allows him to experience inner feelings of emptiness. The therapist cannot fill this emptiness and should avoid false promises. Focus should be on the exploration of feelings of inner emptiness, deprivation, and incompleteness.

■ Parents of the adolescent

If group or individual treatment is selected for the adolescent, the nurse must still consider the family. Many parents overtly claim desire for their adolescent's maturity and independence but unconsciously need to maintain him as a child and covertly undermine growth. Parents may sabotage the adolescent's treatment if they are not helped to understand and accept it. The nurse can work with the parents without revealing confidential material.

Adolescents often try to avoid limits by playing parents against the nurse. If parents are angry with the restriction of their involvement in their child's therapy, there is a greater potential for this. The nurse can encourage healthier aspects of the parent-adolescent relationship and sympathetically accept parental anxieties and needs.

Not all parents need treatment. It is helpful for parents to have treatment if the adolescent is asked to assume an inappropriate destructive role at home, since this interferes with the therapeutic role. If the parents are resistant, the nurse must usually begin with the adolescent until the parents are more receptive.

Telephone contact is a helpful way to ensure cooperation and support by having the parent call when necessary. Parents should tell the adolescent when they call. Parents should be told of normal adolescent behavior they should expect. The nurse should avoid advising the parents about specific actions and focus on attitudes and feelings, especially concerning discipline. Parents can be helped with understanding the purpose of limit setting. Some parents exclude themselves entirely from their adolescent's life. They have brought the adolescent to treatment to ease their guilt by doing all that is possible. They may often want the nurse to take over parenting functions. This should not be permitted, especially during crises. If the adolescent is suicidal or homicidal, the parents are informed and must take the responsibility for action with the nurse's help.

Adolescents often need help in dealing with their parents. At times, late in therapy, it is helpful to verify parental pathological behavior. If done too early in treatment, it can cause the adolescent to see himself as the victim. Later, well into the therapeutic alliance, it permits the adolescent to see his parents realistically, to forgive them, and to work on his own strengths and limitations. Parents should be discussed in an open exploratory manner, with emphasis on them having their own feelings on which their actions are based.

Adolescents can be helped to realize that if their parents are being controlling, adolescents must be free to reject or accept parents' goals according to their own needs and abilities, rather than merely rebelling. Even if the parents treat the adolescent as a child, that does not make him a child. The danger is the adolescent's own childlike wishes.

Sometimes adolescents want to leave home because they hope they will feel more adult away from their parents. It is usually best to support the wish to leave, emphasizing that it must be done in an adult way. If leaving is an impulsive thought with no feasible plan, it will ensure failure, parental rescue, and continued dependency. This is often recapitulated in termination from therapy if the adolescent quits early to avoid the pain of separation that a planned termination would bring.

Evaluation

Problems presented by adolescents, more frequently than those of any other group, activate the nurse's own unresolved conflicts. This countertransference reaction decreases the nurse's usefulness because of anxiety and confusion. The nurse should watch for alignment with either the parents against the adolescent or the adolescent against the parents. Most adults are resistant to reexperiencing the feelings of adolescence and have repressed these experiences. As a result of anxiety, the nurse occasionally may have trouble listening or may encourage the adolescent (for her own unrecognized wishes) to do what the nurse never dared do. The adolescent may be acting as the nurse did during adolescence. The nurse, in an effort to deny this, may see this adolescent behavior as nondeviant. Identification of the nurse with the adolescent can contribute to delays in exploring areas important for psychological growth. The nurse may relate well to the adolescent but because of unresolved, unrecognized conflicts or resentment toward her own parents, may be locked into her own adolescent rebellion. The nurse may overtly or covertly encourage the adolescent to express rage toward his family. Both the adolescent and the nurse then avoid facing the reality of adult burdens. It is easier for the nurse to do this if the adolescent's parents are indeed hostile, rejecting, and irresponsible.

Adults often have motives for emphasizing the inadequacies of adolescents, which can lead to underestimating the adolescent's abilities. These motives are often seen in protective or competitive attitudes of varying degrees, which make it difficult for the nurse to let the adolescent do things on his own. In terminating with an adolescent, as with any valued human relationship, the nurse often has feelings of being abandoned and unappreciated. Many adolescents therefore often seem guilty and apologetic about their wishes to terminate and deal with life on their own. Just as many nurses hold on to adolescents too long, the nurse's unconscious hostile feelings can cause her to claim exaggerated progress. This allows the nurse to disguise unconscious angry rejection and avoid waiting for appropriate termination. Often the nurse's need to achieve quick success causes a superficial handling of necessary therapeutic work. Pressures from the family with financial troubles can hurry an insecure nurse. Fears of erotic feelings stirred up by closeness with the adolescent can lead to a panicked withdrawal and termination motivated by self-preservation.

Nurses owe it to themselves and the adolescents they treat to be honest and rely on intellectual and emotional strengths, using the same exploratory attitude with themselves that is required and encouraged with the adolescents they treat. Errors are unavoidable. Doing therapy should provide a growth experience for the nurse as well as the adolescent. Critical self-evalua-

DIRECTIONS FOR FUTURE RESEARCH

The following are some of the nursing research problems raised in Chapter 31 that merit further study by psychiatric nurses:

1. The relationship between coping skills in early life and later adolescent adjustment
2. The implications of new and blurred sexual roles in increasing anxiety for the adolescent
3. Evidence of an extended adolescence as a result of prolonged economic dependence
4. Indicators of increased depression associated with body image in girls during middle adolescence as compared with older adolescents
5. The effect of the AIDS epidemic on sexual exploration in adolescence
6. Exploration of the relationships between depressed and conduct disordered adolescents and problems with moral and superego development
7. Effective nursing actions for dealing with resistence and negative transference in treatment of the adolescent
8. The effectiveness of limit-setting interventions by nurses in response to selected acting-out behavior in adolescents
9. The relationship between a nurse's comfort with assertive behavior and her effectiveness in setting limits with adolescents
10. The effect of the nurse's own adolescent experiences in creating countertransference problems when working with adolescents.

tion and reassessment of the effectiveness of nursing actions, as well as assessment of the client's progress, are paramount in the treatment of any human being of any age group. Supervision provides an opportunity to explore and evaluate the therapeutic process objectively with an experienced colleague and is a necessary tool to encourage and facilitate this process. Supervision is a necessity for all therapists, no matter how much experience they have, because of the highly emotional nature of the work in treating adolescents.

■ SUGGESTED CROSS-REFERENCES ■

Issues of identity and self-concept are discussed in Chapter 13. Suicide and other forms of self-destructive behavior are discussed in Chapter 15. Problems with the expression of anger are discussed in Chapter 17. Substance abuse is discussed in Chapter 19. Group therapy is discussed in Chapter 28. Family therapy is discussed in Chapter 29.

■ **SUMMARY** ■

1. Adolescence is a movement on a life continuum between the ages of 11 and 20. During this time, shifts in past developmental and learning processes occur.

2. Various theories explain the adolescent's resolution of tasks. The biological theory consists of Gesell's beliefs that adolescence is biologically determined by physical growth changes. Piaget's intellectual development theory bases adolescence on cognitive development. Josselyn sees adolescence as the psychological consequence initiated by the increase in sexual and aggressive impulses causing a psychic restructuring. Blos describes adolescence as the second individuation process. Erikson speaks of adolescence as a normal crisis with a great growth potential in facilitating adjustment to the new environment. Cultural theorists view adolescence as a societal phenomenon induced by society's lack of formal structure for passage into adulthood.

3. An understanding of normal behaviors seen in adolescents reveals basic conflicts adolescents experience. Typical conflicts involve body image, identity, independence, sexuality, social role, and sexual behavior. Body image conflicts reveal behaviors such as self-consciousness, imitativeness, and body concerns. Conflicts concerning identity reveal regressive characteristics, rebelliousness, negativism, confusion, isolation, and depression. Independence versus dependence conflicts lead to behaviors such as independent strivings, inconsistency, intenseness, and defensiveness. Sexuality conflicts produce behaviors attempting to deal with sexual impulses, such as heterosexual relationships, homosexual relationships, and parental rejection. In establishing a social role, adolescents exhibit behaviors involving hero worship, chums, crushes, peer group importance, and acting out. Fantasies, relationships with the opposite sex, masturbation, and homosexual activity reveal sexual behavior conflicts.

4. Various problem areas include the sexually active adolescent, unwed mother, pseudohomosexual, overt homosexual, suicidal adolescent, runaway, conduct disordered adolescent, violent homicidal adolescent, substance abuser, hypochondriac, the adolescent with weight problems, the school phobic adolescent, and the risk-taking behavior of occult involvement. The planning and implementation of various techniques of intervention are presented.

5. Patient education by the nurse of parents, adolescents, and the community are described. Family therapy and group therapy, with its particular advantage to adolescents who can supportively use the peer group, are explored. Individual treatment focuses on establishing an alliance, dealing with transference, and reviewing termination aspects.

6. The special difficulties in dealing with adolescents, including silence, confidentiality, negativism, resistance, limit setting, power struggles, requests for special attention, embarrassment about therapy, bringing friends, and artistic creations, are discussed.

7. Dealing with the adolescent's parents is often a difficult task for the nurse, and some suggestions to facilitate parental support without sabotaging the therapeutic relationship with the adolescent are presented.

8. Evaluation of the nurse's intervention is a necessity. Adolescents arouse feelings within the nurse that must be dealt with if a therapeutic relationship is to be established and maintained.

■ **REFERENCES** ■

1. Addeo E and Addeo J: Why our children drink, Englewood Cliffs, NJ, 1975, Prentice-Hall, Inc.
2. Bandura A and Walters R: Adolescent aggression, New York, 1959, Ronald Press Co.
3. Berkovitz I: Adolescents grow in groups. On growing a group: some thoughts on structure, process and setting, New York, 1972, Brunner/Mazel, Inc.
4. Bhoyrub JP: School phobia, in-patient involvement, Nurs Times 73:1388, 1977.
5. Blos P: On adolescence, New York, 1962, The Free Press.
6. Blos P: The second individuation process of adolescence, Psychoanal Study Child 22:162, 1967.
7. Blumenthal S and Kupfer D: Suicide over the life cycle: risk factors, assessment and treatment of suicidal patients, Washington, DC, 1990, American Psychiatric Press.
8. Brenner C: An elementary textbook of psychoanalysis, New York, 1974, Anchor Press.
9. Erikson E: Childhood and society, ed 2, New York, 1963, WW Norton & Co, Inc.
10. Galanter M: Cults and new religious movements, Washington, DC, 1989, American Psychiatric Press.
11. Gesell A, Ilg F, and Ames L: Youth: the years from ten to sixteen, New York, 1956, Harper & Row, Publishers, Inc.
12. Harley M: Analyst and adolescent at work, New York, 1974, Quadrangle/The New York Times Book Co, Inc.
13. Havighurst RL: Developmental tasks and education, ed 3, New York, 1972, David McKay Co, Inc.
14. Jacobs J: Adolescent suicide, New York, 1971, Wiley-Interscience.
15. Josselyn I: Adolescence, New York, 1971, Harper & Row, Publishers, Inc.
16. Klerman G: Suicide and depression among adolescents and young adults, Washington, DC, 1986, American Psychiatric Press.
17. Laraia M and Stuart G: Bulimia: a review of nutritional and health behaviors, J Child Adolesc Psych Nurs. In press.
18. Marshall R: The treatment of resistances in psychotherapy of children and adolescents, Psychother Theory Res Pract 9(2):143, 1972.
19. Mead M: Culture and commitment: a study of the generation gap, New York, 1970, Basic Books, Inc.
20. Meeks J: The fragile alliance, ed 2, Malabar, Fla, 1980, Robert Krieger Publishing Co.
21. Offer D, Ostrov E, and Howard K, editors: Patterns of the adolescent self-image, San Francisco, 1984, Jossey-Bass, Inc, Publishers.

22. Pfeffer C: Suicide among youth: perspectives on risk and prevention, Washington, DC, 1989, American Psychiatric Press.
23. Piaget J: Six psychological studies, New York, 1968, Vintage Books.
24. Powerd S, Hauser S, and Kilner L: Adolescent mental health, Am Psychol 44(2):200, 1989.
25. Wagner B and Stanley S: Occult involvement as a risk taking behavior by adolescents. Paper presented at Advocates of Child Psychiatric Nursing Conference, New York, Sept 21, 1989.

■ ANNOTATED SUGGESTED READINGS ■

Blos P: The adolescent passage, developmental issues, New York, 1979, International Universities Press, Inc.
  Comprehensive view of adolescence in a developmental perspective.

*Danziger S: Major treatment issues and techniques in family therapy with the borderline adolescent, J Psychosoc Nurs Ment Health Serv 20(1):27, 1982.
  Focuses on five major issues in the treatment of the borderline adolescent and his family: separation-anxiety, lack of control, poor ego boundaries, inability to express feelings, and borderline defense mechanisms. Suggests treatment techniques for each.

*Duffey M: Factors contributing to the development of a cohesive adolescent psychotherapy group, J Psychiatr Nurs 17:21, 1979.
  Describes experiences in setting up an adolescent group. Presents goals, guidelines, and a group contract.

Fishman H: Treating troubled adolescents, New York, 1988, Basic Books, Inc.
  Presents overview of treating adolescents in the context of their family.

*Fox K: Adolescent ambivalence: a therapeutic issue, J Psychiatr Nurs 18(9):27, 1980.
  Explores the dynamics of adolescent ambivalence through clinical examples and suggests related nursing interventions.

Hodgman C: Current issues in adolescent psychiatry, Hosp Community Psych 34(6):514, 1982.
  Reviews selected topics in adolescent psychopathology. Also outlines findings on normal adolescent development and discusses problems of diagnosis.

Jones V: Adolescents with behavior problems: strategies for teaching, counseling and parent involvement, Boston, 1980, Allyn & Bacon, Inc.
  Good overview of dealing with problematic adolescents. Considers such issues as talking to adolescents, understanding their behavior, working with parents, understanding school difficulties, and developing strategies to promote productive behaviors.

*Journal of Child and Adolescent Psychiatric Nursing
  Addresses issues pertaining to adolescent assessment and treatment. Published quarterly since 1988, it should be on the shelf of any nurse interested in working with adolescents.

Manaster G: Adolescent development, Itasca, Ill, 1989, FE Peacock Publishers.
  Discusses developmental facts and theories along with physical and cognitive changes. Excellent overview.

Masterson J and Costelle J: From borderline adolescent to functioning adult, New York, 1980, Brunner/Mazel, Inc.
  Follow-up report to Masterson's Treatment of the Borderline Adolescent.

*McBride A: The secret of a good life with your teenager, New York, 1987, Times Books.
  Explores the key developmental themes that characterize the experience of parents with teenagers. Full of insights, advice, warmth, and humor.

*Mellencamp A: Adolescent depression: a review of the literature with implications for nursing care, J Psychosoc Nurs Ment Health Serv 19(9):15, 1981.
  Treats this important problem in a scholarly, thorough way with clinical application to nursing care. Highly recommended.

*Meyer A: School phobia: care in the community, Nurs Times 73:1393, 1977.
  Describes a nurse's successful work in the community with a 15-year-old adolescent boy who was school phobic for more than 12 months.

*Oehler J and Burns M: Anorexia, bulimia and sexuality: case study of an adolescent inpatient group, Arc Psych Nurs 1(3):163, 1987.
  Describes work with adolescents who have eating disorders and reviews diagnostic classifications, etiology, and rationale for group psychotherapy.

Offer D, Ostrov E, and Howard K, editors: Patterns of the adolescent self image, San Francisco, 1984, Jossey-Bass, Inc, Publishers.
  Second in the New Directions for Mental Health Services Series. Uses the Offer Self Image Questionnaire developed in 1962 in 120 studies on 20,000 adolescents. Reveals that professionals describe adolescents as being in turmoil and disturbed when in fact most are well adjusted, have good relationships with parents and peers, and generally accept societal values.

Pfeffer C: Suicide among youth: perspectives on risk and prevention, Washington DC, 1989, American Psychiatric Press.
  This volume brings together numerous studies on youth suicide integrating risk factors, links with depression, family issues, genetics, and life stress. It is both up-to-date and inclusive.

*Pushkar K, Lamb J, and Martsolf D: The role of the psychiatric/mental health nurse clinical specialist in an adolescent coping skills group, J Child Adoles Psych Mental Health Nurs 3(2):47:1990.
  Describes a nurse-led adolescent prevention program, including the specific adolescent coping skills group format used.

*Scharer K, Challberg C, and Rearick T: Young people and AIDS, J Child Adoles Psych Mental Health Nurs 3(2):41, 1990.
  Reports the development and implementation of a health promotion and AIDS prevention program developed for junior high students, including cognitive and affective learning strategies and the reactions of students, parents and the educational system.

---

*Asterisk indicates nursing reference.

*Schlesinger B: From A to Z with adolescent sexuality, Can Nurse 52:34, Oct 1977.

In this article an attempt is made to understand adolescent motherhood. Schlesinger uses an alphabetical listing to discuss such issues as the double standard for the sexual act (girls responsible, boys not); including fathers in programs; limit setting with adolescents; adults being models, not judges; women's rights; and possible origins for teenage pregnancies.

Valente S and Saunders J: High school suicide prevention programs, Ped Nurs 13(2):108, 1987.

This is a good overview of school programs for all nurses focusing on interventions related to adolescent suicide and its prevention.

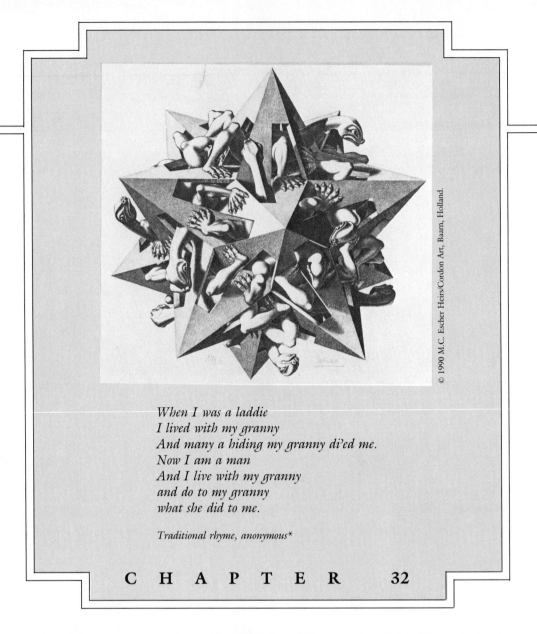

When I was a laddie
I lived with my granny
And many a hiding my granny di'ed me.
Now I am a man
And I live with my granny
and do to my granny
what she did to me.

*Traditional rhyme, anonymous**

C H A P T E R 32

CARE OF VICTIMS OF ABUSE AND VIOLENCE

BARBARA PARKER
JACQUELINE C. CAMPBELL

---

*From Davidson JL: Elder abuse. In Block M and Sinnott J, editors: The battered child syndrome: an exploratory study, College Park, Md, 1977, The University of Maryland Center on Aging.

LEARNING OBJECTIVES

After studying this chapter, the student should be able to:

- identify characteristics frequently observed with violent families.

- compare and contrast theories on the etiology of family violence.

- identify the data base needed for assessment of a violent family.

- formulate individualized nursing diagnoses for survivors of family violence.

- develop short-term and long-term goals for survivors of family violence.

- describe physiological, behavioral, and psychological responses of survivors of family violence.

- identify behaviors and values of nurses that make caring for survivors of abuse a challenge.

- describe nursing actions in the primary prevention of family violence.

- describe common reactions of survivors of rape or sexual assault.

- incorporate assessment of sexual assault into routine nursing assessment.

- identify directions for future nursing research.

- select appropriate readings for further study.

Nurses encounter victims of abuse and violence in a variety of settings. However, since experiencing violence is generally a devastating, overwhelming ordeal, survivors of abuse and violence are frequently seen in psychiatric settings. At times the violence will be openly discussed and recognized as a precipitating event for the current hospitalization, such as a victim of sexual assault treated in an emergency room. Frequently, however, violence will only be disclosed following the establishment of a trusting nurse-patient relationship. Although there are various forms of violence, such as gang behavior and drug-related violence, the types most frequently encountered in the psychiatric setting are family violence and nonfamily rape and sexual assault. Since the dynamics of these two forms of violence are different, they are covered in two separate sections of this chapter. One must remember, however, that rape and sexual assault also can be forms of family violence. In addition, particular attention is given to populations that are particularly at risk for abuse. These include children, spouses, and the elderly.

One issue to confront is the terminology used to describe people who have experienced violence. Tradi-tionally the term "victim" has been used, along with discussions of "syndromes." These labels serve to distance nurses from the person who has experienced abuse as they search for differences between themselves and the survivors to decrease their feelings of vulnerability. Therefore, in this chapter the term "survivor" is used to emphasize that the person who has experienced abuse has many strengths and coping strategies that can be incorporated into the plan of care.

Family violence

Family violence refers to a range of behaviors occurring between family members and includes physical and emotional abuse of children, child neglect, spouse battering, marital rape, and elder abuse. Conceptualizing abuse within families involves several different issues. Although each family is unique, there appear to be certain characteristics common to most violent families. Furthermore, regardless of the type of abuse occurring within a family, all members, including the extended family, are affected. Steinmetz and Straus[97] noted that "any social pattern as widespread and enduring as violence must have fundamental and enduring causes." Family violence, although often unnoted, is at the core of many family disturbances. Violence may be the "family secret" and is often perpetuated through generations.[71,76,77]

Although numerous research studies and theories have been directed toward the causes, treatment, and prevention of family violence, the field has more questions unanswered than answered. Hotaling and Straus[53] note that "the family is the training ground for violence" and ponder why the social group designated to provide love and support is also the most violent group to which most people belong. They point out that behaviors that would be unacceptable between strangers, co-workers, or friends are frequently tolerated within families.

Feminist authors note that most victims of family violence are the most vulnerable and powerless family members: women, children, and the elderly.[17,29] They propose that the root cause of violence is the abuser's need for power and control, which is acted out by violent behavior. The societal context with its historical and current norms supporting or at least allowing male dominance and violence is also considered crucial in the feminist analysis.[108]

Violence and abuse are generally believed to be caused by an interaction of personality, demographic, situational, and societal factors that impact on a family. Many of the unique characteristics of the family as a social group—time spent together, emotional involvement, privacy, and in-depth knowledge of each other—can facilitate both intimacy and violence. A given family can be both loving and supportive as well as violent.

■ **Nursing assessment**

■ **SOCIETAL INFLUENCE ON FAMILY VIOLENCE.** Any attempt to understand violence in American families must consider the influence of the society on the family. The United States has a higher level of violence in comparison to other Western nations,[7] and many believe that societal willingness to tolerate violence sets the stage for family violence. Societal norms are sometimes used to justify violence to maintain the family system. For example, in a number of families the husband's use of violence is considered legitimate if the wife is having an extramarital affair.[32] These authors cite historical attitudes toward women, children, and the elderly; economic discrimination; the nonresponsiveness of the criminal justice system; and the belief that women and children are property as factors maintaining norms allowing violence.[17,20,29] The changing norms regulating our definitions of family privacy and when the state should be allowed to inter-

vene in family matters have also influenced the definitions and recognition of various forms of family violence.[46]

■ **CHARACTERISTICS OF VIOLENT FAMILIES.** There are several factors common to violent families. These include the multigenerational family process, social isolation, the use and abuse of power, and the effect of alcohol and drug abuse.

Multigenerational transmission process. The multigenerational transmission process refers to the prevalent finding that family violence is perpetuated through generations by a cycle of violence. Although several theories have been proposed regarding this phenomenon, the most enduring is that of social learning theory, in which violence is viewed as a learned behavior.

Social learning theory states that a child learns to be violent in a family setting in which a violent parent has been taken as a role model. In this perspective, violence and victimization are behaviors learned through exposure to violence in childhood. This exposure teaches both the means and the approval of violence. Children who witness violence not only learn specific aggressive behaviors but also acquire the belief that violence is a legitimate way to solve problems within a family. When frustrated or angry as an adult, the individual relies on this learned behavior and responds with violence.

Social learning theory was first applied to child abuse when it was noted that many child abusers were themselves abused as children.[60] Numerous studies have suggested the intergenerational transmission of child abuse within families,[27,77,98,99] and this appears to place a parent at risk for abuse. However, other controlled studies[96] examining parental punishment history and current child abuse found no differences between abusive and nonabusive parents. Simply experiencing abuse as a child does not totally determine an adult's later behaviors. Many people who were abused as children are able to avoid violence with their own children. Straus[98] suggests that the key factor may be the age at which the child was abused or which parent was abusive. Experiencing abuse from a father at age 4 years may be totally different than experiencing abuse from one's mother as an adolescent.

A number of authors have also examined the multigenerational process with wife abuse by noting the incidence of violence in the family of both the survivors and the abusers. An extensive literature review conducted by Hotaling and Sugerman[54] identified witnessing parental violence during childhood or adolescence as one of the strongest risk factors for the abuse of wives in adulthood. The case is less persuasive that women learn to be victims of wife abuse from childhood experiences with violence.

To date, there is limited evidence of intergenerational transmission of violence in elder abuse. Pillemer and Suitor,[81] however, suggest that elder abuse could be the result of formerly abused children displaying both retaliatory and imitative behavior or displaying modeling behavior observed between their parents and grandparents.

Many treatment modalities, especially cognitive approaches, are based on the social learning model that violent reactions can be unlearned and replaced with constructive responses to conflict.

Social isolation. Some authors have noted that violent families are also socially isolated, since particular types of violence are considered abnormal or illegitimate and become a "family secret." Exposure of family violence can result in both formal and informal sanctions from other family members, neighbors, the police, or the judicial system; therefore the abuser often purposely keeps the family isolated.[5,74] Social isolation has been found to be a factor in elder abuse,[78,80] wife abuse,[64] and child abuse.[17,58]

Use and abuse of power. An additional commonality within the various forms of family violence is the use and abuse of power. In almost all forms of family violence the abuser has some form of power or control over the victim. For example, with the sexual abuse of children, the abuser is usually a male in an authority position victimizing a young female in a subordinate position.[35,106] A recent study of sexual abuse of children by caregivers[73] also noted the power disparity between the violator and the child victim.

Power issues appear to be a central factor with wife abuse. Many authors have noted that wife abuse is controlling behavior that creates and maintains an imbalance of power within the relationship. Although wife abusers will justify the use of violence for trivial events such as not having a meal ready or not keeping the house tidy, many authors have noted that the violence is related to the husband's need for total domination of his wife. For example, Schechter[90] interviewed a number of wife abusers and survivors and found that for many women, their moves toward self-assertion through jobs or school infuriated their husbands. The women's success or recognition was perceived as threatening to their husbands, who used abuse in an attempt to regain control over their wives. Finkelhor and Pillemer[36] found that the largest single category (60%) of physical abuse of the elderly was actually spouse abuse, thereby incorporating the issues of power and control central in that form of family violence.

Alcohol and drug abuse. The relationship between alcohol and drug abuse and family violence has been studied extensively. Victims of violence frequently report concurrent substance abuse by the abuser. Most researchers, however, deny that substance abuse is a direct causative factor in violence because it does not meet the criteria of stability, consensus, and consistency. That is, people who abuse alcohol are not consistently violent, and people who are violent are not always intoxicated. Instead, it has been suggested that rather than acting violent because one is drunk, the person uses alcohol as a means of deviance disavowal.[6] In this perspective, drinking provides a socially acceptable reason for engaging in otherwise inappropriate behaviors, which the aggressor can later excuse by claiming that he was intoxicated. Family and friends may also attribute the conduct to the effects of alcohol, which to some extent decreases the degree of blame. An additional relationship is that for some people the use of alcohol or drugs reduces fear or inhibitions and creates a lessened perception of the impact of their behavior.

Cross-cultural studies suggest that behavior while drinking varies from culture to culture. In societies where it is believed that alcohol is a disinhibitor, people become disinhibited. If they believe it is a depressant, they become depressed when drinking. If people in America believe that normal rules of behavior are suspended when one is drinking, people will act in an antisocial manner.[40]

Recently Leonard and Jacob[67] conducted an extensive literature review of the relationship between alcohol abuse and family violence. They concluded that there was some evidence implicating alcohol use and alcoholism in marital violence, although the evidence related to child abuse was much weaker. In addition, with marital violence, confounding variables such as the stress of alcoholism on the family system or familial expectations that drinking will increase aggressive behavior have not been adequately controlled.

Connections between drug abuse and family violence have been less well researched. Early research on aggressiveness and illicit drugs has established that marijuana and heroin use are not related to violence. In contrast, drugs such as "crack" cocaine, amphetamines, mescaline, "angel dust" (PCP), and steroids used illegally have been associated with increased violence, but the specific relationships with various forms of family violence are not yet established.[11]

■ **NURSING ATTITUDES TOWARD SURVIVORS OF VIOLENCE.** It can be extremely difficult and frustrating to provide nursing care for survivors of violence. The attitudes nurses bring to these situations help shape their responses. A number of research studies of health care professionals' attitudes indicate that myths about battered women are still accepted even though there is sympathy toward the survivor.[25,89,92] Similarly, nurses have been found *not* to blame rape victims in general. However, the tendency to blame the victim increases when a vignette describes the woman as having gone out late at night, not locked her car doors, or gone shopping for beer rather than milk for the baby.[2,23,24]

Even though most nurses do not actually blame survivors for what has happened to them, they do dislike certain behaviors. They are not happy with sexual assault survivors within and outside the family who do not resist "enough." They have difficulty understanding abused children who want to return to abusive parents. They especially dislike battered women who do not leave their abusers. Kurz[63] published a classic study using qualitative analysis to describe the subtle blaming and distancing of battered women by emergency department personnel, including nurses. Stark and Flitcraft[94] and Stark and Frazier[95] used emergency room chart reviews to document the lack of recognition, negative labeling, and inappropriate treatment that all too often happens to battered women. Other studies describe how survivors find the health care system to be unhelpful and even traumatizing when they have gone for assistance.[9,28] King and Ryan[61] note that nurses most often use a paternalistic and individualistic model of helping in interactions with battered women. In other words, nurses tend to see themselves as more knowledgeable than the woman and place the locus of responsibility for ending the violence with her. Nurses tend to give advice and sympathy rather than respect. An empowerment model that encompasses strategizing with survivors, respecting their competence and experience, sharing knowledge and information both ways, and helping survivors recognize the societal influences on their situations is rarely used. When the paternalistic model is used, the nurse is more likely to be frustrated because the survivor does not follow the nurse's advice. Therefore the empowerment model is not only more helpful to the survivor but also more professionally satisfying for the nurse.

Origins of negative attitudes. There are several theoretic perspectives that can be helpful in understanding nurses' attitudes. The "just world" hypothesis was first advanced by Lerner and Simmons.[68] Basically this refers to the notion that people tend to believe that others generally get what they deserve. Therefore good things happen to good people, and bad things happen to bad people. This belief helps one to regard the world as safe because oneself is seen as basically good and therefore protected. When a person is victimized by violence, a horrible idea to contemplate, one needs to make sense of it. The easiest way is not to see it at all, which explains some of the lack of recognition. However, when family violence is unmistakable, one needs to understand why that particular person is the victim. If bad things happen to bad people, the victimized person must have done something wrong or at least something stupid, something different from what oneself would have done.

The whole process of victim blaming is easier if the victim is of "a type" who is already the focus of bias. It is easier to blame and distance oneself from women or minority groups if there is already bias against them.[89] Conversely, the more the person resembles oneself, the harder it is to recognize the violence at all. Thus it is not reported as often; the abuse is just not "seen" when the people are middle class and especially professionals. Consequently, child abuse is more likely to be reported in the health care system if the family is poor and of a racial minority.[47]

Ryan[88] discusses similar dynamics in the book *Blaming the Victim.* Ryan describes how blaming the victim helps one avoid blaming the system in which this violence is perpetuated. If the battered woman is to blame for at least not ending the violence, society is less at fault for perpetuating the notions that power, aggression, and dominance are the marks of a successful man and a successful country. Consequently the issue can be avoided. If the family who abuses elders is dysfunctional, others need not worry about a society that fails to provide help to the caregivers of the elderly. As another example, consider the family member who has somehow always been considered the most despicable in cases of incest, the "collusive" mother. Despite the lack of research evidence to support this,[33] professionals are still eager to find out the mother's role in sexual abuse of her daughter. They are too sophisticated to blame the child, but they have found another female family member to denigrate rather than trying to understand her normal responses to a horrible dilemma. Even though some of the societal forces that perpetuate incest have been exposed,[86] they are generally unaddressed in recommendations for clinical interventions. Instead, the focus is on the "dysfunctional family unit" rather than calling the issue what it is: a criminal who has violated the safety and health of a child in a society uncomfortable with the attitudes that may encourage such behavior.

Another theoretical perspective, theories of deviance, is especially relevant for nursing. Applying the explanations of Schur,[91] one can understand that making the survivors and perpetrators of violence into objects to be studied or categories with a diagnostic label creates further distance between them and the nurse. This is the problem with the proposed medical diagnosis of "battered woman syndrome" or a psychiatric diagnosis specific to victims of violence.[10,22] If adults receive official diagnoses only because they are abused sometime in their past, the assumption of pathology becomes concrete. The survivor of family violence is officially sick and has the responsibility to become well. There is no chance that her or his responses will be seen as survival strategies or normal reactions; they become symptoms. Both society and the abuser remain undiagnosed, and survivors become a "deviant group" to be studied and "fixed."[69]

It has been suggested that more nurses have been victimized by violence than other groups, which might explain their negative attitudes toward other survivors or their behaviors in other situations. Research has not established whether or not there are more battered women among nurses than among other populations of women. However, Rew[83] found the percentage of nursing students who had experienced childhood sexual exploitation (62%) to be similar to the percentage in another survey of female college students. Regardless of the specific violence experience of nurses, there are certainly power and control and exploitation issues that have shaped the history of the nursing profession and continue to influence nurses' daily reality. Therefore, according to "oppressed group" behavior literature,[38,49] nurses would be predisposed toward negative attitudes toward another oppressed group, the predominantly female victims of family violence.

Overcoming negative attitudes. Exploring ones' own attitudes toward survivors of family violence is an important first step in providing effective nursing care. Understanding the mechanisms that help create such attitudes is also helpful. It has been suggested that nurses who have had clinical experience with survivors and gotten to know them as persons may be less blaming than nurses who have not.[23,55] Therefore it is important to gain this experience either through educational programs or as a volunteer in programs such as rape crisis centers, battered women's shelters, or child protection programs. Formal continuing and in-service education on family violence should be directed toward recognizing and changing feelings, as well as learning facts about violence. Nurses can also increase their own understanding and appreciation of the experience of survivors by reading novels and watching media depictions of these issues.

■ **RESPONSES TO FAMILY VIOLENCE.** There is a growing body of knowledge that documents how people are likely to respond to violence from other family members. Since the definition of nursing is "the diagnosis and treatment of human responses to health problems,"[3] these physical, emotional, and behavioral responses to violence as a major health problem are the primary focus of nursing.

Physical responses to battering. One area of study has been the types and patterns of physical injuries received. A characteristic pattern of injuries, especially to the head, neck/face/throat, trunk, and sexual organs has been found in all forms of family violence.[60] For all groups experiencing family violence, sexual abuse frequently accompanies physical abuse. This has been best documented in battered women; several studies have found that approximately 40% were also sexually assaulted by their partners.[85] All survivors of family violence tend to have injuries at multiple sites in various stages of healing.

Other physical symptoms. Victims of family violence frequently experience a range of physical symptoms not obviously related to their injuries, such as headaches, menstrual problems, chronic pain, and digestive and sleeping disturbances.[10,16,22,43] Frequently, communicable diseases are a problem in shelters for battered women and their children.[52]

Most authors characterize these types of symptoms as evidence of psychopathology, but similar symptoms occur after rape and other forms of violence, as well as in widows and divorcees.[62] Past injuries causing such symptoms as headaches and other forms of chronic pain or the possible effects of stress on the immune system have not been considered as causes of these problems. Thus, rather than thinking of such symptoms as "hysterical," "psychosomatic," or as "evidence of somaticizing," they can be considered as part of a physical stress reaction. Such responses to stress are common to those who have experienced emotional trauma, such as physical attack by a stranger or the loss of a close relationship.

Behavioral responses to battering. Many professionals and researchers have tried to understand the behavior of survivors of family violence, especially in terms of their continued attachment with an abuser. This has been especially damaging in literature addressing the question of why battered women remain in the relationship. There is the assumption that she *should* leave rather than stay. In actuality, when a battered woman leaves, she is in the most danger of being killed by a partner obsessed with power and control.[14,48] Looking at the other end of the continuum, some battered women are able to end the violence but maintain their relationships using a variety of strategies.[8]

However, family violence usually escalates in severity and frequency. In cases where the violence does not end, it is normal and healthy for a battered woman to consider her entire existence and that of her significant others for a long time before ending her most important attachment relationship.[16,65] Constraints that make it difficult to leave include cultural sanctions, an intense attachment to the man, and lack of resources.[100,102] Gilligan's work[41] has demonstrated that the process by which women make moral decisions usually involves weighing the consequences to others more heavily than consequences to themselves. Thus concern for children is a major issue in the woman's decision making.[103]

The majority of battered women eventually leave an abusive relationship if it remains continuously violent, but there is often a pattern of leaving and returning many times before making a final break.[74] Rather than interpreting this behavior as a sign of weakness, it can be viewed as a normal behavioral pattern, influenced by the quality of social support and assistance the woman is given and the behavior of the batterer rather than by the woman's psychological factors.[8] The leaving and returning are done in a purposeful manner to achieve one or more of the following: (1) pressure the abuser into meaningful change, (2) test external and internal resources, and (3) evaluate how the children are reacting without their father.

Similar long processes of ending attachment relationships have been reported for wives of alcoholics, divorced and separated women, and persons experiencing anticipatory grief. A grieving framework can be used to explain some responses, including denial, which is frequently described in battered women.[17] This coping mechanism has been renamed as "forgetting and minimizing" by Kelly[59] in her exploration of responses to sexual violence (rape, incest, battering). The women in Kelly's sample saw this response as generally very useful rather than problematic, as is often implied.

Clinical reports also discuss the reluctance of abused children and elderly family members to leave their families as if this response is pathological rather than normal. When one thinks in terms of normal grief and realistic fear (of foster homes for the children and nursing homes for the elders), these responses seem more understandable and healthy. An important nursing research study by Humphreys[56] also documented that the children of battered women take significant action to try to protect their mothers from abuse. Although these actions are sometimes viewed as unhealthy, Humphreys described them as an instance of Orem's concept of dependent care.[75] This type of reframing of responses to family violence is congruent with nursing's emphasis on physical and mental health.

Psychological responses to battering. More work has been done to explore psychological responses to abuse in battered women than in either child abuse or elder abuse survivors. Most of our knowledge about the emotional responses to incest is in terms of long, delayed responses rather than immediate ones. The psychological responses described and explored most frequently include the cognitive responses of attributions and problem-solving abilities and the emotional responses of depression and lowered self-esteem.

Attributions. Attributions can be defined as the reasoning processes people use to explain events. A relationship to future mental health has been found in a variety of situations, including serious illness.[30] Although it is often said that victims of violence tend to blame themselves, only about 20% of battered women do so when measured in research.[16,39] Battered women tend to blame themselves less over time.[39] In contrast, one report showed that the majority of adult survivors of repeated childhood sexual abuse by a person known to them blamed themselves. However, these women were studied in a clinical setting rather than in the community, which is the usual setting in studies of battered women.[57]

It has been argued that internal attributions (self-blame) either may be adaptive for survivors of violence as a way of maintaining control over their lives[70] or may contribute to long-term depression.[1] To date research has not been definitive on this issue for battered women or for other survivors of family violence. However, there is insufficient evidence to assume that self-blame is either widespread among survivors of family violence or always pathological.[16,21]

Problem-solving techniques. Several studies have found that battered women have trouble in problem solving.[66] School problems have also been reported in abused children.[22,51] Finn[37] compared coping strategies of 56 battered women with instrument norms and found battered women significantly less likely than other women to use three active coping methods (social support, reframing, and spiritual support). However, the researcher failed to consider that (1) the batterer may enforce isolation; (2) avoidance of nonsupportive network members can be adaptive; (3) reframing may minimize the physical danger, thus increasing the risk in a battering situation; or (4) battered women often report clergy to be unhelpful. It is also interesting to note that there was no significant difference between groups in the fourth coping mechanism measured, mobilizing to acquire and accept help.

In contrast, other researchers[8,16,28,39] describe a variety of approaches used and factors considered by battered women that suggest appropriate decision making. Undoubtedly, some battered women, children, and elders are so frequently and severely beaten and controlled that their ability to problem-solve is severely and chronically affected. Techniques of coercive control by batterers, similar to those used by terrorists, have been described in the literature.[74]

Extreme difficulty in problem solving could be explained by "posttraumatic stress disorder," described by the American Psychiatric Association[4] as including symptoms of memory impairment or difficulty concentrating. Problem-solving difficulties have also been noted in widows and divorcees, in which case they were explained as normative responses to loss. Such problems could also be explained as being one of the deficits of learned helplessness (along with depression) or one of the cognitive aspects of depression.

Depression. Depression has been noted by both clinical studies and research instruments (e.g., the Beck Depression Inventory) in many samples of battered women, adult survivors of incest, and abused children.[10,21,72,105,107] Depression has also been noted in survivors of other forms of violence, as well as in divorcees and widows. Interestingly, depression is found more often among young, unemployed, and divorced women in the general population.[84] Since battered women and adult incest survivors are also found most often in these groups, it is difficult to make conclusions about whether depression in adult female survivors of family violence stems from abuse or other factors. Conversely, the greater incidence of depression in these groups may be related to the higher prevalence of violence.

Walker[104,105] hypothesized that learned helplessness was the best explanation of depression in battered women. Although her subsequent research generally supported the model, she found that women who had left the abusive relationship had higher scores on the depression measure than those still with the batterer. This finding may indicate a problem in her assumption that battered women still in the relationship were exhibiting learned helplessness. It could also mean that the depression experienced by the women who left was a result of grief rather than learned helplessness. Campbell[16] found support for both grief and learned helplessness using theory comparison research. However, both models left almost half the variation in depression unexplained. This may reflect the emphasis in both models on the individual situation. The wider influences that contribute to both healthy and unhealthy responses to violence are not included in either model. Furthermore, only a small minority of the battered women in the Campbell sample exhibited all aspects of the syndrome of learned helplessness: depression, low self-esteem, apathy, and difficulty with problem solving.

Self-esteem. Although most research has found low self-esteem in battered women and incest survivors, there have been some exceptions.[10,16,104,105] For instance, Kelly[59] reported that a greater proportion of the incest and battering survivors in her qualitative study felt more "independent and stronger" than more "insecure in self" as a result of the abuse.

One way to resolve these types of discrepancies is to make comparisons between groups who are experiencing the same situational dynamics, except for the violence aspect. Using this approach, Campbell[16] found no significant difference in self-esteem in her comparison of battered women with other women considering leaving an intimate relationship, even though both groups were below norms. Similarly, DiPietro[26] found no significant difference in the self-esteem of incest survivors compared to other young women in treatment for other family problems, although both groups were again lower than norms. However, sexual abuse had a direct detrimental effect on battered women's self-esteem independent of severity and frequency of physical beatings.[16]

In summary, research on responses to family violence can be interpreted as lists of characteristics describing symptoms of pathology of a certain group of people. The same responses also can be interpreted as how normal people respond to an incredible physical and emotional trauma and yet are able to survive. Research regarding this latter approach is beginning to document survivor mechanisms and a recovering process from abuse.[45,64]

■ Preventive nursing interventions

Effectively preventing family violence requires the use of a variety of approaches. These include the primary prevention strategies of changing societal norms and values, programs of preventive education with a variety of populations, and secondary prevention strategies of effective treatment modalities.

■ **PRIMARY PREVENTION.** Primary prevention refers to an activity that stops a problem before it occurs. Changing society's acceptance of violence and abuse is an important first step in prevention. Consider, for example, the changing view of cigarette smoking that has occurred in America in the past 15 years. In less than 2 decades perceptions of cigarette smoking as a attractive, sophisticated behavior have changed to the identification of smoking as a health hazard that is prohibited in most public places.

Effective primary prevention includes eliminating cultural norms and values that accept and glamorize violence. This would begin by severely limiting the amount of violence permitted on television and in other media. The prevalence of violence on television plays a role in creating a social climate that says violence is exciting and appropriate. The average child watches television for 20 hours a week. It has been estimated that American children observe 18,000 killings before they graduate from high school. A recent report summarizing studies on the effect of media violence noted, "Of the 85 major studies into the effects of television violence, only one concluded that television violence did not cause increased aggressiveness in children. It was paid for by NBC."[19]

A related area of primary prevention would be the elimination of pornography, especially violent pornography. Pornography and erotica can be easily differentiated, since pornography depicts the denigration of women (or one of the sexual partners) in some way, whereas erotica is the depiction of sexual pleasure in an egalitarian relationship. Violent pornography has been particularly associated with sexual violence.[93] However, the rates of subscription to even as mild a form of pornography as *Playboy* magazine has been positively correlated with state rape rates.

Primary prevention of abuse also includes strengthening individuals and families so they can cope more effectively with multiple life stressors and competing demands. Nurses can conduct programs in the schools, workplace, or community. Strategies such as nurse-developed educational programs in high-school parenting classes or childbirth education classes can be used to forewarn families of the expected stress of child rearing. These classes could include topics such as normal child development and expectations, basic skills of infant care, and means of disciplining children that do not involve physical punishment. Additional educational strategies include teaching family members that conflict resolution does not always mean one party wins while the other loses and that they should respect individual differences among family members.

Nurses can also be involved in teaching family life and sex education courses in elementary and middle schools. Sexual abuse of children can be prevented or detected when children are taught about inappropriate sexual contact and what they should do if it occurs. Middle-school students need information about how to have heterosexual relationships in which jealousy is not viewed as a sign of love and domination of one partner over the other is not expected. Peer discussions can help counteract the tendencies for manliness being defined in terms of confrontation and control.

Family violence prevention also includes anticipatory guidance while working with families. For exam-

ple, respite care is needed for families with chronically ill or incapacitated family members, including the elderly and children. Planning in advance for relief from responsibility will prevent strained relationships and potential violence or abuse. Families also need to anticipate the difficult developmental stages of children to appreciate that infants are incapable of malicious intent toward parents, that toddlers' obstinance is necessary for independence in later childhood, and that bedwetting is a signal for increased positive attention rather than punishment.

In addition, as a society we must develop programs and policies that support families and reduce internal and external stresses and inequities. This includes adequate and appropriate day care for children and incapacitated elders, equity in salary and wages to make women less financially dependent, public education that ensures an adequate foundation for full employment of all societal members, and sufficient financing of prevention and treatment programs.

■ **SECONDARY PREVENTION.** Secondary prevention of family violence is aimed at its previously discussed cyclic nature. Although there is not a perfect relationship, we do know that children raised in violent, noncaring homes are more likely to become spouse and child abusers. Therefore, one of the most effective methods of preventing violence and abuse in future generations is to stop current abuse effectively.

Even when the violence has ended, those affected will need interventions. The children of battered women and siblings of abused children both are groups who have witnessed violence and are in need of interventions to counteract that learning. Abused children themselves are frequently thought to be "out of the woods" when they have been removed from the home or the family is no longer violent. Even if there are no identifiable long-term effects, there may have been "trauma encapsulation," the effects of which may not be discernible until many years afterward.[13] In addition, there will have been an imprinting of the belief that family members are violent to each other, for which conscious resolve alone may not overcome.[83]

Secondary prevention in family violence also involves the identification of families at risk or those who are beginning to use violence. Table 32-1 lists characteristics common to violent families that can be used for nursing assessment. Additional early indicators of families at risk include violence in the family of origin of either partner, communication problems, excessive family stress such as an unplanned pregnancy, unemployment, or inadequate family resources. The childbearing cycle is an ideal time to identify women at risk to become battered or in the early stages of an

TABLE 32-1

INDICATORS OF ACTUAL OR POTENTIAL ABUSE

Nursing history	Physical examination	Nursing observations
Primary reason for contact	**General appearance**	**General observations**
Vague information about cause of problem	Fearful, anxious, hyperactive or hypoactive	Observations differ significantly from history
Discrepancy between physical findings and descriptions of cause	Poor hygiene, careless grooming	Family members inadequately clothed or groomed
Minimizing injuries	Inappropriate dress	**Home environment**
Inappropriate delay between time of injury and treatment	Increased anxiety in presence of abuser	Inadequate heating
Inappropriate family reactions (e.g., lack of concern, overconcern, threatening demeanor)	Looking to abuser for answers to questions	Inappropriate sleeping arrangements
Information from family genogram	Inappropriate or anxious nonverbal behavior (e.g., giggling at serious questions or questions related to abuse)	Total household disorganization
Family violence in history (child, spouse, elder)		Inadequate food
History of violence outside of home	Flinching when touched	Spoiled food not discarded
Incarcerations	**Vital statistics**	**Family communication pattern**
Violent deaths in extended family	Overweight or underweight	One parent answers all questions
Alcoholism/drug abuse in family history	Hypertension	Looking for approval of other family members before answering questions
Past health history	**Skin**	
History of traumatic injuries	Bruises, welts, edema	Members continually interrupt each other
Spontaneous abortions	Presence of scars and indications of injuries in various stages of healing	Negative nonverbal behavior in other members when one member speaking
Psychiatric hospitalizations		
History of depression	Cigarette burns	Members do not listen to each other
Substance abuse	**Head**	
Sexual history	Bald patches on scalp from pulling hair	Taboo topics (family secrets)
Prior sexual abuse		**Emotional climate**
Use of force in sexual activities	Subdural hematoma	Tense, secretive atmosphere
Venereal disease	**Eyes**	Unhappiness
Child with sexual knowledge beyond that appropriate for age	Subconjunctival hemorrhage	Lack of affection
	Swelling	Apparent fear of other family members
Promiscuity	Black eyes	
Personal/social history	**Ears**	Verbal arguing
Unwanted or unplanned pregnancy	Hearing loss from prior injury or untreated infections	
Adolescent pregnancy		
Social isolation (difficulty naming persons available for help in a crisis)	**Mouth**	
	Bruising	
Lack of contact with extended family	Lacerations	
Unrealistic expectations of relationships or age-appropriate behavior	Untreated dental caries	
	Venereal infection	
Extreme jealousy by spouse	**Abdomen**	
Rigid traditional sex-role beliefs	Intraabdominal injuries	
Verbal aggression	Abdominal injuries during pregnancy	
Belief in use of physical punishment		
Difficulties in school	**Extremities**	
Truancy, running away	Bruising to forearms from attempts to protect self from blows	
Psychological history		
Feelings of helplessness/hopelessness	Broken arms	
Feeling trapped	Radiological indications of previous fractures	
Difficulty making plans for future		
Tearfulness		
Chronic fatigue, apathy		
Suicide attempts		

TABLE 32-1, Cont'd

INDICATORS OF ACTUAL OR POTENTIAL ABUSE

Nursing history	Physical examination	Nursing observations
Financial history Poverty Finances rigidly controlled by one family member Unwillingness to spend money on health care or adequate nutrition Complaints about spending money on family members Unemployment Use of elders' finances for other family members **Family beliefs/values** Belief in importance of physical discipline Autocratic decision making Intolerance of differing views among members Mistrust of outsiders **Family relations** Lack of visible affection or nurturing between family members Extreme dependency between family members Autonomy discouraged Numerous arguments Temporary separations Dissatisfaction with family members Lack of enjoyable family activities Extramarital affairs Role rigidity (inability of members to assume non-traditional roles)	**Neurological** Developmental delays Difficulty with speech or swallowing Hyperactive reflex response **Genital/urinary** Genital lacerations or bruising Urinary tract infections Venereal disease **Rectal** Rectal bruising Bleeding Edema Tenderness Poor sphincter tone	

abusive relationship, as well as to identify infants at risk for abuse. Pregnancy is when healthy women are seen in the health care system most frequently and when a comprehensive assessment should include information about relationships and child-rearing beliefs and practices. It may also facilitate identification early in an abusive relationship before abusive patterns become entrenched. When the nurse hears an indication of risk, this demands immediate nursing intervention. Taking the time to explore the risk factors, to discuss perceptions and attitudes, and to brainstorm with the client about possible alternatives is time well spent.

Special populations

■ Child abuse

The earliest form of family violence that was recognized within the health professional literature was physical abuse to children. Although violence to children was considered to be a social problem in the nineteenth century, it was not until the 1940s that it

was first identified as a medical problem, even a unique "syndrome." In 1962 the classic article by C. Henry Kempe and his associates, "The Battered Child Syndrome," first brought sustained interest in the problem of physical abuse to children. By the end of the 1960s every state had enacted legislation mandating the report of suspected child abuse and neglect.[58] Under current regulations, nurses and any other professionals providing services to children are required to report suspected incidents of child abuse and neglect.

There are many forms of abuse to children, including physical abuse or battering, emotional abuse, sexual abuse, and neglect. Although research on the many forms of child abuse has been extensive, there is still much that is unknown about the causes, treatment, or prevention of child abuse. In addition, research to date has failed to indicate any factors that are present in all abusing and absent in all nonabusing parents.[96]

■ **SEXUAL ABUSE OF CHILDREN AND ADOLESCENTS.** Sexual abuse is defined as the involvement of children and adolescents in sexual activities they do not fully comprehend and to which they do not freely consent.[34] Sexual abuse results in both long- and short-term problems. Short-term physical symptoms include venereal disease or infection; vaginal or rectal bleeding, itching, or soreness; recurrent urinary tract infections; or pregnancy. The presence of any of these symptoms in a child or adolescent should cue the nurse to assess further for sexual abuse, even if it is not readily disclosed by the child. Short-term emotional indicators include behavioral changes, difficulty sleeping, school problems, or chronic fears or unhappiness.

The long-term effects of sexual abuse as a child include sexual problems, difficulty trusting others, anxiety and panic attacks, depression, and substance abuse. A recent study by Feinauer[34] of adult women who had been sexually abused as children found that they experienced more emotional distress and long-term effects when the perpetrator was a person who was known and trusted by them. Feinauer found that the kinship relationship between the victim and the abuser was less important in creating distress than the emotional bond the victim felt toward the perpetrator. Thus a critical factor seems to be the violation of the child's trust, as well as the physical trauma.

■ **NURSING ASSESSMENT.** Nursing assessment of actual or potential child abuse begins with a thorough history and physical examination. Gathering a history of child abuse can be a stressful experience for both the nurse and the family. It is therefore essential that the nurse first examine her or his own values and past experiences to maintain a therapeutic and nonjudgmental clinical approach.

In obtaining a history, it is important to establish an honest, trusting environment that is not intended to punish or shame either the child or the parent.[17] If the nurse recognizes that most abusive parents are genuinely embarrassed about their behavior and would like assistance in developing alternative approaches to discipline, an environment can be established that will facilitate honesty and sharing. The setting for the interview needs to be quiet, private, and uninterrupted.

In general, the initial interview should be conducted by separating the child and the adult(s). This decision, however, depends on the child's age and other extenuating circumstances. The nurse should honestly state the purpose of the interview, type of questions being asked, and the subsequent physical examination. The approach needs to be calm and supportive because both the child and the family will be uneasy.

The interview with the parent(s) can begin with a discussion of the problem that first brought the child to a health care facility. During this discussion the nurse should pay particular attention to the parent's understanding of the problem, discrepancies in the stories, and the parent's emotional responses. The interview can then be expanded to discussions of how the parent "disciplines" the child or spanks the child. The initial interview is not the time to confront the abuser directly, since measures must be taken to document and report the abuse thoroughly to ensure the child's safety.

■ **NURSING INTERVENTIONS.** When child abuse is suspected, the nurse must report her suspicions to protective services. An investigation by the state protective service agency is legally mandated and also serves to reinforce to the family the seriousness of the problem. When protective services are involved, the nurse should explain to the family precisely what will happen in an investigation and the amount of time involved. In addition, the nurse should maintain frequent contact with the assigned worker to ensure a comprehensive, consistent approach. Nurses who work with violent families need to know exactly how protective services work in the community in which they practice. It is extremely valuable to know personally the professionals at the agency in order to remain informed about the policies and reporting protocols and ensure successful coordination and continuity.

Long-term therapy of child-abusing families is a complex process. Psychiatric nurses who wish to engage in such therapy should receive advanced training in courses specifically devoted to this topic.

■ **Wife abuse**

The term "wife abuse" includes all forms of physical violence toward a female partner in an ongoing intimate relationship. The term is also used to refer to emotional degradation and intimidation of female partners, which almost always accompany physical abuse, and to sexual abuse (or marital rape), which is part of the violence in about half the cases of female battering.[16] The violence is part of a system of coercive control that may also include financial coercion, threats against children and other family members, and destruction of property.[90] Wife abuse is the most widespread form of family violence, with at least one in every six wives being hit by a husband sometime during their relationship and at least 1.6 million women each year being severely and repeatedly beaten by their spouses.[99] Although wives do hit husbands, female violence is much more likely to be in self-defense and seldom takes the intentional, repeated, serious, and controlling form characterized by wife abuse. Therefore, to use the terms "spouse abuse" and "domestic violence" obscures the gender specificity of the violence. However, the nurse must be aware that both husband abuse and homosexual partner abuse are possibilities, although rare.

One of the most frightening realities of wife abuse is the potential for lethal outcomes. The majority of female homicide victims in the United States are killed by a husband, lover, or ex-husband or -lover, and the majority of these murders are preceded by wife abuse.[14] In fact, there is evidence that a battered woman is in most danger of homicide when she leaves her abusive partner or makes it clear to him that she is ending the relationship.[48] Battered women also kill their spouses. Many of the risk factors are similar, such as a handgun in the house, a history of suicide threats or attempts in either partner, battering during pregnancy, sexual abuse as part of the violence, severe substance abuse, and extreme jealousy and controlling behavior.[11,15] A frequent statement heard by potentially murderous abusers is, "If I can't have you, no one can."[101]

Stark and Flitcraft[94] assert that battering may be the most important precipitant for female suicide attempts and that 10% of battered women have considered suicide. Therefore, when an abused woman is depressed, suicide potential must be carefully assessed.

■ **NURSING ASSESSMENT.** It has been documented that the most prevalent cause of trauma in women treated in emergency rooms is wife abuse.[43,95] Wife abuse is also a frequent precursor of female visits to psychiatric emergency departments and other mental health treatment centers. It is beginning to be recognized that assessment for all forms of violence is critical information for all nursing histories and that assessment for wife abuse should be mandatory in mental health settings, as well as in emergency rooms, prenatal settings, and primary care facilities.[18,50,87]

When there are no obvious injuries, assessment for wife abuse is best placed within the history about the client's (both genders) primary intimate attachment relationship. Answers to general questions on the quality of that relationship should be assessed for feelings of being controlled or needing to control. A relationship characterized by excessive jealousy (of possessions, children, jobs, friends, and other family members, as well as potential sexual partners) is at risk of also being characterized by violence. The client can be asked about how the couple solves conflicts; one partner needing to have the final say or frequent and forceful verbal aggression also can be considered risk factors. Finally, the client should be asked if arguments ever involve "pushing or shoving." Queries about minor violence within a context of couple relationships help to establish the unfortunate normalcy of wife abuse and to lessen the stigma of disclosure. If the client hesitates or looks away or otherwise displays uncomfortable nonverbal behavior or reveals risk factors for abuse, she or he can be asked again later in the interview about physical violence.

If abuse is revealed, the nurse's first response is critical. It is important that an abused woman realize that she is not alone; important affirmation can be given with a statement about the frequency of wife abuse. The extent of the abuse and what forms are being used need to be elicited and described in the record. Careful documentation using a body map is necessary for potential future legal actions, which are frequently child custody suits as well as criminal actions related to the violence.

The types of responses to the violence the woman has experienced are also a critical area for a mental health assessment. It is important that these responses be interpreted to the woman as normal within the circumstances. Signs of posttraumatic stress disorder, depression, and low self-esteem need to be assessed and recorded. Attribution regarding the abuse is also an important issue. One nursing study[16] revealed that women blaming the abuse on an unchanging personality characteristic within themselves had lower levels of self-esteem and increased depression. It is therefore important that the nurse carefully assess the woman's beliefs regarding the abuse and the responsibility regarding the abuse. Since many wife abusers find an excuse for the violence, the woman may be unnecessarily accepting the blame for his actions.

If the client is an abuser, mental state is also important, with the potential for further violence carefully assessed. The safety of the abused partner is a concern, as is treatment for the abuser. Consultation with other professionals about the nurse's "duty to warn" would be warranted.[48]

■ **NURSING INTERVENTIONS.** Most communities have treatment programs for abusive men, although they have been found to be most effective when the court has ordered treatment with punitive sanctions for noncompliance.[31] Severely abusive men seldom admit they have a problem and frequently need to be mandated into treatment and to remain in treatment. The nurse needs to confront the violence and clarify that the responsibility lies with the abuser. A combination of strategies may be needed to get the abuser into treatment if he is not in the court system.

The type of referral chosen is extremely important. There is a greater likelihood of long-lasting change if the treatment combines behavioral therapy around anger control with a program designed to change attitudes toward women.[44] Traditional marriage therapy or couple counseling as the only treatment is considered potentially dangerous to the woman because of the unequal power in the relationship and the possibility of retaliatory violence.

For an abused woman, empowerment strategies entail first making sure she has the information she needs, such as the illegality of wife assault and the related state and local laws and ordinances. She also needs to be aware of the local battered woman's shelter(s) available for advice, support, and group participation, even if she does not intend to enter the shelter at this time. There is now a national hotline for shelters that women can call and receive information about abuse, including the number of the nearest shelter (1-800-333-SAFE).

Mutual goal setting is particularly important when working with abused women. The nurse can easily be frustrated if she imposes her goals on the woman, who may not be ready for drastic action. It is hoped there will be time for a long-term relationship during which the nurse and client can work through the normal denial and minimization that takes place when the woman's primary attachment relationship is threatened. The nurse and client together can then explore and expand on all the options the woman has thought about and devise others. Dealing with an abusive situation is a recovering process, as detailed by Landenburger,[65] that takes time and ongoing support. The nurse, whether in a short or extended intervention situation, can help the client mobilize both natural and system support so that her economic as well as emotional needs are addressed.

Evaluation of nursing interventions are based on mutual goals rather than on a preconceived notion of what a battered woman should or should not do. Since the majority of abused women eventually leave a seriously violent situation or end the violence in some other way[74] and appropriately seek help when the violence becomes severe,[44] the nurse can be optimistic about the eventual outcome. Her interventions may not result in an immediately happy ending, but they can plant the seeds of empowerment that can facilitate the woman's recovery process.

■ Elder abuse

Estimates of the numbers of elderly persons abused vary widely, from 10% of the adult elderly population (2.5 million) in the United States to 1% in a random sample survey in New Jersey.[42] Using a case-control approach and a stratified random sample, Finkelhor and Pillemer[36] found 32 victims of physical abuse, physical neglect, or chronic verbal aggression per 1000 elderly in Boston. However, the majority of the abuse was committed by spouses (60% of the

physical abuse and 58% of the overall maltreatment). Thus spouse abuse and elder abuse are often overlapping categories.

That the majority of elder abuse is spouse abuse also contradicts the notion that elder abuse is most likely a case of children abusing an elderly parent for whom they are providing physical care. Although caregiver stress is an important nursing concern, it may not play the central role in elder abuse that was previously assumed. In fact, Finkelhor and Pillemer[36] found that an important risk factor for elder abuse was the abuser's financial dependence on the abused. Neither that study nor Phillips' nursing research[78] found abused elders to be more functionally impaired than control groups. Research is thus beginning to indicate that, rather than the condition of the elder, characteristics of the abuser, such as having mental and emotional problems including substance abuse, create a family situation at risk for elder abuse.

■ **NURSING ASSESSMENT.** Based on this information, it would be important to assess for elder abuse in family situations where a client of the mental health care system is financially dependent on elderly parents. Consequently, family interviews would not focus exclusively on the health and welfare of the client, but would also assess the interactions between the client and his or her parents for indications of verbal and physical aggression.

It is difficult for abused elders to admit being physically hurt by a child or spouse. Again, gentle inquiry within the context of normal interactions to resolve interpersonal difficulties is the most useful approach. At least part of this assessment needs to take place with the elder alone. An abused elder may fear being abandoned to a nursing home or a life of total isolation more than he or she fears the violent family member and therefore may be especially reluctant to disclose. Only by establishing a trusting relationship over time or utilizing an already established relationship with someone else will the nurse be able to explore fully the nature of the abusive situation.

Assessment is even more difficult when the elder is severely mentally and/or emotionally impaired. In those cases physical assessment plus careful attention to nonverbal behavior is critical. Bruises to the upper arms from shaking are especially common in elder abuse. Although bruises from abuse are difficult to differentiate from those normal in aging, bilateral upper outer arm bruises are relatively definitive. Lacerations, especially to the face, are relatively infrequent sequelae from falls and should be regarded with suspicion. Vaginal lacerations and/or bruises and twisting bone fractures are particularly indicative of abuse. Signs of neglect are more frequent than those of physical abuse, and determining whether or not the neglect is intentional is the key to determining the nursing course of action.

In all cases where a dependent elderly person is being cared for by another, the interaction between the two will give important clues about the relationship. Flinching or shrinking away by the elder or rough physical treatment accompanied by verbal denigration by the caretaker are possible indicators of abuse. As with all types of family violence, the nurse needs to analyze the data from the history, physical examination, and her own observations to make an assessment of abuse. The decision to report is a difficult one, especially if the eventual outcome of reporting appears likely to be a nursing home placement unwanted by the elder.[79] However, the law in most states is that nurses are among those mandated to report suspected elder abuse.

■ **NURSING INTERVENTIONS.** As with other forms of family violence where reporting is mandatory, the therapeutic relationship with the family will be less damaged if the nurse first discusses her intention to report elder abuse with the family. Deciding whether to discuss reporting beforehand will be influenced by the likelihood of the abusing family member disappearing (or the whole family relocating in a child abuse case) and the severity of the abuse. If the abuse is less severe and/or mainly a neglectful or caretaker stress situation, discussing the intent to report first will make the action seem less a condemnation, allow protective services to be perceived as a helping agency rather than a punitive one, and enhance the possibilities that the nurse will be seen as a continuing source of help. Respite care or other stress relievers may be the key interventions for an overburdened caretaker situation.

In other cases the primary intervention may be therapeutic interventions for the abusers. These may take the form of counseling, therapy for preexisting mental disorders, or substance abuse treatment. The success of various interventions for elder abuse is not yet known, since research into this issue is scant. However, since there is a great overlap with spouse abuse and the dynamics involving noncaretaker elder abusers may be similar, one should assume that the treatment will need to involve specific components aimed at the violence as well as at whatever other problems are involved.

Rape and sexual assault

Rape and sexual assault are concerns for individuals, families, and the community. Sexual assaults against women and children (the most prevalent victims) result in physical trauma, psychic and spiritual disruptions, and deterioration of social relationships. In addition, the fear of rape and sexual assault has major consequences in the lives of women as they restrict their activities in attempts to ensure their safety. Victims of sexual assaults include women and men of all ages, social classes, races, and occupations. Sexual assault causes a disruption in every aspect of the victim's life, including social activities, interpersonal relationships, employment, and career. Although it is recognized that males may be sexually assaulted and women sexual offenders, in this section the victim is referred to as "she" and the offender as "he." It must be recognized, however, that men and young boys are also victimized and that assessment must not be limited to women.

Sexual assault is generally defined as forced perpetration of an act of sexual contact with another person without their consent. This includes the lack of consent because of the victim's cognitive or personality development, her feelings of fear or coercion, or the offender's physical or verbal threats. Most authors agree that sexual assault is not a sexual act but is instead motivated by a desire to humiliate, defile, and dominate the victim. Sexual assault has occurred for centuries but is now recognized as a social and public health problem.

The concept of consent can be conceptualized as a continuum, as seen in the box on page 921. This continuum demonstrates gradations in coercion, including bribery, taking advantage of one's position of power or trust in a relationship, or the victim's inability to consent freely.

In discussing rape and sexual assault, it is important to recognize that most cases of sexual assault do not occur between strangers. Marital rape has recently been recognized in most states, and child sexual abuse by family members, family friends, and caretakers is being reported in record numbers.

Marital rape is frequently reported concurrently with physical abuse. Campbell[16] found that the majority of abused women in her study reported that their husbands believed it was their right to have sex whenever they wanted, including when the women were ill, had recently given birth, or were discharged from a hospital. The women in Campbell's study reported forced vaginal intercourse; anal intercourse; being hit, burned, or kicked during sex; having objects inserted into their vagina and anus; or being forced to perform sexual acts with animals or while their children were observing. Many women were threatened with weapons or beaten when they refused to take part in these activities. Marital rape may be especially devastating

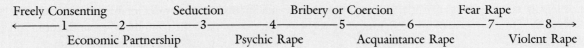

Sexual Behavior: The Force Continuum

Freely Consenting   Seduction   Bribery or Coercion   Fear Rape

←——1——————2——————3——————4——————5——————6——————7——————8——→

Economic Partnership   Psychic Rape   Acquaintance Rape   Violent Rape

1. **Freely consenting.** Partners with equal power mutually choosing sexual activity. Equal power means each partner has equal status, knowledge, and ability to consent. This includes one partner agreeing to engage in sexual activity, even if not interested, as an expression of love and caring for the other person.
2. **Economic partnership.** One person agrees to sexual activity as part of an economic agreement. The type of sexual behaviors permitted are mutually determined as part of the economic agreement.
3. **Seduction.** One party attempts to persuade the other to engage in sexual activities.
4. **Psychic rape.** Assault to another person's dignity and self-respect, such as verbal abuse, street ha-

rassment, or the portrayal of violence or pornography in the media.
5. **Bribery or coercion.** The use of emotional or psychological force to persuade the other to take part in sexual activities. This includes situations of unequal power between the individuals, especially when one person is in a position of authority.
6. **Acquaintance rape.** Sexual assault occurring when one party abuses the trust of a relationship and forces the other into sexual activities.
7. **Fear rape.** When one party engages in sexual activities out of fear of potential violence if she resists.
8. **Violent rape.** When violence is threatened or occurs. This includes forced sexual activity between spouses, acquaintances, or strangers.

---

for the victim, since she often must continue to interact with the rapist because of her dependence on him. In addition, many victims do not seek health care or the support of family members or friends because of embarrassment or humiliation.

Rape and sexual assault are important to nursing because nurses treat victims in the hospital and the community and because they fear for their personal safety. Several aspects of the practice of nursing places nurses at an increased risk for sexual assault by strangers: hours of employment, home visiting in the community, and for some nurses, a reluctance to create a scene or defend themselves aggressively. In recent years nurses who were sexually assaulted in hospital parking lots or on hospital property have successfully sued the hospital for negligence in not providing adequate security.[82]

■ **Nursing care of the sexual assault survivor**

■ NURSING ASSESSMENT. An important consideration in the treatment of victims of rape and sexual assault is the initial assessment. Although most nurses would quickly recognize the woman brought to the emergency department by the police following an attack by a stranger, many victims of sexual assault are

not readily identifiable. Therefore all nursing assessments need to include questions to determine current or prior sexual abuse. Since people have different definitions of rape, the assessment question needs to be broadly stated, such as that suggested by Russell[85]: "Has anyone ever forced you into sex that you did not wish to participate in?" This question may uncover other types of sexual trauma, such as incest, date rape, or sexual abuse as a child. When the answer is affirmative, it can be gently followed with broad questions, such as "Can you tell me more about it?" or "How often has it happened?" Often the response may be an embarrassed laugh or a hesitant or querying response. When this occurs, the nurse can increase the client's comfort by explaining that the question is routinely included because sexual assault is not uncommon and that the nurse is available to assist the woman in obtaining legal or social services.

■ NURSING INTERVENTIONS. When assessment indicates that abuse has occurred, it cannot be ignored. As noted by Campbell,[16] disclosing sexual abuse is an indication of trust. If the nurse responds by immediately referring the client elsewhere, the message given is that the problem is too distasteful or delicate for the nurse to handle or that there are serious psychological implications. Therefore assessment carries a responsibility for immediate intervention of nonjudgmental listening and psychological support. In addition, if a recent attack is disclosed, physical evidence will be needed, the collection of which is an appropriate responsibility for nursing. Later interventions may include referrals to survivors' groups, shelters for battered women (in instances of marital rape), or legal services.

People respond to sexual assault differently depending on their past experiences, personal characteristics, and the amount and type of support received from significant others, health care providers, and the criminal justice system. Burgess[12] describes a two-phase reaction to sexual assault. The acute stage, immediately following the attack, is characterized by extreme confusion, fear, disorganization, and restlessness. Some victims, however, may mask these feelings and appear to be outwardly calm or subdued.

The second phase involves the long-term process of reorganization and generally begins several weeks following the attack. This phase may include intrusive memories of the traumatic event during the day and while asleep; fears; or phobias such as extreme fears of being alone, in a crowd, or traveling. Following a sexual assault, the victim frequently has a sense of living in a dangerous, unpredictable world and may become preoccupied with feelings of victimization and vulnerability. She may encounter difficulties in sexual relationships or her ability to relate comfortably to men. Some victims develop secondary phobic reactions to people or situations that remind them of the attack.

Coping strategies may include changing one's phone number or residence, talking with friends or family, or taking classes in self-defense. Nursing actions to assist the survivor of sexual assault include active listening, empathetic responses, active concern and caring, assistance in problem solving, and referral to sexual assault crisis centers. The box below demonstrates a sample nursing care plan for the victim of sexual assault.

Nursing Care Plan for Rape and Sexual Assault

Case History: Eighteen-year-old Jane visits the student health center at the university, initially complaining of painful urination. As part of the nursing history the nurse learns that Jane was sexually assaulted by her boyfriend last evening. Jane has not told anyone because she feels guilty and "it was partially my fault. We went to a party and I had too much to drink. We were kissing in his apartment and then he wouldn't stop. It's not like I was raped or anything, he didn't use a knife or gun; he just wouldn't take no for an answer. Last night when I got home, I took a hot shower and cried myself to sleep. This morning he acted like nothing happened."

Nursing Diagnosis: Rape-trauma Syndrome

Goals

1. Jane will express feelings related to the assault, including guilt, fear, and vulnerability.
2. Jane will identify supportive people to assist in dealing with this crisis.
3. Jane will receive medical care for vaginal bruising, pregnancy testing, and venereal disease screening.

Interventions

1. Allow Jane to discuss feeling regarding assault.
2. Approach topic of "date rape" to allow Jane to determine if this is what she believes happened to her.

3. Communicate knowledge and understanding of emotional responses to sexual assault (i.e., women often experience various feelings in this situation, such as guilt, shame, embarrassment, and anger) to assist in identification of feelings.
4. Provide anticipatory guidance regarding common physical, psychological, and social responses. The nurse may state, "Even though you feel OK now, you might have a delayed reaction tonight when you will suddenly become fearful or anxious. Do you have a friend whom you can call on if this happens? Can you stay with this friend if you need to?"
5. Explore parental relationships with Jane. Encourage her to discuss the situation with supportive family members.
6. Advise her of the potential for venereal disease or pregnancy and that further medical care is indicated.
7. Support decision making and active problem solving
8. Provide written information regarding community services (e.g., rape crisis center hotlines) and encourage Jane to use them.
9. Plan for a follow-up phone contact within a few days.

DIRECTIONS FOR FUTURE RESEARCH

The following are some of the nursing research problems raised in Chapter 32 that merit further study by psychiatric nurses:

1. The effect of violence during pregnancy on the health of the mother and infant, including the relationship with low birth weight
2. The effects of different cultural group's values and beliefs regarding women, children, and elders on specific forms of family violence
3. The effective coping strategies of survivors of family violence and specific nursing interventions to support effective coping
4. Testing the effectiveness of various nursing interventions for survivors of violence, including group interventions
5. The most effective nursing assessment strategies for survivors and perpetrators of violence
6. Differing responses to rape and sexual assault and the most effective nursing strategies to assist in recovery
7. Short-term and especially the long-term effects of family violence on those not directly victimized (e.g., children of battered women, siblings of abused children).
8. Testing of nursing interventions for primary and secondary prevention of violence in families
9. Developing and testing various strategies for changing attitudes within the health care system toward survivors of violence
10. Ways to enhance identification of victims and perpetrators of violence in the health care system, especially in settings other than the emergency room.

SUMMARY

1. Nursing assessment for all forms of family violence and sexual abuse needs to be incorporated in all nursing histories and physical examinations.

2. There are certain characteristics of abusers that have been identified as risk factors, but very few demographic or personality traits would help identify persons victimized or at risk to be abused.

3. Persons who are physically abused, regardless of age, show a characteristic pattern of injuries: multiple, proximal rather than distal, and in various stages of healing.

4. Whenever one type of abuse is encountered, there needs to be a high index of suspicion for other types of violence occurring, either to the same person or another family member.

5. Sexual abuse must be assessed specifically and separately because such information will not be volunteered.

6. Nursing interventions first must consider the physical safety of those abused and/or sexually assaulted and then interventions for both the survivors and those perpetrating the violence.

7. When the victim is under age 18 or a physically or mentally dependent adult, the law provides that suspected (not necessarily substantiated) *abuse must* be reported by nurses to the local protective services agency. When the violence is severe enough to be a felony (as in all cases of rape, violence involving a weapon, and/or serious injury), all states require reporting to the police regardless of the survivor's age. In some states, all forms of wife abuse must also be reported to the police.

8. Following the determination of the client's safety, responses to the violence can be dealt with. From school age through old age, group interventions have been found to be useful for those experiencing violence.

■ REFERENCES ■

1. Abramson LY, Seligman MEP, and Teasdale JD: Learned helplessness in humans: critique and reformulation, J Abnorm Psychol 87:49-74, 1978.
2. Alexander CS: Blaming the victim: a comparison of police and nurses' perceptions of victims of rape, Women Health 5(1):65-79, 1980.
3. American Nurses' Association, 1980, p 9.
4. American Psychiatric Association: Diagnostic and statistical manual of mental disorders, ed 3, revised, Washington, DC, 1987, The Association.
5. Becker JV and Coleman EM: Incest. In Van Hasselt VB, et al, editors: Handbook of family violence, New York, 1988, Plenum Publishing Corp.
6. Berk R, et al: Mutual combat and other family violence myths. In Finkelhor D, et al, editors: The dark side of families: current family violence research, Beverly Hills, Calif, 1983, Sage Publications, Inc.
7. Bersani C and Chen H: Sociological perspectives on family violence. In Van Hasselt VB et al, editors: Handbook of family violence, New York, 1988, Plenum Publishing Corp.
8. Bowker LH: Beating wife-beating, Lexington, Mass, 1983, Lexington Books.
9. Brendtro M and Bowker HL: Battered women: how can nurses help, Issues Ment Health Nurs 10:169-180, 1989.
10. Briere J and Runtz M: The trauma symptom checklist (TSC-33) early data on a new scale, J Interpersonal Violence 4(2):151-163, 1989.
11. Browne A: When battered women kill, New York, 1987, The Free Press.
12. Burgess A: Rape trauma syndrome: a nursing diagnosis, Occup Health Nurs 33(8):405-406, 419-422, 1985.

13. Burgess AW, et al: Child molestation: assessing impact in multiple victims, Arch Psychiatr Nurs 1(1):33-39, 1987.

14. Campbell JC: Misogyny and homicide of women, Adv Nurs Sci 3(2):67-85, 1981.

15. Campbell JC: Nursing assessment for risk of homicide with battered women, Adv Nurs Sci 8(4):36 51, 1986.

16. Campbell JC: A test of two explanatory models of women's responses to battering, Nurs Res 38:18-24, 1989.

17. Campbell JC and Humphreys JC: Nursing care of victims of family violence, Reston, 1984, Prentice-Hall, Inc.

18. Campbell JC and Sheridan D: Emergency nursing interventions with battered women, J Emerg Nurs 15(1):12-17, 1989.

19. Cannon C: Violent verdict: connecting TV and real-life aggression, The Washington Post, p. D5, 1989.

20. Chapman J and Gates M, editors: The victimization of women, Beverly Hills, Calif, 1978, Sage Publications, Inc.

21. Conte JR: The effects of sexual abuse on children: a critique and suggestions for future research, Victimology: An International Journal, 1-4, 110-130, 1985.

22. Conte JR and Scheurman JR: The effects of sexual abuse on children, J Interpersonal Violence 2:380-390, 1988.

23. Damrosch SP: How nursing students' reactions to rape victims are affected by perceived act of carelessness, Nurs Res 30:168-170, 1981.

24. Damrosch S, et al: Nurses' attributions about rape victims, Res Nursing Health 10:245-251, 1987.

25. Davis LV and Carlson BE: Attitudes of service providers toward domestic violence, Soc Work Res Abstracts 81:34-39, 1981.

26. DiPietro SB: The effects of intrafamilial child sexual abuse on the adjustment and attitudes of adolescents, Violence Victims 2:59-78, 1987.

27. Disbrow M, Doerr H, and Caufield C: Measuring the components of parents' potential for child abuse and neglect, Child Abuse Neglect 1:279-296, 1977.

28. Dobash RE and Dobash RP: Violence against wives, New York, 1979, The Free Press.

29. Dobash RE and Dobash RP: Research as social action: the struggle for battered women. In Yllo K and Bogard M, editors: Feminist perspectives on wife abuse, Newbury Park, Calif, 1988, Sage Publications, Inc.

30. DuCette J and Keane A: Why me? An attributional analysis of a major illness, Res Nurs Health 7:257-264, 1984.

31. Dutton DG: The domestic assault of women, Newton, Mass, 1988, Allyn & Bacon, Inc.

32. Elbow M: Theoretical considerations of violent marriages, Soc Casework 58:515-526, 1977.

33. Faller KC: The myth of the "collusive mother," J Interpersonal Violence 3:190-196, 1988.

34. Feinauer L: Comparison of long-term effects of child abuse by type of abuse and by relationship of the offender to the victim, Am J Fam Ther 17(1):48-56, 1989.

35. Finkelhor D: Common features of family violence. In Finkelhor D, et al, editors: The dark side of families: current family violence research, Beverly Hills, Calif, 1983, Sage Publications, Inc.

36. Finkelhor D and Pillemer K: The prevalence of elder abuse: a random sample survey, Gerontol Soc Am 28(1):51-57, 1988.

37. Finn J: The stresses and coping behavior of battered women, Soc Casework 86:341-349, 1985.

38. Freire P: Pedagogy of the oppressed, New York, 1972, Herder & Herder.

39. Frieze IR: Perceptions of battered wives. In Carroll DB, Carroll JS, and Frieze IR, editors: New approaches to social problems, San Francisco, 1979, Jossey-Bass, Inc, Publishers.

40. Gelles R and Cornell C: Intimate violence in families, Beverly Hills, Calif, 1985, Sage Publications, Inc.

41. Gilligan C: In a different voice, Cambridge, Mass, 1982, Harvard University Press.

42. Gioglio GR and Blakemore P: Elder abuse in New Jersey: the knowledge and experience of abuse among older New Jerseyans, Trenton, New Jersey Department of Human Services, Beverly Hills, Calif, 1983, Sage Publications, Inc.

43. Goldberg WG and Tomlanovich MC: Domestic violence victims in the emergency department, JAMA 251:3259-3264, 1984.

44. Gondolf EW: The effect of batterer counseling on shelter outcome, J Interpersonal Violence 3(3):275-289, 1988.

45. Gondolf EW, Fisher E, and McFerron R: Racial differences among shelter residents: a comparison of anglo, black, and hispanic battered, J Fam Violence 3(1):39-51, 1988.

46. Gordon L: Heroes in their own lives, New York, 1988, Viking Press.

47. Hampton RL and Newberger EH: Child abuse incidence and reporting by hospitals: significance of severity, class, and race. In Hotaling GT, et al, editors: Coping with family violence: research and policy perspectives, Newbury Park, Calif, 1988, Sage Publications, Inc.

48. Hart B: Beyond the "duty to warn": a therapist's "duty to protect" battered women and children. In Yllo K and Bograd M, editors: Feminist perspectives on wife abuse, Newbury Park, Calif, 1988, Sage Publications, Inc.

49. Hedin BA: A case study of oppressed group behavior in nurses, Image 18(2):53-57, 1986.

50. Helton A, McFarlane J, and Anderson E: Battered and pregnant: a prevalence study, Am J Public Health 77(10):1337-1339, 1987.

51. Hoffman-Plotkin D and Twentyman CT: A multimodal assessment of behavioral and cognitive deficits in

abused and neglected preschoolers, Child Dev 55:794-802, 1984.

52. Hollencamp M and Attala J: Meeting health needs in a crisis shelter: a challenge to nurses in the community, J Community Health Nurs 39(40):201-209, 1986.

53. Hotaling GT and Straus M: The social causes of husband-wife violence, Minneapolis, 1980, University of Minnesota Press.

54. Hotaling GT and Sugerman D: An analysis of risk markers in husband to wife violence: the current state of knowledge, Violence Victims 1:101-124, 1986.

55. Humphreys JC: Implications for nursing. In Campbell JC and Humphreys JC: Nursing care of victims of family violence, Norwalk, Conn, 1984, Appleton-Century-Crofts.

56. Humphreys JC: Dependent care with battered women and their children, MAIN Res Rep 1990. (In press).

57. Jehu D: Mood disturbances among women clients sexually abused in childhood, J Interpersonal Violence 4(2):164-184, 1989.

58. Journal of the American Medical Association: AMA diagnostic and treatment guidelines concerning child abuse and neglect, JAMA 254(6):796-800, 1985.

59. Kelly L: How women define their experiences of violence. In Yllo K and Bograd M, editors: Feminist perspectives on wife abuse, Newbury Park, Calif, 1989, Sage Publications, Inc.

60. Kempe CH and Helfer R: The battered child, Chicago, 1980, University of Chicago Press.

61. King MC and Ryan J: Abused women: dispelling myths and encouraging interventions, Nurse Pract 14(5):47-58, 1989.

62. Kitson GC: Attachment to the spouse in divorce: a scale and its application, J Marriage Fam 44:379-393, 1982.

63. Kurz D: Emergency department responses to battered women: resistance to medicalization, Soc Problems 34:501-513, 1987.

64. Landenburger K: Conflicting realities of women in abusive relationships, Communicating Nurs Res 21:15-20, 1988.

65. Landenburger K: A process of entrapment in and recovery from an abusive relationship, Issues Ment Health Nurs 10:209-227, 1989.

66. Launius MH and Jensen BL: Interpersonal problem-solving skills in battered counseling and control women, J Fam Violence 2(2):151-162, 1987.

67. Leonard K and Jacob T: Alcohol, alcoholism, and family violence. In Van Hasselt VB et al, editors: Handbook of family violence, New York, 1988, Plenum Publishing Corp.

68. Lerner JM and Simmons CH: Observer's reaction to the "innocent victim," J Pers Soc Psychol 4(2):203-210, 1966.

69. Loseke DR and Cahill SE: The social construction of deviance: experts on battered women, Soc Problems 31(3):296-310, 1984.

70. Miller DT and Porter CA: Self-blame in victims of violence, J Soc Issues 39:139-152, 1983.

71. Millor G: A theoretical framework for nursing research in child abuse and neglect, Nurs Res 30:78-84, 1981.

72. Murphy SM et al: Current psychological functioning of child sexual assault survivors, J Interpersonal Violence 3:55-79, 1988.

73. Newbern V: Sexual victimization of children and adolescent patients, Image 21(1):10-14, 1989.

74. Okun LE: Woman abuse: facts replacing myths, Albany, NY, 1986, State University of New York Press.

75. Orem DE: Nursing: concepts of practice, ed 3, New York, 1985, McGraw-Hill Book Co.

76. Parker B and Schumacher D:. The battered wife syndrome and violence in the nuclear family of origin: a controlled pilot study, Am J Public Health 67(8):760-761, 1977.

77. Perry M, Wells E, and Doran L: Parent characteristics in abusing and nonabusing families, J Clin Child Psychol 12:329-336, 1983.

78. Phillips L: Abuse and neglect of the frail elderly at home: an exploration of theoretical relationships, J Adv Nurs 8:379-392, 1983.

79. Phillips LR and Rempusheski VF: Decision-making model for diagnosing and intervening in elder abuse and neglect, Nurs Res 34:134-139, 1985.

80. Pillemer K: Social isolation and elder abuse, Response Victimization Women Children 8(5):1-4, 1985.

81. Pillemer K and Suitor J: Elder abuse. In Van Hasselt VB, et al, editors: Handbook of family violence, New York, 1988, Plenum Publishing Corp.

82. Regan W: Rape on hospital property: now you can sue, RN, 69-70, 1983.

83. Rew L: Long-term effects of childhood sexual exploitation, Issues Ment Health Nurs 10:229-244, 1989.

84. Rothblum ED: Sex role stereotypes and depression in women. In Franks V and Rothblum ED, editors: The stereotyping of women: Its effects on mental health, New York, 1983, Springer Publishing Co, Inc.

85. Russell D: Rape in marriage, New York, 1982, Mac-Millan Publishing Co, Inc.

86. Russell D: The secret trauma: incest in the lives of girls and women, New York, 1986, Basic Books.

87. Ryan J and King MC: A study of the health care needs of women experiencing violence in their lives. In Proceedings of Third Nursing Network on Violence Against Women, Concord, Calif, 1989.

88. Ryan W: Blaming the victim, New York, 1976, Vintage.

89. Saunders GD and Rose K: Attitudes of psychiatric and nonpsychiatric medical practitioners toward battered women: an exploratory study, Unpublished doctoral dissertation, University of Wisconsin, 1988.

90. Schechter S: Women and male violence: the visions and struggles of the battered women's movement, Boston, 1982, South End Press.

91. Schur EM: The politics of deviance: stigma contests

and the uses of power, Englewood Cliffs, NJ, 1986, Prentice-Hall, Inc.

92. Shipley SB and Sylvester DC: Professionals' attitudes toward violence in close relationships, J Emerg Nurs 8(2):88-91, 1982.

93. Sommers EK and Check JVP: An empirical investigation of the role of pornography in the verbal and physical abuse of women, Violence Victims 2(3):189-209, 1987.

94. Stark E and Flitcraft AH: Spouse abuse. In Surgeon General's Workshop on Violence and Public Health source book, Atlanta, 1985, US Public Health Service.

95. Stark EF and Frazier W: Medicine and patriarchal violence: the social construction of a "private" event, Int J Health Serv 9(3):461-493, 1979.

96. Starr R: Physical abuse of children. In Van Hasselt VB, et al, editors: Handbook of family violence, New York, 1988, Plenum Publishing Corp.

97. Steinmetz S and Straus M: Intrafamily violence. In Steinmetz S and Straus M, editors: Violence in the family, New York, 1974, Harper & Row Publishing, Inc.

98. Straus M: Stress and child abuse. In Kempe C and Helfer R, editors: The battered child, ed 3, Chicago, 1980, University of Chicago Press.

99. Straus MA and Gelles RJ: Societal change and change in family violence from 1975 to 1985 as revealed by two national surveys, J Marriage Fam 48:465-479, 1986.

100. Strube MJ and Barbour LS: The decision to leave an abusive relationship: economic dependence and psychological commitment, J Marriage Fam 45:785-793, 1983.

101. Stuart EP and Campbell JC: Assessment of patterns of dangerousness with battered women, Issues Ment Health Nurs 245-260, 1989.

102. Torres S: Hispanic-American battered women: why consider cultural differences? Response 10(3):20-21, 1987.

103. Ulrich YC: Cross-cultural perspective on violence against women, Response Victimization Women and Children 12(1):21-23, 1989.

104. Walker LE: The battered women, New York, 1979, Harper & Row, Publishers, Inc..

105. Walker LE: The battered women syndrome, New York, 1984, Springer Publishing Co, Inc.

106. Walsh D and Liddy R: Surviving sexual abuse, Dublin, 1989, Attic Press.

107. Wolfe DA and Mosk MD: Behavioral comparisons of children from abused and distressed families, J Consult Clin Psychol 49:633-640, 1983.

108. Yllo K and Bograd M, editors: Feminist perspectives on wife abuse, Newbury Park, Calif, 1988, Sage Publications, Inc.

■ ANNOTATED SUGGESTED READINGS ■

*Campbell JC: A survivor group for battered women, Adv Nurs Sci 8(2):13-20, 1986.

Describes nurse-facilitated group intervention using Lifton's model to provide affirmation support to battered women. Demonstrates importance of control, body image damage, alternatives to end the violence, and decision making about ending the relationship.

*Campbell JC: Nursing assessment for risk of homicide with battered women, Adv Nurs Sci 8(4):36-51, 1986.

Presents beginning evidence of reliability and validity of an instrument to assess the danger of spousal homicide, a frequent outcome in battering relationships. Designed to increase a battered woman's self-care agency by enhancing her ability to predict whether she was likely to kill or be killed by her abusive partner.

*Campbell JC: A test of two explanatory models of women's responses to battering, Nurs Res 38:18-24, 1989.

Compares battered and nonbattered women also having problems in an intimate relationship. Groups were not significantly different on most measures (e.g., self-esteem, depression, self-blame, self-care agency). Supports both a grief and a learned helplessness model.

*Campbell JC and Alford P: The dark side of marital rape, Am J Nurs 89:946-949, 1989.

Documents the serious physical effects of marital rape. Part of a cooperative effort to change state law.

*Campbell JC and Humphreys JC: Nursing care of victims of family violence, Norwalk, Conn, 1984, Appleton-Century-Crofts.

Only nursing text totally concerned with family violence. Presents theory, research, and nursing care for child abuse, wife abuse, sexual assault, and elder abuse. Discusses the role of nursing in cooperation with the legal and law enforcement systems.

*Corman BJ: Group treatment for female adolescent sexual abuse victims, Issues Mental Health Nurs 10:261-272, 1989.

Describes the dynamics of traumatic sexualization, betrayal, powerlessness, and stigmatization in terms of resulting symptoms and group intervention strategies for each.

*Damrosch S, et al: Nurses' attributions about rape victims, Res Nurs Health 10:245-251, 1987.

Discusses the feelings of registered nurses who were given one of four written accounts of a woman's rape while whe was driving to a drugstore after work.

Dutton DG: The domestic assault of wives, Newton, Mass, 1988, Allyn & Bacon, Inc.

Gives an overview of the recent research on batterers and treatment programs for batterers. Demonstrates that court-mandated treatment is the most effective.

Feinauer L: Comparison of long-term effects of child abuse by type of abuse and by relationship of the offender to the victim, Am J Fam Ther 17(1):48-56, 1989.

---

*Asterisk indicates nursing reference.

Shows that the most devastating psychological effects appear when the victims were abused by a trusted person known to them. Family relationship was less important than the emotional bond violated by the perpetrator.

Gondolf E and Fisher E: Battered women as survivors, Lexington, MA, 1988, Heath & Co.

Based on research with over 6000 survivors of abuse in Texas. Challenges current assumptions regarding abused women as helpless and passive. Describes help-seeking strategies employed by the survivors, a typology of abusers, and policy implications.

*Helton A, McFarlane J, and Anderson E: Battered and pregnant: a prevalence study, Am J Public Health 77(10):1337-1339, 1987.

Reports on percentages of 290 pregnant women receiving prenatal care who reported abuse before, during, after the pregnancy.

*Houck GM and King MC: Child maltreatment: family characteristics and developmental consequences, Issues Ment Health Nurs 10:193-208, 1989.

Presents a comprehensive research review of the cognitive, social, and emotional outcomes for children who have been abused and neglected.

*Landenburger K: Conflicting realities of women in abusive relationships, Communicating Nurs Res 21:15-20, 1988.

Describes stages in the recovering and healing process of women who have survived abusive relationships. Emphasizes that recovery may vary for individual women but often may last for years.

*Lenehan G, Bowie S, and Ruksnaitis N: Rape victim protocol and chart for use in the emergency department, J Emerg Nurs 9(2):83-90, 1983.

Offers a concise guide for the emergency room nurse in dealing with victims of sexual assault. Includes guidelines for collecting evidence, legal considerations of charting, appropriate medications for potential venereal diseases, and special considerations with child and adolescent patients. Includes sample documentation chart.

NiCarthy G: Getting free: a guide for women in abusive relationships, Seattle, 1982, Seal Press.

Assists the woman in objectively evaluating the relationship and her feelings about the abuser. Offers practical advice on such issues as finding shelter; evaluating lawyers, physicians, and counselors; and dealing with the abuser and her children.

*Phillips L: Abuse and neglect of the frail elderly at home: an exploration of theoretical relationships, J Adv Nurs 8:379-392, 1983.

Explores the correlates of elder abuse, such as economic strains, social isolation, and environmental problems within a symbolic interactionist framework.

Walsh D and Liddy R: Surviving sexual abuse, Dublin, 1989, Attic Press.

For survivors of childhood sexual abuse. Includes a summary of the types of assaults, common responses of survivors, strategies for long-term healing and recovery, and case studies and vignettes.

White E: Chain, chain, change: for black women dealing with physical and emotional abuse, Seattle, 1985, Seal Press.

Covers topics such as the psychology of abuse, effects of violence on the children, and dealing with the legal, police, and medical systems from the perspective of black women.

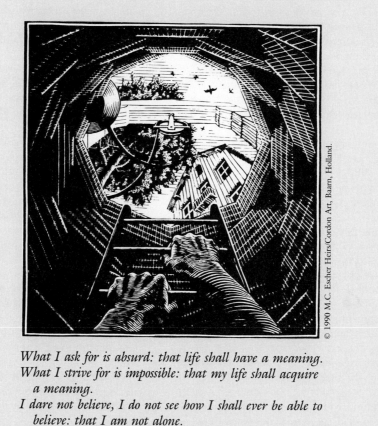

What I ask for is absurd: that life shall have a meaning.
What I strive for is impossible: that my life shall acquire
a meaning.
I dare not believe, I do not see how I shall ever be able to
believe: that I am not alone.

Dag Hammarskjold, Markings*

C H A P T E R 33

CARE OF THE CHRONICALLY MENTALLY ILL PATIENT

RUTH WILDER BELL

SANDRA E. BENTER

*Hammarskjold D: Markings, New York, 1966, Alfred A. Knopf, Inc. (Translated by L Sjoberg and WH Auden.)
Reprinted by permission of Faber & Faber, Ltd, and Alfred A Knopf, Inc.

After studying this chapter, the student should be able to:

- discuss the impact of deinstitutionalization on the care of the chronically mentally ill.

- identify legal issues that have influenced the treatment of the chronically mentally ill.

- describe the evolution of a chronic mental illness, including the development of primary and secondary symptoms.

- assess the nursing care needs of chronically mentally ill patients based on data concerning problem areas and strengths.

- compare and contrast the characteristics of chronically mentally ill young adults with those of older patients.

- describe the elements of psychosocial rehabilitation programs.

- describe the importance of psychoeducation for patients and their families.

- discuss stresses affecting the family with a chronically mentally ill member.

- analyze the role of the nurse caring for seriously mentally disabled patients in community and acute care settings.

- discuss nursing interventions based on the assessed needs of chronically mentally ill people.

- identify directions for future nursing research.

- select appropriate readings for further study.

Before the advent of phenothiazines as treatment for chronically mentally ill patients in the 1950s, these patients lived primarily in large public psychiatric hospitals that were located in rural areas, distant from the populations they served.

The identification and location of the chronically mentally ill and the nurses who care for them is more difficult in the 1990s. In the decade following the CMHC movement of the mid 1960s, the resident population of state and county mental hospitals decreased by two thirds, with less than 4% of those Americans diagnosed as having a severe mental disorder residing in state mental hospitals.[4,6,10,29] While a slight increase in state hospital admissions is projected for the mid 1990s, the vast majority of mentally ill patients will continue to live in the community settings.[24] Nurses now care for the chronically mentally ill in a variety of health care settings: private and public psychiatric hospitals, psychiatric and medical-surgical units in general hospitals, emergency rooms, community-based treatment programs, and patients' homes.

As the "careers" of the discharged chronically mentally ill unfold, there are likely to be periods when they cannot be maintained in the community, and rehospitalization is necessary. As patients alternate between community-based and hospital-based care, nurses in both community-based and inpatient facilities share responsibility for their care. Knowledge of the special needs and characteristics of the chronically mentally ill as a population is important for all nurses who care for these patients, in whatever setting the care may be given.

Social perspective

■ Policy issues

Deinstitutionalization is the term used to describe the process of moving long-term mental hospital patients back into the community, where they are to be supported by a "formal network of clinical, social, and vocational agencies, as well as by an informal network of family, neighbors, and local community resources."[31] Implicit in the concept of deinstitutionalization is the assumption that a network of community resources exists to meet the needs of the chronically ill.

The move to develop resources needed to return

the long-term or chronic psychiatric patient to the community was initiated by a 1961 report of the Joint Commission on Mental Illness and Health. Actual construction of facilities to provide community-based treatment for these patients was made possible by the 1963 Mental Retardation Facilities and Community Mental Health Centers Construction Act. Policy statements by Presidents Kennedy, Johnson, and Nixon further supported the goal of community-based treatment for the mentally ill. President Carter established a second commission on mental health in 1977 to determine and make recommendations about the nation's mental health needs. Two of the many recommendations of the final report of the President's Commission on Mental Health were that a federal grant program be established to develop "comprehensive integrated systems of care" and that the chronically mentally ill be one of the groups receiving funding priority.[38] In the mid 1970s federal initiatives supported the devlopment of the community support program, a program designed to coordinate and provide psychiatric and medical care, housing, and social support for chronically mentally ill individuals.[46]

The development of chronic mental illness

The chronically mentally ill are likely to have both primary and secondary symptoms of their illness. Primary symptoms are those associated with the nature of the illness. For example, hallucinations, delusions, and inappropriate affect are primary symptoms of schizophrenia, and elation and hyperactivity are primary symptoms of manic-depressive illness. Secondary symptoms arise as a consequence of the illness process. They are not only associated with the disability of chronic illness but also perpetuate its existence. The progression from primary to secondary symptoms and ultimately the label "chronically mentally ill" are clarified by more specific examination of the interaction between an individual and his environment.

The behaviors of mentally ill individuals associated with primary symptoms are likely to violate social norms and standards of proper conduct and may be considered deviant behaviors. These deviant behaviors set in motion a social interactive process whereby society protects itself from the deviant person's norm violation. For example, individuals while demonstrating an intellectual understanding of mental illness may oppose the establishment of a group home for the chronically mentally ill in their communities. As this social-interactive process unfolds, individuals increasingly assume the self-identity "mentally ill." They begin to relate to society in terms of this identity rather than in

terms of other available identities, such as wife, mother, husband, father, or worker. The person's ultimate acceptance of the deviant status and his adjustment to society in terms of this role are accompanied by the many secondary symptoms of chronic mental illness.

■ Social interaction model

The interactive process by which society confers and the individual accepts the role of deviant for the chronically mentally ill person has been outlined by Lemert[41] in the following eight steps:

1. Individual instances of deviant behavior; role and status are not defined at this time in terms of a deviant identity
2. Social penalties
3. Further deviant behavior
4. Stronger penalties, and rejection of the individual with the deviant behavior
5. Further deviant behavior, perhaps with hostilities and resentment beginning to focus on those doing the penalizing
6. Crisis reached in society's tolerance quotient, expressed in formal action by the community stigmatizing the deviant
7. Strengthening of the deviant conduct as a reaction to the stigmatizing and penalties
8. Ultimate acceptance of deviant social status, and efforts at adjustment based on an associated role

■ Public health model

As Lemert's social interaction model demonstrates, the disability of chronic mental illness does not suddenly appear, but develops over time as an exchange between an individual with deviant behaviors and the world in which he lives. Similarly, through their attention to the "natural history" of chronic illness, public health epidemiologists view chronic illness not as a state or endpoint but as a process of deterioration. According to the public health model, individuals with chronic illness show increasing symptoms of functional impairment and disability as they move through the four stages of the "natural history" of chronic illness. The first stage, **susceptibility,** is a period of exposure to risk factors. The second stage, **presymptomatic disease,** is the period within which pathological changes begin. The third stage, **clinical disease,** is the period within which primary symptoms of the disease are recognizable. The fourth stage, **disability,** is the period within which there are identifiable changes in both activity level and role perfor-

TABLE 33-1

STAGES OF THE NATURAL HISTORY OF CHRONIC ILLNESS

Stage	Characteristics
Susceptibility	Presence of environmental, biological, behavioral, and emotional risk factors
Presymptomatic disease	No overt symptoms of disease; pathological changes begin; risk factors intensify; behaviors increasing susceptibility solidify and become patterns
Clinical disease	Anatomical and functional changes occur; presence of recognizable disease symptoms
Disability	Disease symptoms increase; anatomical and functional changes produce reduction in activity; impairment of instrumental or expressive function

Modified from Anderson S and Bauwens E: Chronic health problems: concepts and application, St Louis, 1981, Mosby–Year Book, Inc.

mance.[2] Table 33-1 summarizes the characteristics of these four stages. Psychiatric disability occurs because the chronically mentally ill person does not have the skills necessary to meet the environmental role requirements.[38]

Description of the chronically mentally ill

A 1984 survey of clients enrolled in a community support program confirmed that the chronically mentally ill are less likely to be married, have fewer years of education, and with a 25% employment rate, are less likely to be employed than the population at large.[46] Other characteristics influencing the course of their illness are their consistently low self-esteem and preoccupation with avoiding failure rather than with achieving success.[60] The chronically mentally ill, as a group, can be described not only in terms of the problems confronting them but also in terms of their unique strengths and potentials. There is tentative evidence that the kinds of interpersonal strengths available to this population differ from those available to the general population.

■ Activities of daily living

When nurses refer to activities of daily living (ADL), they usually mean the behaviors necessary to maintain independence in personal hygiene, dressing, and grooming. In reference to the chronically mentally ill, the term has an expanded meaning: the skills necessary to live independently as an adult. Professionals who care for the chronically mentally ill also use the broader term **psychosocial rehabilitation** to refer to development of the many skills necessary for independent living.

If one accepts the premise that the chronically mentally ill relate to their world essentially in terms of the role "mentally ill," it follows that these patients have difficulty meeting the multiple functional requirements of an adult. Impairment in instrumental role performance is one of the characteristics of disability, the end stage of the progressive deterioration of individuals with chronic mental illness.[2] As noted by Goldman, individuals are considered legally disabled when their instrumental role performance is impaired in at least three of the following areas: "self-care, receptive and expressive language, learning, mobility, self-direction, capacity for independent living, and self-sufficiency."[28]

■ Interpersonal relations

Over the years, patients in public mental hospitals have been described as apathetic, withdrawn, isolated from other patients and their family, and possessing only the minimum of interpersonal skills. The process leading to impoverished interpersonal relations has been thought to be a secondary symptom resulting from adaptation to life in a rigid and nonstimulating environment. The term **social breakdown syndrome** was coined to describe the progressive deterioration of the social and interpersonal skills of long-term psychiatric patients.[31] However, it is becoming clear that chronically mentally ill patients who have spent most of their lives in the community have the same deterioration of social and interpersonal skills as those who have had long-term hospitalizations. Studies of the social activities of the chronically mentally ill suggest that these patients "lead an unusually barren and isolated existence."[45] A study of all nonhospitalized California residents who received Social Security because of a psychiatric disability showed that fewer than 50% were employed or had any structured activity around which to orient their lives.[29] The question must now be asked whether the social breakdown syndrome of the chronically mentally ill is causally related to long-term hospitalization, or whether there might be another explanation. Minkoff[45] wrote, "Those who tend to be more active socially tend to be less chronic, married, and employed, and characterize a group of high functioning mentally ill whose lives stand apart from the more dreary existence of the rest."

■ Lack of coping resources

The social isolation, lack of support systems, and functional impairment of the chronically mentally ill leave them with minimal skills to use in coping with stress. Social margin, as defined by Segal, Baumohl, and Johnson,[63] is the sum of "all the personal possessions, attributes, or relationships which can be traded on for help in time of need." It is, in effect, the sum of resources available to the individual. With a nearly nonexistent social margin, the chronically mentally ill are likely to respond to stress and the necessity for adaptation as a crisis. (See Chapter 9.)

■ Need for long-term treatment

Implicit in the idea of chronicity is the concept of illness over time. Federal policy makers label patients as having a "chronic mental disability" when they have had either one episode of at least 6 months of continuous hospitalization within 5 years or two or more hospitalizations in a 12-month period.[45] Given the marginal existence of the chronically mentally ill in the community and their vulnerability to stress, it is not surprising that within a year of their discharge from the hospital, 40% are readmitted.[5] Treatment factors that help a patient's remaining in the community are compliance with a medication regimen and involvement in aftercare programs.[45] Because of the need for long-term treatment, the proper focus of treatment for the chronically mentally ill is care and rehabilitation rather than cure.

■ Low self-esteem

Self-esteem is the feeling or sense of regard that accompanies individuals' self-perceptions. It is "the personal judgment of worthiness that is expressed in the attitudes of an individual to himself . . . it indicates the extent to which an individual believes himself to be capable, significant, worthy."[18] Fitts[25,26] found the self-esteem of psychiatric patients to be lower in all areas, especially in the areas of identity and behavior, than the self-esteem of the general population. The self-esteem of the chronically mentally ill parallels that of psychiatric patients,[12] and the chronically mentally

ill suffer from the many perceptual and behavioral difficulties associated with low self-esteem. (See Chapter 13.) A description of the individual with low self-esteem is also a description of the chronically mentally ill individual:

> Persons with low self-esteem . . . have come to believe they are powerless and without resource or recourse. They feel isolated, unlovable, incapable of expressing and defending themselves, and too weak to overcome their deficiencies. Too immobilized to take action, they tend to withdraw and become overly passive and compliant while suffering the pangs of anxiety and symptoms that accompany its chronic occurrence.[18:250]

■ Motivation

As described earlier, the chronically mentally ill have difficulty achieving a level of psychosocial functioning that would allow them to live comfortably in the community. For many patients, success and greater competence result in increased anxiety and symptoms of regression rather than in pride and the sense of improved well-being. Patients attribute their uneasiness with success to the fear that once they succeed, even more will be expected of them, and they may not be able to meet the new expectations.

Chronically mentally ill patients have experienced repeated failures. They have not met the expectations of family, friends, or society. Most important, they have not met their own expectations. They view new experiences as opportunities for further failure rather than as opportunities for growth. Studies of psychiatric patients living both in institutions and in the community support the observation that when compared with the general population, psychiatric patients are more concerned with avoiding failure than with achieving success.[60] This not only leads them to avoid new experiences but also makes it difficult for the chronically mentally ill to acknowledge and assume responsibility for their achievements.

■ Strengths

Rehabilitation of the chronically mentally ill depends on the control of illness, as well as on the development of health potential by mobilizing patients' ego strengths. A strength is an "ability, skill, or interest" an individual has previously used.[48] An emphasis on patient strengths provides hope that improvement functioning is possible.[7] Categories of individual strengths, as derived from work with assumed healthy nonpsychiatric patient groups, are as follows:

Sports and outdoor activities
Hobbies and crafts

Expressive arts
Health
Education, training, and related areas
Work, vocation, job, or position
Special aptitudes or resources
Strengths through family and others
Intellectual strengths
Aesthetic strengths
Organizational strengths
Imaginative and creative strengths
Relationship strengths[49]

Although the assessment and description of patients' strengths are largely an individual matter and the profile of strengths varies from patient to patient, there is evidence that the relationship strengths of the chronically mentally ill differ from those of a nonpatient population.

Porter[55] defined interpersonal strength as a "behavior trait . . . so employed as to enhance the production of mutual gratification between one's self and another person without violating the integrity of either person." According to Porter, interpersonal strengths cluster around three basic motivational patterns, or orientations: "altruistic-nurturing," "assertive-directing," and "analytic-autonomizing" patterns. Associated with each of the motivational patterns are positive goals for interpersonal relationships. Individuals with strengths associated with the altruistic-nurturing motivational pattern report that their goal in interpersonal relations is to be genuinely helpful, with little regard for what they consequently receive from others. Individuals having strengths associated with the assertive-directive pattern desire to lead others in a way that does not interfere with others' rights. The goal behind the strengths associated with the analytic-autonomizing motivational pattern is to create order, becoming self-reliant and independent. The interpersonal strengths of the nonpatient population are evenly divided among the three motivational patterns and represent nurturing strengths, leading strengths, and analyzing strengths (Table 33-2).

Initial evidence suggests that the relationship strengths of the chronically mentally ill are not evenly divided among the three motivational patterns. When interpersonal relationships are going well, chronically mentally ill persons see themselves as mobilizing the nurturing strengths of the altruistic-nurturing motivational pattern. They feel good about themselves when they are caring for someone else with little regard for what they receive in return. In conflict situations their strengths are those of the peacemaker. Aware of the personal cost of their peacemaking efforts, they will insist, probably explosively, that their rights be respected if harmony and peace cannot be restored.[12]

TABLE 33-2

BEHIND THE WEAKNESSES ARE STRENGTHS

Altruistic-nurturing		Assertive-directing		Analytic-autonomizing	
Characteristic strengths	Risks	Characteristic strengths	Risks	Characteristic strengths	Risks
Trusting	Gullible	Self-confident	Arrogant	Cautious	Suspicious
Optimistic	Impractical	Enterprising	Opportunistic	Practical	Unimaginative
Loyal	Slavish	Ambitious	Ruthless	Economical	Stingy
Idealistic	Wishful	Organizing	Controlling	Reserved	Cold
Helpful	Self-denying	Persuasive	Pressuring	Methodical	Rigid
Modest	Self-effacing	Forceful	Dictatorial	Analytic	Nitpicking
Devoted	Self-sacrificing	Quick to act	Rash	Principled	Unbending
Caring	Smothering	Imaginative	Dreamer	Orderly	Compulsive
Supportive	Submissive	Competitive	Combative	Fair	Unfeeling
Accepting	Passive	Proud	Conceited	Persevering	Stubborn
Polite	Deferential	Bold	Brash	Conserving	Possessive
Adaptable	Without principle	Risk taking	Gambler	Thorough	Obsessive

From Porter E and Maloney S: Strength deployment inventory: manual of administration and interpretation, Pacific Palisades, Calif, Personal Strengths Assessment Service, Inc.

The young adult chronically mentally ill patient

■ Characteristics

The characteristics of the chronically mentally ill previously discussed describe such patients regardless of their age. However, the young chronic patient, generally between the ages of 18 and 35, differs in important ways from the chronically mentally ill over 35 years of age. Many of the differences in the two groups can be traced to the deinstitutionalization movement and the development of community-based care.[51]

Generally, chronically mentally ill patients under 35 have not experienced lengthy psychiatric hospitalizations. For those under 35, recurrent short hospitalizations at times of crisis or during periods of acute exacerbation of symptoms have alternated with care in the community. The personal adaptations necessary for long-term hospitalization are different from those necessary for community life interspersed with short hospitalizations.

Patients who have spent years in psychiatric hospitals have been confronted over and over with their personal failure to meet their own, their family's, and society's expectations. In most instances, older chronic patients have traded personal autonomy and adult role functioning for a life of personal dependence and the role of psychiatric patient. Through socialization into this role, chronic patients become compliant and nonassertive, and their social participation becomes limited to the social and geographical boundaries of the hospital or ward where they live. Although such adaptation provides limited potential for growth, it does relieve the patient from seemingly impossible role expectations and continual confrontation with failure.

Younger chronically ill patients do not have such protection from messages about their inadequacy and the resulting sense of failure. Alternating between hospital and community life, they compare themselves with others of their age and continue to expect of themselves behavior similar to that of their nonpatient peers. They expect that they should marry, have children and jobs, and perhaps even acquire advanced education. Given their failure in managing these role expectations and their limited ability to cope with community living, it is not surprising that they are "acutely vulnerable to stress, and are characterized by a high incidence of alcohol and drug abuse, suicide and suicide attempts."[51,52] Generalizing from a study of nearly 300 patients, 42% of this population of young chronic psychiatric patients "present a risk of suicide for reasons that include the simple fact that they see no hope for the future."[51] They cannot see a future in which they will be able to meet the ongoing demands of their daily lives.

Unlike long-term hospital residents, younger chronically mentally ill patients are not characterized by docile, compliant behavior. They do not see themselves as mentally ill but as social casualties, unfortunate victims of social circumstances.[17,51] Not having been hospitalized for long periods, younger chronically ill patients have not been socialized into the compliant, nonassertive behavior associated with older patients. Their self-concepts, accompanied by their particular symptoms, especially disorders of impulse control and disturbances of affect,[62] have important consequences for supporting their marginal life-style.

■ Involvement in treatment

Because they do not see themselves as patients, young patients have little motivation to become involved in aftercare or treatment programs or to comply with a medication regimen. For example, a study of more than 100 young chronically mentally ill patients in New York City found that only 17% complied with their aftercare plan.[16] Aftercare programs and medication regimens have been identified as critical factors for maintenance of the chronically mentally ill in the community.

Further interfering with their involvement in a therapeutic relationship is the general response of anger, which manifests itself in the sarcastic and argumentive manner in which these patients relate to caregivers. Caregivers often report feelings of frustration and helplessness when confronted by the many problems of these patients, and the manner in which they seek help. This behavior has been labeled "help-seeking—help-rejecting behavior."

■ Drug and alcohol abuse

Many patients under 35 years of age have lived primarily in the community during the course of their mental illness and have been exposed to the same health risks as their contemporaries. It is not surprising, then, that young chronically mentally ill patients have a higher incidence of drug and alcohol abuse than older patients.[13,22] A survey of clients in a suburban New York Community Mental Health Center found that 37% of those between 18 and 35 abused alcohol; another 37% abused drugs.[51] Schwartz and Goldfinger documented abuse of multiple drugs by this population.[62] A more recent survey of the characteristics of younger chronically mentally ill patients found that 100% of the records of those under 25 years old referred to incidents involving drugs or alcohol.[17]

Drug and alcohol abuse compound the problems of young chronically mentally ill persons in a variety of ways. Mentally ill patients with an additional diagnosis of alcohol or drug dependence have been less successful in rehabilitation.[11] Young chronically mentally ill patients who abuse drugs or alcohol are more likely to be involved in acting-out behavior, both at home and in the community. Because age itself is not directly related to acting-out behavior, researchers have concluded that drug and alcohol abuse "appear to be largely responsible for the increased acting out" of younger clients.[42] And since psychosis may be drug induced, the problem of determining whether psychotic symptoms result from drug abuse or schizophrenia is difficult and may interfere with planning and implementing treatment.

■ Entry into the mental health system

Because their pathological condition interferes with voluntary involvement in treatment programs and ongoing participation in a therapeutic relationship, younger chronically ill patients are likely to enter the mental health system through hospital emergency rooms or the legal system. Younger patients may seek help from emergency rooms, either voluntarily or at the insistence of family or friends, during times of personal or family crisis. Behavior resulting from poor impulse control is often the precipitating event. Schwartz and Goldfinger[62] reported that although suicidal threats and self-damaging acts are common, impulsive acts against others are less frequent. However, many of these patients enter the mental health system through involvement with the law for offenses such as "minor property damage" and "petty assault." Likewise, Caton[16] found the arrest rate of young chronically mentally ill patients to be eight times that of the general population in the areas in which the patients lived.

Younger chronically mentally ill patients' symptoms and style of interpersonal relationships seem to interfere with their benefiting from present treatment resources. They are characterized by an "unwillingness or inability" to use conventional resources.[17]

■ Strengths

Initial descriptions of this population portrayed a troublesome group with particular deficits that interfered with their adjustment to community life and involvement in a rehabilitation program. More recent research also identifies strengths that are more likely to be available to this population than to the older chronically mentally ill population. In a survey of 844 clients of New York State's Community Support Service pro-

gram, 18% were under 35 years of age. When compared with older clients, younger clients were likely to be

> better educated, more proficient and independent in performing community living skills, actively engaged in significantly more healthy adult leisure activities, more likely to be competitively employed, more capable of living on their own instead of in supervised housing, more likely to be utilizing sheltered workshops and other vocational services, and less dependent on the Community Support System . . . for medical care or transportation.[35:50]

As a group younger patients have been found to be independent in meeting personal care needs and to possess strengths in terms of an ability to shop and travel.

Further description of this rapidly expanding subgroup must continue if programs suitable to their needs are to be developed.

Psychosocial rehabilitation: the Fountain House model

Ronald Peterson, a veteran of 10 years of residence in a state hospital, speaks poignantly of the loneliness and isolation he felt when he left the state hospital to live alone in a small hotel room. Since he had no job, knew no one, and lived on welfare, it never occurred to him that things could be any different. He said, "You take what you can get. There is no choice."[53] Eventually becoming a staff member of Fountain House, a psychosocial rehabilitation program, Peterson spoke for many chronically mentally ill persons trying to adjust to community living when he described their greatest need to be a place where they belong and are needed.

> I think the greatest need is to have a place to go where you are expected each day, a place where you can be with people like yourself and do things that mean something to yourself and others . . . you have to remember that many of us did a lot of things in the hospital. If given a chance we can do lots of things in the community—if we have places to go and can be with people who need us to contribute, to take part, to help, and who notice when we're not present and do something about it.[53:41,42]

In judging the effectiveness of any treatment program for the chronically mentally ill, the program's readmission and employment rates are compared with baseline readmission and employment data.[45] It is expected that 6 months after leaving the hospital, 30% to 40% of the patients will be rehospitalized and that 30% to 50% will be employed. The percentage employed decreases to 20% to 30% after 12 months and to 25% after 3 to 5 years. Despite a lack of adequate follow-up studies, it is generally believed that community-based treatment programs, while increasing in both number and quality, are not adequate to meet needs.

Fountain House, an early psychosocial program, has been described as an excellent program for helping chronically ill psychiatric patients to make a place for themselves in the community. It has been used as a model in developing programs across the country.[3,15,66] Information about rehospitalization of Fountain House participants provides evidence of the program's effectiveness. For the first 5 years after returning to the community, Fountain House members have a 40% lower rehospitalization rate than the baseline percentage. After 9 years, Fountain House's rehospitalization rates are similar to the baseline rate. However, when hospitalization is needed, Fountain House members are hospitalized for only half the usual number of days.[19] Critical to Fountain House's success is attention to psychosocial rehabilitation, especially in facilitating independent living and employment.

Incorporating elements from the medical, rehabilitation, and social support models, psychosocial rehabilitation provides a variety of living and work opportunities to accommodate patients' individual needs and abilities. Staff not only help patients develop necessary skills, but they serve as buffers between the patient and the community. In a sense, they lend their own skills and competency to the patients until the patients can develop these skills for themselves. Compensating for patients' functional inadequacies while encouraging them to assume increasing responsibility allows the patients to experience the pride of achievement rather than the pain and humiliation of failure. Basic to this rehabilitation process is focusing on the strengths of Fountain House members.

Fountain House attributes the state of isolation and alienation of its new members to the process of illness that initially brings the members to Fountain House—but it is the strengths and capabilities of each individual that validate his belonging and are the beginning of the discovery that he is worth something and may be able to achieve at least reasonably full participation in community life.[15:86]

Fountain House functions as a club in which patients are members. The usual hierarchical distinctions between staff (the healthy) and patients (the ill) do not exist. It is a place where members care about each other and pool their resources and abilities as they work toward increasing independence. Thus Fountain House combats loneliness and isolation while providing a variety of living and work situations that require differing levels of functional ability.

The first month at Fountain House is a residential phase, and residents are taught skills necessary for apartment living. Fountain House owns and leases apartments that have staff on call, although not in residence. These supervised apartments allow patients to make a gradual transition to independent living in the community.

Fountain House runs several businesses itself and can provide a protected environment in which patients can develop both self-confidence and job skills. Progressing to a more complex work situation, Fountain House has creatively arranged for transitional employment placements, called TEPs. Recognizing that job interviews are tremendously stressful for recently discharged psychiatric patients, staff, rather than patients, seek out and contract with businesses for jobs. The jobs are assigned to Fountain House rather than to individual patients. Staff are then free to assign a patient to a transitional employment position for as long as needed. The employer is promised that if patients are unable to manage the job or do not show up, Fountain House staff will cover for them. With such an arrangement, the dreaded employment interview is avoided. Fountain House members, who share responsibility for a job with staff, can be given increasing responsibility as they are able to handle it. A TEP can easily be transferred from a member who is ready for a more complex work experience to a member who needs a TEP. Furthermore, employers are satisfied because the quality of work is guaranteed by the staff.

Between 1977 and 1982, Fountain House, with funding from the National Institute of Mental Health, implemented a national training program in the principles of psychiatric rehabilitation upon which the program is based. By 1982, the number of clubhouses based on the Fountain House model had increased from 18 to 148; the number of transitional employment programs from 21 to 102; the number of participating employers from 122 to 507; and the number of job placements from 360 to 1154.[3] Spurred on by mounting evidence that the functional level and quality of life of the chronically mentally ill can be improved by the development of their physical, emotional, and intellectual skills within a supportive environment, clinicians are beginning to use psychiatric rehabilitation principles in designing inpatient programs. There is initial evidence that recidivism decreases and employment and quality of life are positively affected when an inpatient program is based on the principles underlying the Fountain House model.[11,20] More than a decade's experience with model psychosocial rehabilitation programs such as Fountain House has shown that despite variations from one community to another, basic principles underlie effective programs.

Throughout the country psychosocial rehabilitation programs are improving the quality of care for the chronically mentally ill.[17]

Psychoeducation

Psychoeducation is the use of educational methods, techniques, and principles to rehabilitate and treat the mentally ill.[9] Psychoeducation is an important treatment component in psychosocial rehabilitation programs, in which the primary concern is the development of skills rather than the development of insight. In addition to fostering skill development, psychoeducation is used to teach patients about their illness and its management. This information counteracts misconceptions about mental illness and helps patients collaborate and actively participate in their treatment. For example, if patients are taught about the side effects of psychotropic medication, they will be better able to help find the lowest dose that comfortably controls their symptoms; if they are taught about symptoms of their illness, they can recognize early warnings of relapse and ask for help in coping, perhaps avoiding rehospitalization. Psychoeducation is a powerful therapeutic tool in increasing patients' self-esteem and offering hope. When patients are treated as though they are able to learn difficult information and expected to use that information to improve the quality of their lives, they gain some control over their lives and a sense that improvement is possible.[3,9,38] Nurses are increasingly using psychoeducation as an intervention to improve the quality of life for chronically mentally ill clients.[34,47,54]

For families of patients experiencing a first admission, hospitalization provides the hope that "things will be different" in the future. At discharge, however, families express disappointment that the desired changes have not occurred, and they frequently view the patient as not ready for discharge.[40,59] After reviewing a number of studies, Goldman[28] concluded that about 62% of hospitalized psychiatric patients are discharged to their families, and, of these, about 25% are severely ill at the time of discharge. Acknowledging that families are often asked to care for the chronically mentally ill without the necessary expertise, clinicians are beginning to provide psychoeducation for family members, with the hope that families' acceptance and ability to manage the illness will increase. Family sessions usually include information about schizophrenia, its cause and symptoms, treatment approaches, psychotropic medication, management of behavioral problems, and how to deal with crisis.[9] Families can be taught about the consequences of schizophrenia for an individual and how to help patients cope with their environment in a way that minimizes stress on the rest of the family.[33] Family psychoeducation has been successful in decreasing symptoms and avoiding the rehospitalization of chronically ill family members.[23]

Family implications

One aspect of deinstitutionalization receiving increased attention is deinstitutionalization's effect on patients' families. Community care implies increased responsibility and the stress that accompanies that responsibility for families with caregiving roles. Researchers have attempted to identify specific stresses or burdens and have concluded in general it is the unpredictable, embarrassing, threating, violent, and emotionally abusive behaviors that are daily stressors for families of psychiatric patients.[21,32,56,64]

Hatfield[32] describes the needs of family members. She encourages mental health care providers to build alliances with families. She conducted a survey of 89 families of schizophrenic patients. She was able to identify the following patient behaviors or results of behaviors that are most disturbing to families:

1. Tension related to unpredictable behavior
2. Irregular sleep patterns that keep other family members awake as well
3. Mealtime disruptions
4. Argumentativeness
5. Negative relationships with siblings
6. Marital discord between parents

Although one might expect families to be angry at the patient for creating a disrupted family life or guilt for possibly playing a role in the problems, Hatfield elicited more feelings of grief and depression. If anger was present, it was usually directed at fate or the system rather that the patient.

Doll[21] conducted a survey of significant others of psychiatric patients. Whereas the Hatfield group was mostly upper middle class, the Doll group of 125 respondents was a mostly lower middle and lower class. The finding of the two studies were consistent. The Doll group also denied shame or guilt connected to the patient's problem. These families were also able to accept some degree of deviant behavior, although there was a limit to their tolerance. High deviance did eventually lead to a decrease in acceptance of the patient. These families expressed the fear that there would be little or no change in the patient's condition. This was expressed as a feeling of being trapped.

Sources of stress for families of the chronically mentally ill have been reviewed and identified by Baker.[8] A sense of loss of future hopes and goals,[36,57] stigma,[65] guilt,[43] constant realignment of family structure,[43] and depletion of financial resources have been the most frequently cited stresses. Hatfield's study[32] listed the following as the needs most frequently cited by families of psychiatric patients: (a) knowledge; (b) peer support; (c) respite services; and (d) crisis services. Families first and foremost want to be able to understand the patient's behavior and how to repsond helpfully to it (See the section on psychosocial education earlier in this chapter.)

The second need identified by the families in Hatfield's study[32] was to have someone with whom they could talk. Most of the people surveyed were self-help group members and had found that their peer support was helpful to them. The National Alliance for the Mentally Ill has been actively engaged in promoting the development of peer support groups for families of mentally ill people.

The third need was for respite care resources. Respite care provides supervision for the patient in a community setting when the family needs relief from their demands of a mentally ill member. This service allows families to take a vacation or spend a short time away from the patient without feeling guilt that they would if the patient was rehospitalized.

The final need was for crisis services, including home visiting. It can be very difficult for a family to persuade a disturbed member to go to a treatment facility, particularly if the patient has been hospitalized in the past and suspects that he will be again. Families are sometimes forced to wait until the situation becomes so bad that they must call the police to take the patient into custody. Crisis intervention in the home would avert this distressing situation. Home visiting is an acitvity that is generally accepted by nurses, who are in turn usually well received in the community. Home health care and other outreach programs need to be made available to patients who are unwilling or unable to participate in other forms of outpatient care and other outreach programs.

Nursing care of the chronically mentally ill

Although the chronically mentally ill have similar needs whether they are being cared for in inpatient units, community psychosocial rehabilitation programs, or emergency service, the health care setting influences the scope and priorities of nursing care.

■ Psychosocial rehabilitation programs

Nurses working in community-based psychosocial rehabilitation programs are ultimately concerned with helping patients achieve their fullest potential for independent living and interpersonal relations. In this situation, nurses have the opportunity for long-term ongoing relationships with patients and the mutual setting of long-term goals. The nurses' functions will vary. For example, they may be on call to assist patients living in supervised apartments. Others may be active participants in a day treatment milieu, both creating situations for growth and serving as process observers to the patient so that he may analyze his behavior in the therapeutic milieu. Nurses may also provide a formal educational experience, such as teaching patients about community resources, skills necessary for independent living, or self-care behaviors that facilitate health maintenance. They may participate in a variety of work programs with patients or even back a patient up in a transitional work placement. If the nurse has had advanced training and supervision, he or she may function in the expanded role of group leader or co-leader, conduct family meetings, or assume responsibility as the patient's primary therapist.

In most psychosocial rehabilitation programs, the nurse works as a team member with other mental health professionals and nonprofessionals. Although the role and function of the nurse are always bounded by the state nurse practice act, they vary depending on the nature of the program and the available resources. In some programs the nurse may be asked to function as "case manager" for a group of patients. This role is explained in the section below on case management.

■ Acute care settings

Conceptualizing care of the chronically mentally ill as a shared responsibility between the community and residential inpatient facilities means that the focus of care differs in different settings. Because the chronically mentally ill are likely to leave community treatment programs, have difficulties complying with a medication regimen, and are acutely vulnerable to stress, they experience periods of acute exacerbation of symptoms when they need inpatient hospitalization. The goal of care in an acute treatment setting then becomes crisis resolution, with control of acute symptoms. The patient is helped to return to a precrisis level of functioning as quickly as possible, so that he can return to the community, where he can receive support and treatment in a less restrictive environment.

As with any acutely ill psychiatric patient, the nurse, after completing a nursing assessment, makes a nursing diagnosis and plans interventions that help the patient cope with his behavioral responses to his illness. Because chronically mentally ill patients enter inpatient units for crisis intervention, the nurse working in such a setting must thoroughly understand the theory of crisis intervention and be skilled in its implementation. The specific factors to be assessed as the nurse explores the crisis and its effect on the patient are those identified in Chapter 9. That is, the nurse assesses the precipitating event, the patient's strengths and previous coping mechanisms, and the nature and strength of the patient's support systems. Intervention may occur at any of four levels: environmental manipulation; general support; generic intervention, especially grief work; and, particularly, individual intervention. Individual intervention depends on an understanding of the meaning of the precipitating event to the patient at that particular time and an awareness of the resources available. An individual approach, by definition, is idiosyncratic and depends on the development of a competent nurse–patient relationship.

Primary nursing, one of several ways of providing nursing care, has several advantages in meeting the needs of chronically mentally ill patients hospitalized during acute periods.[61] The most obvious advantage is that, once assigned a primary nurse, the acutely ill patient, who is likely to have difficulties establishing interpersonal relationships, knows who is responsible for his care and can focus his energies on developing a trusting relationship with one person. And, because the chronically mentally ill patient is likely to have recurrent inpatient admissions, the same primary nurse can be assigned to him for each admission.

Consistent assignment of patients to primary nurses for each admission has advantages for both patients and nurses. It is probably easier for an acutely ill patient to feel safe when cared for by a nurse he already knows. Prior knowledge of the patient, including the patient's past responses to particular nursing interventions, can expedite nursing care on subsequent admissions. It can also facilitate family and community involvement in the patient's care, since the primary nurse, agency staff, and family members have already established working relationships.

But perhaps an even more important consequence of primary nursing and consistency of assignment is the primary nurse's sense of the patient's progress over time. If the patient has been making incremental gains, however small, in a community rehabilitation program, the goal of crisis therapy during admissions would be return to a steadily increasing functional level. Thus the primary nurse in an acute care setting can document the patient's progress in the community. These observations can then be used to combat the feelings of discouragement and hopelessness that both the nurse and patient sometimes feel. Further discussion of primary nursing is found in Chapter 24.

■ Case management

Since the chronically mentally ill experience periods of symptom exaccerbation and remission, they require a variety of mental health and community services at various points in time. Case management is "a systematic process of assessment, planning, service coordination and/or referral, and monitoring through which the multiple-service needs of clients are met."[50]

Various models of case management for the chronically mentally ill exist in the community, and there is controversy regarding which model is most effective and which category of mental health workers is best qualified to provide the service.[44] Since nurses possess knowledge of the biological and social sciences and can link mental health, health, and community services, they are well equipped to serve as case managers.[67]

The ANA has developed a model for nursing case management that consists of interaction, assessment, planning, implementation, and evaluation. It is the interaction with patients, families, nurses, and other providers that delineates case management as a specific type of psychiatric nursing care. That interaction and coordination assist patients and families in obtaining the appropriate mix of services at any given time.

■ Developing patients' strengths and potentials

Rehabilitation has been described as the "process of actualizing the remaining potentialities and abilities of a handicapped person."[27] Psychosocial rehabilitation programs, such as Fountain House, attribute their success to focusing on patients' strengths. The rehabilitation model of care is concerned both with maximizing wellness and with controlling disease. Nursing also accepts responsibility for promoting wellness and improving patients' health by developing their health potentials. This view of nursing is consistently reflected in the models of nursing that nursing scholars are developing.

The following discussion focuses on nursing interventions that help develop patients' strengths and potentials. Such interventions are part of the nursing process, with the development of an individual plan of care only after completion of a nursing assessment. The principles of developing and implementing nursing care plans for psychiatric patients, as described in this text, also apply in the care of chronically mentally ill patients.

The development of chronically mentally ill patients' strengths and potentials is important for several reasons. Nursing interventions that develop patients' strengths and potentials can help the chronically mentally ill develop their independent living skills, interpersonal relationships, and coping resources, and thus help meet their special needs. Such nursing interventions also help patients alter their motivational style, thus making them more willing to become involved in growth-producing situations. Ultimately, the expected

outcome of such interventions is changes in the patient's self-concept and an increase in self-esteem.

Dr. Vallory Lathrop, a leader in forensic psychiatric nursing, remarked that she would be pleased to receive a nickel from every patient who, when asked to name one of his strengths, responded that he did not have any. The negative self-concept and low self-esteem that characterize the chronically mentally ill interfere with their ability to see themselves as individuals with strengths and potentials.

Rogers[58] wrote that a therapeutic experience was one in which experiences contradictory to the individual's self-concept were brought into awareness and accepted as part of the self. Through experiences of adequacy, self-concept can be altered and self-esteem increased. One nursing intervention that helps patients alter their negative self-perceptions is for the nurse to describe the patient's strengths as the nurse perceives them. Nursing interventions in which patients become aware of their strengths fall into two categories: those which occur spontaneously and those which are planned. The following clinical examples illustrate the nurse's use of two spontaneously occurring situations to increase a patient's awareness of her strengths.

Although the strengths identified in these examples, caring and helping, are consistent with the altruistic-nurturing motivational pattern that is most characteristic of this population, they are not the only strengths which occur spontaneously in the therapeutic milieu. Patients have many opportunities for demonstrating behaviors reflective of strengths in leadership, problem solving, or increased autonomy. A different kind of strength is evident in Clinical example 33-2.

CLINICAL EXAMPLE 33-1

During a 1-hour period a nurse made the following observations. Marie, a frightened 22-year-old young woman who was psychotic as the result of PCP use, was sitting in the craft room. The nurse joined Marie. Janet, another patient, came in and heaped clothes that were still warm from the dryer in Marie's lap. (Janet had voluntarily done Marie's laundry when she noticed Marie having trouble with the dial on the washing machine.)

JANET: **Here are your clean clothes.**

MARIE: Silence, continues drawing.

NURSE: **Do you want some help folding these clothes? It looks hard to draw with such a full lap.**

MARIE: **No, I'm fine, except my head gets dizzy.**

JANET: **That's from your medicine. Didn't you just start on your medicine?**

MARIE: **Yes.**

JANET: **It'll get better soon. It takes a few days to get used to your medicine. You're drawing a Christmas picture. Merry Christmas and Happy New Year. You're thinking about wanting to be home for Christmas aren't you?**

MARIE: **Nods her head yes.**

JANET: **Your picture sure makes me think of how nice home is at Christmas, except we don't have a fireplace. But having a fireplace doesn't make Christmas. Being home with a family you love does.** (Janet continues showing the nurse other artwork that Marie has done, praising her ability.)

Another patient and the recreational therapist came into the room. The therapist changed the music from soul music to a classical symphony. Both Janet and Marie disapproved of the new music. Marie began to look more tense. Janet put her arm around her and said, "Come on. Let's go walk in the hall." They left together.

Later, when the nurse saw Janet in the dayroom, the nurse shared with Janet that she saw her as having been very helpful to Marie. Janet grinned broadly and said "Yeah, I'm a real friend to her. It feels good."

CLINICAL EXAMPLE 33-2

A nurse walking down the hall saw a patient who had made a serious suicide attempt 2 days earlier alone in the kitchen furiously cleaning out the refrigerator. The nurse joined the patient and began to help her. As they talked, the patient expressed concern that many of the feelings that led to the previous suicide attempt were returning. She had initiated the cleaning project to attempt to control her feelings. The nurse defined the cleaning as a strength in that it was more adaptive than another suicide attempt. As the nurse shared this observation with the patient, the patient momentarily looked surprised and then said, "I hadn't thought of it that way. Maybe I am better than I was before."

CLINICAL EXAMPLE 33-3

Theresa, a woman in her fifties, had been in and out of psychiatric hospitals for 30 years and had been living in a supervised apartment in the community for 1 year. One of her nursing diagnoses was difficulty in dealing with interpersonal conflict because of her fear of her aggressive impulses. Theresa shared the apartment with two roommates. She was a talented musician and had her own baby grand piano. Despite her love for classical music, she played only the "oldies and goodies" her roommates preferred. She said that she didn't want to upset her roommates by practicing classical music. She was afraid that if she brought the issue out in the open she might get so upset she would hurt someone. She offered as evidence the numerous times she'd been placed in seclusion rooms for violent behavior. Clearly, keeping peace was her priority.

The nurse and Theresa discussed her strengths as a peacemaker, as well as ways in which she might calmly express her own needs to her roommates. The nurse offered to be with Theresa during the discussion. Declining the nurse's offer, Theresa said that even though she was somewhat anxious, she had a clearer understanding of the abilities she had to use in the situation, and she wanted to try to "pick up" for herself in a situation of interpersonal conflict. She carried out her plan and expressed surprise that her roommates accepted her need and quickly arranged 2 hours a day for her to practice. As she told of her success, Theresa smiled, saying she wondered what would have happened if she

had tried expressing her needs many months earlier.

Cindy, in her early twenties, had recently moved into the supervised apartment with Theresa and one other roommate. One of Cindy's nursing diagnoses was ineffective individual coping related to low self-esteem and feelings of inadequacy. Cindy arrived at the day treatment program crying because she had had a seizure while at her nursing home job the evening before. She felt that in addition to having been embarrassed, she had failed to live up to the trust invested in her by the director of the nursing home. She had decided to quit her job.

The nurse explored with Cindy the meaning of these events in terms of her many strengths in caring for others. Her sensitivity to anticipated criticism and rejection from the director was related to the same sensitivity that allowed her to respond creatively to others' needs. Cindy, at this point, firmly stated that the job was important to her sense of being needed. The nurse encouraged her to call the nursing home, express both her embarrassment and sense of failure, yet state that she wanted to continue working there. Cindy made the phone call with the nurse present for support. Her pleasure at finding out the job was still hers, that she was not viewed unfavorably by the director of nursing, and her sense of personal achievement at having taken a risk and won was so visible and contagious that the other patients staged an impromptu celebration.

Nurses who have an ongoing therapeutic relationship with a small group of patients can provide individualized observations of strengths. These interventions may occur in response to spontaneous behaviors or to a structured growth experience. Clinical example 33-3 is an example of a structured nursing intervention that occurred in a community-based psychosocial rehabilitation program.

An initial research project by Bell[12] provided some support for the premise that educating the chronically mentally ill about their strengths increases their self-esteem. Bell also found that it is important for nurses to understand the meaning of observed behaviors to their patients, rather than to the nurse. For example, one woman who had been out of the hospital for 2 months, after having lived there 20 years, was seen as continually helping others. When the nurse shared this

observation with the patient, the patient responded, "Helping's good, but what really counts is that when I say I'll do something to help someone else, I can count on myself to do what I say." The nurse then redesigned her nursing care plan to include more opportunities for developing the patient's autonomy and independence. As the staff supported the patient's early efforts at independence and autonomy, the patient set increasingly complex goals for herself. As she achieved these goals, she expressed how good it made her feel to be able to maintain herself in an independent living situation after so many years in an institution.

For such interventions to be most effective, the nurse must maintain his or her professional identity and participate in the milieu with the patient. Within the context of a competent, caring nurse–patient relationship, psychiatric-mental health nurses can make

CLINICAL EXAMPLE 33-4

Abdul, the only son of a large and wealthy Middle Eastern family, came to the United States to pursue a graduate degree in engineering at a prominent university. He had been an outstanding student before coming to the United States but struggled all through his graduate education. He gravitated toward other international students, and most of his social activities were with this group of people. He became involved with Ingrid, a graduate student from Germany. When Ingrid became pregnant, they married. Both Abdul and his wife described the discovery of Ingrid's pregnancy as a crisis, but by the time their daughter, Begum, was born, they had reconciled themselves to their situation and, in fact, were excited by the baby's arrival.

Despite the precipitous nature of their marriage, the early years together were pleasant, with Abdul and Ingrid enjoying each other and their daughter. Both parents finished their graduate education, with Abdul finding work as an electrical engineer and his wife finding employment as an assistant professor in the history department of a 4-year college.

By the time the baby, Begum, was 5 years old, Ingrid's parents were living in the United States; there was much visiting between the two families. Since Abdul had not yet introduced Ingrid and Begum to his family, they planned a trip to the Middle East the summer Begum was 5. Abdul's father had a sudden heart attack and died before Abdul and his family arrived. The visit home did not go well. Abdul's family expressed much disappointment in him. They were disappointed that he did not meet the family's standards for material wealth and were even more disappointed that he had not married a Moslem woman. Despite the family's disappointment in Abdul, they exerted much pressure on him to change his plans to return to the United States and remain in the Middle East to assume his proper role as the only son, now the head of the family. At the same time, Ingrid, who was experiencing both culture shock and a feeling of nonacceptance by Abdul's family, insisted on an immediate return to the United States. Abdul returned to the United States feeling disappointed in himself because he had not met his family's expectations and also because he had not been able to speak out in defense of his wife and American daughter.

Life began to deteriorate for Abdul and his family after their return to the United States. Abdul resigned from his engineering position because he believed he wasn't being promoted quickly enough. Although he soon found a position with another reputable company, his work record was increasingly spotty. Some days, Abdul just couldn't make himself get up and go to work. On other days, he'd set out for work, but by midmorning would call Ingrid and tell her he was going to a movie or a museum, followed by a visit to his favorite bar and grill. Abdul found alcohol comforting and began drinking more and more. As Ingrid pressured Abdul to be more responsible about working, Abdul increasingly withdrew and spent much of the time he was home, alone, watching television in his bedroom. Partly in response to her loneliness and sense of helplessness as she watched her husband change, Ingrid overate and began a rapid weight gain, which was accompanied by other physical problems.

After 7 years of university teaching, Ingrid lost her job because she did not meet the requirements for tenure. She began job hunting, but before finding another job, she was involved in a serious car accident and was hospitalized for several weeks. Tension between Abdul and Ingrid increased as a result of the accident. Abdul believed there had been a man in the car with his wife at the time of the accident and accused her of having an affair. This belief was never substantiated, yet Abdul held on to it tenaciously. While his wife was hospitalized, Abdul cared for 7-year-old Begum. However, the day Ingrid returned home from the hospital, Abdul took their car and left, not telling anyone where he was going. After 2 weeks of wandering across the United States, Abdul returned to find he had been fired.

Abdul made no pretense of looking for another job. Welfare funds became the family's sole income. He spent most days alone in his room "tinkering" with one invention or another, listening to Middle Eastern music, or sleeping. Increasingly he slept during the day and stayed up all night. Formerly a fastidious man, he paid little attention to his personal hygiene or nutrition and continued his alcohol consumption. Although he never again left home for any extended time, he periodically disappeared for 2- or 3-day intervals. He always took the family car and was arrested several times for driving without a license or for driving while intoxicated. Invariably Abdul called his wife to rescue him. Ingrid would somehow find money to pay his fine or post bail and would bring him home, where he would once again retreat to his bedroom.

Five years after his visit to the Middle East, Abdul became involved in an altercation with a policeman who stopped him for speeding. As a result, Abdul was convicted of assault and served a brief jail sentence.

Ingrid convinced Abdul to seek psychiatric

CLINICAL EXAMPLE 33-4—cont'd

help after he was released from jail. He was admitted to an inpatient unit of a general hospital. He was given trifluoperazine (Stelazine), desipramine (Pertofrane), benztropine (Cogentin), and diazepam (Valium) and encouraged to participate in the ward milieu. He was not considered ready for discharge when his funds ran out 30 days later. At the encouragement of his psychiatrist, Abdul voluntarily admitted himself to the state mental hospital for continued treatment. Things did not go well for Abdul after his state hospital admission. Worried about Abdul's increasing nonresponsiveness to his environment, Ingrid supported and encouraged Abdul's leaving against medical advice after 3 weeks in the state hospital.

Abdul returned home still receiving medication. He was to attend a medication group at the local CMHC for regulation of his medication. However, he stopped taking his medication soon after he returned home because he did not like the side effects or the feeling that he was being controlled by the medications. He again withdrew to his room, lived a nocturnal existence, and occupied himself inventing electronic gadgets.

In the following year, Abdul made his first suicide attempt. He put a loaded gun into his mouth and pulled the trigger, but the gun didn't fire. He accused "men" who were always aware of his actions of coming into his house and making the gun nonfunctional by jamming it. Abdul was again hospitalized on a psychiatric unit in a general hospital in the community. He was once again given trifluoperazine (Stelazine), desipramine (Pertofrane), and benztropine (Cogentin) and was actively encouraged to participate in the ward milieu. After a month, his seclusive behavior had decreased enough that he was considered ready for discharge. The marital problems identified earlier had intensified sufficiently that couple group therapy was considered the aftercare treatment of choice, along with continuation of drug therapy. After discharge, Abdul unwillingly accompanied Ingrid to their appointments at the CMHC. He never actively participated in the sessions.

Ingrid occasionally sensed her husband's suffering and at those times felt compassion and caring for him. Generally, however, she felt anger toward Abdul and held him responsible for their predicament. She continued to deal with her frustrations by eating and now, because of her obesity, had difficulty getting around. She limited her trips outside the house to those absolutely essential. Because of health limitations and a general sense of despair about the family's situation, Ingrid became increasingly apathetic about the daily maintenance and upkeep of their home. Whenever possible, Begum, now 11, voluntarily accepted responsibility for family chores. She cooked simple meals, did laundry, cleaned house, and cut the grass. The family received some support from the next-door neighbor, who offered to help Begum with the heavy yardwork whenever he saw her struggling. Ingrid had long ago exhausted the support available from her friends and increasingly turned to Begum for companionship and emotional support.

In the next several years, Abdul and Ingrid were not involved in ongoing treatment. Ingrid would call a therapist at the CMHC at times of crisis, generally in response to her concern that Abdul was in physiological danger from not eating. In fact, during this 3-year period, Abdul was admitted five times to general hospitals because of his extreme withdrawal, which resulted in dehydration and other symptoms of malnourishment. Each time he was admitted because of these secondary symptoms, he also spent several weeks on psychiatric inpatient units, where he received treatment for his withdrawal. Abdul's improvement after drug therapy with major tranquilizers or antidepressants was only moderate. Each time Abdul was discharged with these medications, he immediately stopped taking them. On discharge, he would once again return to life in his bedroom and begin another sequence of isolation and progressive deterioration.

One of Abdul's discharge plans included a public health nursing referral. Home visits from the public health nurse helped monitor Abdul's condition but were ineffective in helping him keep his appointments at the CMHC, comply with his medication regimen, and decrease his seclusive behavior. The public health nurse was helpful in arranging for health care for Ingrid and Begum but was not able to help Ingrid alter her self-destructive behavior of using eating as a way of dealing with her own stress and frustration. By now Ingrid weighed over 250 pounds and was having serious health problems of her own.

The summer Begum turned 12, Abdul overheard a neighbor compliment her on her appearance. Abdul misinterpreted the neighbor's remark and accused the neighbor of making sexual advances toward his daughter. A loud argument followed. Abdul threatened his neighbor, telling him that if he ever saw him talking to his daughter again, he would come after him with a gun. As a result of this incident, Abdul and his family were ostracized and ignored by most of their neighbors. With no more help in outside home maintenance,

Continued.

Abdul and Ingrid's home, which was located in an upper middle class neighborhood, became increasingly run down. Abdul rarely went outside the house. Ingrid left home only to take care of essential errands and transport Begum. The years of impoverishment and dealing with chronic mental illness had taken their toll. Ingrid's world was her family, books, and television. No longer were there family outings or visits with friends. The concern had become getting through each day.

As she grew, Begum assumed more and more of the care of her parents. Yet despite her many home responsibilities, Begum did well in school and talked of wanting to be a doctor when she grew up. Begum's physical education teacher took a special interest in her and helped her develop natural gymnastics abilities to the point where she applied for and won a scholarship to a first-rate gymnastics school. Begum quickly made friends with two girls who also attended her gymnastics school and developed strategies to spend time with her friends, away from her home.

The family's life followed much the same pattern until the Christmas Begum was 14. Ingrid and Begum planned to visit Ingrid's parents for several days. Although Abdul had been invited, he refused to accompany his family on their trip. Two days after Ingrid and Begum left, Abdul again made a serious suicide attempt. He cut both wrists and watched them bleed, as he waited to die. Several times, the blood clotted and he had to reopen the wounds for the blood to continue flowing. As he became weaker and started shaking, Abdul feared his suicide attempt would not be successful. He stated that he called the ambulance because he was too weak to hang himself. Abdul was taken to a general hospital for emergency treatment and, after his physiological condition stabilized, he was taken nonvoluntarily to the state psychiatric hospital that served his geographical area.

Immediately on arriving at the state hospital, Abdul was assigned to a nurse who would be his primary nurse while he was on the admission unit. After a first-level assessment, his nurse determined his immediate needs to be care of his bilateral wrist sutures, protection from further self-destructive behaviors, and maintenance of an adequate nutritional intake. Abdul was immediately given suicide precautions, meaning he was always within arm's reach of a nursing staff member, except at night when he slept in an open seclusion room across from the nursing station. The primary nurse was able to spend the first hour of his suicidal precaution time with him. She used this time to begin a

relationship with Abdul, providing an initial orientation to her role as his primary nurse and to the ward, as well as finding out his immediate concerns. Abdul matter of factly expressed annoyance that suicide precaution measures were being used. He stated he was disappointed in himself in that he had not succeeded in killing himself and was determined to succeed on his next attempt.

The nurse also discovered that Abdul had spoken with his wife, who was still out of state, only once since his suicide attempt. The nurse's offer to arrange a phone conversation between Abdul and his wife was met with a positive response and a slight smile from Abdul. Before the nurse left that evening, she had discovered that Abdul, who had barely touched his lunch, preferred small meals to three large ones. In addition to leaving the nursing order that Abdul's nutritional intake be recorded, she requested that he be offered a snack at midafternoon and bedtime. The nurse also alerted the night staff to the possibility that Abdul might have difficulty sleeping because of his history of sleeping during the day and staying awake at night. If he did have difficulty sleeping, his primary nurse requested that staff stay with him and offer him hot chocolate or warm milk.

In the next few days, the primary nurse, in consultation with Abdul and the treatment team, developed a plan of nursing care for Abdul (Table 33-3).

When the nurse first began spending time with Abdul in an effort to develop a trusting relationship, he was unable to tolerate being in an office with her. He would either refuse to come into the office or, after 2 or 3 minutes, would become anxious and leave. The nurse, accepting him where he was, began sitting with him for periods of 10 to 15 minutes in the day hall. Sometimes they would work on a jigsaw puzzle together; sometimes they would carry on a conversation, essentially social in nature, and sometimes Abdul would use the time to sort out his reactions to living in a state hospital. Only rarely would he speak of his past life or personal concerns other than his adjustment to the hospital environment.

As Abdul began to trust the nurse, he accepted her invitation to meet at regular times in her office. Although he was able to stay for only 15 to 20 minutes before getting up and saying "I have to go now," he began to talk about his life and especially about his sense of humiliation at having failed in every area important to him. Despite the nurse's identifying growth he had made in the hospital, Abdul continued to believe there was no hope for the future, and suicide was the only alternative to a life as bleak as his.

Abdul had requested that he not be given medication. Because his history showed poor response to psychotropic medication, the psychiatrist did not order medication. However, after Abdul had been hospitalized 6 weeks, he shared with his primary nurse his belief that during one of his hospitalizations, in a procedure that left no scars, an electrode had been implanted through his nostril into his brain. He believed that his behavior was controlled by laser beams from a radio tower 20 miles away. Because his behavior was under external control, he considered himself to be a robot and thus was not responsible for his behavior. Once the psychiatrist was aware of Abdul's delusional system, intramuscular fluphenazine decanoate (Prolixin) was ordered for him. Seven days after his first injection, Abdul showed significant differences in behavior. He began to initiate conversations with other patients, voluntarily attended ward activities, began to take care of his own hygiene, and expressed an interest in being able to go out for walks. His talk of suicide decreased, and he began to doubt he was controlled by laser beams.

As part of Abdul's treatment plan, the primary nurse and a psychiatric nurse prepared at the master's degree level met with the family weekly to help the family become more functional and again enjoy being together. Interventions were directed toward improving family communication and helping the family reorganize itself so that the parents would assume more parental authority and Begum would become more like the 14-year-old she was, rather than continuing her role as the third adult in the family.

Two critical incidents illustrate the growth of Abdul, Ingrid, and Begum. The first incident occurred 3 months after Abdul's admission. In the family meeting, both Ingrid and Begum were speaking about the disrepair of their home. They focused on their inability, physically and financially, to maintain their home and their embarrassment that their home had become a neighborhood eyesore. Abdul told Begum he did not want her to undertake the heavy yardwork alone. He asked if he might return home to help with the yardwork and fix the plumbing. Although suicide precautions had been dropped only recently and Abdul was not ready for a weekend pass, the primary nurse wanted to support Abdul's initiative in assuming family responsibility. Arrangements were made for the primary nurse and the family therapist to take Abdul home for an afternoon. A potluck supper was planned, with both nurses and all three family members contributing to the effort. Abdul returned

from the trip home with new-found energy and a feeling of self-worth that came from having been needed and the sense of a job well done. The primary nurse capitalized on this experience by helping Abdul examine the sense of well-being, however fragile, that resulted from making a contribution, and suggesting that he become involved in the hospital work program. With much support, Abdul accepted her offer and began working in the hospital horticulture program.

The second incident occurred indirectly as a result of the home visit. After the potluck supper, Ingrid asked the primary nurse to look at some "sores" on her legs. The nurse was concerned not only about the large skin ulcers Ingrid showed her but also about the respiratory distress Ingrid was having. The nurse consulted a social worker who served as a liaison between the hospital and community, and, through the social worker, arrangements were made for Ingrid to be seen by a physician. After her appointment, Ingrid was hospitalized with pulmonary edema and skin ulcers. An old friend with whom Ingrid had recently reestablished contact was able to keep Begum for several days, but there was no one for Begum to stay with over the weekend. Abdul rose to the occasion and said he did not want his daughter home alone. He then marshalled his arguments and asked for a pass to go home and care for Begum. After much consideration, the psychiatrist and the primary nurse decided to let Abdul go home to be with Begum, provided the three following conditions were met: (1) the gun in Abdul's home was to be removed and brought to the hospital for safekeeping; (2) a written contract that specified activities and structure for the time Abdul was home was to be signed by Abdul, the psychiatrist, and the nurse; and (3) Abdul was to return to the hospital Monday morning on the bus. Abdul agreed to these conditions. He returned to the hospital grinning because the weekend had gone better than he had expected. He was especially proud that he had cooked dinner Saturday night and given Begum the best piece of meat.

Abdul's continued improvement was not without setbacks. However, after he had been hospitalized on the admission unit 5 months, he was transferred to an unlocked continued-care ward where rehabilitation would continue until he was ready for discharge. Abdul and his primary nurse met with the social worker who would be coordinating his treatment plan on the new ward to facilitate the transition. While Abdul was in the continued-care area, he worked with vocational rehabilitation and was judged capable of a sheltered workshop placement when he returned to the community. With an

Continued.

eye toward discharge and a desire to increase compliance with an eventual aftercare program, Abdul began making weekly visits home to attend family therapy sessions at the CMHC. On these visits home, he shared with Ingrid his fear that his life was destined to be one of limited functioning and recurrent hospitalizations.

On one of his last weekends before discharge, he had a longer than usual pass because he had a Monday afternoon appointment with the vocational rehabilitation center in the community. Tuesday morning, Ingrid called Abdul's primary nurse on the admissions unit. Abdul was dead. He had hanged himself the night before.

The primary nurse had her own personal grief to confront. Despite her caring and the best efforts of many professionals, the final choice was Abdul's. After struggling for many years, he chose the pain of death over the pain of life. The primary nurse was left with the hope that for a time, however brief, Abdul's life was less painful, that he had a momentary glimmer that life could be different, and that he had experienced the respect and positive regard she had for him. Out of her own grief, respect for Abdul, and continuing concern for his family, Abdul's primary nurse went to his funeral—and cried.

TABLE 33-3

ABDUL'S ABBREVIATED NURSING CARE PLAN

Nursing diagnosis	Intervention	Expected outcome
Inadequate nutritional and fluid intake related to feelings of worthlessness and hopelessness	Monitor input; offer juices; offer snack at 3 and 9 PM	Independent maintenance of adequate nutritional intake
Inadequate personal hygiene related to isolation and feelings of worthlessness and hopelessness	Help patient shave; remind him to bathe; have clean clothes available each day	Independent maintenance of personal hygiene
Sleep pattern disturbance related to withdrawal and isolation	Involve patient in ward activities so he stays awake during day; provide at least one exercise period a day; decrease stimuli and offer bath and warm milk at bedtime	Sleeps at night; stays awake during day
Self-destructive behavior related to feelings of worthlessness and hopelessness	Observe patient closely; be alert for suicidal thoughts; offer hope that future can be different	Investment in future
Social withdrawal related to distrust of others and feelings of inadequacy	Establish therapeutic nurse-patient relationship; invite patient to participate in structured activities, such as cards, chess, walks; help him transfer learnings from nurse-patient relationship to other relationships	Development of relationships with staff and patients
Misinterprets meaning of events in his environment related to social isolation and inadequate feedback	Listen for disorders in logical thinking; matter of factly offer alternate interpretations of events; listen to meaning behind distortions and idiosyncratic interpretation of events	Decrease in idiosyncratic interpretation of events; independence in seeking feedback regarding his interpretation of events
Negative self-concept and low self-esteem related to failure in meeting own and others' expectations	Identify personal strengths with patient; offer alternate view of self based on experiences of patient in milieu; develop nurse-patient relationship to help patient explore his feelings of worthlessness and make choices about future	Self statements reflecting realistic sense of abilities and limitations; willingness to make more productive choices in future

significant contributions to the care of the chronically mentally ill as they support them with one hand and, with the other hand, encourage them to expand their horizons by involvement in growth-producing experiences. As Minkoff[37] stated, "It is only when rehabilitation is not attempted, that hope is truly lost."

Clinical case analysis

Clinical example 33-4 illustrates the development of increasing disability in a chronically mentally ill man. It focuses on several characteristics of chronically mentally ill patients: their low self-esteem, social isolation, involvement with the legal system as a consequence of the secondary symptoms of their illness, and poor coping resources. The example also shows the effect of illness on the patient's family. Particular attention is given to the nursing care the patient received when he was admitted to a state psychiatric hospital after a serious suicide attempt.

DIRECTIONS FOR FUTURE RESEARCH

The following are some of the nursing research problems raised in Chapter 33 that merit further study by psychiatric nurses:
1. Development of psychoeducation programs to increase chronically mentally ill patients' understanding of and participation in self-care related to health promotion
2. Comparison of the quality of life experienced by chronically mentally ill patients residing in institutions and in communities
3. The effectiveness of specific nursing interventions in increasing patients' perceptions of their strengths
4. Evaluation of the integration of principles of psychiatric rehabilitation into the inpatient milieu
5. Evaluation of the effectiveness of the nurse in the role of case manager
6. Comparison of the patient's and nurse's perception of the patient's strengths
7. Nurses' attitudes toward caring for the chronically mentally ill
8. Strategies used by family members in coping with the chronically mentally ill member living at home
9. Comparison of team and primary nursing modalities on patient/family/nurse outcomes.
10. Comparison of quality of life of the chronically mentally ill and other chronically ill populations.

■ SUGGESTED CROSS-REFERENCES ■

The phases of the nursing process are discussed in Chapter 5. Tertiary prevention and rehabilitative psychiatric nursing are discussed in Chapter 10. Problems with self-esteem are discussed in Chapter 13. Legal issues, including commitment proceedings and patient rights, are discussed in Chapter 7. Crisis intervention is discussed in Chapter 9.

■ SUMMARY ■

1. Chronically mentally ill individuals no longer reside primarily in large public psychiatric hospitals. It is estimated that as a result of "deinstitutionalization," the process of moving long-term mental patients into the community to be supported by formal and informal resources, 50% of the chronically mentally ill are now living in local communities.

2. Chronically mentally ill individuals have both primary and secondary symptoms of their illness. Primary symptoms are those associated with the intrinsic nature of their illness. Secondary symptoms develop over time as a consequence of the illness and perpetuate the illness's existence. Chronic mental illness, with its associated secondary symptoms, is not a state or endpoint, but a process of progressive deterioration.

3. The chronically mentally ill have difficulties in activities of daily living and maintaining interpersonal relations, a lack of coping resources, and a need for long-term treatment. Other characteristics influencing the course of their illness are their consistently low self-esteem and their preoccupation with avoiding failure rather than achieving success. As a group, the chronically mentally ill can also be characterized by their unique strengths and potentials.

4. The "young" chronically ill patient, 18 to 35 years old, differs from chronically mentally ill patients over 35 years old. Because of deinstitutionalization and the development of community-based treatment facilities, younger patients have not had to adapt to long-term residence in public psychiatric hospitals. They alternate between inpatient and community-based facilities and maintain age-appropriate role expectations for themselves. Because they cannot meet these expectations, they are continually confronted with their sense of failure. They are likely to enter the mental health system nonvoluntarily, are unlikely to follow through with aftercare plans, have a high suicide rate, and are more likely to abuse drugs or alcohol. They are likely to be better educated and have more independent living skills than older patients. Present treatment resources are inadequate in meeting the needs of this group of patients.

5. Psychosocial rehabilitation programs that incorporate elements of the medical model, rehabilitation model, and social support model have demonstrated their effectiveness in meeting the needs of chronically mentally ill patients. Fountain House, a psychosocial rehabilitation program in New York City, has been used as a prototype for the development of other psychosocial rehabilitation programs. These programs offer their residents choices in living and work situations, but most important, they offer a sense of being needed and a place to belong. Basic to the rehabilitation process is focusing on the strengths of new members.

6. The role and function of the nurse in caring for chronically mentally ill patients are influenced by the setting in which the care is given.
   a. Nurses working in community-based psychosocial rehabilitation programs have the opportunity for long-term ongoing relationships with patients and the mutual setting of long-term goals. In these programs nurses may also be asked to function as case manager, a role that cuts across professional boundaries.
   b. Nurses working in acute care settings often care for chronically mentally ill patients when they are in crisis. Nurses must be able to quickly establish relationships with acutely ill patients and be skilled in applying the principles of crisis intervention. Primary nursing, as a modality of nursing care, offers several advantages when caring for chronically mentally ill patients in acute care settings.

7. In all settings, nurses are responsible for improving their patients' health status by developing the patients' health potentials. Nursing interventions that develop the strengths and potentials of chronically mentally ill patients help them become more competent in meeting the demands of everyday life. Ultimately, the expected outcome of each intervention is a change in the patient's self-concept and an increase in his self-esteem. Nursing interventions in which patients are helped to become aware of their strengths fall into two categories.
   a. Those which occur as a response to the patient's spontaneous participation in the milieu
   b. Those which occur as part of a structured intervention in which experiences are planned to mobilize patients' strengths or develop their potentials

REFERENCES

1. American Nurses' Association: Nursing case management, Kansas City, MO, 1988.
2. Anderson S and Bauwens E: Chronic health problems: concepts and application, St Louis, 1981, Mosby–Year Book, Inc.
3. Anthony W, Cohen M, and Cohen B: Psychiatric rehabilitation. In Talbott J, editor: The chronic mental patient: five years later, New York, 1984, Grune & Stratton, Inc.
4. Bachrach LL: Deinstitutionalization: an analytical review and sociological perspective, US Department of Health, Education, and Welfare Pub No (ADM) 76-351, Washington, DC, 1976, US Government Printing Office.
5. Bachrach LL: A note on some recent studies of released mental hospital patients in the community, Am J Psychiatry 133:73, 1976.
6. Bachrach LL: Deinstitutionalization: what do the numbers mean, Hosp Community Psychiatry 37(2):118, 1986.
7. Bachrach L: The legacy of model programs, Hosp Community Psychiatry 40(3):234, 1989.
8. Baker A: How families cope, J Psychosocial Nursing 27(1):31, 1989.
9. Barter J: Psychoeducation. In Talbott J, editor: The chronic mental patient: five years later, New York: 1984, Grune & Stratton, Inc.
10. Bassuk EL and Gerson S: Deinstitutionalization and mental health services, Sci Am 238:46, 1978.
11. Bell M and Ryan E: Integrating psychosocial rehabilitation into the hospital psychiatric service, Hosp Community Psychiatry 35(10):1017, 1984.
12. Bell R: The effect of interpersonal strengths identification and education on the self-esteem of psychiatric day treatment programs, doctoral dissertation, Washington, DC, 1981, Catholic University of America.
13. Bender M: Young adult chronic patients: visibility and style of interaction in treatment, Hosp Community Psychiatry 37(3):265, 1986.
14. Boss P: The marital relationship: Boundaries and ambiguities. In McCubbin H and Figley C, editors: Coping with normative transitions, New York, 1983, Brunner/Mazel.
15. Brown B: Responsible care of former mental patients. In New dimensions in mental health: report from the director, Washington, DC, 1977, National Institute of Mental Health.
16. Caton D: The new chronic patient and the system of community, Hosp Community Psychiatry 32:475, 1981.
17. Chafetz L: Recidivist clients: a review of pilot data, Arch Psych Nurs 2(1):14-20, 1988.
18. Coopersmith S: The antecedents of self-esteem, San Francisco (1967), 1981, Consulting Psychologists Press.
19. Crossen M: Contemporary models in psychiatric care and rehabilitation: Fountain House, Hoffman-LaRoche Laboratories.
20. Cutler D et al: Disseminating the principles of a community support program, Hosp Community Psychiatry 35(1):51, 1984.
21. Doll W: Family coping with the mentally ill patient: an unanticipated problem of deinstitutionalization, Hosp Community Psychiatry 27:183, 1976.
22. Drake R and Wallach M: Substance abuse among the chronically mentally ill, Hosp Community Psychiatry 40(10):1041, 1989.
23. Falloon H et al: Family management in the prevention of exacerbations of schizophrenia, N Engl J Med 306(24):1437, 1982.
24. Fisher W et al: Projecting inpatient admissions to state facilities in the 1990s, Hosp Community Psychiatry 40(7):747, 1989.
25. Fitts W: Tennessee self-concept manual, Nashville, Tenn, 1965, Counselor Recording and Tests.

26. Fitts W: The self-concept and psychopathology, Nashville, Tenn, 1972, Counselor Recording and Tests.

27. Fitts W et al: The self-concept and self-actualization, Monograph No III, Nashville, Tenn, 1971, Counselor Recording and Tests.

28. Goldman HH: Mental illness and family burden: a public health perspective, Hosp Community Psychiatry 33(7):557, 1982.

29. Goldman H: Epidemiology. In Talbott J, editor: The chronic mental patient: five years later, New York, 1984, Grune & Stratton, Inc.

30. Goldman H, Gattozzi A, and Taube C: Defining and counting the chronically mentally ill, Hosp Community Psychiatry 32:21, Jan 1981.

31. Gruenberg E: The social breakdown syndrome: some origins, Am J Psychiatry 123:1481, 1967.

32. Hatfield AB: The family as partner in the treatment of mental illness, Hosp Community Psychiatry 30:338, 1979.

33. Heinrichs D: Recent developments in the psychosocial treatment of chronic psychotic illnesses. In Talbott J, editor: the chronic mental patient: five years later, New York, 1984, Grune & Stratton, Inc.

34. Holmberg S: Physical health problems of the psychiatric client, J Psychosocial Nursing 26(5):35, 1988.

35. Intagliata J and Baker F: A comparative analysis of the young adult chronic patient in New York State's community support system, Hosp Community Psychiatry 35(1):45, 1984.

36. Kneisman D and Joy V: Family response to the mental illness of a relative: a review of the literature, Schizophrenic Bulletin (10):34-35, 1974.

37. Krauss J: The chronic psychiatric patient in the community: a model of care, Nurs Outlook 28:308, 1980.

38. Krauss J and Slavinsky A: The chronically ill psychiatric patient and the community, Boston, 1982, Blackwell Scientific Pub.

39. Lamb H and Goertzel V: The long term patient in the era of community treatment, Arch Gen Psychiatry 34:679, 1977.

40. Leavitt M: The discharge crisis: the experience of families of psychiatric patients, Nurs Research 24:33, 1975.

41. Lemert E: Secondary deviance and role conceptions. In Farrell R and Swigert V, editors: Social deviance, New York, 1975, JB Lippincott Co.

42. McCarrick A, Manderscheid R, and Bertolucci D: Correlates of acting-out behaviors among young adult chronic patients, Hosp Community Psychiatry 36(8):848, 1985.

43. McFarlane W, editor: Family therapy of schizophrenia, New York, 1983, The Guilford Press.

44. Maurin JT: Case management: caring for psychiatric clients, J Psychosocial Nursing 28(7):7, 1990.

45. Minkoff K: A map of the chronic mental patient. In Talbott J, editor: The chronic mental patient: problems, solutions, and recommendations for a public policy, Washington, DC, 1978, The American Psychiatric Association.

46. Mulkern V and Manderscheid R: Characteristics of community support program clients in 1980 and 1984, Hosp Community Psychiatry 40(2):165, 1989.

47. Nigro A and Maggio J: A neglected need: health education for the mentally ill, J Psychosocial Nursing 28(7):15, 1990.

48. Otto H: The human potentialities of nurses and patients, Nurs Outlook 8:32, 1965.

49. Otto H: Guide to developing your potential, New York, 1967, Charles Scribner's Sons.

50. Parker M and Secord L: Case managers: guiding the elderly through the health care maze, AJN 68:1674-1676, 1988.

51. Pepper B, Kirshner M, and Ryglewicz H: The young adult chronic patient: overview of a population, Hosp Community Psychiatry 32:463, 1981.

52. Pepper B and Ryglewicz H: The young adult chronic patient: a new focus. In Talbott J, editor: The chronic mental patient: five years later, New York, 1984, Grune & Stratton, Inc.

53. Peterson R: What are the needs of chronic mental patients? In Talbott J, editor: The chronic mental patient: problems, solutions, and recommendations for a public policy, Washington, DC, 1978, The American Psychiatric Association.

54. Plante T: Social skills training: a program to help schizophrenic clients cope, J Psych Nurs 27(3):7, 1989.

55. Porter E and Maloney S: Strength deployment inventory: manual of administration and interpretation, Pacific Palisades, Calif, 1967, Personal Strengths Assessment Service, Inc.

56. Pringle J: Schizophrenia: the family burden, England, 1975, National Schizophrenia Fellowship.

57. Raymond M, Slaby A, and Lief J: Familial responses to mental illness, Social Casework 10:492-498, 1975.

58. Rogers C: Client centered therapy: its current practice, implications, and theory, Boston, 1965, Houghton Mifflin Co.

59. Rose L: Understanding mental illness: the experience of families of psychiatric patients, J Adv Nurs 8:507, 1983.

60. Ross G: Attribution retraining of the psychiatrically disabled, doctoral dissertation, Philadelphia, 1978, University of Pennsylvania.

61. Ryan J, et al: A comparative study of primary and team nursing models in the psychiatric care setting, Arch Psych Nurs 2:1, 1988.

62. Schwartz S and Goldfinger S: The new chronic patient: clinical characteristics of an emerging subgroup, Hosp Community Psychiatry 32:470, 1981.

63. Segal S, Baumohl J, and Johnson E: Falling through the cracks: mental disorder and social margin in a young vagrant population, Soc Probl 24:387, 1977.

64. Seymour R and Dawson N: The schizophrenic at home, J Psych Nurs 26(1):28, 1986.

65. Thompson E and Doll W: The burden of families coping with the mentally ill: an invisible crisis, Family Relations 31:379-388, 1982.

66. Turner J and TenHoor W: The NIMH community support program: pilot approach to needed social reform, Schizophr Bull 4:319, 1978.

67. Zander K: Nursing case management: strategic management of cost and quality outcomes, J Nurs Adm 18:23, 1988.

■ ANNOTATED SUGGESTED READINGS ■

Andreasen N: The broken brain, New York, 1984, Harper and Row.

> *Written for the lay person, the reader is given accurate information about the biological revolution in psychiatry and its meaning for patients and their families. Written with sufficient depth to serve as a comprehensive reference for health care personnel.*

Bassuk EL and Gerson S: Chronic crisis patients: a discrete clinical group, Am J Psychiatry 137:1513, 1980.

> *Study of psychiatric patients who made repeated visits to an emergency room in a general hospital; focuses on their nonproductive interaction with the caregivers from whom they seek help. Interventions suggested based on an understanding of patients' help-seeking–help-rejecting behavior.*

*Chafetz L: Recidivist clients: A review of pilot data, Arch Psych Nurs 2(1):14-20, 1988.

> *A survey of 77 recidivist clients provides demographic and clinical data regarding the younger chronically mentally ill patient. The role of nurse case managers in impacting positively on this group is explored.*

Crossen M: Contemporary models in psychiatric care and rehabilitation: Fountain House, Hoffman-LaRoche Laboratories.

> *Provides an overview of the Fountain House program, based on interviews with Fountain House staff and members.*

*deCangas J: Exploring expressed emotion: Does it contribute to chronic mental illness? J Psych Nurs 28(2):31, 1990.

> *The concept of expressed emotion is reviewed with attention to the controversy surrounding its application to the treatment of the chronically mentally ill. The need for further research in this area is identified as essential.*

Falloon H, et al: Family management in the prevention of exacerbations of schizophrenia, N Engl J Med 306(24):1437, 1982.

> *This often-cited research examines the effectiveness of family psychoeducation in reducing family stress and preventing rehospitalization of schizophrenic patients living at home. The family treatment approach was found more effective than individual supportive care in preventing relapse.[2]*

Goldman H, Gattozzi A, and Taube C: Defining and counting the chronically mentally ill, Hosp Community Psychiatry 32:21, Jan 1981.

> *Results of a national study to identify the chronically mentally ill, both descriptively and numerically. The findings provided a foundation for the development of the National Plan for the Chronically Mentally Ill.*

*Kane C: The outpatient comes home: the family's response to deinstitutionalization, J Psychosoc Nurs Ment Health Serv 22(11):19, 1984.

> *An overview of the development of deinstitutionalization as federal policy is followed by a discussion of the effect of this policy on families. Highlighted is the development of the National Alliance for the Mentally Ill, a self-help group expected to have increasing political clout.*

*Krauss J: The three C's and the chronically mentally ill, Arch Psych Nurs 3(2):59, 1989.

> *Makes a case for the power of a caring relationship between a nurse and a chronically mentally ill client and challenges nurses to assume greater leadership in planning and implementing care for this population.*

*Krauss J: When stigma screams, Arch Psych Nurs 3(6):313, 1989.

> *This editorial, in response to public outcry following the stabbing of a 9-year-old girl by an escaped "mental patient," asks difficult questions that challenge a response based on stigma.*

Krauss J and Slavinsky A: The chronically ill psychiatric patient in the community, Boston, 1982, Blackwell Scientific Publications.

> *These authors have provided a comprehensive text on the chronically mentally ill which provides an in-depth analysis of the many issues surrounding this population. While this text is of value to all disciplines involved in the care of the chronically mentally ill, the material on nursing care is most sensitive and thorough.*

*Lenehan G et al: A nurse clinic for the homeless, Am J Nurs 85:1237, 1985.

> *In 1972 a group of Boston nurses began a nursing clinic in a large shelter for homeless men. This article traces the development of that clinic from early beginnings with volunteer staff to its current status with two clinics and paid staff. This clinic is a model for health care for the homeless.*

*Nigro A and Maggio J: A neglected need: health education for the mentally ill, J Psychosoc Nurs 28(7):15, 1990.

> *The authors report on a 4 month health education intervention used in a continuing treatment program. Pre- and post-test evaluation showed an increase in participants' knowledge. It is hypothesized that the changes resulting from the educational experience produce corresponding changes in self-esteem and community living skills.*

Pepper B, Kirshner M, and Ryglewicz H: The young adult chronic patient: overview of a population, Hosp Community Psychiatry 32:463, 1981.

> *Based on a study of nearly 300 patients, 18 to 35 years old, the authors provide a beginning description of the characteristics of this emerging subgroup of the chronically mentally ill.*

Peterson R: What are the needs of chronic mental patients? In Talbott J, editor: The chronic mental patient: problems, solutions, and recommendations for a public policy, Washington, DC, 1978, The American Psychiatric Association.

> *Ronald Peterson, a veteran of 10 years in a state mental hospital, wrote this paper when he was a staff member of Fountain House, a psychosocial rehabilitation program. He provides*

---

*Asterisk indicates nursing reference.

an *"insider's view" of the experience of leaving a state hospital and adjusting to community life. The importance of programs like Fountain House in meeting the needs of the chronically mentally ill is highlighted.*

*Pittman D: Nursing case management: holistic care for the deinstitutionalized chronically mentally ill, J Psychosoc Nurs 27(11):23, 1989.

Provides a brief description of nursing case management for the chronically mentally ill. Rationale for assuming the role of case manager is presented. A case presentation illustrates the implementation of theory into practice.

*Rose L: Understanding mental illness: the experience of families of psychiatric patients, J Adv Nurs 8:507, 1983.

This article reports the results of a qualitative study describing families' experiences when a mentally ill relative is hospitalized for the first time. The process by which the family interpreted and assigned meaning to this experience is described. The process described parallels the stages of the natural history of chronic illness as described in this chapter. Nursing implications are derived.

Schwartz S and Goldfinger S: The new chronic patient: clinical characteristics of an emerging subgroup, Hosp Community Psychiatry 32:470, 1981.

The authors describe their impressions, based on 2 years' clinical work in a general hospital, of the characteristics of younger chronically mentally ill patients. They analyze the interaction of this patient group with present treatment resources and make recommendations for future development of treatment resources.

Sheehan S: Is there no place on earth for me? Boston, 1982, Houghton Mifflin Co.

This journalistic account of the life history of a chronically schizophrenic woman reveals the nature of the mental health care system, including changes initiated by the community mental health movement. The frustration of the patient and her family as they try to find help is clearly communicated to the reader. This book would be particularly worthwhile to the nurse who has had limited contact with chronically mentally ill patients.

Talbott J: The national plan for the chronically mentally ill: a programmatic analysis, Hosp Community Psychiatry 32:699, 1981.

The author summarizes and analyzes the program recommendations in the National Plan for the Chronically Mentally Ill.

Torrey EF: Surviving schizophrenia: a family manual, New York, 1983, Harper & Row.

This book was written for families with the hope that information about schizophrenia, its etiology and treatment, the process and characteristics of psychiatric hospitalization, aftercare, and legal and ethical dilemmas would counteract myths and facilitate family coping. This is a good resource of the beginning psychiatric nurse as well as the family.

Toward a national plan for the chronically mentally ill, US Department of Health and Human Services Pub No (ADM)81-1077, Washington, DC, 1980.

This federal report, originally requested by President Carter's Commission on Mental Health, describes the needs of the chronically mentally ill, analyzes problems in the implementation of deinstitutionalization, and makes recommendations to improve services to this group of patients. Attention is given to fiscal considerations in meeting the needs of the chronically mentally ill.

*Ulin P: Measuring adjustment in chronically ill clients in community mental health care, Nurs Res 30:229, July-Aug 1981.

This study examines the usefulness of the Psychological Mental Health Index (PMHI) in assessing the psychological well-being of chronically ill psychotic patients being cared for in the community.

*Worley N and Albanese N: Independent living for the chronically mentally ill, J Psychosoc Nurs 27(9):18, 1989.

Self Discovery, a nurse-owned and operated residential rehabilitation program for the chronically mentally ill, is described in this article. Nurses are encouraged to become more involved in providing care for this population.

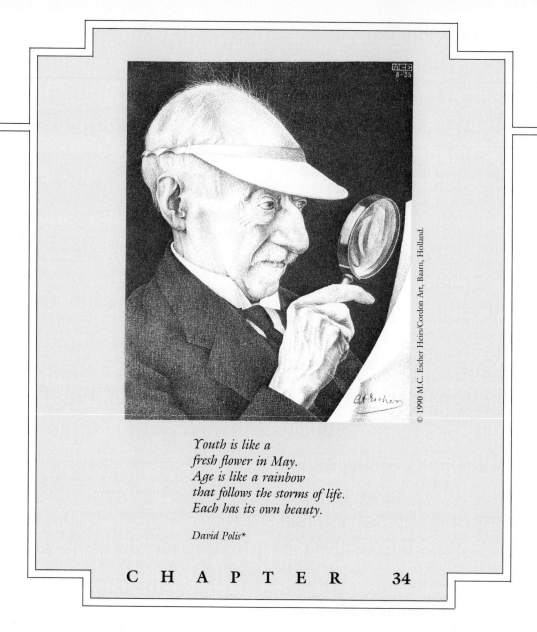

*Youth is like a
fresh flower in May.
Age is like a rainbow
that follows the storms of life.
Each has its own beauty.*

David Polis*

C H A P T E R 34

GERIATRIC PSYCHIATRIC NURSING

BEVERLY A. BALDWIN

After studying this chapter, the student should be able to:

- describe psychiatric disorders associated with aging in relation to the demographic characteristics of the population.

- identify the role and functions of the gerontological psychiatric nurse.

- identify the major biological, psychosocial, and personality theories of aging.

- assess the nursing care needs of the gerontological psychiatric patient.

- assess the nursing care needs of the family of the gerontological psychiatric patient.

- critique assessment tools the nurse may use as one component of data collection.

- analyze the interrelationship of physiological and psychological stressors as they affect the behavior of the aging patient.

- identify intervention strategies appropriate to use with gerontological psychiatric patients.

- identify directions for future nursing research.

- select appropriate readings for further study.

The fastest growing age-groups in the United States are over the age of 65, which now compose almost 13% of the population. One in every nine Americans is 65 or older; in the first half of the twenty-first century, one in five Americans will be over 65. It is estimated that by 2030 there will be 60 million persons over 65—17% to 20% of the total United States population.[42]

Stereotypes and myths often portray the elderly as a homogeneous group. To the contrary, the older adult represents the culmination of multiple interpersonal, developmental, and situational experiences. The complexity and interactive nature of the needs and problems of old age are frequently underestimated and often understated. Mental health in late life depends on a number of factors, including one's physiological and psychological status, personality, social support system, economic resources, and prevailing life-style. It has been estimated that of persons over 65, over 4 million suffer moderate to severe psychiatric impairment resulting from cerebral arteriosclerosis, senile dementia, functional psychosis, alcoholism, or other conditions. The elderly account for over 25% of reported suicides, with the highest rate occurring in white males in their mid-eighties.[6] The extent of mental disorders in the elderly appears to be considerable; therefore, nurses and other health care professionals will be increasingly responsible for caring for older adults with mental and emotional health problems. Helping older adults to maximize their potential can be a challenging and rewarding experience for the nurse. This chapter will address selected aspects of the psychiatric-mental health needs of geriatric patients and their family.

The problem of defining aging and the geriatric patient is complicated. People age in different ways, both psychologically and physiologically; therefore, the chronological demarcation of age 65 is an arbitrary one. As a base for understanding aging and the impact of individual variations, this chapter presents an overview of selected theories of aging. Components of the mental health evaluation of older adults are used to demonstrate how these theories are applied. Although it is acknowledged that assessment of mental health status is but one aspect of assessment of the total person, in this chapter emphasis will be placed on mental and emotional evaluation. By integrating current research findings with the role of the nurse in the care of the geriatric patient, we compare standardized instruments for evaluating mental status with functional and other behaviorally focused measures.

Data obtained from the mental status evaluation, along with a profile of the patient's general status, allow the nurse to develop a working nursing assessment and to plan intervention strategies. For example, memory loss, confusion, or disorientation may represent the older adult's behavioral responses to stress, whether originating internally or externally. The nurse must use knowledge and skill in determining the extent to which the stress is a negative or positive force. Comprehensive evaluation is the first step in that determination.

The next step in nursing care is selecting intervention strategies to meet the patient's needs. An overview of the current techniques in prevention and care of the mentally impaired (or potentially impaired) will focus on clinical research findings. The discussion of intervention strategies will focus on the nurse's role in implementing strategies and assessing their impact on the patient, whether in an individual or group setting.

Evolution of the role of the gerontological psychiatric nurse

Before World War II, the sick elderly were found in general hospitals, their homes, and clinics, but nurses attending them never thought of themselves as geriatric nurses. The passage of the Social Security Act of 1935 had profound effects on the status of the aged. Public assistance funds became available to the needy aged. This hastened the development of profit-making homes, since recipients of monthly stipends could not live in public institutions. Many retired and widowed nurses converted their homes into boarding houses that became, in practice, the first of our present-day nursing homes.[18] Care in the boarding houses for the aged deteriorated as the patients became ill and their needs increased. After World War II, each state established minimum standards for nursing home care, and licensing of homes was introduced. Many of the boarding house nurse-landladies became the administrators of the new federally subsidized nursing homes. With the increase in the number and needs of the patients, it became necessary to employ additional personnel to provide care.[19] The nurse administrator assumed the role of supervisor or manager of nonprofessional personnel, in addition to running the home.

■ Future prospects

The prospects for the future of gerontological/geriatric nursing are encouraging for nurses seeking greater autonomy and control over their practice. Several factors account for the potential for change within this field of nursing. Esther Lucille Brown,[9] in a study of nursing practice in hospitals, extended care facilities, and nursing and retirement homes, notes that except for a few specialists in geriatrics and chronic diseases, the medical profession is largely uninvolved in the problems of aging and care of the older patient who cannot be cured. The functional requirements of physicians in institutions devoted to chronic disease and rehabilitation are minimal. Most of the needs of the elderly in these settings and in community and home care settings result from chronic disability with multiple cause. It is in these settings that the nursing domain may develop and expand.

■ **FUTURE ROLES.** Internally, the field of gerontological/geriatric nursing is changing rapidly. The roles, settings, and focus of practice are unlimited. They will include case management in acute care/trauma settings, chronic disease hospitals, home health and other community care and nursing homes; health assessors with a focus on the interactive nature of functional and medical problems; primary care providers in both institutional and community-based settings; beginning researchers; and private practitioners in sole or group practice with a focus on the elderly and/or their families.

■ **EDUCATIONAL PREPARATION.** As the role of the gerontological/geriatric nurse continues to expand, the educational preparation for this specialty must expand. Presently there are 65 graduate programs offering a concentration or specialty in this area. Preparation at the graduate level includes the clinical specialization, administration, education, and nurse practitioner roles. Also included is preparation of the beginning nurse researcher, the first step toward doctoral preparation. Increasingly, faculty are including more content on gerontological/geriatric nursing in undergraduate curricula. Recognition of the need to prepare nurses to care for the aged continues to grow as the number of elderly persons grows.

Theories of aging

Ways of defining aging and explaining the causes and consequences of the aging process form the basis for the numerous theories of aging. Theories are proposed based on two major conceptual approaches to aging: (1) the causes of the biological and psychological process of aging and (2) the psychosocial results of aging. There is little consensus among gerontologists about the cause and adaptation to aging, and it is unlikely that consensus will be sought. No one theory can take into account all the variables that influence aging and the individual's response to it; these include cultural and ethnic factors, genetic makeup and heritage, physiological conditions at conception and birth, growth and maturation, the environment, the family system, and relationships with significant others. Stages of aging are difficult to differentiate from changes over time that are considered to be secondary to the aging process.

TABLE 34-1

THEORIES OF AGING

Psychobiological theories		Psychosocial theories		Personality theories	
Biological programming	Cell stores memory and capacity for terminating life. Represents entropic explanation of aging.	Disengagement	Elderly people and society mutually withdraw from active exchange with each other. See older adults as homogeneous group.	Ego integrity	Eight stages of humans with specific phases and tasks present at each age. Ego integrity is the last stage and provides a point for reflection on one's life and accomplishments. Assumes normal progression from stage to stage.
Wear-and-tear	Changes occur due to abuse and/or care. Represents decremental model of aging, irreversible decline.	Activity	Aging is but one phase in the developmental process. Recognizes the heterogeneity of all age-groups	Stability of personality	Personality is established by early adulthood and remains fairly stable thereafter.
Stress-adaptation	Stress has both positive and negative consequences for the organism. Represents adaptive-coping model of aging.	Life review	Reminiscence is viewed as a normal life review process. Recognizes need for reintegration of life experiences as preparation for the final stage of life.		

It is difficult to distinguish among stress, disease processes, and specific age-related changes. Selected theories will be discussed to clarify how biopsychosocial manifestations interact in later life. The major theories are summarized in Table 34-1. Theories of aging may further clarify the physiological and mental changes that geriatric patients experience.

■ Psychobiological theories

■ **DELIBERATE BIOLOGICAL PROGRAMMING.** The deliberate biological programming theory has received considerable attention over the last 2 decades. This theory holds that capacity for terminating the life of a cell is stored within the cell itself. Through laboratory studies, Hayflick et al.[33] demonstrated that normal human fibroblasts, when cultured, underwent a finite number of population doublings and then died. The number of doublings is the same in male and female cells. The theory of a human biological clock is an entropic approach to the explanation of aging. The decline of biological, cognitive, and psychomotor function is viewed as inevitable and irreversible, even though modification of diet and prolonged hypothermia may slow up the terminal process. The concept of programmed aging, while answering some questions about the human life span, does not address the intrinsic and external influences on individual variations in aging.

■ **THE WEAR-AND-TEAR THEORY.** The wear-and-tear theory suggests that structural and functional changes may be accelerated by abuse and decelerated by care.[43] From a physiological standpoint, aging is viewed ontogenetically, beginning with conception and leading to decline and death. The pathological consequences of aging are the result of an accumulation of stress, trauma, injuries, infections, nutritional inadequacies, metabolic and immunological disturbances, and prolonged abuse. Although less popular than some current theories, it illustrates the decremental model of aging, leading to irreversible decline. This concept of aging is seen in widely accepted myths and stereotypes regarding the aged, as noted in such phrases as, "He's doing well for his age" or "What can you expect at that age?" Newer research on the value of exercise and cognitive stimulation in later years refutes the basic premise of this theory, since both body and mind seem to benefit from use and stimulation.

■ **THE STRESS-ADAPTATION THEORY.** The stress-adaptation theory emphasizes the positive and negative effects of stress on the individual's physiological and psychological development. Eisdorfer[23] points out that stress is not always a negative experience, contrary to many writings on the subject. Stress may stimulate a person to try new, more effective ways of adapting. Although it is often assumed that stress accelerates the aging process, there is little evidence to substantiate that conclusion. Stress may deplete an individual's reserve capacity, either physiologically or psychologically, thereby making him vulnerable to illness or injury. Some assumptions about stress and adaptation are important for an understanding of the nature of emotional and mental problems in the aged. Although the link between stress and the development of mental illness is unclear, the effect of stress on an individual, and his perception of that stress, play a major role in his ability to cope in adverse situations.

Psychosocial theories

■ **DISENGAGEMENT THEORY.** This controversial theory evolved from studies conducted by the University of Chicago Committee on Human Development.[17] It postulated that older adults and society mutually withdraw from active exchange with each other as part of the normal aging process. The withdrawal was assumed to be characterized by psychological well-being and adjustment on the part of the elder. This theory did not take into account the heterogeneity the elderly and the personality variables important to coping with change. Stereotypes reinforced by this theory include the idea that older people enjoy the company of people their own age exclusively and that retirement facilities should prohibit intergenerational living arrangements. Although many elders may desire such arrangements, others feel isolated and out of the mainstream of society.

■ **ACTIVITY THEORY.** Disputes about the reliability of the disengagement theory led to the development of the currently prevailing view that activity produces the most positive psychological climate for older adults. The activity theory[40] developed as a reaction to the negativistic perspective of disengagement. Many gerontologists champion the idea that aging is but one phase in the developmental process; others contend that old age is only an extension of the middle years and can be modified or abolished by increased activity

levels. The activity theory maintains that the aged should remain active as long as possible. Older adults who must stop working or participating in community activities should find substitutes. This theory emphasizes the positive influence of activity on the older person's personality, mental health, and satisfaction with life.

■ **THE LIFE REVIEW.** The life review was postulated in 1961 by Robert Butler.[12] In elderly persons, reminiscence is viewed as part of a normal life review process brought about by the realization of approaching death. Characteristic of the life review is the progressive return to consciousness of past experiences and the resurgence of unresolved conflicts, which the person examines and reintegrates. Successful reintegration can give meaning to life and prepare one for death by alleviating anxiety and fear. According to the life review theory, this process occurs universally and represents a functional preparation for the final stage of life. Although it occurs in all age-groups to a certain degree, the emphasis and focused concentration are characteristic of the later stage of life. Aged persons have a vivid memory for past events and can recall early life experiences with clarity and imagination. They appear to be reviewing and sorting previous life events to better understand their present circumstances.

The life review may have either positive or negative consequences. Anxiety, guilt, fear, and depression may surface if the person is unable to resolve or accept old unsolved problems. On the other hand, the righting of earlier wrongs can help establish a sense of serenity, pride in working through old conflicts, and acceptance of mortal life. Reflection is thus seen as a positive approach to aging. In addition to offering an explanation for the consequences of aging, reminiscence and the life review have potential for psychotherapeutic intervention. Further discussion of this process is found in the section on strategies for intervening in the mental health problems of the older adult.

Personality theories

■ **ERIKSON'S STAGE OF EGO INTEGRITY.** Erikson's eight stages of humans[24] delineate specific developmental tasks present at each age, based on Freudian dynamics. The last stage of life, which provides a point for reflection on one's life and accomplishments, is one of ego integrity. Erikson maps out a predetermined structural order to development and maturation that progresses by critical or crisis periods and depends on chronological timing and sequence. The rationale for the progression from one stage to the next is unclear; one must assume that biological or psychosocial forces initiate and propel the movement. The concept of ego integrity leaves unanswered many questions, such as the consequences of fixation at one stage of development and individual variation in the complex process of development and maturation.

■ **STABILITY OF PERSONALITY.** Costa and Mc-Crae, as cited by Ehrman,[22] contend that personality is established by early adulthood and remains fairly stable thereafter. Stability of personality has been observed in longitudinal studies of aging individuals at the National Institutes of Health Gerontology Research Center in Baltimore (the intramural research center for the National Institute on Aging). Usually no decline or change in personality, compared with other cognitive changes, is evident. Radical changes in personality in older persons may be indicative of brain disease. Costa and McCrae found that periods of psychological crisis in adulthood do not occur at regular intervals, contradicting some theories, such as Erikson's. Persons with a long history of emotional instability are therefore likely to encounter more crises. However, Costa and McCrae refute the conclusion that individuals are locked into rigid behavior patterns. They note, to the contrary, that changes in roles, attitudes, and situational demands create the need for new behavioral responses. The majority of elderly persons in their studies appear to adapt effectively to those demands.

 # Assessment

The assessment process gives the nurse an opportunity to collect data essential to the development of a nursing diagnosis. The interview and health history constitute a first step in the process. The use of selected standardized assessment tools augments the data the nurse obtains through interviewing the patient or family.

■ The interview

Establishing a supportive and trusting relationship is essential to a positive interview with the geriatric patient. Because the first encounter between the nurse and patient may be uncomfortable for the patient, the nurse must make every effort to put the patient at ease by offering reassurance and positive feedback. It may take repeated contacts and frequent explanations to allay fears and reduce anxiety. The geriatric patient may feel uneasy, vulnerable, and confused in new surroundings or in the presence of strangers. Patience and attentive listening promote a sense of security. The more comfortable the patient, the better able he will be to respond to the interview. The nurse shows respect for the patient by addressing him by his last name: "Good morning, Mr. Smith." The nurse opens the interview by introducing herself and briefly describing the purpose and length of the interview. The patient will respond best when he feels the nurse is concerned about his welfare. The patient should not be rushed or pressed for answers. Direct questions may have to be rephrased in an indirect, less intimidating manner.

■ **THERAPEUTIC COMMUNICATION SKILLS.** Specifying the time allotted and the topic to be discussed at the beginning of the interview orients the patient to its purpose and scope. Reinforcing the amount of time remaining in the interview may help direct a wandering discussion and give the patient the security of knowing the nurse is in control of the situation. Older persons may respond to questions slowly, since reaction time to verbal stimuli lengthens with age. It is important to give the patient sufficient time to formulate answers. Assuming the patient does not know the answer to a question, does not remember, or does not understand because he does not respond immediately can lead the interviewer to false conclusions about the patient's status and mental capabilities.

The manner in which the patient is questioned is important to the outcome of the interview. Older persons often are unfamiliar with new words, slang, or colloquialisms. The nurse should avoid the use of medical abbreviations, terminology, or jargon, and should ask short, concise questions, particularly if the patient has difficulty with abstract thinking and conceptualization. Techniques such as clarification and summarization, described in Chapter 4, are important in validating information obtained. The nurse should rephrase a question if the patient fails to answer appropriately or hesitates when answering.

Concentrated verbal interaction may be uncomfortable for the older person. The nurse can demonstrate interest and support by giving nonverbal cues and responses, such as direct eye contact, sitting close to the patient, and using touch appropriately. Touching the shoulder, arm, or hand of the patient in a firm, purposeful manner conveys support and interest. Avoid stroking or patting the patient, since cultural orientation and alterations in tactile perception may result in misinterpretation.

The ability of the nurse to elicit useful data will depend to a great degree on whether he or she feels comfortable during the interview. The nurse's negative bias toward the aged will surface in an interview. Older people are sensitive to others' lack of interest and impatience.

Although older persons differ in their willingness to reveal life histories and personal experiences, most geriatric patients greatly desire relationships with others and are anxious to share information with interested persons. Elderly patients have much to tell and may offer more information than the nurse needs at a particular time. Older patients often reminisce, and the nurse should encourage this when possible. The patient is concerned with life review or integration of past events with current situations. The life review may serve as an excellent source of data about the patient's current health problems and support resources. Reminiscence and life review may make it difficult to keep the patient focused on the topic at hand; however, they allow the nurse to assess subtle changes in long-term memory, decision-making ability, judgment-making patterns, affect, and orientation to time, place, and person.

Many geriatric patients are aware of changes in their physical or psychological functioning; however, they may hesitate to have their fears confirmed. Consequently, they may minimize or ignore symptoms, assuming they are age related and not relevant to current problems. Often these misconceptions are reinforced by myths about aging and the false assumption of many health professionals that the presenting problems of older persons are irreversible or untreatable.

Contrary to popular myths, most older people do not dwell unrealistically on their health and usually have a physical problem when they describe their health as poor. However, some older persons are preoccupied with the physical decline that occurs with progressing age. It is essential that the nurse observe carefully for clues that allow her to distinguish whether the patient's preoccupation reflects personality factors developed over a lifetime or represents a current distress.

The geriatric patient may misunderstand the purpose of the nurse's questions. He may fail to see the relevance to current health status of questions regarding habits, previous life experience, or social supports. Careful and repeated explanations are necessary if the patient is to cooperate with the nurse. The nurse should never assume that the patient understands the purpose or protocol for the assessment interview. It is wiser to overstate than to increase the patient's anxiety and stress by omitting information. The nurse should take cues from the patient's responses by listening carefully and observing constantly.

■ **THE INTERVIEW SETTING.** The new and unfamiliar surroundings of the hospital or outpatient clinic may impede the initial interview by distracting the patient and increasing his fear of the unknown. The physical environment should be altered as much as possible to promote comfort. Many older persons are unable to sit for long periods because of arthritis or other joint disabilities. Chairs should be comfortable,

and the patient should be encouraged to move about as desired. Changing positions and range-of-motion exercises stimulate circulation and prevent stiffness.

Most older persons experience some form of sensory deficit, particularly diminished high-frequency hearing or changes in vision as a result of cataracts or glaucoma. The environment should be modified to decrease the impact of these deficits. The setting for the interview should be quiet and without peripheral noises. The patient, already under a great deal of stress, may be easily distracted and annoyed by extraneous stimulation. The nurse should speak slowly and in a low-pitched voice. Shouting raises the pitch of the noise and makes hearing more difficult. Because fatigue may contribute to diminished mental functioning, morning is the best time for the interview. Patients not only become tired as the day progresses but also may experience a phenomenon known as **sundown syndrome,**[13] in which cognitive ability diminishes in the late afternoon or early evening. Some patients become disoriented, confused, or apathetic.

The reliability of the data obtained from the assessment interview should be carefully evaluated. If there are questions about some aspects of the patient's responses, the nurse should consult family members or other persons who know the patient well. The nurse should also consider the patient's physical condition at the time of the interview and other variables that may influence his status, such as medications, nutritional state, or level of anxiety.

■ **Functional assessment**

Functional assessment of the gerontological psychiatric patient is not limited to parameters of mental health. Rather, the ability to function emotionally and cognitively depends, to a great degree, on the older person's overall functional capability. Although it is not discussed in this chapter, a comprehensive assessment is considered necessary for an accurate diagnosis. This discussion emphasizes the aspects of the functional assessment that have the greatest impact on mental and emotional status.

■ **MOBILITY.** The loss of mobility and independence are real fears among the elderly. Early in the assessment, the nurse should determine the degree to which the gerontological psychiatric patient can move about unassisted. Restriction of joints may limit ambulation. A plan for range-of-motion exercises or other activity may be needed to ensure that the patient maintains a functional activity level. Patients who use wheelchairs or walkers need help in moving from the bed or chair to standing or walking positions. Orthostatic hypotension is possible when patients move rapidly from a lying to a standing position. The ambulating patient needs secure footwear, because gait may be unsteady and perception of spatial limits altered as a result of visual impairments.

In addition to changes in functional ability caused by changes in physical or psychological status, many medications routinely taken by geriatric patients alter perception and make ambulation and mobility difficult. Of particular significance are the sedatives/hypnotics, tranquilizers, and cardiovascular and hypertensive drugs.[26] Patients should be cautioned about side effects of the medications and encouraged to take plenty of time when ambulating and moving from one position to another. Many falls occur because the patient did not have enough time to adjust to changes in the physical environment (e.g., lighting, texture, or grading of the floor or sidewalk).

■ **NUTRITION.** Many geriatric patients do not require help to eat or determine their nutritional needs. However, gerontological psychiatric patients do have psychosocial problems that precipitate the need for assistance in eating and monitoring of nutritional intake. These include:

1. Depression or loneliness, with a consequent decrease in appetite
2. Changes in cognitive function, such as confusion or disorientation
3. Suicidal tendencies
4. Removal from familiar ethnocultural patterns of eating
5. Fear of hospital routines or procedures

The range of physical problems varies greatly, but some of the areas to be assessed include:

1. Whether the patient has sufficient mobility and strength to open cartons of milk, cut meat, handle utensils
2. The presence of neurological deficits or joint conditions that interfere with hand and arm coordination
3. The presence of visual problems
4. Edentulousness and other losses of chewing ability
5. Problems in swallowing or shortness of breath
6. The presence of ulcerations in the mouth or on the tongue
7. Periodontal disease
8. Dry mouth because of side effects of medications

The nurse should routinely evaluate the patient's needs in eating, because nutritional needs are one of the most significant problems of the institutionalized elderly and can precipitate other problems, such as skin breakdown, inadequate absorption of medications, and diminished wound healing.

■ **ACTIVITIES OF DAILY LIVING.** The assessment of self-care needs and activities of daily living (ADLs) is essential for establishing baseline data on the patient's potential for independence. Activity may be limited because of dysfunctional physical status or psychosocial impairment. ADLs include preparing meals, shopping, eating, bathing, toileting, dressing and other grooming procedures, mobility (e.g., walking, standing, bending, climbing stairs, moving objects from place to place, using a pen or pencil, or other fine-motor skills), and housekeeping chores (e.g., making a bed and washing dishes or clothes). Although geriatric patients should be encouraged to move toward greater independence in self-care, it is unrealistic to expect all patients to function independently. Hospitalization and conformity to the routine and procedures of the hospital environment foster dependence in the patient. Encouraging patients to become involved in their own care is important, because the more independent the patient is, the more his self-esteem will be enhanced. The nurse should establish realistic goals and reevaluate them periodically.

■ **SOCIAL SUPPORT SYSTEMS.** Positive support systems are a critical factor in maintaining a sense of well-being throughout life. Nowhere is this more important than with the gerontological psychiatric patient. Two of every five elderly persons do not spend their final years with a spouse.[34] Therefore, as a person's significant contacts diminish in number, it is important that the remaining support systems be consistent and meaningful.

The patient's ethnic background may be an important factor in identifying support systems and significant others. Strong family and ethnic ties promote feelings of security. Elderly persons who live alone and are also without family ties generally have more serious problems than those who are not isolated. These problems are not limited to financial instability but may affect the patient's desire to get well, be content with his life, and maintain self-care activities whenever possible. When the patient is admitted, the nurse should assess the support systems available to sustain the patient while in the hospital and when he returns home or goes to another institution. Family friends can help reduce the shock and stress of hospitalization and offer reassurance and comfort to the distressed elder.

Studies have shown that relocation is often a traumatic event for the elderly. High morbidity and mortality have been recorded for patients moved from one facility to another or from the familiar home environment to a long-term care facility.[13] The stress of relocation should be anticipated for all geriatric patients, and intervention should be planned to reduce the impact. Allowing the patient to have his own belongings, liberal visiting hours for family or friends, and careful explanations of the purpose and procedures of the institution are a few of the ways in which the stress of hospitalization can be minimized. Establishing an effective support system within the hospital may prevent the negative behavioral responses often observed in isolated elders: apathy, depression, aggression, or hostility.

■ Mental status

Systematic and comprehensive assessment of cognitive function and psychiatric symptoms provides data for drawing diagnostic conclusions and planning intervention strategies. The appropriate use of standardized assessment instruments is an adjunct to the nursing history and interview.

■ **THE MENTAL STATUS QUESTIONNAIRE.** The Mental Status Questionnaire (MSQ)[36] has been extensively used in geriatric research and practice. The questionnaire contains 10 orientation questions about place, date, day of the week and month, age, and birthdate. The last two items cover current events and historical events by questioning the patient's knowledge of the current and past presidents of the United States. Critics of this instrument suggest that the questions about the presidents are irrelevant and inappropriate for some elderly persons, particularly those in institutional settings and those isolated from the news of the day. The number of errors the patient makes in responding to the questions indicates the severity of the brain syndrome, which ranges from none or minimal to severe impairment. The MSQ was not designed to be used alone or as the only indicator of impairment; it provides a gross measure of mental status and change in cognitive function. High reliability has been recorded with other measures of cognitive impairment.

■ **THE SHORT PORTABLE MENTAL STATUS QUESTIONNAIRE.** The Short Portable Mental Status Questionnaire (SPMSQ)[20] is also a 10-item questionnaire that tests orientation, remote and recent memory, practical skills (recalling a telephone number or street address), and mathematical ability (serial subtraction from 20 by 3s). Developed as part of the Older Americans Resources and Services (OARS) program at the Duke University Center for the Study of Aging and Human Development, the SPMSQ has high test-retest reliability. The instrument has been administered on both institutionalized and community-based elders. Scores range from 0 to 10, with four levels of disability (intact, mild, moderate, or severe impairment) defined. Score adjustments are made for race and education.

■ **THE FACE-HAND TEST.** The Face-Hand Test[27] is a test of organicity that has been widely used in gerontological research and practice for the last 20 years. The instrument was developed to distinguish patients with brain damage from those who are psychotic without an organic cause. The test requires that the individual recognize tactile stimulation on the cheek and back of the hand. A rehearsal is allowed so that the individual can become familiar with the procedure. The last 4 of 10 paired stimuli count for the score. The individual sits facing the examiner, with his hands resting on his knees and his feet flat on the floor. The individual is touched simultaneously on one cheek and the dorsum of one hand in a specified order. The test is administered twice, first with the individual's eyes closed, then with them open. The patient must be able to display some degree of concentration and attention to the procedure. Anxiety and distraction by peripheral activities may prevent the patient from following the instructions. The box below describes the order of stimulation used in the Face-Hand Test.

■ **THE MINI-MENTAL STATE EXAMINATION.** The Mini-Mental State Examination[28] is a test of orientation (year, season, date, day, month, state, country, hospital, floor), registration (individually and collectively naming three objects), attention and calculation (counting backward by sevens from 100 or spell-

---

**Order of Stimulation Used
in Face-Hand Test**

1. Right cheek—left hand
2. Left cheek—right hand
3. Right cheek—right hand
4. Left cheek—left hand
5. Right cheek—left cheek
6. Right hand—left hand
7. Right cheek—left hand
8. Left cheek—right hand
9. Right cheek—right hand
10. Left cheek—left hand

Modified from Bender MB, Fink M, and Green M: Arch Neurol Psychiatry 66:355, 1951.

ing "world" backward), recall (repeating three objects named earlier), and language (naming objects, repeating phrases, obeying three-step commands, writing a sentence, and copying a design). This test is presented in the box below. Measurement of cognitive function is the primary focus of the examination, and it is thorough in that area. Because the test requires only 5 to 10 minutes to administer, it is not tiring to the patient. If the patient has difficulty reading or writing, the nurse administering the test may have to make some adjustments, such as using large, bold print when writing out sentences or instructions. This test has been used extensively in distinguishing between patients with dementia, psychosis, and affective disorders (e.g., depression).

■ **THE ZUNG SELF-RATING DEPRESSION SCALE.** The Zung Self-Rating Depression Scale[52] has

the advantage of being a self-report test and the disadvantage of provoking a wide range of interpretation and sensitivity on the part of the patient. The 20-item instrument consists of 10 negatively stated items (e.g., "I feel down-hearted and blue") and 10 positively stated items (e.g., "My mind is as clear as it used to be"). The Likert-type scale ranges from "a little of the time" to "most of the time" and requires the individual to make a choice on each item. If the patient has visual or language problems, the test must be administered orally. Although the test is criticized by some researchers and clinicians as threatening because of the sensitivity of the items, the scale takes minimal time to complete and gives the individual an opportunity to participate in the assessment process.

■ **THE NURSES' OBSERVATION SCALE FOR INPATIENT EVALUATION.** The Nurses' Observa-

Mini-Mental State Examination

Orientation	Maximum score	Score
What is the (year) (season) (date) (day) (month)?	5	(_____)
Where are we (state) (county) (town) (hospital) (floor)?	5	(_____)
Registration		
Name 3 objects: 1 second to say each. Then ask the patient all 3 after you have said them. Give 1 point for each correct answer. Then repeat them until he learns all 3. Count trials and record.	3	(_____)
_____ Trials		
Attention and calculation		
Serial 7s. 1 point for each correct. Stop after 5 answers. Alternatively spell "world" backwards.	5	(_____)
Recall		
Ask for the 3 objects repeated above. Give 1 point for each correct.	3	(_____)
Language		
Name a pencil, and a watch. (2 points)	9	(_____)
Repeat the following "No ifs, ands, or buts." (1 point)		
Follow a 3-stage comment:		
"Take a paper in your right hand, fold it in half, and put it on the floor." (3 points)		
Read and obey the following:		
Close your eyes. (1 point)		
Write a sentence. (1 point)		
Copy design. (1 point)		

TOTAL SCORE _____

Assess level of consciousness along a continuum

Alert   Drowsy   Stupor   Coma

From Folstein MF, Folstein SE, and McHugh PR: J Psychiatr Res 12:189, 1975. Copyright 1975, Pergamon Press, Ltd.

tion Scale for Inpatient Evaluation (NOSIE),[35] developed for use with chronic institutionalized schizophrenics, is based on nursing observation of patient behavior over a 3-day interval. Observable responses of the patient, such as "talks freely with visitors," "hoards things," and "has temper outbursts," are objectively scored using Likert-type choices ("never" to "always"). Factors of social competence, social interest, cooperation, and psychotic depression represent some of the dimensions on the scale. Although only recently used to any extent with a nonpsychiatric geriatric population, the instrument has potential for providing systematic objective ratings of patient behavior. Interrater reliability is high, based on selected studies, compared with other more subjective rating scales.

■ Activities of daily living

Measures of physical functioning in the elderly vary in scope and emphasis. The use of measures of ADLs, along with measures of cognitive function and psychiatric symptoms, enables the nurse to develop a comprehensive database on the patient. These instruments may be used during the initial assessment interview as well as throughout the intervention-evaluation phases of the nurse-patient relationship.

■ **THE KATZ INDEX OF ACTIVITIES OF DAILY LIVING.** The Katz index[37] consists of dichotomous rating of six ADL functions: bathing, dressing, toileting, transfer, continence, and feeding. One point is assigned for each observed item of dependency. The dichotomous dependent-independent categories for each function are defined in observable terms ("gets clothes from closets and drawers"). This widely used instrument has the advantage of measuring change in ADL function over time and as a result of rehabilitation.

■ **PACE II.** PACE II[49] focuses on evaluation of the physical health of nursing home patients. Checklists are used to identify the presence of defined conditions (diagnosed), abnormal laboratory or other findings, risk factors, and other impairments and disabilities. Under each medically defined condition, the duration, type, or location of the problem is specified. Thoroughness of observation is necessary in this patient–care-planning tool, in addition to review and inclusion of the medical history and examination. PACE II has the advantage of providing for interdisciplinary assessment and care planning.

■ Family-patient interaction

The manner in which family members relate to and support (or fail to support) each other has a profound influence on individuals.[8] Nowhere is this influence more evident than when an older adult becomes the central focus of conflict or dysfunction for the family unit. Behavioral problems in the elderly may result from the family's inability to deal with the losses and increasing dependence of an older member.

The importance of including family members or significant others in assessment cannot be overestimated. In addition to verifying information supplied by the patient, the family's perceptions of their relationship with the patient add yet another dimension to the nurse's understanding of the patient's response to his own aging and disability.

The format for assessment of patient-family dynamics varies, depending on the setting (e.g., community clinic, home, or institution) and the patient's behavior and needs. Two instruments for collection of data relevant to this area of assessment are described here.

■ **THE FAMILY APGAR.** The family APGAR[47] is designed to help clinicians systematically assess family function from the perception of individual family members. Categories for rating include adaptation, partnership, growth, affection, and resolve. Sample questions include the following: "I am satisfied with the help that I receive from my family when something is troubling me" (adaptation); "I find that my family accepts my wishes to take on new activities and make changes in my life-style" (growth); and "I am satisfied with the way my family and I share time together" (resolve). Each family member indicates his or her degree of satisfaction or dissatisfaction with each item on a Likert-type 0-to-2 scale ("almost always, hardly ever"). The clinician can also verbally administer each question and score the response. A score of 3 or less (out of 10) indicates high dysfunction for the individual; a score of 4 to 6 indicates moderate dysfunction. Discrepancies or low scores obtained by individual family members indicate problem areas and require further exploration. This practical tool was not developed specifically for assessing families with an older member. As an indication of the patient's and family's perceptions of each other, this instrument has potential for assessing the dynamics of the family's structure and function.

■ **THE SOCIAL BEHAVIOR ASSESSMENT SCHEDULE.** The Social Behavior Assessment Schedule[44] uses the patient's significant relative or friend to elicit information about the patient's social functioning ability. The instrument consists of a semistructured interview schedule focusing on the patient's behavior and psychosocial status. Adverse or dysfunctional effects on family function are explored. Patient behavior, such as withdrawal, forgetfulness, and indecisiveness, are included in the inventory. To rate each behavior, the examiner judges its severity, frequency, and time of onset. Twelve areas of social performance, such as household tasks, household management, and decision making, make up the social functioning rating. The degree of diminished performance and dysfunction is rated in a fashion similar to patient behavior. Additional categories in the instrument query adverse effects of others on the patient's behavior, concurrent events (e.g., physical illness, medications), and support to the informant from neighbors, friends, and other family members. Nurses working with families in the home or community may find this instrument an important measure of the patient's baseline function, as perceived by those involved in his care.

To date, nursing's use of standardized instruments in data collection has been minimal. The selection of a tool depends on the setting, patient population, and purpose of the nursing assessment. The extent to which these tools are used, either alone or in conjunction with other forms of assessment (e.g., physical assessment and evaluation), varies with the presenting problems of the patient. Although the skills required to use the instruments described here are easily learned, the nurse will need practice and verification with others who provide care for the patient is necessary to develop confidence in her findings.

 ## Nursing diagnosis

The nursing diagnosis is the culmination of data collection and analysis of the patient's functional ability and resources. Behavioral interpretation of the patient's presenting needs and problems helps the nurse intervene in dysfunctional or disruptive processes. Both objective and subjective data are required to determine the extent of the patient's functional ability. How the data are used depends on the resources available to the patient and the nurse in collaboratively working toward resolution of the problem or problems.

The medical diagnosis is based on identification of the disease underlying the patient's dysfunctional behavior. The medical diagnosis is complementary to the nursing diagnosis, because psychopathological conditions prevent the patient from functioning at his maximal potential. The relationship between the disease process and the patient's behavioral response is not always clear, because specific behaviors may result from a variety of pathological processes.[45] For example, both depressed patients and patients whose cognitive functions are disrupted because of organic changes, such as Alzheimer's disease, may have mood swings and alterations in mood.

Although older adults may experience a wide range of psychiatric problems, the problems of greatest significance to the nurse and patient in developing a healing therapeutic relationship will be discussed here.

■ Altered thought processes

■ **MEMORY LOSS.** One of the most distressing and frustrating aspects of aging is the potential for progressive memory loss. Although memory loss may result from organic brain disease or depression, it does not necessarily imply an inherent disease process. With age, loss of short-term memory (recall for recent events) is more likely to occur than loss of remote memory (recall for events that occurred in the distant past). The conceptual network of past thoughts, images, ideas, and experiences that makes up memory develops and matures over a lifetime. Primary memory is the conscious control system for memory. It appears to be stable over the life span: there is little difference in primary memory among people of different ages. However, speed of access appears to slow with increasing age.[1] Long-term memory (secondary memory) is the storage system for what is commonly understood as memory. Failure in retrieval, original acquisition, or learning may account for loss in secondary memory.[1]

Many factors contribute to alterations in memory in older adults. Stress or crisis, depression, a sense of worthlessness, loss of interest in present events, cerebrovascular changes that affect cerebral function, loss of neural cells because of disease or trauma, and sensory deprivation or isolation from verbal interactions may all occur with advancing age.[21] Sensory loss, including changes in vision and hearing, makes the older person vulnerable to the environment and to those around him, often resulting in withdrawal into a less-threatening world. The patient may seek comfort in old memories and experiences, which replace the need to remain in touch with the present.

Institutionalized elderly persons appear to have more difficulty with memory than older adults living at home or in other community settings. The institutional geriatric patient is often portrayed as dull, listless, and uncommunicative. The environment often promotes this response and reinforces the "compliant," "cooperative" patient. A stimulating environment and therapeutic regimen can counteract and, in many situations, reverse withdrawal in the gerontological psychiatric patient and revive interest in recall and participation in the present.

■ **WITHDRAWAL.** Multiple losses or fear of loss may precipitate withdrawal. Prolonged grief and hesitation about returning to an active life after the loss of a spouse, sibling, or child predisposes the elder to dysfunctional and nonresponsive behavior. The introverted adult may find it difficult to adjust to change and respond flexibly to new situations with advancing age; therefore, it is important to understand the patient's personality and previous adaptive styles.

Sudden withdrawal and refusal to form relationships with others should alert the nurse to the possibility of physiological factors as potential causes; low-grade infection, pain, and toxicity or side effects of medications are but a few of many possible causes. Careful assessment and evaluation are necessary.

The geriatric patient who is experiencing organic intellectual impairment (e.g., Alzheimer's disease and related disorders) frequently withdraws from social contacts, daily routines, and ADLs. He may deny having a problem or because of difficulties with memory may fear the consequences of these changes. Withdrawal can become a defense mechanism, reinforcing the denial of perceived disability and further loss of functional ability.

■ **CONFUSION.** Confusion has only recently been studied systematically by nurses. The term is used by nurses "to describe a constellation of client behaviors, including inattention and memory deficits, inappropriate verbalizations, disruptive behavior, noncompliance, and failure to perform activities of daily living."[51] Frequently "confusion" is a nonspecific label imposed by staff on apathetic, withdrawn, or uncooperative patients. Wolanin and Phillips[50] suggest that several categories of patients are particularly likely to be labeled as confused: the problem patient, the patient with communication problems (slurred speech, expressive dysphasia), the patient who challenges staff members' personal values, the physically unattractive patient, the depressed patient, and the "troublemaker" (one who does not improve despite nursing interventions and ministrations).

Institutionalized elders are at particular risk of confusion. From 40% to 80% of these patients suffer from some degree of organic brain disease, with concomitant disorientation to time, place, and person, gross remote and recent memory loss, and inability to execute simple calculations. In many long-term care facilities, more than 30% of the patients experience severe confusion.[21] The precipitating factors depend on both the physiological and psychological status of the patient.

Early morning confusion, appearing as a type of **sunrise syndrome,** may result from the hangover effects of sedatives/hypnotics or other nighttime medications that interact with drugs for sleep. Sleep disruptions and insomnia are particularly prevalent in the elderly. Adverse reactions to drugs prescribed for sleep are not uncommon. Increasing disorientation or confusion at night, resulting from loss of visual accommodation, is known as **sundown syndrome.** The nurse

should take special precautions to prevent falls and mobility hazards at these times.

The nurse should never assume that confusion and disorientation are natural consequences of changes in cognitive or physiological status. On the contrary, confusion is reversible in over half the patients who experience it. It is usually transient or of short duration and is one area in which the nurse has primary responsibility. The carefully planned, therapeutic nurse-patient relationship can be a significant factor in preventing and intervening in this distressing condition.

Although the term "disorientation" is often used interchangeably with "confusion," there is a distinction between them. A disoriented patient is not necessarily confused, and a confused patient does not necessarily experience disorientation in all spheres. The mental status tests discussed earlier differentiate disorientation in place, person, and time from components of confusion, such as alterations in memory, judgment, decision making, and problem solving.

■ **PARANOIA.** Some older persons react to loss, isolation, and loneliness with paranoia and fear. Classic psychopathological paranoia, demonstrated by a well-organized and elaborate system of superiority, is rare in older persons. Delusions and disturbances in mood, behavior, and thinking may be transient conditions occurring in reaction to sensory deprivation or sensory loss, isolation from social contacts, or psychotropic or other drugs.[14]

Paranoid symptoms may appear as diffuse or specific. The geriatric patient may perceive threat from certain persons (e.g., family, friends, neighbors) or at certain times (e.g., night). Relocation to a new home, new room, or strange environment precipitates fears, anxiety, and for some, paranoid ideation.

The personality of the aging paranoid patient is characterized by withdrawal, aloofness, fearfulness, oversensitivity, and, often, secretiveness. As long as the patient does not call attention to himself or pose a threat to himself or others, his paranoia may go undetected for a long time. Once he is recognized as a potential threat to himself or others, institutionalization becomes a consideration. Older persons suffering from transient or chronic paranoia are at high risk for victimization by others and self-neglect and abuse (e.g., refusal to eat, take prescribed medications, or attend to hygiene needs).

■ **Changes in affect**

Disturbances in mood, mood swings, or oversensitive emotional reactions are common to persons of all age-groups. The reaction of an older person to physical limitations or disabilities, psychological loss (particularly of a spouse or other significant other), or the possibility of institutionalization depends on his previous coping styles, support systems (especially family), and present psychological and physiological strength.

Radical or abrupt alterations in mood occur in reaction to internal or external stress or as inadequate coping mechanisms in persons confronted with progressive loss or dependency. When this behavior is seen in otherwise content, happy, elderly people, physiological factors, including side effects of cardiovascular or psychotropic drugs, should be considered. Reassurance and support are essential to reducing the patient's anxiety and diminishing the perceived threat.

■ **DYSFUNCTIONAL GRIEVING.** Depression and sadness are sometimes viewed as a natural part of aging, and depression is essentially a disorder of later life. Comfort[16] suggests that scores on the Zung Self-Rating Depression Scale may reflect mild depression in many older people because of instrument bias. The questionnaire emphasizes social usefulness and activity, which may be limited in some older adults. Depression, grief, and loss are common in later life.

Prolonged grief and mourning over a real or imagined loss should be recognized as depression and treated as such. Symptoms common to the depressed geriatric patient include, but are not limited to weight loss; anorexia; undue fatigue; apathy; loss of interest in friends, family, and usual activities; and psychomotor retardation. None of the symptoms are caused by increasing age, and all should be considered problematical.[7]

The older person's attitude toward his own aging and toward death and dying greatly influences whether the depression can be treated. The loss of hope expressed by some older persons, particularly those with increasing disabilities, may precipitate or stem from a depressive reaction.

Undiagnosed depression may have serious consequences for the elderly, since depression always causes physical symptoms. Many of the medications routinely prescribed for older persons can potentiate or enhance depression. Examples include tranquilizers (major and minor), barbiturates, cardiotonics (digoxin), and steroids. A medication history is part of the evaluation and assessment.

When considering mood changes, grief, and depression in the geriatric patient, it is important to understand the patient's and family's attitude toward death and dying. The old differ from the young in their attitudes toward death in several ways: older persons tend to integrate attitudes toward death with their formal religious training, to have experienced the death of significant others, to be more accepting of death, and to approach problems primarily from an internal focus. The state of the older person's health, in addition to what he has learned from observing dying persons, may signal that his life may be coming to an end. Awareness of the older person's "stage of dying" is important to understanding his needs and concerns.

■ **SUICIDE AMONG THE ELDERLY.** Intentional deaths among the elderly are not uncommon. Of all suicides committed in this country each year, over 25% are of persons over the age of 65. White males over the age of 85 are at particular risk. Other high-risk persons include the isolated elderly who have lost family or friends through death; those with changes in body function and decreased independence because of pain, weakness, immobility, or shortness of breath; those with changes in body function because of surgery or stroke; or those with the prospect of a terminal illness. Examples of intentional deaths include excessive risk taking, imprudence in the management of ordinary affairs, refusal to eat, overuse or misuse of alcohol or drugs, and noncompliance with life-sustaining medical regimens, such as refusal to take insulin or digoxin.

Elizabeth Kübler-Ross[38] has described five stages of dying that represent the coping mechanisms of dying persons. Her model is described in detail in Chapter 14. The family and significant others in the patient's life play an important role in the dying process. Nurses can encourage and support increased involvement of these persons in the patient's care. Assessment should be based on the patient's cues that he is ready to talk. Attentive listening alerts the nurse to the patient's need to express feelings or fears. Covert or overt references to death or thoughts about dying are early cues that the patient may be preparing for his own death.

A "living" will has been declared a legal document in over 35 states.[11] This reflects an increasing interest by consumers in how death occurs. It represents a person's choice to refuse heroic measures when he has no reasonable expectation for recovery. On admission, the nurse should ascertain the existence of a living will from the patient, family, or guardian. The nurse should be acquainted with the hospital's policy on such documents and the procedures for informing all staff and for ensuring that the patient's wishes are recognized.

■ **Somatic responses**

■ **HYPOCHONDRIASIS.** There is much overlap between hypochondriasis and depression. Preoccupation with one's physical and emotional health and expression of concern through body complaints are common with depressive and introspective patients but may be present in the absence of a depressed mood.

The patient's hypochondriasis expresses his underlying needs and fears. As a symbol of the geriatric patient's sense of defectiveness and deterioration, somaticism communicates the distress that accompanies a diminished sense of worth. Escape into the sick role is a legitimate and socially acceptable way to deal with stress and anxiety. The patient receives support, concern, and interest and experiences a sense of control.

One of the real problems encountered by the elder with a history of hypochondriasis is health professionals' tendency to label him a "crock" and dismiss his complaints, even if they are based on organic pathological conditions. All the patient's complaints should be taken seriously and investigated thoroughly. One must never assume the problem is "just a response to some emotional distress" and can therefore be dismissed. Whatever its cause, the problem and the patient's discomfort are real.

■ **SLEEP PATTERN DISTURBANCE.** Insomnia may be a symptom or a problem in itself for the gerontological psychiatric patient. Many older adults experience chronic or semichronic sleep problems. Complaints of interrupted sleep, loss of sleep, or "poor sleep," with frequent awakenings and morning exhaustion, are common. Daytime napping and drowsiness add to the problem.

Opinions vary regarding what are normal sleep patterns in older adults. Some researchers suggest that people need less sleep with increasing age. However, chronic fatigue, physical illness, pain, and decreased mobility may result in a need for more sleep. Geriatric patients often express distress over their inability to sleep or stay asleep. Perceived lack of sleep becomes a cyclical reaction. Worry over the lack of sleep prevents the elder from falling asleep. Fatigue, the most common physical complaint of adults over the age of 75, contributes to much of the insomnia of this age-group. Lack of exercise, limited mobility, and side effects of drugs may also contribute to insomnia.

The emotional effects of insomnia vary with the individual, but reinforcement of fatigue and depression is common. Recognizing insomnia as a reaction to emotional and physical disruptions and as a potential cause of other problems is the first step in assessing the problem.

■ **ALTERED NUTRITION: LESS THAN BODY REQUIREMENTS.** Anorexia is common in patients with depression but may also be seen in confused or disoriented patients. Forgetting to eat or being unable to prepare meals may reinforce loss of appetite. Side effects of some drugs (e.g., dry mouth, change in taste) contribute to lack of interest in food. The edentulous patient or the patient with gum disease avoids chewing when possible. The interaction of anorexia and emotional dysfunction should always be considered in the nutritional evaluation. Poor nutrition contributes to fatigue, listlessness, and immobility. Table 34-2 summarizes the categories of nursing diagnoses applicable to the psychogeriatric population.

❧ Planning and implementation

Nursing care strategies have been introduced throughout the chapter as part of the assessment and data collection process. Specific interventions will be considered as part of the total milieu for the patient. The elderly respond well to both individual and group psychotherapy. They need the opportunity to talk, to be supported in their efforts to deal with day-to-day problems, and to plan for a meaningful future.

■ **Approaches to intervention**

■ **LIFE REVIEW THERAPY.** Life review therapy was first described by Butler.[12] It has a positive psychotherapeutic function, providing an opportunity for the individual to reflect on his life and to resolve, reorganize, and reintegrate troubling or disturbing areas. The life review works well in both group and individual settings. Chubon[15] describes an innovative approach to life review with a 65-year-old woman with multiple disabilities. Using a novel about people with lives similar to that of the patient, the therapist helped the patient to identify with the characters, thereby reducing the emotional impact of reliving old conflicts and experiences. In a group setting, members may positively reinforce each other and stimulate mutual learning. Developing individual autobiographies to share with the group is one way to introduce commonalities among the members and put them at ease. The group cohesiveness and sharing can build self-esteem and a feeling of belonging, in addition to the cathartic effect of the review itself.

Ebersole[21] suggests several principles and processes of the life review to guide the nurse. Life review cannot be forced; therefore, when the older adult indicates readiness, its expression should be encouraged. Avoid judgmental interpretations (positive or negative) of the expressions of the elder revealed through life review. Encourage the expressions of feelings and meanings related to the content being presented. Encourage movement from one topic or area to another, rather than promoting the swelling or concentration on a narrow line of memories. The five steps of the process include: (1) ventilation, or the initial attempt at resolution; (2) exploration involves clarification and

TABLE 34-2

NURSING DIAGNOSES

Altered thought processes		Changes in affect		Somatic responses	
Behaviors	Etiologies	Behaviors	Etiologies	Behaviors	Etiologies
Memory loss Recent and/or long-term	Stress, crisis, depression, low self-esteem, cerebrovascular alterations, disease, trauma, sensory deprivation	Disturbed mood Mood swings Overreactions Dysfunctional grieving	Internal or external stress, loss of independence, side effects of drugs, grief, mourning, depression, physiological imbalances	Preoccupation with one's physical and emotional health	Depression, distress, and diminishing sense of worth, sleep pattern disturbance, fatigue, physical illness, alteration in nutrition: less than body requirements, alteration in comfort: pain.
Withdrawal	Multiple losses or fear of loss, grief, resistance to change, infection, pain, toxicity, side effects of drugs, organic impairment				
Confusion	Medication "hangover" (sunrise syndrome), loss of visual accommodation (sundown syndrome), multiple physiological and emotional problems, relocation, loss of family, friends				
Paranoia	Loss, isolation and loneliness, sensory deprivation/loss, adverse drug reactions/toxicity				

articulation of the event; (3) elaboration focuses on more detailed description of the event; (4) catharsis is the expression of suppressed feelings and resulting release of psychic energies; (5) acceptance comes when catharsis is complete or is sufficiently expressed; and (6) integration of the review into one's value system, beliefs, fantasies. The end result of life review is to release energy (emotional and cognitive) and create a sense of self-integrity and integration with the life one has lived. For the older adult, often confronted with time to reflect on a lifetime of memories, this type of approach can have beneficial results.

■ **REMINISCING GROUPS.** Reminiscing groups resemble life review groups in that the focus is on recounting earlier life experiences and events. In reminiscence, people share perceptions, historical life events, and generational attributes. Individual reminiscing should be encouraged as much as possible to help the patient discharge emotional and cognitive energy. Rambling does not constitute a therapeutic reminiscing experience, since the patient's preoccupation with his dissociated thoughts may actually increase anxiety. Reminiscing is a way both of holding on to the past and of letting go.[21] Patients may be encouraged to reminisce by formal story-telling or sharing of news events from an earlier time. Asking group participants to share their experiences of a historical (e.g., D-Day, Lindbergh's flight) or a personal event (e.g., marriage, birth of first child, first day in school) provides a basis for reminiscence.

■ **REALITY ORIENTATION.** Reality orientation was developed as a specific therapeutic program for institutionalized geriatric patients by James C. Folsom and colleagues in 1958.[48] Both 24-hour and classroom (structured) reality orientation have potential for preventing confusion and keeping patients oriented to time, place, person, and situation. The environment reinforces contact with reality, the here and now, when it is kept simple and focused. Helpful physical props include clocks, directional signs, calendars, and orientation boards (season of the year, weather, etc.). The classroom reality orientation consists of an intensive small-group experience, which is especially effective for the moderately to severely impaired elderly. It provides an opportunity to reinforce time, place, and person orientation with patients who have short attention spans and need extra verbal and visual stimulation. Reality orientation, along with a discussion of current events, stimulates the patient to maintain contact with the real world and his place in it. Current events discussions, used alone, may be structured in various ways, such as sharing of newspaper articles or group viewing of television news programs. The scope of the group depends on the patients' abilities and the other therapeutic modalities at hand.

■ **VALIDATION THERAPY.** Although reality orientation is effective for many institutionalized and community-based elderly with confusion and/or disorientation, some evidence indicates that for some older adults, especially those with minimal organic impairment, disorientation may be a form of denial of unpleasant realities. Additionally, these elders may become more anxious or agitated if constantly reminded of environmental realities. An alternate approach to confused and disoriented older adults was developed by Feil[25] and discussed in relation to working with the patient who is nonresponsive to reality orientation. This approach involves searching for the emotion and meaning in the patient's disoriented or confused words and behavior (such as wandering) and validating them verbally with the patient. A series of verbal cues or steps are involved that allow the patient to simply focus on key words or phrases in the confused interaction and the nurse validates by asking for description, more detail, or clarification. What is sometimes categorized as meaningless or incoherent conversation may often have significant meaning for the patient and can be related to current or past events. Validation is being used successfully with both mild and moderately impaired elderly and shows promise for providing an effective avenue for reaching older adults who are experiencing cognitive dysfunction. Little documentation is available on the use of this strategy in group settings or with severely impaired elders.

■ **COGNITIVE TRAINING.** Much research in underway using cognitive training and stimulation. Problem-solving situations, formal or didactic memory training, and selected memory exercises have proved effective in increasing attention span, efficiency of recall, and the ability to learn new skills (i.e., mathemathical calculations and vocabulary). Intelligence does not decline with progressive age but may be dulled by depression, drugs, or lack of use. Cognitive therapy has promise for providing methods for keeping older adults active mentally, which in turn will enhance emotional well-being. The "use it or lose it" adage holds as true for maintenance of intelligence as it does for physical functioning.

Clinical studies and experience to date indicate that cognitive training and therapy may be especially effective for the cognitively intact, motivated elderly persons with minor or major depressions. Cognitive therapy supports higher level defense mechanisms, such as reactionalization and intellectualization, encourages active participation of patients and a highly structured treatment. One positive aspect of this approach is its time-limited nature, which reinforces the goal of a positive change within a specific time period. Use with moderately to severely impaired older persons has not been documented.[39]

Stimulating cognitive skills can challenge the nurse's creativity in relating to gerontological psychiatric patients. To be able to capitalize on the patient's interests and skills, the nurse must be familiar with the patient's past occupation, hobbies, and leisure activities. The nursing interview should focus on gathering as much of that information as possible on admission and adding to the data base as the nurse builds a trusting relationship with the patient.

■ **RELAXATION THERAPY.** Relaxation therapy is another therapeutic modality receiving increasing interest. In addition to promoting a sense of physical well-being, relaxation can release tension and reduce stress, thus reducing barriers to communication. Simple relaxation exercises are described in detail by Wolanin and Phillips and presented in Chapter 11 of this text.[50] Relaxation, combined with mild isometric exercises, increases cardiovascular output, energy, and mobility and reduces stress. Relaxation and exercise strategies, used in group or individual contexts, do not require advanced skills of the nurse or the patient. They may begin with simple tension-releasing muscle exercises, coupled with verbal instructions about breathing and concentration.

■ **SUPPORTIVE AND COUNSELING GROUPS.** Gerontological psychiatric patients respond well to both supportive and counseling groups. These therapeutic outlets may use either a nondirective or unstructured format or a more structured, didactic approach. Group members can ventilate feelings, try out problem-solving approaches, and resolve conflict in a rational systematic manner. These groups may incorporate some aspects of cognitive training or reminiscence, described earlier in this chapter. Older adults respond well to a supportive group structure, which increases self-esteem, self-confidence, risk-taking and empathy for others. Humor may be an effective avenue for reaching the nonverbal or withdrawn elder. The ability to laugh at oneself and see the irony in everyday events provides an effective outlet for frustration, anger, stress, and anxiety. Promoting humor by telling jokes and stories and by watching cartoons or situation-comedies can be therapeutic in either a group setting or with individual patients. Expressions of humor and active laughter allow the older adult an opportunity to step out of his or her situation, thereby releasing some of the psychic energy required in coping with changes accompanying aging. Goodman[30] suggests humor and laughter as both therapeutic and educational activities, since the effects are both a sense of well-being and greater self-awareness and insight.

■ **PATIENT EDUCATION.** Older adults frequently question both physiological and cognitive (memory) changes that occur naturally in aging. Slowed response time, benign memory loss, alterations in gait, and interrupted sleep patterns represent a few of the normal changes of aging that can be interpreted as pathological. The nurse has an opportunity to teach patients about their own developmental changes during the assessment phase of the nurse-patient relationship. Dispelling myths and stereotypes related to the aging process represents a primary goal for patient education.[46]

The depressed older adult is particularly receptive to the educative process, since it is in the depressive state that they are most vulnerable and open to suggestion. Exercises for promoting positive thoughts and images, visualization, and repetitive cognitive games can be used as a basis for teaching new patterns of behavior. Cognitive training, relaxation, and life review approaches are well suited to patient education formats.

■ **FAMILY EDUCATION AND SUPPORT.** Because 80% of the elders living at home are cared for by a spouse, sibling, or adult child, family caregiver education and support groups are becoming essential to the care of the older adult.[2] Many community agencies, clinics, and senior citizen centers are responding to the need of this group with special activities, training classes, and support groups.

Family members often view nurses as the most appropriate health care professional for understanding family relationships, conflicts, needs, and resources. Family education related to the normal aging process, family dynamics and family systems, and stress inherent in the caregiver role can be easily integrated into counseling sessions with family members, referral conferences, or part of the family history on admission of the patient.[3]

A more formal approach to family education can be developed using the numerous books now available commercially that address the caregiving role with older adults. These materials provide practical, step-by-step guides to handling common problems of the frail elderly, including agitation, wandering, withdrawal, resistance, anxiety, insomnia, incontinence, anorexia, and restlessness. These books, which have been written specifically for the consumer, supply the text for nurse-family teaching sessions as well as excellent resource materials for use in the home.[29,32,41]

■ **EVALUATION OF CARE.** Specific nursing interventions designed to promote optimum cognitive function and emotional well-being have been considered as part of the role of the gerontological psychiatric nurse. Increasingly, research is being initiated to determine the most appropriate strategy for the need of the patient and the most effective modality for implementing the strategy.

Hall[31] suggests that evaluation of patient care should be based on a model that explains the progression of dysfunctional behavior from normative to anxious to stress behaviors. The type of care and the evaluation of outcome would be directly related to the level of behavior targeted for intervention.

Beck and Heacock[5] note that the goal of nursing interventions is to promote maximum independence of the older adult, based on capacity and functional abilities. Evaluation of outcomes of nursing care would not be based on reversal of behaviors or elimination of patient needs but on the change the patient demonstrates based on individual abilities. This approach reinforces the emphasis on the individual as a unit for evaluation and allows for patient differences and for the process of change over time.

■ **FUTURE TRENDS.** Gerontological psychiatric nursing offers an exciting and challenging future for nurses interested in working with patients responsive to knowledgeable and creative care. In one sense, most nurses today practice gerontological/geriatric nursing without recognizing it as such, since a growing proportion of patients in all health care settings are elderly. The significance of this growing population will become even more evident as we move toward the twenty-first century. The establishment of chronic disease and other long-term care facilities will supercede the growth of acute care hospitals.[4] The reliance on home care and the use of community resources to meet the health needs of all ages, but particularly the elderly, will grow in the next two decades. Advanced technology will permit shorter stays in acute care hospitals, quicker recovery periods, and less complicated disease courses.

Research in gerontological nursing has grown in the last 15 years. Without research, the direction and impact of practice remain unclear. Burnside[10] suggests several areas for reserach that stem from problems of concern to nurses working with the aged person: continence, sensory stimulation and deprivation, substance abuse, the use of touch and other communicative strategies with the elderly, effectiveness of treatment modalities in senile dementia, and promotion of wellness.

The influence of nursing research on nursing practice will depend on the ability of clinicians and researchers to work together in identifying projects collaboratively to investigate those problems. Only through collaboration will a body of nursing knowledge develop and grow.

Interprofessional activities in gerontology and geriatrics offer yet another avenue for nurses to impact the care of the elderly. The funding by private and federal sources of teaching nursing home demonstration projects with a combined academic, clinical, and research focus promises greater cooperation among nursing, medicine, dentistry, pharmacy, and social work. The extent to which the academic nursing home is successful depends, to a great degree, on the strength of the individual groups participating in the effort.

DIRECTIONS FOR FUTURE RESEARCH

The following are some of the nursing research problems raised in Chapter 34 that merit further study by psychiatric nurses:

1. The relationship between personality factors and coping with loss in increasing age
2. Differentiating depression from dementia
3. Factors contributing to sundown syndrome
4. The effectiveness of nursing actions with agitated elderly
5. Comparison of interventions with confused elderly
6. Preventive measures for disoriented elders
7. The relationship between family stress and elder self-esteem
8. The effectiveness of reminiscence with moderately confused elders
9. The relationship between functional ability and cognitive function
10. Supportive measures to reduce anxiety in the dementia patient
11. The effectiveness of physical exercise with depressed elders
12. The relationship between cognitive function and elder abuse
13. The effectiveness of humor in a regressed group of elders
14. The relationship between elder relocation and changes in recent memory
15. The effectiveness of cognitive therapy with paranoid elders
16. The relationship between staff attitudes toward the elderly and the elderly person's adjustment to an institutional setting
17. The relationship between mental status and cardiovascular response (B/P, P & R)
18. Factors that contribute to withdrawal of the elderly

The growing interest in and focus on gerontological/geriatric nursing as a specialization in nursing education is promising and will assure the nurse of the future an opportunity to offer quality care to this age group.

■ SUGGESTED CROSS-REFERENCES ■

The phases of the nursing process are discussed in Chapter 5. The mental status examination is discussed in Chapter 6. Primary prevention and identification of the elderly as a high-risk group are discussed in Chapter 8. Disturbances of mood are discussed in Chapter 14. Nursing care of the patient with impaired cognition is discussed in Chapter 18.

SUMMARY

1. Sociodemographic factors of aging were presented, with projections for the increase in this minority group over the next 20 years. Psychiatric and related disorders were defined, and the statistical significance was emphasized.

2. The gerontological nurse may function in a variety of roles, including patient-care manager in nursing homes or other long-term care settings, health assessor, primary care provider, independent practitioner, and researcher.

3. Biological theories of aging attempt to explain the reasons the body ages over time. Psychosocial and personality theories of aging focus on emotional response to the aging process.

4. Nursing assessment of the gerontological psychiatric patient is a multifaceted process, consisting of the interview, functional assessment, and evaluation of mental status.

5. Standardized measurement tools for assessing the older adult include the Mental Status Questionnaire, the Short Portable Mental Status Questionnaire, the Face-Hand Test, the Mini-Mental State Examination, the Zung Self-Rating Depression Scale, the the Nurses' Observation Scale for Inpatient Evaluation, the Katz Index of Activities of Daily Living, PACE II, the family Apgar, and the Social Behavior Assessment Schedule. Each tool has advantages and disadvantages as an adjunct to other assessment techniques.

6. Behavioral approaches to nursing diagnosis with assessment and intervention strategies for each include consideration of memory loss, withdrawal, confusion, paranoia, mood swings, grief, loss, depression, perceptions of death and dying, hypochondriasis, insomnia, and anorexia.

7. The life review, as a therapeutic intervention, stresses the idea of context (group versus individual) and innovative approaches to the technique. The similarity of reminiscence groups and the purpose of reminiscence as a therapeutic strategy were discussed.

8. Examples of therapeutic interventions with the elderly include reality orientation, cognitive training, and relaxation and validation therapy.

9. Families and caregivers of the home-bound and home-care elderly respond well to supportive and counseling groups and are receiving increasing attention from nurses and other health care professionals.

10. Humor is an important strategy for use with the elderly, because it both relieves anxiety and stress and provides an acceptable psychological outlet for frustration, anger, and hostility.

11. Patient and family education are important aspects of the gerontological psychiatric nursing role. Both formal and informal teaching should be provided to elders and their families in such areas as normal aging, differentiating normal from pathological states, family dynamics, and relationships.

12. New and innovative approaches to care of the elderly characterize the future of gerontological nursing. The need for clinical research to build a body of nursing knowledge in gerontology is recognized by researchers and practitioners alike. Emphasis is being placed on interprofessional practice approaches to the care of the geriatric patient.

REFERENCES

1. Albert MS: Cognition and aging. In Hazzard WR et al, editors: Principles of geriatric medicine and gerontology, ed 2, New York, 1990, McGraw-Hill Book Co.
2. Baldwin BA: Community management of Alzheimer's disease, Nurs Clin North Am 23:1, 47-56, 1988.
3. Baldwin BA et al: Family caregiver stress: clinical assessment and management, Inter Psychoger 1:2, 185-194, 1989.
4. Baldwin BA: Mental health in nursing homes: barriers and solutions. Testimony before the Joint Hearing before the Subcommittee on Health Services and the Select Committee of Aging, United States House of Representatives, August 3, 1989a. Washington DC, Government Printing Office.
5. Beck C and Heacock P: Nursing interventions with patients with Alzheimer's disease, Nurs Clin North Am 23:1, 95-124, 1988.
6. Blazer DG: The epidemiology of psychiatric disorders in late life. In Busse EW and Blazer DG, editors: Geriatric psychiatry, Washington DC, 1989, American Psychiatric Press.
7. Blazer DG: Affective disorders in late life. In Busse EW and Blazer DG, editors: Geriatric psychiatry, Washington DC, 1989a, American Psychiatric Press.
8. Brody EM: Parent care as a normative experience, Gerontologist 25:19-29, 1985.
9. Brown EL: The professional role in community nursing. II. Nursing reconsidered: a study of change. Philadelphia, 1971, JB Lippincott Co.
10. Burnside I: Gerontological nursing research: overcoming the bias of ageism in long-term care, New York, 1985.
11. Busse EW and Blazer GD: The future of geriatric psychiatry. In Busse EW and Blazer DG, editors: Geriatric psychiatry, Washington DC, 1989, American Psychiatric Press.
12. Butler RN: Re-awakening interest, Nurs Homes 10:8, 1961.
13. Butler RN and Lewis MR: Aging and mental health: psychosocial and biomedical approaches, ed 3, St Louis, 1981, Mosby–Year Book Inc.
14. Christison C, Christison G, and Blazer DG: Late-life schizophrenia and paranoid disorders. In Busse EW and Blazer DG, editors: Geriatric psychiatry, Washington DC, 1989, American Psychiatric Press.
15. Chubon S: A novel approach to the process of life review, J Gerontol Nurs 6:543, 1980.
16. Comfort A: Practice of geriatric psychiatry, New York, 1980, American Elsevier Publishing, Inc.
17. Cumming E and Henry WE: Growing old: the process of disengagement, New York, 1961, Basic Books, Inc.

18. Davis B: A coming of age: a challenge for geriatric nursing, J Am Geriatr Soc 16:1100, 1966.

19. Davis B: ANA and the geriatric nurse, Nurs Clin North Am 3:741, 1968.

20. Duke University Center for the Study of Aging and Human Development: Multidimensional functional assessment: the OARS methodology, Durham, NC, 1978, Duke University.

21. Ebersole P: Caring for the psychogeriatric patient, New York, Springer Publishers, 1989.

22. Ehrman J: Elderly personalities remain stable over time, NIH Record 33:3, Aug 4, 1981.

23. Eisdorfer C and Feidel RO: Cognitive and emotional disturbance in the elderly: clinical issues, St Louis, 1977, Mosby–Year Book, Inc.

24. Erikson EH: Identity and the life cycle: psychological issues, New York, 1959, International Universities Press, Inc.

25. Feil N: Communicating with the confused elderly patient, Geriatrics 39:131-132, 1984.

26. Fielo S and Rizzolo MA: The effects of age on pharmacokinetics, Geriatr Nurs 6(6):328, 1985.

27. Fink M et al: Face-hand test as a diagnostic sign of organic mental syndrome, Neurology 2:46, 1952.

28. Folstein MF et al: Mini-mental state: a practical method for grading the cognitive states of patients for the clinician, J Psychol Res 12:189, 1975.

29. Golden S: Nursing a loved one at home: a caregiver's guide, Philadelphia, 1988, Running Press.

30. Goodman J, editor: Laughing matters: the humor project, Saratoga Springs, New York, Saratoga Institute, 6:2, 44-60, 1989.

31. Hall GR: Care of the patient with Alzheimer's disease living at home, Nurs Clin North Am 23:1, 31-56, 1988.

32. Halpern J: Helping your aging parents: a practical guide for adult children, New York, 1987, McGraw-Hill Book Co.

33. Hayflick L et al: The serial cultivation of human diploid cells, Exp Cell Res 25:585, 1961.

34. Hendricks J and Hendricks CD: Aging in mass society, ed 2, Cambridge, Mass, 1981, Winthrop Publishers, Inc.

35. Honigfeld G and Klett CJ: The nurses' observation scale for inpatient evaluation: a new scale for measuring improvement in chronic schizophrenia, J Clin Psychol 21:65, 1965.

36. Kahn RL: Brief objective measure for the determination of mental status in aged, Am J Psychiatry 117:326, 1960.

37. Katz S et al: Studies of illness in the aged. The index of ADL; a standardized measure of biological and psychosocial function, JAMA 185:914, 1963.

38. Kübler-Ross E: On death and dying, London, 1980, Tavistock Publications, Ltd.

39. Lazarus LW: Psychotherapy with geriatric patients in the ambulatory care setting. In Busse EW and Blazer EG, editors: Geriatric psychiatry, Washington DC, 1989, American Psychiatric Press.

40. Lowenthal MF et al: Four stages of life: a comparative study of women and men facing transitions, San Francisco, 1975, Jossey-Bass, Inc, Publishers.

41. Mace NL and Rabins PV: The 36-hour day, New York, 1984, Warner Books.

42. Moritz DF and Ostfeld AD: The epidemiology and demography of aging. In Hazzard WR, et al, editors: Principles of geriatric medicine and gerontology, ed 2, New York, 1990, McGraw-Hill Book Co.

43. Ochsner A: Aging, J Am Geriatr Soc 24:385, 1976.

44. Platt S et al: Social behavior assessment schedule (SBAS): rationale, contents, scoring and reliability of a new interview schedule, Soc Psychiatry 15:43, 1980.

45. Radar J et al: How to decrease wandering, a form of agenda behavior, Geriatr Nurs July-Aug, 1985.

46. Schwab Sr M, et al: Relieving the anxiety and fear in dementia, J Gerontol Nurs 11(5):8, 1985.

47. Smilkstein G: The family APGAR: a proposal for a family function test and its use by physicians, J Fam Pract 6:1231, 1978.

48. Taulbee L and Folsom J: Reality orientation for geriatric patients, Hosp Community Psychiatry 17:133, 1966.

49. US Department of Health, Education and Welfare: Working-document on patient care management, Washington, DC, 1978, US Government Printing Office.

50. Wolanin MO and Phillips LRF: Confusion: prevention and care, St Louis, 1981, Mosby–Year Book Inc.

51. Yesavage JA et al: Senile dementia; combined pharmacologic and psychologic treatment, J Am Geriatr Soc 29:164, 1981.

52. Zung WWK: A self-rating depression scale, Arch Gen Psychiatry 12:63, 1965.

■ ANNOTATED SUGGESTED READINGS ■

Alzheimer's Disease: Report of the Advisory Panel on Alzheimer's Disease, Washington DC, US Department of Health and Human Services, 1989.

Contains a series of public policy and science policy recommendations for both administrative and legislative action in the areas of biomedical research, health services research, services delivery, and the financing of health care and social services to benefit those suffering from Alzheimer's disease and related dementias and their families.

*Baldwin BA and Stevens G: Family caregiving: education and support. In Eliopoulos C, editor: Caring for the elderly in diverse care settings, Philadelphia, 1990, JB Lippincott.

This chapter describes the recent trends in family caregiving, identifies causes and manifestations of caregiver stress, and discusses ways in which nurses can assist family caregivers through education and support groups.

*Britnell J and Mitchell K: Inpatient group psychotherapy for the elderly, J Psychiatr Nurs 19:19, 1981.

---

*Asterisk indicates nursing reference.

One of the few articles in the nursing literature on group psychotherapy for the elderly. Describes a theoretical framework and applies it to case examples.

*Burnside IM, editor: Working with the elderly: group processes and techniques, North Scituate, Mass, 1978, Duxbury Press.

Volume of papers provides an overview of group work with the elderly, including reminiscence, reality orientation, remotivation, music, and art therapy in a practical "how to" approach.

Busse EW and Blaze DG, editors: Geriatric psychiatry, Washington DC, 1989, American Psychiatric Press.

Reflects the rapidly expanding base of our scientific knowledge of aging and geriatrics. Designed to provide the scholar and clinician with the scientific facts and applied skills and knowledge that are so needed in dealing with the mental disorders of late life.

Comfort A: Practice of geriatric psychiatry, New York, 1980, American Elsevier Publishing, Inc.

Practical approach to geropsychiatry; includes an overview and systematic discussion of every major category of geriatric mental disease. Both diagnostic and therapeutic data are included throughout the text.

Covell M: The home alternative to hospitals and nursing homes, New York, 1985, Holt, Rinehart and Winston.

Describes the impact of home health care on the health care system. A practical guide to care in the home, including care for a mentally ill relative and home care of the older adult. Provides examples of physical and emotional care for teaching families and other caregivers of the home care patient.

Department of Health, Education and Welfare, The Federal Council on the Aging: Mental health and the elderly: recommendations for action, Washington, DC, 1979, US Government Printing Office.

Two reports give an overview of the needs of and resources for the elderly with mental health problems. Recommendations for action in the public and private sector are cited in areas of assessment, treatment, and health care service.

*Ebersole P: Caring for the psychogeriatric client, New York, 1989, Springer Publishers.

Designed for nurses, social workers, counselors, paraprofessionals, and community agency personnel who deal directly with the mental health needs and emotional disorders of the aged. Emphasis is on management strategies shown effective with aged persons demonstrating a variety of emotional and behavioral problems.

Glickstein JK: Therapeutic interventions in Alzheimer's disease, Rockville, MD, 1988, Aspen Publishers, Inc.

Directed toward professionals working with dementia clients, particularly those professionals who are working one-on-one with dementia clients and their caregivers. The overall goal is to provide health care professionals with therapy material that can be used in the development of individualized programs suitable for use with this client population. Contains overview of Alzheimer's disease, workbook with specific lesson plans, and how to suggestions for working with dementia clients.

Hall BA: Mental health and the elderly, New York, 1984, Grune and Stratton, Inc.

Designed for clinical specialists working with elderly patients and students trying to integrate the knowledge gained in specialty areas into their work with the elderly. Focuses on psychosocial aspects of aging, approaches to mental health care of the elderly, aging and death, and models for delivery of care to the elderly.

Kra S: Aging myths: reversible causes of mind and memory loss, New York, 1986, McGraw-Hill Book Co.

Based on scientific findings, author refutes some of the myths regarding age and memory loss. Using a case study approach, the reversible causes of dementia and memory loss are examined, showing that senility is not an inevitable consequence of growing old.

Maclay E: Green winter, New York, 1977, McGraw-Hill Book Co.

A book of poems whose pages surprise with wit, with the unexpected turn of thought and the grit and tenderness of human spirit. A book of celebrations of old age.

Mental illness in nursing homes: agenda for research, National Institute of Mental Health, US Department of Health and Human Services, Public Health Service, Alcohol, Drug Abuse, and Mental Health Administration, Rockville, MD, 1986, DHHS Publication No. (ADM) 86-1459.

Topics include epidemiology of mental illness in nursing homes, research issues and needs, polypharmacy research needs in the nursing home, issues in assessment and evaluation, treatment modalities, outcomes of the conference on mental illness in nursing homes, recommendations for mental health research in nursing homes, and the underrepresentation of minorities in nursing homes.

*National League for Nursing: Overcoming the bias of ageism in long-term care, New York, 1985, NLN.

Contains papers on recruiting and retaining nurses in long-term care, core content in gerontological and geropsychiatric nursing, and research in long-term care.

Psychopharmacology Bulletin: National Institute of Mental Health, Special Issue: Assessment in diagnosis and treatment of geropsychiatric patients, 24:4, 1988.

Designed to assist researchers and practitioners in geropsychiatry by providing a "consumer guide" to instruments that may be of value in the diagnosis and evaluation of treatment effects in the elderly.

Seuss Dr and Geisel AS: You're only old once! New York, 1986, Random House.

Theodor Seuss Geisel, better known as Dr. Seuss, celebrated his eighty-second birthday on March 2, 1986, the publication date of this book. With the humor typical of Dr. Seuss's books, we follow our hapless hero through his checkup with the experts at the Golden Years Clinic.

*Stevens GL and Baldwin BA: Optimizing mental health in the nursing home setting, J Psychosoc Nurs 26:10, 27-31, 1988.

Suggests that the physical and social environment of the nursing home setting can be manipulated by staff to support functional behavior, rather than behavioral decline. Communication and interpersonal skills of nursing home staff can foster resident's sense of worth, a high level of functioning, and an advanced quality of life. A proactive strategy to manage behavior therapeutically and reduce stress for nursing home staff requires anticipating resident needs before behavioral expression is observed.

*Wahl PR: Therapeutic relationships with the elderly, J Gerontol Nurs 6:260, 1980.

Components of a helping therapeutic relationship are posed. Special consideration of the needs of the elderly constitute the discussion of the phases of the relationship, goals, and outcome.

*Wolanin MO and Phillips LRF: Confusion: prevention and care, St Louis, 1980, Mosby–Year Book, Inc.

Using a multidimensional approach to assessment and intervention, the authors emphasize the impact of the diagnosis or misdiagnosis of confusion on treatment selection and outcome for the elderly client.

*Wolanin MO and Phillips LRF: Who's confused here? Geriatr Nurs 1:122, July-Aug 1980.

Use case examples to illustrate how labeling of patient behavior may lead to misinterpretation and misdiagnosis. The consequence of misdiagnosis of confusion in the elderly is addressed, along with suggestions for more accurate assessment and nursing management.

APPENDIXES

A P P E N D I X   A

MENTAL STATUS EXAMINATION

Facility _____
Assessor _____
Date _____

Mental Status Assessment

Appearance and behavior

1. General appearance: physical characteristics, apparent age, peculiarities of dress, cleanliness, use of cosmetics, vocational indicators, appearance of hands
2. Level of consciousness: alert, lethargic, stuporous, comatose
3. Motor
   a. Status: posture (stooped, erect, slouched), gait (shuffling, staggering, stiff, awkward), gestures, tics, grimaces, limpness or rigidity of extremities, tremors, mannerisms
   b. Activity: over- or underactive, purposeful or disorganized, stereotyped, graceful, echopraxia, apraxia
   c. Facial expression: alert, tense, worried, sad, happy, dreamy, frightened, pained, angry, sneering, ecstatic, laughing, smiling, suspicious
4. Behavior: indifferent, frank, friendly, embarrassed, help seeking, evasive, afraid, resentful, sullen, angry, irritable, assaultive, seductive, negativistic, exhibitionistic, dramatic, impulsive
5. Relationship to examiner

Speech

1. Description: soft, loud, stuttering, hesitant, accent, enunciation, dysarthria, mutism, (use test phrases such as Commonwealth of Pennsylvania, Methodist Episcopal, liquid linoleum, third royal riding artillery brigade)
2. Speed and quantity: relationship with motor activity, special topics, or affects; delay in answering questions
3. Aphasias

Feelings

1. Mood: the patient's subjective statement of his feeling state
2. Affect: the feeling state inferred by the examiner on the basis of the patient's statements, appearance, and behavior
   a. Shallowness or flattening of affect: an insufficiently intense emotional display in association with ideas or situations
   b. Inappropriate affect: dissociation or disharmony between affect and thought content
   c. Lability of affect: the degree to which emotional reactions fluctuate during the interview (a certain amount of fluctuation is the norm)
   d. Descriptors: composed, complacent, frank, friendly, playful, teasing, silly, cheerful, boastful, elated, grandiose, ecstatic, tense, worried, anxious, pessimistic, sad, perplexed, bewildered, gloomy, depressed, frightened, aloof, superior, disdainful, distant, defensive, suspicious, irritable, resentful, hostile, sarcastic, angry, furious, indifferent, resigned, apathetic, dull, affectless
3. Signs of biological depression
   a. Appetite and weight changes
   b. Sleep changes
   c. Psychomotor agitation or retardation
   d. Loss of interest and pleasure
   e. Loss of energy; fatigue
   f. Feelings of worthlessness
   g. Subjective or objective difficulty concentrating
   h. Recurrent thoughts of death or suicidal ideation

Perceptions

1. Illusions: misperceptions of external stimuli
2. Hallucinations: false sensory impressions without any external basis in fact; may be formed (e.g., a face) or unformed (e.g., flashing lights)
   a. Visual: flashes, lights, gray patches, whiteness, recognizable persons or things
   b. Auditory: incomprehensive murmurings, voices, voices commenting on one's behavior
   c. Olfactory
   d. Gustatory
   e. Tactile: fornication

Thoughts

1. Content
   a. Note spontaneous trends of thought toward particular topics and preoccupation with these topics; best delineated by giving neutral, simple questions at the beginning of the interview
   b. Delusion: a belief held in the face of incontrovertible evidence to the contrary; different from superstition and religious belief
      i. Delusions of persecution: patient believes he is the object of environmental attention
      ii. Delusions of alien control
      iii. Delusions of grandeur: often associated with elated states
      iv. Somatic delusions of having cancer or other severe illness
2. Progresson: the relatedness of thoughts to each other
   a. Associations: loose associations are demonstrated by illogical, vague, and poorly organized patterns of thought; when extreme, it is referred to as "word salad," where any given word has no relationship to the words that precede or follow it
   b. Circumstantiality: much unnecessary detail given spontaneously; the goal of speech is eventually reached
   c. Blocking: sudden stop in the stream of talk for no apparent external reason
   d. Flight of ideas: clever productivity of talk, which is continuous but fragmentary; connections are often determined by chance associations; a certain amount of coherence is present, but the direction of talk can be influenced by chance external stimuli; may include punning, rhyming, and clang associations (on the basis of similar sounds)

Orientation

1. Time
2. Place
3. Person
4. Self

Memory

1. Remote past recall: the ability of an individual to tell a coherent life story and to remember such questions as time and place of birth, various schools attended, occupational history, date of marriage, number of children and their ages
2. Recent past recall: the ability to tell the history and events leading to hospitalization and treatment
3. Immediate past recall (retention): tests the patient's ability to retain a person's name and three unrelated facts 5 minutes after they have been given; test immediate repetition of digits (digit span) starting with three or four digits until the patient fails twice; read the digits at approximately one per second without rhythmic spacing or vocal inflection; the numbers chosen should not be in their natural order and should not suggest historical dates; also test ability to remember digits backward
4. General grasp and recall can be tested by having the patient read and report his memory of a brief story

Intellectual evaluation

1. General information: examples include the five largest U.S. cities, the capitals of various states, dates of wars and the issues involved, names of the last four presidents, the governor of the state, and differences in abstract words (e.g., idleness and laxiness, poverty and misery, character and reputation)
2. Calculation
   a. Serial sevens: record the answers carefully, including the time taken for the test; do not correct for errors
   b. Ability to make change with money
3. Reasoning and judgment: the patient's ability to estimate correctly and form opinions concerning external objective matters (e.g., what would he do in an emergency situation or if he were given a large amount of money?)
4. Proverb interpretation
5. Similarities

Insight

The degree to which the patient realizes the significance his symptoms and of his current situation; does he consider himself in need of help? Does he understand his physical or emotional affliction? Does he understand how it may affect his life?

MEDICATION AND DRUG ASSESSMENT TOOL

Facility _____

Assessor _____

Date _____

Medication and Drug Assessment

1. Psychiatric medications (for *each* medication *ever* taken by the patient, obtain the following information):
   a. Name of drug
   b. Reason prescribed
   c. Date started
   d. Length of time taken
   e. Highest daily dose
   f. Prescribed by whom
   g. Summarize effects
   h. Side effects or adverse reactions
   i. Was it taken as prescribed? If not, explain.
   j. Other family members prescribed this drug
   k. If so, reason prescribed and effectiveness
2. Prescription (nonpsychiatric) medications (for *each* medication taken by the patient in the past 6 months and for major medical illnesses if more than 6 months ago, obtain the following information):
   a. Name of drug
   b. Reason prescribed
   c. Date started
   d. Highest daily dose
   e. Prescribed by whom
   f. Summarize effects
   g. Side effects or adverse reactions
   h. Was it taken as prescribed? If not, explain.

3. Over-the-counter (nonprescribed) medications (for *each* medication taken by the patient in the past 6 months, obtain the following information):
   a. Name of drug
   b. Reason taken
   c. Date started
   d. Frequency of use
   e. Summarize effects
   f. Side effects or adverse reactions
4. Alcohol and street drugs (see Appendix F for common street names of abused substances)
   a. Name of substance
   b. Date of first use
   c. Frequency of use
   d. Summarize effects
   e. Adverse reactions

PHYSICAL ASSESSMENT TOOL

Facility _____
Assessor _____
Date _____

Physical History

Biographical data

1. Name
2. Age
3. Race
4. Culture
5. Address
6. Marital status
7. Children and family in home
8. Occupation
9. Means of transportation to health care facility, if pertinent
10. Description of home; size and type of community

Reason for visit

One statement that describes the reason for the client's visit, or the chief complaint. State in the client's own words.

Present health status

1. General health status of the client in the past 1 year, 5 years, now
2. Client's current major health concerns
3. If illness is present, include (symptoms analysis) history
   a. When was client last well
   b. Date of problem onset
   c. Character of complaint
   d. Nature of problem onset
   e. Course of problem
   f. Client's hunch of precipitating factors
   g. Location of problem
   h. Relation to other body symptoms, body positions, and activity
   i. Patterns of problem
   j. Efforts of client to treat
   k. Coping ability
4. Current medications
   a. Type (prescription, over-the-counter drugs, vitamins, etc.)
   b. Prescribed by whom
   c. Amount per day
   d. Problems

Current health statistics

1. Immunization status (note dates or year of last immunization)
   a. Tetanus, diphtheria
   b. Mumps
   c. Rubella
   d. Polio
   e. Tuberculosis tine test
   f. Influenza
2. Allergies (describe agent and reactions)
   a. Drugs
   b. Foods
   c. Contact substances
   d. Environmental factors
3. Last examinations (note physician/clinic, findings, advice, and/or instructions)
   a. Physical
   b. Dental
   c. Vision
   d. Hearing
   e. ECG
   f. Chest radiograph
   g. Pap smear (females)

Physical History—cont'd

Past health status

Although each of the following is asked separately, the examiner must summarize and record the data *chronologically*.

1. Childhood illnesses: rubeola, rubella, mumps, pertussis, scarlet fever, chickenpox, strep throat
2. Serious or chronic illnesses: scarlet fever, diabetes, kidney problems, hypertension, sickle cell anemia, seizure disorders, blood infections
3. Serious accidents or injuries: head injuries, fractures, burns, other trauma
4. Hospitalizations: elaborate, reason for, location, primary care providers, duration
5. Surgery: what, where, when, why, by whom
6. Emotional health: past problems, help sought, support persons
7. Obstetrical history
   a. Complete pregnancies: number, pregnancy course, postpartum course, and condition, weight, and sex of child
   b. Incomplete pregnancies: duration, termination, circumstances (including abortions and stillbirths)
   c. Summary of complications

Family history

Family members include the client's blood relatives, spouse, and children. Specifically the interviewer should inquire about the client's maternal and paternal grandparents, parents, aunts, uncles, spouse, and children, as well as about the general health, stress factors, and illnesses of other family members. Questions should include a survey of the following:

Cancer	Retardation
Diabetes	Alcoholism
Heart disease	Endocrine diseases
Hypertension	Sickle cell anemia
Epilepsy (or seizure disorder)	Kidney disease
Emotional stresses	Unusual limitations
Mental illness	Other chronic problems

The most concise method to record these data is by a family tree.

Review of physiological systems

The purpose of this component of the data base is to collect information about the body regions or systems and their function.

1. General—reflect from client's previous description of present health status
   a. Fatigue patterns
   b. Exercise and exercise tolerance
   c. Weakness episodes
   d. Fever, sweats
   e. Frequent colds, infections, or illnesses
   f. Ability to carry out activities of daily living
2. Nutritional
   a. Client's average, maximum, and minimum weights during past month, 1 year, 5 years
   b. History of weight gains or losses (time element; specific efforts to change weight)
   c. Twenty-four-hour diet recall (helpful to mail client chart to fill in before visit)
   d. Current appetite
   e. Who buys, prepares food?
   f. Who does client normally eat with?
   g. Is client able to afford preferred food?
   h. Does client wear dentures? Is chewing a problem?
   i. Client's self-evaluation of nutritional status
3. Integumentary
   a. Skin
      (1) Skin disease or skin problems or lesions (wounds, sores, ulcers)
      (2) Skin growths, tumors, masses
      (3) Excessive dryness, sweating, odors
      (4) Pigmentation changes or discolorations
      (5) Pruritus (itching)
      (6) Texture changes
      (7) Temperature changes
   b. Hair
      (1) Changes in amount, texture, character
      (2) Alopecia (loss of hair)
      (3) Use of dyes
   c. Nails: changes in appearance, texture
4. Head
   a. Headache (characteristics, including frequency, type, location, duration, care for)
   b. Past significant trauma
   c. Dizziness
   d. Syncope
5. Eyes
   a. Discharge (characteristics)
   b. History of infections, frequency, treatment
   c. Pruritus (itching)
   d. Lacrimation, excessive tearing
   e. Pain in eyeball
   f. Spots (floaters)
   g. Swelling around eyes

Physical History—cont'd

h. Cataracts, glaucoma
i. Unusual sensations or twitching
j. Vision changes (generalized or vision field)
k. Use of corrective or prosthetic devices
l. Diplopia (double vision)
m. Blurring
n. Photophobia
o. Difficulty reading
p. Interference with activities of daily living
6. Ears
   a. Pain (characteristics)
   b. Cerumen (wax)
   c. Infection
   d. Hearing changes (describe)
   e. Use of prosthetic devices
   f. Increased sensitivity to environmental noise
   g. Vertigo
   h. Ringing and cracking
   i. Care habits
   j. Interference with activities of daily living
7. Nose, nasopharynx, and paranasal sinuses
   a. Discharge (characteristics)
   b. Epistaxis
   c. Allergies
   d. Pain over sinuses
   e. Postnasal drip
   f. Sneezing
   g. General olfactory ability
8. Mouth and throat
   a. Sore throats (characteristics)
   b. Lesions of tongue or mouth (abscesses, sores, ulcers)
   c. Bleeding gums
   d. Hoarseness
   e. Voice changes
   f. Use of prosthetic devices (dentures, bridges)
   g. Altered taste
   h. Chewing difficulty
   i. Swallowing difficulty
   j. Pattern of dental hygiene
9. Neck
   a. Node enlargement
   b. Swellings, masses
   c. Tenderness
   d. Limitation of movement
   e. Stiffness
10. Breast
   a. Pain or tenderness
   b. Swelling
   c. Nipple discharge
   d. Changes in nipples
   e. Lumps, dimples
   f. Unusual characteristics
   g. Breast examination: pattern, frequency
11. Cardiovascular
   a. Cardiovascular
      (1) Palpitations
      (2) Heart murmur
      (3) Varicose veins
      (4) History of heart disease
      (5) Hypertension
      (6) Chest pain (character and frequency)
      (7) Shortness of breath
      (8) Orthopnea
      (9) Paroxysmal nocturnal dyspnea
   b. Peripheral vascular
      (1) Coldness, numbness
      (2) Discoloration
      (3) Peripheral edema
      (4) Intermittent claudication
12. Respiratory
   a. History of asthma
   b. Other breathing problems (when, precipitating factors)
   c. Sputum production
   d. Hemoptysis
   e. Chronic cough (characteristics)
   f. Shortness of breath (precipitating factors)
   g. Night sweats
   h. Wheezing or noise with breathing
13. Hematolymphatic
   a. Lymph node swelling
   b. Excessive bleeding or easy bruising
   c. Petechiae, ecchymoses
   d. Anemia
   e. Blood transfusions
   f. Excessive fatigue
   g. Radiation exposure
14. Gastrointestinal
   a. Food idiosyncrasies
   b. Change in taste
   c. Dysphagia (inability or difficulty in swallowing)
   d. Indigestion or pain (associated with eating?)
   e. Pyrosis (burning sensation in esophagus and stomach with sour eructation)
   f. Ulcer history
   g. Nausea/vomiting (time, degree, precipitating and/or associated factors)
   h. Hematemesis
   i. Jaundice
   j. Ascites

Physical History—cont'd

k. Bowel habits (diarrhea/constipation)
l. Stool characteristics
m. Change in bowel habits
n. Hemorrhoids (pain, bleeding, amount)
o. Dyschezia (constipation caused by habitual neglect to respond to stimulus to defecate)
p. Use of digestive or evacuation aids (what, how often)
15. Urinary
   a. Characteristics of urine
   b. History of renal stones
   c. Hesitancy
   d. Urinary frequency (in 24-hour period)
   e. Change in stream of urination
   f. Nocturia (excessive urination at night)
   g. History of urinary tract infection, dysuria (painful urination, urgency, flank pain)
   h. Suprapubic pain
   i. Dribbling or incontinence
   j. Stress incontinence
   k. Polyuria (excessive excretion of urine)
   l. Oliguria (decrease in urinary output)
   m. Pyuria
16. Genital
   a. General
     (1) Lesions
     (2) Discharges
     (3) Odors
     (4) Pain, burning, pruritus (itching)
     (5) Venereal disease history
     (6) Satisfaction with sexual activity
     (7) Birth control methods practiced
     (8) Sterility
   b. Males
     (1) Prostate problems
     (2) Penis and scrotum self-examination practices
   c. Females
     (1) Menstrual history (age of onset, last menstrual period [LMP], duration, amount of flow, problems)
     (2) Amenorrhea (absence of menses)
     (3) Menorrhagia (excessive menstruation)
     (4) Dysmenorrhea (painful menses); treatment method
     (5) Metrorrhagia (uterine bleeding at times other than during menses)
     (6) Dyspareunia (pain with intercourse)
17. Musculoskeletal
   a. Muscles
     (1) Twitching
     (2) Cramping
     (3) Pain
     (4) Weakness
   b. Extremities
     (1) Deformity
     (2) Gait or coordination difficulties
     (3) Interference with activities of daily living
     (4) Walking (amount per day)
   c. Bones and joints
     (1) Joint swelling
     (2) Joint pain
     (3) Redness
     (4) Stiffness (time of day related)
     (5) Joint deformity
     (6) Noise with joint movement
     (7) Limitations of movement
     (8) Interference with activities of daily living
   d. Back
     (1) History of back injury (characteristics of problems, corrective measures)
     (2) Interference with activities of daily living
18. Central nervous system
   a. History of central nervous system disease
   b. Fainting episodes
   c. Seizure
     (1) Characteristics
     (2) Medications
   d. Cognitive changes
     (1) Inability to remember (recent vs. distant)
     (2) Disorientation
     (3) Phobias
     (4) Hallucinations
     (5) Interference with activities of daily living
   e. Motor-gait
     (1) Coordinated movement
     (2) Ataxia, balance problems
     (3) Paralysis (partial vs. complete)
     (4) Tic, tremor, spasm
     (5) Interference with activities of daily living
   f. Sensory
     (1) Paresthesia (patterns)
     (2) Tingling sensations
     (3) Other changes
19. Endocrine
   a. Diagnosis of disease states (thyroid, diabetes)
   b. Changes in skin pigmentation or texture
   c. Changes in or abnormal hair distribution
   d. Sudden or unexplained changes in height and weight
   e. Intolerance to heat or cold

Physical History—cont'd

f. Exophthalmos
g. Goiter
h. Hormone therapy
i. Polydipsia (↑ thirst)
j. Polyphagia (↑ food intake)
k. Polyuria (↑ urination)
l. Anorexia (↓ appetite)
m. Weakness

20. Allergic and immunological (Optional; use if client indicates allergic history. Note precipitating factors in each case.)
a. Dermatitis (inflammation or irritation of skin)
b. Eczema
c. Pruritus (itching)
d. Urticaria (hives)
e. Sneezing
f. Vasomotor rhinitis (inflammation and swelling of mucous membrane of nose; nasal discharge)
g. Conjunctivitis (inflammation of conjunctiva)
h. Interference with activities of daily living
i. Environmental and seasonal correlation
j. Treatment techniques

21. Does client have any other physiological problems or disease states not specifically discussed? If so, explore in detail (e.g., fatigue, insomnia, nervousness).

Health maintenance efforts

1. General statement of client's own physical fitness
2. Exercise (amount, type, frequency)
3. Dietary regulations; special efforts (describe in detail)
4. Mental health; special efforts such as group therapy, meditation, yoga (describe in detail)
5. Cultural or religious practices
6. Frequency of physical, dental, and vision health assessment

Environmental health

1. General statement of client's assessment of environmental safety and comfort
2. Hazards of employment (inhalants, noise, heavy lifting, psychological stress, machinery)
3. Hazards in the home (concern about fire, stairs to climb, inadequate heat, open gas heaters, inadequate toilet facilities, concern about pest control, inadequate space)
4. Hazards in neighborhood (noise, water, and air pollution, inadequate police protection, heavy traffic on surrounding streets, isolation from neighbors, overcrowding)
5. Community hazards (unavailability of stores, market, laundry facilities, drugstore; no access to bus line)

From Thompson J and Bowers A: Clinical manual of health assessment, ed 3, St Louis, 1988, Mosby–Year Book, Inc.

A P P E N D I X   D

FAMILY ASSESSMENT TOOL

Facility _____

Assessor _____

Date _____

Guide to Family Analysis

Family genogram

1. Names, ages, ethnic and religous affiliation of all family members
2. Exact dates of birth, marriage, separation, divorce, death, and other significant life events
3. Notations with dates about occupation, grade in school, places of residence, illness, and changes in life course on the genogram itself
4. Information on three or more generations
5. Notation about frequency and type of contact (mail, telephone, visit, marriage, and funerals only)
6. Notation about closest and most distant relationships

Description of home environment

1. Characteristics of neighborhood, type of housing, ownership of housing, car
2. Adequacy of housing (safe, healthy, privacy, food preparation, temperature, space for children to play, yard)
3. Family satisfaction with housing, community
4. How does the family perceive the community's "attitude" toward it?
5. What are the private and public transportation facilities for the family? Are they a help or hindrance to their way of living?
6. What beauty exists in their environment? What efforts have they made to add beauty to the home?

Health and related factors

1. Physical level of growth and development, including developmental lags in the past
2. Past physical problems, including genetic and accidents

3. Current physical problems
4. Status of immunizations
5. Special physical abilities or hobbies (e.g., mechanical, gardening, sewing)
6. What treatment does he rely on before calling a physician?
7. How does he utilize medical resources (episodic or preventive)?
8. What is the family's usual source of health care, single or multiple?
9. What does the family's nutritional assessment reveal?
10. How susceptible to illness does the identified patient think he is? Does the family agree?
11. What is the identified patient's theory about his illness (i.e., to what does he attribute it)? What is the family's theory?
12. How has the identified patient's illness changed the family's functioning? Who has been most involved in the care? Who has been most affected?
13. Mental abilities (social and/or academic performance, particular philosophical outlook, thought or language disorder)
14. Sense of self-esteem of family members
15. Sense of humor of family members
16. Personal appearance and hygiene of family members

Financial status

1. What is the family's annual income? Who earns it? Where?
2. What work and homemaking skills are available to each person?
3. How is money managed in this family?
4. If the family does not have an adult who is working, why is the adult not able to work and earn a living? (There is usually more than one reason.)

3. How is money managed in this family?

4. If the family does not have an adult who is working, why is the adult not able to work and earn a living? (There is usually more than one reason.)

5. What consumer skills are available in the family? (Do they know how to comparison shop?) (Do they now how to determine what they need?) (Can they do home repair, sew, can food?)

6. Are there financial constraints on seeking health care?

Developmental state in family life cycle

1. Is the family in a normative crisis of transition?

2. Are there outstanding emotional tasks from previous stages unsuccessfully completed and impeding current family functioning?

3. What are the major emotional tasks confronting the family at this stage in the family life cycle?

4. How is the identified patient's illness influencing the emotional process of the family life cycle?

Family structure

1. Are the boundaries in the family clearly delineated or diffuse between the following:
   a. The marital subsystem
   b. The parental subsystem
   c. The sibling subsystem
   d. Individual subsystems
   e. The grandparent subsystem
   f. The sexes

2. Are there identifiable coalitions or alliances? What are the key family triangles?

3. Are authority and responsibility clearly defined and/or delegated? Does the responsibility to the delegated member exceed his physical or maturational capacities?

4. Are subsystem functions being performed and subsystem interpersonal skills being developed?

Intrafamily relationships

1. How do family members converse with each other? Is communication direct, clear, tangential, amorphous, covert? What kind of information is communicated? Is there a "central switchboard"?

2. How are decisions made (about vacations, discipline, large purchases, personal problems)?

3. How do they have fun together? Do they share time, space, money?

4. How do family members encourage separateness, recognize privacy, among members?

5. How is nurturance, recognition, support given to each other?

6. How is the marital relationship (emotionally and sexually satisfying or distant and conflictual)?

7. How does each parent relate to the children? What child-rearing skills do the parents have or lack?

8. How are children being taught to problem solve, to develop independence and self-reliance?

9. How do family members interact with the outside world (neighbors, schools, work, agencies, church)?

10. What is the nature of extended family relationships? (Is one side or both distant or cut off? Is contact formal and obligatory? Is contact open, regular, and emotionally meaningful even if infrequent?)

11. Who are the most significant members in the extended families? How are they significant?

Sociocultural family context

1. What is the ethnic or cultural background of the family? In what ways is this apparent in their way of living? In household furnishing?

2. Is there a religious belief? Affiliation? How does this influence each one or the family?

3. Have members in any way altered the cultural, ethnic, or religious practices or beliefs? What has been the result of these changes?

4. What are the dominant attitudes toward health, the community, achievement in school and career, toward life?

5. What dominant stereotyped sex-role expectations are expressed or demonstrated between husband and wife, between parents and children?

Strengths and weaknesses of the family

1. As seen by the family
2. As seen by the nurse

Problems identified

1. By the family
2. By the nurse
3. Solutions tried by the family to resolve the problems

From Helm PE: Guide to family analysis, New Haven, Conn, 1982, Yale University School of Nursing.

PSYCHIATRIC NURSING ASSESSMENT

Facility _____

Assessor _____

Date _____

Name _____ Age _____ Sex _____

Address _____ Telephone _____

Significant other _____ Telephone _____

Date of admission _____ Medical diagnosis _____

Allergies _____ Detention: Yes _____ No _____

Legal proceedings pending: Yes _____ No _____

Nursing Diagnosis
(Potential or Altered)

COMMUNICATING ▪ A pattern involving sending messages

Verbal: Presence of: (circle) thought blocking, flight of ideas, perseveration, circumstantiality, punning, rhyming, tangential blocking, loose association

Speech impaired _____

Verbal coherence _____ Aphasia _____

Mutism _____ Echopraxia _____

Rate _____ Volume _____ Intonation _____

Nonverbal: Posture _____ Facial expression _____

Gesture _____ Eye contact _____

Read, write, understand English (circle) _____

Other languages _____

Physical impairment affecting communication _____

Alternate form of communication _____

Grooming and dress _____

General appearance _____

Other observations _____

Communication
Verbal
Nonverbal

KNOWING ▪ A pattern involving the meaning associated with information

Orientation

Level of alertness _____

Orientation: Person _____ Place _____ Time _____

Appropriate behavior/communication _____

Orientation
Confusion

Psychiatric Nursing Assessment—cont'd

Nursing Diagnosis
(Potential or Altered)

Memory
Memory intact: yes/no Immediate _____ Recent _____   Memory
Remote _____
Level/fund of knowledge _____
Ability to abstract _____
Current physical health problems _____   Knowledge deficit
Previous illnesses/hospitalizations/surgeries _____
_____

History of the following problems:
Heart _____
Peripheral vascular _____
Lung _____
Liver _____ Kidney _____
Cerebrovascular _____
Thyroid _____
Diabetes _____ Medication _____
Substance abuse _____
Alcohol use _____
Other _____
Current medications _____
_____

Perception/knowledge of planned therapy _____
_____
Expectations of therapy _____
_____
Misconceptions _____
Rediness to learn _____
Request information concerning _____   Thought processes
Educational level _____   Impaired problem
Learning impeded by _____   solving

EXCHANGING · A pattern involving mutual giving and receiving
Hormonal/Metabolic Patterns

Hematocrit _____ Hemoglobin _____ Platelets _____   Menstrual patterns
NA _____ K _____ Cl _____ Glucose _____   Premenstrual
Medications that potentiate blood dyscrasias _____   syndrome
Other laboratory tests _____
Menstrual patterns _____
BCP _____ Other methods _____
Physical Integrity

Tissue integrity _____ Rashes _____ Lesions _____   Impaired skin
                                                                                     integrity
Petechiae _____ Bruises _____   Impaired tissue
                                                                                     integrity
Abrasions _____ Lacerations _____   Violence

Surgical incisions _____ Scars _____   Injury
                                                                                     Trauma

Psychiatric Nursing Assessment—cont'd

Nursing Diagnosis
(Potential or Altered)

Circulation
  Neurologic changes/symptoms _____   Cerebral tissue
  Glascow Corna Scale total _____   perfusion
  CT scan _____ MRI _____
  ECG reading _____ Heart rate _____   Nutrition
Nutritional
  Eating patterns
    Number of meals per day _____
    Special diet _____
    Where eaten _____
    Food preferences/intolerances _____
    Food allergies _____
    Caffeine intake (coffee, tea, soft drinks, chocolate)
    _____
    Appetite changes _____
    Nausea/vomiting _____
    Anorexia _____ Bulimia _____
    Other observations: _____
  Condition of mouth/throat _____   Oral mucous
     membranes
    Height _____ Weight _____   More/less than body
    Weight loss/gain _____   requirements
Physical Regulation
  Immune
    Lymph nodes enlarged _____ Location _____   Infection
    WBC count _____   Hypothermia
  Body temperature   Hyperthermia
    Temperature _____ Route _____   Ineffective
  Medications with anticholinergic action _____   thermoregulation
  History of malignant neurolepsis syndrome _____
  History of extrapyramidal symptoms _____

Oxygenation
  Smoker _____ Number per day _____ How long _____   Ineffective airway
    clearance
  Color of nail beds _____ Nicotine stain _____   Ineffective breath-
    ing patterns
  Complaints of dyspnea _____ Precipitated by _____   Impaired gas
  Rate _____ Rhythm _____ Depth _____   exchange
  Labored/unlabored (circle) Chest expansion _____
  Cough: productive/nonproductive _____
  Sputum: Color _____ Amount _____ Consistency _____
  Breath sounds _____
Elimination
  Gastrointestinal/bowel   Bowel elimination
    Usual bowel habit _____   Constipation
    Alterations from normal _____   Diarrhea
    Laxative use _____   Incontinence
    Incontinence _____

Psychiatric Nursing Assessment—cont'd

	Nursing Diagnosis (Potential or Altered)

Abdominal physical examination _____ GI tissue perfusion

Renal/urinary

   Usual urinary pattern _____ Urinary elimination

   Alteration from normal _____   Incontinence

   Color _____ Appearance _____   Retention

   Urine output: 24 hours _____   Enuresis

   Intake _____

   Bladder distention _____ Renal tissue

   _____   perfusion

Toxicology screen _____

BUN _____

Lithium/other medications _____

MOVING · A pattern involving activity

Activity

History of physical disability _____ Impaired physical

_____   mobility

Verbal report of fatigue or weakness _____

_____

Motor activity: Tics _____ Tremors _____

   Gait disturbances _____ Agitation _____ Activity intolerances

   Compulsive behavior _____ Lethargy _____

   Retardation _____

   Hyperactivity _____

   History of medications related to involuntary movements _____

   _____

   Other observations _____

Rest

Hours slept/night _____ Feels rested: yes/no Sleep pattern

  disturbance

Sleep aids (pillows, medications, food) _____   Hypersomnia

Difficulty falling/remaining asleep _____   Insomnia

Changes from usual sleep patterns _____   Nightmares

Other observations _____

Recreation

Leisure activities _____

Increase/decrease from usual _____

Social activities _____ Diversional activity

Other observations _____   (deficit)

Environmental Maintenance

Home maintenance management

   Size and arrangement of home (stairs, bathroom) _____

   _____ Safety needs _____

Access to firearms/weapons _____ Violence

Limitations in daily activities _____ Injury

Exercise habits _____

Psychiatric Nursing Assessment—cont'd

Nursing Diagnosis
(Potential or Altered)

Home responsibilities _____

_____

Impaired home
maintenance
management
Safety hazards

Other observations _____

Health Maintenance
Health insurance _____

Regular physical checkups _____

Other observations _____

Health maintenance

Self-Care
Ability to perform activities of daily living: Independent _____ Dependent _____

Specify deficits _____

Discharge planning needs _____

Self-care
  Feeding
  Bathing/hygiene
  Dressing/
  grooming
  Toileting

PERCEIVING • A pattern involving the reception of information

Sensory Perception
Vision _____ Last examination _____ Glasses/contacts _____

Auditory _____ Last examination _____ Hearing aid _____

Prostheses _____

Gustatory _____ Changes in taste _____

Tactile examination _____ Numbness _____

Olfactory examination _____ Changes in smell _____

Reflexes: Grossly intact _____

Content of thought: Intact memory _____ Obscessions _____

  Hallucinations _____ Phobias _____

  Delusions _____ Other _____

Sensory/perceptual
Visual
Auditory
Kinesthetic
Gustatory
Tactile
Olfactory

Attention
Patient's ability to follow directions _____

_____

Responds to verbal cues _____

Responds to visual cues _____

Unilateral neglect
  Distractibility
  Hyperalertness
  Inattention
  Selective
  attention

Self-Concept
Patient's description of self _____

Negative self-concept _____

Poor self-esteem _____

Perceived strengths _____

Perceived weaknesses _____

Self-concept
Body image
Self-esteem
Personal identity
Growth and
development
Socialization

Meaningfulness
Verbalizes hopelessness/powerlessness _____

Perceives/verbalizes loss of control _____

Verbalizes suicidal ideations _____

Hopelessness
Powerlessness

Verbalizes violent intentions _____

Verbalizes homicidal intentions _____

Engages in self-destructive acts _____

Awareness of values _____

Violence
Injury

Psychiatric Nursing Assessment—cont'd

Nursing Diagnosis
(Potential or Altered)

Awareness of conflicts _____
Desired/stated goals of hospitalization/treatment _____
_____

RELATING ▪ A pattern involving establishing bonds

Role

Marital status _____   Role performance
Age and health of significant other _____   Parenting
_____   Work
Number of children _____ Ages _____   Family
Role in home _____   Social/leisure
Multiple roles _____
Role-related problems _____
Financial support _____
Occupation _____   Family processes
    Job satisfaction/**concerns** _____
Sexual relationships (satisfactory/unsatisfactory) _____   Sexual dysfunction
    Physical difficulties related to sex _____   Sexuality patterns

Socialization

Patient's identification of additional significant others
_____

Quality of relationships with others _____   Impaired social
Patient's description _____   interaction
Significant others' descriptions _____
Staff observations _____
Verbalizes feelings of being alone _____   Social isolation
Loneliness attributed to _____   Social withdrawal
Level of trust in relationships _____
Level of dependence/independence _____
_____

FEELING ▪ A pattern involving the subjective awareness of information

Comfort

Pain/discomfort: yes/no   Comfort
    Onset _____ Duration _____   Pain/chronic
    Location _____ Quality _____ Radiation _____   Pain/acute
    Associated factors _____   Discomfort
    Aggravating factors _____
    Alleviating factors _____
Altered Emotional Integrity States
Recent stressful life events _____
Verbalizes feelings of anxiety _____   Anxiety
Source of anxiety _____   Fear
Object of fear _____

Psychiatric Nursing Assessment—cont'd

Nursing Diagnosis
(Potential or Altered)

Usual method(s) for coping with anxiety/fear _____
Physical manifestations: Muscle tension _____
   Dry mouth _____ Skin pallor _____ Nausea/vomiting _____
   Difficulty sleeping _____ Unsteady voice _____
   Increased pulse rate _____ Increased respiratory rate _____
Other observations _____

Cognitive manifestations: Narrowed sensory perception _____

Anxiety
   Selective inattention _____ Blocking of words _____

Fear
   Difficulty concentrating _____ Defensiveness _____
Social manifestations: withdrawal _____
Demanding or aggressive behavior _____
Other observations _____
Event that precipitated anger _____

Anger
Usual method for coping with anger _____

Violence
Manifestations: Flushed face _____

Aggression
   Shallow breathing _____ Sweating _____
   Use of sarcasm _____ Argumentative _____

Disorganized
    behavior
   Fault finding _____ Dominating _____

Compulsive
    behavior
   Use of violence _____
Other observations _____
Event that precipitated guilt/envy/shame _____
Usual method of coping with guilt/envy/shame _____

Guilt/envy/shame
   Manifestations: Embarrassment _____ Regret _____
    Inappropriate affect _____ Self-punishing thoughts _____
    Preoccupation with what "should" have been _____
    Isolation _____
    Lack of self-forgiveness _____
Other observations _____
Event that precipitated sadness _____

Sadness
Usual method of coping with sadness _____
   Manifestations: Emptiness _____ Unworthiness _____
    Helplessness _____ Powerlessness _____
    Hopelessness _____ Withdrawal _____
    Suicidal ideas _____
Other observations _____

CHOOSING ▪ A pattern involving the selection of alternatives

Coping
   Patient's usual coping methods _____

Ineffective
  individual coping
_____

   Family's usual coping methods _____

Ineffective family
  coping
_____

   Patient's usual defense mechanisms: Rationalization _____

Impaired
  adjustment
   Conversion _____ Sublimation _____ Regression _____

Impaired problem
   Introjection _____ Projection _____ Denial/repression _____
  solving

Psychiatric Nursing Assessment—cont'd

Nursing Diagnosis
(Potential or Altered)

Participation

   Compliance with past/current health care regimens _____   Noncompliance
   Conflicts/obstacles _____
   Noncompliance _____
   _____   Ineffective
   Willingness to comply with future health care regimen _____   participation
   _____
   Family's ability to support patient _____   Family processes

Judgment

   Decision-making ability: Judgment
     Patient's perspective _____   Indecisiveness
     Others' perspectives _____

VALUING · A pattern involving the assigning of relative worth

Religious preference _____   Spiritual distress
Important religious practices _____
   Does religion/spirituality offer comfort/hope? _____
   Or guilt and fear? _____
Changes in religious practices _____
Cultural practices _____   Despair
Important life values _____
Influence of illness on values _____
Creativity _____
Aesthetic sense _____

Prioritized nursing diagnosis/problem list

1. _____
2. _____
3. _____
4. _____
5. _____

Signature _____   Date _____

From Guzetta C et al: Clinical assessment tools for use with nursing diagnoses, St Louis, 1989, Mosby–Year Book, Inc.

APPENDIX F

DRUG ABUSE TERMS

This glossary* contains street language regarding the drugs of abuse. The same term may have different meanings in different areas.

a-boot Under the influence of drugs

Acapulco gold Mexican marijuana that contains about 1% or less of tetrahydrocannabinol (THC)

ace A marijuana cigarette

acid LSD (lysergic acid diethylamide)

acid head A user of LSD

ad Refers to an addict

all lit up Under the influence of a drug

amys Amyl nitrite ampules

angel dust Parsley leaves covered with phencyclidine, finely powdered hashish

Are you anywhere? Do you use marijuana?

around the turn Having gone through withdrawal period

artillery Equipment used for injecting and dissolving a powdered drug, or a solution of drugs

baby Marijuana

bad trip/bad acid An unpleasant reaction caused by a hallucinogenic drug, usually LSD; may be caused by taking a mixture of chemicals, resulting from an attempt at synthesis; emotions are dreadful and horrible; the images can be terrifying

bag (1) A package of drugs, usually marijuana or heroin; (2) a person's favorite "thing" or drug

bagman A person who supplies narcotics or other drugs; a pusher

ball Absorption of stimulants and cocaine through the genitalia

balloon A penny balloon that contains narcotics

bambita Desoxyn or amphetamine derivative

bammies A poor quality of marijuana

bang The injection of narcotics, usually heroin

banging Under the influence of drugs

barb(s) Barbiturates

barrels LSD tablets

batted out Apprehended by law

bean A capsule containing drugs

beat the gong Smoke opium

bedbugs Fellow addicts

behind the iron house Staying in jail

belongs On the habit

belted Under the influence of a drug

bending and bowing Under the influence of drugs

---

*From the Office of Training and Education for Addiction Services of the Maryland Department of Health and Mental Hygiene.

bennies Benzedrine tablets (amphetamines)

Bernice Cocaine

Bernie's flake Cocaine

bhang Marijuana

big bloke Cocaine

big C Cocaine

big D LSD

big John Police, law

big man A person who supplies drugs

big O Opium

bindle A package of narcotics (usually contains an ounce)

bingle A supplier of drugs

bingler A person selling narcotics

bingo The injection of drugs

biz Utensils used in dissolving and injecting narcotics and other drugs

black beauties Biphetamine capsules (amphetamines)

black magic LSD

black stuff Opium

blank Container of nonnarcotic powder that is sold as heroin

blast (1) Party, (2) a strong effect resulting from drug usage

blasted Under the influence of a drug

blow (1) To miss a vein when injecting, (2) to move from a place

blow Charlie or snow Sniff cocaine

blow horse Sniffing heroin

blow (pot) Smoke a cigarette that contains marijuana

blow your mind (1) To be high from a hallucinogenic drug, (2) to achieve a particular ecstatic mental level or high

blue acid LSD

blue angels, blue clouds, blue devils, blue heaven Amytal (amobarbital sodium) capsules

blue cheer LSD, methamphetamine, and strychnine tablets

blue heaven LSD

blue morphine Numorphan tablets (no longer made)

blue velvet (1) A mixture of Terpin Hydrate and Codeine Elixir and Pyribenzamine (tripelennamine) (antihistamine), (2) a mixture of paregoric and antihistamine

bluebirds Amytal (amobarbital sodium) capsules

blues Amytal (amobarbital sodium)

bo bo bush Marijuana

bomb Heroin that is highly potent and relatively undiluted

bombida Methamphetamine

bombita An amphetamine injection, occasionally with heroin

boost Robbery

boxed Confined in jail

boy Heroin

brain pills Amphetamines

bread Money

brick Compressed block made of marijuana

broker A person who peddles dope to addicts

brown dots LSD

browns Multicolored capsules that are long-acting amphetamine sulfate

bull (1) A federal narcotics agent, (2) a police officer

bum trip A bad experience with psychedelics

bummer Another word for a "bad trip"

burn transaction Selling a substance as a certain drug when actually it is something else (e.g., goldenrod for marijuana)

burned Getting cheated during a drug transaction

bush Marijuana

business Equipment used when injecting drugs

businessman's trip Dimethyltryptamine (DMT)

busted Arrested for possession of drugs

buttons Peyote buttons

buy A purchase of drugs

buzz Mild euphoric reaction to a drug

C Cocaine

C-joint A place where cocaine can be bought

cabbage head An individual who will use or experiment with any kind of drug

caca (1) Heroin; (2) an inferior quality of hashish, heroin, or LSD; (3) imitation or counterfeit heroin

cadet A new addict

California sunshine LSD

can A container that holds marijuana

candy Barbiturates

candy man A pusher

cannabis Marijuana

cap A gelatinous capsule that contains heroin or other drugs (usually 1 ounce or less)

Carrie Cocaine

cartwheels Amphetamine tablets

cashing a script Obtaining drugs by getting an illegal prescription filled

catch up A process of withdrawal

caught in a snow storm Being drugged by cocaine

CB Doriden (glutethimide) tablet

Cecil Cocaine

charge A quick drug effect

charged up Under the influence of drugs

chicken powder Some amphetamine powder

chief LSD

chip Use small injections occasionally

chipping Irregular use of small amounts of drugs

chocolate chips LSD

Cholley Cocaine

Christmas trees Tuinal (secobarbital sodium and amobarbital sodium) or Eskatrol (dextroamphetamine sulfate and prochlorperazine)

Cibas Doriden (glutethimide)

Cibees Doriden (glutethimide)

clean Not using drugs any longer

cleared up A withdrawal method

clipped Getting arrested

coasting Under the influence of drugs

coast-to-coast Long-acting amphetamines

coffee habit A beginner in the use of narcotics

coke Cocaine

cokie Cocaine addict

cold turkey Sudden withdrawal from narcotics

coming down Recovering from a drug experience or trip

connect To make a purchase of drugs

connection A drug supplier

contact lens LSD found on round gelatin flakes

cooker Bottle cap or spoon needed for heating and dissolving heroin in preparation for injection

cop To obtain drugs

cop a deuceway To buy a $2 pack of narcotics

cop man A supplier

cop out (1) Running away, (2) to leave, (3) to inform, (4) not participating, (5) to defect

cop-a-sneak To leave a place

copilots Amphetamine tablets

Corrine Cocaine

cotton shot When water is added to cotton to attempt to get remaining heroin out

crank Methamphetamine crystals

crashing Withdrawing from a drug experience

crashing pad Place where a user recovers from amphetamine use

crinic, cris, Cristina Methamphetamine

croaker A physician

croaker joint A hospital

crossroads Amphetamine tablets

crusher A police officer

crutch A device for holding a marijuana cigarette butt

crystal Methamphetamine (Methedrine), cocaine

crystal palace A room, location, or house where methamphetamine is injected

cube juice Morphine

cubehead A person who uses LSD frequently

cupcakes LSD

cut (1) To dilute a powder drug, usually a narcotic; (2) to dilute the potency of marijuana

cut out To leave a certain place

D Doriden (glutethimide) tablets

dabble To use small amounts of drugs infrequently

dead on arrival Phencyclidine base

dealer (1) A person who supplies drugs, (2) a pusher

deck A package of narcotics (usually an ounce)

dexies Dexedrine (dextroamphetamine sulfate) tablets or capsules (amphetamines)

diet pills Include amphetamine tablets or capsules

dime bag $10 purchase, usually marijuana

dirty Have drugs on you; can be arrested if searched

do a bit To spend time in jail

do righters Nonaddicts

DOA Phencyclidine base

doin' Using some kind of drug, such as "He is doin' cocaine"

dollies Dolophine (methadone) tablets

DOM STP (2,5-dimethoxy-4-methylamphetamine)

domes LSD tablets

domino To complete a purchase of drugs

doojee Heroin

dope Includes any narcotics, sometimes extended to other drugs

dope fiend A heroin addict

doper Someone who uses drugs regularly

double trouble Tuinal (secobarbital sodium and amobarbital sodium) capsule

down, downer, downie (1) Barbiturates, (2) tranquilizers

down it To swallow a pill or capsule

dream Cocaine

dried up Off drugs, especially heroin

dripper Eyedropper

drop To take a capsule or tablet orally

drop acid To take LSD

drop out To leave a place

dujie Heroin

dummy (1) A purchase in which there are no narcotics, (2) a poor quality of merchandise

dust Heroin, cocaine

dust of angels Phencyclidine base

dynamite (1) A high quality of heroin and cocaine taken together, (2) a strong drug

eighth Heroin (⅛ ounce) that is diluted with some inert powder

emsel Morphine

eye openers Amphetamines

factory The equipment used when injecting drugs

fall To be arrested

fall out When an addict nods or falls asleep on and off after injecting

far out (1) Out of touch with reality, (2) under the influence of drugs

Feds Federal agents

fine stuff Marijuana that is finely cut or manicured

fix An injection of a narcotic

fixed Under the influence of a drug

flake Cocaine

flash A euphoric feeling following an injection

flashback When a previous drug user hallucinates without taking the drug again

flats LSD tablets

flea powder Poor-quality heroin or heroin that is greatly diluted

flip Become psychotic

floating Under the influence of drugs

flying high Under the influence of marijuana

fold up A withdrawal procedure

folding stuff Money

foolish powder Heroin

footballs Amphetamine tablets or capsules that are oval shaped

freak A regular user of a particular drug (e.g., acid freak)

freakout An experience that is unpleasant and frightful, resulting from the use of a drug

freeze When a sale is turned down

fresh and sweet A person coming out of jail

front of the bread The money is put up first for a drug purchase

fu Marijuana

Fuzz (1) A policeman, (2) a detective

Fuzzy tail Police

gage Marijuana

garbage A poor-quality drug

gazer A federal agent

GBs Seconal (secobarbital), Tuinal (secobarbital and amobarbital), or Doriden (glutethimide)

gear Refers to drugs in general

gee head A person who uses paregoric

geetis Money

geezer A needle shot of any type of narcotic

get beat To buy a package that does not contain any heroin

get a gift To obtain some narcotics

get high To smoke a cigarette containing marijuana

get off To inject or use drugs

get the wind To leave a place or area

gimmicks Equipment with which a person injects drugs

girl Cocaine

give wings Give the first heroin injection to a friend

glad rag A handkerchief or cloth saturated with substances to be inhaled

glass eyes A narcotic addict

glued Arrested

gluey An individual who sniffs glue vapors

G-man A federal agent

go in sewer Inject a drug into a vein

gold A Mexican marijuana that has 1% or less of tetrahydrocannabinol (THC)

gold dust Cocaine

good go Purchase a fair amount of narcotics for the money

good trip Psychedelic drugs that cause good emotional feelings and pleasant imagery

goods (1) Narcotics, (2) includes any drugs

goofball Barbiturate

gorilla pills Doriden (glutethimide)

gow head Addict

gram The cube form of hashish

grape parfait LSD

grass Marijuana

green domes LSD tablets

greenies The mixture of barbiturates and amphetamines found in a green heart-shaped tablet

griefo Marijuana

gun (1) Eyedropper, (2) syringe, (3) hypodermic needle

H Heroin

hack Physician

hairy Heroin

half spoon Half a teaspoonful of heroin

hand-to-hand Paying for drugs when they are delivered

hang-up (1) A personal problem or personality problem, (2) a withdrawal

happy dust Cocaine

hard narcotics Includes all addicting narcotics

hard stuff Includes any addicting narcotic (e.g., heroin, morphine)

harness bull Police
Harry Heroin
hash Hashish
hassle The procedure of buying drugs, preparing them, and taking the injection
Hawaiian sunshine LSD
hay Marijuana
head A person who depends on drugs
hearts Amphetamine tablets that are heart shaped
heat The police
heaven dust Cocaine
heavenly blue Morning glory seeds
heavy man Someone who possesses narcotics
hemp Marijuana
high Under the influence of drugs
hit To make a purchse of drugs
hitting the pipe, hitting the steam Smoking opium
hitting the stuff Under the influence of drugs
hitting up The act of injecting drugs
hocus Morphine
hog Vegetable material that has phencyclidine in it
holding To have drugs in one's possession
hooked Dependent on drugs
hop Opium
hop head A narcotic addict, mainly an opium addict
hoppie A narcotic addict
horner One who sniffs narcotics
horse Heroin
hot (1) Sought by police, (2) stolen articles, merchandise
hotshot A fatal injection of heroin, that may have been intentional
hot sticks Marijuana cigarettes
hustle (1) Prostitution, (2) any activity used to obtain money for heroin
hustler Prostitute
hype Addict
ice-cream habit Nonregular drug user
iced In jail
I'm beat I need a marijuana cigarette
I'm holding I am carrying drugs
I'm way down I need a marijuana lift
in high Under the influence of drugs
in a jam Wanted by the police
Indian bay, Indian hay Marijuana
into Involved with a drug (e.g., "She is into acid")
jab (1) To inject a drug, (2) a hypodermic shot
jag (1) Under the influence of drugs, (2) under the influence of amphetamines
jay Marijuana cigarette
jelly beans Tuinal (secobarbital sodium and amobarbital sodium)
jive Marijuana
jive sticks, joints Marijuana cigarettes
jolly beans Pep pills
Jones A habit
joy popping (1) Subcutaneously injecting a drug, (2) irregular drug habit

joy powder Cocaine
jump skid To leave a place
junk (1) Heroin, (2) can denote any drug
junker, junkie Addict (heroin)
kee A kilogram of a drug, usually heroin
keif Hashish
kick To get rid of a habit
kick the habit To stop using narcotics or drugs in general
kick sticks Marijuana cigarettes
kicking A withdrawal process
kicking the gong To be around an area where narcotics are sold
kilo A kilogram of drugs equivalent to 2.2 pounds
kit Equipment used when injecting drugs
knocking on the door When an addict is trying to stay away from other addicts while attempting to quit a habit
LA turnabouts Various-colored capsules that are long-acting amphetamine sulfate
lay out (1) Equipment for injecting drugs, (2) opium smoker's outfit
laying on the hip Smoking opium
laying the hypo Receiving or taking a shot of narcotics
LBJ-336-JB-336 Methyl piperidyl benzilate (hallucinogen)
leader User of cocaine
leaping Under the influence of drugs
lemonade Poor-quality heroin or any merchandise
lettuce Money
lid A measure of marijuana in a sale
lid poppers Amphetamines
lid proppers Amphetamines
lie down To smoke opium
light artillery A hypodermic addict
Lipton tea Poor-quality merchandise
lit up Under the influence of drugs
load A quantity of 25 bags of heroin
loco weed Marijuana
log Marijuana cigarette
long green Money
love drug (1) MDA (methylene dioxyamphetamine), (2) methaqualone (soapers)
love weed Marijuana
LSD Lysergic acid diethylamide
m Morphine
machinery Utensils used when injecting drugs
magic mushroom A mushroom containing psilocybin
magic pumpkin seed An STP (2,5-dimethoxy-4-methylamphetamine) tablet shaped like a pumpkin seed
mainlining Shooting or injecting a drug directly into a vein
maintaining Keeping a particular level of a drug effect
make a croaker To trick a physician into giving narcotics
make a meet To make a buy
make a reader To get a physician to fill out a prescription
make the turn A withdrawal process
man (1) Policeman, (2) detective
manicure Removal of seeds, dirt, and stems from dried marijuana
Mary Jane, Mary Warner Marijuana

merchandise Narcotics or any drug in general

mese Mescaline (hallucinogenic drug from the peyote cactus)

meth (1) Methamphetamine, (2) methadone, (3) methedrine, (4) methaqualone

meth head A regular use of methamphetamine

meth run Constant intravenous injection of methamphetamine

Mexican horse Mexican (brown) heroin

Mexican reds Secobarbital capsules

mezz Marijuana

Mickey Chloral hydrate

Mickey Finn The mixture of chloral hydrate plus alcohol

micro dots LSD

mikes Micrograms (millionths of a gram)

mind benders, mind blowers Hallucinogens

Miss Emma Morphine

MJ Marijuana

monkey A drug habit in which there is a physical dependence

monster Methamphetamine

mootos Marijuana cigarettes

mor-a-grifa Marijuana

morph, morphie, morpho Morphine

mouth worker A narcotic addict who swallows his drugs

Mr. Whiskers Federal agents

mud Asthmador mixed with a carbonated cola beverage

muggles Marijuana cigarettes

mule A supplier of drugs

mutah Marijuana

nail Needle

nailed Arrested

narc, narco Federal, state, or local narcotic officer

needle The syringe for injecting drugs

needle freak A person who enjoys using a needle

nibies Nembutal (pentobarbital sodium)

nickel bag (1) A $5 purchase of marijuana, (2) a measure of heroin

nimby Nembutal (pentobarbital sodium)

noise Heroin

nose candy Cocaine

OD An overdose of drugs or narcotics, resulting in death or a coma

OJ Opium joint, a marijuana cigarette that has been dipped or smeared in opium

on ice In jail

on the beam Feeling good

on the blues Using Numorphan (oxymorphone hydrochloride)

on the bricks, on the ground Out of jail

on the nod The cycle of dozing and awakening when using heroin

on the street Out of jail

on a trip Under the influence of LSD

orange wedges LSD

oranges Heart-shaped amphetamine tablets containing Dexedrine (dextroamphetamine sulfate)

out of it Nonaddict

outfit Equipment used when injecting drugs

over the hump The completion of withdrawal

Owsley's acid LSD

pad A person's habitat or room

Pam freak Person who inhales aerosolized products

Panatella A large, strong marijuana cigarette

panic man Addict who has lost his source of drugs

paper (1) A package of drugs (usually a quantity of 1 ounce), (2) prescription

PCP Phencyclidine

PCPA p-Chlorophenylalanine

peace (1) LSD tablets, (2) STP (2,5-dimethoxy-4-methylamphetamine)

peace pill Phencyclidine

peace tablet LSD tablets

peaches Benzedrine (amphetamine sulfate) tablets

peanuts Barbiturates

pearly gates Morning glory seeds

peddler Dealer in drugs

pee Heroin powder

pep pills Amphetamine capsules or tablets

Pepsi Cola habit A small habit

Peter Chloral hydrate

PG, PO Paregoric

pickup To buy drugs

piece (1) A measure of narcotics, (2) a holder of drugs

pig Policeman

piki A person who smokes opium

pillhead A person who often uses drugs, usually amphetamines and barbiturates

pillows Sealed polyethylene bags that contain drugs

pin yen Opium

pinks Seconal (secobarbital sodium) capsules

pipe (1) To look, (2) an opium utensil

plant A place to hide drugs

play around Irregular use of drugs

pod Marijuana

pop To inject drugs, usually below the skin

poppers Amyl nitrite ampules

pot Marijuana or hashish

pothead Marijuana user

product IV Combination capsules of PCP and LSD

purple barrels, purple haze, purple ozone LSD

purple rock A mixture of caffeine, barbiturates, heroin, and strychnine

push shorts To cheat a buyer of drugs; to sell short amounts of drugs

pusher A person who peddles drugs, narcotics, marijuana

R and R, ripple and reds Taking secobarbital capsules when drinking Ripple wine

rainbows Tuinal (secobarbital sodium and amobarbital sodium) capsules

red birds, red devils, red lilies, reds Secobarbital capsules

red rock Mixture of heroin and strychnine, barbiturates, and caffeine

reefer Marijuana cigarette

riding the wave Under the influence of narcotics

roach A marijuana cigarette butt

roach clip A device that holds a marijuana cigarette butt

robe Robitussin A-C cough syrup (guaifenesin and codeine phosphate)

robo, romo Codeine

rope Marijuana

roses Benzedrine (amphetamine sulfate) tablets

run Continuing the injection of methamphetamine

Sam Federal agent

satch cotton Cotton used to strain drugs before injection

sativa Marijuana

scag Heroin

scene Place where a person can buy drugs

schmack (1) Heroin, (2) cocaine

schoolboy Codeine

score To purchase drugs

scrap iron A bootleg drink made with a hypochlorite solution, alcohol, and mothballs

scratch Prescription

script Physician's prescription

script writer A person who forges prescriptions

seccy, seggy Seconal (secobarbital sodium) capsules

seeds Morning glory seeds

serenity, tranquility, and peace STP (2,5-dimethoxy-4-methylamphetamine)

sewer Vein

sex drug Methaqualone (soapers) or STP (2,5-dimethoxy-4-methylamphetamine)

sex juice An aphrodisiac

sharps Needles

shit (1) Heroin; (2) poor-quality heroin, hashish, or LSD; (3) drugs

shoot up To inject drugs

shooting The injection of drugs

shooting gallery Location, room, or house where drugs are injected

short go To take a small portion of narcotics

shot down Under the influence of drugs

shrink Psychiatrist

sizzling Sought by police

skee Opium

skid (1) Heroin, (2) to leave a place

skin popping The injecting of a narcotic underneath the skin

slammed In jail

sleepers, sleeping pills Barbiturates

sleigh ride Under the influence of drugs

smack (1) Heroin, (2) cocaine

smash Marijuana that has been cooked with acetone, the oil residue of which is added to hashish

smears LSD

smoke (1) Wood alcohol, (2) marijuana

snappers Amyl nitrite ampules

sniffer A narcotic addict who takes drugs through his nose

sniffing Inhaling solvents, cleaning fluid, etc.

snort The inhalation of cocaine or heroin through the nose

snorter A person who sniffs drugs through his nose

snow Cocaine crystals

snowbird Cocaine addict

soapers Methaqualone (sleeping pill)

sound Benactyzine

spaghetti sauce Robitussin A-C cough syrup (guaifenesin and codeine phosphate)

speed Amphetamines, usually methedrine

speed demon Methamphetamine user

speed freak Frequent methamphetamine user

speedball A mixture of heroin and cocaine that is taken intravenously

spike Hypodermic needle

splash Amphetamine powder

splim Marijuana

split To leave a place

splivins Amphetamine powder

spoon (1) A measure of heroin, (2) the spoon used for dissolving heroin over heat

spots Dextroamphetamine

square An individual who does not use drugs

squirrels LSD

star dust Cocaine

stash A safe place to keep drugs

station worker A user of narcotics who injects into his arms or legs

stick Marijuana cigarette

stinking Under the influence of drugs

stoned (1) Under the influence of drugs, (2) a relaxed, pleasant state of mind

stoolie Informer

stoppers Barbiturates

straight (1) Not using any drugs, (2) not having any drugs in one's possession

strawberry field LSD

street market Black market

strung out An amphetamine overdose

stuff Narcotics

stumblers (1) Barbiturates, (2) tranquilizers

sunshine LSD

superman pills Amphetamines

sweet Lucy Marijuana

swing man A supplier of drugs

syrup Codeine

TMA A combination of mescaline, LSD, and tetrahydrocannabinol

T-man A federal agent

take a powder, take the wind To leave a certain area

taking a main Injecting directly into the vein

tar Opium

taste A small amount of narcotics

tea Marijuana

tea pad The place where a group of people smoke marijuana

tea party A party where mostly everyone is smoking marijuana

teed up Intoxicated by a large quantity of drugs

Texas tea Marijuana

the bag The bag used to sniff airplane glue or cleaning fluid

the confidence drug Amphetamine

the one A material like hashish, supposedly natural tetrahydrocannabinol

thing A person's particular interest, often refers to a specific drug

three-day-habit The irregular use of drugs

TNT Heroin

to be off A process of withdrawal

toak (toke) A drag off a marijuana cigarette

toke pipe A short-stem pipe used for smoking marijuana

tooies Tuinal (secobarbital sodium and amobarbital sodium) capsules

tools Equipment used when injecting drugs

toy A small container of drugs

tracks Needle scars that result from frequent injecting of drugs

tranquility STP (2,5-dimethoxy-r-methylamphetamine)

travel agent LSD pusher

trey A purchase worth $3

trip A hallucinogenic drug experience

tripping out Under the influence of any hallucinogen

truck drivers Amphetamine tablets

tuies Tuinal (secobarbital sodium and amobarbital sodium)

turkey The absence of drugs or narcotics

turkey trots Scars and marks left from the use of a hypodermic needle

turn off To quit using drugs

turn on (1) To introduce a person to the use of drugs, (2) any stimulating experience caused by the use of drugs

turn up To feel the influence of a drug

turned on Under the influence of drugs

turps Terpin Hydrate and Codeine Elixir (a cough syrup)

twenty-five LSD

twist A marijuana cigarette

twisted Intense sedation caused by the use of drugs

uncle, Uncle Sam Federal narcotics agent

unkie Morphine

upper, ups Amphetamine tablets

viper's weed Marijuana

wake ups, washed ups Amphetamines

washed up A withdrawal process

wasted Under the influence of drugs

wedges (1) Dexedrine (dextroamphetamine sulfate) tablets, (2) LSD tablets

weed Marijuana

weekend habit The irregular use of drugs

wen shee Gum opium

whickers Federal agents

white junk Heroin

white lightning LSD

white merchandise, white stuff Morphine

whites Amphetamines

whiz bang A combination of morphine and cocaine, or heroin and cocaine, used by the old addicts

window glass A square gelatin flake that contains LSD

work the leather To leave an area

works Equipment used when injecting drugs

yellow birds Nembutal (pentobarbital sodium)

yellow dimples LSD

yellow jackets, yellow submarines, yellows Nembutal (pentobarbital sodium) capsules

yen hook The utensil used when smoking opium

yen shee The ashes from opium

yen sleep A period of restlessness and drowsiness during a withdrawal process

FREQUENTLY USED BEHAVIORAL RATING SCALES

The Beck Depression Inventory[1,4]

The Beck Depression Inventory consists of 13 multiple choice clinical items. This is a self-report scale, designed to measure the depth of depression as well as to screen depressed patients rapidly. The Beck is applicable to psychiatric and medical patients with depressive illness. It covers the time span at the rating session (i.e., "right now"). The items measure sadness, pessimism, sense of failure, dissatisfaction, guilt, self-dislike, self-harm, social withdrawal, indecisiveness, self-image change, work difficulty, fatigability, and anorexia.

Brief Psychiatric Rating Scale (BPRS)[4,8]

The 18 items of this rating scale provide rapid and efficient evaluation of treatment response in both clinical drug trials and routine clinical settings; its focus is primarily adult inpaitent psychopathology, although it has been used in outpatient settings. It is designed to be scored after a 45-minute interview by a clinician on a Likert-type scale (0, not assessed, to 5, extremely severe). Span of 1 week between interviews is suggested. The scale items are somatic concern, anxiety, emotional withdrawal, conceptual disorganization, guilt feelings, tension, mannerisms, grandiosity, depressive mood, hostility, suspiciousness, hallucinatory behavior, motor retardation, uncooperativeness, unusual thought content, blunted affect, excitement, and disorientation.

Clinical Global Impressions (CGI)[4]

This rating scale consists of three global items that are for use in all research/psychiatric populations and designed to be administered by a clinician with at least some clinical experience. The first two items are rated on a 7-point scale, whereas the third item requires a rating of the interaction of drug therapeutic effectiveness and adverse reactions. The items of the CGI are (1) severity of illness (1, normal, not ill, to 7, among the most extremely ill patients);(2) global improvement: (1, very much improved, to 7, very much worse); and (3) efficacy index, rated on the basis of

drug effect only (therapeutic improvement as compared with severity of side effects). Severity of illness is rated pre- and posttreatment and at the discretion of the clinician. It measures the time period of "now, or within the last week." Global improvement requires no pretreatment measurement; a posttreatment measurement is done, as are more frequent measurements at the discretion of the clinician. It measures the time period "since admission to the study (program, or unit)." Efficacy index is rated similar to global improvement, but the time period is "now, or within the last week."

Hamilton Anxiety Scale (HAM-A)[4,6]

This 14-item scale was designed for use with patients already diagnosed as suffering from anxiety. The scale uses a five-point scale (0, not present, to 4, very severe), with the highest score rarely applicable in outpatient settings. The scale places great emphsis on the patient's subjective state, and the scale questions are answered by directly eliciting the patient's subjective feelings. In treatment the patient's subjective state takes first place both as a criterion of illness, which brings the patient for treatment, and as a criterion of improvement. The scale items measure anxious mood, tension, fears, insomnia, intellectual (cognitive) difficulty, depressed mood, general muscular somatic complaints, general sensory somatic complaints, cardiovascular symptoms, respiratory symptoms, gastrointestinal symptoms, genitourinary symptoms, autonomic symptoms, and patient's behavior during interview. The HAM-A can be used as frequently as the clinician thinks necessary.

Hamilton Psychiatric Rating Scale for Depression (HAM-D)[4,5]

The 21 items of this rating scale provide a simple way of quantitatively assessing the severity of an adult patient's condition and showing changes in that condition. It is not to be used as a diagnostic instrument. It is useful as both an inpatient and an outpatient scale; it is designed to be scored after a 45-minute interview by a clinician. The scoring is multiple choice. A span of 3 to 7 days between interviews is suggested. It is desirable to supplement information the patient gives by questioning significant others and other staff. The scale items measure depressed mood, guilt, suicide, insomnia, work and activities, retardation, agitation, anxiety, somatic symptoms, genital symptoms, hypochondriasis, weight loss, insight, diurnal variation, depersonalization and derealization, paranoid symptoms, and obsessive/compulsive symptoms.

Manic-State Rating Scale[2]

This rating scale is a quantitative measure of manic symptomatology. Each of 26 items is rated with a Likert-type scale on two parameters:frequency of observed behavior (0, none, to 5, all) and intensity of behavior (1, very minimal, to 5, very marked). The scale is designed to be used by clinical staff trained to work with manic patients and has good interrater reliablility. Beigel, Murphy, and Bunney[2] suggest that the scale can be used as frequently as every 8 hours on an inpatient service because it measures overt behavior, and manics frequently have mood swings. The items cover looks depressed, talking, moving, threatening, poor judgment, inappropriate dress, happy and cheerful, seeks out others, distractable, grandiose, irritable, combative or destructive, delusional, verbalizes depressed feelings, active, argumentative, talks about sex, angry, careless in dress and grooming, poor impulse control, suspicious, verbalizes feelings of well-being, makes unrealistic plans, demands contact with others, sexually preoccupied, and jumps from one subject to another.

Nurses' Observaion Scale for Inpatient Evaluation (NOISE)[4,7]

This 30-item scale was designed for the assessment of adult and geriatric ward behavior by nursing personnel. It provides measures of the patient's strengths as well as pathology. It uses a five-point Likert-type scale (0, never, to 5, always). The items are written in simple language and ask for ratings based on the direct observation of behavior. The scale clusters into three positive factors: social competence, social interest, and personal neatness; and four negative factors: irritability, manifest psychosis, retardation, and depression. It is useful to include the observations of many ward personnel. A span of 3 to 7 days between ratings is suggested.

Self-Report Symptom Check List   90 (SCL-90)[3,4]

This 90-item scale was designed to be rated by the patient. It presents a list of problems and complaints that people sometimes have and asks the patient to rate "how much that problem has bothered or distressed you during the past week, including today." This tool uses a five-point Likert scale (0, not at all, to 4, extremely). Patients obviously have to be well enough to do the scale and should be encouraged not to take too long on any one item. The scale should take 15 minutes to complete. The items cluster into nine subscales that measure somatization, obsessive-compulsive, interpersonal sensitivity, depression, anxiety, anger-hostility, phobic anxiety, paranoid ideation, and psychoticism. The scale is designed for adults in psychiatric and nonpsychiatric outpatient settings and should be used at least pre-and posttreatment. Many clinicians use it weekly.

■   REFERENCES   ■

1. Beck AT and Beamesderfer A: Assessment of depression: the depression inventory. In Pichot P, (editor:) Psychological measurements in psychopharmacology, vol 7, Basel, 1974, Karger.
2. Beigel A, Murphy MD and Bunney WE Jr: The Manic-state rating scale, Arch Gen Psychiatry 25:256, 1971.
3. Derogatis LR et al: Dimensions of outpatient neurotic pathology: comparison of a clinical vs. an empirical assessment, J Consult Clin Psychol 34:102, 1970.
4. Guy W: ECDEU assessment manual for psychopharmacology, revised, Rockville, Md, 1976, US Department of Health, Education, and Welfare, National Institute of Mental Health, Psychopharmacology Research Branch, Division of Extramural Research Program.
5. Hamilton M: Development of a rating scale for primary depressive illness, Br J Soc Clin Psychol 6:278, 1967.
6. Hamilton M: Diagnosis and rating of anxiety. In Lader MD, editor: Studies of anxiety, Br J Psychiatry 3:76, 1969.
7. Honigfeld G and Klett C: The Nurses' Observation Scale for Inpatient Evaluation (NOSIE): a new scale for measuring improvemenmt in chronic schizophrenia, J Clin Psychol 21:65, 1965.
8. Overall, JE: The Brief Psychiatric Rating Scale in psychopharmacology research, Psychometric Laboratory Reports, no,. 29, Galveston, 1972, University of Texas.

GLOSSARY

abreaction Ventilation of feelings that takes place as an individual verbally recounts emotionally charged areas.

absolute discharge A final and complete termination of the patient's relationship with the hospital.

abuse An act of misuse, exploitation, deceit; wrong or improper use or action so as to injure, damage, maltreat, or corrupt.

accountability Self-regulation and responsibility for the quality of one's nursing care.

acrophobia Fear of high places.

acting out Indirect expression of feelings through behavior, usually nonverbal, that attracts the attention of others.

action cues A category of nonverbal communication that consists of body movements; sometimes referred to as *kinetics*.

activities of daily living When applied to the chronically mentally ill, refers to the skills necessary to live independently as an adult.

adolescence The period from the beginning of puberty to the attainment of maturity. The transitional stage during which the youth is becoming an adult man or woman. This period is described in terms of development in many different functions that may be reached at different times. Only conventional limits may be stated: 12 to 21 years, girls; 13 to 22 years, boys.

adventitious crisis Accidental, uncommon, and unexpected crisis that may result in multiple losses and gross environmental changes.

advocacy One method by which patients, mental health professionals, attorneys, and concerned citizens can work together to improve and protect the rights of all citizens to high-quality mental health care that is clinically and constitutionally appropriate.

affect Feeling, mood.

aggression Mental drive to action that encompasses both constructive and destructive activities.

agonist In pharmacology, a substance that acts with, enhances, or potentiates a specific activity.

agoraphobia Overwhelming symptoms of anxiety, often leading to a panic attack in a variety of everyday situations (e.g., standing in line; eating in public; being in crowds of people, on bridges, in tunnels; driving) in which a person might have an attack and be unable to escape or get help and be embarrassed.

akathisia Motor restlessness ranging from a feeling of inner disquiet, often localized in the muscles, to inability to sit still or lie quietly; a side effect of some antipsychotic drugs.

alcohol withdrawal delirium A medical diagnosis for a serious alcohol withdrawal syndrome that is characterized by delirium and autonomic hyperactivity occurring within 1 week of reduction of alcohol intake.

alcoholic hallucinosis A medical diagnosis referring to an alcohol withdrawal syndrome that is characterized by auditory hallucinations in the absence of any other psychotic symptoms.

alcoholism Any degree of dependency, physical or psychological, on alcohol to the extent that it interferes with normal life activities.

alexithymia The inability to experience and communicate feelings consciously.

alliance A relationship based on shared common interests.

altruism A sense of concern for the welfare of others that can be expressed at the level of the individual or the larger social system.

ambivalence An inability to make decisions based on double approach-avoidance conflict feelings.

amino acids Any organic acid containing one or more amino groups; they are integral parts of proteins and are precursors of brain neurotransmitters.

amnesia Loss of memory for a specific period of time or a loss of all past memories.

anaclitic depression A deprivational reaction in infants separated from their mothers in the second half of the first year of life. The reaction is characterized by apprehension, crying, withdrawal, psychomotor slowing, defection, stupor, insomnia, anorexia, and gross retardation in growth and development.

anger A feeling that is an expression of the anxiety aroused by a real or perceived threat to one's rights, possessions, values, or significant others.

anorexia nervosa An eating disorder in which the person experiences hunger but refuses to eat based on a distorted body image leading to a self-perception of obesity. Starvation ensues.

antagonist A substance or a drug that reduces or blocks the action of another substance or drug; by competing with another substance for the same receptor site, one of the substances is prevented from binding to the receptors and thus its effects are prevented.

anticipatory guidance Information and advice given to patients for future therapeutic purposes.

antisocial personality A personality disorder characterized by manipulativeness, disregard for social norms, and a lack of concern for others.

anxiety A diffuse apprehension that is vague in nature and is associated with feelings of uncertainty and helplessness. It is an emotion without a specific object, is subjectively experienced by the individual, and is communicated interpersonally. It occurs as a result of a threat to the person's being, self-esteem, or identity.

ascribed role An assigned role, such as age and sex, about which the individual has no choice.

assertiveness Behavior that is directed toward claiming one's rights without denying the right of others.

assertiveness training An application of the behavioral model of psychiatric care. The patient is taught to stand up for his rights while not infringing on the rights of others.

assessment A phase of the nursing process in which information about the health status of a patient is systematically obtained, communicated, and recorded. Also known as the *nursing assessment*.

associationist model of learning A theory that defines learning as behavioral change resulting from reinforced practice.

assumed role Role the individual selects or achieves by choice, such as occupational or marital roles.

attachment State of being emotionally attracted to a person and highly dependent on that person for emotional satisfaction.

attention The element of cognitive functioning that refers to the maintenance of mental focus on a specific issue, activity, or object.

authority A relation between two or more persons such that the commands, suggestions, or ideas of one of them influence the other(s).

authority figure Person(s) who by virtue of status, role, or recognized superiority in knowledge, strength, etc., exerts influence in the authority relation.

autism A preoccupation with the self and with inner experiences.

autistic thought Ideation that has a private meaning to the individual.

autonomy The socially sanctioned condition that allows for the definition and control over one's work domain, achieved through a negotiated process.

autonomy drive The tendency for the individual to attempt to master the environment and to impose his purposes on it.

aversion therapy An application of the behavioral model of psychiatric care. A painful stimulus is given to create an aversion to another stimulus, which leads to a behavior the individual wishes to change.

baseline behavior (or operant level) Specified rate (frequency and form) of a particular behavior during preintervention or preexperimental conditions.

baseline condition Environmental condition during which a particular behavior reflects a stable rate of responding, before the introduction of intervention or experimental conditions.

battered wife Any woman who is beaten by her mate, regardless of the legality of the marital relationship.

behavior Any observable, recordable, and measurable act, movement, or response of an individual.

behavior hierarchy A graded list of behavioral segments, beginning with the baseline behavior and gradually moving up to the terminal behavior.

behavior modification Changing and controlling behavior through the application of techniques derived from learning theory.

benzodiazepines A group of chemically related antianxiety drugs.

biofeedback A method of tension reduction in which electrodes are attached to the person's forehead, and he is then instructed to concentrate on relaxing, which will reduce the pitch of the biofeedback tone created by his tension. The lower the tone, the greater the muscle relaxation.

biological psychiatry A school of psychiatric thought that emphasizes physical, chemical, and neurological causes and treatment approaches.

biopolar affective disorder A subgroup of the affective disorders that is characterized by at least one episode of manic behavior, with or without a history of episodes of depression.

biopolar affective disorder A subgroup of the affective disorders that is characterized by at least one episode of manic behavior, with or without a history of episodes of depression.

bisexuality Sexual attraction to persons of both sexes and engagement in both homosexual and heterosexual activities.

blocking An interruption in the flow of speech caused by the intrusion of distraction thoughts.

blood levels The concentration of a drug in the plasma, serum, or blood. In psychiatry, the term is most often applied to levels of lithium or some tricyclic antidepressants. Maximum clinical responses to these agents have been correlated with specific ranges of blood levels.

board and care home A site for housing discharged patients that may provide a shared room, three meals a day, the dispensing of medication, and minimum staff supervision.

body image Sum of the conscious and unconscious attitudes the individual has toward his body. It includes present and past perceptions, as well as feelings about size, function, appearance, and potential.

body language The transmission of a message by body position or movement.

borderline personality An individual with instability of mood, interpersonal relationships, and self-image, with a marked lack of a sense of identity.

buccolinguomasticatory triad A complex of lips, tongue, jaw, and head movements that are associated with tardive dyskinesia.

bulimia An eating disorder that is characterized by uncontrollable binge eating alternating with vomiting or dieting.

burnout A syndrome of physical and emotional exhaustion, involving the development of negative self-concept, negative job attitudes, and loss of concern and feeling for clients. It may lead to physical illness, irritability, cynicism, fatigue, and withdrawal from one's nursing work.

butyrophenones A group of chemically related antipsychotic drugs.

camisole restraint A straitjacket; a shirtlike garment that restrains the arms.

case management The assignment of a mental health care provider to assist a patient in assisting the health care and social services systems and to ensure that all required services are obtained.

case manager A clinician who accepts responsibility for identifying, securing, and coordinating all the resources necessary for a mentally ill client to live in the community.

catatonic A state of psychologically induced immobilization at times interrupted by episodes of extreme agitation.

catatonic excitement A state of extreme agitation that occurs when a person is unable to maintain catatonic immobility.

catatonic stupor An apparently unresponsive state that is related to a fear of loss of impulse control.

catharsis Release that occurs when the patient is encouraged to talk about things that bother him most. Fears, feelings, and experiences are brought out into the open and discussed.

cathexis Freud's term for the attachment of psychic energy (libido) to an object or mental construct.

certification The successful outcome of a formal review process of the clinical practice of a nurse who is required to show a high degree of proficiency in interpersonal skills, use of the nursing process, and psychiatric psychological, and milieu therapies.

child An individual who is prepubscent (in infancy, of preschool age, of school age, or preadolescent).

child abuse Physical injury or sexual or emotional abuse that occurs when children are ignored, isolated, or continually shamed and demeaned.

chronic illness The process of progressive deterioration, with increasing symptoms, functional impairment, and disability over time.

chronic mental disability A label applied to an individual who has had either one continuous psychiatric hospitalization within the past 5 years or two or more psychiatric hospitalizatons in a 12-month period.

circumstantial speech Inclusion of many nonessential details in a response.

clang association A speech pattern characterized by rhyming.

claustrophobia A fear of closed places.

client-centered mental health consultation A format through which the consultant focuses on helping the consultee find the most effective treatment for a client.

clinical nurse specialist A master's degree–prepared nurse with a concentration in a specific area of clinical nursing.

coalition A power relationship composed either of two like partners joined together against an unlike opponent or an unlike partner joined together against an opponent who is like one of the partners. Partners can be differentiated by gender or generation.

cognition The ego function that relates to the process of logical thought.

cognitive model of learning A theory that defines learning as behavioral change based on the acquisition of information about the environment.

cohesiveness Force that attracts members to a group and causes them to remain in the group.

coitus Sexual intercourse with a partner of the opposite sex.

cold, wet sheet pack A form of somatic therapy in which the patient is swathed in cold, wet sheets, which then are warmed by body heat. The warmth and immobilization are soothing to very agitated people.

collective bargaining The use of collective action in negotiating patient care and economic issues with one's employer, including wages, hours, and conditions of work.

commitment Involuntary admission in which the request for hospitalization did not originate with the patient. When he is committed, he loses the right to leave the hospital when he wishes. It is usually justified on the grounds that the patient is dangerous to self or others and needs treatment.

community mental health A treatment philosophy based on the social model of psychiatric care that advocates a comprehensive range of mental health services that are to be made readily available to all community members.

compensation Process by which a person makes up for a deficiency in his image of himself by strongly emphasizing some other feature that he regards as an asset.

competent community A population of persons who are aware of resources and alternatives, can make reasoned decisions about issues facing them, and can cope adaptively with problems. It parallels the concept of positive mental health.

compromise A task-oriented coping reaction that involves changing one's usual way of operating, substituting goals, or sacrificing aspects of one's personal needs. Compromise reactions are usually constructive and are frequently employed in approach-approach and avoidance-avoidance situations.

compulsion A recurring irresistible impulse to perform some act.

concrete operation A thought process based on a concrete rather than abstract point of reference.

concreteness Use of specific terminology rather than abstractions in the discussion of the patient's feelings, experiences, and behavior.

conditional discharge A specified leave of absence or liberty from a psychiatric hospital in which certain things are expected from the patient and during which the commitment order is still in effect.

confabulation The manufacture of a response that is inaccurate but sounds appropriate. This is done to avoid embarrassment about memory loss.

confidentiality The ethical principle in the nurse-patient relationship, founded on trust and respect, that prohibits disclosure of privileged information without the patient's informed consent.

conflict Clashing of two opposing interests. The person experiences two competing drives and must choose between them.

confrontation An expression by the nurse of perceived discrepancies in the patient's behavior. It is an attempt by the nurse to bring to the patient's awareness the incongruence in his feelings, attitudes, beliefs, and behaviors.

confusion Constellation of behaviors, including inattention, memory deficits, inappropriate verbalizations, disruptive behavior, noncompliance, and failure to perform activities of daily living.

congruent communication A communication pattern in which the sender is comminicating the same message on both verbal and nonverbal levels.

consensual validation Ensuring understanding of the communication of another person by reaching agreement on the meaning of the message.

consequences Stimulus events following a behavior that strengthen or weaken the behavior. These are either reinforcers or punishers.

consultation A process of interaction between two professional persons—the consultant, who is a specialist, and the consultee.

context Setting in which an event takes place.

continuous reinforcement A schedule of reinforcement in which each emission of a response is followed by the reinforcer.

conversion disorder A somatoform disorder characterized by a loss or alteration of physical functioning without evidence of organic impairment.

coping mechanisms Any effort directed at stress management. They can be task-oriented and involve direct problem-solving efforts to cope with the threat itself or be intrapsychic or ego defense–oriented with the goal of regulating one's emotional distress.

coping resources Characteristics of the person, group, or environment that are helpful in assisting individuals in adapting to stress.

coping style The cognitive, affective, or behavioral response of a person to a problematic or traumatic life event.

coprolalic A person who obtains sexual pleasure from using filthy language.

countertransference An emotional response of the nurse that is generated by the qualities of the patient and is inappropriate to the content and context of the therapeutic relationship or inappropriate in the degree of intensity of emotion.

criminal prosecution The filing of a complaint in a criminal court for an alleged criminal or felonious act against a perpetrator; a guilty or not guilty verdict is delivered by either a judge or a jury, and the perpetrator, if convicted, is sentenced for the offense.

crisis An internal disturbance that results from a stressful event or perceived threat to self.

crisis intervention A short-term active mode of therapy that focuses on solving the patient's immediate problem and reestablishing psychological equilibrium.

cult A specific complex of beliefs, rites, and ceremonies maintained by a social group in association with some particular person or object. Cult is usually considered as having magical or religious significance.

cultural relativism The idea that health and normality emerge within a social context and that the content and form of mental health and mental illness will vary greatly from one culture to another. Differences result from variations in stressors, symbolical interpretation, acceptance of expression and repression, and cohesion of social groups and their tolerance of deviation.

cunnilingus Oral stimulation of the female genitalia.

data base Sum total of information from which the patient's problems can be identified.

date/acquaintance rape The perpetration of a sexual assault or rape on a person by someone known to the victim; may include dates, casual acquaintances, therapists, employers, friends, etc.

daydream A reverie while awake; usually the unfulfilled wishes of the dreamer are imagined as fulfilled. Wishes are not disguised and fulfillment is imagined as direct, without repression. Not inherently pathological.

defense mechanisms Coping mechanisms of the ego that attempt to protect the person from feelings of inadequacy and worthlessness and prevent awareness of anxiety. They are primarily unconscious in nature and involve a degree of self-deception and reality distortion.

deinstitutionalization At the individual patient level, the transfer to a community setting of a patient who has been hospitalized for an extended period of time, generally many years. At the mental health care system level, a shift in the focus of mental health care from the large, long-term institution to the community, accomplished by discharging long-term patients and by avoiding unnecessary admissions.

delayed treatment seeker A person who delays seeking mental health intervention for a problematic life event (e.g., sexual assault/rape) and seeks treatment months or years after the event, usually following a precipitating event.

deliberate biological programming Memory and the capacity for terminating the life of a cell is stored within the cell itself (one theory of psychobiological aging).

delinquency A relatively minor violation of legal or moral codes, especially by children or adolescents. Juvenile delinquency is such behavior by a young person (usually under 16 or 18 years) that brings him to the attention of a court.

delirium The medical diagnostic term that describes an organic mental disorder characterized by a cluster of cognitive impairments with an acute onset and the identification of a specific precipitating stressor.

delirium tremens A medical diagnostic term that has been replaced with the diagnosis of alcohol withdrawal delirium

delusion A fixed false belief. It may be persecutory, grandiose, nihilistic, or somatic in nature.

delusion of grandeur The false belief that one has great money, power, and prestige. It is frequently manifested in the belief that the individual is a famous person.

delusion of poverty The false belief that one is impoverished.

dementia The medical diagnostic term that describes an organic mental disorder characterized by a cluster of cognitive impairments that are generally of gradual onset and irreversible. The predisposing and precipitation stressors may or may not be identifiable.

denial Avoidance of disagreeable realities by ignoring or refusing to recognize them.

depersonalization A feeling of unreality and alienation from oneself. It is associated with a panic level of anxiety that produces a blocking off of awareness and a collapse in reality testing. The individual has difficulty distinguishing self from others, and one's body has an unreal or strange quality about it. It is the subjective experience of the partial or total disruption of one's ego and the disintegration and disorganization of one's self-concept.

depot injection Intramuscular injection of medication in an oil suspension that results in sustained release over a period of several days.

depression An abnormal extension of overelaboration of sadness and grief. The term "depression" can be used to denote a variety of phenomena—a sign, symptom, syndrome, emotional state, reaction, disease, or clinical entity.

detoxification The removal of a toxic substance from the body, either naturally through physiological processes, such as hepatic or renal functions, or medically by the introduction of alternative substances and gradual withdrawal.

developmental tasks Hierarchy of age-appropriate behaviors to be mastered as an individual matures.

deviancy Failure to comply with a social norm.

differentiation Sufficient separation between intellect and emotions so that one is not dominated by the reactive anxiety of the family's emotional system.

direct nursing care functions Liaison nurse activities that are focused on a particular client and his family or on a group for whom the nurse is directly responsible and accountable.

direct self-destructive behavior (DSDB) Suicidal behavior.

disability Impairment of instrumental role performance in at least three of the following areas: self-care, receptive and expressive language, learning, mobility, self-direction, capacity for independent living, and self-sufficiency.

discharge plan A formal written document that describes in detail the transition of the patient from one level of the mental health care system to another.

disengaged A transactional style in a family reflecting inappropriately rigid boundaries requiring a high level of individual stress to activate family response.

disengagement theory Individuals and society mutually withdraw as part of normal aging.

disorientation Inability to identify correctly the self in relation to time, place, or person.

displacement Shift of an emotion from the person or object toward which it was originally directed to another usually neutral or less dangerous person or object.

dissociation The separation of any group of mental or behavioral processes from the rest of the person's consciousness or identity.

dissociative reaction Process by which a person blocks off part of his life from conscious recognition because of the threat of overwhelming anxiety.

diurnal mood variation Changes in mood that are related to the time of day.

divorce therapy A type of counseling that attempts to help couples disengage from their former relationship and malicious behavior toward each other or their children.

double bind Simultaneous communication of conflicting messages in the context of a situation that does not allow escape. (See *incongruent communication*.)

dream analysis A psychoanalytical therapeutic technique that requires the patient to report his dreams to the analyst, who then interprets the meaning of the dream symbolism to assist the patient in understanding his unconscious mental functioning.

drug abuse Use of any chemical substance for reasons other than medical treatment.

drug-induced parkinsonism A reversible syndrome resembling the disease parkinsonism, resulting from the dopamine-blocking action of antipsychotic drugs.

drug interaction The effects of two or more drugs being taken simultaneously, producing an alteration in the usual effects of either drug taken alone. The interacting drugs may have a potentiating or additive effect, and serious side effects may result.

drug tolerance Repeated use of some substance or drug (e.g., narcotics) so that larger and larger doses are required to produce the same physiologic and/or psychologic effect obtained previously by a smaller dose.

drug trial The time it takes to administer a drug at adequate therapeutic doses for a sufficient period to determine its efficacy for a particular patient. The trial culminates with (1) acceptable clinical result, (2) intolerable adverse effects, and (3) poor response after an appropriate blood level is reached, or the drug is administered for a time period specific for the illness (3 weeks for antidepressants; 3 to 6 weeks for antipsychotics).

DSM-III Diagnostic and Statistical Manual of Mental Disorders standard nomenclature of emotional illness used by all health care practitioners; DSM-III-R is a revised version published in 1987; it updates and classifies mental illnesses, as well as presents guidelines and diagnostic criteria for various mental disorders.

dyspareunia Recurrent or persistent genital pain occurring before, during, or after intercourse (male or female).

dystonia Acute tonic muscle spasms, often of the tongue, jaw, eyes, and neck, but sometimes of the whole body. Sometimes occurs during the first few days of antipsychotic drug administration.

echolalia Repeating exactly whatever is heard.

echopraxia Imitation of the body position of another.

ego The I, self, or individual that is postulated as the "center" to which all a person's psychological activities and qualities are referred. The aspect of the psyche that is conscious and most in touch with external reality. An aspect of the personality that is in contact with the external world by means of perception, thought, and reality.

ego boundaries An individual's perception of the boundaries between himself and the exteral environment.

ego defense mechanisms Coping mechanisms of the ego that attempt to protect the person from feelings of inadequacy and worthlessness and prevent awareness of anxiety. They are primarily unconscious in nature and involve a degree of self-deception and reality distortion.

ego deficit/strength The inability or ability of the ego to test reality and maintain that function under stress and anxiety.

ego interpretive techniques A milieu management technique that helps the child gain ego strength through insight into his maladaptive behavior.

ego state A transactional analysis term that refers to the role behaviors an individual assumes in a particular unit of communication. They may be adult, parent, or child.

ego supportive techniques A milieu management technique for dealing with a child in the early phase of treatment in which the child is helped to regain self-control and reenter the daily routine from a panic-aggressive state.

ejaculatory imcompetence Inability of a man to ejaculate intravaginally. It is also known as retarded ejaculation.

electroconvulsive therapy (ECT) Artificial induction of a grand mal seizure by passing a controlled electrical current through electrodes applied to one or both temples. The patient is anesthetized and the seizure attenuated by administration of a muscle relaxant medication.

empathic understanding Ability to view the patient's world from his internal frame of reference. It involves the nurse's sensitivity to the patient's current feelings and the verbal ability to communicate this understanding in a language attuned to the patient.

enabler The role that is frequently assumed by the significant others of substance abusers, characterized by covert support of the substance-abusing behavior.

encopresis Repeated voluntary or involuntary passage of feces of normal or near-normal consistency into places not appropriate for that purpose, and not caused by any physical disorder.

encounter group therapy An application of the existential model of psychiatric care in a group setting. The focus is on here-and-now experience and the expression of real feelings verbally and nonverbally as members react to events in the group.

endorphins Naturally occurring peptides that have been found in the central nervous system and have a physiological effect similar to that of opiates.

endogenous Developing or originating within the organism, or arising from causes within the organism.

enkephalins Naturally occurring peptides that have been found in the central nervous system and have a physiological effect similar to that of opiates.

enmeshed A transactional sytle in a family reflecting diffuse subsystem boundaries resulting in stress in one family member emotionally reverberating quickly and intensely throughtout the family system.

enuresis Repeated involuntary voiding of urine during the day or at night, after an age at which continence is expected, that is not caused by any physical disorder.

environment The circumstances, objects, or conditions that surround and have an internal influence on the life and effective functioning of the family and its members.

environmental change Activities that have a social setting focus and require the modification of an individual's or group's immediate environment or the larger social system.

ethic A standard of valued behavior or beliefs adhered to by an individual or group. A goal to which one aspires.

ethical dilemma An issue for which moral claims conflict with one another. It can be defined as (1) a difficult problem that seems to have no satisfactory solution or (2) a choice between equally unsatisfactory alternatives.

ethnocentrism A threat to the therapeutic relationship by imposing one's own views and standards on other cultural groups and desiring to change the way of life of others to be consistent with one's own.

evaluation A phase of the nursing process in which the patient's progress or lack of progress toward goal achievement is determined by the patient and nurse. This determination directs reassessment, reordering of priorities, new goal setting, and revision of the plan of nursing care.

exhibitionism Intense sexual arousal or desire and acts, fantasies, or other stimuli involving exposing one's genitals to an unsuspecting stranger.

existentialism A school of philosophical thought that focuses on the importance of experience in the present and the belief that persons finds meaning in life through their experiences.

exogenous Developing or originating outside the organism.

expert witness A person qualified by experience and or education to form a definition and objective opinion based on scientific opinion or medical theory.

extinction Withholding reinforcement that was previously provided.

extrapyramidal syndrome A variety of signs and symptoms, including muscular rigidity, tremors, drooling, shuffling gait (parkinsonism); restlessness (akathisia); peculiar involuntary postures (dystonia); motor inertia (akathisia); and many other neurological disturbances. Results from dysfunction of the extrapyramidal system. May occur as a reversible side effect of certain psychotropic drugs, particularly antipsychotics.

face-hand test A psychomotor test used to assess the presence of organic mental disorders.

family A group of people living in a household who are attached emotionally, interact regularly, and share concerns for the growth and development of individuals and the family.

family Apgar An evaluation tool that focuses on family function as viewed by each member.

family projection process Transmission of anxiety of one or both parents onto a target child establishing an overly protective or conflictual relationship with the child, resulting ultimately in impairment of the child.

family structure The way in which the family is organized according to roles, rules, power, and hierarchies, including generational boundaries.

family style Those pervasive patterns characteristic of the family's interaction (e.g., chaotic, rigid, enmeshed, conflictual).

family system Those individuals who contribute to the functional state of the family as a unit.

family therapy The focus of family therapy is to treat as the primary unit a social system, rather than an individual member who has been defined as a "patient".

family violence The physical, psychological, sexual, material, or social violation or exploitation of a person by a family member or their delegate; the mode by which a given family system expresses its dysfunction.

fellatio Oral stimulation of the male genitalia.

female orgasmic dysfunction Inability of a female to achieve orgasm that may be primary or situational in origin.

female sexual arousal disorder Either (1) persistent or recurrent partial or complete failure to attain or maintain the lubrication-swelling response until completion of sexual activity or (2) persistent or recurrent lack of a subjective sense of sexual excitement and pleasure in a female during sexual activity.

fetishism Intense sexual arousal or desire and acts, fantasies, or other stimuli involving nonliving objects by themselves.

fixation A psychoanalytical term that refers to a failure to resolve the conflicts inherent in a particular stage of psychosocial development. Psychological energy (libido) is invested in these conflictual areas, thus inhibiting the person's ability to grow beyond that point.

fixed interval (FI) reinforcement Specific lapse of time required for reinforcement.

fixed ratio (FR) reinforcement Specific number of responses required for reinforcement.

flashback A phenomenon experienced by individuals who have taken hallucinogenic drugs in which they unexpectedly reexperience the effects of the drug.

flight of ideas A pattern of speech characterized by a rapid transition from one topic to another, frequently without completing the original thought. This behavior is characteristic of manic states.

Food and Drug Administration (FDA) One of a number of health administrations under the Assistant Secretary of Health of the U.S. Department of Health, Education and Welfare (in April 1980, Department of Health and Human Services) to set standards for, to license the sale of, and in general to safeguard the public from the use of dangerous drugs and food substances.

free association A psychoanalytical therapeutic technique that requires the patient to repeat all his thoughts without censorship, drifting naturally from one thought to the next.

freebasing A chemical process that is applied to cocaine to amplify the effect of the drug. The cocaine is then smoked.

frotteurism Intense sexual arousal or desire and acts, fantasies, or other stimuli involving rubbing against a nonconsenting person.

frustration A feeling that results when something interferes with one's ability to attain a desired goal, satisfaction, or security.

functional disorder A mental or emotional impairment that is believed to be psychosocial in origin.

fusion A blurring of self-boundaries in a highly reactive emotional relationship with another.

game In the context of transactional analysis, repetitive sets of ulterior transactions that are psychologically gratifying.

genuineness A quality of the nurse characterized by openness, honesty, and sincerity. The nurse is self-congruent and authentic and relates to the patient without a defensive facade.

geriatric patient Adult recipient of health care services, who is, chronologically, 65 years of age or older.

gerontology The study of the phenomenon of aging.

gestalt therapy A therapeutic approach based on the existential model of psychiatric care. It was developed by Perls and focuses on the development of enhanced self-awareness.

grief An individual's subjective response to the loss of a person, object, or concept that is highly valued. Uncomplicated grief is a healthy, adaptive, reparative response.

group A collection of three or more individuals who have a relationship with one another, are interdependent, and may share some common norms.

group-centered mental health consultation A format through which the consultant meets with a group to provide guidance regarding the consultees' work encounters.

group maintenance Group functions directed toward satisfaction of members' psychosocial or emotional needs.

group therapy A form of psychiatric treatment in which six to eight patients attend a specified number of meetings that are conducted by a therapist. Examples of some common inpatient groups are remotivation groups, problem-solving groups, supportive groups, and reeducation groups.

habeas corpus A right retained by all psychiatric patients that provides for the release of an individual who claims he is being deprived of his liberty and detained illegally. The hearing for this determination takes place in a court of law, and the patient's sanity is at issue.

half-life The amount of time it takes the body to excrete approximately half of an ingested drug; after this time the effects of the drug usually begin to deteriorate.

hallucination A sensory experience that is not the result of an external stimulus; it may be visual, auditory, tactile, olfactory, or gustatory.

hallucinogens A class of abused drugs that cause a psychotic-like experience.

health education A nursing intervention that involves increasing a person's awareness of health issues, understanding of the dimensions of possible stressors and outcomes, knowledge of how to acquire needed resources, and actual coping responses.

helplessness A person's belief that no one will do anything to aid him.

homicide The illegal killing of one human being by another.

homosexual One who is motivated in adult life by a definite preferential erotic attraction to members of the same sex and who usually (but not necessarily) engages in overt sexual relations with them.

homosexual panic A state of extreme agitation resulting from fear related to awareness of previously repressed homosexual impulses.

hopelessness An individual's belief that neither he nor anyone else can do anything to aid him.

hostility A feeling of anger and resentment characterized by destructive behavior.

hyperactive Unusually or excessively active.

hypoactive sexual desire disorder Persistently or recurrently deficient or absent sexual fantasies and desire for sexual activity.

hypochondriasis A somatoform disorder characterized by the belief that one is ill without evidence of organic impairment.

hypomania A clinical syndrome that is similar to, but less severe than, that described by the term "mania" or "manic episode."

id Element of the personality described by Freud that represents one's instinctual drives and primitive impulses and is largely unconscious in nature.

identification Process by which a person tries to make himself like someone else whom he admires by taking on the thoughts, mannerisms, or tastes of that individual.

identity Organizing principle of the personality system that accounts for the unity, continuity, uniqueness, and consistency of the personality. It is the awareness of the process of "being oneself" that is derived from self-observation and judgment.

identity confusion Lack of clarity and consistency in one's perception of the self, resulting in a high degree of anxiety.

identity diffusion An individual's failure to integrate various childhood identifications into a harmonious adult psychosocial identity.

identity foreclosure Premature adoption of an identity that is desired by significant others without coming to terms with one's own desires, aspirations, or potential.

idiopathic pain disorder A somatoform disorder characterized by pain as its only symptom and no evidence of organic impairment.

illusion Misinterpretation of a sensory input.

immediacy State that occurs when the current interaction of the nurse and the patient is focused on.

implementation A phase of the nursing process in which nursing actions are carried out that assist the patient to maximize his health capabilities and provide for patient participation in health promotion, maintenance, and restoration.

impotence Failure to achieve an erection.

incest Act of having sexual relations with a close relative, such as one's mother, daughter, or son.

incompetency A legal status that must be proved in a special court hearing. As a result of the hearing the person can be deprived of many of his civil rights. Incompetency can be reversed only in another court hearing that declares the person competent.

incongruent communication A communication pattern in which the sender is communicating different messages on the verbal and nonverbal levels and the listener does not know to which level he should respond. (See *double bind*.)

indirect nursing care functions Liaison nurse activities used to problem solve with consultee who is responsible and accountable for implementing and evaluating any recommended changes to effect problem resolution.

indirect self-destructive behavior (ISDB) Any activity that is detrimental to the well-being of the person and potentially has the outcome of death, accompanied by lack of conscious awareness of the self-destructive nature of the behavior.

individual psychotherapy A formal one-to-one therapeutic relationship in which the patient is encouraged to develop insights into the soruces of his thoughts, feelings, perceptions, and behavior. By developing these insights, the patient is better able to deal with stress and maintain effective interpersonal relationships.

informal admission A type of admission to a psychiatric hospital in which there is no formal or written application and the individual is free to leave at any time.

informed consent Disclosure of a certain amount of information to the patient about the proposed treatment and the attainment of the patient's consent, which must be competent, understanding, and voluntary.

inhibited female orgasm Persistent or recurrent delay in or absence of orgasm in a female following a normal sexual excitement phase during sexual activity that is judged by the clinician to be adequate in focus, intensity, and duration.

inhibited male orgasm Persistent or recurrent delay in or absence of ejaculation in a male following a normal sexual excitement phase during sexual activity that is judged by the clinician to be adequate in focus, intensity, and duration.

insanity defense Legal defense proposing that a person who has committed an act that in a usual situation would be criminal should be held not guilty by reason of "Insanity."

institutional syndrome Characterized by lack of initiative, apathy, withdrawal, and submissiveness to authority.

insulin shock therapy Induction of a coma by administration of insulin. The comatose state is allowed to last up to an hour and is then reversed by the administration of glucose or glucagon.

intellectualization Excessive reasoning or logic used to avoid experiencing disturbing feelings.

intermittent reinforcement Noncontinuous reinforcement in which not every response is reinforced. Some emissions of a particular behavior are reinforced; others are not.

interpersonal strength A behavioral characteristic of an individual that when used in an interpersonal relationship, enhances mutual enjoyment of the relationship, without interfering with the integrity of either person.

introjection An intense type of identification in which the person incorporates qualities or values of another person or group into his own ego structure.

involuntary admission See *commitment*.

involuntary patient A patient admitted to a psychiatric facility through the commitment process.

isolation Splitting off of the emotional component of a thought. It may be temporary or long term.

joining The process of the therapist gaining entry into a family system by recognizing family strengths, respecting existing hierarchies and values, and confirming individual members in their sense of self.

judgment The ability to make logical, rational decisions.

judicial discharge A discharge granted by the courts.

Katz Index of Daily Living An instrument that is used to measure the individual's ability to bathe, dress, toilet, transfer, and feed himself and remain continent.

la belle indifference Term used to describe the patient's lack of concern or anxiety regarding his physical illness. It is used to describe the bland attitude characteristic of hysteria or conversion reactions.

labile Subject to frequent or unpredictable changes.

latency Psychosexual stage of development first identified by Freud in which the child's ego has developed considerable impulse control and energy is focused on learning and more organized play.

learned helplessness A behavioral state and personality trait of a person who believes that he is ineffectual, his responses are futile, and he has lost control over the reinforcers in his environment.

learning A relatively stable, observable change in the frequency or form of behavior resulting from interaction with environmetal antecedent and consequences.

least restrictive alternative Providing patients with the greatest freedom from restriction, especially that of long-term hospitalization.

legal responsibilities Include expectations of a mental health professional in (1) documenting the signs and symptoms of a person in response to a life event and (2) giving testimony in criminal and civil litigation proceedings.

lesbian A woman whose sexual preference is for another woman.

lethality An estimation of the probability that a person who is threatening suicide will succeed based on the method described, the specificity of the plan, and the availability of the means.

liaison nurse A master's degree–prepared nurse clinician who provides psychiatric nursing services in nonpsychiatric settings.

liaison nursing A professional process between two systems in which one of the systems (the user) has a current work-related problem and voluntarily requests help from an outside system (the provider) who is perceived to have a specialized competency in a defined area.

libido Freud's term for psychic energy.

life review Progressive return to consciousness of past experiences.

life space interview An interaction between a child and adult that takes place outside the context of individual therapy. The focus is on improving the child's sense of self-identity and ego functioning with the developmental process.

limbic system An area in the brain associated with the control of emotion, eating, drinking, and sexual activity.

limit setting Act of making a person aware of his rights and responsibilities, while communicating the expectation that he will respect the rules. Also, the application of appropriate sanctions if the person does not obey the rules.

living will Determining in advance one's participation in heroic measures during the dying process.

logotherapy An approach to psychotherapy based on the existential model and developed by Frankl. The focus is on the search for meaning in present experiences.

loose associations A communication pattern characterized by lack of clarity of connection between one thought and the next.

male sexual arousal disorder Either (1) persistent or recurrent partial or complete failure in a male to attain or maintain erection until completion of the sexual activity or (2) persistent or recurrent lack of a subjective sense of sexual excitement and pleasure in a male during sexual activity.

malingering Deliberate feigning of an illness.

malpractice Failure of a professional person to give the kind of proper and competent care that is given by members of his profession in the community, which causes harm to the patient.

mania A condition that is characterized by a mood that is elevated, expansive, or irritable.

manipulation Controlling the behavior of others to achieve one's own goals.

marital rape The perpetration of a sexual assault or rape on a partner by one's spouse.

mashochism Intense sexual arousal or desire and acts, fantasies, or other stimuli involving being humiliated, beaten, bound, or otherwise made to suffer (real or simulated).

masturbation The induction of erection and the obtaining of sexual satisfaction in either sex, from manual or other artificial stimulation of the genitals. Usually is self-induced.

maturational crisis Transitional or developmental periods within a person's life when his psychological equilibrium is upset.

mechanical restraints Any of several means of restricting a patient's freedom of movement. Includes camisoles, wrist and ankle restraints, sheet restraints, and sheet packs.

medical diagnosis The independent judgment of a physician of the health problems or disease states of the patient.

meditation A technique of tension reduction in which the person closes his eyes, relaxes the major muscle groups, and repeats a cue word silently to himself each time he exhales.

memory The ability to recall past events.

menarche First menstruation of a woman, which indicates that she may be capable of conceiving.

mental health consultation nurse A master's degree–prepared nurse whose scope of practice includes the health illness continuum as it applies to psychosocial aspects of health care.

mental status examination A formal exploration of data relative to a patient's mental functioning in which information is collected about the patient's sensorium and intelligence, thought processes, mood and affect, and insight.

message A unit of communication.

metacommunication Messages about a communication pertaining to both the relationship and the informational aspects.

milieu therapy A scientific manipulation of the environment aimed at producing changes in the personality of the patient.

Mini-Mental State Examination A brief psychological test designed to differentiate between dementia, psychosis, and affective disorders.

model A means of organizing a complex body of knowledge.

monoamine oxidase (MAO) inhibitors A group of chemically related antidepressant medications.

mood A prolonged emotional state that influences one's whole personality and life functioning.

mourning Includes all the psychological processes set in motion within the individual by a loss. The process of mourning is resolved only when the lost object is internalized, bonds of attachment are loosened, and new object relationships are established.

multidisciplinary health care team A group of health care workers who are members of different disciplines, with each one providing specific services to the patient.

multigenerational transmission process The repetition of relationship pattterns and anxiety associated with toxic issues passed through generations in a family.

multiple personality The existence within an individual of two or more distinct personalities or personality states, each having its own pattern of perceiving, feeling, and thinking.

mutual support groups A type of group in which members organize themselves to solve their own problems. They are led by the group members themselves, who share a common experience, work together toward a common goal, and use their own strengths to gain control over their lives.

myth A false belief not supported by empirical facts.

narcissism An exaggerated sense of self-importance manifested as extreme self-absorption.

narcotics A class of drugs that have powerful analgesic and euphoria-inducing properties.

National Institute of Mental Health (NIMH) Responsible for programs dealing with mental health, NIMH is an institute within the Alcohol, Drug Abuse, and Mental Health Administration (ADAMHA). ADAMHA, an agency in the U.S. Department of Health and Human Services, provides leadership, policies, and goals for the federal effort to ensure the treatment and rehabilitation of persons with alcohol, drug abuse, and mental health problems; this agency is also responsible for administering grants to advance and support research, training, and service programs.

National Organization of Victims Assistance A private, nonprofit organization of victim and witness assistance practitioners, criminal justice professionals, reserachers, former victims, and others committed to the recognition of victim's rights; four purposes are national advocacy, victims aid, service to local programs, and membership support.

necrophile A person who is sexually aroused by thought of death or sexual activity with a dead person.

need-fear dilemma An approach-avoidance conflict related to the need to experience closeness coupled with fear of the experience.

negative identity Assumption of an identity that is at odds with the accepted values and expectations of society.

negative punishment Removal of something following operant, decreasing probability of operant's recurrence.

negative reinforcement Refers to the procedure whereby the removal or termination of an aversive stimulus contingently follows the emission of a response and results in an increase in the rate responding.

negative reinforcer A stimulus that, when presented immediately following the occurrence of a particular behavior, will decrease the rate of responding of that behavior. If antecedent to the emission of a particular behavior and terminated by that response, it will increase the rate of responding of that behavior.

neglect Condition that occurs when a parent is unable to or fails to provide minimum emotional and physical care to a child.

neologisms Words that are invented by the person and understood only by him.

networking A process of linking individuals or agencies with mutual interests to form a coalition and thereby more effectively bring about social change.

neurasthenia A type of disorder chacterized by chronic mental and physical fatigue and a variety of vague aches and pains, including weakness, headaches, and back pain. This reaction is not caused by overwork but is an attempt to reduce or mask areas of conflict.

neuron Nerve cell; both an electrical and a chemical unit; neurons are separated from each other by spaces called synapses. They are the basic function units of the nervous system.

neurotic behavior A behavioral dysfunction that is characterized by anxiety, but in which there is no distortion of reality.

neurotic disorders A category of health problems that are distinguished by the following characteristics: symptoms that are distressing and unacceptable to the individual, grossly intact reality testing, behavior that does not violate gross social norms, a disturbance that is relatively enduring or recurrent without treatment, and no demonstrable organic etiology.

neurotransmitter A chemical found in the nervous system (e.g., norepinephrine, serotonin, dopamine) that facilitates the transmission of impulses across synapses between neurons. Disorders in the brain physiology of neurotransmitters have been implicated in the pathogenesis of several psychiatric illnesses, particularly affective disorders and schizophrenia.

nihilistic delusion The false belief that the self, part of the self, or another object has ceased to exist.

noncompliance The failure of the individual to carry out the self-care activities prescribed in a health care plan.

nonverbal communication Transmission of a message without the use of words. It involves all five senses.

norm A culturally defined standard of behavior.

nuclear family emotional system Patterns of interaction between family members and the degree to which these patterns promote fusion.

nurse practice act A state law that defines the legal limits of nursing practice and that must be adhered to by all licensed nurses.

nurses' observation scale for inpatient evaluation (NOSIE) A systematical, objective behavioral rating scale applied by nurses to patients' behavior.

nursing The diagnosis and treatment of human responses to actual or potential health problems.

nursing audit A type of clinical evaluation of nursing care that may focus on a nursing activity (process audit) or on the behavior of a patient in response to the nursing care that has been provided (outcome audit).

nursing diagnosis The independent judgment of a nurse of the patient's behavioral response to stress. It is a statement of the patient's nursing problems, which may be overt, covert, existing, or potential, and includes both the behavioral disruption or threatened disruption and the contributing stessors.

nursing problems Aspects of the patient's health that may need to be promoted or with which the patient needs help in his biopsychosocial adaptation to stress.

nursing process An interactive problem-solving process used by the nurse as a systematical and individualized way to fulfill the goal of nursing care. It includes the components of data collection, formulation of the nursings diagnosis, planning, implementation, and evaluation.

nursing therapeutic process The process by which the nurse strives to promote and maintain the adaptive coping responses of the patient. It involves the establishment of a therapeutic nurse-patient relationship and the use of the nursing process.

obesity A condition in which the individual weighs at least 20% more than his ideal weight.

object cues A category of nonverbal communication that includes the speaker's intentional and nonintentional use of all objects, such as dress, furnishings, and possessions.

observers Adults or children in the nuclear and extended family who neither perpetrate nor are victims of the family abuse or violence by an offender.

obsession A recurring thought that is unwanted but that cannot be voluntarily excluded from consciousness.

oculogyric crisis A side effect of antipsychotic medication that is characterized by the uncontrollable rolling upward of the eyes.

offenders Adults or children who perpetrate any type or form of abuse or violence on family members of other persons.

operant Behavior maintained or changed by its consequences.

operant behavior Behavior whose strength is controlled by the stimulus events that precede and follow it.

operant conditioning Modification of operant behavior by systematical manipulation of antecedents and consequences.

operant level Frequency or form of a performance under baseline conditions before any systematical conditioning procedures are introduced.

organic disorder A mental or emotional impairment that is believed to be physiological in origin.

orientation The ability to relate the self correctly to time, place, and person.

orthostatic hypotension A drop in blood pressure related to change in position. A common side effect of psychotropic medications.

PACE II An evaluation tool that focuses on the physical health of nursing home patients.

panic An attack of extreme anxiety that involves the disorganization of the personality. Distorted perceptions, loss of rational thought, and an inability to communicate and function are evident.

paranoia A behavioral manifestation representatie of the unconscious operation of the mechanism of projection whereby the person attributes his ego-alien thoughts and impulses to others; a feeling of extreme suspicion.

paranoid delusion The false belief that one is being persecuted.

paraphilias Characterized by sexual arousal in response to objects or situations that are not normally arousing for affectionate sexual activities with human partners (pedophilia, exhibitionism, zoophilia, etc.).

parent education Any educational experience geared toward the thoughtful conveyance of information enabling the parent to provide quality childrearing.

parkinsonian equivalents Side effects of antipsychotic medications that are behaviors characteristic of Parkinson's disease, including fine tremors, pill-rolling tremor of the fingers, drooling, and petit pas gait.

passive Behavior that subordinates the individual's own rights to the demands of others.

passive-aggresive Term describing indirect expression, verbal or nonverbal, of angry feelings.

paternalism The ethical principle that provides for the regulation of the activities of another in the same manner in which a benevolent parent regulates the activities of a child.

pedophilia Intense sexual arousal or desire and acts, fantasies or other stimuli involving one or more children 13 years of age or younger.

peer A person deemed an equal for the purpose at hand. A companion or associate on roughly the same level of age or endowment, an age mate.

peer group The group with whom a child associates on terms of approximate equality. Usually very heterogenous.

peer review Review of clinical practice with peers, supervisors, and/or consultants.

perception Sensory reception of a stimulus; meaning one attributes to a situation.

perseveration Repetition of a single word or phrase over and over.

pharmacokinetics The study of the process and rates of drug distribution, metabolism, and disposition in the organism.

phenothiazines A group of chemically related antipsychotic medications.

phobic reaction A persistent fear of some object or situation that presents no actual danger to the person or in which the danger is magnified out of proportion to its actual seriousness.

physical dependence A characteristic of drug addiction that is present when withdrawal of the drug results in physiological disruptions.

physical restraint Limitation of the individual's freedom of movement by immobilizing all or part of the body or by restricting the person to a confined space.

planning A phase of the nursing process in which goals are derived from the nursing diagnosis, priorities are set, and nursing approaches or measures to achieve the goals are prescribed.

play therapy The utilization of child's play as a mode of self-expression and communication to work through conflicts with an adult therapist.

polypharmacy Use of combinations of psychoactive drugs in a patient at the same time; more than one drug may not be more effective than a single agent, can cause drug interactions, and may increase the incidence of adverse reactions.

positive punishment A punishment procedure in which the presentation of an aversive stimulus immediately following the occurrence of a particular behavior results in a decrease in the rate of responding of that behavior.

positive reinforcement Presentation of environmental event as a consequence of operant, increasing probability of operant's recurrence.

possession The belief that one has been taken over by some spirit or person.

postvention Therapeutic intervention with the significant others of an individual who has committed suicide.

preadolescence The arbitrarily distinguished period of 10 to 12 years of age, the 2 years before puberty.

predisposing factors Conditioning factors that influence both the type and the amount of resources that the individual can elicit to cope with stress. They may be biological, psychological, and sociocultural in nature.

premature ejaculation Ejaculation occurring with minimum sexual stimulation, or before, on, or shortly after penetration, and before the individual wishes it.

primary appraisal of stressor An evaluation of the significance of an event for one's well-being that takes place on the cognitive, affective, physiological, behavioral, and social levels.

primary gain A decrease in anxiety resulting from the individual's efforts to cope with stress.

primary nursing A modality of care delivery characterized by the assignment of one nurse to coordinate the total nursing care of a patient from admission to discharge.

primary prevention Biological, social, or psychological intervention that promotes health and well-being or reduces the incidence of illness in a community by altering the causative factors before they have an opportunity to do harm.

primary process thought Primitive thought process that is normally kept unconscious by use of the coping mechanism of repression; impulsive infantile ideation.

primary symptoms Symptoms that are intrinsically associated with the disease process.

privileged communication A legal term that applies only in court-related proceedings and means that the right to reveal information belongs to the person who spoke, and the listener cannot disclose the information unless the speaker gives permission. It exists between a patient and health professional only if a law specifically establishes it.

professionalization Evidence of a continuous attempt of a group in any community or society to gain more and more control over certain resources related to an occupational area.

program-centered consultation A format through which the consultant focuses on broader organizational and program areas in an attempt to help the consultee solve institution-wide issues.

projection Attributing one's own thoughts or impulses to another person. Through this process the individual can attribute his own intolerable wishes, emotional feelings, or motivations to another person.

pseudodementia A depressive condition of the elderly that is charcterized by impaired cognitive functioning.

psychiatric nursing An interpersonal process that strives to promote and maintain behavior that contributes to integrated functioning. It employs the theories of human behavior as its science and purposeful use of self as its art. Psychiatric nursing is directed toward both preventive and corrective impacts on mental disorders and their sequelae and is concerned with the promotion of optimum mental health for society, the community, and those individuals who live within it.

psychoanalysis A therpaeutic approach based on the belief that behavioral disorders are related to unresolved, anxiety-provoking childhood experiences that are repressed into the unconscious. The goal of psychoanalysis is to bring repressed experiences into conscious awareness and to learn healthier means of coping with the related anxiety.

psychobiological resilience A concept that proposes that there is a recurrent human need to weather periods of stress and change throughout life. The ability to weather each period of disruption and reintegration successfully leaves the person better able to deal with the next change.

psychodrama A modality of therapy that uses structured and directed dramatizations of a patient's emotional problems and experiences.

psychoeducation The use of the principles and methods of education to facilitate the rehabilitation and treatment of the mentally ill.

psychogenic amnesia Temporary inability to recall important personal information that is too extensive to be explained by ordinary forgetfulness.

psychogenic fugue Sudden, unexpected travel away from home or one's customary place of work, with an inability to recall one's past.

psychological autopsy A retrospective review of the individual's behavior for the time preceding his death by suicide.

psychological dependence A characteristic of drug addiction that is manifested in a craving for the abused substance and a fear that it will not be available in the future.

psychological factors affecting physical condition A category of psychophysiological disruptions in which organic impairment is evident. Examples include migraine headache, asthma, hypertension, colitis, and duodenal ulcer.

psychological testing A diagnostical tool used by the psychologist to aid in assessment of the patient. It includes administration of a battery of cognitive and projective tests.

psychomotor retardation A slowing of motor activity related to a state of severe depression.

psychoneuroimmunology The scientific field exploring the relationship between psychological states and the immune response.

psychopharmacology Drugs that treat the symptoms of mental illness, and whose actions in the brain provide us with models to understand better the mechanisms of mental disorders.

psychosocial rehabilitation The process of development of the many skills necessary for the chronically mentally ill patient to live independently.

psychosomatic reactions Disorders in which the emotional tension is not discharged outwardly but is instead unconsciously channeled through the visceral organs.

psychosurgery Surgical interruption of selected neural pathways that involve the transmission of emotional impulses in the brain.

psychotherapy group A group developed for the purpose of treating emotional distress and disorder through means of a group method and group process.

psychotic behavior Severely dysfunctional behavior characterized by a panic level of anxiety, personality disintegration, and regressive behavior. The person experiences a reduced level of awareness and has great difficulty functoning adequately.

psychotic disorders A category of health problems that are distinguished by the following characteristics: severe mood disorder, regressive behavior, personality disintegration, reduced level of awareness, great difficulty in functioning adequately, and gross impairment in reality testing.

psychotomimetic Imitating a psychosis; refers to the effects of hallucinogenic drugs.

puberty The period during which the generative organs become capable of functioning and the person develops secondary sex characteristics in the female, its onset is marked by the beginning of menstruation; in males, one fairly reliable sign is the pigmenting of underarm hair.

punishment Procedures that decrease probability that operant will recur.

quality assessment measures Formal, systematic, organizational evaluation of overall patterns or programs of care, including clinical, consumer, and systems evaluation.

quality assurance activities Clinical evaluation of ongoing programs that include both evaluation and corrective action.

rape Legally defined as the forcible perpetration of the act of sexual intercourse on the body of a woman not one's wife. A more contemporary definition would include acts of oral and anal sodomy and allow for its occurrence within marriage as well.

rational-emotive therapy A therapeutic approach based on the existential model of psychiatric care and developed by Ellis. The emphasis is on risk taking and the assumption of responsibility for one's behavior.

rationalization Offering a socially acceptable or apparently logical explanation to justify or make acceptable otherwise unacceptable impulses, feelings, behaviors, and motives.

reaction formation Development of conscious attitudes and behavior patterns that are opposite to what one really feels or would like to do.

reality orientation Formal process of keeping an individual alert to events in the here-and-now.

reality testing The ego function of determining the objective reality of experience or a nursing action that validates objective reality for a patient who is unable to do so.

reality therapy A therapeutic approach based on the existential model of psychiatric care and developed by Glasser. The focus is on recognition and accomplishment of life goals with emphasis on development of the capacity for caring.

reasoning The ability to consider facts and arrive at a logical conclusion.

receptor A specialized area on a nerve membrane, a blood vessel, or a muscle that receives the chemical stimulation that activates or inhibits the nerve, blood vessel, or muscle.

reciprocal inhibition A behavior modification technique that attempts to substitute a more adaptive behavior for a symptom by learning an alternative means of reducing anxiety.

reframing To change the conceptual and/or emotional viewpoint in relation to which a situation is experienced and to place it in a different frame that fits the "facts" of the concrete situation equally well, thereby changing its entire meaning; often imputing positive motivations behind undesirable behavior constitutes reframing.

regression A retreat in the face of stress to behavior characteristic of an earlier level of development.

reinforcement Process in which operant consequences increase probability operant will recur.

reinforcer Consequence that increases probability that operant will recur.

relatedness Process of establishing intimate relationships with others, including a meaningful balance among dependence, independence, and interdependence.

relaxation response A protective mechanism against stress that brings about decreased heart rate, lower metabolism, and decreased respiratory rate. It is the physiological opposite of the fight or flight, or anxiety, response.

relaxation therapy A behavior modification approach based on the principle of reciprocal inhibition. Consciously induced relaxation is experienced in conjunction with actual or fantasied anxiety-provoking experiences.

reminiscence Recounting early life experiences and events.

repression Involuntary exclusion of a painful or conflictual thought, impulse, or memory from awareness. It is the primary ego defense, and other mechanisms tend to reinforce it.

residual Remaining, or left behind; those symptoms that remain after treatment has reached its maximum effect.

resistance Attempt of the patient to remain unaware of anxiety-producing aspects within himself. Ambivalent attitudes toward self-exploration in which the patient both appreciates and avoids anxiety-producing experiences that are a normal part of the therapeutic process.

respect An attitude of the nurse that conveys caring for, liking, and valuing the patient. He is regarded as a person of worth and is accepted without qualification.

respite care The provision of temporary supervision in a community setting for a psychiatric patient who lives with his family to provide the family with relief from the demands of his care.

response Cost category of negative punishment in which reinforcer is lost or withdrawn following operant.

reversible brain syndrome Also known as delirium, or acute brain syndrome, this disorder is related to a variety of biological stressors and is characterized by a disruption of cognition. Recovery is possible.

role ambiguity A type of role strain that occurs when shared specifications set for an expected role are incomplete or insufficient to tell the involved individual what is desired or how to do it.

role clarification Gaining the knowledge, information, and cues needed to perform a role.

role conflict Frustration experienced by the individual because of role demands that are incompatible or incongruent or confusing regarding appropriate role behavior.

role overload A type of role strain that occurs when a person is faced with a role set that is too complex or overwhelms available resources.

role playing Acting out of a particular situation. It functions to increase the person's insight into human relations and can deepen one's ability to see a situation from another point of view.

role strain Stress associated with expected roles or positions, experienced as frustration.

roles Set of socially expected behavior patterns associated with one individual's function in various social groups. Roles provide a means for social participation and a way to test out identities for consensual validation by significant others.

sadism Intense sexual arousal or desire and acts, fantasies, or other stimuli involving the inflicting of real or simulated psychological or physical suffering.

Sandoz Clinical Assessment—Geriatric An examination of psychological functioning that is administered to the elderly to assist in the diagnostical process.

schizophrenia A manifestation of anxiety of psychotic proportions, primarily characterized by inability to trust other people and disordered thought process, resulting in disrupted interpersonal relationships.

school phobia A child's state of anxiety related to separating him from his parents by his attending school. It is a form of separation anxiety; the child is not afraid of school per se.

script A transactional analysis term that refers to a life plan that originates in childhood perceptions and experiences.

seclusion A form of physical restraint in which the individual is placed in a single room, which may be locked, to decrease stimuli and allow the agitated patient to gain control of his behavior.

secondary appraisal of coping resources An evaluation of one's coping resources or strategies that involves cognitive, affective, physiological, behavioral, and social responses.

secondary gain Advantages other than a decrease in anxiety that are associated with the sick role (e.g., dependency need gratification, relief from responsibilities).

secondary prevention A type of prevention that seeks to reduce the prevalence of illness by interventions that provide for early detection and treatment of problems.

secondary process thought Conscious thought processes that are under the control of the ego and are characterized by logic.

secondary symptoms Symptoms that are not intrinsically associated with the disease process but are a consequence of the illness process.

security operations A term related to the interpersonal model of psychiatric care that refers to mental mechanisms developed to deal with anxiety-provoking experiences.

self-actualization The process of fulfilling one's potential.

self-concept All the notions, beliefs, and convictions that constitute an individual's knowledge of himself and influence his relationships with others.

self-destructive behavior Any behavior, direct or indirect, that if uninterrupted, will ultimately lead to the death of the individual.

self-disclosure Revelation that occurs when a person reveals information about himself, his ideas, values, feelings, and attitudes.

self-esteem The individual's personal judgment of his own worth obtained by analyzing how well his behavior conforms to his self-ideal.

self-help group An organization of people who share a similar problem and meet to receive peer support and encouragement.

self-ideal The individual's perception of how he should behave based on certain personal standards. The standard may be either a carefully constructed image of the kind of person one would like to be or merely a number of aspirations, goals, or values that one would like to achieve.

self-system A term related to the interpersonal model of psychiatric care that refers to the self as perceived by the individual.

senility A nonspecific term that refers to impaired cognitive functioning in the elderly and is usually used in a derogatory sense.

sensitivity training group A group developed for the purpose of increasing self-awareness, increasing understanding of group process, or increasing awareness of the effects of one's behavior in groups.

separation-individuation A process whereby the child achieves a state of psychological separateness from the mother and develops a sense of identity.

set A predisposition to behave in a certain way

sexual assault/rape The forcible perpetration of an act of sexual contact on the body (male or female) of another person without his or her consent; legal criteria vary among the states.

sexual aversion disorder Persistent or recurrent extreme aversion to and avoidance of all or almost all genital sexual contact with a partner.

sexuality Broadly defined as a desire for contact, warmth, tenderness, or love.

Short Portable Mental Status Questionnaire A short tool used to screen for cognitive impairment.

situational crisis Crisis that occurs when a specific external event upsets an individual's psychological equilibrium.

Social Behavior Assessment Scale A semistructured interview guide that elicits information from significant others regarding the patient's functioning.

social breakdown syndrome Progressive deterioraton of social and interpersonal skills of long-term psychiatric patients.

social learning theory A theory that explains the development of aggressive behavior as part of the socialization process.

social margin The sum total of all the resources—material, personal, and interpersonal—available to assist an individual in coping with stress.

social networks See *social support systems.*

social support systems Those members of one's social environment who are perceived by the individual as "significant others" and who provide some degree of emotional support, task-oriented help, feedback and evaluation, social relatedness and integration, and access to new information.

society A nation, community, or broad grouping of people who establish particular aims, beliefs, or standards of living and conduct.

somatic delusion The false belief that all or a part of the body is impaired in some way.

somatic therapies Treatment affecting one's physiological functioning.

somatization disorder A somatoform disorder characterized by multiple physical complaints with no evidence of organic impairment.

somatoform disorder A category of psychophysiological disruptions with no evidence of organic impairment.

somnambulism Dissociative manifestation of sleepwalking.

specialist in psychiatric and mental health nursing A psychiatric nurse who is characterized by graduate education, supervised clinical experience, and depth of knowledge, competence, and skill in practice.

splitting Viewing people and situations as either all good or all bad. Failure to integrate the positive and negative qualities of oneself.

steady state The body has reached a state of drug level equilibrium: a drug has been taken long enough that the amount of drug excreted equals the amount ingested. This occurs in approximately four to six half-lives.

stigma An irrational attribution of negative worth based on a person's behavior or experiences.

stimulus Any physical or environmental object, event, or condition, including one's own behavior and the behavior of others, that does or can influence.

strength An ability, skill, or interest an individual has previously used.

stress-adaptation theory Stress depletes the reserve capacity of individuals, thereby placing them in a vulnerable position for disease or illness.

stressors Stimuli that the individual perceives as challenging, threatening, or harmful. They require the use of excess energy and produce a state of tension and stress within the individual.

sublimation Acceptance of a socially approved substitute goal for a drive whose normal channel of expression is blocked.

substance abuse The use of any mind-altering agent to such an extent that it interferes with the individual's biological, psychological, or sociocultural integrity.

subsystems Smaller components of the larger system composed of individuals or dyads, formed by generation, gender, interest, or function.

suicide Self-inflicted death.

suicide attempt Any action deliberately undertaken by the individual that, if carried to completion, will result in his death.

suicide gesture A suicide attempt that is planned to be discovered in an attempt to influence the behavior of others.

suicide threat A warning, direct or indirect, verbal or nonverbal that the individual plans to attempt suicide.

sundown syndrome Cognitive ability diminishes in the late afternoon or early evening.

sunrise syndrome Unstable cognitive ability on rising in the morning.

superego Element of the personality described by Freud that represents one's conscience and culturally acquired restrictions.

supervision A process whereby a therapist is helped to become a more effective clinician. The nurse supervisor serves as a provider of theoretical knowledge and therapeutic techniques, validates the use of the nursing process, and supports the working through the transference and countertransference reactions.

suppression A process that is the conscious analogy of repression. It is the intentional exclusion of material from consciousness.

symptom-bearer The family member frequently seen as the psychiatric patient who is functioning poorly because of family dynamics that interfere with his functioning at a higher level.

synapse The gap between the membrane of one nerve cell and the membrane of another. The synapse is the point at which the transmission of nerve impulses occurs.

synergistic A reaction between two or more substances in which, after introduction into the body, the physiological effect of each is enhanced by the other.

systematical desensitization A technique of behavior therapy that involves the paring of deep muscle relaxation with imagined scenes depicting situations that cause the patient to feel anxious. The assumption is that if the person is taught relaxation rather than anxiety while imagining such scenes, the real-life situation that the scene depicted will cause much less anxiety.

systems evaluation An evaluation of the organization of the health care delivery system that includes the components of systems analysis, economic analysis, and operations research. It is a supplement to clinical evaluation.

tangential speech Loss of goal direction in communication. Failure to address the original point.

tardive dyskinesia Literally, "late-appearing abnormal movements"; a variable complex of choreiform or athetoid movements developing in patients exposed to antipsychotic drugs. Typical movements include tongue writhing or protrusion, chewing, lip puckering, choreiform finger movements, toe and ankle movements, leg jiggling, or movements of neck, trunk, and pelvis.

target symptoms Symptoms of an illness that are most likely to respond to a specific treatment, such as to a particular psychopharmocologic drug.

tertiary prevention Measures designed to reduce the severity, disability, or residual impairment resulting from illness through rehabilitation.

testamentary capacity A person's competency to make a will, which requires that he knows he is making a will, the nature and extent of his property, and who his friends and relatives are.

thanatology The study of dying and death.

themes Underlying issues or problems experienced by the patient that emerge repeatedly during the course of the nurse-patient relationship.

therapeutic community A concept proposed by Maxwell Jones in which the patient's social environment would be used to provide a therapeutic experience for him by involving him as an active participant in his own care and the daily problems of his community.

therapeutic group A group developed for the purpose of preventing emotional turmoil or disturbances through prevention, education, and providing support.

therapeutic impasses Roadblocks in the progress of the nurse-patient relationship. They arise for a variety of reasons and may take different forms, but they all create stalls in the therapeutic relationship.

therapeutic nurse-patient relationship A mutual learning experience and a corrective emotional experience for the patient, in which nurses use themselves and specific clinical techniques in working with the patient to bring about behavioral change.

therapeutic touch The nurse's laying of hands on or close to the body of an ill person for the purpose of helping or healing him.

third-party reimbursement Payment for health services by a government or private health insurance program.

time-out Category of negative punishment in which reinforcer is lost or withdrawn following operant.

token economy A behavior modification approach that uses positive reinforcement in the form of a tangible object to promote positive behavioral change.

tolerance In pharmacology, progressive decrease of the effects of a drug during continued use of the same dose; this accounts for a decease in some side effects and also some therapeutic effects.

tort A civil wrong for which the injured party is entitled to compensation.

trance An altered state of consciousness with markedly diminished responsiveness to the environment.

transactional analysis A therapeutic modality based on the communications model of psychiatric care and developed by Berne. Therapy takes place through the identification and interpretation of communication units (transactions), leading to understanding of interpersonal games that underlie behavioral disturbances. The goal is to develop the ability to communicate directly without using games.

transference An unconscious response of the patient in which he experiences feelings and attitudes toward the nurse that were originally associated with significant figures in his early life.

transitional employment placement (TEP) A job that belongs to a psychosocial rehabilitation program rather than to an individual and that is assigned by program staff to a particular patient (member) for the time period that patient (member) needs it. When no longer needed by that patient (member), the TEP is assigned to someone else.

transsexual A person who is genetically an anatomical male or female and who expresses, with strong conviction, that he or she has the mind of the opposite sex, part time or full time, and seeks to change his or her sex legally and through hormonal and surgical sex reassignment.

transvestism Condition in which a male has a sexual obsession for or addiction to women's clothes.

triangle A predictable emotional process that takes place when there is difficulty in the relationship. Triangles represent dysfunctional efforts to reduce fusion or conflict in a relationship. The three corners of a triangle can be composed of three people, two people and an object or group or issue.

tricyclics A group of chemically related antidepressant medications.

undoing An act or communication that partially negates a previous one.

unidisciplinary health care team A group of health care workers who are all members of the same discipline.

urologic A person who receives sexual stimulation from acts involving urine, such as watching people urinate or wishing to urinate on another.

vaginismus Involuntary contractions of the outer third of the vagina that prevent insertion of the penis.

value clarification A method whereby a person can assess, explore, and determine his personal values and what priority they hold in his personal decision making.

values The concepts that a person holds worthy in his own personal life. They are formed as a result of one's life experiences with family, friends, culture, education, work, and relaxation.

variable interval (VI) reinforcement Specific lapse of time required for reinforcement.

variable ratio (VR) reinforcement Various numbers of responses required for each reinforcement.

verbal communication Written or spoken transmission of a message.

victims Adults or children who are the target or scapegoat of family abuse or violence perpetrated by an offender and dysfunctional family system.

violence The exertion of extreme force or destructive action so as to injure or hurt; discordance, outrage, and sudden intense activity to the point of loss of control.

visualization The conscious programming of desired change with positive images.

vocal cues A category of nonverbal communication that includes all the noises and sounds that are extraspeech sounds. They are sometimes referred to as paralinguistic cues.

voluntary admission A type of admission to a psychiatric hospital in which the individual applies in writing and agrees to receive treatment and abide by the hospital rules. If the patient wishes to be discharged, he must give written notice to the hospital.

voluntary patient A patient who chooses to be admitted to a psychiatric facility of his own free will.

voyeurism Intense sexual arousal or desire and acts, fantasies, or other stimuli involving observing unsuspecting people who are naked, in the act of disrobing, or engaging in sexual activity.

wear-and-tear theory Structural and functional changes of a person may be accelerated by abuse and decelerated by care.

withdrawal An adaptive or coping mechanism that involves physically pulling away from or psychologically losing interest in others and the environment.

withdrawal syndrome Constellation of behaviors that occurs when use of an abused substance is terminated. Behaviors are specific to the abused substance.

word salad A communication pattern characterized by a jumble of disconnected words.

working through Process by which repressed feelings are released and reintegrated into the personality.

young adult chronically mentally ill patient A chronically mentally ill person beween 18 and 35 years of age.

zoophilia Intense sexual arousal or desire and acts, fantasies, or other stimuli involving animals.

Zung Self-Rating Depression Scale An instrument administered to determine the presence of depression.

Index

NANDA - APPROVED NURSING DIAGNOSES

Activity intolerance
Activity intolerance, potential
Adjustment, impaired
Airway clearance, ineffective
Anxiety
Aspiration, potential for
Body image disturbance
Body temperature, altered, potential
Breastfeeding, effective
Breastfeeding, ineffective
Breathing pattern, ineffective
Cardiac output, decreased
Communication, impaired verbal
Constipation
Constipation, colonic
Constipation, perceived
Coping, defensive
Coping, family: potential for growth
Coping, ineffective family: compromised
Coping, ineffective family: disabling
Coping, ineffective individual
Decisional conflict (specify)
Denial, ineffective
Diarrhea
Disuse syndrome, potential for
Diversional activity deficit
Dysreflexia
Family processes, altered
Fatigue
Fear
Fluid volume deficit (1)
Fluid volume deficit (2)
Fluid volume deficit, potential
Fluid volume excess
Gas exchange, impaired
Grieving, anticipatory
Grieving, dysfunctional
Growth and development, altered
Health maintenance, altered
Health seeking behaviors (specify)
Home maintenance management, impaired
Hopelessness
Hyperthermia
Hypothermia
Incontinence, bowel
Incontinence, functional
Incontinence, reflex
Incontinence, stress
Incontinence, total
Incontinence, urge
Infection, potential for
Injury, potential for

Knowledge deficit (specify)
Mobility, impaired physical
Noncompliance (specify)
Nutrition, altered: less than body requirements
Nutrition, altered: more than body requirements
Nutrition, altered: potential for more than body requirements
Oral mucous membrane, altered
Pain
Pain, chronic
Parental role conflict
Parenting, altered
Parenting, altered, potential
Personal identity disturbance
Poisoning, potential for
Post-trauma response
Powerlessness
Protection, altered
Rape-trauma syndrome
Rape-trauma syndrome: compound reaction
Rape-trauma syndrome: silent reaction
Role performance, altered
Self-care deficit, bathing/hygiene
Self-care deficit, dressing/grooming
Self-care deficit, feeding
Self-care deficit, toileting
Self-esteem, disturbance
Self-esteem, chronic low
Self-esteem, situational low
Sensory, perceptual alterations (specify) (visual, auditory, kinesthetic, gustatory, tactile, olfactory)
Sexual dysfunction
Sexuality patterns, altered
Skin integrity, impaired
Skin integrity, impaired, potential
Sleep pattern disturbance
Social interaction, impaired
Social isolation
Spiritual distress (distress of the human spirit)
Suffocation, potential for
Swallowing, impaired
Thermoregulation, ineffective
Thought processes, altered
Tissue integrity, impaired
Tissue perfusion, altered (specify type) (renal, cerebral, cardiopulmonary, gastrointestinal, peripheral)
Trauma, potential for
Unilateral neglect
Urinary elimination, altered patterns
Urinary retention
Violence, potential for: self-directed or directed at others

From the Proceedings of the Ninth National Conference of the North American Nursing Diagnosis Association, March 1990.